KIRK'S
GENERAL SURGICAL OPERATIONS

Raymond Maurice (Jerry) Kirk

Jerry Kirk was born and brought up in Nottingham. While he was still at school the Second World War began, and after a brief interim as a bank clerk he served as an ordinary seaman in the famous cruiser, HMS Ajax, during Operation Torch – the first combined American–British landings in North Africa – and ended up in charge of a minesweeper in the Mediterranean Sea. After demobilisation, and financed by an ex-service grant, Jerry attended medical school at King's College London and Charing Cross Hospital. He became an anatomy lecturer at King's College London and went on to work for Professor Ian Aird at the Royal Postgraduate Medical School, Hammersmith Hospital. He held registrar posts at Charing Cross Hospital and, subsequently, the Royal Free Hospital, where he became a consultant general surgeon in 1964 and remained throughout his career. He was also a member of the Council of the Royal College of Surgeons of England, and devised the original basic surgical skills (BSS) course, as well as the first minimal access course, alongside Professor Sir Alfred Cuschieri. As Director of the Overseas Doctors Training Scheme he was proud to see trainees return home with greater confidence and competence to deal with the surgical challenges in their homelands.

Jerry Kirk was privileged to work with a series of wonderful teachers, colleagues, students and patients. Notable among these were Ian Aird, a scintillatingly brilliant intellect, and Norman Tanner who, from modest beginnings, became internationally celebrated as a pioneer of standardized, safe gastric surgery, resulting in outstanding long-term outcomes. A third giant was the eminent oesophageal surgeon, Hiroshi Akiyama of Tokyo, who could have been a twin brother of Tanner in character, both matching each other in talent, commitment, honesty and teaching by example. All three left Jerry recognising the privilege of being a teacher.

After retiring from clinical surgical practice in 1989, Jerry was appointed an honorary consulting surgeon at the Royal Free Hospital and Honorary Professor of Surgery at University College London teaching anatomy, basic surgical skills and essential clinical insights. As well as being former President of the Surgical Section of the Royal Society of Medicine, the Medical Society of London and the Hunterian Society, he was Editor of the Annals of the Royal College of Surgeons and has also written and edited numerous books for surgeons in training including *Basic Surgical Techniques*, *Clinical Surgery in General* and *General Surgical Operations*. He holds honorary fellowships of the Association of Surgeons of Poland and the College of Surgeons of Sri Lanka. He is a Fellow of the Royal Society of Medicine.

For Elsevier

Content Strategist: Laurence Hunter
Content Development Specialist: Helen Leng
Project Manager: Vinod Kumar Iyyappan
Designer/Design Direction: Christian Bilbow
Illustration Manager: Jennifer Rose
Illustrator: Robert Britton/Martin Woodward

KIRK'S GENERAL SURGICAL OPERATIONS

SIXTH EDITION

EDITED BY

RICHARD NOVELL MChir FRCS

Consultant Colorectal Surgeon, The Royal Free London NHS Foundation Trust; Honorary Senior Lecturer, University College London, London, UK

DARYLL M. BAKER BSc PhD BM Bch FRCS FRCS

Consultant General and Vascular Surgeon, The Royal Free London NHS Foundation Trust, London, UK

NICHOLAS GODDARD MBBS FRCS

Consultant Orthopaedic Surgeon, The Royal Free London NHS Foundation Trust, London, UK

EDITOR EMERITUS

R.M. KIRK MS FRCS

Honorary Professor of Surgery, University College London School of Medicine; Honorary Consulting Surgeon, The Royal Free London NHS Foundation Trust, London, UK

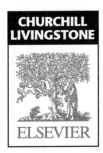

CHURCHILL LIVINGSTONE

ELSEVIER

Edinburgh   London   New York   Oxford   Philadelphia   St Louis   Sydney   Toronto   2013

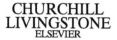

CHURCHILL
LIVINGSTONE
ELSEVIER

First edition 1978   Fourth edition 2000
Second edition 1987   Fifth edition 2006
Third edition 1994   Sixth edition 2013

ISBN 978-0-7020-4481-6
International ISBN 978-0-7020-4482-3

British Library Cataloguing in Publication Data
A catalogue record for this book is available from the British Library

Library of Congress Cataloging in Publication Data
A catalog record for this book is available from the Library of Congress

Notices
Knowledge and best practice in this field are constantly changing. As new research and experience broaden our understanding, changes in research methods, professional practices, or medical treatment may become necessary.

Practitioners and researchers must always rely on their own experience and knowledge in evaluating and using any information, methods, compounds, or experiments described herein. In using such information or methods they should be mindful of their own safety and the safety of others, including parties for whom they have a professional responsibility.

With respect to any drug or pharmaceutical products identified, readers are advised to check the most current information provided (i) on procedures featured or (ii) by the manufacturer of each product to be administered, to verify the recommended dose or formula, the method and duration of administration, and contraindications. It is the responsibility of practitioners, relying on their own experience and knowledge of their patients, to make diagnoses, to determine dosages and the best treatment for each individual patient, and to take all appropriate safety precautions.

To the fullest extent of the law, neither the publisher nor the authors, contributors, or editors, assume any liability for any injury and/or damage to persons or property as a matter of products liability, negligence or otherwise, or from any use or operation of any methods, products, instructions, or ideas contained in the material herein.

your source for books, journals and multimedia in the health sciences
www.elsevierhealth.com

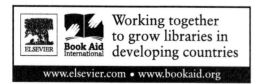
Working together to grow libraries in developing countries
www.elsevier.com • www.bookaid.org

The Publisher's policy is to use paper manufactured from sustainable forests

Contents

CONTENTS

Foreword

Many of the operations I performed alone as a trainee surgeon were new to me. It was then customary practice. I relied on operative textbooks, frequently dashing to the library between operations. In the books were listed the sequential steps for each procedure. They did not provide advice on likely difficulties and hazards - how to anticipate, avoid, identify or respond to them. This book was a response to them. Experts who write textbooks have, over years, often armed themselves, almost unconsciously, with the required precautions. They are then no longer aware of their intuitively acquired knowledge. I believe it is the duty of experienced surgeons to identify and articulate their hard-won skills.

If you have difficulty with a manoeuvre, watch and question an expert whenever possible. In the absence of advice and guidance, you may nevertheless succeed with a struggle. Recall your actions and carefully record the circumstances and the steps. If your method proves effective, let others know. Similarly, if you face a decision that does not meet the guidelines and so demands an unorthodox solution, carefully record it. Question it as though you will need to justify it. In doing so, you may uncover a worthwhile modification to the guidelines. Although objective, evidence-based knowledge is rightly pre-eminent, all human activities are partly governed by intuition. It is in this area that you may identify a possible advance. Rational, objective thought does not provide all the answers.

The intuitive mind is a sacred gift and the rational mind is a faithful servant. We have created a society that honours the servant and has forgotten the gift. Attributed to Albert Einstein.

What is the relevance of a textbook covering most of the generality of surgery? It is valuable for intending surgeons to rotate, see and understand a variety of possible attractive careers. Too narrow concentration of interests blunts the appreciation of translating techniques across specialities. Even in highly organized countries, emergencies in the form of natural and deliberate disasters may create emergencies in which a soundly trained surgeon may act as a substitute for an unavailable colleague. Finally, there are still some surgeons working from choice or necessity in constrained circumstances. They may offer the only hope for saving life, limb or a special sense.

R.M. Kirk
London, 2013

Preface

A good surgeon knows how to operate
A better surgeon knows when to operate
The best surgeon knows when not to operate

Welcome to the Sixth Edition of this much-loved textbook which has guided most of us through the uncharted waters of surgical training for the past 35 years. Much has changed since the last edition, a mere seven years ago, and in an era which is increasingly defined by instantaneous access to information via the world-wide web the question must be asked: is there still a need for a comprehensive overview of operative general surgery, a specialty whose very existence is threatened by relentless subspecialisation? The answer is, we believe, emphatically 'Yes'. As Jerry Kirk argued in his preface to the previous edition, the new generation of surgeons are trained within a narrower field, but in many countries limited manpower has resulted in only a partial implementation of specialization: surgeons dealing with emergency admissions are frequently required to provide urgent care for conditions outside their sphere of expertise. Indeed, we in the UK are seeing the emergence of a new breed of general surgeon specialising in emergency surgery, with a practice characterized by breadth rather than depth of knowledge. Natural disasters, terrorist bombs and civil war have no respect for specialties and it is more vital than ever that those surgeons managing such patients are familiar with the broad spectrum of conditions and surgical techniques contained herein.

When we were asked to take over the editorship of *General Surgical Operations*, we were faced with a dilemma: how to make it relevant to a new readership, many of whom are familiar with the latest high-tech, minimally invasive techniques, whilst still retaining the practical, 'cottage industry' approach of which Jerry is rightly proud. The results, we hope, speak for themselves. The involvement of no less than 42 new contributors has meant that 33 chapters from the previous edition have been completely rewritten. Laparoscopic surgery is gaining in popularity and is now often the gold standard in management: the six chapters dealing with laparoscopic techniques have therefore been incorporated into those dealing with the relevant system. The remaining 15 chapters have been revised and in many cases invigorated by new co-authors. The illustrations have been redrawn in a new half-tone style which has greatly improved their clarity.

Readers who are nostalgic for previous editions need not fear: we have retained the standardized style and headings to allow ease of reference. Each section covers patient selection, pre-operative preparation, surgical access, assessment of the situation, a detailed description of the operative technique, aftercare and potential complications. *General Surgical Operations* continues to be aimed at a broad readership: the candidate preparing for the Intercollegiate FRCS in General Surgery or international equivalents; the trained surgeon faced, through necessity, with undertaking an infrequently performed procedure; and the many surgeons working in hospitals throughout the world without access to specialist services. It remains above all a practical text which will guide the surgeon in training or one unfamiliar with a procedure on how to perform it, but more importantly on how to manage the uncertainties which so often arise.

The successful accomplishment of major surgical procedures is based on sound surgical technique: those in the earlier stages of their training are encouraged to consult *Basic Surgical Techniques* (6th Edition), also published by Elsevier.

The editorial team's enthusiasm for this project has been matched by our many contributing authors. We are grateful to Laurence Hunter, Sally Davies and Helen Leng at Elsevier who have guided three novice editors over many hurdles during the last two years. Most importantly, we would like to thank Jerry Kirk whose contribution as Emeritus Editor has been invaluable and whose achievement is reflected in the book's new title.

Richard Novell
Nicholas Goddard
Daryll Baker
London, 2013

Contributors

The late Hiroshi Akiyama MD PhD FACS FRCS
Formerly President Emeritus, Toranomon Hospital, Tokyo, Japan

Shaun G. Appleton MS FRCS
Consultant Surgeon, Wycombe Hospital, High Wycombe, UK

Daryll M. Baker BSc PhD BM Bch FRCS FRCS
Consultant General and Vascular Surgeon, The Royal Free London NHS Foundation Trust, London, UK

Richard N. Brueton MA MD FRCS
Honorary Consultant Orthopaedic Surgeon, The Royal Free London NHS Foundation Trust, London, UK

Peter E.M. Butler FRCSI FRCS
Consultant Plastic Surgeon, The Royal Free London NHS Foundation Trust, London, UK

Hester Y.S. Cheung FRACS, FHKAM
Consultant Surgeon, Department of Surgery, Pamela Youde Nethersole Eastern Hospital, Hong Kong

Adrian B. Cresswell MBChB FRCS
Consultant Hepatopancreatobiliary Surgeon, The Basingstoke Hepatobiliary Unit, Hampshire Hospitals NHS Trust, Basingstoke, UK

Osama Damrah MD FRCS
Senior Clinical Fellow, The Royal Free London NHS Foundation Trust, London, UK

Clare Davey MSc MBBS FRCS FRCOphth
Consultant Ophthalmologist, The Royal Free London NHS Foundation Trust, London, UK

Brian R. Davidson MBChB MD FRCPS FRCS
Professor of Surgery, University Research Department of General Surgery, University College London Medical School, London, UK

Meryl Davis BSc MBBS FRCS
Consultant Vascular Surgeon, The Royal Free London NHS Foundation Trust, London, UK

Khaled I. Dawas MBBChir MA MD FRCS
Senior Lecturer and Consultant Oesophago-gastric Surgeon, University College Hospital, London, UK

Rovan E. D'Souza FRCS MS DNB
Consultant General and Vascular Surgeon, The Royal Free London NHS Foundation Trust, London, UK

James A. England MB ChB FRCS
Consultant ENT-Thyroid Surgeon, Castle Hill Hospital, Hull, UK

Debashis B. Ghosh MS FRCS FRCS FEBS
Consultant Breast Surgeon, The Royal Free London NHS Foundation Trust, London, UK

Nicholas Goddard MBBS FRCS
Consultant Orthopaedic Surgeon, The Royal Free London NHS Foundation Trust, London, UK

Nigel J. Hall MRCPCH FRCS PhD
Clinical Lecturer in Paediatric Surgery, University College London Institute of Child Health, London, UK

Mo Keshtgar BSc MBBS FRCSI FRCS PhD
Consultant Surgical Oncologist, The Royal Free London NHS Foundation Trust, London, UK

Edward Kiely MB FRCSI
Consultant Neonatal and Paediatric Surgeon, Great Ormond Street Hospital for Children, London, UK

Dae S. Kim MBChB BDS MSc FRCS PhD
Consultant ENT and Thyroid Surgeon, Queen Alexandra Hospital, Portsmouth; Honorary Senior Lecturer, Cancer Sciences, University of Southampton, UK

R.M. Kirk MS FRCS
Honorary Professor of Surgery, University College London School of Medicine; Honorary Consulting Surgeon, The Royal Free London NHS Foundation Trust, London, UK

Rahul S. Koti MD FRCS
Honorary Lecturer in Surgery, The Royal Free London NHS Foundation Trust and University College London School of Medicine, London, UK

Tom R. Kurzawinski PhD FRCS
Consultant Pancreatic and Endocrine Surgeon, University College London Hospital Foundation Trust and Great Ormond Street Hospital, London UK

Roger J. Leicester OBE MB FRCS
Consultant Colorectal Surgeon and Director of Endoscopy Services, St George's Hospital, London, UK

Michael K.W. Li MBBS MRCS LRCP FRCS FRCS FCSHK FHKAM
Professor of Surgery, University College London, United Kingdom; Honorary Consultant in General Surgery, Director of Minimally Invasive & Robotic Surgery Development, Hong Kong Sanatorium & Hospital, Hong Kong; Consultant Surgeon (Department of Surgery), Advisor of Minimal Access Surgery Training Centre, Pamela Youde Nethersole Eastern Hospital, Hong Kong

Eric K.S. Lim MBChB MD MSc FRCS
Consultant Thoracic Surgeon, The Royal Brompton Hospital, London, UK

Adam Magos BSc MBBS MD FRCOG
Consultant Gynaecologist and Honorary Senior Lecturer, The Royal Free London NHS Foundation Trust, London, UK

Arundathi O. Mahendran BSc MBBS MRCS MEd
Fellow in Abdominal Transplant Surgery, Columbia University/New York-Presbyterian Hospital, New York, USA

Sue Mallett FRCA
Consultant in Anaesthesia, The Royal Free London NHS Foundation Trust, London, UK

Nimalan Maruthainar MBBS FRCS
Orthopaedic Surgeon, The Royal Free London NHS Foundation Trust, London, UK

Robert C. Mason BSc MBChB ChMMD FRCS
Professor of Gastrointestinal Surgery, St Thomas' Hospital, London, UK

Peter McDermott BDS MBBChir FDS RCS FRCS
Consultant Maxillofacial Surgeon, Barnet and Chase Farm Hospitals NHS Trust, Enfield, UK

Konstantinos G. Miltsios MD FRCA
Consultant Anaesthetist, The Whittington Hospital, London, UK

Afshin Mosahebi MBBS FRCS MBA PhD
Consultant Plastic Surgeon, The Royal Free London NHS Foundation Trust, London, UK

Richard Novell MChir FRCS
Consultant Colorectal Surgeon, The Royal Free London NHS Foundation Trust; Honorary Senior Lecturer, University College London, London, UK

Olagunju A. Ogunbiyi MD FRCS
Senior Lecturer/Consultant Colorectal Surgeon, The Royal Free London NHS Foundation Trust, University College London, London, UK

Simon Pridgeon FRCS PhD
Urology Specialty Registrar, North Thames Rotation, UK

Jeremy Prout BSc MBBS MRCP FRCA FRCS
Consultant Anaesthetist, The Royal Free London NHS Foundation Trust, London, UK

Sakhawat H. Rahman MBChB FRCS MD
Consultant Pancreaticobiliary Surgeon, The Royal Free London NHS Foundation Trust, London, UK

Keith Rolles MA MS FRCS
Consultant Surgeon and Lead Clinician, Liver Transplant Unit, The Royal Free London NHS Foundation Trust, London, UK

Debabrata Roy MBBS MS FRCS FRCS
Specialist Registrar, Oxford, UK

Amir Sadri BSc MBChB MRCS
Core Surgical Trainee, Academic Division of Thoracic Surgery, The Royal Brompton Hospital, London, UK

Gillian Smith MD FRCS
Consultant Urologist, The Royal Free London NHS Foundation Trust, London, UK

Joel A. Smith BmedSc MBChB FRCS
Speciality Registrar and Research Fellow, University of Birmingham, Birmingham, UK

Michael P. Stearns MBBS BDS FRCS
Consultant Otolaryngologist/Head and Neck Surgeon, The Royal Free London NHS Foundation Trust, London, UK

Vijay Sujendran MD FRCS
Consultant Upper Gastrointestinal Surgeon, Addenbrookes Hospital, Cambridge, UK

Nigel R.M. Tai MBBS MS FRCS RAMC
Consultant in Trauma and Vascular Surgery, The Royal London Hospital, London; Senior Lecturer, Academic Department of Military Surgery and Trauma, Royal Centre for Defence Medicine, Birmingham, UK

Benjamin R. Thomas MA BM BCh MRCOG
Consultant Gynaecologist and Obstetrician, Stanger Hospital, KwaZulu-Natal, South Africa; Honorary Clinical Lecturer, Nelson Mandela School of Medicine, KwaZulu-Natal, South Africa

Lewis W. Thorne FRCS
Consultant Neurosurgeon, The National Hospital for Neurology and Neurosurgery, Queen Square and The Royal Free London NHS Foundation Trust, London, UK

Harushi Udagawa MD DMSc FACS
Head of Gastroenterological Surgery, Toranomon Hospital, Tokyo, Japan

Christopher E.G. Uff FRCS PhD
Specialist Registrar in Neurosurgery, The Royal Free London NHS Foundation Trust, London, UK

Carolynne Jane Vaizey MD FRCS FCS
Consultant Surgeon, St Mark's Hospital, London, UK

Peter Veitch MBBS BMedSci FRCS
Consultant Surgeon, The Royal Free London NHS Foundation Trust, London, UK

Nicholas J. Ward MD MRCS
Specialty Registrar in General Surgery, Norfolk and Norwich University Hospital, Norwich, UK

Janindra Warusavitarne FRACS PhD
Consultant Colorectal Surgeon, St Mark's Hospital, Harrow, UK

John C. Watkinson MSc MS FRCS DLO
Consultant ENT/Head and Neck and Thyroid Surgeon, Queen Elizabeth Hospital, Birmingham, UK

Douglas E. Whitelaw MBChB FRCS FRCS
Consultant Laparoscopic Surgeon and Lead Clinician for Obesity, Luton and Dunstable University Hospital, Luton, UK

Marc C. Winslet MS FRCS
Professor of Surgery, The Royal Free London NHS Foundation Trust, London, UK

Choose well, cut well, get well

R.M. Kirk

CONTENTS

This three-point dictum, probably coined in the early 20th century, was never intended as a simple three-step sequence. 'Choose well' extends throughout, leading the celebrated American surgical teacher Frank C. Spencer, to claim that good surgery is 20–25% manual dexterity and 70–75% decision-making.[1]

CHOOSE WELL

'Not everything that counts can be counted and not everything that can be counted, counts.'

Notice on the Princeton University office wall of Albert Einstein
Choosing – decision-making – is not a once and for all action. It incorporates continuous anticipation, identification and interpretation of change, and intelligent, timely response to it throughout. We treat the whole patient, and all the separate activities interact. We proceed through the steps in assessment, preparation, operation and subsequent management and aftercare, performing the procedures partly in series, partly in parallel. Remember that within the sequence of complex decisions and actions, each single one 'carries' the whole and it requires only a single error to threaten the whole procedure.

'Choose well', was originally directed only at the surgeon. The 1948 United Nations Declaration of Human Rights and subsequent legislation have emphasized the paramount rights of the fully informed patient[2] to control what is done. Complex decisions, in particular those involving alternative or adjuvant (Latin: ad = to + juvare = to assist) therapies, intended to supplement effectiveness, are increasingly made at multidisciplinary meetings seeking a formalized consensus.

BACKGROUND KNOWLEDGE

1. Make decisions on the basis of critical reading of up-to-date reports, observation, copying successful colleagues, and following your patients in order to learn as you acquire experience. Test your decisions by presenting them to respected colleagues. As you organize the information you often recognize strengths and weaknesses.

2. Statistical analysis of the gathered experience from a large number of patients has profoundly influenced practice. Prospective, double-blind, controlled clinical trials, meta–analysis of the results of different studies,[3] and application of Bayesian logic (a means of quantifying uncertainty as fresh information accumulates[4]), may offer guidance for treatment.

3. Decision analysis offers a means of weighing all the factors and possible outcomes[5] (Fig. 1.1). The subjective assessments of satisfaction values are termed utilities, an unexpected term for anticipated benefit. Decision analyses are published for a number of common conditions. Computerized decision-support systems exist, offering advice and information which can be incorporated into subsequent judgements.[6]

4. The patient's valuation must prevail, and patients may measure their satisfaction with treatment using criteria that differ from those of you, the surgeon. Dignity and quality of life weigh heavily with patients alongside life expectancy. A number of terms are used in assessing this: one measure is the quality-adjusted life-year (QALY).[7] One year of life in perfect health is 1 QALY; a lower figure is allocated for a portion of a year in perfect health or a full year spent with a disability.

5. There are many general reviews such as evidence-based Cochrane Collaboration reports,[8] and Clinical Knowledge Summaries commissioned by the National Institute for Health and Clinical Excellence,[9] Centers for Disease Control and Prevention[10] and Health and Safety Executive.[11]

6. Economic cost–benefit analysis must be added, usually as a rule by economists and health management organizations.

7. In balancing variable evidence, numerical indicators are preferred over analogue terms because numbers can be manipulated and compared. Ensure that what is chosen to be measured is valid, and not selected merely because it can be assigned a number.

8. As new methods become available, conflicting evidence emerges about effectiveness and safety compared with existing practice. Enthusiasm of originators and early promoters of treatments may lead them to confuse placebo effect with successful treatment. In case of doubt, wait for confirmation from a source unconnected with inaugurating the procedure. The eminent London physician Sir William Whithey Gull (1816–1890) humorously and cynically stated, 'Make haste and use all the new remedies before they lose their effectiveness.'

9. It is claimed that the tradition of doctors to customize treatments on an individual patient basis is detrimental to establishing the best method of management. Evidence-based medicine requires that fragmentation should be selectively replaced by standardization based on scientifically valid knowledge: an example cited is the success of well-vetted guidelines. Current methods of ranking outcome results for reporting to the public are imperfect, but transparency based on improved analyses should be the aim.[12]

10. 'Choose well' thus incorporates a complex challenge even before you face your patient.

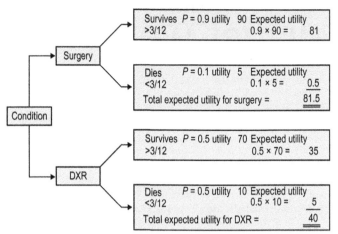

Fig. 1.1 Decision analysis, taking only short-term survival into account. The probability (*P*) of each outcome following surgery or deep X-ray therapy (DXR) is calculated from published results and local experience. The utility of each outcome is given a value between 0 (worst) and 100 (best). The expected utility is the product of probability and utility for each outcome. The sum of the expected utilities for each decision is compared with those of the other decisions. The highest scoring decision offers the best outcome. The square node is a 'decision node'; the circular nodes are 'chance nodes'.

INDIVIDUAL PATIENTS

1 In spite of increasing standardization and however much evidence is available, there are many factors that must be understood and negotiated with the patient (and often with multidisciplinary teams). Much of this information is subjective and may be difficult to identify, quantify or weigh. Each decision is a best guess, so it is valid only for the time it is made and must be flexible. Your initial plan is comparable to the strategy (Greek: stratos = army + agein = to lead; the overall plan) of a general before battle. Once battle is enjoined, he needs to monitor progress and alter his tactics (Greek: tassein = to arrange), responding to opportunities and threats.

2 We cannot always concentrate on a single patient when many people are ill. This is particularly true in wartime or following a civilian disaster. You must make urgent, sometimes agonizing, decisions. This process of triage (Old French = to pick, select) involves choosing to treat first those whose lives can be saved by quick action, whilst deferring treatment of those with peripheral, less lethal injuries: 'Life comes before limb.'

3 Particularly in acute conditions, the features may change rapidly. Take your own history and only then read the existing notes and letters. They often differ. In case of doubt, when possible defer a decision. After an interval take a fresh history and thoroughly re-examine the patient. It is remarkable how often discrepancies are then revealed.

4 Do not be too proud to take advice. The very action of arranging and presenting the problem to another person often clarifies it.

5 Choose investigations carefully from those available after asking yourself 'What do I expect to be revealed by the result?' Prefer investigations that confirm or exclude a diagnosis, or clarify the extent of disease. Avoid 'trawling' – performing a battery of tests in the hope that something emerges: as the French chemist Louis Pasteur (1822–1895), stated, 'Chance favours the prepared mind.' If the results of investigations conflict with carefully and confidently obtained clinical findings, trust your clinical judgement. Many investigations are operator dependent: be prepared to confer with the person who has performed them.

LEARNING

1 Even if you are a trainee, not permitted to make and act on your decision, do not ignore the opportunity to increase your experience. Commit yourself: mentally consider the possible options as though you do have the responsibility and are defending your proposed course of action. Follow the patient to determine the outcome. Do not be an onlooker – learn from the encounter.

2 Try to consider the possibilities – the 'what ifs. . . .' and how you would modify your management in each circumstance. Take up every opportunity to present your decision and be willing to offer the evidence to justify it.

■ If you avoid committing yourself to a decision, planning a course of action and following the patient to determine the outcome, you are wasting your time.
■ *'Experience is as to intensity, not as to duration'* (adapted from Thomas Hardy (1840–1928), poet and novelist).

CUT WELL

A good surgeon knows how to operate
A better surgeon knows when to operate
The best surgeon knows when not to operate

It is estimated that approximately 230 million surgical procedures are performed each year worldwide.[13] Operative techniques are undergoing remarkable changes as the result of technological improvements, particularly in three-dimensional imaging and minimally invasive surgery, which permits improved access to the target structures requiring surgical intervention while causing minimal damage to the interposed tissues. Many previously sacrosanct 'rules' of procedure no longer apply, but one tradition remains inviolate. Following the successful demonstration of general anaesthesia with inhaled ether in 1846 and the development of antiseptic, then aseptic, surgery from 1867, three visionary surgeons and friends, Theodore Kocher of Berne (1841–1917), William Halsted of Baltimore (1852–1922) and Harvey Cushing of Yale (1869–1939), pioneered the era of gentle, deliberate, aseptic, painstakingly haemostatic technique, completed with accurate apposition of viable, tension-free tissues. All subsequent technological refinements are merely instruments designed to reduce to a minimum the threat to living tissues. You cannot make the tissues heal but your disregard for them can prevent them from doing so.

■ *'I dressed his wounds, God healed him'*. Ambroise Paré (1510–1590) French surgeon

Your commitment to performing operations carefully and skilfully does not appear automatically as you enter the operating theatre. You bring it with you, by acquiring the habit in everyday life of striving to perform every activity carefully, faultlessly and to completion, so that it becomes second nature.[14]

Just as the most excellent operation can be prejudiced by poor selection, preparation and after-care, so can excellent general management be wasted if the operation is imperfectly or inappropriately performed.

PREPARE

Preoperative preparation varies for different procedures. Employ a checklist to ensure that every requirement has been considered. Patients often forget events of major importance unless they are prompted, because they are at the time of surgery existing in an artificial, confusing environment. Do not take anything for granted:

1 Make sure that the patient is correctly identified, labelled and listed.

2 Re-assess the condition requiring surgery and check for any previous operations – and any untoward reactions. Identify and personally mark unilateral conditions.

3 Obtain a list of routine drugs being taken.

4 Identify any co-morbidity such as infection, diabetes, allergies or drug reactions.

5 In appropriate circumstances screen the cardiorespiratory, peripheral vascular, haematological, urogenital, endocrine, digestive and neurological systems. Check the nutritional state and fluid and acid-balance.

6 If the patient will require special treatment postoperatively, for example care of a stoma or a limb prosthesis, they should receive preoperative specialist instruction and reassurance.

7 Check the psychological state.

8 Make sure that the patient gives informed consent.

9 Arrange for appropriate corrections to be made to make the patient fully fit for surgery, including prophylactic antibiotics, prevention of thrombo-embolic complications, necessary modifications in the presence of prostheses and dealing with conditions normally treated with regular drugs.

10 Arrange for preparations appropriate to the procedure, such as bowel preparation. Shaving is employed much less frequently than formerly and is usually carried out immediately preoperatively or replaced by the use of depilatory preparations.

PRACTISE

1 It is now widely accepted that as far as possible you should find alternative methods of learning skills before performing them on patients. Attend courses, operate on simulations, virtual reality trainers, and the tissues of cadavers or dead animals to gain familiarity with the necessary sequence of activities. Use every opportunity to develop your skills to the point where you automatically perform each action gently and accurately. In many countries, including the United Kingdom, you are permitted to operate on living animals to practise technique only in exceptional circumstances, but even in countries where practice on anaesthetized living animals is permitted you cannot replicate the textural changes produced by disease and injury. These artificial representations are imperfect but they offer practice in familiarizing yourself with the instruments and equipment. When you operate on patients, your attention can be focused on the target structures, since you can relegate the manipulation of instruments to a subsidiary focus.[15]

2 Assiduously watch experts and copy them. Concentrate not only on the limited area of the procedure but also observe the peripheral details. Practise the manoeuvres. Practice is different from exercise, which is repeating the same manoeuvre over and over until it becomes automatic: this precludes improvement. In contrast, during practice each attempt differs from the last, to determine if it can be improved, made smoother, feel more natural or more perfect. Only then is it converted into an exercise. Musicians and instrumentalists, even at the peak of their careers, continuously practise to improve their technique and to identify and correct acquired bad habits.[16]

3 Even if you are already highly skilled, do not despise creating a simple simulation in order to perfect an otherwise difficult manoeuvre. Again, note that professional musicians are willing to practise challenging sections right up to the moment of performance. Lord Moynihan (1865–1936), much admired for his gentle technique, always carried a length of thread with which he practised tying knots with consummate perfection.

4 Know the anatomy. Learn it thoroughly, not just from books but by every available means. Know it extensively and in three dimensions, not just locally.

5 Exploit your acquired knowledge of inter-related structures and the (usually potential) spaces between them. Avoid wandering inadvertently away from the target structures but, in contrast, gain in confidence when you need to explore away from them.

6 Be aware that the planes of contact change between structures as a result of postural changes.

> ■ Missiles, injuries, infections, neoplasms do not respect anatomical boundaries.
> ■ The relationship between structures does not always conform to the relationships found in standard dissected bodies.
> ■ Posture at the time of sustaining injury may not correspond with the posture you encounter.

7 Handle living tissues with meticulous gentleness. Every thoughtless grasp, even with fine dissecting forceps, exerts a powerful crushing force per unit area.

8 Scrupulously observe the best aseptic techniques.

9 Achieve and maintain absolute haemostasis while avoiding excess burning, strangulation of tissue and insertion of foreign materials.

10 Appose the tissues perfectly with the minimum distortion and constriction.

11 Be aware that visual assessment of tissue vitality is notoriously unreliable. When wounds are closed, within the now closed compartment the interstitial oxygen concentration falls initially.[17,18]

SET UP

1 Inexperienced and overconfident surgeons, anxious to demonstrate that they are expeditious, rush to start the operation. Do not. Carefully check that you have all the components required for smooth, calm, progression. Ask yourself again:

■ Correct patient, correct operation site?
■ Correct instruments and equipment checked and confirmed to be working?
■ Colleagues and assistants all in attendance, fully informed and acquiescent?

2 As soon as you expose the operation site, stop and gently assess the situation. In the presence of susceptible infection or neoplasia, start at a distance and work towards the diseased centre in order to avoid spreading micro-organisms or malignant cells.

3 Do not proceed until you are confident in your decision and your ability to achieve your intention.

IMPROVE PATIENT SAFETY

Healthcare has traditionally been proudly delivered on an individual basis. The variations of treatment make it difficult to compare outcome results. Powerful arguments are now advanced for acceptance of standardized methods of delivering healthcare to facilitate measurement, with general adherence to the proven most successful methods. When scientifically validated standardized treatments are available, rigid adherence to treating each patient on an individual basis is compared with cottage industry practice.[12]

■ We are no longer independently employed craftsmen.
■ Surgery is no exception to the general call for transparency.[19]

It is estimated that the perioperative death rate is 0.4–0.8% and that at least half of these deaths are avoidable.[20] Adverse events must be reported, often with the hope of modifying the system rather than merely blaming the operator.[21] With the intention of reducing errors, checking of action sequences is being widely and rapidly introduced (WHO Guidelines for Safe Surgery):[22]

1 When preparing to perform an emergency procedure, do not rush to get started before you have calmly and fully considered what you should do, how you intend to achieve your objective, what essential equipment you will require and whether it is in proven working order. Have you considered the possibilities of unexpected findings and difficulties, and how will you deal with them?

2 Consider if your decision can be modified with the help of carefully selected available investigations.

3 Should you make written and photographic records of the preoperative situation?

4 Do not hurry for any reason that you cannot fully justify. When you hurry, the skilful actions that you have learned to perform perfectly and automatically are transferred to your conscious focus, distracting your prime concentration from awareness of the whole situation. You can demonstrate this to yourself: type information hurriedly into your computer and note the rise in the error rate – you become clumsy.

5 As you perform an emergency operation, never lose sight of your intentions. Carry out the procedure that will, as simply and safely as possible, correct the problem for which you embarked on the operation. Do no more unless you encounter a new threat. Subsidiary and unnecessary 'just in case' actions are potent causes of complications.

■ At an emergency operation never forget your initial intentions.
■ Do not indulge in unnecessary 'extra' procedures: you may later need to justify them to your patient, your peers and to your conscience.

6 As you proceed through the operation, performing the required actions partly in series, partly in parallel, remember that within the sequence of complex decisions and actions, it needs but one imperfect component to threaten the success of the procedure. For example, once you think you have identified a structure it is tempting not to challenge the assumption. During laparoscopic surgery in particular, misperception has been identified as a potent contributor to errors.[23]

7 Never relax your vigilance over the wound, instruments, swabs and other materials placed into the wound. Use as few swabs as possible and always use the largest ones compatible with the task. Avoid burying all of a swab or pack in the wound; leave a portion, or attached tape, protruding to be clipped to the wound towels. There is no single, once-and-for-all action that will prevent articles from being left inside: check everything, every time. Involve as many others as possible in the check: they may save you from a momentary lapse.

8 If you repeatedly encounter difficulty and have to rectify it, what steps have you taken to ensure that you confidently perform smoothly and faultlessly at the next initial attempt?

■ Get it right first time.
■ *'Man who leaves luck out of plans usually finds it'* (Chinese proverb).

PREVENT OR COMBAT INFECTION

1 Surgical infection is not static and changes continuously as a result of multiple factors. Ensure you are aware of current practice by frequently consulting the bacteriologists and regularly searching the published literature including bulletins from the Health Protection Agency and the Surgical Site Infection Surveillance Service.[24,25]

2 Standard practices to combat infection are complimented by the skill with which you operate, reducing trauma, tissue de-vitalization and contamination to a minimum.

3 Wounded tissues resist infection with non-specific immunity provided by neutrophils. These cells depend on a high partial pressure of oxygen, from which superoxides are catalysed in their cellular membranes, and these are bactericidal. Wound oxygen tension depends on full blood perfusion and high arterial oxygen partial pressure. It is reduced by vasoconstriction, as from exposure to cold, sympathomimetic effects, including failed pain relief and by hypovolaemia. The use of peri-operative high fractional inspired oxygen has been reported to be beneficial.[26]

4 Administer prophylactic antibiotics 30 minutes before the operation in order to gain the highest level of protection.

GET WELL

1 You have not yet fulfilled your commitment to the patient when you have completed the correct operation skilfully. In former circumstances a familiar team would take over the care of the patient. Teams now work in timed shifts and those who replace the ones you have advised need to receive written instructions that they can consult and pass on. Clearly and fully record what should be monitored, what to expect and how to react. Organize aftercare meticulously or risk undoing the benefits of all your preceding planning and efforts.

2 Always make a full record as soon as possible of the operative findings, giving details of the procedure carried out and any special points such as the insertion of drains. Be prepared to provide a sketch of the incisions and of attached drains, cannulae or other apparatus, with instructions about the management of each one: in complicated cases ensure that drains are labelled.

3 Especially following a major operation, or one carried out on a poor-risk patient, inform the relatives and the general practitioner as soon as it is convenient, personally or by telephone. It is usually best to defer passing on the full impact of distressing news to relatives until you can speak under less stressful circumstances.

RECOVERY PHASE

Regard the patient who has just been submitted to an operation in the same light as one brought into the hospital following trauma or an acute illness.

Monitor

1 Airway, Breathing, Circulation (ABC) are vital functions to observe during the recovery from anaesthesia.

2 Regularly review the pulse, blood pressure chart, respiration rate and temperature chart to pick up the trend.

3 Order frequent checks of the consciousness level by noting the response to stimuli, such as calling the patient's name. In case of doubt ask for pupillary and other reflexes and peripheral muscular tone to be tested.

4 Do not take a fixed attitude to the amount of pain the patient is likely to suffer. Order small, repeated doses of analgesics if the recovering patient suffers pain.[27]

5 Give appropriate orders for checks of the wound and drains, especially if blood emerges from an abdominal or chest drain.

6 Restlessness of the patient may have other causes than wound pain, such as an overfilled bladder, uncomfortable position or pressure from sharp or hard apparatus.

7 Ensure that as soon as the patient is responsive they are given information, which is as reassuring as possible, about the operation and the present situation.

8 The wakened patient needs to breathe deeply, cough and exercise the legs within the limits posed by the procedure.

INTERMEDIATE PHASE

1 Regularly check not only the patient but also the pulse, temperature and respiration rate.

2 Mobilize the patient as quickly as possible. Order breathing and coughing exercises, leg and foot movement to reduce venous stasis, frequent changes of posture and walking as soon as possible.

3 Achieve and maintain fluid, electrolyte and acid–base balance and nutritional requirements.

4 Frequently check the wound, infusion sites, drains and the function of the system subjected to operation.

5 Bear in mind co-morbidities including insulin-dependent diabetes, depression, drug abuse and long-term therapeutic drugs. Patients with prosthetic heart valves who are temporarily on heparin usually require warfarin therapy to be reinstated postoperatively.

6 If the patient's condition deteriorates, first carry out a thorough systematic examination and carefully selected investigations. Do not restrict your survey to the operative condition and thereby miss an overlooked co-morbidity.

7 If you initiate non-specific supportive treatment and the patient improves do not assume that the problem is solved. Placebo effects may mislead you. Remain vigilant and anticipate possible deterioration (see Fig 1.2).

DAY CASE SURGERY

1 Monitor the recovery from a general anaesthetic as thoroughly as for an inpatient. Sedation with benzodiazepines and administration of analgesics may depress respiration: monitor breathing rate and depth for 2 hours.

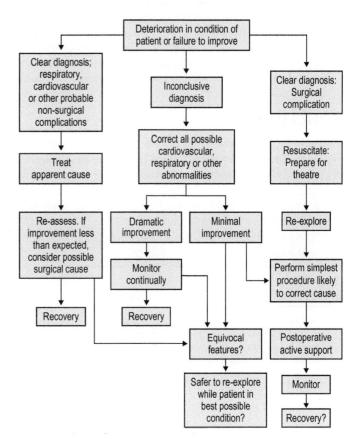

Fig. 1.2 Scheme for management of a patient who develops a complication or fails to recover. (Adapted with permission from Kirk RM 1990 Reoperation for early intra-abdominal complications following abdominal and abdominothoracic operations. Hospital Update 16:303–310).

2   Even though you are compressing the assessment of recovery into a shorter period, ensure that the cardiovascular and respiratory functions are normal before discharging the patient.

3   Check the wound.

4   Fully inform the patient of the procedure, the likely sequelae, danger signs and what to do about them. If possible, give written instructions for later reference.

5   If a follow-up appointment is to be given, arrange it now.

6   Ensure that those who have had a general anaesthetic or sedation are accompanied home.

7   Record the findings and procedure immediately. Day case patients are often admitted, treated, monitored and discharged in sequence. It is easy to confuse their details if these are not recorded individually between procedures.

AUDIT

1   Well organized audit (Latin: audire = to hear; a hearing, a trial) is a powerful driver for improvement. Identifying problems is only the beginning of the process: it is vital that this is followed by solutions. 'Closing the circle' describes the need to identify why outcomes are poor, what practical solutions can be implemented, implementing them – and demonstrating that the introduction has corrected the results.[28]

2   The improvement achieved by the Great Britain and Ireland Society of Cardiac Surgeons is remarkable.[29] They have compiled a database of 400 000 patients over a 15-year period, demonstrating a 21% reduction in mortality when compared to previous outcomes. In particular, they have devised methods of incorporating and accounting for many of the variations from standard scenarios, and have thrown down a challenge to the remainder of surgical specialties to achieve comparable success in surveillance and transparency.

CONCLUSION

Choose well, cut well, get well remain three elements in our treatment of patients. They were never truly discrete, but then neither is surgery a discrete specialty apart from other aspects of medical and social care.

> ■ A true professional sees every commitment through to completion.
> ■ 'Choose well' begins the process and remains vital through to the last.

REFERENCES

1. Spencer FC. Teaching and measuring surgical techniques – the technical evaluation of competence. Bull Am Coll Surg 1978;63:9–12.
2. Doyal L. Consent for surgical treatment. In: Kirk RM, Ribbans WJ, editors. Clinical Surgery in General. 4th ed. Edinburgh: Churchill Livingstone; 2004. p. 155–64.
3. Ng TT, McGory ML, Ko CY, et al. Meta–analysis in surgery: methods and limitations. Arch Surg 2006;141:1125–30.
4. Freedman L. Bayesian statistical methods. BMJ 1996;313:569–70.
5. Kirk RM, Cox K. Decision making. In: Kirk RM, Ribbans WJ, editors. Clinical Surgery in General. 4th ed. Edinburgh: Churchill Livingstone; 2004. p. 144–51.
6. Wyatt JC. Decision support systems. J R Soc Med 2000;93:629–33.
7. Langenhoff BS, Crabbe PFM, Wobbes T, Ruers TJM. Quality of life as an outcome measure in surgical oncology. Br J Surg 2001;88:643–52.
8. www.cochrane.org.
9. www.nice.org.uk/search/guidance.
10. www.cdc.gov.
11. www.hse.gov.uk.
12. Swenson SJ, Mayer GS, Nelson EC, et al. Cottage industry to post-industrial care – the revolution in health care delivery. N Engl J Med 2010;362:e12.
13. Weiser TG, Regenbogen SE, Thompson KD, et al. An estimation of the global volume of surgery: a modelling strategy based on available data. Lancet 2008;372:139–44.
14. Kirk RM. Basic Surgical Techniques. 6th ed. Edinburgh: Churchill Livingstone; 2010.
15. Polanyi M. Two Kinds of Awareness. Personal Knowledge. London: Routledge and Keegan Paul; 1958. p. 55–7.
16. Kirk RM. Surgical skills and lessons from other vocations. Ann R Coll Surg Engl 2006;88:95–8.
17. Chang N, Goodson III WH, Gottrup E, Hunt TK. Direct measurement of wound and tissue oxygen tension in postoperative patients. Annals Surgery 1983;197:470–8.
18. Ueno C, Hunt TK, Hopf HW. Using physiology to improve surgical wound outcomes. Plast Reconstr Surg 2006;117(7S) Supplement: 595–715.
19. O'Neil O. A question of trust. The Reith Lectures 2002. Cambridge Cambridge University Press; 2002.
20. Gawane AA, Thomas EJ, Zinner MJ, et al. The incidence and nature of surgical adverse events in Colorado and Utah in 1992. Surgery 1999;126:66–75.
21. Reason J. Human error; models and management. BMJ 2000;320:768–70.
22. WHO. Guidelines for Safe Surgery 2009: safe surgery saves lives. Geneva: World Health Organization; 2009.
23. Way L, Stewart L, Gantert W, et al. Causes and prevention of laparoscopic bile duct injuries: analysis of 252 cases from a human factors and cognitive psychology perspective. Annals Surgery 2003; 237:460–9.
24. www.hpa.org.
25. Reilly J, Kilpatrick C. Preventing surgical wound infection: evidence based practice for surgical wound care. Nurse 2 Nurse 2002;2: 47–50.
26. Greif R, Akca O, Horn E-P, et al. Supplemental peri-operative oxygen to reduce the incidence of surgical wound infection. N Engl J Med 2000;342:161–7.
27. Sodhi V, Fernando R. Management of postoperative pain. In: Kirk RM, Ribbans WJ, Clinical Surgery in General. 4th ed. Edinburgh: Churchill Livingstone; 2004. p. 357–69.
28. Davidson B, Schneider HJ. Audit. In: Kirk RM, Ribbans WJ, editors. Clinical Surgery in General. 4th ed. Edinburgh: Churchill Livingstone; 2004. p. 428–36.
29. Bridgewater B, Kinsman R, Walton P, Keogh B. UK 'Blue Book'@ 2009. The 6th National Adult Cardiac Surgical Database Report. Oxon: Dendrite Clinical Systems; 2010. ISBN:1-903968-23-2.

2

Anaesthesia-related techniques

J. Prout, S. Mallett, K. Miltsios

INTRODUCTION

The practice of anaesthesia is not merely confined to the operating theatre, but includes preoperative assessment and, importantly, risk stratification of surgical patients, continuing through to postoperative care, be this in a ward setting or on a high-dependency or intensive care unit. In many respects, the role of the anaesthetist has extended to that of a perioperative care physician.

Today there is an emphasis on multidisciplinary care, and it is essential for surgeons to be conversant with the role of anaesthesia in overall patient care and outcome.

The aim of the following chapter is to summarize some of the most important aspects of anaesthetic care and practical techniques that have direct relevance to the practice of surgery.

TECHNIQUES TO ASSESS PERIOPERATIVE RISK

Appraise

Background

A fundamental role of both surgeon and anaesthetist is to seek to identify patients who may be at increased risk of mortality or serious morbidity following surgical intervention.

Perioperative *cardiovascular* events are a major source of adverse outcomes. The incidence of death following major non-cardiac surgery in the United Kingdom is 0.5–1.5% (approximately 25 000 deaths per year). A further 2–3.5% of patients suffer major cardiac complications. A major focus of ongoing research is concerned with how to identify this high-risk subgroup of patients and what interventions may minimize the risk.

Aims of preoperative assessment in respect of the high-risk patient

- To quantify known disease, and to identify subclinical disease, aiming to intervene and optimize where possible
- To facilitate informed patient consent: a better appreciation of risk allows patients and clinicians to discuss the risk–benefit ratios of alternative procedures and/or conservative treatment
- To assist in appropriate allocation of critical care or high-dependency beds
- To assist decision-making in respect of both anaesthesia and surgery: for example, in deciding between open or laparoscopic surgery, or whether to use regional techniques as an adjunct or alternative to general anaesthesia.

Assess

Cardiac risk indices

The time-honoured approach to patient assessment is based upon history, examination and investigations. In the past, several scoring systems have emerged based on this principle.

The first widely used cardiac risk index was that proposed by Goldman et al in 1977.[1] Nine independent criteria were identified as indicators of increased risk (Box 2.1). The Goldman Index has been revised by subsequent workers, notably Detsky[2] and Lee.[3]

In 2007, the American College of Cardiology (ACC) and American Heart Association (AHA)[4] sought to stratify apparent cardiac risk factors into three categories – those that require further investigation, and others that may or may not actually impose increased risk (Box 2.2).

A step-by-step approach to risk assessment

Subsequent guidelines propose a stepwise approach to the evaluation of a potential high-risk surgical patient. The aim is to assist in creating an individualized cardiac risk assessment, and to suggest appropriate interventions before surgery in terms of optimization. The process is summarized in Box 2.3 and expanded upon in the sections that follow.

Assessing the risk of the surgical procedure

The risk of serious cardiac complications following surgery depends not only on the presence of risk factors, such as those described above, but also varies according to the type of surgery performed. Surgery induces a physiological stress response, with sympatho-humoral activation, increased myocardial oxygen demands and hypercoagulability. With regard to cardiac risk, surgical interventions fall into one of three categories: low, intermediate or high-risk, according

TABLE 2.1 Risk of MI/cardiac death within 30 days of surgery

Low risk (<1%)	Intermediate risk (1–5%)	High risk (>5%)
Breast	Abdominal	Aortic and major vascular surgery
Dental	Carotid	Peripheral vascular surgery
Endocrine	Endovascular aneurysm repair	
Eye	Head and neck	
Gynaecology	Neurosurgery	
Plastic/reconstructive	Major orthopaedic	
Minor orthopaedic	Renal transplant	
Minor urology	Major urology	

to the risk of myocardial infarction (MI) and cardiac death within 30 days of surgery (Table 2.1).

Action

Tests of functional capacity including cardiopulmonary exercise testing

A potential consequence of the physiological response to major surgery is an imbalance between oxygen supply and demand: hence the interest in measuring a patient's exercise capacity as an index of *global* cardiorespiratory reserve. Tests of *individual* components of exercise capability (e.g. exercise electrocardiography (ECG), pulmonary function tests) have shown poor correlation as predictors of postoperative problems.

A careful history may, of course, give some indication of a patient's exercise tolerance, but may not be accurate. Efforts to make this more objective have included structured questionnaires, such as the *Duke Activity Status Index*, which grades exercise tolerance according to the ability to perform tasks ranging from washing and dressing through to strenuous activities such as tennis.

In the *shuttle walk test*, the patient is observed walking back and forth between two fixed points, usually 10 m apart, against a timed bleep which is made progressively shorter as the test continues. The completed distance within the allowed time is taken as a measure of exercise ability and has shown reasonable correlation with postoperative mortality and morbidity after major surgery.

Cardiopulmonary exercise (CPEX) testing is increasingly regarded as a gold-standard for preoperative exercise testing, yielding considerable data on oxygen uptake and utilization. CPEX testing is cheap and relatively non-invasive, and aims to determine the patient's anaerobic threshold. Since it evaluates both the cardiovascular and respiratory systems, it is ideal for investigation of the patient with exertional breathlessness. The patient exercises on a bicycle ergometer, with measurement of gas exchange at the mouth together with ECG monitoring. CPEX detects the change from aerobic to partial anaerobic metabolism (Fig. 2.1): at the anaerobic threshold (AT), production of CO_2 relative to consumption of O_2 increases. An AT of less than 11 ml/min/kg has been associated with a higher perioperative cardiovascular mortality.

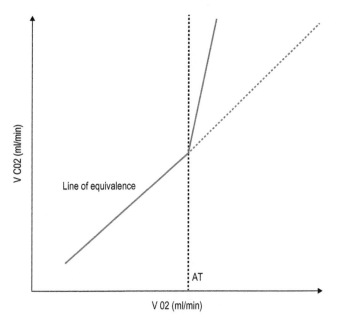

Fig. 2.1   CPEX testing and anaerobic threshold.

Other cardiac investigations

Electrocardiography

The 12-lead ECG is widely performed as part of the preoperative cardiovascular risk assessment. Whilst it may yield important prognostic information in patients with ischaemic heart disease, the ECG may be normal or show only non-specific changes in patients with both ischaemia and infarction, so results need to be interpreted with caution. Nonetheless, an abnormal ECG is a predictor of a higher incidence of cardiovascular death in surgical patients.

Assessment of resting left ventricular function

Trans-thoracic echocardiography and radionuclide angiography can be used to measure resting left ventricular (LV) function. Although an association has been demonstrated between poor LV ejection fraction (<40%) and an increased risk of adverse perioperative cardiac events, the predictive value of such tests is increased if dynamic images are taken under stress.

Dobutamine stress echocardiography

This has been demonstrated to be a superior investigation in predicting postoperative cardiac events. Increased heart rate and myocardial oxygen demands may induce regional wall motion abnormalities in patients with ischaemic heart disease which precede the onset of ECG changes or anginal symptoms. Dobutamine stress echocardiography (DSE) also has a particularly high negative predictive value, such that a normal result is associated with a very low incidence of cardiac events.

It is, however, a subjective test that requires a high degree of operator skill.

Coronary angiography

Although well-established as an invasive diagnostic procedure, coronary angiography is rarely indicated to assess the risk of non-cardiac surgery. Patients with acute myocardial infarction, unstable angina or with poorly controlled angina despite maximal medical therapy should undergo angiography.

Aftercare

Pharmacological strategies to reduce risk

Pharmacological interventions to reduce perioperative risk have been the focus of much interest and research. A number of classes of drug have been investigated.

β-blockers

Part of the physiological stress response to surgery is a catecholamine surge with increased heart rate and myocardial oxygen consumption. In surgical patients with known ischaemic heart disease, Mangano et al[5] reported a reduced *2 year* mortality after 7 days' perioperative β-blockade.[1] These findings were swiftly incorporated into new guidelines recommending use of β-blockade in patients with overt ischaemic heart disease or with risk factors. Subsequent studies produced more equivocal results and a more cautious approach followed, recommending use of β-blockers in *high-risk* patients rather than in all patients at risk.

Then came the POISE (PeriOperative Ischaemia Study Evaluation) study,[6] which measured 30-day mortality and morbidity after oral metoprolol. There was a significant reduction in the number of cardiac events, but the overall mortality rate actually *increased*, with a significant excess of strokes – possibly because of the excess of patients suffering from hypotension and bradycardia amongst those treated.

More recent work again suggests that high-risk patients benefit from β-blockade – and certainly that withdrawal of established therapy is dangerous.

Close monitoring of blood pressure and heart rate intra- and post-operatively is, however, essential.

Other drugs

Angiotensin converting enzyme inhibitors (ACEI) are of proven benefit in reducing disease progression in patients with cardiac failure and it is postulated they may improve postoperative outcomes. They may, however, interact with anaesthesia to cause significant hypotension – hence common practice is to discontinue ACEI therapy 24 hours preoperatively, especially when prescribed for hypertension. In patients with stable chronic heart failure, it may be preferable to continue ACEI *throughout* the perioperative period, with appropriately close haemodynamic monitoring.

Statins are widely used in patients with cardiovascular disease because of their lipid-lowering effect. They also have plaque-stabilizing properties and have been postulated to reduce the incidence of perioperative myocardial infarction. Several studies have confirmed benefit, and it is recommended that statins be started preoperatively in high-risk surgical patients, and be continued throughout the perioperative period.

Myocardial revascularization

Patients with *unstable* angina who require non-cardiac surgery are high-risk. The mainstays of management are antiplatelet anticoagulant therapy and beta-blockade, proceeding to prompt revascularization. Most patients will undergo a percutaneous coronary intervention (PCI), often with bare-metal stents (see below) if the proposed surgery is urgent.

The evidence differs, however, in respect of surgical patients with *stable* ischaemic heart disease. Coronary artery bypass grafting

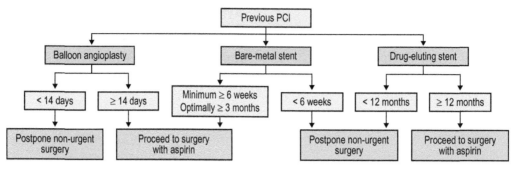

PCI = percutaneous coronary intervention

Fig. 2.2 Recommendations for timing of surgery after PCI (from Poldermans et al Guidelines for pre-operative cardiac risk assessment and perioperative cardiac management in non-cardiac surgery. European Heart Journal 2009: 30(22): 2769–2812).

(CABG) improves prognosis and relieves symptoms in patients with significant left main-stem disease and/or significant triple vessel disease, especially when there is poor left ventricular function, and in patients with other categories of lesion PCI is now a valuable alternative. Nonetheless, evidence is lacking that prophylactic revascularization reduces perioperative mortality in stable cardiac patients undergoing non-cardiac surgery.

Management of antiplatelet therapy

An increasing number of patients now present for non-cardiac surgery having previously undergone myocardial revascularization. Most will be receiving single or dual antiplatelet therapy.

Two sorts of stent are commonly employed: bare-metal stents have generally been superseded by drug-eluting stents which carry a reduced risk of re-stenosis but a higher risk of stent thrombosis. Drug eluting stents require continuous dual antiplatelet therapy (aspirin + clopidogrel) for at least 12 months after implantation. It is now generally accepted that elective surgery should not take place within 12 months of drug-eluting stent implantation. After 12 months, surgery can proceed, but with *at least* continuation of aspirin therapy. It is no longer acceptable simply to discontinue all antiplatelet therapy in all patients, and discussion between surgeon, anaesthetist and cardiologist is to be recommended. The recommendations in respect of the timing of non-cardiac surgery after PCI are summarized in Figure 2.2.

REFERENCES

1. Goldman L, Caldera DL, Nussbaum SR, et al. Multifactorial index of cardiac risk in noncardiac surgical procedures. N Engl J Med 1977;297 (16):845–50.
2. Detsky AS. Cardiac assessment for patients undergoing non cardiac surgery: a multifactorial clinical risk index. Arch Intern Med 1996;146 (11):2131–4.
3. Lee TH. Derivation and prospective validation of a simple index for prediction of cardiac risk of major noncardiac surgery. Circulation 1999;100:1043–9.
4. Fleisher LA. ACC / AHA 2007 Guidelines on perioperative cardiovascular evaluation and care for noncardiac surgery. J Am Coll Cardiol 2007;50 (17):e159–242.
5. Mangano DT, Layug EL, Wallace A, et al. Effect of atenolol on mortality and cardiovascular morbidity after noncardiac surgery. Multicenter Study of Perioperative Ischaemia Research Group. N Engl J Med 1996;335(23):1713–20.
6. POISE Study Group. Effects of extended-release metoprolol succinate in patients undergoing non-cardiac surgery (POISE trial): a randomised controlled trial. Lancet 2008;371:1839–47.

FURTHER READING

Atkinson D, Carter A. Pre-operative assessment for aortic surgery. Current Anaesthesia and Critical Care 2008;19:115–27.
Foex P, Sear JW. Challenges of β-blockade in surgical patients. Anesthesiology 2010;113:767–71.
Poldermans D, Bax JJ, Boersma E, et al. Guidelines for pre-operative cardiac risk assessment and perioperative cardiac management in non-cardiac surgery. Eur Heart J 2009;30(22):2769–812.

OXYGEN THERAPY

Appraise

Rationale for oxygen therapy

Mild-to-moderate hypoxaemia during the postoperative period is extremely common and may contribute to poor outcome in a variety of areas (Box 2.4).

Certain patient groups are at particular risk from hypoxaemia: these include patients at extremes of age, pregnant women, obese patients, smokers and those with pre-existing cardiorespiratory disease.

Factors contributing to postoperative hypoxaemia

From first principles, adequate tissue oxygenation depends on:

- adequate alveolar ventilation
- diffusion of oxygen across alveolus into the pulmonary capillaries
- delivery of arterial blood to the tissues and uptake of oxygen.

Box 2.4 Potential adverse consequences of hypoxaemia

Reduced resistance to infection

Delayed wound healing

Anastomotic breakdown

Loss of GI mucosal integrity: may result in bacterial translocation and sepsis

Diminished cognitive function: may contribute to postoperative delirium

Potential adverse cardiovascular effects: including hypertension, ischaemia and arrhythmias

Increased incidence of postoperative nausea and vomiting.

Box 2.5 Factors contributing to postoperative hypoxaemia

CNS depression
Opioids/residual anaesthetic agents/sleep apnoea

Peripheral nervous system pathology
Residual neuromuscular block/myasthenia gravis, etc.

Chest wall pathology
Trauma/pneumothorax/poor analgesia after thoracic surgery

Airway compromise
Diminished conscious level/obstruction/bronchospasm, etc.

Diaphragmatic splinting
Abdominal distension/poor analgesia after abdominal surgery

Alveolar pathology
Atelectasis/infection/pulmonary oedema/pleural effusion

Shunt
Hypovolaemia/pulmonary embolism

Anaesthesia and surgery may disrupt each of these processes. The main factors that contribute to postoperative hypoxaemia are conveniently classified anatomically from respiratory drive onwards, and are summarized in Box 2.5.

Assess

Assessment and detection of hypoxaemia

Mild-to-moderate hypoxaemia is difficult to detect by purely clinical methods. More profound cases may result in:

- altered mental state (disorientation, confusion, etc.)
- dyspnoea or tachypnoea (difficulty completing sentences, use of accessory muscles, etc.)
- cyanosis (often difficult to detect clinically)
- cardiovascular: tachycardia/hypertension/arrhythmias
- vasodilatation (headache/bounding pulses) if accompanying hypercarbia.

A high index of clinical suspicion is required, and pulse oximetry should be routinely available, with a low threshold for arterial blood gas analysis to confirm a hypoxic state.

Pulse oximetry

This has rightly become a routine component of basic nursing observations. It is, however, important to recognize one *fundamental* limitation – that it will not detect hypoventilation. Measuring the respiratory rate is an integral and essential part of respiratory observations. Arterial gas analysis (see below) will confirm hypoventilation.

Various factors make pulse oximetry unreliable. These include: movement artefact, cool extremities, exogenous or endogenous pigments (e.g. nail varnish, jaundice) and high levels of carboxy- or methaemoglobin.

Arterial gases

These are essential to confirm hypoventilation (producing a raised arterial PCO_2) as a cause of hypoxaemia. They also very helpfully reveal metabolic disturbance (electrolyte imbalance, metabolic acidosis, etc.), although the latter will also be revealed by *venous* gases, the collection of which is less traumatic for the patient. Use of a small

dermal injection of local anaesthetic (lidocaine) greatly facilitates obtaining an arterial gas sample from the radial artery: it greatly reduces discomfort, and makes the process much easier for both patient and operator!

Action

Oxygen therapy devices

Increasing the inspired concentration of oxygen provides a higher gradient for diffusion of oxygen from the alveolar gas into the pulmonary capillary blood. Two sorts of device are available – variable and fixed performance (Fig. 2.3).

Variable performance devices

The Hudson mask is a variable performance device in that air is entrained around the sides of the mask in proportion to the peak

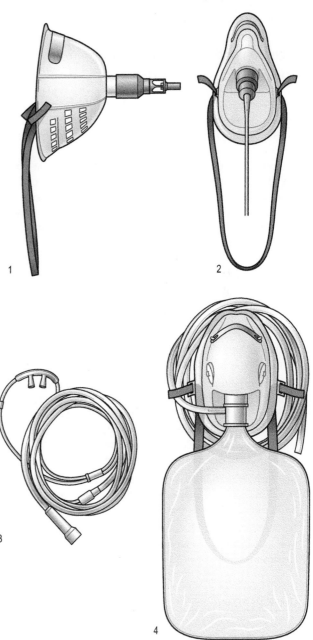

Fig. 2.3 Oxygen delivery devices. 1. Venturi mask. 2. Hudson mask. 3. Nasal cannulae. 4. Reservoir bag and mask.

inspiratory flow rate, such that the inspired concentration of oxygen is diluted.

The addition of a reservoir bag increases the amount of inspired oxygen, up to about 80%.

Nasal cannulae are often used on the wards at low flow rates (2 l/min) to provide supplemental oxygen whilst allowing patients to eat and drink.

Fixed performance devices

Venturi masks entrain a fixed percentage of oxygen (up to 60%) according to the O_2 flow rate and the size of the orifice of the colour-coded adaptor.

Concern is frequently expressed about patients with chronic obstructive airways disease and CO_2 retention – in practice, this is relatively uncommon, but a Venturi device will allow delivery of 24% or 28% oxygen in the minority of patients with *chronic* hypercarbia who are truly dependent upon hypoxic drive.

Recognition and management of respiratory failure

Respiratory failure is defined as a failure of oxygenation of arterial blood to achieve a partial pressure of oxygen (PaO_2) of 8kPa breathing room air at sea level. Two types are described: in type 1, ventilation is preserved ($PaCO_2 < 6.5$ kPa). In type 2 respiratory failure, there is a failure of both oxygenation *and* ventilation ($PaCO_2 > 6.5$ kPa).

The common causes in surgical patients are as listed in Box 2.5 and the clinical manifestations are as described above. In terms of investigations, these should include arterial blood gas analysis and an urgent chest X-ray (CXR). It is important to note that arterial gases do *not* require to be taken on air for a diagnosis to be made – this is dangerous, and may provoke severe desaturation.

The initial management of the hypoxaemic patient is high-flow oxygen therapy: as explained above, the scenario of the patient with chronic CO_2 retention losing his or her hypoxic drive in response to oxygen therapy is not common. If there is *any* doubt, high-flow oxygen should be given pending a respiratory opinion.

If, despite oxygen therapy, the oxygen saturation cannot be maintained above 92% (or the PaO_2 above 9 kPa), then further respiratory support may be required. In essence, this may be one of three types:

- *Continuous positive airways pressure (CPAP):* delivered via a close-fitting mask, maintaining a positive expiratory pressure of 5-15 cm H_2O. It increases FRC and reduces the work of breathing. The increase in intrathoracic pressure reduces cardiac preload and afterload and hence CPAP may be of great benefit in acute heart failure. Gastric distension may be a problem.

- *Non-invasive ventilation (NIV):* this applies a positive *inspiratory*, as well as expiratory, pressure (e.g. BiPAP), and is particularly useful in the presence of raised $PaCO_2$.

- *Invasive ventilation:* requires sedation and endotracheal intubation and may supervene from BiPAP in a patient whose gases are deteriorating or who is becoming exhausted.

FURTHER READING

Burt CC, Arrowsmith JE. Respiratory failure. Surgery 2009;27(11):475–9.
Strachan L, Noble DW. Hypoxia and surgical patients – prevention and treatment of an unnecessary cause of morbidity and mortality. J R Coll Surg Edinb 2001;46:297–302.

PERIPHERAL VENOUS ACCESS

Appraise

Peripheral venous access is used for fluid and intravenous drug administration. When selecting an appropriate cannula (Fig. 2.4), it is important to remember that flow rates increase in proportion to the fourth power of the radius (Poiseuille's law). Hence volume resuscitation requires a large-bore (14 G or 16 G), short cannula. Smaller diameter devices are suitable for maintenance fluids and/or drug administration.

Action

Having selected a cannula of suitable size, according to the indication, an appropriate site should be chosen. This will usually be the upper limb and, most conveniently, the dorsum of the hand or the radial border of the forearm (cephalic vein). It is preferable to avoid insertion sites over the wrist and elbow joints.

Venous access in the lower limb is generally avoided and carries a greater risk of thrombosis.

A meticulous aseptic technique should be employed, preparing the skin with 2% chlorhexidine. It should be routine practice to use 1% or 2% lidocaine (via a 25 G needle) to reduce discomfort when inserting cannulae of sizes larger than 20 G.

A few tips for successful peripheral venous cannulation are given in Box 2.6.

Aftercare

The cannula site should be covered with a transparent, semi-permeable dressing and inspected daily for signs of inflammation. An entry should be made within the clinical notes documenting the date of insertion. It is usual to change the cannula site every 48–72 hours to reduce infection risks.

Where possible, potassium-containing solutions should be avoided peripherally, owing to the risk of thrombophlebitis. Cannulae should always be removed as soon as they are no longer needed.

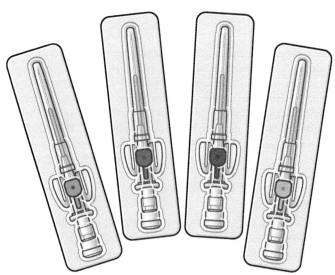

Fig. 2.4 Peripheral intravenous cannulae.

Try not to be rushed: allowing time for adequate venous distension from a proximal tourniquet will increase the chances of success.

Try to immobilize the vein distally with the free hand.

Keep the angle of insertion *low* (essentially parallel to the vein), making puncture of the posterior wall of the vein less likely.

Remember that the needle extends several millimeters beyond the tip of the cannula: rather than 'freezing' when a flashback is obtained, instead aim to confidently insert the needle/cannula assembly in one movement such that *both* are within the lumen: the needle can then be withdrawn slightly and the device advanced easily along the vein.

CENTRAL VENOUS ACCESS

Appraise

Central venous lines are usually multichannel devices comprising three to five lumens (ranging from 20 G to 14 G size). Indications for central venous access are summarized in Box 2.7.

Central lines allow simultaneous infusions of multiple drugs and fluids, in addition to measurement of central venous pressure. Single-lumen catheters are sometimes used for administration of total parenteral nutrition, since the risk of catheter-related sepsis is less compared to multi-lumen devices.

Traditional central venous lines are unsuitable for large volume resuscitation since flow rates decrease with increasing length. Special rapid infusor central lines are available if potential volume requirements exceed what can be provided through large-bore peripheral cannulae. There are essentially three possible approaches: internal jugular, subclavian and femoral.

Prepare

A central venous line insertion is by no means a risk-free procedure, and it is therefore important to take certain precautions. Any pre-existing coagulopathy should be corrected, especially if using a subclavian approach, where direct pressure cannot be applied. When preparing for an internal jugular or subclavian approach, it is important to exclude abnormalities on the *contra-lateral* side (such as pneumothorax or

Box 2.7 Indications for central venous access

Monitoring of central venous pressure

Administration of irritant or potent drugs (e.g. inotropes, K$^+$)

Administration of total parenteral nutrition

Difficult peripheral venous access

As a conduit for:
- renal replacement therapy
- pulmonary artery catheter insertion
- transvenous cardiac pacing.

haemothorax) – otherwise a complicated line insertion may result in *bilateral* pathology and a risk of significant cardiorespiratory compromise.

Informed consent should be obtained, and full monitoring applied (3-lead ECG, pulse oximetry and non-invasive blood pressure monitoring).

Central venous lines remain the commonest source of hospital-acquired bloodstream infections, and an aseptic insertion technique (gown, gloves, mask, sterile drapes and 2% chlorhexidine skin preparation) is mandatory. A ready-made sterile pack containing gown, drapes, syringes, etc., is helpful.

Local skin infiltration with 1% or 2% lidocaine is required in the awake patient – who must be able to lie flat throughout the duration of the procedure.

To promote venous distension and to reduce the risk of air embolism, the patient may be placed in a head-up (femoral) or head-down (subclavian/internal jugular) tilt.

INSERTION TECHNIQUE

All multi-lumen lines are inserted using a Seldinger technique (needle, guidewire, dilator, line). The skin incision should be kept superficial but sufficiently generous to allow easy passage of the dilator – it is imperative not to use undue force.

Ultrasound guidance (Fig. 2.5) is strongly recommended for internal jugular lines, and has been demonstrated to reduce the incidence of complications. The surface landmark for the vein lies over a triangle formed from the two heads of sternomastoid (medial and lateral) and the clavicle (inferior). In the absence of ultrasound, the needle should be advanced at an angle of about 30^0 towards the ipsilateral nipple. A high approach reduces the risk of pneumothorax but increases the risk of arterial puncture – the converse is true of a low approach.

A subclavian approach tends to be more comfortable for the patient but carries a greater risk of pneumothorax and haemothorax. Ultrasound visualization is less reliable than with the internal jugular route and an inadvertent arterial puncture is not amenable to direct pressure. The needle entry point should be about one finger's breadth inferior to the clavicle, at the junction of the outer and middle thirds, aiming towards the suprasternal notch (i.e. perpendicular to the sagittal plane of the body). It is important to begin sufficiently distant from the clavicle as to be able to pass

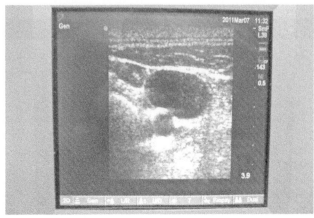

Fig. 2.5 Ultrasound image of internal jugular vein.

Box 2.8 Complications of central venous line insertion

Early:
  Arterial puncture (leading to haemorrhage/ischaemia/ thromboembolism)
  Damage to other adjacent structures (e.g. pneumothorax, thoracic duct injury)
  Air embolism
  Cardiac arrhythmia.
Late:
  Infection (catheter-related sepsis)
  Venous thrombosis
  Perforation of right atrial wall (leading to pericardial tamponade)
  Chylothorax

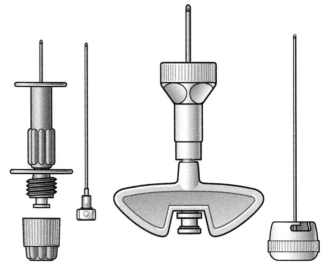

Fig. 2.6   Intraosseous devices.

under it with the needle almost horizontal – in so doing, the risk of pneumothorax will be reduced.

A CXR should be obtained after internal jugular or subclavian cannulation: the tip of the line should reside above the pericardial reflection, within the superior vena cava (*not* the right atrium): this corresponds to the level of the carina on the CXR.

A femoral line insertion is again facilitated by ultrasound guidance, and may be preferred in the presence of coagulopathy.

COMPLICATIONS OF CENTRAL VENOUS ACCESS

The most important complications are *immediate* damage to adjacent structures (manifesting as haemothorax, pneumothorax, etc.) and *later-onset* infection (Box 2.8).

Strategies to reduce the risk of complications are listed below:

- Is the line really indicated?
- What is the most appropriate site? (check vein patency with ultrasound if previous insertions)
- Always use a strict aseptic technique
- Use ultrasound guidance wherever possible
- Always request (and review) a CXR immediately following the procedure.

INTRAOSSEOUS ACCESS

In cases where immediate resuscitation is required in the absence of intravenous access, intraosseous access may be life-saving, most especially in children (Fig 2.6).

The commonest insertion site is the anterior surface of the tibia, 2–3 cm below the tibial tuberosity. After skin preparation, the needle and trocar kit is advanced until cortical penetration occurs. The trocar is removed and the needle aspirated. Fluid injection should not encounter resistance.

Intraosseous access can be used for fluid resuscitation and drug administration. Possible complications include osteomyelitis and compartment syndrome. The device should be removed as soon as adequate intravenous access has been obtained.

GENERAL ANAESTHESIA TECHNIQUES

Appraise

Within the operating theatre, the primary responsibility of the anaesthetist is to ensure patient safety during surgical procedures. Self-evidently, this involves measures to relieve pain and discomfort, but fundamentally, anaesthesia aims to minimize the physiological disturbance from surgery and to support vital functions – respiratory, cardiovascular, metabolic and so on, whilst providing suitable operating conditions for the surgeon.

Anaesthesia may be general, regional or local, and sometimes a combination of these: a careful preoperative visit will inform the decision-making process.

There is certainly evidence, for example, that combining epidural anaesthesia with general anaesthesia reduces respiratory complications after major abdominal surgery and promotes faster recovery of gut function, though no overall mortality benefit has been demonstrated.

In medically unstable or high-risk patients, evidence supports a period of 'pre-optimization', usually in an intensive care or high-dependency environment, with correction of fluid deficits *prior* to anaesthetic induction.

Action

Basic principles of general anaesthesia

General anaesthesia is a balanced technique comprising a *triad* of analgesia, hypnosis (unconsciousness) and muscle relaxation. The balance varies according to circumstances: these include factors relating to the patient (e.g. size, co-morbidity) and to the operation (e.g. surgery on the extremity as opposed to within a body cavity).

Induction of anaesthesia

General anaesthesia may be induced by either an intravenous or inhalational technique.

The intravenous route is most commonly employed, and provides a swift and smooth induction with minimal excitation. It is also suitable for 'rapid-sequence' induction (in the presence of a full stomach), but carries the potential for rapid loss of airway control (for instance in cases of upper airway obstruction).

An inhalational technique is often preferred in small children, and is sometimes advocated in difficult airway situations since spontaneous breathing may be maintained until control of the airway is assured. In the latter situation, an awake fibreoptic intubation may be a safer technique: anaesthesia is induced *after* the airway has been secured.

Airway management

The unconscious patient requires support of the airway, which will otherwise become obstructed. To achieve airway patency requires 'head tilt-chin lift' and 'jaw thrust' procedures. The airway may then be maintained through a variety of techniques:

- Holding a facemask (with or without airway adjuncts such as an oropharyngeal airway)
- Inserting a laryngeal mask airway
- Endotracheal intubation.

Holding a facemask

The ability to maintain the airway with a facemask is an essential skill that can only be acquired with practice. When other techniques prove difficult, it is the fundamental default position: patent facemask ventilation is infinitely preferable to prolonged and unsuccessful attempts at intubation. During short procedures in a spontaneously breathing patient, the airway may be managed solely by holding a facemask.

The laryngeal mask airway

The laryngeal mask airway (LMA) is a remarkable device that has greatly facilitated airway management in both elective and, sometimes, in emergency situations. It is very frequently used to support the airway during anaesthesia with spontaneous breathing. It may also be used during positive pressure ventilation if inflation pressures are low, although it cannot fully protect against the possibility of aspiration. In the emergency situation of failed intubation and difficult facemask ventilation, it may offer a route to restore airway patency.

Endotracheal intubation

Endotracheal intubation provides the 'definitive' airway and is required if there is a significant risk of aspiration, or if positive-pressure ventilation requires high inflation pressures (for example, in the obese patient). Intubation is usually performed via the oral route, but nasal intubation may be indicated for oro-facial procedures or to allow longer-term ventilation, especially in children.

A key aspect of the preoperative assessment is an evaluation of the likely difficulty or otherwise of endotracheal intubation (and, even more importantly, of mask ventilation). Certain clinical features predict possible difficulty (Box 2.9).

Failed intubation

Failed intubation is defined as the inability to intubate the trachea during direct laryngoscopy. In any situation, *the priority is to maintain oxygenation*. The most senior available help should be sought at an early stage. Algorithms exist to guide management, but the basic pathway is thus:

- Reattempt intubation under optimal conditions: improved head and neck position; different laryngoscope blade; gum-elastic bougie
- Insert an LMA (which will usually re-establish the airway and may itself provide a conduit for intubation)

Box 2.9 Clinical predictors of difficult intubation
Altered body habitus: obesity, short neck, large breasts
Prominent upper incisors
Reduced mouth opening (less than three fingers' breadth)
Limitation of neck extension
Reduced jaw protrusion/prominent overbite/receding mandible
Short thyro-mental distance (<6 cm)
Oropharyngeal infection or tumour
Presence of stridor
Trauma/obstetric patient.

- If now able to ventilate but unable to intubate, consider waking the patient and postponing surgery
- In a 'can't intubate, can't ventilate' scenario, proceed without delay to cricothyroidotomy.

Ventilation during anaesthesia

Following anaesthesia induction and after establishing a stable airway, ventilation must be continued throughout surgery: either a spontaneous or a controlled ventilation technique may be used.

Spontaneous ventilation is typically employed in slim patients requiring relatively minor and superficial procedures of short duration, and the airway is usually maintained with an LMA.

Controlled breathing, usually with neuromuscular blockade, is generally used in longer, more major procedures, in obese patients and in those with poor respiratory reserve. It is also required when there is a surgical need for full muscle relaxation (e.g. intra-abdominal surgery) or when tight control of the arterial $PaCO_2$ is indicated (e.g. to control intracranial pressure). In appropriate situations, an LMA may be employed during controlled ventilation: for instance, when the anaesthetist wishes to avoid a hypertensive response to intubation in a relatively short procedure and when the patient's anatomy is favourable.

Principles of monitoring
Essential requirements

The Association of Anaesthetists of Great Britain and Ireland (AAGBI) have published clear guidelines regarding minimum standards of monitoring (Box 2.10).[1]

Indications for invasive monitoring

In complex cases, an enhanced level of monitoring may be indicated. An **arterial line** allows continuous, beat-to-beat recording of the arterial blood pressure (Box 2.11). Further advanced cardiovascular monitoring may include measurement of cardiac filling pressures (most commonly the central venous pressure), cardiac output and mixed venous oxygen saturation.

Measurement of **central venous pressure** (CVP) gives an estimate of the cardiac pre-load, but becomes unreliable in the presence of impaired cardiac function. Nonetheless, observation of the *trend* in CVP and its response to fluid challenges provides useful information in respect of volume status both in the operating theatre and in intensive care.

Box 2.10 Monitoring requirements during induction and maintenance (AAGBI guidelines 2007)

Essential monitoring during induction and maintenance:
    Pulse oximeter
    Non-invasive blood pressure (NIBP) monitoring via cuff
    Electrocardiogram
    Airway gases: oxygen, carbon dioxide, anaesthetic vapour
    Airway pressure

The following must also be available:
    Nerve stimulator (when muscle relaxants are used)
    A means of measuring the patient's temperature.

Box 2.11 Indications for invasive arterial pressure monitoring

Haemodynamically unstable patient, e.g. shock/polytrauma

Significant pre-existing cardiovascular disease

Raised intracranial pressure

Major surgery: cardiac/thoracic/ hepatobiliary/major vascular.

Box 2.12 Levels of postoperative care

Level 0
For patients whose needs can be met through normal ward care in an acute hospital

Level 1
For patients at risk of deteriorating (or after recent transfer from a higher level of care) whose needs can be met on an acute ward with advice/support from ITU team

Level 2
For patients requiring more intensive observation monitoring (e.g. invasive BP) and/or single organ support (not mechanical ventilation)

Level 3
For patients requiring mechanical ventilation and/or support of other organs

---

Measurement of **cardiac output** may be extremely useful in both anaesthesia and intensive care. A variety of techniques are available: the pulmonary artery flotation catheter provides much haemodynamic information, but it is an invasive procedure and some controversy persists as to whether it confers a survival benefit.

More recently, less invasive techniques have emerged based on arterial pulse contour analysis, for example the PiCCO (using thermodilution) and the LiDCO (uses lithium dilution).

The oesophageal Doppler has been used successfully to guide fluid therapy, with demonstrable improvements in outcome amongst surgical patients. Trans-oesophageal echocardiography is a semi-invasive procedure requiring a high degree of operator skill, but gives information regarding filling status and contractility in addition to revealing structural abnormalities such as valve lesions or pericardial collections.

There is increasing interest in the use of central and mixed **venous oxygen saturation** (SvO2) to guide perioperative interventions. Venous oxygen saturation reflects the relationship between global oxygen delivery (reflecting cardiac output + arterial oxygen content) and consumption. A high SvO_2 may reflect increased O_2 delivery (e.g. inotrope therapy) or reduced O_2 utilization (e.g. sedation/hypothermia/sepsis). Conversely, a low SvO_2 reflects increased tissue O_2 extraction (e.g. anaemia/hypoxia) or reduced O_2 delivery (e.g. hypovolaemia/pulmonary embolism/heart failure).

Aftercare

The recovery room

The anaesthetist is responsible for the safe transfer of patients to the recovery room for continued care and 1:1 nursing following a detailed handover of all pertinent information including the procedure performed, analgesic/fluid therapy and nil by mouth status. Tracheal extubation requires the presence of the anaesthetist, and it is usually safer for this to take place in theatre before transfer. LMAs are more usually removed in recovery. Monitoring of oxygen saturation and NIBP are essential, as are facilities for more intensive monitoring if required. The recovery bed space should contain all essential airway equipment.

With guidance from the anaesthetic and surgical teams, the recovery nursing staff will monitor the patient's vital signs and operative site, and attend to common postoperative problems such as pain and nausea. A further detailed handover should take place between the recovery and ward nursing staff.

Levels of postoperative care

An ever-increasing number of patients undergo day case surgery or are discharged from hospital within 24 hours. For those who require inpatient management postoperatively, several levels of care are defined (Box 2.12).

Analgesic techniques

A robust strategy for managing postoperative pain is essential since untreated pain has a variety of adverse consequences (Box 2.13).

The pharmacological management of acute pain includes:

- Classical analgesics: simple analgesics, NSAIDs, opioids
- Local anaesthetics: neuraxial, regional and local blocks
- Adjuvant drugs: clonidine, ketamine, pregabalin, amitriptyline, etc.

Box 2.13 Adverse effects of postoperative pain

Psychological
Anxiety/distress/sleep disturbance/loss of confidence in healthcare team

Physical
Cardiovascular: hypertension/tachycardia, etc.
    Respiratory: poor cough/retained secretions/basal atelectasis/chest infections

Socio-economic
Prolonged hospital stay/delayed rehabilitation and return to work.

Pre-emptive analgesia (i.e. *before* the skin incision) may have an impact on postoperative pain.

Most acute hospitals run an acute pain service, under the guidance of a consultant anaesthetist and usually run by a clinical nurse specialist. The team predominantly looks after patients with epidurals and patient-controlled analgesia (PCA) devices, but also offers staff education and training, and provides advice in difficult situations.

The analgesic ladder

This was originally introduced by the World Health Organization[2] as a guide to the management of patients with malignancy. It comprises three steps:

- Mild pain: non-opioid (paracetamol) ± NSAID ± adjuvant
- Moderate pain: weak opioid (e.g. codeine) + paracetamol ± adjuvant
- Severe pain: strong opioid + paracetamol ± adjuvant.

Pain relief should be provided on a *regular*, rather than 'as required' basis with regular assessment by scoring systems such as a verbal rating (mild-moderate-severe or 0-10) or visual analogue (distance along a line measured in millimetres) scale.

REFERENCES

1. AAGBI. Recommendations for standards of monitoring during anaesthesia and recovery. London: AAGBI; 2007.
2. World Health Organization. The analgesic ladder. Geneva: World Health Organization; 1997.

FURTHER READING

Spoors C, Kiff K, editors. Training in Anaesthesia; the Essential Curriculum. Oxford: Oxford University Press; 2010.

LOCAL ANAESTHESIA TECHNIQUES

Local anaesthesia is widely used, as a sole technique or as an adjunct to general anaesthesia. Local anaesthetic agents are potentially dangerous, and a knowledge of safe doses and of the management of suspected toxicity is paramount. These subjects are discussed, together with examples of a few blocks in common use.

Appraise

Operative procedures are frequently undertaken under local anaesthesia (LA), both in and out of theatre. LA techniques are well suited to minor procedures, and cause less systemic upset than general anaesthesia.

LA agents may be administered in a variety of ways according to the required area of analgesia:

- *Topical anaesthesia:* application of LA to the skin, and to the mucous membranes of the conjunctival sac, mouth, nose, tracheobronchial tree and urethra
- *Local infiltration:* direct injection of LA into the operative site
- *Field block:* injection of LA around the operative site, so as to create an analgesic zone
- *Individual peripheral nerve blocks:* e.g. median, ulnar, femoral or pudendal nerves
- *Regional block:* injection of LA around nerve trunks supplying the region to be operated upon, e.g. brachial plexus block

- *Neuroaxial blocks:* spinal and epidural anaesthesia
- *Intravenous regional anaesthesia:* injection of a large, dilute LA volume into the veins of a previously exsanguinated limb.

LOCAL ANAESTHETIC AGENTS

Various LA agents are available, and are classified into two groups – esters and amides – according to the structure of their carbonyl linkage group. The agents in most common clinical use (lidocaine, bupivacaine and prilocaine) are all amides.

LAs block sodium channels to cause a reversible interruption of nerve impulse conduction. Most are weak bases and will exist in both ionized and unionized forms according to the pH of the tissue fluid. LAs are relatively ineffective in an acid pH (e.g. inflamed or infected tissues), in which the ionized (non-lipid soluble) form predominates.

Addition of a vasoconstrictor (e.g. adrenaline (epinephrine)) prolongs the duration of action of LAs. Epinephrine is added to LA in concentrations ranging from 1:80 000 to 1:300 000. The commonest strength is a 1:200 000 (5 µg per ml) concentration of adrenaline (epinephrine) (Box 2.14).

Adrenaline (epinephrine) may cause tachycardia and hypertension, and should be used with caution in patients with cardiovascular disease. The use of adrenaline (epinephrine) is absolutely contraindicated in areas supplied by end arteries (e.g. digits, penis).

Important features of the different LA agents are summarized in Table 2.2.

It is always sensible to calculate the maximum safe dose for the individual patient: for example, the maximum safe dose of lidocaine is 3 mg/kg without adrenaline (epinephrine) and 7 mg/kg with adrenaline (epinephrine). In a 70 kg adult, therefore, the maximum safe dose of plain lidocaine is 210 mg. This equates to 21 ml of a 1% solution (10 mg/ml). If larger volumes are required, the concentration should be reduced, or adrenaline (epinephrine) added.

LOCAL ANAESTHETIC TOXICITY

All local anaesthetics may exert toxic effects if administered in excess of the safe maximal dose. Systemic absorption is influenced by the site of injection (more rapid in vascular tissues, e.g. intercostal blocks) and by the addition of adrenaline (epinephrine) (slows absorption). Inadvertent *intravascular* injection may cause rapid cardiovascular and central nervous system collapse.

Strategies to reduce the risk and/or impact of LA toxicity include:

- Ensure patent IV access, availability of resuscitation equipment and presence of a trained assistant *before* LA administration

---

Box 2.14 Preparation of LA solutions

0.25% bupivacaine contains **0.25** g per **100** ml solution, i.e. 2.5 mg per ml

Adrenaline (epinephrine) 1:1000 contains **1** g of adrenaline (epinephrine) in **1000** ml of solution, i.e. 1 mg/ml

To prepare a 1:200 000 solution, the 1:1000 solution must be diluted 200 times. This can be achieved by taking 0.1 ml (= 0.1 mg) and adding 19.9 ml of LA solution

TABLE 2.2 A comparison of commonly used local anaesthetic agents

	Lidocaine	Bupivacaine	Prilocaine
Onset	Rapid onset	Slower in onset	Intermediate
Duration	Short-acing	Longer acting	Short-acting
Preparations	0.5–2% (5–20 mg/ml) for infiltration 4% (40 mg/ml) topical	0.25–0.5% (2.5–5 mg/ml)	0.5% (5 mg/ml) for intravenous regional anaesthesia (IVRA) 0.5–1% for infiltration 1–2% for blocks
Maximum safe dose	3 mg/kg (plain) 7 mg/kg (with adrenaline (epinephrine))	2 mg/kg (with or without adrenaline (epinephrine))	6 mg/kg (plain) 8 mg/kg (with felypressin)
Typical uses	Local infiltration Treatment of arrhythmias	Nerve blocks/epidurals	IVRA
Adverse effects		Most cardiotoxic	Methaemoglobinaemia

- Use the least toxic drug, in the lowest dose, and reduce doses in the elderly and frail
- Calculate the dose *carefully* (this point cannot be overstated!)
- Inject slowly, aspirating during injection in case of inadvertent vascular puncture.

LA toxicity typically presents with clinical features relating to the central nervous and cardiovascular systems:

- *CNS:* lightheadedness, dizziness, taste disturbance, tinnitus, circumoral paraesthesiae; progressing to agitation, convulsions, coma and respiratory arrest
- *CVS:* hypotension, myocardial depression, arrhythmias and cardiac arrest.

Initial management

- Stop injecting the LA and call for help
- Assess patient according to ABC principles
- Maintain the airway: if necessary, secure it by endotracheal intubation
- Give 100% oxygen and ensure adequate ventilation
- Confirm or establish IV access: administer fluids ± vasopressors
- Control seizures with thiopentone or benzodiazepines
- If the patient is in cardiac arrest, perform cardiopulmonary resuscitation (CPR) according to ALS protocol.

Use of Intralipid®

The use of Intralipid® may reverse LA toxicity. CPR should be continued throughout treatment with lipid emulsion. Recovery may take more than an hour. The Association of Anaesthetists of Great Britain and Ireland has produced comprehensive guidelines (2010)[1] detailing the management of severe local anaesthetic toxicity and the use of lipid emulsion:

- Immediately:
  - give an initial intravenous bolus injection of 20% lipid emulsion in a dose of 1.5 ml/kg over 1 min
  - start an intravenous infusion of 20% lipid emulsion at 15 ml.$kg^{-1}.h^{-1}$

- After 5 min:
  - give a maximum of two repeat boluses (same dose, 5 min apart) if circulation not restored
  - continue infusion (doubling the rate if stability not restored) until stable or maximum dose ($12 \ ml.kg^{-1}$) is reached.

CERVICAL PLEXUS BLOCK

This technique is used for awake carotid artery surgery, and may combine deep and superficial plexus blocks:

- *Deep:* identify the lateral border of the sternomastoid at the level of the thyroid cartilage (C4) and feel for the interscalene groove. Aim the needle in a caudal and medial direction 10–20 mm towards the contralateral elbow, until paraesthesiae are felt or contact made with the C4 transverse process. *After aspiration,* inject 8–10 ml of LA solution. Complications include blockade of the phrenic nerve, recurrent laryngeal nerve and stellate ganglion
- *Superficial:* the superficial plexus is blocked by a 10 ml 'sausage-shaped' injection along the posterior border of sternomastoid.

INTERSCALENE BLOCK

This block is useful for shoulder and upper arm surgery. The needle passes between the anterior and middle scalene muscles and achieves a high brachial plexus block.

Identify the posterior border of sternomastoid at the level of the cricoid cartilage (C6). The interscalene groove is just behind sternomastoid. Introduce the needle slightly caudad, medial and posterior, *to a depth of no more than 1–2 cm* and, after aspiration, inject 30 ml of LA solution. Phrenic nerve block is a frequent occurrence, and caution should be exercised in patients with respiratory disease.

FEMORAL NERVE BLOCK

This block is used in knee and anterior thigh surgery. Locate the groin crease (1 cm below the inguinal ligament) and insert the needle 1 cm lateral to the femoral pulse and 45° cephalad, to a depth of 3–5 cm. Inject a volume of 25–30 ml.

Box 2.15 Technique for intravenous regional anaesthesia

- Insert two IV cannulae, one into each hand
- Exsanguinate limb with Esmarch bandage
- Apply double cuff proximal tourniquet and inflate upper cuff to 100 mHg above systolic pressure then remove Esmarch bandage
- Inject LA solution slowly into exsanguinated limb via cannula
- After 10 minutes, inflate lower cuff to above systolic pressure then release upper cuff (improves patient comfort, since the arm beneath the lower cuff will now be anaesthetized)
- Pay *constant* attention to cuff inflation throughout the procedure
- At the end of the procedure, after a minimum of 20 minutes, deflate lower cuff.

USE OF PERIPHERAL NERVE STIMULATORS AND ULTRASOUND

The use of nerve stimulators and, more recently, ultrasound, has improved the accuracy and safety of regional techniques, and hence their popularity. It remains imperative, however, to have a sound knowledge of the underlying anatomy.

INTRAVENOUS REGIONAL ANAESTHESIA

Intravenous regional anaesthesia (IVRA) was first described for forearm anaesthesia (Bier's block), but can also be used on the lower limb and for sympathetic blocks in chronic pain states.

A dilute solution of LA is injected intravenously into an exsanguinated limb kept isolated by a tourniquet cuff from the rest of the circulation.

The block is technically simple (Box 2.15) yet potentially dangerous: escape of LA into the systemic circulation may cause severe toxicity. Prilocaine 0.5% (without adrenaline (epinephrine)) is thought to be the safest agent (maximum 6 mg/kg or up to 300 mg).

The most important potential complication is systemic LA toxicity from cuff failure. The tourniquet may produce pressure-related damage. The technique is not suitable in the grossly obese, in hypertensive patients (systolic BP > 200 mmHg) or in those with peripheral vascular disease.

REFERENCE

1. AAGBI. Management of Severe Local Anaesthetic Toxicity (AAGBI Safety Guideline). London: AAGBI; 2010.

CENTRAL NEURO-AXIAL BLOCKS

Spinal or subarachnoid block and epidural blocks are the major neuro-axial techniques.

SPINAL ANAESTHESIA

The introduction of LA solutions into the cerebrospinal fluid (CSF) produces spinal anaesthesia. The LA does not have to cross tissue barriers and the central attachments of the ventral and dorsal nerve roots are un-myelinated, which allows for a rapid uptake of the LA drug. There is a rapid onset of effect (within a few minutes with lidocaine but up to 20 minutes for bupivacaine) and the dose of drug required is small (2 to 4 ml). Lidocaine (5%) or heavy bupivacaine (0.5%) are commonly used. This is a 'one-shot' technique and the duration of action should be adequate to perform the intended surgery. Offset may be as rapid as 30–40 minutes following lidocaine and 90–120 minutes following bupivacaine, although the addition of adrenaline (epinephrine) will prolong the duration of the block. Spinal anaesthetics are useful for urological and gynaecological procedures, lower limb surgery and also obstetric procedures.

EPIDURAL ANAESTHESIA

This can be used as a sole anaesthetic for procedures involving the lower limbs, perineum, pelvis and lower abdomen. It is possible to perform upper abdominal and even thoracic procedures under epidural anaesthesia alone, but the height of the block required, with its attendant side-effects, makes it difficult to avoid patient discomfort and risk. The advantage of epidural over spinal anaesthesia is the ability to maintain continuous anaesthesia after placement of an epidural catheter, thus making it suitable for procedures of a longer duration. This feature also enables the use of the technique into the postoperative period for analgesia, using lower concentrations of local anaesthetic drugs or in combination with different agents, usually opiates.

Technique

The tip of a hollow bored needle with a bevelled end (Tuohy needle) is introduced into the epidural space, after it has passed through the ligamentum flavum. The epidural space is really only a potential space, as the dura and ligamentum flavum are usually closely adjacent. The epidural space contains adipose tissue, lymphatics and the epidural veins. The space has to be carefully identified as the bevel of the needle passes through the ligamentum flavum as the dura will be penetrated shortly after if the needle is advanced any further. The most common method used is pressure applied to a syringe attached to the Tuohy needle, and a sudden loss of resistance is felt as soon as the epidural space is entered. Saline or sometimes air is used in the syringe. The block is usually performed with the patient awake and in the sitting position or sometimes the lateral decubitus position.

The quality and extent of the block is determined by the volume as well as the total dose of the drug. The spread of the block may be more extensive in pregnancy as the volume of the space is reduced by venous engorgement.

INDICATIONS FOR EPIDURAL ANAESTHESIA/ANALGESIA

1. **Hip and knee surgery:** Internal fixation of a fractured hip is associated with less blood loss when central neuro-axial blocks are used. The incidence of deep vein thrombosis is reduced in patients undergoing total hip and knee replacement under an epidural technique.

2. **Vascular reconstruction of the lower limbs** and endovascular arterial reconstructions: Epidural anaesthesia improves distal blood flow and can be used as the sole anaesthetic technique. Patients undergoing lower limb amputation may have a reduced incidence of phantom limb pain if neuro-axial blockade is established before surgery.

3 **Postoperative pain relief following abdominal and thoracic surgery:** Low concentration bupivacaine (0.125%), often in combination with an opioid such as fentanyl or preservative-free morphine provides effective pain relief. It also minimizes the effects of surgery on cardiopulmonary reserve, such as diaphragmatic splinting and the inability to cough effectively. This is especially important in patients with compromised respiratory function, e.g. chronic obstructive airways disease, morbid obesity and the elderly. Adequate analgesia allows better cooperation with chest physiotherapy. Epidural analgesia also facilitates earlier mobilization and reduces deep vein thrombosis.

EFFECTS ON ORGAN SYSTEMS

Cardiovascular: Sympathetic blockade (sympathetic outflow T1–L2) results in vasodilatation of resistance and capacitance vessels, causing relative hypovolaemia and tachycardia, with a resulting fall in blood pressure. This is managed with fluid loading and/or a vasoconstrictor. If the block is as high as T2 the sympathetic supply to the heart (T2–T5) is also interrupted, leading to bradycardia.

Respiratory: Usually unaffected, unless the blockade is high enough to affect the intercostal muscle nerve supply (thoracic nerve roots) leading to reliance on diaphragmatic breathing alone.

Gastrointestinal: Blockade of the sympathetic outflow to the GI tract leads to a predominance of parasympathetic (vagus and sacral parasympathetic) tone, with active peristalsis and relaxed sphincters and a small contracted gut which can enhance surgical access. Urinary retention is a common problem with epidural anaesthesia.

CONTRAINDICATIONS

Absolute

1 *Patient refusal:* A primary absolute contraindication

2 *Coagulopathy:* Clotting abnormalities may lead to the development of a large haematoma and spinal cord compression. In warfarinized patients the international normalized ratio (INR) should be below 1.4 prior to catheter insertion. A platelet count below 100 000 is a relative contraindication

3 *Skin infection at proposed injection site:* Insertion of an epidural needle through an area of skin infection may introduce pathogenic bacteria into the epidural space, leading to abscess formation or even meningitis

4 *Raised intracranial pressure:* Accidental dural puncture in patients with raised ICP may lead to brainstem herniation (coning).

Relative

1 *Bacteraemia:* Some may consider this an absolute contraindication. Epidural abscesses have been described occurring de novo, even when no epidural has been inserted

2 *Fixed cardiac output states:* E.g. severe aortic stenosis, hypertrophic cardiomyopathy, complete heart block. These patients are unable to increase their cardiac output to compensate for the peripheral vasodilatation that occurs and can develop profound circulatory collapse. Hypovolaemia is also a relative contraindication

3 *Neurological disorders:* E.g. multiple sclerosis – since any new neurological symptoms may be ascribed to the epidural.

EPIDURALS AND ANTICOAGULANT THERAPY

The incidence of epidural haematoma is unknown but it has increased since the use of low-molecular-weight heparin (LMWH) therapy for thromboembolic prophylaxis. Over 80% of epidural haematomas are related to haemostatic abnormalities or procedural difficulties with catheter insertion.

Antiplatelet therapy

Current guidelines are that clopidogrel should be stopped for a minimum of 5 days prior to epidural catheter insertion. Low-dose aspirin is not a contraindication.

Low-molecular-weight heparin

The timing of catheter insertion and removal is critical. For prophylactic therapy at least 12 hours should have elapsed from when the last dose of LMWH was given before the epidural catheter is inserted or removed. For treatment doses of LMWH it is recommended that there is a delay of 24 hours from the last dose before catheter removal. Caution is advised in the elderly and those with impaired renal function, if they have had repeated doses of LMWH, as they may still have some drug present even at this time interval. With unfractionated heparin this interval can be reduced to 4 hours.

MANAGEMENT OF SURGICAL PATIENTS RECEIVING LONG-TERM ANTICOAGULANT OR ANTIPLATELET THERAPY

Increasing numbers of patients are receiving anticoagulant or antiplatelet therapy. When such patients require surgery, a balance of risks must be considered:

■ The risk of thromboembolic events if anticoagulant or anti-platelet therapy is interrupted

■ The risk of bleeding if therapy is continued.

ANTICOAGULANT THERAPY

There are a number of indications for long-term anticoagulant therapy, including the presence of atrial fibrillation, a prosthetic heart valve or a history of arterial or venous thromboembolism.

Patients treated with a vitamin K antagonist (VKA) may require interruption of anticoagulation prior to surgery. Frequently, either LMWH or unfractionated heparin (UFH) is used to bridge the gap in therapy since these agents have a relatively rapid onset and offset of action compared to warfarin.

Patients on oral anticoagulants undergoing elective surgery

The key issues are:

■ Identifying patients who can safely undergo an invasive procedure whilst *continuing* their VKA

■ Identifying patients who are at high risk of thromboembolism and who require bridging therapy with UFH or LMWH when the VKA is stopped

■ Determining the optimal dose and timing of parenteral anticoagulants during the perioperative period.

The difficulties presented by these issues are reflected in the current wide variation in practice regarding bridging therapy for perioperative anticoagulation.

Procedures which do not require warfarin interruption: Patients on warfarin may undergo minor procedures such as dental extraction without discontinuing their treatment, provided their INR is in the therapeutic range and they receive tranexamic acid mouthwashes.[1]

For minor dermatological and ophthalmological (e.g. cataract extraction) procedures, it is also recommended that patients do not stop their VKA therapy.

Stratification of thromboembolism risk

- **Atrial fibrillation:** approximately 50% of *all* patients receiving warfarin therapy have atrial fibrillation (AF) which is, therefore, the most common clinical condition requiring a decision about bridging therapy. The average risk of perioperative stroke in patients with AF who do not receive antithrombotic therapy is 4.5%. The risk can be further stratified based on a 'CHADS' score (1 point each for congestive cardiac failure, hypertension, age > 75 years and diabetes, and 2 points for history of stroke or transient ischaemic attack). The American College of Physicians recommends low dose LMWH or no bridging for a score of 0–2, and bridging with therapeutic LMWH or UFH for CHADS scores of 4 and above. Intermediate levels of risk can be managed with higher prophylactic doses of LMWH.

- **Mechanical heart valves:** the risk of thromboembolism is such that bridging therapy is essential. The risk varies according to the type of valve and also its position (mitral > aortic). If the patient's target INR is 3, then bridging therapy with therapeutic/full-dose LMWH is required. If the target INR is 2.5, then low-dose LMWH bridging is sufficient. Whenever surgery is planned, the risk of procedure-related bleeding must be balanced against the possible risk of thromboembolic events.

- **Venous thromboembolic disease (VTE):** therapeutic dose bridging is recommended for high-risk patients. These include patients who have suffered an episode of VTE within the previous 3 months, or those with known thrombophilia (such as deficiency of Protein S, Protein C or antithrombin III, or the presence of antiphospholipid antibodies). Moderate-risk patients (e.g. those with VTE within 3–12 months or with Factor V Leiden mutation) also require full-dose bridging therapy. Low-risk patients require either no bridging or prophylactic dose LMWH only.

Bleeding risk with bridging therapy: The risk of surgery when a patient is on full-dose bridging therapy varies markedly with the type of surgery. The risk of major bleeding is low for minor surgery such as inguinal hernia repair, but for major surgery, including knee and hip replacement, the risk of major bleeding is significantly greater. LMWH bridging therapy should be stopped 24 hours before surgery and therapeutic doses resumed 24–48 hours postoperatively. Low-dose LMWH may be considered as an alternative option during resumption of anticoagulant bridging after major surgery. LMWHs are very dependent on adequate renal function for their elimination, and reduced doses may be required in the presence of renal impairment or in the very elderly. In general, monitoring of LMWH activity is not required, but factor Xa levels can be measured where necessary.

A scheme for management of perioperative bridging therapy according to the risk of thromboembolic events is presented in Table 2.3.

New oral anticoagulant drugs

Warfarin has a variable dose–response, a narrow therapeutic index and numerous drug and dietary interactions, and requires frequent monitoring.

Recently, new oral anticoagulant drugs have been developed for the prevention and treatment of thromboembolic disease and also for the prevention of stroke in patients with atrial fibrillation. These drugs are given once a day, have a wider therapeutic index and do not require monitoring:

Rivaroxaban: Is a direct inhibitor of factor Xa. It has been licensed for the prevention of VTE following major joint replacement surgery. There is no specific reversal agent for this drug. It is recommended that this drug be discontinued 24 hours prior to surgery. If it is used for postoperative VTE prophylaxis 24 hours should elapse before epidural catheter removal.

TABLE 2.3 Management of bridging therapy according to thromboembolism risk

Thromboembolism risk	Example	Preoperative management	Postoperative management
Low	Atrial fibrillation	Stop warfarin 4 days prior to surgery Check international normalized ratio (INR) on admission INR should be < 1.6	Restart warfarin on night of surgery Add prophylactic low-molecular-weight heparin (LMWH) until INR > 2
Medium	Previous venous thromboembolic disease (VTE)	Stop warfarin 4 days prior to surgery Check INR on day of surgery	Restart warfarin on night of surgery LMWH (e.g. enoxaparin 40 mg od) until INR > 2
High	Mechanical heart valves High-risk VTE, e.g. Budd Chiari syndrome	Stop warfarin 4 days prior to surgery When INR < 2 start **either:** treatment dose LMWH (stop 24 hours preop) **or:** unfractionated heparin (UFH) (maintain activated partial thromboplastin time (APTT) 1.5–2.5 and stop 4–6 hours preop	Restart warfarin when taking oral medication Restart UFH after 6–12 hours or treatment dose LMWH 24 hours postop, if not bleeding, until INR > 2 For patients at high risk of bleeding: give low-dose LMWH and wait 48 hours to start full dose

Dabigatran: Is a direct thrombin inhibitor. Both the INR and aPTT are prolonged by the drug, but not in a dose-dependent manner. The thrombin clotting time (TT) is highly sensitive for quantifying its anticoagulant effects. It is almost entirely dependent on renal excretion for its elimination. There is no reversal agent for this drug.

Emergency surgery in patients on anticoagulant therapy

For patients on warfarin therapy requiring urgent surgery or if there is life-threatening bleeding (e.g. intracranial) give prothrombin concentrate concentrate (PCC) 20–50 units/kg and 5 mg of vitamin K intravenously. PCC contain factors II, VII, IX and X and produces rapid and effective reversal. Fresh frozen plasma is no longer recommended as a means of reversing warfarin therapy. UFH can be readily reversed with protamine (50 mg), but protamine is far less effective at reversing the anticoagulant effects of LMWH. There is no reversal agent for the new oral anticoagulant drugs – however, recombinant VIIa (NovoSeven™) 90 μg/kg, has been suggested as a possible agent in these circumstances. It is advisable to seek guidance from a haematologist.

ANTIPLATELET THERAPY

The two most commonly used antiplatelet drugs are **aspirin**, which irreversibly inhibits platelet cyclo-oxygenase-1 (COX-1), and **clopidogrel**, which binds irreversibly to the platelet ADP P2Y12 receptor. Dual therapy is known to provide more effective platelet inhibition, as the effects are synergistic and is routine therapy in patients who have received drug eluting stents (DES). These drugs inherently increase bleeding risk but discontinuing them will in many patients lead to an increased risk of thrombosis.

Stratifying the bleeding risk: Because there is considerable inter individual variability in response to both aspirin and, especially, clopidogrel therapy, some patients may be at greater risk than others for adverse bleeding outcomes. It is now becoming apparent that the degree of platelet inhibition in patients treated with the same antiplatelet regime is highly variable and up to 30% of patients may show no demonstrable platelet inhibition on standard therapy. This has implications not only for the risks of recurrent ischaemic events in 'hypo-responders', but at the other end of the spectrum for bleeding risks in 'hyper-responders'. In terms of antiplatelet therapy there is undoubtedly an optimal therapeutic window, but there are many challenges left to define the best method for monitoring platelet function and to identify 'cut-off' values where the risk of ischaemic events or bleeding becomes a significant risk. There is accumulating evidence that bleeding risk increases as the degree of irreversible platelet inhibition increases. Prasugrel is a third generation thienopyridine that achieves 4–5 times more potent ADP P2Y12 receptor blockade than clopidogrel. It significantly reduced ischaemic events in the TRITON – TIMI trial but the occurrence of major bleeding was also significantly increased. Prasugrel is increasingly used in patients with coronary stents who have had a poor response to conventional therapy. Point of care platelet function monitoring as a means of assessing the efficacy of these drugs is still under evaluation, but the most promising techniques in terms of assessing bleeding risk are platelet mapping™, which is a modification of the thromboealstographic technique and the Multiplate® analyser.

Perioperative management: It is currently recommended that patients on aspirin as primary prevention should continue therapy up until the day of surgery and those on clopidogrel should discontinue treatment at least 5 days prior to surgery. However, there are serious thrombotic risks associated with the discontinuation of these agents when they are used for secondary prevention of vascular disease or after coronary revascularization. It is generally agreed that aspirin should never be discontinued before surgery unless the risk of bleeding is thought unacceptable, e.g. intracranial surgery. Clopidogrel alone appears to increase the bleeding risk more than for aspirin alone. Dual therapy increases the relative risk of bleeding by 50% and the absolute risk by 1%. This risk remains increased in patients who stopped clopidogrel less than 5 days before surgery.

The difficulty is how to manage patients who have to stay on their antiplatelet therapy because they have coronary stents (see also management of antiplatelet therapy in previous section) or who currently are on treatment because they are presenting as an emergency or have been asked to stop their therapy prior to elective surgery and have forgotten to do so. A multidisciplinary approach to this problem is essential, with discussion between the patient's cardiologist, surgeon and anaesthetist. Prior to surgery, patients on dual therapy should always continue their aspirin until the day of surgery. If it is felt prudent to discontinue clopidogrel, bridging therapy with UFH or LMWH will be necessary.

In patients on antiplatelet therapy requiring urgent surgery, platelet concentrates should be ordered and available for transfusion if required. Without assessment of the degree of platelet inhibition, the increased risk of perioperative bleeding is undefined and prophylactic transfusion is generally unjustified. Patients who are taking Prasugrel will almost certainly have significant platelet inhibition and would probably benefit from platelet transfusion prior to surgical procedures with a high risk of bleeding.

REFERENCE

1. British committee for standards in haematology (BCSH). Guideline details. London: BCSH; 2006.

3

The severely injured patient

N.R.M. Tai

INTRODUCTION

This chapter concerns the surgical management of injury – in particular the operative management of major torso trauma. The frequency with which general surgeons are called upon to deal with major injury depends upon their professional circumstances. If you are a surgeon who regularly participates in an emergency roster or acute surgical 'take', you must be familiar with the tenets of damage control surgery and modern resuscitative practice. Your skills in dealing with the sickest trauma patient may be called upon at any moment – be this the cyclist with the crushed pelvis, a school boy with a penetrating injury to the heart, or the work-man who has sustained a fall from height – usually individually but occasionally as part of the response to a mass casualty incident. In treating such patients it is often a serious error to rely upon the dictums of elective surgical practice – where time is used to secure absolute technical perfection, and restoration of anatomical congruity is paramount – to guide your hand. In the unstable patient, the over-riding imperative is one of ensuring that the surgery you undertake is just sufficient to stop bleeding and control contamination, such that dwindling patient reserves are not exhausted by overly long surgical strategies. As with other spheres of surgical practice, successful operative management of injury is based around decision-making as much as technical proficiency. In major trauma, your decisions are often time-critical. Your first goal is to decide if the patient is physiologically unstable. Take the following as indicating continued bleeding: any evidence of lower-than-expected blood pressure, tachycardia, tachypnoea or acidosis (as judged by arterial blood gas measurement of base excess or lactate). Next determine the likely source of bleeding – whether from pelvis, thorax, abdominal cavity, junctional areas or extremities. Make this decision within the resuscitation bay using your interpretation of the history, mechanism of injury, and relevant physical findings, plus special investigations such as plain radiography, focused assessment by sonography for trauma (FAST) or diagnostic peritoneal lavage (DPL). Reserve computed tomography (CT) for those patients who are physiologically unchallenged. Having 'triaged the body cavities' decide upon the best way to address the injuries,

factoring in other associated trauma and your institution's capabilities. For instance, where protocols and facilities allow, some injuries may be amenable to interventional radiological techniques (such as angio-embolization). In the absence of these, surgical control of haemorrhage remains the default action.

The guidance in this chapter assumes that the patient has been fully assessed, resuscitation is ongoing and you have made a decision to operate. Techniques relevant to initial resuscitation (Advanced Trauma Life Support®) such as chest drainage, cricothryroidotomy and pericardiocentesis are not described. Rather, those surgical techniques relevant to the damage control approach are emphasized and discussed in detail.

PRINCIPLES OF DAMAGE CONTROL

1. Damage control surgery (DCS) is a well-established suite of techniques relevant to the management of severely injured patients.

2. The essence of the damage control approach is to tailor the *extent* of the surgical intervention to that which will most rapidly restore physiological normality in the patient. Control of haemorrhage takes precedence, with completeness of surgical reconstruction sacrificed, in order that the physiological burden of surgery is as light as possible. Keep the first operation (DCS phase one) short, completing the procedure within 60–90 minutes, and deferring definitive closure of body cavities if required. After a period of time in intensive care (DCS phase two – which may be hours or days depending on how rapidly the patient can be returned to physiological normality), the patient may be transferred back to theatre for re-inspection and completion of surgery plus closure if appropriate (DCS phase three).

3. Patients with serious injury, particularly when shocked, are at risk of acute coagulopathy of trauma (ACoT). Hypoperfusion and tissue damage, exacerbated by hypothermia and acidaemia, can serve to disable the normal clotting pathways, leading to continued haemorrhage (often from multiple sites) and a lethal outcome. By choosing a damage control approach, you can rapidly reduce the chance of ACoT developing, or mitigate the extent of ACoT if it is already present. An important and recently developed adjunct to damage control is the use of matched ratios of blood (packed cells) and plasma during initial and ongoing fluid resuscitation efforts. Published experience from the wars in Iraq and Afghanistan, combined with data from civilian centres, supports early use of equal or near-equal ratios (1:1–1:2) of packed cells and plasma in reducing mortality, organ failure rates and ongoing need for blood transfusion, especially if used in conjunction with aggressive, early use of platelet transfusion. Damage control resuscitation (DCR) is the overarching term used to describe this haemostatic transfusion strategy plus damage control surgery to

optimally treat the major trauma patient. As a practitioner of damage control surgery, you must be conversant with modern fluid resuscitation in order to ensure that your anaesthetic colleagues and other members of the trauma team are optimally managing the patient's physiological requirements.

4 Having decided on which cavity or body area requires initial attention, you next need to determine whether the patient will tolerate a definitive repair of their injury complex, or whether damage control mode needs to be selected. This can only be answered by rigorously seeking information from other members of the trauma team – particularly the anaesthetist – as to the current and anticipated physiological state of the patient. Remember that this state is dynamic, and although a patient may appear to be stable on cursory assessment, never underestimate the ability of fit young patients to compensate for severe haemorrhage until they enter a rapid and unanticipated phase of terminal decline. Always be prepared to 'course-correct' according to new information that is presented to you.

> ### ▶ KEY POINTS Deciding to use damage control surgery

Mechanism of injury:	Multi-storey fall from height
	High energy-exchange road traffic collision
	Severe crush injury to pelvis (cyclist trapped under goods vehicle)
	High energy weapon system (hunting rifle, military rifle)
	Explosion
Injury pattern:	Cross-torso penetrating/perforating trauma
	Multiple torso penetrations/perforations
	Presence of multiple system injury
Physiological trends:	Shock that does not rapidly respond to volume resuscitation
	Acidaemia
	Hypothermia
	Coagulopathy

Prepare

1 Ensure that you have gained sufficient information from physical examination and relevant investigations to undertake the operation you deem necessary. Whilst a thorough physical examination is required (always examine the back), this does not mean exhaustive special investigations, particularly when you suspect haemorrhage. There is a danger in utilizing additional investigations as a means of 'opting out' (or deferring) decision-making in trauma, particularly when faced with the prospect of performing an unfamiliar surgical intervention in unfamiliar clinical circumstances. Transfer for surgical control of haemorrhage is occasionally indicated very early on in the primary survey – sometimes as part of 'C' (Circulation) – so address it before making the rest of the assessment.

2 Ensure rapid transport to the operating theatre. Activate the hospital's massive transfusion protocol. Relay your intentions to the anaesthetic and scrub teams, stating what you expect to find,

what you plan to do about it, and your back-up plan. Give your anaesthetic colleagues an opportunity to do the same. Ensure that all relevant surgical sets, equipment and sutures are available, including two suckers and multiple large packs. Call for assistance from colleagues early, particularly if you require specialist assistance. Alert intensive care and ensure that they are updated regularly with the progress of the case. In cases of competing injury sets (e.g. abdominal haemorrhage plus open femoral fracture; pelvic fracture plus knee dislocation with lower limb ischaemia) decide upon surgical priority with relevant colleagues before beginning operation.

3 Supervise the transfer of the patient on to the operating table and ensure adequate access. The standard patient position for truncal trauma is supine with arms outstretched at 90 degrees (cruciform position). Ensure ECG leads and tubing (ventilation, urethral catheter, chest drains) are routed away from your preparation area. Place a warming blanket over the extremities and the head; adjust operating room temperature upwards to mitigate hypothermia.

4 Prepare the entire torso from the level of the mid thighs to the clavicles. Lay drapes, covering the groin with a separate towel. If necessary, control active bleeding (from a neck or groin wound) with a sponge stick during the preparatory phase.

Access

1 Make all surgical incisions in trauma patients large enough to allow full access to the relevant cavity or structure that is injured. Incisions should be *extensile,* i.e. amenable to elongation along an appropriate axis. The workhorse incisions for torso trauma are full-length midline laparotomy (abdominal and pelvic trauma), left/right anterolateral thoracotomy – proceeding to clamshell thoracotomy if required (thoracic trauma), and median sternotomy (control of aortic arch vessels). Any of these incisions can be combined with other incisions – for instance, laparotomy may be combined with a right anterolateral thoracotomy in cases of severe liver injury – if that is what is required to effect rapid visualization and control.

Assess

1 The keys to making an accurate assessment of the injury set and determining the source(s) of haemorrhage are:
   ■ Rapid evacuation of all free blood
   ■ Identification of the zone from which most bleeding is apparent (finding the 'compelling' source of bleeding)
   ■ Thorough and systematic examination of all areas and visceral contents for subsidiary injuries once the majority of bleeding has been controlled.

2 If the degree of bleeding is not consistent with the degree of physiological instability, you must ensure that another cavity does not harbour the primary source of shock. For instance, if you performed a laparotomy, but are unconvinced that the degree of haemorrhage encountered explains the shock, search for bulging of the diaphragm and check chest drainage output as a means of re-assessing the thoracic cavity.

Action

1 Having identified the bleeding organ or vessel, first control the haemorrhage. Initially you should use your hands to accomplish this, judiciously applying direct pressure (e.g. to a bleeding

vessel), pinching tissue (such as the hilar vessels supplying a bleeding spleen or liver), or packing around a bleeding structure (such as the liver) in order to diminish blood loss and give yourself a little time to organize yourself and your team.

2 Whilst performing this initial manoeuvre, think: *'Is my incision large enough for what I wish to accomplish? Have I got the correct retractors? Have I deployed my assistants correctly to use them properly? Are the lights angled correctly to give maximum illumination? What clamps/sutures/needle-holders/forceps do I need? Are the instruments the scrub team has laid out for me sufficient?'* Getting these factors addressed – setting yourself up correctly for success – is easier whilst maintaining digital haemorrhage control.

3 Communicate with the anaesthetist and explain what the source of the bleeding is, what you plan to do about it, and allow him or her a short period of time to optimize the requirements before removing your hands and proceeding.

4 Typically, gaining definitive control requires definitive visualization, often preceded by some dissection, and application of a clamp or haemostatic sutures, and/or resection of tissue or organ removal. These steps in haemostatic control may be made difficult by excessive haemorrhage, distorsion of normal anatomy by haematoma, and unfamiliarity with the procedure or anatomy. Your difficulties may be compounded by your natural anxiety at, and awareness of, the time-critical nature of the procedure. In such circumstances, energy and visual focus may become funnelled in to a particular task (*'I must correctly clamp the thoracic aorta'*) at the expense of overall situational awareness (*'The internal mammary arteries, sectioned on entry to the chest, are still bleeding and need to be ligated'*). Furthermore, under excessive stress, you lose creativity, so surgical technique and action resort to stereotype (*'This haemostatic suture has not worked; I shall ask for another suture and repeat the manoeuvre until something changes, even though this technique did not work the first time round'*) – a phenomenon that Mattox and Hirschberg aptly describe as 'flailing'. Be aware of this phenomenon, monitor yourself and the success of the manoeuvre you are employing to dissect/control/clamp/suture – above all, maintain situational awareness.

Checklist

1 DCS laparotomy is always accompanied by temporary means of abdominal cavity closure in order to diminish (but not abolish) the risk of abdominal compartment syndrome and to allow for easy re-exploration in DCS phase three. Similarly, when operating on the injured extremity, the likelihood of compartment syndrome is significantly reduced by adequate fasciotomy. Have a very good reason NOT to leave the operated cavity open.

2 Having completed the surgery, consider and plan for the actions needed so that the patient can be eventually returned to the theatre for completion of surgery.

> ▶ KEY POINTS Post damage control surgery

Generic checklists:
- Has the swab and instrument count been clearly documented, with special attention to residual (intra-cavity) swabs?
- Are supplementary means of haemorrhage control required (e.g. transfer to interventional radiology for embolization of internal iliac vessels in major pelvic trauma)?
- Have the primary and secondary surveys been completed?
- Has all radiology been completed (plain films, CT)? Will completion of these surveys benefit the patient at this time, and is the patient fit for transfer to radiology?
- Have the other injuries (e.g. orthopaedic) been identified and has a plan been made to address these with other members of the multidisciplinary team?
- Does the operation note record a plan for scheduled take-back?
- Have you briefed the on-coming surgical and critical care staff as to the nature of the patient's injuries, possible complications ahead, and an action plan in the event of deterioration?

NECK AND THORACIC OUTLET

Appraise

1 Penetrating trauma to the neck is more likely to require intervention than blunt trauma. The key decision you need to make is: does the patient need to go to theatre immediately or not? Patients who need urgent surgical exploration are those who display active arterial bleeding, have an expanding haematoma, or are shocked with poor response to haemostatic resuscitation. If your patient does not fall in to this category, examine the wound and determine if it has breached the platysma. You should be able to do this without formally exploring the wound. If the wound is superficial to platysma, simply close the skin. If the platysma is breached, investigate with imaging to exclude damage of the vascular or visceral structures. Contrast enhanced multi-detector CT has largely replaced screening by formal selective arteriography and barium contrast swallows for penetrating neck injuries. Reviewing the images, you should be able to follow the track of any penetrating mechanism and account for the integrity of all structures in the path, marrying up structural information with clinical features such as haemoptysis, haematemesis, neurological injury, or an obvious air leak, to enhance diagnosis.

2 Injuries to the lateral aspect of the neck, related to the thoracic outlet, may be associated with vascular compromise to the upper limb (damaged subclavian or axillary vessel) and damage to the brachial plexus. Endovascular stent grafting of these vessels may be an acceptable alternative to open surgery.

3 You must ensure that the airway is definitively controlled in the unstable patient. In the stable patient it is also wise to default to early intubation and ventilation when you have sufficient information to predict that the patient will require surgery.

Prepare

1 When operating on injured structures in the neck, be aware of the zone of likely injury and ready yourself accordingly. Zone I injuries (inferior to the cricoid cartilage) are likely to require a median sternotomy to gain access to the proximal aortic

branches. Zone III injuries, superior to the angle of the mandible, prove problematic in gaining distal control of the internal carotid and may require manoeuvres such as dislocation of the mandible to gain access.

2 Ensure that your preparation and draping takes account of these issues. In general, have the patient's head rotated away from the side of the injury to gain better access to the carotid sheath.

Access

1 When exploring the neck for possible vascular injury, begin by making a full-length incision along the anterior border of the sternocleidomastoid muscle, from mastoid process to jugular notch. Retract the SCM muscle laterally as you deepen the incision. The first structure you encounter is the internal jugular vein. Divide the facial vein and the omohyoid muscle, stretching across the carotid artery, to gain access to this vessel and its bifurcation. Divide the stylohyoid muscle in the superior part of the wound to gain access to the higher internal carotid. Be wary of the XII nerve as it crosses the internal carotid artery (see Chapter 23).

2 Be prepared to commence exploration of a Zone I injury by performing a median sternotomy (see Chapter 27), particularly if the patient is unstable. Open the pericardium and identify the aortic origin, then follow the vessel as it curves upwards and posteriorly, giving off the brachiocephalic, left common carotid and left subclavian arteries. Dividing the innominate vein gives better access; it can be repaired at the completion of the procedure if circumstances permit (Fig. 3.1).

3 Expose the 2nd part of the subclavian artery by a supraclavicular incision that runs above the medial two-thirds of the clavicle. Cut through platysma and the clavicular head of the sternocleidomastoid. Sweep the scalene fat pad laterally and palpate the anterior scalene muscle, running supero-inferiorly. Divide this muscle, sparing the phrenic nerve lying on the anterior surface, to reveal the subclavian artery lying in the base of the wound.

4 Having gained proximal and distal control, consider your options. Simply ligate veins. Repair damaged arteries if possible. Always repair the common or internal carotid. Excise injured arterial tissue and tack down the intima if there is a danger of a flap. Close simple lacerations transversely to avoid luminal narrowing. Usually, a patch of vein or Dacron is required. Prefer to repair segmental loss with an in-situ graft. In patients unable to tolerate definitive repair, then shunt the vessel with a commercial shunt or a short segment of diameter-matched IV tubing. You may safely ligate the external carotid artery. Haemorrhage from the vertebral artery is usually more difficult to deal with. Obtain access by retracting the carotid sheath medially and incising the prevertebral tissue plane so revealed. Beware of the prevertebral venous plexus which adds to the haemorrhage if damaged. You may achieve haemostasis using bone wax and pressure but otherwise control the artery above and below the injury by removing the costal face of the appropriate cervical transverse processes with bone nibblers. Repair of the vessel is technically difficult and ligation or clipping is usually the most practical option.

5 Explore tracheal wounds through a transverse skin crease incision or, if associated with a carotid injury, via medial dissection from the standard anterior sternocleidomastoid approach. You can normally repair the trachea using a single layer of absorbable

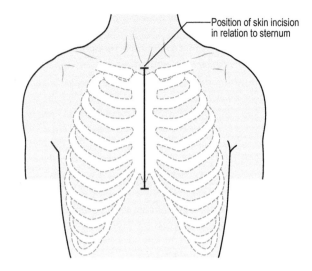

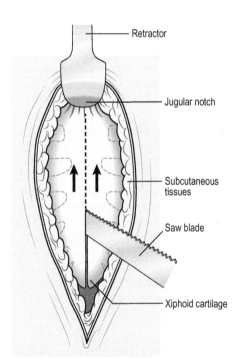

Fig. 3.1 The midline sternotomy for access to all chambers of the heart, the pulmonary vessels and the arch of the aorta. You may use a Gigli saw if you do not have a powered sternal saw available.

material over the endotracheal tube. Check for associated pharyngeal injuries and repair them in two layers. Ensure that the two repairs are separated, to avoid a fistula forming. A mobilized length of strap muscle serves this purpose well.

CHEST

In civilian trauma the mainstay of treatment of chest trauma, blunt or penetrating, is effective intercostal chest drainage (for pneumothorax or haemothorax), analgesia (to allow for proper ventilation) and supplementary oxygen. Thoracotomy, although infrequently required, is relatively straightforward to perform. Thoracotomy is not an end of itself but merely a means to access the thoracic viscera in order to control haemorrhage or air leak, or relieve tamponade (French = plug).

THORACOTOMY

Appraise

1. Perform thoracotomy for trauma under emergent or urgent conditions. Undertake emergency thoracotomy on an *in-extremis* casualty who has no detectable circulation. The patient's condition usually precludes transport to the operating theatre and for this reason the surgery is often performed in the Emergency Department. The outcome is far better following penetrating trauma than after blunt trauma. Survivors of emergent thoracotomy are generally those patients who have sustained a small stab wound to the front of the heart where loss of circulation has occurred in the presence of the trauma team. Factors mitigating against successful outcome include blunt mechanism of injury without evidence of tamponade, exsanguinating hypovolaemia, and prolonged 'downtime' (absence of circulation) prior to presentation to hospital. Tamponade is the injury pattern most amenable to emergency thoracotomy. Always search for it in the *in-extremis* or unstable casualty with thoracic trauma. This is particularly so when the injury is to 'The Box' of the anterior chest wall – an area demarcated superiorly and inferiorly by horizontal planes passing through the xiphisternum and jugular notch respectively, and bounded laterally by vertical planes passing through each nipple. Ultrasound scan is the most useful emergency department tool for detecting tamponade.

2. Urgent thoracotomy is usually performed in the operating theatre on a casualty who is unstable but exhibiting spontaneous circulation and has yet to decompensate. The diagnosis is usually either massive haemothorax or cardiac tamponade, but there is more time for you to plan your approach. In circumstances other than emergencies always ensure you have addressed the fundamental principles of current trauma management in Advanced Trauma Life Support® protocols, including appropriate imaging and correctly sited chest drainage.

▶ KEY POINTS Indications for thoracotomy

Emergent:	Penetrating trauma to chest with loss of cardiac output in the previous 10 minutes; cardiopulmonary resuscitation maintained throughout 'downtime'
	Blunt trauma to chest with loss of cardiac output in the previous 10 minutes; cardiopulmonary resuscitation maintained throughout 'downtime' AND evidence of cardiac tamponade on FAST scanning
Urgent:	Blunt or penetrating trauma to chest with evidence of cardiac tamponade
	Blunt or penetrating trauma to chest with evidence of massive haemothorax (>1.5L initial ICD drainage), ongoing losses (>200 ml/hour for 4 or more hours) and deteriorating physiological state
	Blunt or penetrating trauma to chest with evidence of massive air leak and inability to ventilate the patient.

Prepare

1. Double lumen tubes are seldom required for these patients. Do not allow the search for double lumen tubes or a 'cardiac anaesthetist' familiar with double lumen intubation to delay surgery.

2. Standard trauma preparation and drape; cruciform position. Preparation consists of pouring of antiseptic skin solution onto the chest in the emergent situation.

Access

1. For suspected tamponade, perform a left anterolateral thoracotomy (Fig. 3.2). Identify the fifth interspace immediately inferior to the male nipple, or by counting down from the angle of Louis (2nd costal cartilage meets sternum at this point). Make a bold transverse incision from the midline of the sternum, curving posteriorly and superiorly, following the fifth interspace as far back as the space between the mid and anterior axillary lines (Fig. 3.2). Deepen the incision. Retract the lowermost portion of pectoralis major superiorly or cut through these inferior fibres to reach and swiftly divide intercostal muscle with knife or scissors. Cleave the muscles toward the lower rib and avoid the intercostal bundle.

2. Prior to perforating the pleura, ask the anaesthetist to disconnect the patient from the ventilator in order to drop the lung away

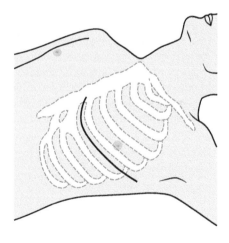

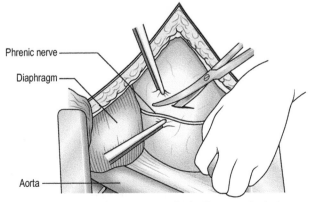

Phrenic nerve

Diaphragm

Aorta

Fig. 3.2 Left anterior thoracotomy, which allows ready drainage of the pericardium in tamponade. Avoid the phrenic nerve.

from the knife. Extend the perforation medially and laterally with scissors prior to re-ventilation.

3 Place the blades of a Finnecetto retractor in the wound and open up the incision to expose the pleural contents. Obtain maximal exposure. If time allows, examine the medial (sternal) portion of the wound as you widen the retractor, clamping and ligating the ipsilateral internal mammary artery.

Assess

1 Examine the thoracic cavity. Quickly evacuate any clot. Keep the operative field clear with effective and intelligent retraction and suction. Gently push the left lung down (inferiorally) and identify the pericardial sac and phrenic nerve running supero-inferiorally. A bulging, purple pericardial sac indicates tamponade. Open the pericardium correctly by grasping it at least 2 cm anterior to the phrenic nerve with long-handled haemostats, then incising this tented portion with scissors. If it is difficult to gain purchase with haemostats on a very tense sac, carefully perforate the pericardium with an 11 bladed scalpel, avoiding the heart itself. Generously lengthen the incision supero-inferiorally so that the clot can be evacuated and the heart delivered.

2 Usually a bleeding wound is observed on the front aspect of the heart. Control it digitally whilst optimizing access. If you are inexperienced in cardiac repairs it is advisable to convert the left anterolateral thoracotomy into a clamshell thoracotomy (Fig. 3.3). Perform a mirror incision on the right chest wall and thence a right anterolateral thoracotomy. Expeditiously divide the sternum with a Gigli saw, a set of bone cutters, a Lebske knife, or a pair of paramedic 'tough-cut' scissors. Reposition the Finnecetto retractor or insert a second one, to maximize exposure. Throughout this manoeuvre, be sure that you, or your assistant, have digital control of the myocardial wound.

3 Even when performing a thoracotomy for massive haemothorax or air leak, open the pericardium to ensure that you have not missed a tamponade.

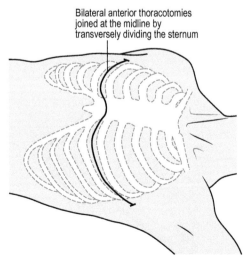

Bilateral anterior thoracotomies joined at the midline by transversely dividing the sternum

Fig. 3.3 The clamshell incision for access to both thoracic cavities and the mediastinum. A common error is to transect the sternum immediately above the xiphisternum. This makes subsequent closure difficult.

Action

1 Temporarily control myocardial wounds of the atrial appendages using a side-biting vascular clamp. Under-run (beneath the clamp limbs) a 3/0 polypropylene stitch in a haemostatic 'sewing machine' continuous suture technique, prior to removing the clamp. Add a second layer of 'over and over' sutures using the remainder of the polypropylene. For atrial wounds temporize (gain time) by using a Foley catheter. Insert a collapsed Foley catheter into the wound, after ensuring that you have clamped off the urinary channel. Inflate the balloon and pull it gently against the inner edges of the defect. Place a purse string suture around the wound, avoiding inadvertant bursting of the balloon and loss of control. Tighten the purse string, deflate the balloon and withdraw the catheter. For ventricular lacerations use interrupted, deeply-placed pledgetted sutures, maintaining digital control between needle placement. Use a large, curved, round bodied needle of 2/0 or 3/0 prolene. Avoid entrapment of the coronary vessels when dealing with injuries adjacent to these structures. When suturing myocardium, a large curved round-bodied needle (2/0 or 3/0 prolene) is valuable, particularly when dealing with injuries adjacent to the left anterior descending artery.

2 If a coronary vessel has been transected, and cardiac by-pass/cardiothoracic assistance is not immediately available, prefer ligation rather than attempting inexpert repair.

3 Now examine the other structures of the chest, including lungs, diaphragm, chest wall, and mediastinum.

4 When performing a thoracotomy for massive haemorrhage, evacuate the clot and blood and determine the source. In penetrating trauma check for bleeding from the chest wall (intercostal artery, internal mammary artery), the lung (parenchyma, hilar vessels), the mediastinum (superior vena cava, inferior vena cava, azygous vein, aortic arch vessels, aorta) and diaphragm (intra-abdominal source demanding exploratory laparotomy). If the lung is bleeding from a tract, or bubbling air and blood due to a major airway injury, you need to mobilize the lung by dividing the inferior pulmonary ligament (investing the hilar vessels like a cuffed sleeve of pleura). If the air leak or bleeding is particularly severe you will then be in a position to control the hilum, either between fingers and thumb, or by using a curved atraumatic vascular clamp (or even a non-crushing bowel clamp). Alternatively, temporarily twist the lung through 180 degrees, bringing the apex downwards and the lower lobe into the superior part of the pleural cavity, to lock off the hilum. These manoeuvres render the patient into a one-lung state, producing considerable right heart strain. Ensure that the anaesthetist is fully aware of your plans.

5 Never simply oversew the bleeding tract. Open it up by the technique of 'tractotomy'. Pass the limb of a linear-cutter stapler device down the tract to its natural extent. Now apply compression of the intervening parenchyma with the opposite limb. Activate the device and the tract is opened up to allow visualization and under-running of the bleeding vessel. If a stapler is not available, undertake the technique using two straight clamps (Fig. 3.4). Divide the intervening tissue bridge with a knife to open the tract and visualize bleeding vessels. Be sure to oversew the edges of the tract following haemostasis of the tract and clamp removal or the cut edges will bleed.

6 In blunt trauma, discrete areas of haemorrhage easily amenable to control are not usually found. Instead, you often see multiple

7 When performing thoracotomy in a patient who has no circulatory output, ensure that, following rapid application of one of the preceding manoeuvres (rapid control of myocardial bleeding, application of a hilar clamp) you reassess the contractile state of the heart and augment cardiac output if required. This is best done between two hands with your thenar and hypothenar eminences in opposition; the heart itself lying between the flat surfaces offered by your palm and extended digits. Undertake compressions in a way that ensures that blood is moved from the apical parts of the ventricles toward the outflow tracts in a coherent manner. Rate of compression is affected by how quickly the heart refills following each compression, but should not be less than 60 beats per minute. Recognize arrhythmia and treat ventricular fibrillation with appropriate defibrillation – internal paddles oriented across the heart, 10–30J DC. External paddles can be used across the chest wall in the conventional way using standard charges if no internal paddles can be located. Treat pulseless electrical activity primarily by continued attempts to volume-load the circulation, guided by your observations as to how 'full' the heart is. Gauge this as you apply internal cardiac massage. Effective massage results in endotracheal carbon-dioxide (ETCO2) readings of >3.0.

8 During such efforts, manually applying pressure to the distal thoracic aorta (lying in the left posterior mediastinum immediately anterior to the vertebral bodies) ensures maximal pre-load and re-distribution of blood to the cerebral and coronary circulation. If the patient fails to return a spontaneous cardiac output despite this manoeuvre, and you have transfused the patient to the extent that there is a 'full heart', further resuscitative effort is futile.

Checklist

Do not close the chest until you have ensured that all major bleeding has been controlled and that you have restored the patient's physiological trajectory toward normality.

Closure

1 The techniques of formal thoracotomy closure in the trauma patient are no different from those used in elective procedures (see Chapter 27). Always leave the pericardium open. Insert two large wide-bore, fenestrated chest drains to each pleural cavity.

2 There are infrequent occasions (transfer to another facility, worsening of instability on attempting chest wall closure) when the chest should be temporarily left open. Achieve this by means of a Bogota bag, stapled to the skin edges, or simply invest the wound with wet swabs and place an over-sized sterile adherent plastic drape over the chest.

Postoperative

1 Ensure that the patient is carefully monitored in a critical care unit. Complications such as atelectasis and chest infection must be anticipated and avoided by vigorous physiotherapy, regular airway suctioning, appropriate antibiotic therapy and early extubation if possible.

2 Order an echocardiogram in those with myocardial trauma to exclude valvular damage or dysfunction.

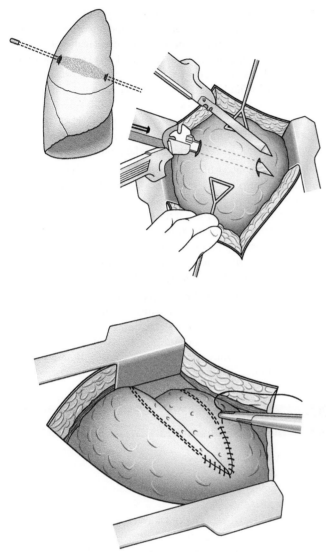

Fig. 3.4 Tractotomy using a linear cutting stapler.

areas of fractured ribs or traumatized chest wall in association with contused segments of lung. Bleeding intercostal vessels may be difficult to control with sutures, especially when located posteriorly. Incise and dissect off the parietal pleura overlying the intercostal space and visualize the vessel before applying a ligaclip to stem the haemorrhage. With massive chest wall trauma, maintain firm manual compression through large swabs for at least 20 minutes while anaesthetic efforts are made at 1:1 resuscitation to encourage haemostasis. Resect areas of irretrievably damaged lung that are bleeding in non-segmental, lung-sparing fashion, using linear-cutter stapler devices. Request suspension of ventilation. Compress the injured lung tissue between your hands. Apply the stapler across the injured portion of lung where you judge the line of demarcation to be. Resect the injured portion before resuming ventilation. Rarely, the lung is so damaged, or there is such severe haemorrhage from torn hilar vessels, that the only viable manoeuvre is pneumonectomy. Clamp the hilum as described and apply and activate a linear stapler device across the hilum, sectioning the tissue on the lung side of the device with a long-handled knife before disengaging the stapler. Oversew the staple line with continuous 3/0 polypropylene for added security.

Complications

1 Check for cessation of haemorrhage by gauging chest drain output and normalization of physiological trends. If, in spite of aggressive haemostatic resuscitation, the chest drain output continues to exceed 250 ml per hour, or the patient's haemoglobin level continues to drop, or the need for inotropic support becomes more pronounced, then you should re-open the chest. Visually confirm that you have addressed all the potential sources of bleeding.

2 Infection of the thoracotomy incision or of sustained entry and exit wounds is common, particularly if resources are constrained. Employ first principles, including re-opening the wound, draining any pus and giving appropriate antibiotics.

3 Intrathoracic infection usually presents later as an empyema, presenting as swinging fever and evidence of a pleural effusion. Prevent this by aggressively tapping any residual signs of retained haemothorax under ultrasound control. If this proves ineffective, proceed to video-assisted thoracoscopic surgery (VATS) – washing out the retained blood and repositioning fresh chest drains. Prefer to treat an established empyema by posterolateral thoracotomy and decortication of the fibrous membrane, which encapsulates the intra-pleural collection of pus, plus drainage.

4 Continuing air leak is common following lung parenchymal injury. Provided the lung is fully expanded it stops spontaneously over 24–48 hours. Leaks beyond this point may be associated with previously unrecognized bronchial or even tracheal injury. Consider this if the lung fails to expand despite the presence of two large drains and suction.

ABDOMINAL TRAUMA

LAPAROTOMY

Appraise

1 The indications for laparotomy can be categorized according to whether the patient is unstable (physiologically unwell, transiently or not responding to IV fluids) or stable (normal or near-normal physiology, sustained response to IV fluid resuscitation). The threshold for proceeding to laparotomy in a stable patient is higher than in an unstable patient and you may use the time to characterize the injury better and determine if laparotomy might be avoided.

2 The exact criteria that warrant laparotomy in stable patients depend upon your work environment. There are two broad and complementary strategies of management. The first is to image the entire torso with multi-detector CT. In penetrating trauma, CT allows you to determine the trajectory of the wound track and to decide if the peritoneum has been breached. If the wound track is followed in to a solid organ (such as the liver), but does not exit the organ, and there is little evidence of ongoing haemorrhage (in the form of a contrast blush) then conservative management is often possible. Conversely, if there is blush then the patient requires angio-embolization or surgical haemostasis. If the breach does not overlie a solid organ then there is a much higher risk of visceral perforation and the threshold for laparotomy drops accordingly. In blunt trauma, multi-detector CT

allows you to determine if there is intra-peritoneal fluid and to check for solid organ damage. Again, solid organ trauma without active extravasation may be managed conservatively, although evidence of bleeding demands action. If there is intra-peritoneal fluid without solid organ trauma then you must explain the source of the fluid. Has the bladder been ruptured, is there a mesenteric laceration (with risk of bowel ischaemia), or is there a perforation of the bowel (with liberation of bowel content)? The presence of free intra-peritoneal gas suggests the latter. The safest way to exclude these injuries is via laparotomy.

3 The second strategy of managing stable patients with abdominal trauma is to place the casualty in a high-dependency area and ensure repeated re-examination at 6-hourly intervals. Follow conservative management if the patient does not develop peritonitis, maintains stability (with little need for ongoing fluid therapy), and records no drop in the serum Hb. If these criteria are not fulfilled the patient requires a laparotomy. Treat such an event not as a failure but as a declaration of the need for surgery.

4 There is little place for digital exploration of abdominal wounds in the emergency department, since failure to palpate a breach within the peritoneum does not mean that no breach exists. The abdominal wall consists of a series of moveable baffles, which interfere with apparent wound trajectory and make the information gained from exploration unreliable.

> **KEY POINTS** Preconditions for successful conservative management of abdominal trauma

- Physiological stability
- Conscious, cooperative patient
- Availability of high-dependency area where patient can be accurately monitored
- Availability of experienced surgical staff with time to regularly review patient
- CT evidence of lack of ongoing bleeding (no active contrast extravasation, absence of layered/sedimented contrast surrounding the bleeding organ).

Prepare

There is always time to prepare and drape the abdomen properly before laparotomy. If the patient is unstable, defer inserting a urinary catheter and nasogastric tube until the end of the procedure.

Access

The default incision is a long midline incision. Ensure that you have thoroughly examined every component of the abdominal viscera. A long midline incision affords this. Have no hesitation in opening the abdominal cavity from xiphisternum to pubis if necessary.

Assess

Examine all viscera systematically, explore the lesser sac, identify all sources of bleeding and be certain to account for the state of all organs.

Action

1 Control of haemorrhage is the first priority within the abdomen. As soon as the peritoneum has been opened fully pack the abdomen in quadrants with large abdominal packs, starting from the left upper quadrant and moving clockwise around the abdominal cavity. Then remove the packs, starting from the least likely source, removing the packs from the 'compelling' source of bleeding last.

2 Splenectomy is the safest approach to the ruptured spleen. Sweep your hand between the diaphragm and the spleen to break down any adhesions and deliver the spleen medially and forwards into the wound. Clamp and divide the gastrosplenic and lienorenal ligaments, avoiding the tail of the pancreas and the greater curvature of the stomach. Resect the spleen and suture-ligate the pedicles with heavy absorbable ligatures. Control oozing from disrupted adhesions by packing. It usually stops without further attention; if it does not, use diathermy current coagulation.

3 Splenic salvage surgery may spare the patient from splenectomy. It involves applying haemostatic agents to the injury such as microfibrillar collagen or Vicryl mesh bags, together with diathermy coagulation and oversewing of the defect. Alternatively, pack the spleen with the intent to remove the packs within 48 hrs. Pursue conservative management or splenic salvage surgery in children who are haemodynamically stable. They are more likely than adults to develop overwhelming post-splenectomy infections. Remember to arrange for immunization against encapsulated cocci and long-term antibiotics if the spleen must be resected.

4 Hepatic tears are often mild. Bleeding may already have ceased by the time you perform the laparotomy. Larger lacerations are generally controllable with appropriate packing. First appraise the site and orientation of the tears, then determine the direction of the pressure needed to establish apposition of parenchymal surfaces. In severe tears use your hands to compress the liver directly along this pressure vector. Evaluate how your packs need to lie to continue exerting sufficient pressure. This dictates whether you need to take down any of the triangular ligaments to accommodate your packs. It is unusual to require much mobilization. Place folded abdominal packs into the various spaces adjacent to the liver – laterally, superiorly, inferiorly – to re-oppose planes of cleavage. If there is substantial haemorrhage from the liver use the manoeuvre described in 1908 by the Glaswegian surgeon J. Hogarth Pringle (1863–1941) (Fig. 3.5). Place a non-crushing clamp across the portal triad, with one blade through the foramen of Winslow into the lesser sac. This compresses the hepatic artery and portal vein while you assess and repair the liver damage. If bleeding continues after clamping, it is from the hepatic veins or inferior vena cava. Do not leave the clamp in place for more than 45 minutes. Suture liver tears using a large blunt needle, taking care to prevent the needle from moving laterally in the parenchyma and so increasing the tear. Be aware that the deeper portions of the tear may not be encompassed, leaving a space for haematoma to accumulate and setting the conditions for liver abscess. Over-tight sutures devitalize liver parenchyma, leading to the same complication.

5 Damage to the retrohepatic inferior vena cava is particularly challenging as efforts to lift or rotate the liver in order to address the area usually result in torrential bleeding. Ensure your Pringle

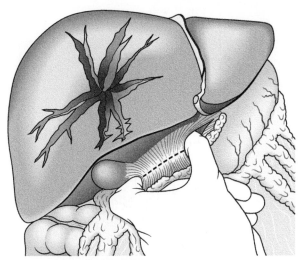

Fig. 3.5 Pringle's manoeuvre. A soft bowel or vascular clamp can be readily applied following digital control.

manoeuvre is applied. Attempt to press down on the liver in the antero-posterior plane and maintain compression using aggressive packing. You may succeed in controlling smaller tears in the retrohepatic inferior vena cava in this way, although at the expense of significant reduction in cardiac output secondary to very reduced venous return. Inform your anaesthetist before contemplating this manoeuvre. AP compression may allow you time to complete haemostatic resuscitation and seek expert help. If this fails, ready yourself for exploration of the retrohepatic area. First, medially rotate the viscera from the right and 'Kocherize' the duodenum to expose the suprarenal IVC and clamp it. This isolates the liver from below and may diminish the bleeding sufficiently to allow full mobilization, taking down the liver's peritoneal attachments and 'medializing' it to expose the hepatic veins and retrohepatic inferior vena cava. However, controlling the IVC from below infrequently slows the haemorrhage sufficiently enough to allow accurate visualization of the bleeding point. In such cases, control from above is often required to 'isolate' the liver. Do this by extending your laparotomy incision into a right anterolateral thoracotomy. Open the pericardium, find the intra-pericardial inferior vena cava and control it. Expect profound reduction in cardiac filling and output. Injuries requiring this manoeuvre are very often fatal.

6 Repair diaphragmatic injuries with non-absorbable interrupted mattress sutures. Facilitate the repair by grasping the apices of the defect with long-handled artery forceps and applying traction to bring the mobile diaphragm in to a more superficial position.

7 Retroperitoneal injury usually presents as a haematoma sited centrally, laterally, or in the pelvis (Fig. 3.6). There are two absolute indications for exploring retroperitoneal haematoma. Firstly, visible expansion associated with physiological instability, irrespective of the site of the haematoma or the mechanism of injury. Secondly, central haematomata caused by a penetrating mechanism (associated with a high risk of damage to a major branch or tributary of the aorta or inferior vena cava). A penetrating mechanism indicates potential loss of tamponade, underlining the early need to seek definitive control.

8 Characterize central haematoma as lying to the left or right of the midline. Right-sided haematomata are more likely to be due to

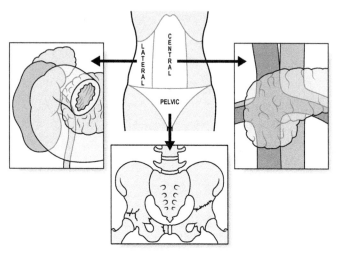

Fig. 3.6   Classification of retroperitoneal haematomas.

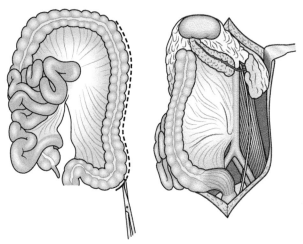

Fig. 3.8   Medial visceral rotation from the left.

caval injury. Achieve access to the inferior vena cava on the right of the abdomen by dividing the congenital adhesions in the right paracolic gutter and sweeping the entire right colon together with the duodenum to the left in an extended kocherization manoeuvre (medial visceral rotation from the right – Fig. 3.7). You can then control the cava proximally and distally with swab-sticks and suture a tear with 3/0 polypropylene. In the case of a through and through injury, open the anterior laceration as much as is required to inspect and repair the posterior surface from within the lumen. Never try to rotate the inferior vena cava to achieve this or you risk avulsing lumbar veins with disappointing results. Central haematomas that are to the left of the midline are best explored by rotating the left-sided abdominal viscera to the midline. Divide the congenital adhesions in the left paracolic gutter and swing the entire left colon, including if necessary the spleen and left kidney, to the right (Fig. 3.8). In this way you can expose, control and deal with injuries to the suprarenal and coeliac levels of the aorta. High, tense central haematomas, lying in the supracolic compartment above the mesentery of the transverse colon, demand control of the suprarenal aorta before beginning the rotation manoeuvre. Achieve this by retracting the liver toward the patient's right shoulder, counter-tracting the stomach toward the left hip. Bluntly pierce the stretched lesser omentum between liver and stomach and expose the peritoneum overlying the conjoined crura (median arcuate ligament) of the diaphragm. Feel for the aortic pulse and make a vertical incision in the overlying peritoneal membrane to reveal the fibres of the crura, encircling

the supracoeliac aorta as it transits from the thoracic cavity into the abdomen. These muscular fibres can be spread apart in the plane of orientation using long-handled dissecting scissors, to reveal the pearly white adventitia of the aorta. Develop a plane either side, extending down to the prevertebral fascia, to accommodate the limbs of a straight vascular clamp which can be positioned prior to opening the haematoma from the left during your rotation manoeuvre. Ligate all bleeding branches of the aorta save the superior mesenteric artery. Repair this if possible, as injury can result in midgut infarction.

9 Exploration of supracolic, central haematomas may also reveal trauma to the pancreatic–duodenal complex. Biliary discoloration in the region of the duodenum usually indicates a duodenal or extra-hepatic biliary tract disruption. Mobilize the duodenum by Kocher's manoeuvre to examine its posterior surface. If possible, repair it rather than resect it. Most duodenal tears can be repaired primarily or patched with a loop of jejunum. Protect an extensive repair by undertaking a diversionary gastrojejunostomy, having closed off the pylorus from within via a purse string of absorbable suture. Extensive damage to the bile duct can be temporized by crossing the damaged area with the long limb of a T-Tube, inserted via a distal incision in to normal adjacent duct, or by widely draining the affected area. Manage head of pancreas injuries similarly with haemostatic sutures and wide drainage. Deal with superficial injuries to the body and tail of the pancreas with debridement and drainage combined with judicious suture repair. Treat more extensive trauma by distal resection using a transverse linear cutter-stapler device.

10 Lateral haematomas usually indicate renal trauma. Avoid opening these unless the patient is unstable or the haematoma is growing before your eyes. Use the relevant left or right medial visceral rotation procedure to expose the kidney, then incise Gerota's (Bucharest anatomist 1867–1939) fascia vertically, releasing the haematomata and delivering the kidney. If there is profound haemorrhage, control the hilum between finger and thumb and then apply a vascular clamp while you assess the damage. Repair renal lacerations using pledgeted absorbable monofilament sutures. A damaged pole can be filleted and then closed in 'fishmouth' fashion. Be aware of the intolerance of renal parenchyma to warm ischaemia and remove any hilar clamp within 15 minutes of application. Overwhelming renal trauma necessitates nephrectomy, best done by individual suture ligation of the

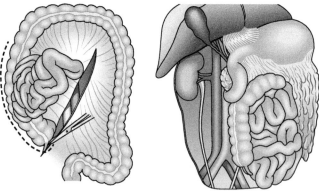

Fig. 3.7   Medial visceral rotation from the right.

pedicle vasculature using polypropylene but mass ligation is preferred when time does not permit a nuanced approach. In such circumstances, manually confirm the presence of the contralateral kidney – there is no role for on-table intravenous urography in the shocked patient – although note that congenital absence of the contralateral kidney does not change the indication for nephrectomy in a patient unable to tolerate prolonged attempts at renal salvage.

11 The excellent vascularity of the stomach means that it usually tolerates repair of injury well. Close lacerations in two layers with absorbable sutures. Small bowel injuries are generally easily dealt with. It is not uncommon for a single stab wound to traverse several loops of small bowel. Carefully oversew all penetrating wounds or tears in a single layer of extra-mucosal absorbable sutures. Consider resection if there are a large number of tears in a short length of bowel, or if you are in doubt about viability. If operating in damage control mode, simply isolate segments of damaged bowel by placing them into discontinuity using a linear cutter stapler. Defer re-anastomosis until phase three of the DCS process.

12 The large bowel is less tolerant of poorly executed repair, particularly if the patient has been shocked. Always mobilize the relevant segment of large bowel fully to exclude through and through injury. Beware of overlooking injuries around the hepatic and the splenic flexure. Repair small penetrating wounds, particularly on the right side of the colon, by freshening up the edges of the laceration and closing them carefully with interrupted sutures. Treat larger defects or areas of significant tissue loss by resecting the affected area in the standard manner (right hemicolectomy, extended right hemicolectomy, left hemicolectomy). Perform a primary anastomosis if the patient's physiological state is normal. If not, leave the bowel ends in discontinuity, deferring restoration or stoma formation until DCS phase three. Treat the right side of the colon by right hemicolectomy and primary anastomosis. Injuries which declare themselves after a period of initial conservatism (or neglect) may be associated with significant contamination – do not be tempted to repair anything definitively other than the simplest lacerations in these circumstances.

13 Treat intra-peritoneal rectal injuries in the same way as left colon injuries. Treat discrete extra-peritoneal injuries by defunctioning the sigmoid colon. Extensive dissection around the extra-peritoneal rectum may compromise vascularity. Also, avoid damaging the neurological supply of the sphincter unless there is significant disruption, as with high energy transfer missile trauma.

14 Repair injured ureters and bladder primarily, using absorbable sutures. Insert a single layer to the ureter over a double 'J' stent or neonatal feeding tube. Insert a double layer into the bladder. For small lacerations a suprapubic catheter is not usually necessary if a large bore urethral catheter is in place. Larger disruptions have a greater propensity for leakage and combined suprapubic and per-urethral catheter drainage is advisable.

Checklist

1 Check that you have secured haemostasis and that you have 'run the bowel' adequately to exclude all injuries.

2 Make sure that the peritoneal cavity is well washed out and confirm that all the viscera are viable once they have been returned to the abdomen.

3 Specific drainage is not usually required if the abdomen is being managed with topical negative pressure dressings. Drains to biliary or pancreatic injuries are wise if you intend to close the abdomen.

Closure

1 If you are in DCS mode leave the abdomen open (Table 3.1).

2 If DCS is not required, close the laparotomy wound using a mass closure technique, usually with a single layer looped no. 1 nylon

TABLE 3.1 Management of the open abdomen		
Technique	Method	Comments
Bogota bag	Open up a sterile 1 L bag of crystalloid. Overlay bowel and suture the outer margin to circumferential skin of the laparotomy wound using continuous nylon.	Readily available materials and easy technique. Leaks fluid ++.
Topical negative pressure wound dressing (e.g. Opsite®-sandwich)	Encapsulate a large, opened abdominal pack (or sterile dressing towel) between two sterile adhesive transparent plastic drapes. Using a blade, perforate this several times and place the fenestrated 'sandwich' over the bowel (and well under the circumferential wound margins). Place suction tubing over the exterior surface of the sandwich and bring out via a separate stab incision cephalad to the laparotomy incision. Place fluffy gauze (e.g. Kerlix®) over the sandwich and the drains, then seal in the Opsite sandwich, drains and gauze by overlaying a generously sized adhesive drape over the laparostomy wound. Connect the drains to negative pressure at 100 mg Hg and seal any residual airleaks with further adhesive dressings.	Readily available materials; inexpensive. Significantly less leakage than the Bogota bag. Slower to configure than commercial variants; less control of amount of pressure. Pack count may be confused with use of abdominal packs in 'sandwich'.
Commercial vacuum-therapy (VAC®) dressing	Open VAC consumable pack; tuck in the pre-perforated plastic sheeting; trim VAC sponge to match size of laparostomy; staple to edges of wound; apply overlying adhesive dressing; perforate and apply connector to negative pressure system.	Quick to set up; negative pressure can be readily controlled. More costly than improvised variants. May not be readily available in some institutions.

thread. Very heavy contamination is an indication for leaving the superficial tissues and skin open, to be addressed later at delayed primary closure.

3 DCS laparotomy mandates transfer of the patient to the intensive care unit for continued haemostatic resuscitation. It is usually necessary to maintain sedation and continued ventilation throughout this period until such time that physiological normality has been attained and the patient can be submitted to scheduled definitive surgery.

Postoperative

1 Perform definitive or second-look surgery when the patient is fit enough and you have gathered the requisite theatre time, equipment and expertise sufficient to ensure optimal outcome. It is essential to ensure that any specialist help you require is available, and that you have factored in other procedures such as orthopaedic or plastic surgery, that may be undertaken at the same operation. It may not be possible to formally close the abdomen at this time due to visceral oedema, in which case you should plan to re-dress the laparostomy until such time that you can effect closure. Techniques used to definitively cover the bowel include mesh coverage followed by interval split skin grafting, use of composite or allograft materials, progressive advancement of the rectus sheath through incrementally tensioned sutures, or components separation procedures.

Complications

1 The most important postoperative complication is bleeding. It demands re-laparotomy.

2 Occasionally, an imperfect seal in the laparostomy dressing requires buttressing with further transparent adhesive dressings. Escape of bowel demands removal of the original dressing and re-application – which can be readily undertaken on the intensive care unit.

3 Despite laparostomy, the complication of abdominal compartment syndrome may still develop due to the constraining effect of the adhesive drapes or Bogota bag. Avoid this by insisting on regular measurements of intra-abdominal pressure via the urinary catheter. Pressures greater than 25 mmHg merit re-laparotomy.

4 Sepsis is a potent cause of collapse after 48–72 hours. Immediate postoperative temperature increase is nearly always respiratory. Actively treat the patient with physiotherapy and appropriate antibiotics and with suction if the patient is on a ventilator. Abdominal causes of sepsis tend to be related to intra-peritoneal collections 2–7 days post closure of the abdomen. Contrast enhanced CT is the prime mode of investigation. Re-laparotomy may be required in the setting of sepsis and an identified abscess cavity related to adjacent and probably leaking anastomosis. Isolated pelvic or subphrenic collections may be amenable to image-guided percutaneous drainage, avoiding re-laparotomy.

PELVIS

Appraise

1 In some circumstances the source of shock in a polytrauma patient will be from retroperitoneal haemorrhage following major pelvic injury. The pelvic ring may be disrupted secondary to force vectors applied across the antero-posterior (AP) plane (causing 'open book' type distraction of the pelvic ring), transversely across the lateral plane (with lateral compression (LC) fractures), or in the supero-inferior axis, with vertical displacement of elements of one hemi-pelvis compared to the other (vertical shear fractures). Each mechanism involves disruption of the venous plexus and tributaries, plastered to the side walls of the pelvis, draining in to the internal iliac vessels. According to the type of injury, damage may be sustained by the arterial branches of the internal iliac artery, with vertical shear fractures often associated with combined arterial and venous trauma.

2 You should ensure that all patients with a mechanism of trauma consistent with pelvic trauma have had their legs brought together in the neutral position and that a pelvic binder or sheet has been correctly applied (with the equator of the binder superimposed over a transverse plane drawn across the greater trochanter of the femurs). If the patient is responsive to resuscitation and remains well, then you can take the patient for multi-detector CT scanning and interrogation of the torso and pelvis. Any contrast blush in association with a pelvic haematoma indicates an ongoing haemorrhage and needs to be addressed via interventional radiology and urgent embolization.

3 Management of the shocked, unstable patient with a major pelvic ring fracture – diagnosed on gentle clinical palpation (once only!) or (preferably) by plain radiography – calls for urgent decision-making. You need to stop the haemorrhage from the pelvis and address other areas of co-incident bleeding. If the chest X-Ray and FAST scan are grossly clear, and you have the services of an interventional radiologist and an on-site endovascular suite immediately available, then the whole trauma team may transport the patient for selective angiography of the internal iliac arteries and embolization. If these services are not available, or the patient is decompensating, or if you envisage having to make other rapid surgical interventions such as a laparotomy for a positive FAST scan, then it is better to take the patient to theatre and address the pelvic haemorrhage using the technique of extra-peritoneal packing (EPP).

Prepare

1 Ensure that you have a laparotomy set open and that there is a vascular set ready. You do not need an external fixator set if the pelvic belt is correctly positioned and adequately (but not over-) tightened.

2 Standard trauma cruciform position and preparation. Ensure that the anaesthetic team is following DCR principles and that the scrub team is forewarned of your intent to perform EPP. Alert the interventional radiology team, which should be mustered toward the end of the procedure.

Access

1 EPP is usually performed in the context of a deteriorating patient where there is little tolerance to missed sources of haemorrhage. For this reason, even if your FAST scan was negative, perform a midline laparotomy in the standard fashion. The lowermost part of the incision may reveal haematoma spreading up and around from the pelvic fracture but this is not of major concern.

Assess

1   If there is major intra-abdominal haemorrhage, deal with it expeditiously but do no more than what is required (packing, organ removal). Turn your attention to the pelvis. The haematoma is largest on the side of maximal disruption, and may have tracked upward into the peri-renal tissues, displacing colon anteriorly.

Action

1   Apply two haemostats to the anterior edge of the cut peritoneum in the lower portion of your laparotomy wound on the side of the haematoma. Using scissors, rapidly develop the plane in front of the grasped peritoneum. You quickly encounter more haematoma as you work your way at first laterally and then posteriorly into the true pelvis. The dissection rapidly becomes easier as the haematoma has already dissected the plane for you, and you can then use your hand to sweep the peritoneum medially, liberating much of the haematoma as you do so. Now develop the plane posteriorly as far as the sacro-iliac joints, and you feel bony fragments as you encounter the fracture line (Fig. 3.9).

2   Take a large, open abdominal swab and, using a pair of forceps, push it into the furthest reaches of this plane, whilst retracting the peritoneum and viscera with your non-dominant hand. Be sure that this initial swab is as posterior and as deep as possible, abutting the fracture line. Lowering the operating table, or calling for a step, facilitates this process. Then take a second and then a third swab and sequentially pack on top of the initial swab. Take down the peritoneum on the contralateral side and repeat the packing process. The two sets of swabs should efface each other posteriorly, much like a pair of boxer's gloves pushed against each other at the knuckles.

3   Now focus on the superficial, lower portion of the laparotomy incision. Hitch up the medial edge of the peritoneal shelf (where you placed your haemostats when 'taking down' the peritoneum initially) against the medial edge of the rectus muscles with absorbable sutures. This 'seals' the extra-peritoneal space and helps prevent swab migration.

Closure

1   Leave open as this is a DCS procedure and there is often a high risk of abdominal compartment syndrome. However, several interrupted sutures to the lower rectus sheath are helpful in restoring the constraining/tamponading effect of the lower abdominal wall on the pelvic haematoma.

Postoperative

1   This is a temporizing manoeuvre ('a bridge to embolization'). Ensure that, unless there are competing priorities, the patient is transferred to the interventional radiology suite for follow-on embolization.

2   The scheduled re-look and pack-removal procedure should involve your orthopaedic colleagues, preferably within 24 hours. Make sure that image intensification is available. Take down the peritoneum again by cutting your sutures and remove the packs under copious warm saline. If there is no further bleeding your orthopaedic colleague can assess the suitability for internal fixation or external fixation. Close the abdomen, remove the belt and stabilize the pelvic ring. If you encounter further bleeding, re-pack and schedule further inspection and attempted pack removal in 48 hours' time.

Complications

1   EPP patients are amongst the sickest trauma patients you encounter as the injury set includes profound haemorrhage often associated with severe injuries to multiple body regions. Expect prolonged ICU and inpatient stay with a protracted rehabilitation process.

2   Patients are usually bed-bound for many weeks. Introduce aggressive anti-thrombo-embolism measures within 24 hours of pack removal.

SOFT-TISSUE WOUNDS

Appraise

1   In general, wounds caused by handguns do not require formal surgical excision, but you do need to clean and dress them. Administer a broad-spectrum antibiotic and tetanus prophylaxis, assuming that the missile track has not crossed into a body cavity, a joint, a vascular structure or the thecal sac.

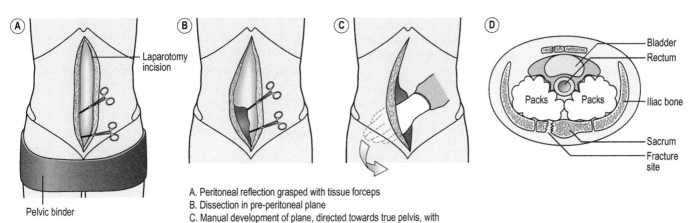

A. Peritoneal reflection grasped with tissue forceps
B. Dissection in pre-peritoneal plane
C. Manual development of plane, directed towards true pelvis, with liberation of haematoma
D. Cross-section of pelvis after packing. Note position of packs, abutting each other and fracture sites

Fig. 3.9   Extra-peritoneal packing of the pelvis.

2 Wounds caused by missiles from military assault rifles require full exploration, due to the higher energy exchange between the round and the tissue, potentially damaging structures beyond the wound track. With few exceptions, leave the wound open. Perform delayed primary closure after 4–7 days.

3 Soft-tissue wounds associated with significant disruption of the long bones require special attention as these are frequently limb-threatening wounds. Use the BOAST4 guidelines (see Further reading) to guide your management.

Prepare

1 Prepare the wounded area and a large enough surrounding area to allow for a necessary, but unplanned, extension of the skin incision.

Access

1 You usually need to enlarge the wound in order to obtain adequate access to damaged structures. Further enlargement may be necessary later during definitive repair.

2 Digital exploration may indicate the direction of the wound but cannot reliably reveal its depth or eventual extent. The most direct way of doing this is usually to incise tissue immediately overlying the track. Bear in mind the site and extent of the resulting wound, particularly if it needs to be extended as part of the definitive procedure, or if it crosses major skin creases. However, cosmesis (the future appearance) is not of primary concern during life-saving surgery. Whenever possible, incise in the long axis of a limb. In some circumstances be willing to make counter-incisions.

Assess

1 Explore the wound in layers. Follow any puncture wound through the layers, opening each in turn until you can detect no further penetration. Remember that the tissues may no longer be in the same relationship that they were at the time of the injury, and a penetrating wound may seem to take a different course from that expected. The tissue layers form a series of baffles, as in the abdomen, mentioned above.

2 Identify neurovascular bundles in the wound track and note any damage, but you need not dissect out nerves. The majority of nerve injuries are neuropraxias [Greek: *neuron* (= nerve) + *a* (= not) + *prassein* (= to do)], described by H.J. Seddon as temporary paralysis without degeneration, and recover spontaneously. If a nerve appears to be injured, requiring later exploration, mark its position with a non-absorbable suture.

Action

1 Arrest haemorrhage, temporarily compressing the bleeding point with swabs, controlling major vessels proximally and distally with slings or with arterial clamps. Do not apply haemostatic arterial clamps indiscriminately but capture and ligate small bleeding vessels under vision as you encounter them.

2 Once you have achieved this, start by cleaning the wound. Irrigate it with copious quantities of saline followed by aqueous antiseptic. This removes most superficial foreign material and improves visualization. Remove deeper contaminants as the exploration progresses.

3 It is not necessary to remove every piece of metal or glass visible on a radiograph. Use your clinical judgment. Vegetable material or slivers of wood form potent sources of chronic infection. Remove them.

4 Identify and rigorously excise dead muscle, which is pale, non-contractile, mushy and does not bleed when incised. Inspect for tendon damage. Tendon repair need not be performed initially. Trim tattered ends and mark them with a non-absorbable suture as for nerves (see above).

5 Pay particular attention to comminuted bony injuries. Clean contaminated bone but do not remove it if it is still attached to viable periosteum or healthy muscle. Discard small detached bony fragments, which contribute to postoperative wound infection. Ensure that the skeleton is stabilized after restoring limb perfusion. Temporize by using a vascular shunt prior to external or definitive fixation, then complete the vascular repair in definitive fashion.

6 Identify injuries to joints and clean them rigorously. Cover exposed cartilage with at least one layer of healthy tissue, ideally with synovium.

7 Irrigate the wound again at the end of the repair procedure. Secure haemostasis before dressing an open contaminated wound or before closing a clean one.

Checklist

1 Make sure that all dead tissue has been removed, that an open wound is open enough to drain and that haemostasis is secure.

2 Always check distal limb viability before leaving the operating theatre, particularly in the presence of constrictive dressings.

Open wound

Dress an open wound with lightly fluffed gauze to allow free drainage. Avoid tight packing.

Closure

1 Do not close a wound unless you are sure it is recent, clean and healthy. Use delayed primary closure if in doubt. Approximate tissue loosely during closure, never under tension, and in its natural layers. It is seldom necessary to repair muscle, but approximate subcutaneous tissue with absorbable sutures, preferably interrupted, to reduce the risk of tissue fluid collecting in dead spaces.

2 Close the skin with interrupted non-absorbable sutures, trimming the edges where required to reduce bevelling.

3 Consider the use of primary split-skin grafting in addition to suturing at delayed primary closure, particularly when there has been tissue loss.

Postoperative

1 Immobilize the injured soft tissue with cotton wool, conforming bandages and, if necessary, a splint, even in the absence of bony injury.

2 Watch for the signs of postoperative limb ischaemia, haemorrhage and sepsis (fever, worsening limb pain and swelling) and ensure that antibiotics are continued until definitive wound coverage has been achieved, or after 72 hours, whichever is the sooner.

FURTHER READING

British Orthopaedic Association and British Association of Plastic, Reconstructive and Aesthetic Surgeons. Standard for Trauma – 2009. BOAST4: The management of severe open lower limb fractures. Available at http://www.boa.ac.uk/.

Brohi K, Cohen MJ, Ganter M, et al. Acute traumatic coagulopathy: initiated by hypoperfusion: modulated through the protein C pathway? Ann Surg 2007;245:812–8.

Holcomb JB, Jenkins D, Rhee P, et al. Damage control resuscitation: directly addressing the early coagulopathy of trauma. J Trauma 2007;62:307–10.

Maier RV (Ed). Trauma care today. Surg Clin North America 2007;87: 1–278.

Mattox K, Hirschberg A. Top Knife: the Art and Craft of Trauma Surgery. TFM Publishing; 2004.

Milia DJ, Brasel K. Current use of CT in the evaluation and management of injured patients. Surg Clin North Am 2011;91:233–48.

Rossaint R, Bouillon B, Cerny V, et al. Management of bleeding following major trauma: an updated guideline. Crit Care 2010;14:(R52) Available at: http://ccforum.com/content/14/2/R52.

Rotondo MF, Bard MR. Damage control surgery for thoracic injuries. Injury 2004;35:649–54.

Shapiro MB, Jenkins DH, Schwab CW, Rotondo MF. Damage control: collective review. J Trauma 2000;49:969–78.

Starnes BW, Beekley AC, Sebasta JA, et al. Extremity vascular injuries on the battlefield: tips for surgeons deploying to war. J Trauma 2006;60 (2):432–42.

Tai NRM, Dickson EJ. Military junctional trauma, JRAMC 2009;115: 285–92. Available at: www.ramcjournal.com/2009/dec09/tai3.pdf.

Tisherman SA, Bokhari F, Collier B, et al. Clinical Practice Guidelines: Penetrating Neck Trauma. Clinical Practice Guidelines of the Eastern Association for the Surgery of Trauma; 2008. Available at http://www.east.org/tpg.asp.

Totterman A, Madsen JE, Skaga NO, Røise O. Extraperitoneal pelvic packing: a salvage procedure to control massive traumatic pelvic haemorrhage. J Trauma 2007;62:843–52.

4

Laparotomy: elective and emergency

R.E. D'Souza, R. Novell

CONTENTS

INTRODUCTION

Laparotomy (from the Greek laparos = soft, referring to the abdomen) is a skill every surgeon caring for general surgical patients should possess and master to a level which makes him or her confident to perform whenever called upon. The approach to a patient with abdominal pathology has undergone significant changes due to advances in both diagnostic techniques and treatment options. Rapid progress in endoscopic and imaging techniques has led to better preoperative assessment of the abdomen, thereby enabling surgeons to make a more confident decision on the necessity and timing of laparotomy. Minimal access surgery (laparoscopy) has added to the repertoire, aiding both in diagnosis of the acute abdomen[1] and in therapeutic procedures. As a result of these changes diagnostic laparotomy is now a rarity. Better understanding of many disease processes, such as peptic ulcer and pancreatitis, and improvements in their pharmacotherapy have led to a significant decrease in patients undergoing laparotomy for these conditions.

Although preoperative investigations may give you more information about the intra-abdominal pathology, do not overlook clinical assessment of the patient. An accurate and detailed history and examination, hallmarks of an astute clinician, are still paramount in surgical practice and will guide you towards fewer, more focused investigations. At times, be willing to repeat investigations after an interval to establish a diagnosis.

Surgical approaches to the abdomen are undergoing continuous change and procedures such as single incision laparoscopic surgery (SILS)[2] and natural orifice endoscopic surgery (NOTES),[3] whilst still in their infancy, are gaining popularity.

OPENING THE ABDOMEN

Preparation

1 Ideally, see the patient in the ward before their arrival in the operating theatre. Explain the procedure along with the options available and associated risks. Clearly explain any possibility of additional procedures to ensure informed consent. Review the case notes and arrange to display relevant imaging in the operating room.

2 The WHO surgical safety checklist[4] is now universally employed in the UK and in many other countries. Follow it meticulously in every case to prevent mishaps arising from human error.

3 Give prophylactic antibiotics at this stage (if not already started), according to hospital guidelines.[5]

4 Palpate the patient's abdomen after induction of general anaesthesia. Previously impalpable or indistinct masses may be more evident, such as an appendix mass or empyema of the gall bladder, or less evident, for example an incisional hernia that has spontaneously reduced following muscle relaxation.

5 Consider the patient's position on the operating table before commencing the procedure. If a lateral tilt is required, secure the patient adequately. Employ a Lloyd-Davies position for all procedures likely to involve the pelvic organs or left colon, to allow access to the rectum.

6 Prepare the skin with an antiseptic solution such as 10% povidone-iodine, 1:5000 chlorhexidine or 1% cetrimide, provided there is no known allergy to any of these agents, using a swab on a sponge holder.[5] For a laparotomy, prepare the skin from the nipples to the mid thigh. Alcohol-based antiseptics give superior bactericidal results, but remove any excess (which often pools around the flanks) if diathermy is to be used on the skin or subcutaneous tissues to prevent burns.

7 Drape the patient with sterile drapes, adequately exposing the area of interest. An adhesive plastic drape, such as Opsite™ or Steridrape™ may be used on the exposed skin after the drapes are placed. Make the skin incision through this adhesive drape.

Incisions

1 Principles influencing the choice of incision are adequate exposure, minimal damage to deeper structures, ability to extend the incision if required, sound closure and, as far as possible, a cosmetically acceptable scar. Placement of stomas and the need to access the abdomen quickly may also dictate the choice of incision: thus for abdominal trauma and major haemorrhage always use a midline incision.

2 Placement of the incision depends on the planned procedure: a roof top incision is ideal for surgery on the liver, a left subcostal incision for an elective splenectomy and McBurney's incision for appendicectomy. Cosmesis is important, but not at the cost of adequate, safe exposure of the relevant structures. Consider achieving a sound repair at the end of the procedure at this stage. There is no conclusive evidence that transverse incisions heal better than vertical incisions but reports support a non-statistical advantage for the former.[6]

3 **Midline laparotomy** (Fig. 4.1) is the default incision for most procedures on the abdomen: the extent will vary according to the exposure required. The incision traverses a relatively avascular field (the linea alba). As the peritoneum is exposed, the falciform ligament comes into view in the upper abdomen. This can be ligated and divided or avoided by deepening the incision to one or other side of the ligament. Curve the incision around the umbilical cicatrix to avoid dividing it. Close the midline incision by a single layer mass closure technique using No.1 nylon, polypropylene or PDS. In the lower one-third of the abdomen the posterior rectus sheath is deficient: ensure adequate bites of tissue when closing this part of the incision.

4 **Paramedian incision** (Fig. 4.1). This gives comparable exposure to the midline incision but is time-consuming to create and close, gives an inferior cosmetic result and carries a greater risk of postoperative dehiscence, therefore use a midline incision wherever possible. Make the skin incision 2–3 cms lateral to the midline and incise the anterior rectus sheath along the skin incision. Retract the rectus muscle laterally and incise the posterior rectus sheath and peritoneum in the midline. Close the abdomen in layers: close the peritoneum and the posterior rectus sheath either with Vicryl, PDS, polypropylene or nylon. Allow the rectus muscle to fall back in place and close the anterior rectus sheath. Perform skin closure as usual.

5 **Oblique subcostal incisions** (Fig. 4.2) are used to access the upper abdomen, for example the liver and gall bladder on the right (Kocher's incision, after the Nobel prize winner Theodore Kocher, 1841–1917) and the spleen on the left. They may be extended across the midline as a roof top incision if required, for example, in surgery of the liver and pancreas. Make the incision over the area of interest, about two finger breadths below the subcostal margin and towards the xiphisternum. Deepen the incision to expose the external oblique and the anterior rectus sheath. Divide these layers and the rectus muscle and incise the internal oblique muscles with diathermy. It is helpful to insert a long artery forceps such as Robert's or Kelly's under the muscle belly to facilitate this. Divide the posterior rectus sheath and transversus abdominis aponeurosis to expose the pre-peritoneal fat and open the peritoneum in line with the incision. Take care to spare the ninth costal nerve, which is visible at this stage. A midline superior extension through the linea alba to form a 'Mercedes Benz' incision provides further access if required.

6 **The Rutherford Morrison** (1853–1939) incision (Fig 4.2) starts about 2 cm above the anterior superior iliac spine and extends obliquely down and medially through the skin, subcutaneous tissues and external oblique along its fibres, cutting the underlying internal oblique and transversus abdominis and the peritoneum along the line of the skin incision. Use an extra-peritoneal approach to place a transplanted kidney in the iliac fossa or to expose the iliac artery during vascular operations. Use a shorter incision, centred over McBurney's point and splitting the external oblique, internal oblique and transversus abdominis muscles along the direction of the fibres (*the grid iron incision*) in conventional appendicectomy. This incision can be extended laterally and medially if required to convert into a Rutherford Morrison incision.

7 **Transverse incisions** (Fig. 4.2) provide the best cosmetic scars. They can be used above or below the umbilicus depending on requirements. Ramstedt's pyloromyotomy and transverse colostomy are performed via incisions above the umbilicus. Lanz incision (Otto Lanz, 1865–1935) is used for appendicectomy and the Pfannenstiel incision (Hermann Johannes Pfannenstiel, 1862–1909) is used for operations on the uterus, urinary bladder and the prostate. The Pfannenstiel incision is a slightly curved horizontal incision about 2–3 cm above the pubic symphysis. Incise the anterior rectus

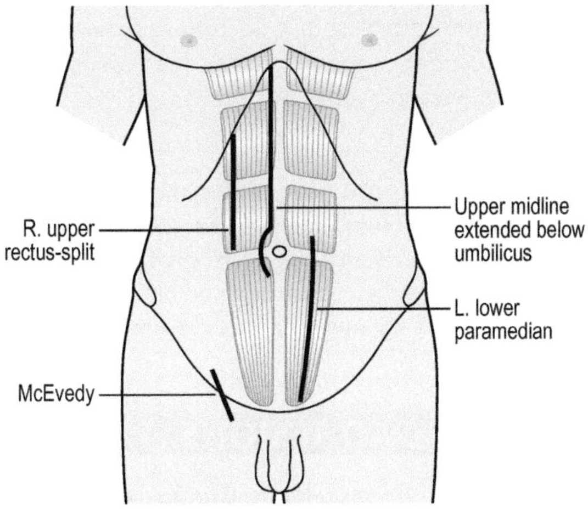

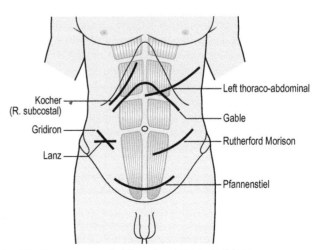

Fig. 4.1 Vertical laparotomy incisions.

R. upper rectus-split

Upper midline extended below umbilicus

L. lower paramedian

McEvedy

Kocher (R. subcostal)

Gridiron

Lanz

Left thoraco-abdominal

Gable

Rutherford Morison

Pfannenstiel

Fig. 4.2 Transverse and oblique laparotomy incisions.

sheath along the skin incision and retract the rectus and the pyramidalis muscles laterally. Incise the peritoneum vertically. Close the peritoneum in the midline using polyglycolic acid sutures and close the rectus sheath with polypropylene, PDS or nylon. The Lanz incision starts 2 cm below and medial to the right anterior superior iliac spine and extends medially for 5–7 cm. The rest of the exposure is similar to the grid iron incision.[7]

8 **Thoraco-abdominal incisions** usually follow the line of a rib and extend obliquely into the upper abdomen, dividing the cartilaginous cage protecting the upper abdominal viscera. Alternatively, you may convert a vertical upper abdominal incision into a thoraco-abdominal approach by extending it in the line of a rib across the costal margin. Radial incision of the diaphragm towards the oesophageal hiatus (left) or vena cava (right) converts the abdomen and thorax into one cavity and provides unparalleled access for oesophago-gastrectomy and right hepatic lobectomy. Thoraco-laparotomy may also be indicated for removal of a massive tumour of the kidney, adrenal or spleen.

9 **Posterolateral incisions** for approach to the kidney, adrenal and upper ureter are described in the relevant chapters.

Making the incision

1 Make the incision with the belly of a no. 20/22 scalpel, holding the knife as you would a table knife and using controlled movements. Once you have cut the skin pass the knife back to the scrub nurse in a kidney dish.

2 Alternatively, use a cutting diathermy spatula. Despite early concerns that the use of diathermy to incise skin and subcutaneous tissue might affect wound healing, it provides superior haemostasis and does not appear to adversely influence wound infection or cosmesis.

3 Deepen the incision using either a scalpel or cutting diathermy spatula. Control any ensuing bleeding from subcutaneous or intramuscular vessels with forceps and diathermy or suture. Use a unipolar or bipolar diathermy forceps, taking care not to burn the adjacent skin. Ligate vessels larger than 2 mm with an absorbable suture.

4 Apply wound towels to the wound edges and clip the tails of these towels with a Dunhill clip so that they are not lost. Change these towels if they become contaminated with infected abdominal contents.

5 Cut, split or retract the muscles of the abdominal wall as required and dictated by the incision that you use. Pick up the peritoneum with Dunhill or Fraser-Kelly artery forceps and tent it up to ensure no bowel is caught. Incise the tented peritoneum to enter the abdominal cavity. In patients with intestinal obstruction, bowel may lie close to the peritoneal incision or, in case of a previous laparotomy, may be adherent to it. Take the utmost care to avoid making an enterotomy which, even if noticed and repaired, may result in subsequent complications.

RE-OPENING THE ABDOMEN

Appraise

1 If the previous incision coincides with the site chosen for present access, use it. If not, use a new incision.

2 A longer incision may be required than was necessary for the initial operation.

> ### ▶ KEY POINT Old or new incision?

> ■ If the previous incision is convenient there is little advantage in creating a fresh incision. When a new incision is made parallel to the old one, it will result in a strip of denervated (and possibly devascularized) skin between the two scars.

Access through the old incision

1 If the old scar is acceptable make your incision through this without any attempt to excise it. If the scar is ugly or stretched, excise it by making an incision on either side of the scar.

2 For a paramedian scar the dissection is deepened in the line of the skin incision without any attempt to dissect the rectus sheath.

3 Open the peritoneum with great care as adhesions are common and bowel is often adherent to the old scar. It is wise to approach a virgin area first (hence a longer incision than before), then proceed towards the scarred area. Another alternative is to open the peritoneum to one side of the previous scarring and then dissect the scarred area under direct vision. Time spent here is amply justified.

4 Plan a secure closure at the time of the incision, as in a first-time laparotomy. Make sure that adequate abdominal wall and peritoneum remain and are free of adherent viscera.

> ### ? DIFFICULTY

> 1. If mobilization of fixed viscera is difficult, skirt around them, leaving them attached to one side of the wound, or open the other end of the wound and approach them from a different direction.
> 2. Carry out all sharp and blunt dissection under direct vision.
> 3. If there is inadvertent damage to bowel, repair it immediately if possible. Reassess the damage at the time of closure.

Access through a new incision

> ### ▶ KEY POINT Ubiquitous adhesions

> ■ Although this approach may be initially easier, viscera may be adherent to the parietal peritoneum in areas distant from the previous incision.

Once the abdomen is opened, gently retract the abdominal wall and divide any adhesions by blunt and sharp dissection, making use of tactile sensation and direct vision. If necessary, change position or side to get a better view of the adherent structures before dissecting them out safely. Be willing to tilt the operating table to one side or the other.

ABDOMINAL ADHESIONS

1 Adhesions occur in 90–95% of patients undergoing an invasive procedure on the abdomen, irrespective of the operative approach.[8,9]

They are a cause of much morbidity: 35% of patients with a prior laparotomy will be re-admitted to hospital an average of two times with adhesion-related complications.[10] In 1992, a UK survey reported 12 000 to 14 400 cases of adhesive small-bowel obstruction annually; in the USA in 1988, 950 000 days of inpatient care were required for adhesiolysis at a cost of 1.18 billion dollars.[11]

2 Intra-abdominal trauma or invasion of the peritoneal cavity, infection, bleeding and foreign material (glove powder, fibre from surgical swabs, suture materials, etc.) and intra-peritoneal chemotherapeutic agents are all thought to be responsible for increased formation of adhesions.

3 The most frequent sites are omentum (68%), small-bowel (67%), abdominal wall (45%) and colon (41%).

Prevention of adhesions

1 Meticulous haemostasis, prevention of intra-peritoneal spillage of intestinal contents, minimal handling of bowel, use of powder-free gloves, glove cleansing using a 10% solution of povidone-iodine in a non-toxic detergent base and not closing the peritoneum have all been advocated to prevent adhesion formation.

2 Seprafilm™ (hyaluronate-carboxymethyl cellulose membrane, Genzyme) has been reported to reduce the incidence of adhesions and the number of patients requiring surgery for small-bowel obstruction. However, the incidence of intra-abdominal abscesses and anastomotic leaks was higher in the Seprafilm group compared to controls. Adept™ (icodextrin 4% solution) has been shown to be safe and effective in reducing adhesions during laparoscopy. Interceed™ (oxidized regenerated cellulose, Johnson & Johnson) is another anti-adhesion barrier that has gained popularity among gynaecological surgeons. None, however, have found widespread acceptance, due in part to their cost. A cheaper alternative is liberal irrigation with Ringer lactate solution, which has been reported to decrease adhesions in experimental animal models.

Division of adhesions

1 It is futile to divide every single adhesion as, once divided, they are likely to form again, so divide adhesions only if they are causing a problem. Patients with recurrent adhesive small-bowel obstruction benefit from adhesiolysis and restoration of the bowel anatomy. However, it may be safer to leave the adhesions alone when they are dense but still allow intestinal contents to pass freely.

2 If in the process of releasing the adhesions the bowel is injured, perform a meticulous repair. Minimize contamination of the abdominal cavity by liberal suctioning and lavage.

3 The aims of the operation should be:
- To allow adequate exploration
- To permit safe closure without fear of damaging the viscera
- To prevent subsequent kinking or herniation of the bowel
- To minimize iatrogenic injury and complications.

EXPLORATORY LAPAROTOMY

1 Exploration of the abdomen was used extensively and routinely in the past. Each time an abdomen was opened, the surgeon meticulously and methodically examined every organ to ascertain the cause of the patient's symptoms. Improvements in diagnostic and imaging methods (in particular endoscopy and computed tomography) have made this unnecessary in most cases. However, exploration is still important in emergencies affecting the abdomen where a clear diagnosis may not be available due to the emergent nature and need to operate without thorough investigation. Knowledge of exploratory laparotomy is, therefore, still important, particularly for surgeons in training.

2 The advent of intra-operative ultrasound, endoscopic ultrasound and in some centres even on-table CT scan and angiography are welcome additions to the surgeon's armamentarium and may improve the assessment of deeper organs and intraluminal pathology. However, these modalities are not widely accessible and even if the technology is available, the expertise may not be.

> ### ▶ KEY POINT Full abdominal examination
>
> ■ It is useful to do a routine examination of the abdominal viscera as often as possible to familiarize yourself with the normal abdominal structures, so that if there is an abnormality you will be able to identify it. Moreover, if the symptoms persist or new symptoms arise, it is reassuring to know the normal exploratory findings.

3 Despite advances in investigative technology, exploration of the abdomen is still occasionally carried out as an elective 'final' diagnostic procedure in patients with inexplicable, distressing or sinister symptoms. However, such instances are becoming increasingly rare: one such example is small-bowel tumours, which were traditionally confirmed at laparotomy but can now be diagnosed on capsule endoscopy. Diagnostic laparoscopy has largely replaced laparotomy in these difficult cases.

4 Symptoms arising from the abdominal wall may confuse the diagnosis. A careful examination performed with the abdomen relaxed and a trial of local anaesthetic may help. Beware of referred pain from the spine and *Herpes Zoster* infection.

5 In patients with suspected mesenteric ischaemia and possible intra-abdominal sepsis, make an early decision on operative intervention. Diagnostic laparoscopy in the former and a CT scan in the latter may be helpful.

> ### ▶ KEY POINTS The need for laparotomy
>
> ■ In an emergency, while resuscitating the patient it is useful to repeat clinical assessment. The features may change and at times you may make the decision to defer operation.
> ■ When in doubt, trust your clinical acumen rather than the results of investigations that are at odds with your clinical findings.

Access

1 The principles governing incisions were addressed at the beginning of this chapter and will be re-addressed in chapters dedicated to the relevant organs. When the diagnosis is in doubt

TABLE 4.1 Rutherford Morrison incisions to expose abdominal viscera		
Midline	Upper	Hiatus, oesophagus, stomach, duodenum, spleen, liver, pancreas, biliary tract
	Central	Small-bowel, colon
	Lower	Sigmoid, rectum, ovary/tube/uterus, bladder and prostate (extraperitoneal)
	Throughout	Aorta
Paramedian (incl. rectus split)	Upper	Biliary tract (right), spleen (left), etc.
	Central	Small-bowel, colon
	Lower	Pelvic viscera, lower ureter (extraperitoneal)
Oblique	Subcostal	Liver and biliary tract (right), spleen (left)
	Gable (bilateral subcostal)	Pancreas, liver, adrenals
	Gridiron	Caecum–appendix (right)
	Rutherford Morison	Caecum–appendix (right), sigmoid (left), ureter and external iliac vessels (extraperitoneal)
	Posterolateral	Kidney and adrenal (extraperitoneal)
Transverse	Right upper quadrant	Gallbladder, infant pylorus, colostomy
	Mid-abdominal	Small-bowel, colon, kidney, lumbar sympathetic chain, vena cava (right)
	Lanz	Caecum–appendix (right)
	Pfannenstiel	Ovary/tube/uterus, prostate (extraperitoneal)
Thoraco-abdominal	Right	Liver and portal vein
	Left	Gastro-oesophageal junction, enormous spleen

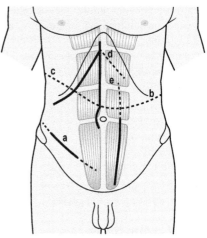

Fig. 4.3   Methods of extending abdominal incisions. a, gridiron incision extended laterally and (to a greater extent) medially; b, midline incision with T extension into left upper quadrant to deal with profuse splenic haemorrhage; c, midline incision with T extension into the right chest for ruptured liver; d, Kocher incision with left subcostal extension for major hepatic procedures; e, left lower paramedian incision extended upwards for mobilization of left colic flexure.

performed to facilitate appropriate surgery and adequate lavage of the abdomen.

4   Figure 4.3 displays the different techniques to extend incisions in order to deal with unexpected findings or intra-operative difficulties.

5   A wide range of retractors is available. The Goligher, Bookwalter and the Omni-tract retractors greatly facilitate access during a difficult laparotomy and should be kept available. Make sure they can be fixed to the operating table. Proper and liberal use of retractors frees an assistant to be used in other crucial steps.

6   Adjust the patient's position when required to improve exposure to an organ or area. Tilt the patient away from the area of interest so that bowel falls away, giving a better exposure. This is particularly important in laparoscopic surgery where a tilt of about 20 degrees can make a great difference.

Assess

1   Have the theatre nurse clear all unnecessary instruments from the operative field. Transfer sharp instruments in a kidney dish and not directly, to avoid injuries.

2   Carry out a systematic examination of the abdomen and its contents by feel and visually after ensuring that lighting is optimal. It is recommended that a set sequence is followed in examining the abdominal viscera so that no structure is missed (Fig. 4.4):
- Right lobe of liver, gallbladder, left lobe of liver, spleen
- Diaphragmatic hiatus, abdominal oesophagus and stomach: cardia, body, lesser curve, antrum, pylorus and then duodenal bulb
- Bile ducts, right kidney, duodenal loop, head of pancreas; the transverse colon is drawn out of the wound towards the patient's head
- Body and tail of pancreas, left kidney
- Root of mesentery, superior mesenteric and middle colic vessels, aorta, inferior mesenteric artery and vein, small-bowel and mesentery from ligament of Treitz to ileocaecal valve

select a midline incision, which is quick, versatile and allows access to the whole abdomen, which affords the luxury of almost unlimited extension from thoracic cavity to pelvis. Other incisions mentioned earlier may be used in specific conditions (Table 4.1).

2   In patients with a previous laparotomy scar, favour the same scar to enter the abdomen, but not at the cost of urgency, exposure or safe closure. Try to avoid an area where a stoma will need to be sited.

3   When the findings on entering the abdomen are different from those suspected preoperatively, the incision may have to be extended or even closed and another incision made. For example, if a duodenal perforation is discovered at appendicectomy, the Lanz incision may have to be closed and a midline incision

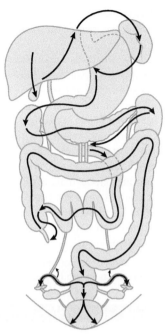

Fig. 4.4 The order of examining the abdominal contents at exploratory laparotomy.

- Appendix, caecum, colon, rectum
- Pelvic peritoneum, uterus, tubes and ovaries in the female, bladder
- Hernial orifices and main iliac vessels on each side: the ureters can sometimes be seen in thin patients, or if they are dilated.

3 Record the findings of this exploration in detail at the end of the operation. You may be able to dictate the findings to an observer for direct entry into the operation notes.

Complete exploration of the abdominal viscera is not possible in every case. In patients having an appendicectomy through an incision in the right iliac fossa or a Ramstedt's pyloromyotomy through a transverse scar, exploration may be limited to the area exposed. In situations where further exploration of the abdomen is futile, such as in carcinomatosis peritonei, make a gentle search for the primary tumour and biopsy any visible metastatic lesions. Perform a palliative procedure such as a stoma or entero-enteric bypass if necessary.

4 In the presence of a tumour it is usual to adopt a no touch or minimal touch technique, although there is no firm evidence that this improves survival.[12]

5 In emergency laparotomy immediate action may be required, for example to stop bleeding or close a perforation. Thereafter, perform a methodical examination of the other viscera unless the patient's general condition precludes it. Note the nature and amount of any free fluid, collecting some for chemical, cytological and microbiological examination.

Action

1 Make a decision on any definitive procedure: consider the preoperative diagnosis, operative findings and the patient's condition. In elderly or sick patients control of the emergency condition takes precedence over the complete eradication of disease. Inform the anaesthetist as soon as you decide a course of action.

2 Incidental findings such as gallstones, diverticula, fibroids or ovarian cysts do not automatically call for action unless they pose an immediate threat to health or offer a better explanation for the patient's symptoms than the original diagnosis. Similarly, during a laparotomy for another condition, do not perform an appendicectomy without an indication. The patient's prior consent is unlikely to have been obtained, so any adverse outcome may be more difficult to defend. By contrast, ordinarily remove an unsuspected neoplasm, if necessary through a separate incision, provided the patient's condition allows. Whatever course you adopt, meticulously record the findings in the operation notes.

3 The contents of the distal small-bowel and the entire large-bowel are unsterile. Visceral contents that are normally sterile such as bile, urine and gastric juice may also become infected as a result of inflammation and obstruction. Before opening the bowel or other potentially contaminated viscera, isolate the area from contact with the wound and other organs by using moist abdominal swabs. Apply non-crushing clamps to occlude the lumen and ensure that an efficient suction apparatus is available to remove any contents that spill. Following closure of the viscus discard all instruments and swabs used on opened bowel and change gloves.

4 The risk of infection depends on the degree of contamination. Healthy tissues can normally cope with a small number of organisms but are overwhelmed by heavy contamination or re-infection. Logically, reducing bacterial contamination reduces infection.

5 Patients with impaired local host defences, such as those on immuno-suppressants, steroids and diabetic patients, are susceptible to a wide range of organisms including fungi, particularly if they have previously had antibiotics. When there is gross infection (peritonitis) or spillage into the peritoneal cavity, liberally irrigate with warm saline or diluted povidone-iodine to reduce the bacterial load.

6 With the increased use of intestinal staplers, bowel clamps are infrequently used in some centres. It is, however, useful to know the types of bowel clamp and when they should be used. Intestinal clamps are of two types: crushing and non-crushing:
- *Crushing* clamps are applied to seal the bowel when it is cut. Payr's powerful double-action clamps are most frequently used, but Lang Stevenson devised a similar clamp with narrow blades. Cope's triple clamps allow the middle clamp to be removed, so that the bowel can be divided through the crushed area, leaving its ends sealed. These clamps are useful in partial gastrectomy.
- *Non-crushing* clamps have longitudinal ridges and control the leakage of bowel contents without causing irreversible damage to the gut. Lane's twin clamps, which can be locked together, allow two segments of intestine to be occluded and held in apposition for anastomosis. Pringle's clamps hold cut ends of bowel securely, and the lightly crushed segment is so narrow that it can safely be incorporated in the anastomosis.

7 We are all familiar with stories of instruments and swabs left inside the abdomen and this represents one of the surgeon's worst nightmares. There is no single routine that entirely guards against this mishap. Use the minimum number of instruments and the largest swabs, which should remain attached to large clips lying outside the abdominal wound. Avoid using small

swabs deeply within the abdomen. If possible, use long-handled instruments on tissues and structures when prolonged use is anticipated. Although the primary responsibility of leaving a swab or an instrument in the abdomen rests with you as the operating surgeon, encourage the entire team to take an active role in preventing it. The scrub nurse counts the instruments and swabs before the procedure and before closure of the operative wound. He or she also counts any extra instruments, needles or swabs used during the procedure. If the scrub nurse reports a missing swab or instrument while closing the abdomen, carry out a thorough search of the abdomen and vicinity. If all else fails, perform an abdominal X-ray before waking the patient from the anaesthetic.

> ▶ KEY POINT Avoid needless procedures
>
> ■ If this is an exploration for undiagnosed acute or chronic symptoms and the expected diagnosis is not confirmed and no cause is found, so be it. Resist the desire to 'do something.' It provides a false sense of security and may be the cause of further complications or confusion in the diagnosis. Having made sure you have overlooked nothing, close the abdomen and record your findings clearly.

PERITONEAL LAVAGE

1 The peritoneal cavity has a remarkable ability to combat sepsis. Nonetheless, spillage of contaminated contents, such as faeces or infected bile, may lead to early septicaemia and late abdominal abscess.

2 Where local peritonitis is marked, carry out peritoneal lavage with warm saline, sucking out the fluid and inserting a drain. The theoretical risk of disseminating the infection throughout the peritoneal cavity does not appear to hold true in practice.

3 In generalized peritonitis, wash out the peritoneal cavity with warm saline (1–2 L or more) at the end of the operation. In very severe cases (e.g. pancreatic necrosis, faecal peritonitis), be prepared to insert one or two drainage tubes for postoperative lavage. Place one drainage tube in the abscess cavity and one in the pelvis: soft, wide-bore silicone tubes or sump drains are appropriate. Irrigate with warmed (37 °C) peritoneal dialysis fluid (Dialaflex 6 L) with added potassium at a rate of 50–200 ml/hour, depending on the extent of sepsis. A water-tight closure of the abdominal wound is essential, so initially perfuse a small amount of dialysate (50 mL/hour) overnight until the peritoneum seals any defects. Postoperative lavage is well tolerated and does not seem to interfere with intestinal motility. Continue the treatment until there is clinical improvement and the effluent becomes clear.

CLOSING THE ABDOMEN

1 The scrub nurse will check counts of swabs, instruments and needles to confirm that they are correct.

2 To drain or not to drain? Leaving a drain in the abdomen following a major laparotomy has been frequently questioned. There is no evidence to support their use in every case and in elective abdominal surgery most studies have found no benefit from drainage.[13] A selective use policy is more appropriate, and indications for draining the peritoneal cavity may include the following:

■ Operations on the bile ducts or pancreas where there is potential leakage of bile or pancreatic juice

■ Where there is a localized abscess

■ After suture of a perforated viscus where the tissues are friable, or when a controlled fistula is planned

■ When there is a large raw area from which oozing can occur. Meticulous haemostasis is preferable.

In all other patients drains are of no use. Bacteria may enter from outside through an open drain, especially if nursing care is poor, or the drain may erode a vessel or a suture line, especially if it is left in for a long time. When you must use a drain it should be a closed drain, and if suction is to be used employ a low-pressure system.

3 Carefully return abdominal viscera to the abdominal cavity, taking care there are no twists in the bowel.

> ▶ KEY POINT Avoid needle-stick injury
>
> ■ Take every precaution to avoid transmitting infection through needle-stick injuries. Many such injuries are sustained during abdominal wall closure. Avoid hand-held needles. Even when using curved needles held in a needle holder, there is a danger of injury. A valuable development is the introduction of blunt-tipped (often called 'taper-point') needles, which pass through the tissues but penetrate gloves and skin only if pressed hard against them.

4 There are several different techniques for abdominal closure with no consensus on which is best.[14] The choice depends upon the type of incision, the extent of the operation, the patient's general condition and your preference. It is a common error among surgical trainees to sew up the abdomen too tightly. Wounds swell during the first 3–4 postoperative days, oedema makes the sutures even tighter and there is a risk of tissue necrosis and subsequent dehiscence:

■ Mass closure technique is currently used by most surgeons with evidence that this technique is associated with the lowest incidence of wound dehiscence.[15] It is usually used following midline laparotomy, but can used with subcostal or transverse abdominal incisions.

■ Close the abdomen with No.1 nylon, polypropylene or polydioxanone (PDS). There is evidence that PDS causes fewer stitch sinuses than non-absorbable sutures.

■ A continuous stitch is more secure than interrupted stitches. Place the sutures 1 cm away from the wound edge and at 1-cm intervals.

■ The length of the suture used should be four times the length of the wound.[16]

■ There is disagreement about the use of tension sutures. In the presence of risk factors for poor healing such as a distended or obese abdomen; if the wound is infected or likely to become so; if the patient is malnourished, jaundiced or suffering from advanced cancer, consider using these sutures. However, they cause ischaemia and necrosis of the tissues, resulting in delayed wound healing and severe pain, and may contribute to respiratory compromise and abdominal compartment syndrome. Most surgeons reserve them for the repair of complete abdominal dehiscence ('burst abdomen').

■ Subcutaneous sutures are generally not necessary. There is no evidence that suturing this layer affords any benefit.[17]

Mass closure

1 As a rule, use this technique for closing a midline laparotomy wound or a laparotomy through a previous scar. It can also be used in oblique or transverse incisions.

2 The peritoneum need not be sutured. Peritoneal closure is thought to predispose to adhesion formation.

3 Pick up the linea alba with a Kocher's or Lane's forceps to clearly define the apex and the lower end. Using a No.1 nylon/polypropelene/PDS suture on a blunt or taper-cutting needle, approximate this layer with a continuous running stitch using a 1:4 wound-to-suture length ratio, ensuring that no intra-peritoneal contents are caught in the stitch. When half the length of the wound is approximated, commence suturing from the other end and tie the two sutured segments in the middle with a secure knot. Bury the knot under the fascial layer so that it does not lie subcutaneously and cause discomfort.

4 Secure haemostasis in the subcutaneous fat using diathermy or ligatures as required. This layer is usually not approximated but if it is very thick, 2/0 or 3/0 polyglactin (Vicryl) interrupted sutures may be used to obliterate the potential dead space. An inverted suture, starting and ending in the depth of the wound buries the knot, giving a better result.

5 Approximate the skin with 3/0 or 4/0 undyed polyglactin (Vicryl) or polygecaprone (Monocryl) subcuticular sutures. When the wound is contaminated, use staples or interrupted non-absorbable sutures such as 3/0 nylon or polypropylene. When the wound is dirty, you may leave open the skin and subcutaneous fat, undertaking delayed primary closure 5 days later.

Layered closure

1 The peritoneum is left to heal by mesothelial regeneration, thereby reducing the chances of adhesion formation.

2 In paramedian, oblique and transverse incisions the posterior rectus sheath/tranversus aponeurosis/internal oblique muscles are sutured using polyglactin 910, PDS no.1 or nylon/polypropylene no.1.

3 The muscle layer can safely be left alone without suturing, especially when it is split and not cut.

4 The anterior rectus sheath/external oblique aponeurosis is sutured with a no.1 PDS, nylon or polypropylene continuous suture.

5 Subcutaneous fat and skin are then dealt with as described above.

Tension sutures

1 Use tension sutures in patients who have risk factors predisposing to wound dehiscence (vide supra) and in patients with established full thickness wound dehiscence ('burst abdomen').

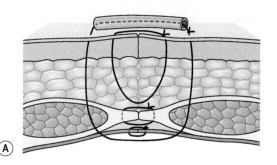

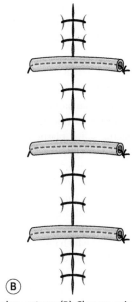

Fig. 4.5 (A) Deep tension suture; (B) Closure using deep tension suture.

2 Use No.1 or 2 nylon or polypropylene full-thickness interrupted sutures which include all layers of the abdominal wall including the skin. They can be placed as vertical simple or mattress sutures (Fig. 4.5A). Avoid using horizontal mattress sutures as they cause ischaemia of the tissue within the stitch. Thread small 4 to 5-cm segments of plastic or rubber tubing on to the sutures on one side and leave them ready to tie. Perform mass closure of the abdomen as described above and tie the tension sutures sequentially as the mass closure progresses (Fig. 4.5B).

3 Approximate the skin if it is clean or relatively clean, using interrupted 3/0 nylon or polypropylene.

Removal of skin sutures

As a rule in a healthy individual, remove abdominal skin sutures on day 7–10 postoperation. In debilitated individuals, it is preferable to leave the stitches or staples for at least 2 weeks. If at this stage the wound has not healed, there is no point in leaving the sutures longer. Look for a cause for delayed healing: a deep-seated collection is the usual culprit.

The difficult closure

1 At times closure of the abdomen may be the most difficult part of the operation, even to an experienced surgeon. Inadequate closure can be disastrous, but take the utmost care to make sure there is no injury to the bowel.

2 Relaxation of the abdomen is extremely important throughout a laparotomy and this applies equally during closure of the abdomen. Maintain good communication with the anaesthetist.

3 It is good practice to place the omentum over exposed bowel in the wound when possible.

4 Place an abdominal swab over the bowel and omentum to help prevent them from being caught in the suture during abdominal closure. Remove the swab before inserting the last few sutures.

5 If there is too much tension in the middle of the wound, it is easier to stitch the wound alternately from either end, slowly advancing towards the centre. Use interrupted sutures in this situation as they help to reduce the tensile force on the suture. Unlike a continuous suture, if one stitch subsequently fails the other sutures will hold.

6 If the wound cannot be closed despite these simple steps, you may use a variety of different materials including bio-prostheses to obtain a tension-free closure.[18,19]

7 In an emergency and when biomaterials are not available, temporary abdominal closure can be achieved using a Bogota bag.[20] Empty a large sterile saline plastic bag, open it and suture the edges to the rectus sheath to close the abdomen, or use an Opsite 'sandwich' vacuum dressing.[21] These are commonly used in the grossly infected abdomen to allow drainage of sepsis prior to a delayed closure.[22] Newer (and more costly) alternatives include Strattice (Lifecell Corporation),[23] a biocompatible tissue matrix which allows ingrowth of healing tissue, the ABRA system (Canica Design Inc.),[24] which uses tensioned silicone elastomers to re-approximate the edges of the fascial defect allowing delayed primary closure in 60% of cases, and the V.A.C. system (KCI Medical Ltd.). The latter uses a permeable membrane and porous foam dressing in combination with a closed, low-pressure suction drainage system which removes exudate from the wound whilst preventing retraction of the wound edges, and has been shown to reduce mortality compared to conventional treatment methods.[25] Be aware in patients with a newly fashioned anastomosis that a higher rate of anastomotic leakage has been reported following V.A.C. therapy.

Delayed closure

1 If the abdominal cavity is grossly contaminated, as in faecal peritonitis, some degree of wound sepsis is almost inevitable. One option is to close the superficial tissues lightly around a drain. Another is delayed primary suture, leaving the skin and subcutaneous tissue widely open. In either case give parenteral antibiotics and drain the peritoneal cavity.

2 Suture the musculo-aponeurotic layers of the abdominal wall with a continuous monofilament nylon suture, taking care not to draw the edges together too tightly as considerable swelling can be anticipated. Superficial to this layer, loosely pack the wound with gauze swabs wrung out in saline. Change these packs and inspect it daily. Perform delayed closure when the condition of the wound improves, usually at around 5 days.

3 If peritonitis is particularly severe, for example after a major colonic perforation or infected pancreatic necrosis, some surgeons prefer to leave the abdomen completely open as a 'laparostomy', employing a Bogota bag and sometimes a zip fastener, with daily irrigation of the peritoneum. The drawbacks of this approach are lateral retraction of the rectus sheath with fusion of the small-bowel to the wound edges, high metabolic demands (malnutrition and fluid losses) and an increased risk of enteric fistulae.[26] If the patient survives, late closure of the large incisional hernia is usually required and is frequently challenging. In our opinion it is advisable to avoid the technique wherever possible.

Abdominal dressings

The UK National Institute for Clinical Excellence (NICE) guidelines[27] recommend an appropriate dressing depending on the nature of the wound and anticipated discharge. A plastic spray may be used if the wound is not expected to discharge much; use a more absorbent dressing when you expect discharge from the wound (for example after a laparotomy for peritonitis or in a patient with ascites).

ABDOMINAL COMPARTMENT SYNDROME

1 Abdominal compartment syndrome may be primary (intra-abdominal peritonitis, mesenteric ischaemia, obstructed bowel or intra-abdominal bleeding), or secondary to causes outside the abdomen, such as sepsis elsewhere, causing paralytic ileus[28] or colonic pseudo-obstruction.

2 The consequences of a raised intra-abdominal pressure are:
- Respiratory failure and the need for higher ventilator pressures in mechanically ventilated patients
- Decreased venous return due to compression of the inferior vena cava
- Decreased renal perfusion causing acute renal failure
- Reduced splanchnic (G splanchnon = visceral, intestinal) perfusion causing intestinal ischaemia.

3 Intra-abdominal pressure is usually measured using a Foley catheter in the bladder primed with 50 ml of fluid. However, there are concerns that measurement of bladder pressure may overestimate abdominal pressure, and the results should be taken in the context of other parameters such as respiratory pressures and oxygen saturation, renal function and urine output, lactate levels and abdominal distension.

Prevention

When there is grossly distended bowel and the abdominal closure is judged to be under undue tension, you may leave the abdomen open as a laparostomy using either a Bogota bag or 'sandwich' dressing. Avoid this if possible (vide supra), and close the skin only after placing the omentum over the viscera.

Treatment

Treatment may be:
Medical:
- Correction of electrolyte imbalance or other causes of paralytic ileus
- Neostigmine – contraindicated in presence of mechanical bowel obstruction or a bowel anastomosis
- Colonoscopic decompression if the large-bowel is distended.
Surgical:
- Drainage of haemoperitoneum and control of intra-abdominal bleeding

- Drainage of ascites
- Laparostomy with delayed closure of the abdomen (vide supra).

BURST ABDOMEN

This is full thickness dehiscence of a laparotomy wound. The incidence of burst abdomen ranges from 0.6% to 6% and mortality is around 10-40%.[29] Predisposing factors for wound dehiscence are anaemia, hypoalbuminaemia, malnutrition, malignancy, jaundice, obesity and diabetes, male gender, elderly patients and emergency laparotomy:[30]

1 Dehiscence usually declares itself on the 6th to 15th postoperative day[31]. It may be preceded by low-grade pyrexia and there may be delay in the return of bowel sounds.

2 In 85% of patients impending full thickness dehiscence presents with a salmon pink serous exudate from the wound.

3 Wound disruption may occur without warning following straining or removal of the sutures. The dehiscence may be associated with evisceration of abdominal contents, although sometimes the bowel does not eviscerate, leaving an open abdomen with adherent bowel visible in the depths of the wound.

Management

1 Reassure the patent and provide adequate analgesia and sedation. A burst abdomen, particularly with evisceration of the bowel, is a frightening experience for the patient and relatives. If the wound is relatively clean and if the bowel is eviscerating undertake immediate repair of the wound to prevent bowel injury or strangulation.

2 Fluid resuscitation is important as exposed bowel tends to lose large amounts of fluid rapidly. Administer broad-spectrum antibiotics if not already prescribed.

3 Make an attempt to reduce the exposed bowel back into the abdomen and dress the wound with a non-adhesive dressing. If the bowel cannot be reduced, cover it with an empty sterile 3 L saline bag and make arrangements to transfer the patient urgently to theatre.

4 During closure of the burst abdomen take a swab for microbiology and use liberal amounts of warm saline to wash out the peritoneal cavity. Make no attempt to mobilize densely adherent bowel as there is high risk of bowel injury at this stage. If there is an anastomotic dehiscence, deal with it by exteriorization or re-anastomosis (ideally with a covering stoma). Close the abdomen with interrupted polypropylene or nylon no.1 sutures, supported by deep-tension sutures. Close the skin if the wound is clean, leave it open if the wound is grossly contaminated. If the abdomen cannot be closed and the linea alba is retracted too far laterally, resort to temporary closure using the techniques described above, leaving the wound to heal by secondary intention. Repair the ensuing incisional hernia electively. Various other techniques that are used to achieve closure of a burst abdomen include biosynthetic or synthetic mesh,[18] component separation[32] or a combination of these techniques.

5 While suturing the abdominal wall, take care not to use excess force as the sutures will tear out of the inflamed tissues.

LAPAROTOMY FOR TRAUMA

See Chapter 3.

LAPAROTOMY FOR PERITONITIS

APPRAISE

1 Intra-abdominal sepsis in critically ill patients carries a significant mortality (32% in patients with an APACHE score of more than 10).[33] Features of peritonitis develop when the parietal peritoneum is irritated either by an inflamed organ such as appendix, gall bladder, colonic diverticulitis or fallopian tube or by chemical contact with gastric juice, bile, activated pancreatic enzymes, bowel contents or blood. The features may be localized over the inflamed structure or generalized, depending on the patient's capacity to contain the inflammation with the help of the omentum and surrounding bowel.

2 A patient with generalized peritonitis presents with sudden-onset abdominal pain, worse on movement. On examination the patient is tachycardic, tachypnoeic and pyrexial with generalized tenderness, rigidity and rebound tenderness. If the inflammation is localized, the abdominal signs are also localized to that area. A patient who develops septicaemia may become hypothermic instead of pyrexial.

3 It is good practice to re-examine the patient after an interval. The features of generalized pain may have localized, as in the case of appendicitis or cholecystitis, or a localized pain may have become generalized as in the case of appendicular perforation. In patients with a duodenal perforation, pain that is excruciating may completely wane and re-appear later. This is due to the different phases of peptic ulcer perforation: the initial chemical peritonitis due to gastric acid or bile leaking into the peritoneum leads to a peritoneal reaction and features of peritonitis. This in turn leads to fluid exudation, thus diluting the gastric acid or bile, and the pain wanes. Infection secondary to bacterial contamination results in further pain and the patient again exhibits features of peritonitis.

4 Perform a urine examination and a pregnancy test in women of child-bearing age. Order blood tests including haemoglobin, white cell count, platelet count, renal function, liver function, amylase, pancreatic lipase and a blood gas. Erect chest X-ray or lateral decubitus abdominal X-ray may demonstrate signs of free intra-peritoneal air. If available, order a CT scan of the abdomen, which will usually reveal the cause of the peritonitis and will also differentiate pancreatitis and may avoid an unnecessary laparotomy.

5 Immunocompromised patients (those with AIDS or transplant patients on immunosuppressants) may present with particular diagnostic problems such as toxic megacolon, appendicitis caused by cytomegalovirus (CMV), spontaneous bacterial peritonitis or atypical mycobacterial infection.

6 Exclude medical conditions such as diabetic keto-acidosis, Henoch-Schonlein purpura, porphyria, sickle cell crisis, basal pneumonia and pyelonephritis, which may mimic peritonitis.

7 Critically ill patients who develop an acute abdomen present a diagnostic challenge. An urgent CT scan of the abdomen will

usually provide a diagnosis. Acalculous cholecystitis is common in acutely ill patients in the intensive care setting: order an ultrasound scan, which can be performed at the bedside, in septic patients with right upper quadrant signs to confirm the diagnosis.

8 Very occasionally, generalized peritonitis develops in the absence of any overt visceral pathology. Primary peritonitis, commonly due to *Streptococcus pneumoniae*, can occur spontaneously in children and in patients with ascites, nephrotic syndrome and in patients undergoing continuous ambulatory peritoneal dialysis (CAPD).

9 Diagnostic laparoscopy is used increasingly in assessment of the acute abdomen. It can be very helpful in equivocal cases but is unnecessary if there is clear evidence of generalized peritonitis.

Decision

1 It is often valuable for an individual or a small group to sit down and review what has been discovered, what it means and what should be done about it before taking a decision on treating a patient with an acute abdomen. Operative intervention may not always be the correct course.

2 Re-examining the patient after an interval may give new clues to the diagnosis or the diagnosis may become more apparent. If the patient's condition permits, go back after a few hours and re-examine them, looking for any new signs.

3 A decision to treat a patient conservatively is always provisional and subject to monitoring and repeated examination. If the patient is not responding to the treatment regime consider changing the strategy. Diagnostic imaging may be required or the patient may need an operation.

4 When clinical findings and investigations do not match, trust your clinical findings provided they are based on a thorough and accurate clinical examination.

Prepare

1 Correct any fluid, electrolyte or acid–base imbalance intravenously.

2 Pass a nasogastric tube and aspirate the stomach.

3 As far as possible assess and correct incidental medical conditions, in particular cardiorespiratory disease.

4 Start parenteral broad-spectrum antibiotic therapy, such as a third-generation cephalosporin with an aminoglycoside and metronidazole, according to your hospital protocol. A wide spectrum of pathogens may be encountered, particularly in critically ill or immune-suppressed patients, including *Candida albicans*, *Enterococcus* sp. and *Staphylococcus epidermidis*.

Access

1 Examine the abdomen under anaesthetic. It may reveal an unsuspected mass. If there are no localizing signs, use a midline incision centred on the umbilicus. Be prepared to extend it in either direction once the cause is evident.

2 If peritonitis follows a recent operation, re-open the previous incision (vide infra).

Assess

1 Note any free fluid or pus and take a specimen for laboratory examination.

2 After a rapid preliminary examination of the abdomen, carry out a methodical exploration.

Action

1 Make sure that the incision, the assistance, the lighting and the instruments available are adequate for the proposed procedure.

2 Resect an inflamed, perforated appendix or Meckel's diverticulum. Undertake cholecystectomy for a perforated empyema of the gallbladder; if dissection proves difficult due to dense fibrosis or bleeding, drain the gallbladder using a Foley catheter as a cholecystostomy. Close a perforated peptic ulcer using a Graham's omental patch.

3 Treat localized injuries to the small-bowel by primary repair, provided soiling is not excessive. Resect gangrenous or ischaemic small-bowel but undertake primary anastomosis only if the proximal and distal margins are healthy and viable.

4 Resect perforated colon, but be very cautious about restoring intestinal continuity without a proximal diverting colostomy. Resection with exteriorization of the bowel ends is an even safer option. Sigmoid diverticulitis with purulent peritonitis can often be treated by lavage and drainage without resection of the diverticular segment, but resect perforated carcinomas if possible.

5 Recognize acute pancreatitis by a bloodstained effusion, discoloration of the retroperitoneum and the presence of whitish patches of fat necrosis. In salpingitis, the uterine tubes are reddened, swollen and oedematous, often discharging pus from the abdominal ostia. Crohn's disease of the terminal ileum manifests as inflamed, thickened bowel and mesentery, typically with 'fat wrapping' of the bowel. In these conditions do not undertake any resection, but close the abdomen and institute appropriate medical therapy.

6 Make sure no dead or devitalised tissue remains and remove any foreign bodies from the peritoneal cavity. Drain abscesses and institute copious lavage with warm normal saline if there is infection or contamination by intestinal contents.

7 Your priority throughout the operative procedure is to identify the cause of the patient's condition and deal with it, in order to avoid the need for re-operation. In patients in whom a single surgical intervention is performed the mortality rate is 27%, compared with 42% for subjects undergoing multiple laparotomies.[33,34] The role of planned re-laparotomy in critically ill patients with abdominal sepsis has been questioned: the use of predictive indices, used to guide decisions on re-laparotomy, has been shown to reduce mortality.[35]

Checklist

1 Has the laparotomy achieved its purpose? If not, and the patient requires re-operation, the chance of recovery will be seriously prejudiced.

2 Ensure that any postoperative sequelae which may occur are not the result of some overlooked, correctable lesion.

LAPAROTOMY FOR INTESTINAL OBSTRUCTION

Appraise

1. Patients with intestinal obstruction have a varied presentation ranging from colicky abdominal pain and distension to strangulated bowel with peritonitis. Classically there are four cardinal features—colic, distension, vomiting and constipation—but the prominence of each of these is affected by the site and type of obstruction: for example a high intestinal obstruction presents with profuse vomiting and pain in the absence of abdominal distension.

2. Small-bowel obstruction is most commonly secondary to adhesions resulting from a previous laparotomy. Examination of the hernia orifices (inguinal, femoral, umbilical and incisional) is vital. Missing an obstructed inguinal or femoral hernia might subject a patient to an unnecessary laparotomy when a simple hernia reduction and repair would suffice. Conversely, a missed hernia treated conservatively will put the patient in danger of early strangulation and rapid deterioration.

3. Large-bowel obstruction is frequently caused by a tumour and presents with abdominal distension and a change in bowel habit, depending on the site of obstruction. Classically, left-sided large-bowel obstruction presents with constipation or overflow diarrhoea. Right-sided lesions may present with anaemia or as small-bowel obstruction or with a palpable mass. Perform a digital examination of the rectum in every patient with abdominal distension to assess if there is a rectal mass, faecal impaction or an extraluminal mass or abscess. Large-bowel obstruction is often insidious in onset, and there is usually time to investigate the cause and to differentiate mechanical obstruction from pseudo-obstruction: CT scanning is the investigation of choice.

4. Other causes of large-bowel obstruction include stricture secondary to diverticulitis, ischaemic colitis or rarely Crohn's disease, and volvulus of the sigmoid colon (and, rarely, of the caecum). Abdominal X-ray shows the classical coffee bean sign in a sigmoid volvulus. Diagnosis of a caecal volvulus is more difficult but a plain X-ray of the abdomen shows dilated caecum in the middle and left side of the abdomen. Volvulus may present fulminantly or subacutely. In subacute sigmoid volvulus a phosphate or gastrografin enema may relieve the obstruction; failing this, employ flexible sigmoidoscopy to decompress the sigmoid colon. Depending on the patient's general condition and co-morbidities, definitive surgery may be required to fix or resect the redundant bowel to prevent recurrence. In fulminant volvulus perform an emergency laparotomy, resecting the gangrenous sigmoid colon and bringing the proximal end out as a stoma (Hartmann's resection). This can be reversed at a later date if the patient's condition permits.

5. Mesenteric ischaemia may present as a catastrophe or as a slowly evolving process. A history of atrial fibrillation or atherosclerotic disease elsewhere is often present in mesenteric arterial occlusion; venous occlusion is rarer and occurs in fulminant pancreatitis and prothrombotic states. A high index of suspicion is necessary for diagnosis, especially in an emergency setting. Sudden onset abdominal pain without signs of peritonism, bleeding per rectum or malaena, metabolic acidosis and rising lactate levels are all suggestive of mesenteric ischaemia and further investigation with a CT angiogram should be done on an emergent basis.

6. Crohn's disease may cause obstruction through a variety of mechanisms:
   - Inflammation and oedema may obstruct the lumen in active disease: most patients respond to conservative treatment with steroids.
   - Adhesions between affected segments and other structures may require surgical intervention.
   - Longstanding disease may result in a stenosed, fibrotic segment causing chronic obstruction and proximal stagnation.
     Diagnosis is by contrast-enhanced CT scan or MR enterography. If these modalities are not available, order a conventional small-bowel enema using gastrografin or dilute barium. Treat stenosed segments by resection or stricturoplasty.

7. Radiation enteritis results from progressive vascular and interstitial cellular damage and is dose-related. It most frequently affects the rectum following pelvic irradiation, causing rectal bleeding which is rarely profuse. Small-bowel involvement typically results in chronic strictures and subacute obstruction: the symptoms can be delayed for several years. Treatment is conservative wherever possible, as operative treatment carries a high morbidity and mortality due to poor healing of irradiated tissues.

8. Sclerosing peritonitis was historically associated with the beta-blocker practolol, which is no longer used. It is now mainly seen in patients on long-term peritoneal dialysis and, in the tropics, due to tuberculous peritonitis. In some patients no cause may be found (idiopathic sclerosing peritonitis; G idios = one's own + pathos = suffering). The small-bowel is thickened and encased in a matrix of dense, fibrotic connective tissue, resulting in episodes of subacute obstruction. Once again, pursue conservative management wherever possible as surgery is technically difficult, demanding the utmost patience and skill. The bowel is often oedematous and friable, and there is a significant risk of perforation while attempting to free the matted bowel loops. Plication of the small-bowel in a step ladder fashion has been described with some success in recurrent small-bowel obstruction (Fig. 4.6).

9. Pseudo-obstruction (*Ogilvie's syndrome*) presents with episodes of large-bowel obstruction in the absence of a mechanical cause. The cause is not known, although various theories have been proposed. In 1948, Sir Heneage Ogilvie first postulated an imbalance between the sympathetic and parasympathetic nervous systems, and more recent authors have suggested excessive sympathetic tone, decreased parasympathetic tone or a combination of the two. The use of epidural and spinal anaesthesia to relieve pseudo-obstruction supports this theory, as does the beneficial therapeutic effect of guanethidine and neostigmine. Pseudo-obstruction may develop in a wide variety of clinical settings, including:
   - Intra-abdominal surgery, including urological and gynaecological surgery
   - Spinal surgery, spinal cord injury and retroperitoneal trauma
   - Sepsis and viral infections such as herpes or varicella zoster
   - The elderly patient
   - Neurological disorders, hypothyroidism, electrolyte imbalances such as hypokalaemia, hypocalcaemia, and hypomagnesaemia, cardiac disorders (myocardial infarction, cardiac surgery) and respiratory disorders (pneumonia), renal insufficiency

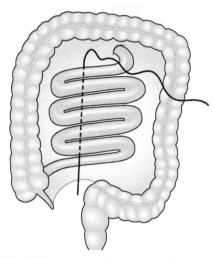

Fig. 4.6 Childs-Phillips method of plication of bowel to prevent recurrent adhesions.

■ Medications such as narcotics, tricyclic antidepressants, phenothiazines, antiparkinsonian drugs, and anaesthetic agents.

The clinical presentation may be acute or chronic. Acute colonic pseudo-obstruction has an underlying cause in 95% of patients:[36] it typically presents with acute, painless and massive distension of the abdomen. Abdominal tenderness may indicate bowel ischaemia or perforation. Plain X-ray of the abdomen will demonstrate dilated colon and CT scan of the abdomen with contrast or gastrograffin enema confirms the diagnosis.

Initially, try conservative treatment with nasogastric decompression, correction of fluid and electrolyte imbalance and aggressive treatment of any sepsis. Neostigmine has been used successfully in pseudo-obstruction, although it can induce cardiac arrhythmia and haemodynamic instability and should be used with caution. Colonoscopic decompression is also effective in the short term, although recurrent distension is common. Resort to surgical intervention only in patients with signs of peritonism, bowel ischaemia or toxic megacolon. Laparotomy in a patient with uncomplicated pseudo-obstruction will not cure the problem, and the patient is at risk of abdominal compartment syndrome and wound dehiscence.

10 Intestinal obstruction following laparotomy may result from temporary oedema of a recently fashioned stoma, a localized collection of fluid, blood or pus, a segment of bowel rendered ischaemic at the operation, an anastomotic leak, wound dehiscence or paralytic ileus. Be prepared to repeat investigations and invite a second opinion from a colleague or senior.

Investigations

1 Blood tests should include a haemoglobin, white cell count, renal function, electrolytes, and liver function tests. Tumour markers (carcino-embryonic antigen and CA 19-9) may be helpful if you suspect colonic cancer. A rising lactate level may indicate strangulated bowel or perforation.

2 Abdominal X-ray and an erect chest X-ray are helpful in determining the presence of bowel obstruction and perforation, respectively.

3 A CT scan usually shows the level and cause of obstruction. In a left-sided large-bowel obstruction, a gastrografin study shows the obstructing lesion and may temporarily relieve the obstruction. You may then undertake colonoscopy and biopsy of the lesion if the patient remains stable with no signs of peritonism or impending perforation.

Prepare

1 In a patient with a distended abdomen that is non-tender and soft, have a nasogastric tube inserted to decompress the bowel. Stop feeding and keep the patient on intravenous fluids and potassium supplements. Introduce a urinary catheter to assess urine output and closely monitor the fluid balance. If there is no improvement in 48 to 72 hours or if there are signs of deterioration (increasing pain, tenderness or peritonism), favour laparotomy. If the condition improves, with decreasing pain and distension, decreasing NG aspirate or passage of faeces and/or flatus, spigot the nasogastric tube, start the patient on a liquid diet and monitor for symptoms or signs of recurrent obstruction.

2 Re-examine the patient after relieving the distension to exclude a mass that was obscured by the tensely distended abdomen.

3 Suspect strangulated bowel in a patient with a tender abdomen, raised inflammatory markers and lactate levels. Be prepared to perform early operative intervention. Carry out urgent laparotomy for closed loop obstruction resulting from an obstruction at two sites (usually a tumour in the distal colon with a competent ileocaecal valve).

4 If the nasogastric aspirate is faeculant or stagnant small-bowel contents, commence broad-spectrum antibiotic cover as these patients are at risk of developing pneumonia.

Access

1 Access the abdomen through a midline incision. If there is an old scar of a previous laparotomy, make the incision through this scar if it is convenient, extending the incision to a non-scarred area where there is less chance of adherent abdominal viscera.

Assess

1 On entry into the peritoneal cavity, note any free fluid and collect some for bacteriology and, if indicated, for cytology.

2 Introduce a hand into the abdominal cavity, taking care not to injure the distended bowel. Examine the caecum. If it is collapsed the obstruction lies proximally in the small-bowel.

3 Deliver the distended bowel through the wound, ensuring that it is supported at all times by an assistant to avoid traction on the mesentery.

4 Trace the bowel distally to the level of obstruction, dividing any significant bands you encounter.

5 If the vascular supply to the bowel is compromised by a band adhesion, strangulation of a hernia, a volvulus or a closed loop, venous outflow is first impeded while higher pressure arterial inflow continues. Capillaries and venules dilate with stagnating blood losing its oxygen. Eventually small vessels rupture, allowing extravasation visible in the visceral sub-peritoneum. The appearance resembles a bruise. Like a bruise it will take days to be absorbed. As the swelling increases, arterial inflow is halted. The bowel layer with the highest metabolic demand is the mucosa.

This becomes porous to fluid and bacteria which rapidly multiply when bowel content stagnates. The submucous, muscular and peritoneal coats survive while the mucosa undergoes necrosis. This is most critical at the constriction rings created by the neck of a hernia – the point at which the vascular restriction and eventual occlusion occurs. Palpable arterial pulsation in the mesentery up to the bowel and a shiny appearance of the visceral peritoneum are reassuring signs.

> ### ▶ KEY POINT
>
> ■ The crucial sites to examine are constriction rings which remain white.

Action

1. If the obstruction is due to a band adhesion, divide it. Carefully assess the viability of the involved small-bowel, indicated by a return of the normal pink colour. If the bowel is bruised (vide supra) it may still be viable. Wrap a swab soaked in warm saline around the bowel and administer 100% oxygen for 10 minutes, then reassess viability. When in doubt resect the segment and perform an anastomosis rather than risk leaving ischaemic bowel. If there is extensive bowel involvement, or the patient's condition precludes resection so that bowel of doubtful viability is left behind, be willing to carry out re-exploration at 24–48 hours to reassess the segment in doubt.

2. If you encounter generalized adhesions, carefully begin to divide them by sharp dissection with scissors, taking care not to damage the bowel loops. Any serosal tears should be repaired immediately with interrupted absorbable sutures (2/0 Vicryl or 3/0 PDS). Continue gentle dissection until the site of obstruction is reached and filling of the collapsed distal bowel is observed: patient dissection will usually lead you into the true peritoneal cavity, rendering further dissection easier. You may encounter very dense adhesions, particularly in the pelvis following previous peritonitis, anastomotic leakage or radiotherapy. In these circumstances it may be better to bypass an obstructed loop lying deep in the pelvis rather than attempt a difficult and potentially hazardous dissection. Occasionally you will encounter a 'hostile' abdomen where the peritoneal cavity is completely obliterated by dense, fibrotic adhesions, for example following multiple laparotomies, sclerosing peritonitis or radiotherapy (vide supra). Dense, generalized adhesions rarely result in closed loop obstruction and prolonged attempts at dissection are likely to result in a fistula. Attempt a trial dissection of the most accessible bowel loop: if you have made no progress within 20 minutes it is safer to close the abdomen and treat the obstruction conservatively with nasogastric aspiration and parenteral feeding.

3. If the obstruction is due to a missed external hernia, reduce the bowel, confirm its viability and repair the hernial defect. A knuckle of bowel from an internal or external hernia may reduce spontaneously during the laparotomy. If on examining the bowel, there is a constriction ring suggesting this, search for the offending hernia and repair it.

4. Resect a frankly ischaemic segment of bowel or a tumour and undertake anastomosis if the margins are viable and healthy.

5. Bypass an obstructing lesion that cannot be resected. Construct a gastrojejunostomy to relieve pyloric or duodenal obstruction and an entero-enteric anastomosis to bypass a fixed and unresectable small-bowel tumour. Take a biopsy when possible.

6. Treat roundworm bolus conservatively with anti-helminthics. Some authors advocate a hypertonic saline small-bowel enema to purge the worms into the large-bowel: do so cautiously to avoid causing hypovolaemia or bowel perforation. Operate on patients with rectal bleeding (rectorrhagia; G –rhegnynai = to burst) or toxicity and in those who are unresponsive to medical treatment. Massage the bolus of worms towards the colon to relieve the obstruction. You may need to perform an enterotomy to deliver the bolus when there is a volvulus of the bowel, since attempts to milk the worms distally in this situation may cause bowel perforation. Similarly, other intraluminal causes of obstruction such as food bolus, phytobezoar (Greek: phytos = plant) or gallstone will often require an enterotomy to remove the obstructing lesion.

7. When intussusception is the cause of obstruction, reduce it if possible by milking the apex proximally between the thumb and index fingers. If this is not possible or the bowel is not viable, resect the intussuscepted segment. Always look for an underlying cause, such as a polyp or tumour, and remove it.

8. Resect lesions in the right or transverse colon, constructing an end-to-end anastomosis if the patient's condition and the status of the bowel permit. If left-sided obstruction is diagnosed early, perform a primary resection, on-table lavage[37] and primary anastomosis with or without a covering ileostomy. If the obstruction is well-established and the proximal bowel grossly distended and poorly perfused perform a Hartmann's resection, bringing out the proximal end as a stoma. Close the distal end and leave it in the abdomen. If the tumour is not resectable, create a defunctioning stoma proximal to the obstruction. When gaining consent from a patient to operate for bowel obstruction, always discuss the possibility of stoma formation.

9. To perform on-table lavage, pass a large Foley catheter through the appendix or directly into the caecum (Fig. 4.7). Secure it with a purse-string suture. Distally, tie a length of corrugated anaesthetic tubing into the bowel at the site of proximal resection and connect it to a large plastic bag, forming a closed effluent system. Install normal saline solution via the Foley catheter, milking the bowel contents distally until there are no remaining palpable faecal masses and the effluent is clean. Take down the lavage system and perform a sutured end-to-end anastomosis.

10. Management of bowel obstruction in neonates is described in later chapters.

Closure

1. Inform the anaesthetist before attempting to close the abdomen, since adequate relaxation of the abdominal musculature is essential to achieve a sound repair.

2. While dealing with the obstruction you should have achieved decompression of the bowel. If distension remains it is still possible to decompress the bowel by milking the contents proximally into the stomach. Use a nasogastric tube to aspirate the stomach contents.

3. Consider inserting tension sutures, particularly in obese patients.

Aftercare

1. Closely monitor the fluid, electrolyte and acid–base balance.

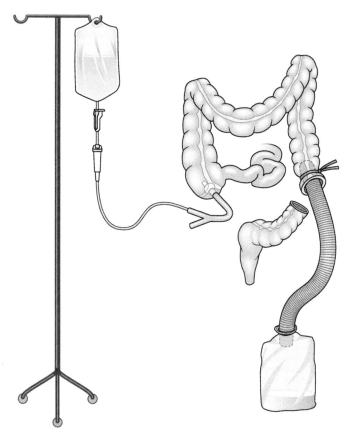

Fig. 4.7   On-table lavage.

2   Leave a nasogastric tube in-situ, aspirating at 4-hourly intervals. Remove it as soon as the aspirate diminishes: there is no evidence that leaving an NG tube for a longer time improves outcomes.[38] Encourage early feeding as soon as it is tolerated. Re-insert the nasogastric tube if the patient vomits or abdominal distension recurs.

3   Consider giving parenteral (Latin: para = beside + enteron = intestine) nutrition to patients whose dietary intake has been poor for more than a week and in those in whom functional recovery of the intestines may be prolonged.

LAPAROTOMY FOR GASTROINTESTINAL BLEEDING

Assess

1   Assess patients with gastrointestinal bleeding according to ALS protocols, applying a systematic approach to airway, breathing and haemodynamic stabilization. If the patient is bleeding profusely resuscitate aggressively, initially with crystalloid fluids, but give blood transfusion in patients who have lost more than 30% of their circulating volume.[39] If the patient remains haemodynamically unstable order an urgent CT angiogram and embolization of the bleeding vessel.

2   Patients with gastrointestinal (GI) bleeding rarely need surgery, and most settle down with conservative measures. Classify them into upper or lower intestinal bleeding; further classify those with upper gastrointestinal bleeding into variceal and non-variceal bleeding. The role of surgery for variceal bleeding has diminished with the advent of potent medications such as somatostatin and the use of transjugular intrahepatic portal systemic shunt (TIPS). Variceal bleeding is not considered further in this chapter.

NON-VARICEAL UPPER GASTROINTESTINAL BLEEDING

1   Common causes include peptic ulceration, gastritis and lower oesophageal (Mallory-Weiss) tear. If these patients with peptic ulcer bleed remain unstable despite resuscitation they need urgent intervention. Coffee ground vomiting suggests a slowly bleeding lesion, whereas fresh blood suggests a peptic ulcer that is bleeding at a rapid rate.

Action

1   If the patient is unstable despite resuscitation or requires transfusions to maintain a normal blood pressure, undertake an urgent endoscopy in the operating theatre. If you can identify the bleeding point and have the appropriate expertise, use injection of adrenaline, diathermy or clips to control it. If a bleeding peptic ulcer is unresponsive to endoscopic measures, proceed to emergency laparotomy (see Fig. 4.8 for guidelines in the management of patients with upper GI bleeding).

2   For a duodenal ulcer, open the pylorus and proximal part of the first part of the duodenum with a longitudinal incision along the outer border of the duodenum. Identify the bleeding point, control it with a finger or a swab on a sponge holder and aspirate the remaining blood from the surgical field. At this stage confirm control of the bleeding source by stabilization of the patient's condition following continued resuscitation. Under-run the bleeding ulcer using a 2/0 Prolene, Vicryl or PDS suture. Confirm that the bleeding has stopped. Close the pylorus and duodenum transversely as a pyloroplasty using interrupted 3/0 Vicryl or PDS sutures.

3   Gastric ulcers rarely bleed. It is more common for gastric erosions to bleed and these almost always stop with conservative treatment. If a bleeding ulcer does not respond to radiological or endoscopic measures, open the stomach along the greater curvature, identify the bleeding point and under-run it as for a duodenal ulcer. Close the gastrotomy with 2/0 Vicryl or PDS. If you suspect malignancy perform a sleeve resection of the ulcer-bearing area and close the defect as for a gastrotomy. Erosive bleeding which fails to respond to conservative measures requires gastrectomy (partial or total as the situation demands).

4   Continue pantoprazole or omeprazole intravenously for the first 48–72 hours. Commence eradication treatment for *H-pylori*.

LOWER GASTROINTESTINAL BLEEDING

Action

1   Bleeding per rectum causing haemodynamic instability may be due to upper GI or lower GI pathology, therefore carry out an urgent upper gastrointestinal endoscopy to exclude a bleeding peptic ulcer. Bleeding from the lower bowel may be altered or fresh and is usually due to diverticular disease (see Table 4.2 for common causes of lower GI bleeding). Perform digital rectal

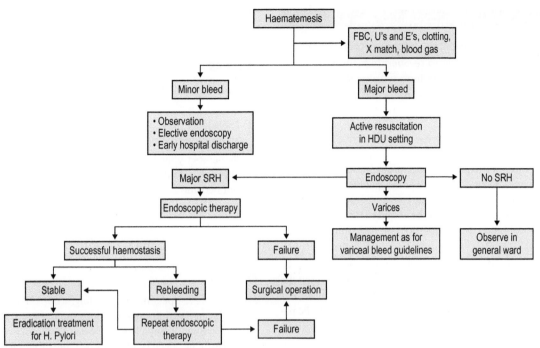

Fig. 4.8   Algorithm showing management pathway for upper GI bleed (Adapted from British Society of Gastroenterology Guidelines[39]). SRH - stigmata of recent haemorrhage.

TABLE 4.2 Major causes of colonic bleeding
Diverticular disease
Vascular malformations (angiodysplasia)
Ischaemic colitis
Haemorrrhoids
Inflammatory bowel disease (e.g. ulcerative proctitis, Crohn's disease)
Neoplasia (carcinoma or polyps)
Radiation enteropathy

examination, proctoscopy and sigmoidoscopy to seek causes such as haemorrhoids, polyps, diverticulosis or cancer. Resuscitate the patient with fluids and blood products and correct coagulopathy. In 80% of patients with lower GI bleeding the haemorrhage stops spontaneously and you need only to transfuse blood if necessary and closely monitor the patient.

2 Urgent colonoscopy in acute bleeding is technically difficult, as altered blood in the bowel lumen absorbs light, resulting in poor visualization, and has not been shown to confer any survival benefit.[40] For this reason most endoscopists decline to perform a colonoscopy in an acutely bleeding patient. In a haemodynamically stable patient, a nuclear scan (^{99m}Tc sulphur colloid or ^{99m}Tc labelled RBC scan) is useful when the bleeding rate is as slow as 0.05–0.1 ml per minute, but the test lacks specificity.

3 If the patient is unstable order a CT angiogram. If this demonstrates a bleeding point, proceed to conventional angiography and embolization of the bleeding vessel. The bleeding rate must be at least 1–1.5 ml per minute to be detected on angiography. The procedure may need to be repeated if the patient re-bleeds.

4 If the bleeding site is not identified, you may be left with no alternative to laparotomy. Be willing to carry out on-table enteroscopy; if this is unavailable, create a transverse colostomy and perform on-table irrigation of the colon to determine whether the bleeding is right or left-sided. Proceed to segmental resection of the appropriate hemicolon. Lower gastrointestinal bleeding is further discussed in Chapter 13.

LAPAROTOMY FOR EARLY POSTOPERATIVE COMPLICATIONS

1 If the postoperative course is not as expected, look for general as well as abdominal causes. Inspect the wound, looking for redness and swelling and gently palpate for tenderness. If in doubt, insert a needle and syringe through the scar and aspirate for haematoma, seroma or pus.

▶ KEY POINTS Develop and utilize basic clinical skills

- If you are uncertain, repeat the complete examination after an interval; it is remarkable how rapidly the physical findings can change.
- You are most likely to make an accurate assessment if you have acquired experience by always carrying out regular postoperative examinations in your patients, as you will then learn what is within normal limits and what is suspicious.

2 Ultrasound scans, CT and endoscopy may be valuable in localizing or excluding pathology. However, whenever clinical findings and investigations are in opposition, trust your clinical judgement.

▶ KEY POINTS Early operation is often wise

- Do not hope for the best. If you suspect a catastrophe do not put off the decision to re-operate by ordering unnecessary investigations. Patients with sepsis or ischaemic bowel can deteriorate very rapidly.
- In these cases remember the aphorism, 'It is better to look and see than wait and see'.

3 Not all complications require immediate operation. Manage conservatively an entero-cutaneous fistula in a patient who is otherwise well. This allows time for the cause to be investigated and the nutritional status of the patient to be corrected. Provided the fistula output continues to reduce do not rush into operative management.

4 Do not be too proud to call in someone more experienced to assist at re-exploration. You may feel that since you performed the first operation it is your responsibility to correct whatever has gone wrong. Your primary responsibility is to ensure that the patient has the best chance of recovery.

5 The most frequent complication requiring early re-operation is haemorrhage which may be continuing, primary bleeding or reactionary haemorrhage, which occurs when the patient's blood pressure rises and dislodges an occluding clot, or a cut artery comes out of spasm. Secondary haemorrhage usually occurs after 7–10 days and is due to clot digestion by proteolytic enzymes from infecting micro-organisms. Early detection of continuing primary or reactionary haemorrhage may be difficult as the vital signs vary during the immediate postoperative period for a variety of reasons including pain, analgesia and vascular dilatation as the patient is warmed.

▶ KEY POINT

- Do not rely upon intra-abdominal or intra-luminal drains to detect bleeding.

Prepare

1 It is very rare that you cannot spend even a few minutes improving the patient's general condition before embarking on a second operation.

2 Start broad-spectrum antibiotics and ensure that blood is cross-matched.

3 Pass a nasogastric tube so that the stomach can be emptied.

4 Warn the theatre staff of the likely findings, procedure and equipment required.

Access

1 Have the dressings and skin sutures removed. Alternatively, wear two pairs of sterile gloves and discard the outer pair after removing the skin sutures yourself.

2 After cleansing the skin, gently separate the wound edges and remove the deep sutures.

3 Open up the peritoneal cavity with care, using a fingertip to break through the healing peritoneum.

Assess

1 Note any gas, blood or other fluid, and take a specimen for microscopy and culture.

2 Expose the site of the previous operation and look for bleeding, anastomotic dehiscence, infection or ischaemia.

3 Remember your objective and aim is to carry out the simplest effective procedure(s) that will allow the patient to recover. Do not become side-tracked by other issues.

4 If the patient does not recover satisfactorily, will you wish that you had chosen another procedure? If so, why are you not planning to carry out that procedure now?

Action

1 If you are re-operating for bleeding, scoop out any blood clot and wash out the abdomen with large quantities of warmed normal saline. Identify any bleeding vessels and under-run them using a 2/0 Prolene, Vicryl or PDS suture. If the bleeding is from a splenic injury (for example following gastrectomy or left hemicolectomy) it may be possible to control it using 2/0 PDS sutures buttressed with omentum, or by wrapping the organ in an absorbable polyglycolic mesh bag. If in doubt perform a splenectomy.

2 If you encounter generalized peritonitis, perform copious lavage with warmed normal saline, seek the source of the infection and control it. Repair gastro-duodenal perforations using an omental patch; exteriorize or defunction injured small or large-bowel. If you find a localized abscess and this is compatible with the clinical picture, drain the sepsis and avoid further exploration, which may spread the infection more widely. Be careful not to disturb anastomoses that appear to be healing satisfactorily.

3 Anastomotic leaks may result from tension, inadequate blood supply, poor technique, impaired healing or distal obstruction, or a combination of these factors. It is sometimes possible to repair a limited leak, but more usually it is necessary to refashion the anastomosis after resecting devitalized tissue and carrying out further mobilization to avoid tension. When refashioning a gastrointestinal anastomosis ensure that there is no distal obstruction (e.g. from adhesions).

4 If extensive contamination has occurred, the most careful re-anastomosis will fail and you will probably do more harm than good. Small leaks are best accepted but must be adequately drained and defunctioned. If you cannot exteriorize, resect or bypass the leak, reduce the inflow by proximal aspiration or a stoma, insert a sump drain near the defect and commence gentle continuous suction. If possible, institute distal enteral feeding through a feeding jejunostomy (Fig. 4.9). A bypass procedure may help to protect a re-anastomosis, for example gastrojejunostomy following repair of a duodenal leak.

5 Repair a leaking ureteric anastomosis over a double-J stent. Treat a leaking biliary anastomosis by inserting a T-tube.

6 Evacuate any residual blood, pus or other intra-abdominal fluid and provide adequate drainage to the operation site.

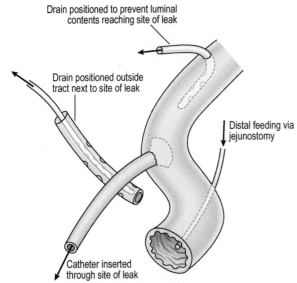

Drain positioned to prevent luminal contents reaching site of leak

Drain positioned outside tract next to site of leak

Distal feeding via jejunostomy

Catheter inserted through site of leak

Fig. 4.9 Draining a leak which cannot be closed. (Adapted with permission from Hospital Update).

Checklist

1 Have you dealt adequately with the complication?

2 Check the area of the operation thoroughly to ensure that all is well.

3 Replace the viscera in their anatomical position.

Closure

1 Use the simplest and most effective means of closing the abdomen. Like burst abdomens, re-opened wounds seldom break down completely, though superficial dehiscence may complicate infection.

2 Record the details in the operation note immediately after the operation.

REFERENCES

1. Memon MA, Fitzgibbons Jr RJ. The role of minimal access surgery in the acute abdomen. Surg Clin North Am 1997;77:1333–53.
2. Cuscheiri A. Single-incision laparoscopic surgery. J Minim Access Surg 2011;7(1):3–5.
3. Flora ED, Wilson TG, Martin IJ, et al. A review of natural orifice transluminal endoscopic surgery (NOTES) for intra-abdominal surgery: experimental models, techniques, and applicability to the clinical setting. Ann Surg 2008;247(4):583–602.
4. Haynes AB, Weiser TG, Berry WR, et al., for the Safe Surgery Saves Lives Study Group. A surgical safety checklist to reduce morbidity and mortality in a global population. N Engl J Med 2009;360:491–9.
5. Alexander JW, Solomkin JS, Edwards MJ. Recommendations for control of surgical site infections. Ann Surg 2011;253(6):1082–93.
6. Brown SR, Tiernan J. Transverse versus midline incisions for abdominal surgery. Cochrane Database Syst Rev 2011;(6).
7. O'Neill S, Abdelaziz EA, Andrabi SI. Modified Lanz incision – the surgical trainee's best friend. Int J Surg 2010;8:56–7.
8. Stanice D, Menzies D. The magnitude of adhesion-related problems. Colorectal Dis 2007;9(s):35–8.
9. Liakakos T, Thomakos N, Fine PM, et al. Peritoneal adhesions: aetiology, pathophysiology and clinical significance. Recent advances in prevention and management. Dig Surg 2001;18(4):260–73.
10. Ellis H, Moras BJ, Thompson JN, et al. Adhesion-related hospital re-admission after abdominal and pelvic surgery: a retrospective cohort study. Lancet 1999;353(9163):1476–80.
11. Jeekel H. Cost implications of adhesions highlighted in European study. Eur J Surg 1997;579(s):43–5.
12. Atkin G, Chopada A, Mitchell I. Colorectal cancer metastasis: in the surgeon's hands? Int Semin Surg Oncol 2005;2:5.
13. Pai D, Sharma A, Kanungo R, et al. Role of abdominal drains in perforated duodenal ulcer patients: a prospective controlled Study. ANZ J Surg 1999;69(3):210–3.
14. Rahbari NN, Knebel P, Diener MK, et al. Current practice of abdominal wall closure in elective surgery - is there any consensus? BMC Surg 2009;9:8.
15. AdilCeydeli A, Rucinski J, Wise L. Finding the best abdominal closure: an evidence-based review of the literature. Curr Surg 2005;62(2):220–5.
16. Millbourn D, Yucel Cengiz Y, Israelsson LA. Effect of stitch length on wound complications after closure of midline incisions. A randomized controlled trial. Arch Surg 2009;144(11):1056–9.
17. Paral J, Ferko A, Varga J, et al. Comparison of sutured versus non-sutured subcutaneous fat tissue in abdominal surgery. A prospective randomized study. Eur Surg Res 2007;39:350–8.
18. Dunn RM, Pickett LC, Rivadeneira DE. Challenges in complex ventral hernia repair: examining the role of specialized techniques and mesh materials. A supplement to American College of Surgeons Surgical News. Elsevier; 2009.
19. Bellows CF, Alder A, Helton WS. Abdominal wall reconstruction using biological tissue grafts: present status and future opportunities. Expert Rev Med Devices 2006;3(5):657–75.
20. Hensbroek PBV, Wind J, Dijkgraaf MGW, et al. Temporary closure of the open abdomen: a systematic review on delayed primary fascial closure in patients with an open abdomen. World J Surg 2009;33:199–207.
21. Navsaria PH, Bunting M, Omoshoro-Jones MJ, et al. Temporary closure of open abdominal wounds by the modified sandwich–vacuum pack technique. Br J Surg 2003;90:718–22.
22. Myers JA, Latenser BA. Non-operative progressive Bogota bag closure after abdominal decompression. American Surgery 2002;68:1029–30.
23. Harper JR, McQuillan DJ. A novel regenerative tissue matrix technology for connective tissue reconstruction. Wounds 2007;19(6):163–8.
24. Reimer MW, Yelle J, Reitsma B, et al. Management of open wounds with a dynamic fascial closure system. Can J Surg 2008;51(3):209–14.
25. Miller PR, Meredith JW, Johnson JC, Chang MC. Prospective evaluation of vacuum-assisted fascial closure after open abdomen. Ann Surg 2004;239(5):608–16.
26. Kaplan M, Banwell P, Orgill DP, et al. Guidelines for the management of the open abdomen. Supplement to wounds: a compendium of clinical research and practice, October 2005.
27. Prevention and treatment of surgical site infection. NICE, October 2008.
28. Schein M, Whittmann DH, Aprahamian CC, et al. The abdominal compartment syndrome: the physiological and clinical consequences of elevated intra-abdominal pressure. J Am Coll Surg 1995;185:745–53.
29. Carlson MA. Acute wound failure. Surg Clin North Am 1997;77:607–36.
30. Sorensen LT, Hemingsen U, Kallehave F, et al. Risk factors for tissue and wound complications in gastrointestinal surgery. Ann Surg 2005;241:654–8.
31. Spiliotis J, Tsiveriotis K, Datsis AD, et al. Wound dehiscence: is still a problem in the 21st century: a retrospective study. World J Emerg Surg 2009;4:12–6.
32. Ramirez OM, Ruas E, Dellon AL. Component separation method for closure of abdominal wall defects: an anatomic and clinical study. Plast Reconst Surg 1990;86:519–23.
33. Christou NV, Barie PS, Dellinger EP, et al. Surgical Infection Society intra-abdominal infection study. Prospective evaluation of management techniques and outcome. Arch Surg 1993;128(2):193–8; discussion 198–9.

34. Anderson ID, Fearon KC, Grant IS. Laparotomy for abdominal sepsis in the critically ill. Br J Surg 1996;83(4):535–9.

35. Pusajo JF, Bumaschny E, Doglio GR, et al. Postoperative intra-abdominal sepsis requiring reoperation. Value of a predictive index. Arch Surg 1993;128(2):218–22; discussion 223.

36. Vanek VW, Al-Salti M. Acute pseudo-obstruction of the colon (Ogilvie's syndrome). An analysis of 400 cases. Dis Colon Rectum 1986;29:203.

37. Gramegna A, Saccomani G. On-table colonic irrigation in the treatment of left-sided large-bowel emergencies. Dis Colon Rectum 1989;32(7):585–7.

38. Cheatham ML, Chapman WC, Key SP, Sawyers JL. A meta-analysis of selective versus routine nasogastric decompression after elective laparotomy. Ann Surg 1995;221(5):469–78.

39. British Society of Gastroenterology Endoscopic committee. Non-variceal upper gastrointestinal haemorrhage: guidelines. Gut 2002;51 (Suppl. IV):iv1–6.

40. Green BT, Rockey DC, Portwood G, et al. Urgent colonoscopy for evaluation and management of acute lower gastrointestinal hemorrhage: a randomized controlled trial. Am J Gastroenterol 2005;100(11):2395–402.

Principles of minimal access surgery

P.S. Veitch, A.O. Mahendran

GENERAL PRINCIPLES OF LAPAROSCOPY

1 The aim of minimal access surgery is to cause the least anatomical, physiological and psychological trauma to the patient.

2 Patient expectations have moved with the new technology, leading to profound changes in patient selection, consent and management.

3 This chapter outlines the basic principles of laparoscopy. Almost all general surgical procedures can be performed with minimal access techniques. This includes surgeries involving the chest and pelvis. We shall describe them in detail under appropriate chapter headings (Table 5.1).

4 Minimal access surgery has implications for hospital budgets. Capital equipment is expensive and requires updating at intervals. Consumables are particularly expensive and re-usage of disposable equipment is inadvisable. Theatre times are increased initially, although they decrease as surgeons gain experience. Short-stay and 5-day wards with rapid turnover reduce 'hotel' costs, free up main ward beds and help to reduce waiting lists.

5 The success of MAS is largely founded on the team based approached. Complicated procedures are performed with complex equipment that requires constant maintenance and upkeep. In addition, during a surgery, multiple intraoperative adjustments of the equipment (camera, monitors) are required which demand a skilled and collaborative theatre team that work in a coordinated fashion to ensure patient safety and excellent outcomes. Discuss Box 5.1 with PSV.

6 Increasing familiarity with the laparoscopic approach has led to its use in many situations previously contraindicated. Table 5.2 indicates common absolute and relative contraindications for laparoscopy.

Preparation

1 **Admission:** Ideally plan admission for the day of surgery following appropriate investigation and work up. Evaluate patients to see if they can be managed on a day-case basis.

2 **Consent:** Obtain informed consent, including permission to convert to open surgery if necessary and quote a percentage probability. Warn patients about postoperative shoulder-tip pain and surgical emphysema. Always explain the commonly occurring

risks, how they present and how they are managed. Explain the benefits of laparoscopic surgery, which include; small scars, quicker recovery and a reduction in post-operative pain.

3 **Prophylaxis:** Evaluate the thromboembolism risk and arrange prophylaxis accordingly (typically low-dose heparin and compression stockings). Prescribe prophylactic antibiotics if appropriate (e.g. biliary and bowel surgery). Bowel preparation is unnecessary except for some colorectal procedures.

4 **Analgesia:** Evaluate the likely postoperative analgesia requirements. Most anaesthetists avoid premedication in patients admitted on the day of surgery. Patients undergoing major laparoscopic procedures may still need opiates, albeit in reduced dosage. Their requirements may be further reduced by the use of intraperitoneal local anaesthesia or abdominal wall nerve blocks. Patient-controlled analgesia (PCA) is appropriate following major procedures; however, for lesser procedures simple analgesics such as intravenous paracetamol, oral non-steroidal anti-inflammatory drugs and weak analgesics are usually effective.

5 **Equipment:** Make sure every member of the surgical team is fully familiar with the basic equipment for laparoscopy.

> ► KEY POINT Basic equipment for laparoscopy
>
> You must be familiar with **all** of the following equipment *without exception*:
>
> Monitor
> Light source
> Insufflator
> Camera
> Diathermy/irrigation

Basic laparoscopic equipment (excluding instruments)

1 **Laparoscopic theatre:** Modern laparoscopic suites incorporate core equipment (monitor, insufflators, screens) within a mobile, ceiling-mounted console that can be maneouvred quickly to ensure rapid equipment adjustment throughout a procedure, ease of movement of the theatre staff, improved ergonomics and an efficient operating room.

2 **Monitor:** In the absence of an integrated theatre use a large monitor with high resolution screens. This can be mounted on mobile trolleys with a light source, insufflator and camera (Fig. 5.1).

3 **Light source:** Illumination of the image is dependent on the light cable and light source. Damage to the optical fibres in the cable will dull the light. Xenon or halogen bulbs are used to create high

TABLE 5.1 Examples of minimal access operations

Basic	Advanced
Diagnostic laparoscopy	Nissen fundoplication
Cholecystectomy	Repair of perforated duodenal ulcer
Appendicecomy	Heller's serocardiomyotomy
Hernia repair	Gastrectomy
Adhesiolysis	Hepatectomy
Arthroscopy	Adrenalectomy
	Splenectomy
	Nephrectomy
	Oophorectomy
	Hysterectomy
	Prostatectomy

Box 5.1 Advantages and disadvantages of minimal access surgery

Advantages

Smaller incisions with less postoperative pain and disability

Improved cosmesis

Decreased wound-related pathology, such as wound infection and hernia

Decreased tissue trauma

Decreased physiological insult

Earlier return to full activity

Significantly reduced hospital stay, improving cost-effectiveness

Improved visualization of the operative field for the whole surgical team including trainees and students

Decreased contact with pathogens such as human immunodeficiency virus (HIV) and hepatitis B virus (HBV) for the surgical team

Use of video records aids communication with patients and their families.

Disadvantages

Loss of tactile feedback from tissues and instruments

Potential difficulty in controlling major bleeding which may be associated with a rapidly deteriorating visual field

Longer procedure times, especially on the initial slope of the surgical learning curve

Requirement for specialist instrumentation and an appropriate surgical skill set

Greater potential for iatrogenic damage either through surgical disorientation (e.g. bile duct injury) or unrecognized visceral injury (e.g. missed bowel perforation)

intensity light, however they also generate high heat which can injure the patient and surgeon through direct contact with the source or the tip of the light cable. Light is absorbed by blood, therefore in a situation of bleeding, the image can become dark quickly.

TABLE 5.2 Contraindications to laparoscopic surgery

Absolute contraindications	Relative contraindications
Generalized peritonitis	Gross obesity. Simple overweight is no contraindication; such patients suffer less from postoperative respiratory complications than they would following open operation
Intestinal obstruction	Pregnancy
Major clotting abnormalities	Multiple abdominal adhesions. Provided the first instrument port is inserted by an open technique, laparoscopy can be safely performed on patients with moderate adhesions following, for example, previous surgery
Liver cirrhosis/portal hypertension	Organomegaly (enlarged liver or spleen)
Failure to tolerate general anaesthesia	Abdominal aortic aneurysm
Uncontrolled shock	
Patient refusal	

4 **Insufflator:** This delivers carbon dioxide from a high pressure cylinder at a high flow rate but a low accurately controlled pressure, to create the pneumoperitoneum. Ensure that it is positioned within your view so that you can monitor the pressures and flows. Familiarity in changing the gas cylinder is important as cylinders may empty at a critical point in surgery, with loss of pneumoperitoneum as a result.

5 **Camera:** The video camera head, either a single chip or a superior three-chip instrument, is attached to the laparoscope to form an electrical–optic interface. The camera is connected by cable to a video processor, which interprets and modifies the signal and transmits it to the monitors. Most systems incorporate a 'white balance' function, which can be calibrated to represent colours accurately. Some newer camera systems dispense with the laparoscope by placing the microchip on the end of a 10-mm rod (chip-on-a-stick).

6 **Laparoscope:** The standard laparoscope measures 24 cm in length and contains a series of quartz optical rods and focusing lenses that conduct the image to the eyepiece. The telescope can have a flat end with a straight on view (0 degree) or can be angled with an oblique view (30 or 45 degree). The 30 degree scope can provide a much greater fieldview compared to the 0 degree scope. The telescopes can vary in diameter from a 5 mm to a 10 mm (the latter providing the brighter image and more visual acuity). The 10 mm 30 degree telescope is used for most procedures.

▶ **KEY POINTS Instrument & Team Check**

■ Meticulously check every piece of equipment (monitor, light source, insufflator, camera, diathermy and suction/irrigation) prior to each and every surgery.

■ Malfunction of any piece of equipment midway through a surgery endangers a patient. For example; failure of suction/irrigation while trying to achieve haemostasis.

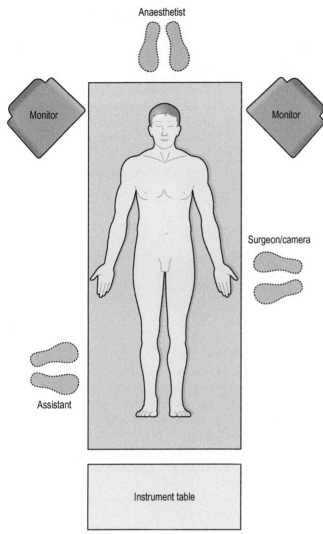

Fig. 5.1 Diagram showing the positioning of the patient, surgeon, assistant and video monitors for a laparoscopic cholecystectomy.

■ Ensure that the camera operator is aware of camera etiquette – obeys clear instructions, keeps the area of interest in the centre of the field of view, maintains stability and orientation and is aware of additional functionality, such as angled scopes as well as zoom, white balance, picture and video buttons.

7 **Suction/irrigation** is performed usually through a disposable or reusable 5-mm instrument. The hand piece is connected to a pressurized reservoir of warm saline as well as the suction. Both are controllable by buttons on the hand piece. The disposable instruments tend to be more ergonomic and often come with a mechanical irrigation feed.

8 **Ports** provide passages through which to insert instruments, which can be disposable or reusable. The more expensive disposable ports have the advantage of being more ergonomic (Greek: ergon = work + nemein = to manageable: easy to use) as well as being radiolucent and sterile. They may have blunt ends for open induction of pneumoperitoneum or be fitted with a sharp, spring-loaded trocar with a plastic guard that projects beyond the point as soon as

the trocar enters the peritoneal cavity. Some of the blunt ended ports are designed so that the tip expands rather than divides while passing through abdominal wall structures. Ports are presented in a range of sizes to accommodate various instruments. Large ports can be fitted with 'sizers' to reduce the lumen. Alternatively, some disposable large ports have an inbuilt diaphragm permitting the introduction of a number of instrument diameters without loss of pneumoperitoneum. All have attachments to allow insufflation, and valves to prevent gas leaks. Some have collars, allowing them to be secured in position (Fig. 5.2). It is good practice to rehearse port requirements for specific procedures with the surgical team. This ensures appropriate port availability and avoids the expense of opening unnecessary disposable ports.

9 **Instruments:** Laparoscopic instruments come in a standard length (30 cm long shaft). However, bariatric surgeries require longer instruments (45 cm in length). Most instruments come in a variety of handles with different locking handles. Instruments can be wholly disposable or reusable but may also be a combination of a reusable hand piece/shaft with a disposable tip. Many reusable instruments are of a modular design with separate hand pieces and shafts (Box 5.2). In any specific procedure a variety of types may be in use. Instrument selection is often dictated by a number of factors, which include procedure-specific requirements, personal preference and cost. Most surgical units possess a number of identical basic trays of non-disposable instruments for laparoscopic procedures. Multidisciplinary input from the surgical and scrub teams is important when there is an opportunity to influence the specification of such trays. Since disposables are expensive, either specify which ones are required beforehand or ensure that they are opened only when needed. A combination of reusable and disposable items (ports and instruments) are usually required.

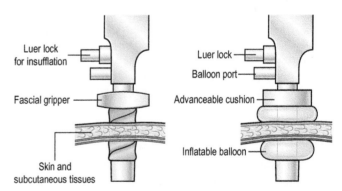

Fig. 5.2 Diagram of two types of laparoscopic port, one with a screw collar and the second with inflatable balloons. Both help to prevent gas leaks around the ports.

Box 5.2 basic laparoscopic instrument tray (reusable items)
■ Basic set of open surgical instruments
■ Light cable, camera and laparoscope
■ Veress needle (Fig. 5.3), gas supply and gas extract tubing
■ Laparoscopic instruments +/− reusable ports
■ Monopolar and bipolar diathermy cables, diathermy hook and bipolar forceps
■ Suction/irrigation tubing and probe

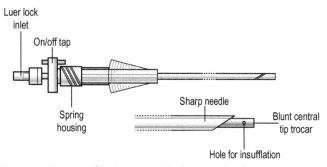

Fig. 5.3   Diagram of a Veress needle showing the device in its entirety, and the spring-loaded tip.

Have a large range of graspers available on the basic laparo-scopic tray. A range is available, including atraumatic graspers (Johan DeBakey, Desplanter) and others (Babcock).

Consider incorporating a range of dissectors from those available, such as Maryland, Mixter.

For instruments that are likely to degrade with use, such as scissors and diathermy hooks, wholly disposable or disposable-tipped are preferable. Always check the insulation integrity of instruments equipped for electrocautery.

Plan ahead to ensure you have a clean laparoscope lens. Avoid fogging by warming the laparoscope: use a thermos of warm sterile water or other proprietary system. Do not insufflate cold carbon dioxide through the same port as the camera. Rehearse a routine with the camera holder for efficient cleaning of a contaminated lens, such as washing in warm water followed by a wipe with a dry swab.

10 **Anaesthesia:** General anaesthesia is usually augmented with muscle relaxation, intubation and ventilation so that a pneumoperitoneum can be induced without causing cardiorespiratory embarrassment. Abdominal distension affects venous return, heart rate and consequently blood pressure. A profound bradycardia is not uncommon even in fit individuals, particularly on induction of the pneumoperitoneum. Abdominal distension also affects chest-wall compliance and the ease with which patients can be ventilated. Aim to use the lowest pre-set intra-abdominal pressure compatible with adequate surgical exposure.

Access

1 **Patient positioning:** Patients are placed in a supine position with the legs either abducted (allowing the surgeon to operate from between the legs, for example in a hepatectomy) or elevated in stirrups (for access to the pelvis), or in the lateral decubitus position (access to the retroperitoneum when performing a nephrectomy). All pressure points must be adequately padded to prevent neuropathies and skin damage and strapping may be used to stabilise the patient especially when the table is tilted. The arms are usually tucked to the sides to allow ease of movement of the surgeon as she lines up instruments with target tissue.

> ▶ KEY POINT Insert instruments carefully

> ■ Instruments must be inserted under direct vision. Blind introduction risks injury to underlying viscera (bowel, bladder) or even deeper structures (aorta, vena cava).

2 **Port placement:** The camera port is usually at the umbilicus or at a site which is directly opposite the target tissue of interest. Subsequent ports are inserted after a pneumoperitoneum has been established and under direct camera vision. This minimises iatrogenic injury as the trocars pass into the abdominal cavity. The ideal port orientation creates an equilateral triangle between the surgeon's left and right hand, with the telescope positioned at the apex of the triangle. The left and right hand ports should be approximately 10 to 15 cms apart for optimum instrument use.

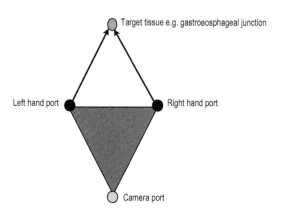

3 **Camera Holder:** The surgeon stands behind the telescope. The camera holder may be required to reach between the Surgeon's hands to guide the telescope to the area of interest. The ergonomics of this arrangement are sometimes better facilitated if the camera holder is seated on a stool next to the Surgeon.

4 **Pneumoperitoneum:** Induce a pneumoperitoneum. The initial penetration of the abdominal cavity to produce a pneumoperitoneum can be a hazardous task in laparoscopic surgery. Once the first port is established you can introduce additional ports under direct vision and with relative safety. There are open and closed methods of producing a pneumoperitoneum:

■ The open (Hasson) method of port insertion is safer, especially if there has been previous surgery. Make a 1–2-cm infraumbilical incision, deepening it to the linea alba. Observe the transverse fibres of the linear alba at the base of the umbilical ligament. Incise the linea alba at this point between two stay sutures and open the peritoneum under direct vision. The stay sutures can be tied together to close the port site at the end of the procedure, by using a box stitch (Fig. 5.4). If you have difficulty locating the linea alba in an obese patient, evert the base of the umbilical ligament upwards, using a clip. This brings the linea alba to the surface (Fig. 5.4A). Insert a finger to sweep away any adhesions around the insertion site before introducing a blunt-tipped trocar. Connect the gas supply and establish a pneumoperitoneum. The main disadvantage of this method is the increased incidence of gas leaks around the port. Special ports with sealing balloons have been developed to prevent this.

■ The closed (Veress needle) technique is also commonly used. As before, make an infra-umbilical skin incision. Apply a 20–30° Trendelenburg tilt to the patient. Together with your assistant, grasp the anterior abdominal wall and lift it up. Insert a Veress needle (Fig. 5.5) perpendicular to the abdominal wall until it penetrates the linea alba and the peritoneum. As soon as you feel the 'click' as the needle enters the peritoneal cavity, direct the needle downwards towards the pelvis to avoid damaging the great vessels. When the abdomen is fully distended and tympanitic to percussion, withdraw the Veress needle and enlarge the superficial part of the incision to accommodate the cannula. Insert a 10-mm trocar and cannula, aiming the tip anterior to the sacral promontory, parallel to the aorta. Use a drilling action from the wrist while lifting up the abdominal wall below the insertion site.

► KEY POINTS Check the position of the Veress needle tip

- Is the needle tip freely mobile?
- Does a drop of saline placed on the Luer connector of the Veress needle fall freely into the abdomen, where the pressure is subatmospheric?
- Aspirate to check that you do not obtain bowel content or blood
- Inject 5 ml of saline; it should flow freely through the needle
- Imperative that surgeon monitors the flows and pressures during initial insufflation to create the pneumoperitoneum. This will confirm appropriate intraperitoneal needle placement

? DIFFICULTY IN CREATING PNEUMOPERITONEUM

A rapid rise in pressure above the pre-set level?
A lack of tympanitic, symmetrical distension of the abdomen?
No loss of liver dullness on percussion?
At this point:
1. Stop insufflation
2. Check port/needle positioning
3. Check that the gas tubing is not obstructed and that the control taps are on
4. If there has been too much gas introduced into the abdomen, let some gas out via one of the ports
5. Liaise with the anaesthetist in case there has been a loss of muscle relaxation.

- There are alternative access techniques which, although less commonly used, can be helpful in certain situations. Following previous surgery, particularly through a vertical midline incision, avoid the umbilical region. Use a modified Hasson technique to access the peritoneum, by performing a cut-down through the various layers of the abdominal wall through a small laterally placed skin incision. Alternatively, insert a Veress needle through a laterally placed incision. Here you must be aware that there are often two 'clicks' on the needle before it is in position. The first is as the tip perforates musculature, then as it perforates the peritoneum. When you expect multiple intraperitoneal adhesions consider using the laparoscope to provide visual passage of the tip of the trocar though abdominal wall structures. Effect this by using a hollow trocar to accommodate the laparoscope and a see-through blunt plastic tip. Other proprietary devices on the market perform a similar task.

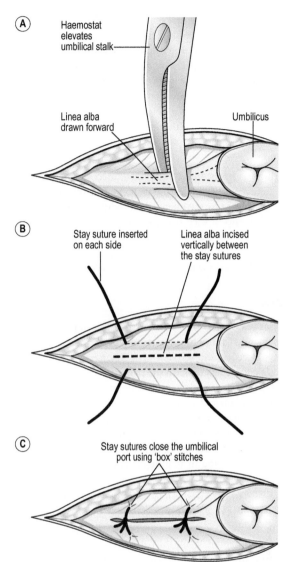

Fig. 5.4 Insertion of a Hasson port just below the umbilicus. (A) Shows the vertical incision made just below the umbilicus, dissected down to the linea alba. (B) Longitudinal absorbable stitches (Vicryl) have been inserted on each side of the midline; the vertical midline incision will be made between them, through which the Hasson port will be inserted. (C) On completion and removal of the port, close the defect by tying the sutures across to produce a 'box' or 'mattress' stitch.

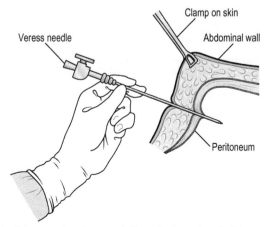

Fig. 5.5 Diagram showing a technique for inserting the Veress needle into the abdominal wall and the layers the needle passes through.

5 **Inspection:** With the first port connected to the insufflator wait until the pre-set pressure is achieved, then insert the warmed laparoscope. Observe the view on insertion to ensure the viscera are not at risk. Inspect the abdomen immediately below the first port to identify structures that could have been damaged. Perform a general laparoscopy looking for any expected or un-expected pathology (see below). The inspection helps general orientation as well as the identification of safe sites for additional ports. Secure ports using either a threaded collar or stay sutures.

6 **Additional ports:** Insert these under direct vision. Prior to incision infiltrate the skin with local anaesthetic. The sites, size and number are determined by the intended procedure. Instruct the assistant to follow the tip of each trocar carefully to detect potential visceral damage. In more obese individuals these additional ports often need be passed obliquely through the abdominal wall, so lying in the direction in which they are most useful during the procedure.

Assess

1 **Upper abdomen:** Now survey the abdomen prior to performing the intended procedure. Be systematic in identifying landmarks and inspecting the relevant area. Locate the ligamentum teres and falciform ligament. In the right upper quadrant visualize the liver, gallbladder and the underside of the right hemidiaphragm. Now manipulate the laparoscope under the ligamentum teres to look at the left lobe of the liver and the spleen. Change the patient's position using table tilt and aid visualization by moving the bowel. Inspect both the left and right paracolic gutters, facilitating the exposure by inserting an atraumatic grasper to manipulate the bowel if necessary.

2 **Lower abdomen and pelvis:** Place the patient in the Trendelenburg position to locate the caecum and appendix. Insert an atraumatic grasper to manoeuvre the bowel while you examine it from distal to proximal. While the patient is in the head-down position, examine the pelvis; this is especially important in female patients presenting with lower abdominal pain of unknown cause. You can directly visualize the ovaries, uterus and vermiform appendix.

3 In order to inspect organs such as the pancreas, additional manipulation and dissection may be necessary.

Safe use of diathermy

1 **Burns:** Carefully identify the correct structure. The most common diathermy injury (monopolar and bipolar) results from misidentification and a burn to the wrong structure.

▶ KEY POINT Beware diathermy burns

■ Diathermy, used inappropriately during laparoscopic surgery, can cause unrecognized, inadvertent and fatal injury.

2 **Inadvertent activation:** Inadvertent activation of the diathermy pedal risks damaging other structures in the abdominal cavity, especially when the electrode is outside the field of view.

3 **Insulation failure:** Abrasive cleaning, particularly of old instruments, may lead to an insulation failure. It is then possible for a conducting surface other than the electrode to come into contact or create an arc with an adjacent viscus. If burning does not directly cause a perforation, it may lead to necrosis and perforation at a later date.

4 **Direct coupling:** Current may flow from the active electrode of a monopolar instrument to a contiguous conducting instrument; this is an example of direct coupling. The result is poor function at the active electrode and an unnoticed burn from the second instrument.

5 **Residual heat:** After use, diathermy electrodes can remain sufficiently hot to cause burns. After use, withdraw the electrode or keep it in view.

6 **Current concentration:** As in open surgery, monopolar diathermy of a pedicle concentrates the current density. This may lead to inadvertent heating of other structures, for example heat injury at laparoscopic cholecystectomy can lead to a late stricture of the common bile duct.

7 **Capacitative coupling:** Alternating currents can pass through insulating materials, as occurs in devices called capacitors. During laparoscopy a capacitor may be formed inadvertently so current induced in a metal port then flows into neighbouring bowel and causes a burn. Avoid capacitative coupling by using a non-conducting electrode. If you are using a metal port ensure that it makes good contact with the abdominal wall. Avoid open-circuit activation and high-voltage diathermy such as fulguration.

Dissecting technique

1 **Challenges:** As in open surgery a safe and effective approach to tissue dissection is crucial to patient outcome. However, there are additional challenges during laparoscopy. In the main these relate to a loss of tactile feedback from tissues and instruments, challenges in exposure/retraction and difficulties in maintaining haemostasis.

▶ KEY POINT Try to maintain a dry surgical field

■ Significant bleeding rapidly leads to a degradation of the image. The area of interest becomes obscured by blood and the image darkens because of light absorption by blood.

2 **Tactile feedback:** Laparoscopic instruments do provide tactile feedback but you need to spend time either on a simulator or in a mentored environment acquiring sensitivity to the feel and handling of tissues, needles and sutures. Remember that the body wall acts as a fulcrum and forces applied at the hand piece are modified as they are transmitted to tissues at the tip.

3 **Instrumentation:** Developments in surgical approaches and laparoscopic instrumentation have to a degree mitigated some of the problems associated with dissection techniques. There are a range of purpose built, mainly disposable instruments, that now enable you to develop tissue planes and transect structures without the penalty of major delays in maintaining haemostasis.

4 **Effective combinations:** There are certain instrument combinations that have proved to be reliable and effective for dissection. The choice of any particular combination depends on the specific procedure, personal preference, instrument availability and cost as follows:

- Monopolar diathermy hook in your dominant hand complements atraumatic graspers in your non-dominant hand. This is the classic combination for laparoscopic cholecystectomy, while occasionally exchanging the hook diathermy for a dissector.
- Monopolar diathermy scissors in your dominant hand can be used while atraumatic forceps are held in your non-dominant hand. This is a low-cost combination and it can be remarkably effective for some of the simpler procedures such as appendicectomy and adhesiolysis.
- Monopolar diathermy scissors held in your dominant hand make an effective combination with bipolar diathermy forceps controlled by your non-dominant hand. The bipolar forceps act both as atraumatic graspers and diathermy for small vessels. It is a demanding combination since you need a degree of ambidexterity.
- Ultrasonic shears in your dominant hand can complement an atraumatic grasper held in your non-dominant hand. This combination is very useful for more complex procedures. Ultrasonic shears require a separate generator and are manufactured as a disposable item by a number of companies. All have both a 'cut' and a 'coagulation' mode. You can safely transect vessels up to a diameter of 4–5 mm. It is easy to become overconfident with the instrument as it is so effective at rapidly transecting tissue and leaving behind an avascular plane.

> **KEY POINT** Caution

- Beware retained heat in the instrument tip

- Tissue-sensing bipolar diathermy forceps in your dominant hand as a counterpart to an atraumatic grasper in your non-dominant hand. The tissue-sensing control system for this bipolar instrument adjusts to differences in tissue impedance. It provides 'cut' and 'coagulation' modes. Like the ultrasonic instruments it can handle vessels up to 4–5 mm in diameter. Retained heat is not a problem, but the instrument is slightly slower than the ultrasonic shears.
- Robotic assisted surgery offers major advantages. The precision of movement includes elimination of tremor and movement scaling. The robotic arm is also able to mimic certain hand movements that are not reproducible by conventional laparoscopic instruments. Various instrument combinations are available. Cost and training issues remain a major obstacle to its wider usage.

Exposure

1 **Gravity:** Gravity can be a useful adjunct to aid exposure in laparoscopic surgery. This starts with patient positioning, followed by appropriate table tilt. For each of the commoner procedures there are standard positions for patient, table and surgeon. For procedures requiring prolonged exposure in an extreme Trendelenburg position care must be taken to avoid the risk of retinal vein thrombosis.

2 **Retraction:** There are a large number of disposable and reusable designs of retractor for specific laparoscopic procedures. Most are 5-mm or 10-mm instruments, which have intra-abdominal parts that are deployed after insertion. Avoid retractors with sharp edges. Favour using fixed table clamps for retractors that are likely to remain in place for long periods during the procedure.

HAEMOSTASIS

1 **Small vessels:** As in open surgery, applying heat to achieve tissue desiccation, either generated by diathermy or ultrasound, secures most small vessels. All the instruments described above have limitations; adhere to them. Use them to best advantage. They all require a degree of sophistication in handling. In particular, avoid haste when using the ultrasonic shears and tissue sensing bipolar diathermy. In both, the effect on tissues is time dependent. In addition care must be exercised in selecting the appropriate mode (i.e. cut for relatively avascular structures and coagulation for specific vessels).

> **KEY POINT** Haemostasis

- Employ modern haemostatic aids appropriately, otherwise they are ineffective and potentially damaging.

2 **Larger vessels and pedicles:** There are a number of methods of securing larger vessels and pedicles as follows:
- Although ligatures remain the cheapest option they are more difficult to secure in laparoscopic surgery compared with open surgery. Knots can be formed in both an extracorporeal and intracorporeal fashion. Both need considerable dexterity to be used quickly and effectively. A preformed Roeder knot mounted on a disposable pusher remains a simple solution to ligation provided it can be passed over the tissue in question, such as an appendix stump or oedematous cystic duct.
- Laparoscopic clips are available in non-absorbable and absorbable materials. The non-absorbable clips are usually titanium and mostly 5 mm or 10 mm. They come in a variety of shapes and sizes, with single fire and multi fire disposable and reusable applicators. Prefer metal clips that are difficult to dislodge inadvertently and for enhanced security always consider using two clips rather than one on a particular structure. Absorbable clips are available in a range of sizes and usually for single fire with a reusable applicator. Most have some form of locking design for added security. They are particularly effective on the ureter and medium-sized vessels. Fatalities have been reported resulting from dislodgement following their use on the renal artery during live donor nephrectomy.
- Laparoscopic staplers and stapler cutters are relatively expensive disposable items but they are often the only safe option for transecting major pedicles and large vessels during more complex surgery. Most are available as 10-mm, 12-mm and 15-mm instruments. The suppliers take great care to ensure their safety and reliability. Many have safety lock-out features preventing inadvertent activation. All have a sequential action that must be followed by the operator from cartridge loading through to eventual firing.

> **KEY POINT** Stapling devices

- It is incumbent on you to be fully familiar with all the features incorporated in laparoscopic staplers and staple cutters. You invite disaster by ignoring this.

Select the appropriate cartridge carefully, such as including vascular load when transecting a vessel. In spite of these safety features there have been numerous reports of stapler cutter failures, sometimes with catastrophic consequences. Common causes of instrument misfires include attempts to transect heavily calcified or atherosclerotic vessels, the inadvertent incorporation of metal clips between the instrument jaws, inappropriate cartridge selection and faulty cartridge loading.

- Laparoscopic suturing is technically challenging but you may need to oversew vessels, particularly if other attempts at control have not been unsuccessful. As a general rule, if you are embarking on complex laparoscopic surgery where the control of major vessels may be required you ought to be competent at laparoscopic suturing. Do not underestimate the amount of practice required to achieve this level of competence. High-end laparoscopic simulators with suturing modules are ideal training platforms for this task; however, a lot can be achieved with simpler models.

3 **Coping with haemorrhage:** Ability to cope with degrees of haemorrhage is an essential accomplishment in all surgery. The challenge is greater in laparoscopic procedures and best avoided if at all possible by using a more measured approach to dissection. Nevertheless, bleeding occurs from time to time, particularly in complex procedures. This often arises from a single bleeding point. As in open surgery, the correct sequence of applying immediate tamponade, followed by suction/irrigation to clear the field, completed by the definitive step of securing the source of the bleed, is usually effective. A helpful adjunct is to apply tamponade with small swabs over which you can use suction to improve the field of view. Additionally, you may use additional ports through which an assistant can independently control suction and irrigation. This tactic frees both of your hands to effect control. Bleeding can also occur on removal of ports with damage to the inferior epigastric vessels. Application of direct pressure using a Johann or other laparoscopic instrument will buy you time. A suture applied across the vessel and abdominal wall should suffice to stem the bleeding. Alternatively in cases of catastrophic bleeding, a foley catheter can be placed through the trocar site and inflated to create a balloon tamponade effect.

4 **Surface control:** Controlling haemorrhage on the surface of a raw area is an occasional problem. Typically, this occurs on a friable organ such as liver, perhaps in the gall bladder bed, or the spleen following a capsular tear. Applying a monopolar diathermy instrument effectively produces an area of desiccation, but the eschar may then be torn away as you withdraw the tip of the diathermy instrument. Occasionally, bipolar diathermy is more effective in this situation but is less efficient when you need to control a large area. Such an area can be approached using monopolar diathermy set on 'fulguration' (Latin: fulgur = lightning) in which the electrical spark arcs without tissue contact. Be careful to adjust the setting of the electro-cautery device at a safe level. If it is available, use an argon beam diathermy delivered via a laparoscopic probe to control large surface areas. Care needs to be taken in using this instrument as large volumes of argon gas are injected into the pneumoperitoneum at high pressure. Vent this gas via a port to prevent overpressure and argon gas embolus.

> ▶ KEY POINTS Surface bleeding

- Select complex methods of controlling surface bleed with care.
- Contact-free electro-cautery and argon-beam diathermy are effective but potentially dangerous if they are used inexpertly.

Conversion

1 **Indications:** Do not view conversion to open surgery as a failure on your part. View it as an act performed in the patient's best interests. There are a number of indications for conversion, including failure to make progress, unsuspected pathology, uncontrolled haemorrhage, technical difficulties and equipment failure.

2 **Timing:** Uncontrolled haemorrhage is the single commonest reason for rapid conversion. Fatalities have been reported following failure to appreciate the urgency for conversion, particularly following aortic or caval trauma during first port insertion.

> ▶ KEY POINTS Retroperitoneal bleeding

- Beware missing a major retroperitoneal haemorrhage
- You may detect the rapid fall in blood pressure and the impression of increasing fullness in the retroperitoneal space
- You may not appreciate that there can be remarkably little intraperitoneal blood.

Most other conversions are semi-elective in nature when you have time to plan the subsequent incision and exposure. Consider incorporating port wounds in the incision to improve cosmesis. Postoperatively, take care to explain to the patient the decision-making process that led up to the conversion, illustrated by any video footage if this is thought to be helpful.

Closure

1 Before removing the ports, ensure that you have achieved complete haemostasis. Ensure that there are no retained foreign bodies in the abdomen such as spilt gallstones, small swabs, needles. Wash out any blood remaining in the peritoneal cavity. Remove all laparoscopic instruments and ports under direct vision while checking for port-site bleeding. Make sure no intra-abdominal structures have become trapped in the ports or port sites. Remove the final port slowly, while the laparoscope is still inside so you can finally check for bleeding.

2 Gas can be removed by using the suction device or expelled through palpation of the abdomen. Midline 10 mm port incision should be closed using a 2 o'vicryl suture or PDS mounted on a J needle. A crochet needle may also be applied for a closure technique. Ensure that fascia is taken with each suture bite and triangulate the port defect. Take care not to pick up bowel in the suture. This allows a mass closure of the abdomen and prevents future port site hernia with potential for incarceration.

TABLE 5.3 Some complications common to laparoscopy and pneumoperitoneum

During pneumoperitoneum induction	Related to port placement	During procedure	Patient-related complications
Damage to viscus or vessels	Damage to underlying structures	Diathermy-related injuries	Obesity: makes operation more difficult, increasing operating time, and may require special instruments
Misplacement of the gas	Be poorly placed	Inadvertent organ ligation or division	Ascites causes oozing from port sites, increasing the risk of port-site damage
Insufflation of the bowel lumen	Haemorrhage	Unrecognized haemorrhage	Organomegaly increases the risk of organ damage
Carbon dioxide embolus and metabolic acidosis may complicate pneumoperitoneum			
Over-insufflation of the peritoneal cavity may cause cardiorespiratory problems	Herniation		Clotting problems may result in haemorrhage, or conversely in deep vein thrombosis
			Following operation for malignant disease, cancer cells may be transferred to the port site, resulting in metastases

Postoperative

1 Monitor all patients as following an open laparotomy, with regular observations. Remind the patients of referred shoulder tip pain following pneumoperitoneum. Mobilize them early and encourage them to eat and drink.

2 Most patients can be discharged within 24 hours of laparoscopy; the length of stay increases with more extensive procedures.

Complications

Since laparoscopic surgery usually requires a general anaesthetic, patients are susceptible to the usual complications related to this. Table 5.3 lists complications common to laparoscopy and pneumoperitoneum. Unrecognized bowel injury is a particular worry following any laparoscopic procedure and should be suspected in any patient in whom there is no reasonable explanation for a slow or delayed recovery on their first or second postoperative day.

Natural Orifice Transluminal Endoscopic Surgery (NOTES)

Advances in MAS include the development of NOTES, the introduction of a flexible endoscope through the GI, urinary or reproductive organs in order to enter the peritoneal cavity, mediastinum or chest. The procedure is aided by the use of a laparoscope to ensure safety and has led to the transgastric and transvaginal removal of the gallbladder, for example. NOTES may well be applied in the future to staging of intraabdominal malignancies, ablation of Barrett's oesophagus and gastrojejunostomy to name but a few, where the goal is consistent with the aims of MAS; surgical procedures performed with minimal tissue trauma, reduced pain and less disability to patients.

FURTHER READING

Darzi A, Monson JRT. Laparoscopic inguinal hernia repair. Oxford: ISIS Medical Media; 1994.

Darzi A, Talamini M, Dunn DC. Atlas of laparoscopic surgical technique. London: Saunders; 1997.

Goldfaden A, Birkmeyer JD. Evidence-based practice in laparoscopic surgery: Perioperative care. Surg Innov 2005;12: 51–61.

Hasson H. Open laparoscopy: A report of 150 cases. J Reprod Med 1974;12:234–8.

Herron DM, Gagner M, Kenyon TL, et al. The minimally invasive surgical suite enters the 21st century. A discussion of critical design elements. Surg Endosc 2001;15:415.

Hunter JG, Jobe BA. Chapter 14. Minimally Invasive Surgery, Robotics, and Natural Orifice Transluminal Endoscopic Surgery. In: Brunicardi FC, Andersen DK, Billiar TR, Dunn DL, Hunter JG, Matthews JB, Pollock RE, editors. Schwartz's Principles of Surgery. 9th ed. New York: McGraw-Hill; 2010.

Hurd WW, Amesse LS, Gruber JS, et al. Visualization of the epigastric vessels and bladder before laparoscopic trocar placement. Fertil Steril 2003;80:209–12.

Larsen JF, Svendsen FM, Pedersen V. Randomized clinical trial of the effect of pneumoperitoneum on cardiac function and haemodynamics during laparoscopic cholecystectomy. Br J Surg 2004;91:848–54.

Lowry PS, Moon TD, D'Alessandro A, Nakada SY. Symptomatic port-site hernia associated with a non-bladed trocar after laparoscopic live-donor nephrectomy. J Endourol 2003;17:493–4.

Mishra RK. Textbook of practical laparosocpic surgery. Mc-Graw Hill-Medical. 2nd ed. 2009.

Vernon AH, Hunter JG. Chapter 44. Fundamentals of Laparoscopic Surgery. In: Ashley SW, Zinner MJ, editors. Maingot's Abdominal Operations. 11th ed. New York: McGraw-Hill; 2007.

6

Abdominal wall and hernias

D.M. Baker

CONTENTS

GENERAL ISSUES IN HERNIA SURGERY

1 **Definition:** A hernia is an abnormal protrusion of a viscus (Latin: internal organ) through its containing wall. Abdominal wall hernias are very common, especially in the groin (inguinal hernias) and umbilical area.

2 **Diagnosis:**
   - Consider whether there is another cause for the patient's symptoms. Groin pain may be due to osteoarthrosis of the hip or a groin strain, rather than the obvious inguinal hernia. Epigastric pain may be biliary colic or a symptom of peptic ulcer and not a consequence of the epigastric hernia.
   - The hernia may not be evident in the anaesthetized patient so mark the site (and side) preoperatively.

3 **Indications to treat:** Most hernias are operated on to ensure they do not enlarge, become uncomfortable, and to avoid the risk of strangulation. Reserve non-operative management for asymptomatic direct inguinal hernias, particularly in elderly, inactive or terminally ill patients and those who will not consent. The few who do not have an operation are best left without a truss, which is uncomfortable and difficult to manage.

4 **Repair:** There are three steps to a hernia repair:
   - Herniotomy: remove the hernia sac
   - Herniorraphy: close the hernia neck or wall defect
   - Hernioplasty: support the defect, usually using a prosthetic mesh.

5 **Select the approach** (open or laparoscopic): This depends on the hernia site, your surgical expertise, operating facilities, the patient's anatomy and wishes. Laparoscopic repair requires different surgical skills, may be more expensive for the hospital than an open repair and cannot be undertaken under local anaesthetic.

6 **Consent:** Ensure the patient has given full consent to the operation and understands the circumstances under which it will be performed. Provide full information on discharge arrangements.

7 **Suture** the repair with a non-absorbable monofilament suture on a curved, round-bodied needle, polyamide (nylon) and polypropylene being the most popular. Remember the following:
   - Monofilament sutures require extra knots for security.
   - Handle synthetic monofilament suture material with care. Do not hold it with instruments or jerk it when tying knots or it will be seriously weakened.
   - Do not drag the fine suture through the tissues, since it will cut them, enlarging the holes.
   - Do not tie the sutures too tightly. They will either cut out now or strangulate the tissues and weaken them later and may also increase the risk of troublesome neuralgia.
   - Do not take even bites of the tissues. Although this looks neat, evenly inserted stitches tend to detach a strip of aponeurosis. Therefore, take successive bites at differing distances from the edge.

8 **Prosthetic mesh in hernia repair:** If you use prosthetic mesh for the repair, give a prophylactic dose of antibiotic at induction. Always administer this in operations for strangulated hernia as the wound may be contaminated.

   Prosthetic mesh is an integral part of almost all hernia repairs as it often makes hernia surgery quicker and easier and reduces recurrence rates. There are many materials available, with several factors influencing choice:
   - *Strength/stiffness* results not only from the intrinsic strength of the mesh, often related to the density of prosthetic material, but also from the resulting in-growth of fibrosis, which is greater with smaller pore sizes.
   - *Flexibility/elasticity:* meshes should be flexible enough to conform to the abdominal wall movements on a long-term basis. It is increasingly apparent that current polypropylene meshes

may be unnecessarily strong, resulting in pain and the sensation of stiffness when compared with lighter-weight open-weave or compound meshes (e.g. Vypro, Ethicon).

- *Size and shape:* all prostheses shrink as part of the process of scar maturation. Therefore allow a minimum overlap of the hernial defect by the mesh of 2–3 cm for initial fixation and long-term coverage. For laparoscopic ventral hernia repair, favour a 5-cm overlap. Various preformed meshes are now available for some hernia sites.
- *Expense* often limits the use of newer, composite meshes.
- *Adhesion formation* remains a problem, particularly with intra-peritoneal implantation. Two-sided meshes, with one side engendering tissue ingrowth, the other inhibiting it (e.g. DualMesh, Gore, Proceed, Ethicon), reduce this risk.
- *Infection:* systemic prophylactic antibiotics have been shown to reduce the risk of wound infection.

9 **Local anaesthesia** is suitable for many groin hernia repairs and some other hernias. Young adults may not tolerate it alone and may require the addition of sedation. There are economic benefits, particularly for day-case surgery and in the elderly. Its use carries its own risks and the following general considerations apply:

- Monitor the blood pressure, pulse rate and oxygen saturation.
- Know the appropriate resuscitation procedures in case the patient develops an adverse reaction.
- For effective anaesthesia give a sufficient volume. Use either 0.5% lidocaine with adrenaline (epinephrine) 1 in 1 000 000 or bupivacaine (0.25%). Select your choice of local anaesthetic for hernia operations and do not vary, to avoid confusion.
- Do not exceed the safe dose of local anaesthetic: for lidocaine with adrenaline (epinephrine) this is 70 mg lidocaine per kg, approximating for an average adult to 5000 mg, equivalent to 100 ml of a 0.5% solution.
- Clearly record in the notes the dose of local anaesthetic and other drugs.

10 **Close the skin** with sutures, clips, staples or adhesive strips. Continuous, absorbable subcuticular stitches provide a very neat result and avoid the discomfort and cost of suture removal.

11 **Provide adequate postoperative analgesia.** Inject local anaesthetic into the wound. Prescribe preoperative analgesics such as IV paracetamol and regular postoperative oral medication such as non-steroidal anti-inflammatories or co-codamol for 2 days.

12 **Wound complications:**

- Reduce bruising and haematoma formation by achieving meticulous haemostasis and judiciously inserting suction drains.
- Wound infection rarely requires more than drainage of any collection. Sinus formation is rare with the use of monofilament sutures but occasionally requires removal of suture knots or mesh.

13 **Hernia recurrence** is related to technical failure, including a missed hernial sac and inadequate placement or sizing of the mesh.

INGUINAL HERNIA

Appraise

1 Most inguinal hernias are repaired.

2 **Repair techniques:** There are several open and laparoscopic techniques described to repair an inguinal hernia:

- The Lichtenstein mesh repair, developed by Irving Lichtenstein (1920–2000) of Los Angeles, in 1984; in 1989 he reported no recurrences in 1000 patients after 1–5 years. It is the most popular open technique, relatively easy to master and has a low recurrence rate Other open techniques repair the posterior wall of the inguinal canal by suturing the conjoint tendon to the inguinal ligament (Bassini repair) or by overlapping the transversalis fascia (Shouldice repair).
- Through a laparoscopic approach a synthetic mesh can be placed in the pre-peritoneal space from the midline medially to a point close to the level of the anterior superior iliac spine laterally, thus covering the whole extent of the inguinal canal including the internal ring and the area medial to the inferior epigastric vessels where direct hernias originate, as well as covering the internal opening of the femoral canal. The pre-peritoneal space can be reached either via a total extra-peritoneal (TEP) approach which should not involve entry into the peritoneal cavity, or via a transabdominal pre-peritoneal (TAPP) approach. For inguinal hernia repairs the TEP requires more surgical experience, but is considered safer as the peritoneum is not breached.

3 Selecting the correct approach to repair an inguinal hernia.

- Familiarize yourself with all techniques and adapt them according to the patient's anatomy and wishes, rather than be compromised by lack of surgical expertise or equipment. The two approaches (open and laparoscopic) require very different surgical skills.
- The laparoscopic approach has slightly less postoperative pain, a faster return to work, a lower incidence of chronic groin pain and fewer wound complications. Long-term recurrence rates are similar for both methods. Laparoscopic repair costs more and carries a very small risk of serious injury to the intestine or major blood vessels, especially if the TAPP approach is adopted.
- The open operation has the advantage of being feasible under local anaesthesia. It is also cheaper and simpler to learn, and is currently recommended by NICE as the procedure of choice for primary, unilateral inguinal hernia in the UK. Consider especially women with primary unilateral inguinal hernias for open surgery.
- Repair a recurrent inguinal hernia through unscarred tissue: that is, if an open repair has recurred consider a laparoscopic approach, but if a laparoscopic repair has recurred consider an open approach.
- Bilateral inguinal hernia repairs are usually repaired laparoscopically as the operation is quicker. When repaired openly at the same time, the results are slightly inferior to separate repairs.
- For obese patients laparoscopic inguinal hernia repair is often easier.
- Undertake open repairs of large indirect inguinoscrotal hernias and urgent operations for hernias which may have strangulated.
- Avoid a laparoscopic approach if there has been previous lower abdominal surgery as a clear pre-peritoneal plane is difficult to find. Avoid it following previous open prostatectomy or procedures for urinary incontinence, but previous appendicectomy does not usually preclude it. A TAPP repair may be difficult or even hazardous if there are intra-peritoneal adhesions following previous lower abdominal surgery.

■ Select an open approach if there is an increased risk of bleeding such as anticoagulant therapy (even if was stopped preoperatively) or anti-platelet therapy such as clopidogrel, since bleeding can be more difficult to control than during the open operation.

Inspect

1 The diagnosis of groin swellings is notoriously difficult. Experienced as well as inexperienced surgeons make frequent mistakes. Do not accept the diagnosis of the referring doctor, but take a fresh history and carry out a complete examination. Is there another possible cause for the patient's symptoms apart from the hernia? If a clear history of a reducible intermittent lump in the groin is accompanied by a negative examination, a hernia will be found on exploration; if in doubt, consider herniography.

2 Palpation is not the only or even the most important method of examination. Look with the patient standing and again with the patient supine. If you see a lump, ask yourself 'Where is it?' If it is reducible, where does it first reappear on coughing or straining? A cough impulse may be absent, especially over a femoral hernia in which a small sac is covered by much fatty extra-peritoneal tissue. Conversely, a cough impulse is present over Malgaigne's (Parisian surgeon 1806–1856) bulging, or a saphena varix.

3 Always examine the scrotum and its contents in male patients. If there is a swelling, ask yourself the fundamental question 'Can I get above it?' Occasionally you discover undescended testes; deal with them at the same procedure.

4 Finally, examine the other hernial orifices.

Prepare

1 Obtain the patient's signed consent, warning of the possible complications of haematoma (especially for large inguinoscrotal hernias), ischaemic orchitis, persistent groin pain, hernia recurrence, wound and mesh infection, and damage to local structures, which can be more significant with a laparoscopic approach. In laparoscopic surgery obtain consent for conversion to open repair if necessary. Discuss with the patient what action you should take, if, at operation for unilateral hernia, an unexpected, asymptomatic contralateral hernia is revealed. Record the agreed consent on the form.

2 Mark the hernia side.

OPEN MESH INGUINAL HERNIA REPAIR (Lichtenstein Repair)

Local anaesthesia for inguinal hernia repair

1 Follow the instructions for local anaesthesia.

2 Inject 20 ml along the line of the proposed incision using a fine needle to raise a continuous bleb within the epidermis.

3 Replace the needle with a larger one to inject deeply and along the same line superficial to the anterior wall of the canal.

4 Blunt the needle to improve the 'feel' of passage through the aponeurosis and inject 5 ml of fluid 2 cm above and medial to the anterior superior iliac spine deep to the external oblique to block the iliohypogastric and ilioinguinal nerves.

5 Reserve about half the volume of anaesthetic to inject under the external oblique aponeurosis, around the neck of the sac and into other sensitive areas during the operation.

Access

1 Start the incision a finger's breadth above the palpable pubic tubercle within the skin crease which is often present (as opposed to parallel to the inguinal ligament) and extend this to two-thirds of the way to the anterior superior iliac spine. Incise the fascia to expose the external oblique aponeurosis, ligating and dividing two or three large veins that cross the line of the incision. Avoid cutting into the hernial sac and spermatic cord at the medial end of the incision.

2 Expose the glistening fibres of the external oblique aponeurosis and identify the external inguinal ring, which confirms the line of the inguinal canal.

3 With a scalpel split the external oblique aponeurosis in the line of the fibres. Enlarge the split medially and laterally by pushing the half-closed blades of the scissors in the line of the fibres. At the medial end of the split you open the external inguinal ring. Ensure that you do so. Do not allow curved blades of scissors to skirt around the crura of the ring. Preserve the ilioinguinal nerve, lying under the external oblique, to minimize the risk of postoperative numbness and pain.

4 Apply artery forceps to the edges of the aponeurosis and gently elevate each side. As you evert the upper leaf, look for the arching lower border of internal oblique muscle, with the cord below it. As you evert the lower leaf, sweep loose tissue from the deep surface of the inguinal ligament.

Assess (Fig. 6.1)

▶ KEY POINT Confirm the diagnosis

■ Do not rely on preoperative findings of the type of inguinal hernia; determine this during mobilization.

1 Start to mobilize the cord by incising, just above and lateral to the public tubercle, the 'mesentery' of fascia and fibres of cremasteric muscle that extends downwards from the medial part of the conjoint tendon to envelop the cord. Deepen this small incision behind the cord, drawing the latter downwards while passing the index finger from below against the pubic tubercle, to develop a plane to encircle the cord and apply a hernia ring.

2 Now dislocate the cord laterally and downwards by incising the coverings along lines just above and below it. This exposes a direct hernia, which can be freed from the cord.

3 Carefully divide the fibres of cremaster just distal to the internal ring, ensuring haemostasis.

4 Even though a direct hernia is evident, examine the cord. Normally it is about the thickness of a pencil. It is markedly distended by an unreduced, sometimes adherent or sliding, hernia. A thickened sac results from a longstanding indirect hernia. Cord lipomata produce thickening, as does an encysted hydrocele of the cord (in females a hydrocele of the canal of Nuck). To exclude an indirect sac, open the spermatic fascia covering the cord and identify the edge of the peritoneum deep to the internal ring.

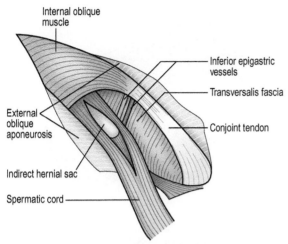

Fig. 6.1 Exposure of the right inguinal canal. The cremasteric fascia is split to show an indirect hernial sac.

5 Identify the lower arching fibres of the internal oblique muscle, becoming tendinous at the conjoint tendon, and examine the posterior wall below this. A direct hernia may be a large bulge, a diffuse weakness of the whole posterior wall or, less often, a funicular hernia through a small localized defect (Ogilvie's hernia).

6 If you have any concern that a femoral hernia may be present, incise the transversalis fascia to expose the upper aspect of the femoral canal. If a femoral sac is present, deal with it via a High approach repair (Lothiesen procedure, see later).

7 The cremasteric vessels pass medially from the inferior epigastric vessels adjacent to the cord. If the internal ring is enlarged it may be necessary to carefully identify, isolate, ligate and then divide the cremasteric vessels to facilitate a snug repair at the internal ring. If they are injured more medially, ligate them proximally and distally to the damage.

Hernia sac

Indirect sac

1 With the left thumb in front, gently stretch the previously mobilized cord over the left index finger, which is placed behind the cord. Make a short split with a knife, in the line of the cord, through the cremasteric and internal spermatic fascial layers. Continue the split proximally to the internal ring using scissors, first with their blades on the flat, separating fascia from deeper layers, then splitting the fascia.

2 Look for the sac. A white curved edge may be seen if the hernial sac is small (Fig. 6.1); if it is large it will be obvious as the fascial layers are separated. Using the point of the scalpel, gently incise the fibres crossing the fundus or the side edges of the sac. Unless it is very adherent it will then be possible to peel the sac out of the cord with the aid of a few further strokes of the blade. The sac is then dissected back to the level of the abdominal peritoneum, using a combination of wiping with a gauze swab and snipping firm attachments with scissors. Keep the dissection close to the sac and avoid damaging other structures in the cord.

3 Pick up the sac with two artery forceps and open it between the forceps with a scissors. Note any contents of the sac and return them to the peritoneal cavity. Adherent omentum may be freed, or ligated and excised. Be sure this is not part of a sliding hernia (see below).

4 While the empty sac is held vertically by means of the artery forceps, transfix its neck with a polyglactin (Vicryl) suture. Tie the ends of the suture-ligature into a half hitch, completely encircle the neck of the sac and tie a triple-throw knot to ligate the neck of the sac. If contents tend to bulge into the sac, gently hold them back using non-toothed dissecting forceps, sliding them out as the ligature is tightened.

5 Do not let your assistant cut the ends of the ligature. First excise the sac 1 cm distal to the ligature. Examine the cut end to ensure that only sac is seen, it does not bleed and the suture is secure, then cut the ligature yourself. The stump of the sac should retract through the internal ring.

6 Alternatively, fully mobilize and simply invert the sac. It need not be ligated for this.

7 If the margins of the internal ring have been stretched by the indirect hernia, narrow the gap in the posterior wall using a non-absorbable suture to approximate the attenuated margins of the transversalis fascia medial to the cord.

8 If there are large extra-peritoneal lipomata, carefully isolate, ligate and excise them but do not try to dissect out all the fatty tissue.

Large indirect sac

1 Complete hernias, or scrotal funicular hernias, have no distal edge to the sac as seen at the level of the pubic tubercle. Attempts to dissect out the whole sac cause the scrotal part of the sac and the testis to be drawn into the wound, increasing the risk of haematoma or ischaemic orchitis.

2 Purposefully divide the sac straight across within the inguinal canal. Isolate the proximal portion up to the internal ring, and leave the distal portion open. In this way the dissection is kept to a minimum.

3 If the sac is adherent, open it in front and place artery forceps at intervals round the inside as markers. Lift up two forceps, stretch the portion of sac between them, separate the sac from the cord and cut it distal to the forceps. Take the next two forceps and repeat the manoeuvre. Continue in this manner until the proximal circumference of the sac is completely sectioned, with the edges still held in the forceps.

4 After stripping the proximal part of the sac to the inguinal ring, transfix and ligate the neck.

5 Leave the distal part of the sac open.

Sliding indirect sac

1 In some hernias, retroperitoneal structures slide down to form part of the sac wall, chiefly the sigmoid colon, bladder or caecum. Always be on the look-out for sliding hernia.

2 You discover the sliding component when you attempt to empty and free the sac.

3 If the sac is intact, do not open it. If the sac has been opened, mark the fringe of peritoneum on the viscus with artery forceps and close the sac. Ensure that closure is complete.

4 Make sure that neither the organ nor its blood supply was damaged before the true situation was recognized. If the bladder was damaged, repair the wall and remember to insert an indwelling urethral catheter at the end of the operation.

5 Fully mobilize the entire hernia sac and sliding viscus from the cord and replace it in the abdomen. If the sac is inguinoscrotal, divide and close it below the sliding viscus and return it to the abdomen.

Direct sac

1 Always look for an indirect sac.

2 If the direct sac is funicular, resulting from a localized defect in the posterior wall, isolate it, empty it, then transfix, ligate and divide it at the neck. Define the margins of the posterior wall defect. If the hole is small and it can be closed without tension, suture it now, with non-absorbable material on a fine, curved, round-bodied needle.

3 More often the sac is diffuse and associated with a general weakness of the posterior wall. Do not open it. Push it inwards and maintain the invagination with a running suture of absorbable or non-absorbable suture, carried across the stretched transversalis fascia so as to flatten the bulge without tension. The sutures must not bite deeply or the bowel or bladder may be damaged.

Combined direct and indirect sac

1 Such hernias protrude on either side of the inferior epigastric vessels. They are sometimes likened to the legs of pantaloons.

2 Isolate each sac and deal with it separately.

> **? DIFFICULTY**
>
> 1. If you cannot find the sac or recognize the tissues, first find the vas deferens, which can be felt as a string-like structure towards the back of the cord. The testicular vessels lie near the vas and, once these are separated, the rest of the cord may be cautiously divided, starting at the front, while keeping in mind that abdominal organs may be encountered. If a structure seems to be the sac, cautiously open it after tenting a portion between two artery forceps. Look for a glistening inner surface and insert a finger to determine if the sac communicates with the peritoneal cavity.
> 2. *Torn neck of sac?* Carefully free peritoneum from the abdomen to form a new neck.

Posterior inguinal canal wall repair

The Lichtenstein repair is the mainstay of all open inguinal hernia repairs and employs a sheet of polypropylene mesh covering the posterior wall of the inguinal canal and extending, for security, over adjacent structures, with a hole to transmit the cord. It is a 'tension-free repair'. Additionally, or alternatively, a mesh 'plug' may be inserted into the defect.

Action

1 The mesh should have overall dimensions of 11 cm × 6 cm. To accommodate this, separate the external oblique aponeurosis from the deeper layers superiorly and medially and from the muscular part of internal oblique laterally to create an adequate pocket to receive the mesh.

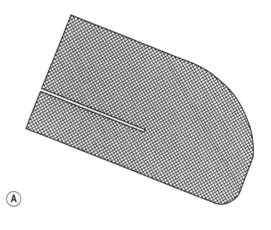

(A)

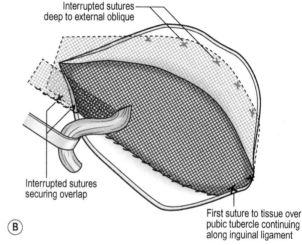

Interrupted sutures
deep to external oblique

Interrupted sutures
securing overlap

First suture to tissue over
pubic tubercle continuing
along inguinal ligament

(B)

Fig. 6.2 Lichtenstein repair: (A) mesh cut to shape; (B) mesh sutured in place.

2 Prepare the polypropylene mesh as indicated in Figure 6.2A. The lower medial corner is slightly rounded, the upper medial corner rather more so. The mesh is then incised from its lateral margin, placing the cut one-third of the distance from the lower edge. The cut extends for approximately half the length of the mesh, depending upon the size of the patient; it may need to be extended when the mesh is in place. In small patients the upper edge may need to be trimmed slightly.

3 Place the mesh in its final position (Fig. 6.2B). Lift the cord and bring the narrow lower tail through under it, below the internal ring. Then tuck the lateral end under the external oblique; the lower edge of the mesh now lies along the inguinal ligament. Now insert the upper two-thirds of the mesh so that it lies under the external oblique aponeurosis superiorly and medially, ensuring that there is a good overlap on the rectus sheath medially. Tuck the wide upper tail under the external oblique laterally, with its lower edge over the lower tail. Insert your fingers under external oblique superiorly and laterally to ensure that the mesh lies quite flat in the peripheral part of the pocket, though there may be a slight bulge centrally.

4 The mesh does need to be secured in place across the posterior wall of the inguinal canal. Although most use polypropylene sutures, it is possible to use staples or glue. Start the fixation by passing a 2/0 polypropylene stitch through the mesh and the tissues overlying the pubic tubercle and tying this. Use this to form a

continuous locking suture between the lower edge of the mesh and the inguinal ligament, working from medial to lateral, extending to at least 2 cm lateral to the internal ring. Take irregular bites of the inguinal ligament to avoid splitting it and do not allow the lower leaf of the external oblique to roll in and be included in the sutures; if this happens, there will be no external oblique left to close. For the medial part of this suture line it is best to retract the cord downwards. Then, as the suture approaches the internal ring, move the cord cephalad and pass the needle under it to continue laterally. When suturing immediately in front of the femoral vessels be careful to take only the ligament and not a bite of a major vessel!

5 If the slit in the mesh is too short extend it so that the cord passes directly from the internal ring to the opening in the mesh. A bulky cord may be accommodated by making a small cut in the mesh at right-angles to the slit. If you made too long a cut, all is not lost; simply shorten the slit with one or two sutures.

6 Overlap the tails of the mesh by bringing the lower edge of the upper portion in front of the lower tail and securing it to the inguinal ligament with two interrupted sutures (or by including it in the lateral part of the continuous suture). The resulting opening in the mesh should be a snug, but not a tight, fit around the cord (Fig. 6.2B).

7 Now secure the medial and upper margins of the mesh with about six interrupted sutures, avoiding the nerves (Fig. 6.2B). These are most conveniently placed 0.5 cm away from the edge, so that the mesh lies flat on the underlying aponeurosis or muscle. The medial sutures are particularly important as there is less overlapping of the mesh there, making it a potential site for recurrence.

8 The mesh repair is now completed. It appears slightly redundant centrally but that does not matter.

▶ KEY POINT Sound repair?

■ Provided there is sufficient overlap medially, superiorly and laterally, with a good suture line inferiorly, the fibrosis induced by the polypropylene (Prolene) mesh will produce a sound result.

9 Replace the cord in the inguinal canal.

10 Wash the inguinal canal with any remaining local anaesthetic, making sure not to remove it too quickly.

11 Close the external oblique aponeurosis with a synthetic absorbable suture, starting laterally and ending medially to reform the external ring snugly but not tightly around the emerging cord. Once again, take care to take bites at unequal distances from the edges; otherwise you will pull from the cut edges a strip of aponeurosis.

12 Appose the subcutaneous fascia with fine absorbable stitches and close the skin wound (see above).

Postoperative management

1 Following repair of inguinal hernia under local anaesthesia, allow the patient to leave the operating theatre on foot. This is good for confidence.

2 Encourage patients to mobilize immediately after recovery from general anaesthesia.

3 Activities should be limited only by the patient's comfort.

Complications of open inguinal hernia repair

In addition to the complications mentioned in the section on general issues, there are others specific to the groin:

1 *Scrotal complications:* Ischaemic orchitis is an uncommon complication presenting as pain and swelling in the first few days after hernia repair. In a proportion of cases it results in testicular atrophy. Damage to the vas should be recognized and repaired at the time of hernia repair. Hydrocele formation is more common after transection of the sac and resorbs spontaneously in most cases. Genital oedema, relatively common in the first 3 days, settles spontaneously, requiring reassurance only.

2 *Haematoma:* Bruising can be significant, often involving the scrotum, to the alarm of the patient, developing a couple of days after surgery. Even significant haematomas can be left to resolve, although this may take months and does increase the risk of orchitis, mesh infection and possibly recurrence and groin pain.

3 *Wound infections:* Reddening of the wounds is not uncommon, but frank purulent discharge is. If this persists, be concerned about a mesh infection and consider removing the mesh.

4 *Nerve injury:* Some degree of transient numbness below and medial to the incision is very common and may persist with little disability. Of much more significance is the incidence of chronic residual pain that occurs in at least 3% of conventional hernia repairs.

5 *Urinary problems:* Make sure you are aware of the possibility of bladder injury and recognize it at the time of surgery. Treat it by primary repair and insert an indwelling catheter until a cystogram demonstrates healing. Postoperative urinary retention becomes more common with age, after general anaesthesia and following bilateral hernia repair and usually resolves following a 24-hour period of catheterization.

6 *Impotence:* This is an occasional complaint for which there does not appear to be an organic basis.

OPEN RECURRENT INGUINAL HERNIA REPAIR

Appraise

1 Consider laparoscopic repair to avoid the adherent tissues.

2 For open operations, take considerable time to define the anatomy. This is difficult as there is distortion from the previous repair and all structures tend to be encased in fibrous tissue.

3 Once the anatomy is defined, secure the posterior wall and undertake a mesh repair as described.

4 Orchidectomy need not be considered, but warn the patient of the increased risk of ischaemic orchitis.

Access

1 Incise or excise the previous skin scar.

2 Deepen the incision at a higher or more lateral level than the previous approach, so that unscarred external oblique aponeurosis is encountered first.

3 Display the external oblique aponeurosis downwards to the inguinal ligament.

4 Re-open the inguinal canal through the scar in the external oblique aponeurosis. Avoid damaging the contents of the canal, which will be adherent.

5 Elevate the upper and lower leaves of the external oblique aponeurosis until you reach unscarred tissue.

6 Isolate the spermatic cord below the pubic tubercle and follow it up to the internal ring. It may lie in an unusual place or be adherent and the vas may have been separated from the vessels.

Assess

1 Look for an indirect recurrence. If you find a sac, isolate it, empty it, then transfix, ligate and divide it at the neck.

2 Look for a direct recurrence. If the recurrence is funicular, isolate it, empty it, then transfix, ligate and divide it at the neck. If it is a diffuse bulge, invert the sac with a running suture to maintain the invagination.

Repair

1 Almost always, the repair should be a mesh repair as outlined above.

2 Occasionally, for a small well defined direct defect, a 'plug' repair can be undertaken. Insert a bunched-up piece of polypropylene mesh through the small defect into the extra-peritoneal space and secure it with a few sutures across the open defect.

? DIFFICULTY

The dissection described for a recurrent hernia assumes that the anatomical relationships have not been altered by previous operations. There are several findings that may perplex you:

1. In the Halsted method, the posterior wall was reinforced by closing the external oblique aponeurosis behind the cord, thus superimposing the internal and external rings. A recurrence may appear alongside the cord, leaving the rest of the repair sound. Deal with the sac and define the edges of the stretched ring. This is one circumstance in which it may be best, with the patient's prior permission, to divide the cord so that the ring may be closed, but there is a 15% risk of ischaemic orchitis.

2. The previous use of a plastic mesh or tantalum gauze insert may result in dense fibrosis, making dissection difficult. Where this is known it is best to arrange for a laparoscopic repair.

3. Recurrences following darns with non-absorbable material are often local defects, suitable for the underlay mesh repair. Leave the sound parts undisturbed.

OPEN STRANGULATED INGUINAL HERNIA REPAIR

Appraise

1 Most operations listed as strangulated hernia are carried out for painful, irreducible or obstructed hernias.

2 An open approach to the strangulated inguinal hernia repair is easiest and most common,

3 Strangulation results from venous obstruction, a rise in capillary hydrostatic pressure, transudation of fluid, exudation of protein and cells, and eventual arterial obstruction. Alternatively, the pressure of a sharp constriction ring at the neck of the sac may cause local necrosis of the bowel wall.

4 Once diagnosed, try to reduce the hernia, making emergency surgery unnecessary and allowing for an early elective operation. The effect of reassuring the patient, who is laid supine in the head-down position, encourages spontaneous reduction. Try to gently reduce the hernia, making sure not to hurt the patient. There is a slight but real risk that you may reduce the hernia en masse: that is, the hernia remains within the peritoneal sac, the neck of which remains as a constriction, so the strangulation is not relieved. Some hernias reduce spontaneously when the patient is sedated prior to operation, or when anaesthesia is induced.

Prepare

1 Do not rush patients with strangulated hernias to the operating theatre. Make sure you know any reason (such as urinary outflow obstruction or a chest infection) why the patient has developed strangulation now. Identify coincidental disease that may make general anaesthesia and operation hazardous.

2 If strangulation has been present for some time, the patient requires fluid and electrolyte replacement. This takes priority over the operation. It is likely, in such cases, that bowel in the hernia will already be irreversibly ischaemic, so little is lost by the delay.

Access

1 The approach is open and identical to that for an elective operation.

Assess

1 If the history was short, the sac will frequently be empty by the time you expose it. The relaxation produced by the anaesthetic often succeeds when other conservative methods have failed to reduce a hernia. There is then no merit in exploring the abdomen. Repair the hernia as though this were an elective operation.

2 If bowel is present in the sac, do not let it slip back into the abdomen but gently draw it down into view. The bowel is likely to have suffered the greatest damage where it was trapped at the neck of the sac.

3 Feel the margins of the neck of the sac with a fingertip.

4 In Richter's hernia, a knuckle of the bowel wall is trapped. The bowel lumen is thus not obstructed but the knuckle may become gangrenous and perforate.

5 Maydl's strangulation is very rare. Two loops lie in the sac but the blood supply to an intermediate loop within the abdomen may be prejudiced so that it is gangrenous.

▶ KEY POINTS Is the bowel viable?

■ If there is a sheen to the bowel wall, if it is pink or becomes pink after release, if the arteries pulsate, if peristalsis is seen, replace the bowel with confidence.

■ If the wall is black, green or purple, with no sheen, if there is no pulsation in the mesenteric vessels or it is malodorous, resect it.

■ If the bowel is congested, bluish or plum-coloured and still has a sheen, but vascular pulsations cannot be felt, then its viability is doubtful. Remember, however, that blood extravasated subperitoneally cannot be reabsorbed immediately so the colour may not change. Cover the bowel with warm moist packs for 5 minutes and re-examine it. If it has improved in appearance and mesenteric arterial pulsations are palpable it is probably viable.

■ The critical areas are the constriction rings at the point of entrapment. These are white when the bowel is first drawn down but may be greenish or black if they are obviously necrotic. Re-examine doubtful rings after an interval to see if the blood supply returns. If it does not, the bowel must be resected. Occasionally it is possible to invaginate and oversew a doubtful ring.

■ Experienced surgeons probably resect bowel less frequently than those who are inexperienced. The mucosa is more vulnerable than the seromuscularis to the effects of ischaemia and, if the outer layers survive, the mucosa may slough to leave an annular ulcer. When this heals a constriction may develop – the intestinal stenosis of Garré. The patient presents after an interval of weeks or months with incipient small-bowel obstruction. Provided this is recognized, a simple elective resection can be carried out.

Action

1 If the neck of the hernia sac is constricted, first draw down healthy bowel, then place an index fingertip on each side of the contents, nails facing outwards. Gently dilate the neck of the sac (Fig. 6.3). Make sure the bowel does not slip back. Draw it out to ensure that there is no peritoneal constriction and to expose healthy bowel.

2 If the bowel is viable, return it to the abdomen.

3 If necessary, resect a gangrenous segment of bowel, performing an end-to-end anastomosis.

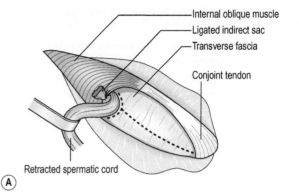

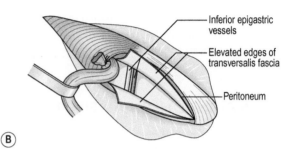

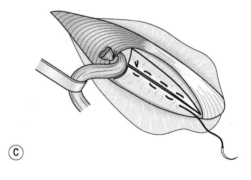

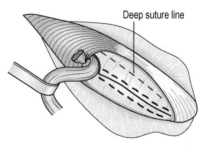

Fig. 6.3 Shouldice repair: (A) the broken line is the incision in transversalis fascia and around the internal ring; (B) the upper and lower flaps have been elevated; (C) the lower flap is sutured to the undersurface of the upper flap; (D) the upper flap is sutured over the lower flap. Finally, the conjoint tendon is sutured to the inguinal ligament.

Repair

After opening the sac and dealing with the contents, repair the hernia as though this were an elective operation, but if possible avoid the use of mesh if there has been bowel content spillage.

1. Sometimes the bulk of tissues contained in the hernial sac makes reduction seem impossible. Provided the margins of the neck are defined, gentleness, patience and persuasion will succeed. If only a little at a time is reduced do not despair, because the reduction must get progressively easier.
2. A large mass of fibrotic greater omentum may be adherent within the sac. Do not hesitate to excise the mass, provided the neck of the sac can be isolated, the bowel is not damaged and every blood vessel is safely ligated.
3. If gangrenous bowel slips back into the abdomen and cannot be recovered, repair the hernia, then open the abdomen through an appendix incision, following the terminal ileum proximally until the affected bowel can be delivered, wound protection applied and the gangrenous segment resected.

OPEN INGUINAL HERNIA REPAIR IN WOMEN

1. In primary inguinal hernias, prefer an open approach. The technique is similar to that employed in men. The sac is almost invariably indirect.
2. The round ligament of the uterus lies in the position of the male spermatic cord. Ligate and excise it at the level of the internal ring to allow closure of the latter.
3. Recognize and isolate the sac, then transfix, ligate and divide it at its neck.
4. If the hernial sac is small, herniotomy is sufficient, combined with closure of the internal ring. For a larger hernia, repair the posterior wall with a mesh as in a male.

OPEN INGUINAL HERNIA REPAIR IN INFANTS

1. Open surgery remains the approach of choice.
2. Infants' tissues are not suitable for handling by impatient or rough surgeons.
3. Make an incision in the skin crease just above the superficial inguinal ring. The well-developed deep fascia is easily mistaken for the external oblique aponeurosis.
4. The internal and external rings are almost superimposed in infants and it is therefore unnecessary to split the external oblique aponeurosis.
5. Isolate the cord just distal to the external ring, open the external fascial layers of the cord longitudinally and look for the sac. Pick up each layer with two pairs of fine artery forceps and open it between the forceps in the line of the cord. A short sac can be recognized by the white curved distal edge. The easy movement of the slippery internal surfaces of a large sac helps in identifying it. Make sure you are in the correct layer. When the sac is opened, the inner wall is shiny and the tips of the forceps can be passed into the peritoneal cavity.
6. Take great care in dissecting the fragile sac proximally; avoid tearing or splitting it or damaging the inconspicuous and adherent

vas deferens. The sight of extra-peritoneal fat confirms that the neck has been reached. If the hernia is complete (i.e. it extends down to the testis), do not dissect it distally. Carefully free it circumferentially just distal to the external ring, either from the outside if it is unopened or from within if it is open. Transect the sac, leave the distal end open and dissect the proximal sac. At the external ring, transfix, ligate and divide the neck of the sac. Do not twist the sac, because the vas may be inadvertently twisted with it and damaged.

7. In an infant or child with a small indirect hernia, herniotomy is all that is required. If the external ring has been stretched by a large hernia, narrow it with one or two absorbable synthetic stitches. No other repair is necessary in an infant. Do not use a mesh.
8. Close the subcutaneous layers with fine absorbable sutures. Close the skin with a fine absorbable subcuticular suture.

LAPAROSCOPIC INGUINAL HERNIA REPAIR

Prepare

1. Do not shave the abdomen.
2. Ensure that the patient empties the bladder before the operation. Do not routinely pass a urinary catheter. If preliminary laparoscopic assessment reveals that the bladder is full, pass a catheter before proceeding further with the operation.
3. Place the anaesthetized patient supine on the operating table with arms by the side as they sometimes interfere with the operation if they are folded across the chest.
4. Clean the abdomen with povidone-iodine 10% alcoholic solution or other antiseptic.
5. Drape the whole abdomen to give adequate exposure for the placement of port sites.
6. As the lead surgeon, stand on the side opposite the inguinal hernia, or the hernia which is largest (Fig. 6.4). An assistant and/or 'scrub' nurse stands on the other side (Fig. 6.5).
7. Position television monitors at the foot of the patient. Although one screen is sufficient, a second screen helps the assistant.

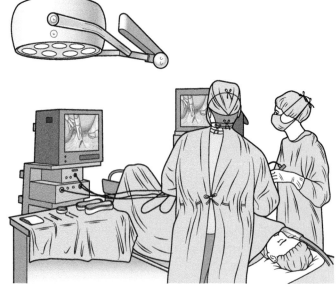

Fig. 6.4 Laparoscopic repair in progress.

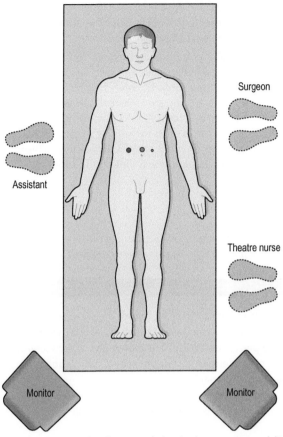

Fig. 6.5   The theatre plan for transabdominal pre-peritoneal (TAPP) repair.

8 Ensure that you can observe the carbon dioxide insufflator to monitor gas flow and intra-abdominal pressure.

9 Do not have a screen between you and the anaesthetist as this interferes with your manipulation of instruments.

TOTALLY EXTRA-PERITONEAL HERNIA REPAIR

Access

1 Make a transverse incision exactly 1.5 cm from the midline immediately below the umbilicus on the side of the hernia. Make the incision to the side of the larger of the hernias when bilateral hernias are to be repaired (Fig. 6.6).

2 Deepen the incision to the rectus sheath using small retractors to facilitate dissection.

3 Incise the rectus sheath for about 1 cm.

4 Identify the medial border of the rectus muscle and retract it laterally. Access has now been gained to the space within the rectus sheath.

5 In order to fashion a pre-peritoneal space, pass a 10-mm trocar and cannula with a balloon at its tip into the rectus sheath and guide it downwards until it reaches the pubic symphysis and then angle the tip to a position just behind the symphysis (Fig. 6.7).

> ▶ KEY POINT Caution
>
> ■ Take great care not to angle the cannula in such a way that it might damage the peritoneum and enter the peritoneal cavity, as carbon dioxide gas entering the peritoneal cavity could lead to difficulty maintaining access for TEP repair.

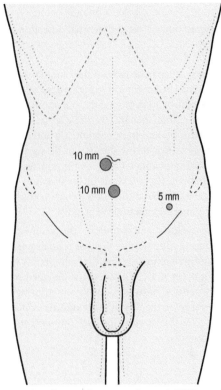

Fig. 6.6   Trocar sites for total extra-peritoneal (TEP) repair of right inguinal hernia.

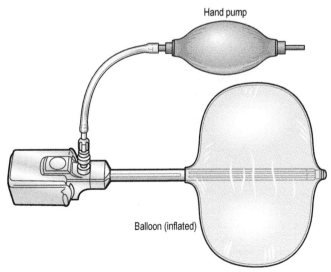

Fig. 6.7   An example of a disposable trocar. Prior to inflation, the balloon is placed through the subumbilical incision and used to initiate the dissection of the pre-peritoneal space.

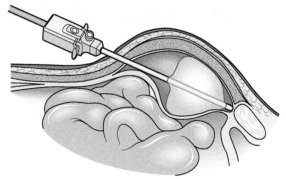

Fig. 6.8 A diagrammatic view of the initial dissection of the pre-peritoneal space.

6 Insert a 30 degree laparoscope into the cannula and maintain the tip of the cannula at a point immediately deep to the pubic bone. Gently inflate the balloon around the end of the cannula until the pubic bone is visible, thereby creating a space between the peritoneum posteriorly and the rectus muscle anteriorly. The lower edge of the posterior rectus sheath can be seen (arcuate line). Inflate the balloon under direct vision and resist the urge to pump the balloon up quickly as this will reduce the likelihood of bleeding. Ensure that the balloon inflates completely. Approximately 30 pumps are required (Fig. 6.8).

7 Deflate the balloon and withdraw the cannula. Replace the 10-mm cannula with another that has a small retaining balloon at its tip and inflate this so that the balloon sits just inside the rectus sheath (Fig. 6.9). The cannula is designed so that there is very little extension beyond the balloon, ensuring that the cannula does not get in the way of the two further cannulas that will be needed. Pass the laparoscope back into position through the umbilical cannula.

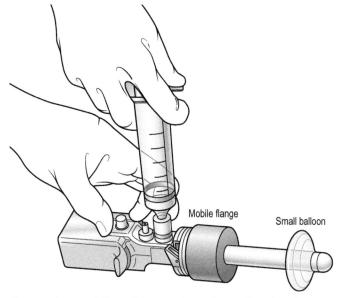

Mobile flange

Small balloon

Fig. 6.9 A second disposable cannula used to replace that shown in Figure 6.7 after the initial pre-peritoneal dissection has been completed. The small balloon at the tip of the cannula can be inflated to retain the cannula within the pre-peritoneal space. The mobile flange is passed distally along the cannula so that the abdominal wall is gripped between the distal balloon and the flange. The laparoscope is then passed through the trocar.

8 Attach the gas lead to the cannula and inflate with carbon dioxide up to a pressure of 8–10 mmHg. Note the partially created pocket in the pre-peritoneal space. Further dissection is now required.

9 Place a second 5-mm trocar and cannula under laparoscopic vision in the pre-peritoneal space already created using a 1-cm midline incision approximately three fingerbreadths below the umbilical cannula at the level where the posterior rectus sheath becomes deficient. This ensures that the second cannula is placed as high as possible in order to facilitate further dissection of the pre-peritoneal space, but is not placed too close to the umbilical cannula, which would cause technical difficulties.

Assess

1 Place a blunt-ended 5-mm dissector in the second (subumbilical) cannula and enlarge the pre-peritoneal space by blunt dissection.

? DIFFICULTY

If gas escapes into the peritoneal cavity via a small hole in the peritoneum, place a Veress needle in the left upper quadrant of the peritoneal cavity. This allows gas to escape and prevents distension of the peritoneal cavity, obscuring the view for TEP repair.

Convert to open repair or TAPP repair if a very large tear in the peritoneum prevents completion of TEP repair.

2 Clarify the anatomy. Note the pubic bone medially. Identify the inferior epigastric vessels, which are normally visible at this stage (Fig. 6.10).

3 Strip the peritoneum downward away from the anterior abdominal wall. Do not start at the internal ring but dissect laterally and medially first.

4 Commence the dissection laterally in the region of the anterior superior iliac spine and ensure that the epigastric vessels do not come down with the dissected peritoneal sac but remain up on the anterior abdominal wall.

5 Coagulate small blood vessels and do not rush this phase of the operation.

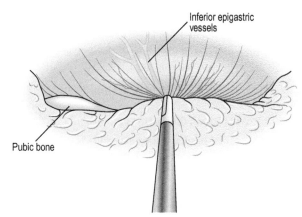

Inferior epigastric vessels

Pubic bone

Fig. 6.10 The dissecting instrument is stripping the intact peritoneal sac away from the anterior abdominal wall and the inferior epigastric vessels are in view.

6 Continue to strip the fat and areolar tissue and the peritoneal sac downwards and backwards in the lateral part of the dissection to reveal a portion of the psoas muscle.

7 Identify the pubic bone medially and gently strip the peritoneum down from this area. The bladder will be seen below the pubic bone near the midline and is gently stripped downwards and backwards. Look for the sac of a direct inguinal hernia, which will be seen attached to the white fold of transversalis fascia.

8 Note an indirect sac as it passes forwards into the internal ring close to the lower end of the inferior epigastric vessels.

Action

1 Create a space for an additional 5-mm cannula by enlarging the pre-peritoneal pocket by blunt stripping of the peritoneum away from the muscles of the anterior abdominal wall on the side of the hernia.

2 Identify the point of insertion by placing the scope near the abdominal wall and seeing the light shine through. Then insert a needle through the abdominal wall and confirm this by seeing it in the extra-peritoneal space. Inject some local at this time. Place the 5-mm trocar and cannula under laparoscopic vision at a point 2 cm medial to the anterior superior spine on the side opposite the hernia. Use this cannula to pass the 5-mm forceps.

3 Retract and free a direct hernia sac by stripping it away from the white fold of transversalis fascia using blunt and occasional scissors dissection. Make sure the sac is completely freed from its coverings and the pre-peritoneal space can be enlarged below it.

4 Turn your attention to the region of the internal ring.

5 Using a mixture of blunt and, if necessary sharp, dissection carefully dissect the tissues in the region of the internal ring and identify any hernia sac.

6 Grasp an indirect sac with the left-hand grasper and pull it backwards, stripping tissue away from it with the right-hand instrument. As you withdraw the sac place the right-hand forceps beyond the left-hand forceps and further retract the sac with the right hand using the left-hand instrument to strip tissue away from it. Large sacs can usually be withdrawn in this way (Fig. 6.11).

7 As the indirect sac is gradually withdrawn, look for the vas deferens or round ligament (passing medially) and the gonadal vessels (passing laterally). These structures are applied to the deep surface of the peritoneum at the internal ring.

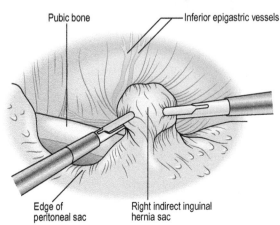

Pubic bone — Inferior epigastric vessels

Edge of peritoneal sac   Right indirect inguinal hernia sac

Fig. 6.11 The right indirect inguinal hernial sac is being retracted from the inguinal canal.

A very large indirect sac may be difficult to withdraw. Although transection of such a large sac with closure of the peritoneal defect may be possible, it may prove technically difficult. In case of technical difficulties convert to an open or TAPP repair.

8 Using blunt and sharp dissection separate the vas deferens and gonadal vessels from the peritoneum of the sac so that the latter can be fully withdrawn (Fig. 6.12).

9 When you have withdrawn the sac fully, strip the peritoneum back further from the internal ring to enlarge the pre-peritoneal pocket. The edge of the peritoneum should be at least 3–4 cm distant from the internal ring (Fig. 6.13).

10 Avoid injury to the iliac vessels, which lie deep to the triangle between the vas deferens and the gonadal vessels. Do not tamper with the fatty tissue deep to these structures as they protect you from damaging the iliac vessels

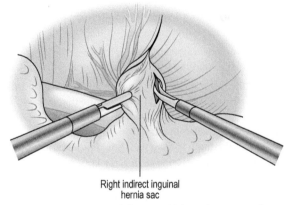

Right indirect inguinal hernia sac

Fig. 6.12 Using a mixture of sharp and blunt dissection, the sac is separated from the vas deferens and the spermatic vessels.

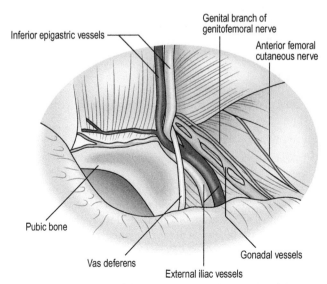

Inferior epigastric vessels

Genital branch of genitofemoral nerve

Anterior femoral cutaneous nerve

Pubic bone

Vas deferens

External iliac vessels

Gonadal vessels

Fig. 6.13 The anatomy of the groin has been displayed and the intact visceral sac has been stripped away from the interior of the groin.

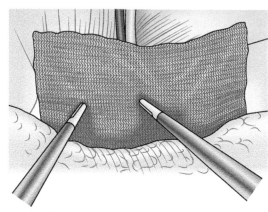

Fig. 6.14 The 15 cm × 10 cm mesh has been placed to cover the hernia defect and extends laterally from the midline. It is being held in place by two forceps as the extra peritoneal space is allowed to deflate. In this case, the mesh has not been stapled in place.

11 Prepare a similar pocket in the pre-peritoneal space on the opposite side if you are repairing bilateral hernias.

12 For unilateral hernias prepare a 15-cm × 10-cm patch of polypropylene mesh. To orientate the mesh correctly mark the long axis of the mesh by drawing a line on it.

13 Grasp the mesh with forceps and insert it into the pre-peritoneal space using the midline subumbilical cannula.

14 Position the mesh so that it covers the inguinal region from the midline, passing laterally for 15 cm. Ensure that it covers the region of the internal ring, the region medial to the inferior epigastric vessels and the femoral canal and that it reaches the midline. Ensure that the mesh is lying flat against the anterior abdominal wall and on the psoas muscle (Fig. 6.14).

15 Staple or glue the mesh in position. Do not leave it unfixed. If you are using staples, secure the lower medial part of the mesh to Cooper's ligament or the pubic bone first, then fix the upper border of the mesh to the abdominal wall. Do not place staples elsewhere.

16 Place a second mesh in a similar fashion if treating bilateral hernias. It is important that the right- and left-sided meshes overlap the midline.

Checklist

1 Check that there is no bleeding and control it with diathermy or clips.

2 Remove any staples that have fallen loose.

3 Place a large volume of low concentration local anaesthetic into the pre-peritoneal space.

Disconnect the insufflation and, as the pre-peritoneal space 'collapses', ensure that the mesh remains flat against the anterior abdominal wall. It is important that the lower edge of the mesh is not lifted up by the peritoneum as the pre-peritoneal space collapses.

4 Remove the cannulas and check that there is no bleeding.

5 Close the anterior rectus sheath as hernias can develop here. Close the skin incision with a single polypropylene 3/0 suture

TRANSABDOMINAL PRE-PERITONEAL INGUINAL HERNIA REPAIR

Access

1 Create a pneumoperitoneum using an open (Hasson) technique (see Chapter 5).

2 Make a vertical 1-cm incision from the centre of the umbilicus towards the symphysis pubis. Incise down to the rectus sheath. Open it to enter the peritoneal cavity under direct vision.

3 Insert a 10-mm blunt-tipped trocar and cannula into the peritoneal cavity under direct vision.

4 Attach the lead from the insufflator to the cannula and rapidly create a pneumoperitoneum up to a maximum pressure of 13–14 mmHg.

5 First 'white-balance' the video camera. Remove the trocar and pass a laparoscope into the cannula and into the abdomen. Prefer a 30-degree scope. Direct the laparoscope towards the groin.

6 Adjust the operating table so that the patient is positioned head-down and allow the intestines and omentum to fall away from the groin area to facilitate your view of the hernia orifice.

7 Under direct vision, create two new ports. Insert a 5-mm trocar and cannula at the level of the umbilicus lateral to the lateral border of the left and right rectus muscle (Fig. 6.15).

Assess

1 If adhesions obscure your view of the inguinal region, divide them carefully using scissors and diathermy. If they are very dense, consider conversion to open hernia repair.

2 Now establish the anatomy as it relates to the hernia (Fig. 6.16). Starting at the midline, identify the bladder and the median

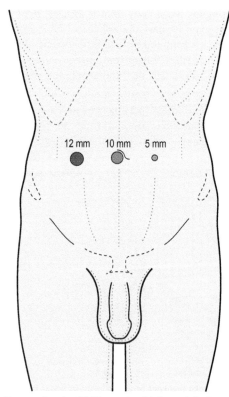

Fig. 6.15 Trocar sites for TAPP repair of left or right inguinal hernia.

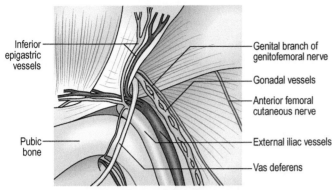

Fig. 6.16 The anatomy of the right groin in relation to TAPP repair. The shaded area has been called the 'triangle of doom' and is bounded by the vas deferens medially and the spermatic vessels laterally. In the floor of the triangle the external iliac vessels can be seen. The femoral nerve is not shown as it is on a deeper plane lateral to the vessels. The genitofemoral and anterior cutaneous nerve of the thigh are shown.

umbilical ligament (obliterated urachus) on the inner aspect of the lower abdominal wall. Check that the bladder is not full and catheterize the patient if it is.

3 Moving away from the midline, identify the medial umbilical ligament (obliterated umbilical artery). Immediately lateral to this is the area through which a direct inguinal hernia may pass. Lateral to this, note another ridge, the inferior epigastric vessels that form the lateral umbilical ligament. Lateral to this again is the internal ring through which an indirect inguinal hernia may pass.

4 Moving yet further laterally, compress the abdominal wall at the anterior superior iliac spine and note the lateral extent of the dissection for the TAPP repair.

5 Locate the region of the internal ring by looking for two divergent structures which emerge from it. Passing medially, particularly in thin patients, identify the vas deferens (round ligament of the uterus in females) beneath the peritoneum. Passing laterally from the internal ring is a less distinct ridge caused by the gonadal vessels. Between the diverging vas and the gonadal vessels is the 'triangle of doom' containing the external iliac vessels.

6 Identify whether the hernia is direct (medial to the inferior epigastric vessels) or indirect (lateral to the inferior epigastric vessels).

7 The steps involved in the repair of direct and indirect hernias are essentially the same. However, whereas a direct hernia sac is normally easy to retract, a large indirect hernia sac may be difficult to retract from the scrotum and may need to be divided at or distal to the internal ring. Check that there is not an unexpected hernia on the other side. Now decide whether your repair will be unilateral or bilateral.

8 Do not be alarmed if you find a sliding hernia, as you should not separate the colon from the peritoneal sac. The colon will be retracted with the sac when you are dissecting a pre-peritoneal pocket in which to place the mesh.

? DIFFICULTY

If you encounter any potentially dangerous and unexpected findings, such as a large iliac artery aneurysm, remove your instruments, deflate the abdomen.
Proceed to a standard open mesh repair.

Action

1 Ensure that any contents of the hernia sacs are reduced. Omentum adherent to the inside of the sac can be separated with scissors and diathermy. If the contents cannot be reduced laparoscopically, convert to an open repair.

2 Prepare a pre-peritoneal pocket between the peritoneum and the abdominal muscles in which to place the artificial mesh. The pocket should extend from the midline medially to approximately the level of the anterior superior iliac spine laterally. For bilateral hernias, pockets need to be fashioned on both sides and become continuous across the midline. A single large mesh or two individual meshes can be used for bilateral hernias.

3 Pick up the peritoneum 1–2 cm above the hernial orifice and make a short incision through the peritoneum using scissors with diathermy attached for haemostasis (Fig. 6.17). Gas may now enter the pre-peritoneal space and help to lift the peritoneum away from the underlying fascia and muscles.

4 Extend the incision laterally to a level below the anterior superior iliac spine, carefully avoiding the inferior epigastric vessels, and medially into the peritoneal fold of the medial umbilical ligament. It is seldom necessary to fully divide this ligament, which sometimes bleeds.

5 By blunt and sharp scissors dissection (with diathermy), separate the peritoneum below the initial incision away from the underlying fascia and muscle.

6 Deepen the pre-peritoneal pocket medially and laterally before separating the peritoneum from the internal ring where the peritoneum will be at its most adherent and there will be a risk of injury to the gonadal vessels and the vas deferens.

7 Strip the peritoneum medially downwards and inwards. In the case of a direct hernial sac it usually retracts out of the hernia orifice with traction and with a little blunt and sharp dissection so that the whole sac is freed from the transversalis fascia. The latter appears as a white fold attached to the sac. Identify the shining white appearance of the superior ramus of the pubic bone and gently strip the tissues downwards away from the pubic ramus, extending the dissection 1–2 cm beyond the midline. The bladder is seen below and behind the area of dissection.

8 Fashion the lateral part of the peritoneal pocket by stripping the peritoneum downwards and away from the abdominal wall. Below the level of the inguinal ligament, branches of the genitofemoral nerve may be seen lying on the psoas muscle and should be carefully preserved.

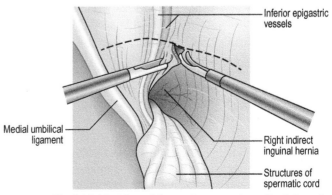

Fig. 6.17 The initial incision of the peritoneum above the internal opening of a right indirect inguinal hernia.

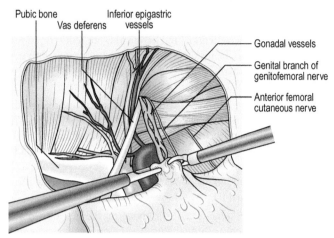

Fig. 6.18 The indirect sac has been withdrawn and the pre-peritoneal space prepared prior to insertion of the mesh in transabdominal pre-peritoneal (TAPP) repair.

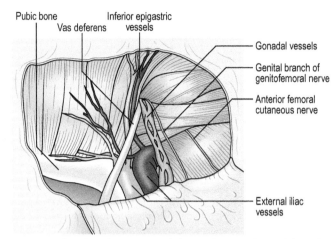

Fig. 6.19 The view during transabdominal pre-peritoneal (TAPP) repair immediately before positioning the mesh.

9 Now separate the peritoneum, or an indirect sac if present, from the structures at the internal ring (Fig. 6.18). If there is no indirect sac, separate the peritoneum, using a mixture of blunt and sharp dissection, from the vas deferens or round ligament passing medially and from the gonadal vessels passing laterally from the internal ring. The round ligament is often very adherent to the peritoneum and may be divided.

10 Retract an indirect sac or transect it if it is large. The sac lies anterior to the vas deferens and the gonadal vessels. Retract it progressively from the inguinal canal using a grasper held in the left hand. Control scissors in the right hand for blunt and sharp dissection, to strip away the coverings of the sac. As the dissection proceeds, look for the gonadal vessels laterally and the vas deferens medially. Dissect the peritoneum away from these structures.

11 A large sac is difficult to reduce, so transect it. Withdraw the sac partially into the abdomen and divide around its circumference, taking care posteriorly where the vas deferens and the gonadal vessels are closely applied. The distal sac retracts back into the inguinal canal. Dissect the transected proximal sac away from the gonadal vessels and vas deferens. Control bleeding with diathermy.

12 Transection of the indirect sac results in a hole in the mobilized peritoneum that requires closure when the mesh has been placed.

13 Now check that the depth of the pre-peritoneal pocket is sufficient to accommodate a 10-cm deep mesh extending for 15 cm from the midline laterally towards the anterior superior iliac spine. Divide any strands of tissue that would get in the way and prevent the mesh from lying flat (Fig. 6.19).

14 If you are repairing bilateral hernias, repeat the dissection of the pre-peritoneal pocket on the other side. The resultant pocket extends from one anterior superior iliac spine to the other. It is not usually necessary to divide the peritoneum above the bladder, nor is it necessary to divide either of the medial umbilical ligaments unless access is difficult.

15 Cut the synthetic mesh to the required dimension. For a unilateral hernia this is normally 15 cm × 10 cm. Bilateral hernias can be repaired using two separate 15-cm × 10-cm patches or by one large 28-cm × 10-cm mesh; this is stronger but more difficult to place. The latter is more difficult to orientate within the abdomen but is aided by cutting off the corners along one of the long sides of the mesh or by drawing a line on the mesh to indicate the long transverse axis.

16 Take hold of one corner of the mesh with a strong grasper and pass it through the 12-mm port under vision into the region of the pocket you have created.

17 Orientate the mesh so that it covers the groin from the midline to the anterior superior iliac spine within the pocket in front of the peritoneal flap, using graspers in each hand. Ensure that the mesh is lying flat and covers the hernial orifice.

18 If you are repairing bilateral hernias with a 28-cm × 10-cm mesh, pass it behind the midline peritoneum, which has been left undivided, and position it to lie flat and cover the relevant areas on both sides. Alternatively, place two 15-cm × 10-cm meshes meeting in the midline.

19 Most surgeons staple or glue the mesh in position. Take great care where you put staples. Place three to five staples spaced across the upper border of the mesh, attaching it to the abdominal muscles. Two or three staples may be used to fix the mesh to Cooper's ligament on the superior aspect of the pubic bone medially. No other staples are required (Fig. 6.20).

▶ KEY POINTS Anatomy

■ Never staple in the region of the lateral cutaneous nerve of thigh laterally.
■ Avoid the area around the femoral vessels and adjacent nerves.
■ Staples placed too low risk causing serious injury to the great vessels. Persistent genitofemoral neuralgia and even femoral nerve paralysis have been reported.

20 Cover the mesh with the peritoneum forming the pocket. Pick up the upper border of the peritoneum with a grasper in the left hand and staple the flap of peritoneum to the abdominal wall, covering the mesh completely. Alternatively, place a running suture between the peritoneum above the mesh and the free peritoneal flap. Ensure complete coverage of the mesh in order to avoid small-bowel adhesion and possible small-bowel obstruction (Fig. 6.21).

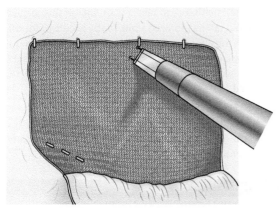

Fig. 6.20 The 15-cm × 10-cm mesh is being stapled into place. Note the three medial staples anchoring the mesh to Cooper's ligament and the pubic bone. Staples are also placed along the superior border of the mesh but nowhere else.

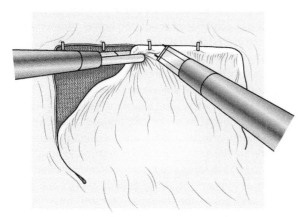

Fig. 6.21 The mesh is being covered completely by replacing the peritoneum.

21 Repair any hole in the peritoneal covering of the mesh either with staples or by suturing. Such a hole might permit small bowel to pass into the pre-peritoneal space you have created and give rise to small-bowel obstruction.

Check

1 Check that there is no bleeding. Control bleeding from damaged inferior epigastric and gonadal vessels using haemostatic clips. Gonadal injury is unlikely unless previous surgery has been performed, compromising alternative blood supply.

2 Remove any staples that have fallen loose.

3 Check that there are no defects in the peritoneal covering of the mesh. If the peritoneum is thin and tending to tear, staple the margins of the defect in the peritoneum to the mesh, thereby reducing the likelihood of small-bowel herniation.

4 If you have repaired a sliding hernia, carefully check that the colon has not been injured in any way.

5 Disconnect the insufflation and allow the abdomen to deflate.

6 Remove the 5-mm cannulas under direct vision and check that there is no bleeding. Control any bleeding and, in the case of unexpected brisk bleeding from the deep part of the port site, pass a

Foley catheter into the abdomen through the port site and blow up the balloon. Exert traction on the catheter, thus compressing the port site. The balloon can be left in position and removed later on the ward if necessary.

7 Do not remove the 10-mm cannula until the pneumoperitoneum has been evacuated lest a knuckle of small bowel be forced into the port site.

8 Close the rectus sheath in the 10-mm port sites using 2/0 multifilament synthetic absorbable sutures. Close the skin incisions with polypropylene 3/0 sutures.

FEMORAL HERNIA

Appraise

1 Repair all femoral hernias because of the high risk of strangulation.

2 One of the reasons for offering surgical repair freely is that an open operation can be accomplished easily using local anaesthesia.

3 Laparoscopic femoral hernia repair is not advocated as an alternative to open femoral hernia repair. A co-existing femoral hernia may be repaired at the same time as an inguinal hernia using the laparoscopic route.

4 Be aware of the prevascular femoral hernia; its neck extends laterally in front of the vessels.

5 Be skilled in each of the three current open approaches for femoral hernia repair (Fig. 6.22). They all have merits and they are all safe, provided the operation is skilfully performed. In general, the low approach is used for elective operations and McEvedy's for strangulated hernias.

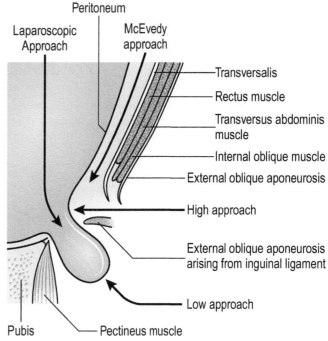

Fig. 6.22 Femoral hernia. A sagittal section through the hernial sac shows the various approaches.

LOW APPROACH (LOCKWOOD)

Access

1 Make an incision 4–5 cm long in the crease of the groin, below the medial half of the inguinal ligament.

2 Cut the superficial tissues over the hernia in the line of the skin incision. Look out for the small veins running into the long saphenous vein; ligate and divide them as necessary.

Action

Hernial sac

1 Expose the fat-covered hernial sac. Often, what appears to be a large swelling is mostly extra-peritoneal fat, in which lies a small sac. Clean the sac so that it may be traced proximally beneath the inguinal ligament.

2 Cautiously open the sac by incising it while it is held up between two artery forceps. Remember that the bladder may form the medial wall of the sac. Recognize the inside of the sac by seeing free fluid, a glistening surface and contents that may be reduced into the main peritoneal cavity.

3 Pick up the open edges of the sac with three equally spaced artery forceps, then sweep away the external fat to expose the neck, lying between the inguinal ligament anteriorly and the pectineal ligament posteriorly in the same horizontal plane. Note how deeply the neck of the sac lies.

4 Identify the femoral vein lying just laterally and preserve it from damage.

5 Empty the sac, transfix and ligate the neck with 2/0 absorbable suture; it should retract.

6 Excise the sac 1 cm distal to the ligature.

Repair

1 The inguinal and pectineal ligaments meet medially through the arched lacunar ligament. The object of the repair is to unite the ligaments for about 1 cm laterally, without producing constriction of the femoral vein (Fig. 6.23).

2 Use 2/0 monofilament nylon or polypropylene, on a small needle. Many use a J-shaped needle.

3 Place a small curved retractor over the femoral vein to protect it and draw it laterally. Insert a stitch deeply into the inguinal ligament and use this to draw the ligament upwards, while the needle

is insinuated behind it, to take a good bite of the pectineal ligament. Avoid taking too deep a bite or the needle point will break as it strikes the pubic crest. One, two or three stitches may be used but, for ease of access, insert all the stitches before tying any. As the stitches are tightened, ensure that the femoral vein is not constricted.

4 Alternatively, the femoral canal may be occluded with a 'plug' of rolled mesh, secured with three sutures. This technique is simpler to perform, less likely to result in compression of the femoral vein and less prone to recurrence.

? DIFFICULTY

1. *Can you not identify the sac in the fatty lump?* Remember that most of the lump may be pre-peritoneal fat. Gently and carefully incise it and separate it. When the peritoneum is incised you can usually see glistening visceral peritoneum or lobulated omental fat. If the sac contains free fluid it appears bluish and may be confused with the appearance of congested bowel. When the sac is carefully incised the fluid escapes, revealing the contents.

2. If you inadvertently tear the neck of the sac, gently free peritoneum from the peritoneal cavity so that it can be drawn down to form a new neck.

3. If the femoral vein is torn, control the bleeding with pressure from gauze packs for 5 minutes. Meanwhile, order blood, arterial sutures, tapes, bulldog clamps and heparin solution, and summon assistance. Expose the vein; do not hesitate to approach it from above and below the inguinal ligament. Apply bulldog clamps and tapes above and below the damaged segment. Insert fine 5/0 sutures set 1 mm apart, 1 mm from the torn edges, to evert them and close the hole. Flush with heparin at intervals. Release, then remove the clamps and tapes.

4. It is not possible to suture the whole of a prevascular defect. Insert a piece of mesh and suture the opening medial to the vein.

Closure

Unite the subcutaneous tissues with fine absorbable stitches and close the skin, preferably with an absorbable subcuticular suture.

HIGH APPROACH (LOTHIESEN)

Appraise

1 The advantage of this approach is that it can be used for repairing co-existing inguinal and femoral hernias.

2 For femoral hernia alone it has the disadvantage that it damages the inguinal canal and could lead to a subsequent inguinal hernia.

Access

1 Expose the inguinal canal and dislocate the cord, as for operation for inguinal hernia.

2 Incise the transversalis fascia.

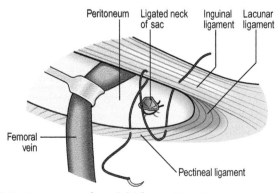

Peritoneum   Ligated neck   Inguinal   Lacunar
             of sac   ligament   ligament

Femoral vein

Pectineal ligament

Fig. 6.23   Low approach to right femoral hernia.

Action

Hernial sac

1 Identify the neck of the sac and the external iliac vein.

2 Isolate the neck of the sac and gently withdraw the fundus. If there is difficulty, have the lower skin flap retracted downwards, incise the cribriform fascia and isolate, open and empty the sac from below.

3 Ensure that the sac is empty and that the bladder is not adherent, then transfix, ligate and divide the neck of the sac.

Repair

1 With the index finger, feel the margins of the femoral canal. In front is the inguinal ligament, medially the lacunar ligament, posteriorly the pectineal ligament and laterally the femoral vein.

2 Narrow the triangular gap by inserting non-absorbable sutures of 2/0 monofilament nylon or polypropylene between the pectineal ligament and the inguinal ligament.

3 If the upper approach was selected because there is also an inguinal hernia, deal with an indirect sac now.

4 Either close the incision in the posterior wall transversalis fascia with a non-absorbable suture or carry out a mesh Lichtenstein repair.

Closure

Close the inguinal canal, subcutaneous tissue and skin as for an inguinal hernia.

McEVEDY'S APPROACH

Appraise

1 Use this approach for strangulated hernias as it provides excellent access for assessment of bowel and if necessary for resection.

2 The skin incision, as originally described, left an ugly scar, but this can be avoided by placing it more horizontally.

3 A urinary catheter inserted preoperatively, reduces the risk of damage to the bladder.

Access

1 Make an incision from 3 cm above the pubic tubercle running obliquely upwards and laterally for 7–8 cm, crossing the lateral border of the rectus muscle, which lies more vertically. Reflect the skin flaps so as to display the lateral part of the rectus sheath.

2 Incise the lower rectus sheath about 1–2 cm from, and parallel to, its lateral border. The lateral edge may tend to separate into its two anatomical layers.

3 Lift the lateral edge of the sheath and incise the thin transversalis fascia from about 2.5 cm above the pubic tubercle to mobilize the lower lateral edge of the rectus medially. Ligate and divide the inferior epigastric vessels which cross this line low down. The neck of the hernia is now in view as it enters the femoral canal.

Action

1 Retract the lower skin flap and isolate the sac.

2 Reduce the sac, manipulating it from above and below. Open and empty it, then transfix, ligate and divide the neck of the sac.

3 For a strangulated hernia (which is the reason for using this approach) the peritoneum may be opened above the neck to facilitate assessment of the bowel and any necessary resection.

4 Repair the canal from above.

5 Close the incision in the rectus sheath with 0 nylon or polypropylene.

6 Appose the subcutaneous layers and close the skin.

UMBILICAL HERNIA

ADULT UMBILICAL HERNIA

Appraise

1 Most hernias in adults are para-umbilical, protruding adjacent to the cicatrix. The contents are most frequently omentum, which is often adherent to the interior of the sac.

2 Some adults, especially of African origin, have true umbilical hernias that have been present throughout life.

3 Repair umbilical hernia by early operation for fear of strangulation. In particular operate on strangulated, painful (reducible or not) hernias, especially those with small, hard margins. However:
  ■ Small para-umbilical hernias (less than 1 cm) can be left untreated if asymptomatic.
  ■ Many patients are grossly obese and elderly, with cardiovascular or respiratory disability and a longstanding hernia that has not been troublesome. Adjure such patients to lose weight and hesitate before offering operation.
  ■ Ascites may provoke umbilical hernia. Find the cause and treat it. In some cases there is extensive malignant disease, when surgery is rarely indicated.

4 An open or laparoscopic approach can be used. With an open approach a mesh is placed either extra-peritoneally, deep to the abdominal wall, or as an onlay mesh anterior to it, often in association with a traditional double breasted 'Mayo's repair'. With a laparoscopic approach the mesh is secured intra-peritoneally against the defect with staples or sutures. For small primary umbilical hernias an open approach is recommended. For recurrent or periumbilical incisional hernias a laparoscopic approach may be considered.

5 In large hernias which distort the entire umbilicus, the possibility of excising and refashioning the umbilicus should be discussed preoperatively.

OPEN ADULT UMBILICAL HERNIA REPAIR

Access

1 Make a curved incision in the groove above or below the hernia. If necessary extend the cut transversely outwards on each side, for 2–4 cm.

2 Deepen the incision, identify the aponeurosis and expose it around the adjacent half of the circumference of the hernia.

3 If the hernia is small, preserve the umbilical skin by dissecting it off the hernia as a flap. If the hernia is large, make a spindle-shaped incision to include the umbilicus, excising the stretched skin.

4 Expose 2 cm of aponeurosis around the remainder of the margin of the hernia.

Action

1 Cut through the thinned-out edge of aponeurosis to expose the peritoneum and gradually work round to display the whole circumference of the neck of the sac.

2 Clear the sac of fatty tissue and cut it right round, at least 2 cm distal to the neck if possible. The contents of the sac are less likely to be adherent here than in the fundus, but free them if necessary. Mark the peritoneal edges with artery forceps.

3 If the contents of the sac are free, reduce them. If they are adherent to the fundus of the sac, free them and return them to the peritoneal cavity. If there is a mass of fibrous omentum, excise it with the fundus of the sac but take care to ligate all the bleeding omental vessels and avoid damaging the transverse colon.

4 Separate the peritoneum from the under-surface of the rectus sheath all round, without tearing it.

5 Close the peritoneal neck of the sac with a continuous 2/0 synthetic absorbable suture, producing a transverse linear suture line.

Repair

Extra-peritoneal mesh repair

1 For the underlay repair of a small, well-defined direct defect, take a piece of polypropylene mesh 2 cm larger in diameter than the defect. At each quadrant insert a 2/0 polypropylene suture through the intact tissue about 8 mm from the edge of the defect, pick up a small bite of the mesh and pass the needle back out through the intact tissue of the posterior wall, close to the point of entry. Hold the suture with an artery forceps and repeat the manoeuvre at each quadrant of the defect. Then parachute the mesh through the defect into the extra-peritoneal space and tie the four sutures. Additionally, suture the edge of the defect to the surface of the mesh with continuous polypropylene.

2 Throughout the procedure, ensure that the peritoneum is not breached, as placing 'ordinary' mesh in contact with abdominal wall contents increases the risk of adhesions and fistulation. If this occurs, consider converting to a Mayo's repair with onlay mesh placement.

Mayo's repair (Fig. 6.24)

1 Consider this repair if the peritoneum has been breached, or the wound is possibly contaminated, as in urgent cases. If this is likely consider avoiding an adjunct onlay mesh.

2 Attempt the repair staying in the extra-peritoneal approach, but often the peritoneum is breached.

3 Place a series of horizontal mattress sutures using 0 or 1/0 polypropyline sutures, without tying them. Each stitch penetrates the upper leaf of the rectus sheath 3 cm from the edge, passes beneath it to catch the lower leaf 1 cm from the edge and passes back 3 cm from the edge. When the stitches are tied they draw the lower leaf underneath the upper leaf.

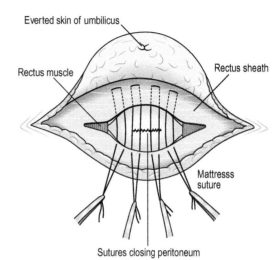

Fig. 6.24 Mayo's repair.

Onlay mesh repair

1 Place the mesh over the defect, the peritoneum having been closed as above. Secure the mesh into good tissue with 2/0 polypropylene sutures allowing a 2-cm margin.

2 Consider using a vacuum drain, as this procedure with its undermining of the skin and placement of a foreign body is at risk of seroma formation. Remove the drain early if there is no leakage.

3 In all repairs instil local anaesthetic into the wound.

Closure

1 If the skin over the fundus was preserved, pick up the undersurface of the navel with a synthetic absorbable stitch and sew it to the rectus sheath to produce a dimple. Suture the skin as a curved line above or below the newly fashioned umbilicus.

2 If the umbilicus was excised, close the subcutaneous fat and the skin as a transverse suture line.

? DIFFICULTY

1. The hernia may be a true umbilical one, hidden within the cicatrix.
2. Divide the upper or lower edge of the cicatrix to find it.
3. If present, the congenital defect will be obvious and can be closed with interrupted non-absorbable sutures or a Mayo's repair.

LAPAROSCOPIC UMBILICAL HERNIA REPAIR USING INTRA-PERITONEAL ONLAY MESH

Appraise

Intra-peritoneal onlay polypropylene mesh in contact with the viscera of the abdominal cavity adheres to omentum and bowel because of its macroporous nature. The risk of enterocutaneous or intra-abdominal fistula from intra-peritoneal placement of polypropylene mesh is reduced by ensuring omental coverage. Use composite meshes in large defects, but they are more expensive. Addition of polyglactin to the polypropylene mesh does not reduce adhesions, although coating with titanium significantly reduces its inflammatory reaction. Polytetrafluoroethylene, as a composite with polypropylene with the polytetrafluoroethylene side in contact with the viscera, significantly lowers the incidence of adhesions.

Preparation

1 Place the anaesthetized patient supine on the operating table with their arms by their side.

2 Clean the abdomen with povidone-iodine 10% alcoholic solution or other antiseptic.

3 Drape the whole abdomen to give adequate exposure for the placement of port sites.

4 Stand on the same side as the assistant and/or 'scrub' nurse. Position television monitors on the opposite side of the patient. Sometimes with mesh placement it is easier to move around the patient and so it is therefore useful to have a monitor on both sides.

Access

1 Obtain access in an area away from any previous incision and away from the hernia, both of which are usually in the midline. Previous incisions may have adhesions or bowel adherent to them, presenting an inherent risk of damage, so gain access to the abdominal cavity as far back laterally as is safe on the insufflated abdomen. Use either an open (Hasson) technique or a closed technique using a Veress needle. The left subcostal area is often suitable for initial insufflation with a Veress needle.

2 Insert a 10-mm trocar and cannula through the initial incision as described, far back laterally on the abdomen. Use a 'Visi' port if possible, as entry can be watched.

3 Remove the trocar and introduce a laparoscope through the cannula into the abdomen.

4 Assess the abdomen and select a suitable position to insert a 5-mm trocar and cannula to the left of the laparoscope and another 5-mm trocar and cannula further left of the laparoscope, both under direct vision (Fig. 6.25).

5 Place ports to access midline hernias either on the right and/or the left of the abdomen, depending on your preference. Add an extra-port if access is difficult.

Assess

If adhesions obscure your view of the hernia, divide them carefully using scissors and diathermy.

> ? DIFFICULTY

If initial access to the abdomen is difficult, try placing a 5-mm trocar and cannula in the left subcostal position, then select suitable positions for the lateral insertion of the trocars and cannulas into the abdomen under direct vision.

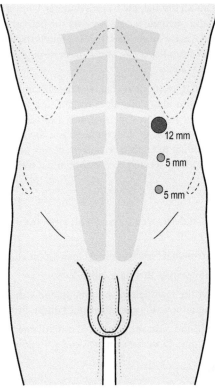

Fig. 6.25 Trocar sites for intra-peritoneal incisional hernia repair.

> ▶ KEY POINTS Respond to potential difficulties

- Giant incisional hernias and those resulting in a substantial abdominal wall defect are probably better converted to open surgery.
- If adhesions are very dense, consider conversion to open hernia repair.
- Convert to open surgery if bowel is adherent within the hernia.

Continue to divide any adhesions to allow visualization of the anterior abdominal wall for an area large enough to enable placement of a flat mesh of sufficient size. Adhesions around the neck of the hernia are often very adherent and may bleed.

Action

1 Define the margins of the hernia defect and ensure that any adhesions are cleared for at least 5 cm from the edge of the hernial defect.

2 Reduce the contents of the hernia sac using graspers and diathermy scissors. If this is not possible, convert to an open repair.

3 Leave the peritoneal sac in situ. It is very difficult to dissect a sufficiently large pre-peritoneal pocket into which a mesh can be placed in such a way that it is extra-peritoneal.

4 Assess the size of mesh required to give a minimum of a 4-cm overlap of the hernial defect on all sides. Cut the mesh in a circle shape to give an equal overlap on all sides. Mark the centre of the mesh with a marker pen to aid orientation inside the abdomen and ensure you position it centrally over the hernia defect.

5 Insert the mesh through the 12-mm cannula. Unfold it, using two graspers, and orientate it centrally over the hernial defect, ensuring equal coverage on all sides. This is sometimes helped by passing a suture from the centre of the mesh through the umbilicus. Remove this later.

6 Make sure that the mesh lies flat over the abdominal wall. Staple it into position along all sides. Try and use absorbable tacks. Although they are more expensive and more difficult to handle, they reduce the risk of adhesions. If you are inserting a large mesh, be willing to apply a second inner row of staples around the defect to fix it securely to the abdominal wall.

Checklist

1 Is the hernial defect well covered with mesh overlapping at least 4 cm all round?

2 Check any residual bleeding, using laparoscopic clips if necessary.

3 Remove any staples that have fallen loose.

4 Disconnect the insufflation equipment, allow the abdomen to deflate and remove the cannulas under direct vision.

5 Close the 12-mm port site using a 2/0 multifilament synthetic absorbable suture. Close the skin incisions with polypropylene 3/0 sutures.

INFANTILE UMBILICAL HERNIA

Appraise

1 Repair infantile umbilical hernia via an open approach.

2 Most infantile umbilical hernias protrude through the incompletely closed cicatrix. They occur more frequently in infants of African origin. Most of them close spontaneously without surgical repair, especially if the neck is less than 2 cm in diameter, so wait for 1–2 years. Repair them only if they increase in size.

3 Infants infrequently develop a supra-umbilical hernia. It will not close spontaneously, so repair it locally through a transverse incision sited directly over the defect.

Access

1 Approach the hernia through a transverse incision curved beneath the everted umbilicus.

2 Preserve the umbilical skin by turning it upwards as a flap.

Action

1 Expose the aponeurosis and the neck of the sac, which is within the cicatrix. The separation is much easier than in acquired hernias.

2 Open the sac, empty it, then close it by suture or transfixion ligature.

Repair

1 Edge-to-edge repair of the aponeurosis is effective.

2 Make sure the peritoneum is separated sufficiently to allow good bites of sheath to be taken, without piercing the peritoneum.

3 Create a transverse suture line using polypropylene or nylon, inverting the knots.

Closure

1 Suture the deep surface of the umbilical skin to the aponeurosis with fine absorbable synthetic material.

2 Close the skin to leave a curved transverse wound, using an absorbable subcuticular stitch.

OMPHALOCELE

Carry out closure with the minimum delay after birth; otherwise infection supervenes and the neonate will die (see Chapter 34).

UMBILICAL INFECTIONS, TUMOURS, FISTULAS AND SINUSES

Appraise

1 Neglected or imperfectly treated umbilical sepsis in infants can progress to septicaemia, distant pyogenic infections, pylephlebitis, liver suppuration and fatal jaundice.

2 An enteroteratoma is the remnant of the vitellointestinal duct forming a raspberry tumour. Cauterize it to destroy the mucosa.

3 Persistent discharge from the umbilicus in infants, children and young adults is likely to result from a congenital abnormality. An MRI (magnetic resonance imaging) scan may show the connecting track:

- *Congenital faecal fistula* results from persistence of the whole vitellointestinal duct. Faecal staining may be temporary if the fistula closes spontaneously. If there is distal obstruction, relieve this at the same time as closing the fistula.

- *Patent urachus* is persistence of the allantois (Greek: allos = sausage + eidos = form) usually associated with membranous obstruction of the urethra. Deal with the urinary obstruction at the time of closing the fistula.

4 In adults, infection is often the result of aggregated keratin forming an 'omphalolith' (Greek: lithos = stone), which can be lifted out of a deep umbilicus without anaesthesia. Persistent omphalitis stimulates granulation tissue, treated by cautery. Recurrent infections may require a minor plastic procedure to reduce the depth of the umbilicus.

5 The umbilicus is a rare site for pilonidal sinus, treated by excision.

6 Endometrioma at the umbilicus classically bleeds at the time of the menses.

7 Squamous epithelioma may develop at the umbilicus and subsequently can involve the inguinal lymph nodes. Excise the umbilicus and, if indicated, carry out bilateral block dissection of the inguinal nodes (vide infra).

8 Secondary carcinoma from the liver or porta hepatis may reach the umbilicus along the ligamentum teres. This presents as Sister Joseph's nodule (first noticed by an observant nun and immortalized by the famous surgeon and author Hamilton Bailey 1894–1961).

9 A port-site metastasis may occur after laparoscopic surgery for malignancy.

EPIGASTRIC HERNIA AND PORT-SITE HERNIA

Appraise

1 In an epigastric hernia a small knuckle of extra-peritoneal fat insinuates itself through a vascular opening in the linea alba. It rarely has a peritoneal sac or contains bowel.

2 Port-site hernias occur after laparoscopic surgery. Repair is similar to that for epigastric hernia.

3 Laparoscopic repair is an alternative to the open operation, but for small hernias has no advantages.

Action

1 Make a transverse incision through the skin and deepen it down to the herniated fat.

2 Define the margins of the defect and reduce the hernia. If there is a peritoneal sac, simply invaginate it into the peritoneal cavity.

3 Suture a small (less than 1 cm) defect with a good rim using non-absorbable stitches, inverting the knots. Otherwise place a piece of polypropylene mesh 2 cm larger than the defect in each direction in the extra-peritoneal plane and secure it, as described for the underlay repair of a well-defined inguinal defect.

4 Close the skin, using a synthetic, absorbable subcuticular suture.

INCISIONAL HERNIA

Appraise

1 Incisional hernia is a deep disruption of the abdominal wound while the superficial layers remain intact (if the superficial layers also separate then a burst abdomen results).

2 Herniation may occur early, while the patient is still in hospital. More usually it develops during the following months or years.

3 Incisional hernias are associated with careless suturing, the use of rapidly absorbable instead of non-absorbable material, haematomas and infection, the insertion of drains through the main incision and damage to abdominal nerves. Jaundice, malnutrition, obesity, postoperative distension and re-exploration through the same incision after a short interval are other contributory factors, as are steroids and immunosuppression. Incisional hernia may follow delayed healing of a laparostomy.

4 Incisional hernias rarely strangulate; therefore do not rush to re-operate. Repairs have a high recurrence rate, reduced by the use of mesh, but this increases the risk of persistent infection or intestinal fistula.

5 If the patient is overweight, advise reduction before surgery. Ensure that infection has completely resolved before proceeding.

6 If mesh is to be used, give perioperative antibiotic cover.

7 Laparoscopic mesh repair is an alternative.

OPEN INCISIONAL HERNIA REPAIR

Appraise

1 Large defects are best repaired using a composite mesh to reduce the risk of bowel adhesions (see laparoscopic umbilical hernia repair, above). Infected defects can be repaired using biological meshes such as Permacol or Strattice (Lifecell Corporation) but these are very expensive.

Access

1 Excise the old scar.

2 If the skin and peritoneum are fused, excise an ellipse of skin wide enough to expose subcutaneous tissue.

3 Dissect back the skin on each side until unscarred subcutaneous tissue is reached beyond the margins of the defect.

Action

1 Deepen the incision until you reach aponeurosis or muscle, then work towards the margins of the defect.

2 Dissect the edges cleanly and separate the peritoneum from the deep surface all around unless you intend placing mesh intra-peritoneally.

3 If possible, invaginate the sac with a continuous suture. However, adherent contents and a narrow neck may require that the sac be opened to achieve reduction; if practicable close it.

4 Multiple defects in the abdominal wall ('buttonhole tears') are most conveniently managed by uniting them and repairing the resulting larger defect.

5 The cavity from which the sac has been stripped out often oozes, so meticulously apply haemostasis to minimize the risk of haematoma or seroma formation.

Repair

1 There is no advantage in attempting to define the layers of the abdominal wall.

2 Suture small defects, less than 4 cm, using non-absorbable material (0 or 1 G), but this does introduce tension adjacent to the repair so it is suitable only if the edge is strong.

3 Large defects, or poor tissue, are best repaired with a synthetic patch, to avoid a recurrence rate of 40–50%. The mesh may be applied at three levels in the abdominal wall, as described below (Fig. 6.26). Wherever it is placed it must extend at least 2 cm beyond the margin of the defect.

4 There are also methods that attach a piece of mesh to each side of the defect and then suture the two together or sandwich the abdominal wall between two layers of mesh.

Action

Onlay patch repair

1 This is the simplest method, placing a patch anterior to the aponeurosis and the defect, which may or may not have been sutured. Polypropylene mesh is most suitable as it is rapidly incorporated in scar tissue. It should extend 4 cm beyond the edge of the defect.

2 Secure the edge of the mesh with interrupted 2/0 polypropylene sutures at 2-cm intervals, reinforced with a continuous over-and-over stitch.

3 Place another continuous suture to fix the mesh where it lies over the edge of the defect. This is important to prevent herniation of bowel beneath the mesh.

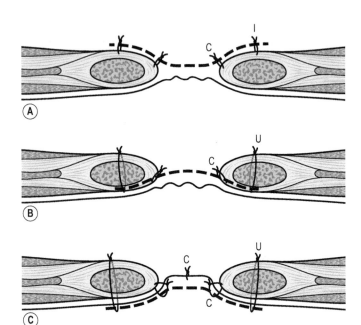

Fig. 6.26 Three alternative levels for placement of mesh in incisional hernia repair: (A) onlay; (B) extra-peritoneal; (C) intra-peritoneal. Transverse section through abdominal wall. i, interrupted sutures; c, continuous suture; u, 'U' sutures.

Extra-peritoneal mesh repair

1 This is suitable for midline hernias.

2 The peritoneum, plus the posterior rectus sheath if above the arcuate line, is dissected off the posterior aspect of the rectus muscle laterally and from the aponeurosis in the midline, for about 3 cm.

3 Polypropylene mesh will incorporate more rapidly but polyester is easier to position as it can deform on the bias.

4 Cut a piece of mesh 2 cm larger than the defect at each margin.

5 The mesh is drawn into the space deep to the abdominal wall by interrupted 'U' sutures of 2/0 polypropylene at 2-cm intervals. Each passes in through the anterior rectus sheath and rectus, picks up the edge of the mesh and returns to be tied externally.

6 Then suture the margin of the defect to the surface of the mesh with a continuous over-and-over suture.

Intra-peritoneal mesh repair

1 Open the sac and free any adhesions for 4 cm around the rim.

2 Cut a piece of polyester mesh 2 cm larger than the defect in each direction (polypropylene is liable to cause dense intestinal adhesions).

3 Draw the margin of the mesh under the rim of the defect with a series of 'U' sutures of 2/0 polypropylene. These penetrate the peritoneum 2–3 cm from the rim. First place four cardinal sutures and hold them with forceps, adjusting the size of the mesh so that it fits the opening. Then insert more 'U' sutures at 1-cm intervals between one pair of cardinal sutures and tie these. Repeat this for the other three sections.

4 Pick up the mesh and the overlying rim with a continuous over-and-over suture, taking care to avoid the bowel.

CLOSURE

1 Drain the large subcutaneous space with one or two suction drains. The tubing tends to curl up in one corner; prevent this by tunnelling the tube under the fascia at one or two points.

2 Appose the subcutaneous fat.

3 Close the skin with an absorbable subcuticular suture.

Aftercare

1 Leave the drains until the daily loss is less than 30 ml.

2 Any subsequent collection should be aspirated, with sterile precautions.

3 In the event of a wound infection, do not rush to remove the mesh, almost inevitably resulting in re-herniation; it may survive.

SPIGELIAN HERNIA

Appraise

1 Described by Adriaan van der Spieghel (Spigelius) of Padua (1578–1625), herniation is at the lateral margin of the lower rectus sheath and often expands beneath the external oblique aponeurosis.

2 Repair may be by open operation or laparoscopically. The latter facilitates accurate diagnosis.

Action

1 At open operation, make a skin crease incision over the lump and open the external oblique aponeurosis in the line of its fibres, extending the incision medially to open the anterior rectus sheath.

2 Once dissected, invert the sac and develop the pre-peritoneal space, allowing a check along the lateral edge of the rectus for other defects. Then place a mesh extra-peritoneally. The layers of the abdominal wall can usually be closed without tension using a 0 Prolene suture.

PARASTOMAL HERNIA

Appraise

1 Stomas leave weak areas in the abdominal wall. The whole area around the stoma may bulge diffusely or a segment of bowel may herniate. In addition, the stoma itself may prolapse.

2 Some parastomal hernias can be accepted, in particular diffuse hernias that are not troublesome, since they are unlikely to produce obstruction.

3 Re-siting the stoma, usually on the opposite side of the abdomen, is an effective treatment but involves a laparotomy and has a high rate of re-herniation.

4 The best method is to repair the hernia with polypropylene (or Vypro) mesh, either at laparotomy or by a local approach through a curved skin incision lateral to the stoma.

5 The mesh may be placed either extra-peritoneally or on the outside of the abdominal wall. Cut a hole in the mesh for the bowel, with a slit to enable it to be inserted without detaching the stoma from the skin. The slit is then sutured. The risk is wound infection, minimized by antibiotic prophylaxis and by sealing the stoma with plastic film.

NON-HIATAL DIAPHRAGMATIC HERNIA

Appraise

1. Neonatal diaphragmatic hernia must be repaired immediately because the lungs cannot expand since the chest cavity is filled with abdominal viscera. It is generally diagnosed on ultrasound scan before delivery so that specialist paediatric care can be arranged. There is no hernial sac because the defect is the persistent pleuroperitoneal canal – the hernia of Bochdalek (Vincent Bochdalek 1801–1883, Prague anatomist).

2. Adults occasionally present with acute obstruction within a persistent pleuroperitoneal canal, almost always on the left side. It may also follow thoracoabdominal surgery.

3. Reduction from below is easy, unless the abdominal viscera are adherent within the chest.

Action

Persistent pleuroperitoneal canal (hernia of Bochdalek) in adults:

1. By whatever approach is favoured, reduce the abdominal viscera.

2. Trace out the margins of the defect and close it using non-absorbable sutures. The margins usually come together more easily than anticipated.

Hernia of the foramen of Morgagni

1. An abdominal approach is best for this rare hernia, which passes between the costal and xiphoid slips of the diaphragm.

2. Define and repair the defect.

Eventration of the diaphragm
(Latin: e = out + venter = belly; protrusion of the belly)

1. A thinned-out leaf of the diaphragm is found, with good muscle at the periphery.

2. Plicate the diaphragm by gathering up a fold and suturing the base of the fold. Lay the fold flat and stitch it down flat, using non-absorbable suture material.

Traumatic hernia

1. An abdominal approach is usually satisfactory and the viscera can be replaced within the abdomen, but a laparoscopic approach is beneficial for postoperative respiratory function in patients who may have lung injury from the trauma.

2. The margins of the defect are nearly always easy to define and repair using non-absorbable suture material.

3. Laparoscopic tensioning of the knots is facilitated by use of braided non-absorbable sutures. Buffers do not appear to be necessary.

LUMBAR HERNIA

Appraise

1. This may emerge spontaneously through the triangle of Petit (Jean Louis Petit 1674–1741, Parisian surgeon), bounded by the iliac crest, the posterior edge of the external oblique and the anterior edge of the latissimus dorsi muscles.

2. Lumbar hernia complicates renal incisions in the loin, drainage of lumbar abscess, trauma or paralysis of the muscles in the lumbar region.

3. Operative repair is rarely required.

OBTURATOR HERNIA

Appraise

1. This is rare. Most occur in females aged over 50 years, and on the right side.

2. Most are admitted with small-bowel obstruction, which, at operation, is discovered to be from an obturator hernia, sometimes of Richter's type. A possible clinical clue is radiation of pain down the inner thigh to the knee. CT is diagnostic.

3. If diagnosed preoperatively it can be repaired laparoscopically by extending the pre-peritoneal TAPP (transabdominal pre-peritoneal hernia) or TEP (totally extra-peritoneal hernia) dissection inferiorly to include the obturator canal.

Action

1. Assuming the operation is being performed for intestinal obstruction and the small bowel is found to be tethered in the region of the obturator canal, improve the access by carrying the incision down to the pubis. A catheter should already be draining the bladder.

2. Identify the canal with the nerve entering it from the anteromedial aspect; the artery is posterolateral.

3. Gently free the bowel and inspect it to determine if it is viable.

4. Either make no attempt to repair the defect or suture peritoneum over a mesh patch.

GLUTEAL AND SCIATIC HERNIA

Appraise

1. Gluteal hernia emerges above or below the pyriformis muscle through the greater sciatic notch.

2. Sciatic hernia emerges through the lesser sciatic notch.

3. These hernias are usually discovered at exploratory laparotomy for intestinal obstruction and rarely produce a palpable swelling in the buttock.

PELVIC FLOOR HERNIA

This may occur spontaneously, accompanying a cystocele, rectocele or rectal prolapse. It most frequently follows surgery of the pelvic floor, including abdominoperineal resection and hysterectomy.

INTERNAL HERNIA

Appraise

1. Internal hernias present as intestinal obstruction. Most follow abdominal or abdominothoracic operations, the most common mechanism being a band adhesion. Intestine may herniate

behind an anterior gastroenterostomy, through a transverse mesocolic defect following posterior gastroenterostomy or beside an abdominal stoma if the lateral space is not closed.

2 Internal hernias also occur at anatomical openings, such as the foramen of Winslow (Jacob Winslow 1669–1760, Danish anatomist) or the paraduodenal fossae, and through defects in the falciform ligament, the mesentery or the broad ligament. Think before dividing the 'band', as it may contain an important structure such as the portal triad! After dealing with the bowel the defect must be closed.

HAEMATOMA OF THE RECTUS SHEATH

Appraise

1 A sudden strain may rupture one of the inferior epigastric vessels entering the lower rectus abdominis muscle, producing pain. It is more common in patients who are anticoagulated.

2 On the right side, the localized pain and tenderness may be misdiagnosed as appendicitis. However, the patient does not have systemic or gastrointestinal symptoms, pyrexia or leucocytosis. Furthermore, the local tenderness in the right iliac fossa is greater when the patient puts the muscles under tension.

3 Ultrasound or CT (computed tomography) confirms the diagnosis and management is then conservative.

4 If you operate thinking the patient has appendicitis and discover a haematoma lying behind the lower rectus muscle, evacuate it. If there is a suspicion of continuing bleeding, isolate and ligate the inferior epigastric vessels in continuity.

ABDOMINAL WALL SEPSIS

WOUND INFECTION

Appraise

1 Wound contamination and haematoma are the major factors leading to wound infection. Following abdominal surgery a variety of organisms may be responsible. Multifilament stitches may perpetuate a wound infection, so prefer monofilament materials for non-absorbable sutures.

2 Prophylaxis for potentially contaminated wounds comprises perioperative antibiotics, scrupulous haemostasis in the abdominal wall and covering the wound edges with Betadine (povidone-iodine)-soaked swabs or plastic wound protectors.

3 The infection may be a localized wound abscess or an abscess occupying the whole wound, with or without surrounding cellulitis, or there may be cellulitis without an abscess (yet). The wound is hot, red and swollen and the patient is pyrexial and may be toxic.

ACTION

1 The mainstay of treatment is drainage. Often it is possible to achieve this on the ward by removing a suture from the softest part of the wound, followed by probing with forceps. If the wound has discharged spontaneously, consider enlarging the opening to provide adequate drainage. Where an absorbable

subcuticular suture has been inserted, cut it. This risks inadvertently opening up the whole wound. It can be prevented by inserting a skin suture under local anaesthesia, on either side of the site of the opening. Be prepared to open the whole length of the wound for a severe infection. Always send a specimen for bacteriology.

2 Normally, do not administer antibiotics for wound infection unless there is cellulitis or the patient is already septic or at risk from immune deficiency, cardiac disease or prosthetic heart valves.

3 Sometimes when you open the wound you discover severe tissue necrosis. Do not then make the error of leaving a small hole and inserting a drain (see Necrotizing fasciitis, below).

4 Following drainage of a wound abscess, a chronic stitch sinus may persist. Explore the sinus with a pair of fine, sterile mosquito forceps, or a sterile crochet hook, to extract the stitch if possible. If the sinus persists, explore it under local or general anaesthesia to remove the suture material. Usually you find a knot of non-absorbable suture material. If you remove it now you may weaken the whole wound. Delay the removal for up to a year.

SYNERGISTIC SPREADING GANGRENE

Appraise

1 This is usually named after Meleney, the New York surgeon who described it in 1933. When it affects the scrotum it is called Fournier's gangrene (Jean Fournier 1832–1914, Parisian dermatologist). It may result from the synergistic effects of a number of micro-organisms, or from a single organism.

2 The nature of an operation or injury, and the patient's general condition, may predispose to the condition. Exclude diabetes, immunosuppression, uraemia and hepatic disease.

3 It develops as a slowly extending area affecting the whole thickness of the skin. The advancing edge is typically serpiginous and leaves dead, sloughing skin that separates to expose unhealthy granulation tissue.

Action

1 Start the patient immediately on broad-spectrum antibiotics, such as a cephalosporin and metronidazole, pending the result of bacteriology.

2 The essential action in controlling the infection is to excise all the necrotic tissue, exposing healthy, clean tissue. Leave the wound open and dress it frequently, repeating the excision of any developing necrotic tissue.

3 When the infection has been completely controlled, plan to resurface the denuded area with partial thickness skin grafts.

NECROTIZING FASCIITIS

Appraise

1 This spreading gangrene primarily affects the abdominal fascia. It may follow surgical operations or injury. It is predisposed to by general disease, particularly diabetes. Subsequently the overlying

skin is also affected, but the skin involvement may not indicate the extent of the fascial infection. The mortality rate is 30%.

2 Management is with broad-spectrum antibiotics and immediate radical excision of all the necrotic tissue to leave healthy living tissue (in the limbs this may involve amputation).

GAS GANGRENE

Appraise

1 Clostridial infection of abdominal wounds is remarkably rare, considering that the organisms can be recovered from normal faeces.

2 The patient rapidly develops pyrexia, toxicity and hypotension.

3 The discoloured wound edges are crepitant and may discharge thin pus, described as smelling 'mousy'.

Action

1 Administer 1 million units of benzylpenicillin and continue high doses thereafter.

2 As far as possible, and as rapidly as possible, correct the patient's general condition.

3 Under general anaesthesia radically excise the whole area, back to clean, living tissue. Thoroughly wash the raw area with hydrogen peroxide (20 vols).

4 Hyperbaric oxygen at 3 atmospheres has been recommended.

DESMOID AND OTHER ABDOMINAL WALL TUMOURS

Appraise

1 Desmoid tumours are non-encapsulated tumours that develop in the muscle intersections. They are classified as fibromatoses. Hyperplastic connective tissue infiltrates locally, but does not metastasize. Most occur in women, especially those who have borne children. Remove abdominal wall desmoids completely or they recur.

2 Patients with familial adenomatous polyposis may also develop desmoids within the abdomen. These generally surround the mesenteric vessels and so are irremovable.

3 Carcinoma of intra-abdominal structures may directly invade the abdominal wall. If the tumour is otherwise resectable do not hesitate to excise a portion of the abdominal wall en bloc with the primary neoplasm.

Action

1 Concentrate on excising the tumour with adequate clear margins and depth. In the case of a desmoid tumour do not fail to cut through healthy muscle and connective tissue all the way round.

2 If the abdominal wall is invaded from its deep surface, excise the peritoneum and the deep part of the muscle wall, but leave intact the superficial muscle layer. Do not attempt to repair the defect, which will peritonealize.

3 Close a small full-thickness defect layer by layer.

4 A large defect can often be closed by creating a flap of anterior rectus sheath based on its medial edge to swing to the opposite side, or a layer of lateral muscle may be swung over.

5 If you cannot close the defect with muscle or aponeurosis, the best alternative is to use a myocutaneous flap from the chest or thigh. Unless you are skilled in preparing such flaps, obtain the help of a plastic surgery colleague.

6 If you are completely unable to close the defect, consider inserting a polypropylene mesh or other plastic sheet until you can obtain help and advice.

7 When you cannot close the skin defect by any other means, create a large skin flap based laterally that you can slide over to cover the defect, applying split skin grafts to the donor site.

BLOCK DISSECTION OF GROIN LYMPH NODES

Appraise

1 Radical groin dissection is carried out for resection of proven or suspected malignant lymph nodes.

2 In general surgery, the operation is employed most frequently to excise metastatic melanoma deposits from primary sites in the leg, perineum and gluteal regions.

3 The inguinal nodes may be involved by epidermoid carcinoma of the external male or female genitalia, or of the anal skin. In these cases the nodal dissection is usually accomplished in continuity with excision of the primary lesion.

INGUINAL NODES

Access

1 Make a linear incision, 2.5 cm below and parallel to the inguinal ligament.

2 Alternatively, make a spindle-shaped incision, so that skin overlying involved glands can be excised en bloc.

Action

1 Raise the upper skin flap so that the superficial and deep fascia can be incised 2–3 cm above and parallel to the inguinal ligament to display the lower fibres of the external oblique aponeurosis. Sweep the connective tissues downwards, leaving the lower portion of external oblique stripped clean.

2 Dissect the lower flap to reach the fascia lata over the lateral edge of the sartorius muscle and incise it here, preparing to sweep it medially with the superficial fascia. Look for, and preserve if possible, the lateral and intermediate cutaneous nerves of the thigh.

3 At the medial border of the sartorius muscle, the dissection extends into the femoral triangle as you display in turn the femoral nerve, femoral artery and femoral vein. In the groin, identify, doubly ligate and divide the superficial circumflex iliac, superficial epigastric and superficial external pudendal vessels, to avoid tearing their junctions with the main vessels.

4 Ligate and divide the saphenous vein at the lower extremity of the clearance and again as it joins the femoral vein, so that you remove the segment within the femoral triangle with the specimen.

5 Sweep the superficial tissues and lymph nodes medially as far as possible then incise the fascia lata vertically over the adductor magnus muscle.

6 The specimen is still attached by the fat and lymphatic tissue entering the femoral canal. Gently draw down the lymph node lying within the canal and remove it with the specimen.

Closure

1 Insert one or two suction drains.
2 Close the skin.

ILIAC NODES

This dissection may be made in continuity with the inguinal node dissection, before or after the groin clearance.

Access

1 For a combined approach, make a vertical incision, starting superiorly at the midpoint of a line joining the umbilicus and anterior superior iliac spine and finishing inferiorly at the apex of the femoral triangle. The incision follows a gentle 'S', lest a future contracture restrict hip movements.

2 Alternatively, perform a laparoscopic iliac node dissection.

Action

1 Enter the iliac region through the inguinal ligament, by dividing the ligament over the femoral canal or detaching it from the pubic tubercle.

2 Incise the external oblique, internal oblique and transversus abdominis muscles 1–2 cm above and parallel to the inguinal ligament, so that the inguinal ligament can be swung laterally.

3 Doubly ligate and divide the inferior epigastric vessels.

4 Sweep up the intact peritoneum from the iliac vessels, making sure that the ureter remains attached to the peritoneum and is thus preserved from damage. Divide the obliterated umbilical artery.

5 Starting in the hollow of the sacrum, sweep out the connective tissue and lymph nodes from the iliac vessels and their branches, including the obturator vessels and nerve. Remove glands along the obturator vessels and nerve and at the obturator foramen.

6 Strip out the loose tissue and lymph nodes from the femoral canal.

Closure

1 Re-attach or repair the inguinal ligament and abdominal muscles. Insert one or more suction drains.
2 Close the skin.

Aftercare

1 Minimize oedema of the leg by elevation then mobilize in a supporting stocking.
2 Remove the suction drains when the loss is less than 30 ml/day.

Appendix and abdominal abscess

D.E. Whitelaw, N.J. Ward

CONTENTS

OPEN APPENDICECTOMY

Appraise

1 Acute appendicitis is essentially a clinical diagnosis. A detailed history and careful examination of the patient carry more weight in making the diagnosis than embarking on radiological investigations, although these investigations can be useful to rule out alternative diagnoses.

2 Although appendicectomy is still the most common reason for laparotomy, remember the following:
   - Young children and the elderly may have atypical presentations of appendicitis and also have a higher mortality and morbidity from this condition.[1]
   - Female patients may have a gynaecological cause for pain and tenderness in the right iliac fossa rather than appendicitis. Order a pelvic ultrasound scan and consider carrying out a diagnostic laparoscopy in such cases.
   - There is good evidence that in female patients, appendicitis, even when perforated, does not adversely affect fertility, so you need not perform a mandatory appendicectomy in equivocal cases.[2]
   - Although elderly patients do develop appendicitis, consider other pathology such as perforating carcinoma of the caecum and diverticulitis, which may mimic its presenting features. In case of doubt, use a midline incision so you can carry out a full examination of the peritoneal cavity.
   - Computed tomography (CT) is the most sensitive imaging technique for diagnosing appendicitis.[3] In view of the radiation dose, reserve this investigation for those in whom a negative laparotomy represents an unjustifiable risk.

3 Tend to treat conservatively a patient with symptoms for 5 or more days in whom you find a mass in the right iliac fossa. Give a 7-day course of intravenous antibiotics such as co-amoxiclav and metronidazole, withhold oral feeding and replace fluid intravenously. Mark the extent of the mass on the abdominal wall. Perform an ultrasound or CT scan to exclude the presence of a large abscess that can be drained percutaneously. Carefully monitor the patient and perform an operation only if:
   - The mass increases in size despite antibiotics
   - The patient develops features of bowel obstruction or peritonitis
   - The patient develops worsening toxaemia or septic shock.

As a rule, in patients over the age of 40 years, order a barium enema X-ray, CT colography or colonoscopy when the mass has settled to exclude caecal carcinoma. It has been conventional practice to re-admit patients for 'interval' appendicectomy 1–2 months later, but the number of patients developing recurrent appendicitis is small, so it may be justifiable to defer operation indefinitely, but warn the patient to seek medical attention if symptoms recur.

4 Some surgeons carry out diagnostic laparoscopy whenever they suspect appendicitis, proceeding to laparoscopic appendicectomy if the diagnosis is confirmed.

5 Avoid removing a normal appendix incidentally during other operations, such as cholecystectomy. It is a possible cause of complications such as wound infection and subsequent adhesive intestinal obstruction.

PREPARE

1 Wound infection is the most common complication following operation for acute appendicitis, so routinely give 500 mg of metronidazole and a broad-spectrum antibiotic (e.g. co-amoxiclav) intravenously at induction of anaesthesia.

2 In patients with clinically severe acute appendicitis who are demonstrating signs of systemic sepsis, commence intravenous metronidazole and a broad-spectrum antibiotic as soon as the decision to operate is made.

3 Patients who have a perforated appendix require a full 5-day course of broad-spectrum antibiotic and metronidazole.

> ▶ KEY POINTS Antibiotic usage
>
> - Where the diagnosis of appendicitis is equivocal, avoid starting antibiotic therapy, as this will mask developing signs and symptoms of the disease, thus making surgical exploration mandatory. Antibiotics should only be commenced once the decision to operate has been made.
> - Traditionally, cephalosporins have been combined with metronidazole for treatment of intra-abdominal sepsis. They have, however, been linked with antibiotic-associated infective colitis and many hospitals have now developed guidelines discouraging the widespread use of cephalosporins. Always use local prescribing guidelines when choosing antibiotic therapy, or consult with a microbiologist.

■ Always re-examine the abdomen when the patient is anaesthetized. You may feel the inflamed appendix in the relaxed abdomen, which was impalpable beforehand. This is a valuable general rule before any abdominal operation, and may help you determine the best site for the incision.

Access

1 As a routine employ a Lanz incision in a skin crease. This modification of the gridiron incision transversely crosses McBurney's point – the junction of the middle and outer thirds of a line joining the anterior superior iliac spine and the umbilicus. The incision starts 2 cm below and medial to the right anterior, superior iliac spine and extends medially for 5–7 cm. It may be possible to site it lower in a young girl so that the scar lies below the waistline of a bikini.

2 Alternatively, use the traditional gridiron incision, 5–8 cm long, in line with the external oblique fibres if you anticipate the need to extend the exposure (Fig. 7.1). The incision crosses McBurney's point at right-angles to the spino-umbilical line, one-third above, two-thirds below. If necessary, the external oblique muscle and aponeurosis can be split in both directions and the internal oblique and transversus muscles can be cut to convert the incision into a right-sided Rutherford Morrison incision.

3 If appendicitis is one of a number of likely diagnoses, opt for a lower midline incision.

Opening the abdomen

1 Incise the skin cleanly with the belly of the knife. Divide the subcutaneous fat, Scarpa's fascia and subjacent areolar tissue to expose the glistening fibres of the external oblique aponeurosis. In the gridiron approach these fibres run parallel to the skin incision.

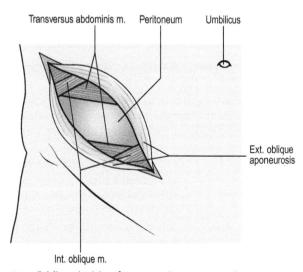

Transversus abdominis m.   Peritoneum   Umbilicus

Ext. oblique aponeurosis

Int. oblique m.

Fig. 7.1   Gridiron incision for appendicectomy. In the Lanz modification the skin incision is transverse but the abdominal muscles are similarly split in the line of their fibres.

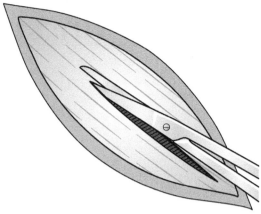

Fig. 7.2   Appendicectomy. Regardless of which skin incision is used, the external oblique aponeurosis is split by pushing partly closed scissors in the line of the fibres.

2 Stop the bleeding. Incise the external oblique aponeurosis in the line of its fibres. Start with a scalpel, then use the partly closed blades of Mayo's scissors (Fig. 7.2) while your assistant retracts the skin edges.

3 Retract the external oblique aponeurosis to display the fibres of the internal oblique muscle, which run at right-angles. Split internal oblique and transversus abdominis muscles, using Mayo's straight scissors (Fig. 7.3). Open the blades in the line of the fibres and use both index fingers to widen the split. Provided the scissors are not thrust in violently, the transversalis fascia and peritoneum are pushed away unopened.

4 Stop the bleeding. Have the muscles retracted firmly to display the fused transversalis fascia and peritoneum.

5 Pick up a fold of peritoneum with toothed dissecting forceps and grasp the tented portion with artery forceps. Release the dissecting forceps and take a fresh grasp to ensure that only the peritoneum is held. Make a small incision through the peritoneum with a knife. Allow air to enter the peritoneal cavity, so that the viscera fall away. Use scissors to enlarge the hole in the line of the skin incision. Now protect the wound edges with swabs or skin towels.

Assess

1 Look. Is there any free fluid or pus? If so, take a specimen for microscopy and culture.

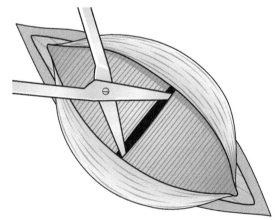

Fig. 7.3   Appendicectomy. The internal oblique muscle is split by opening Mayo's straight scissors in the line of the fibres.

2 Find the caecum, identify a taenia and follow it distally to the base of the appendix. Insert a finger and lift out the appendix by pushing from within, not by pulling from without.

> ▶ **KEY POINT** Manipulate the inflamed appendix with care

> ■ Never pull on the appendix if the distal end is stuck. If it is gangrenous it will tear and release infected material into the peritoneal cavity. Improve your view if necessary by extending the incision.

3 If the appendix is not evident, push your index finger posteriorly until it comes to lie on the peritoneum over the psoas muscle. Then, maintaining contact with the posterior peritoneum, draw your finger to the right until it can go no further. The caecum should now lie between the 'hook' of your finger and the right limit of the iliac fossa, and may be gently pushed out onto the surface. In some cases you may need to mobilize the caecum by incising the parietal peritoneum in the paracolic gutter, in order to raise the caecum on its mesentery, especially if the appendix is adherent retro-caecally. If the caecum is not evident, remember that it sometimes lies quite high, under the right lobe of the liver.

> ? **DIFFICULTY**

> There is no appendix? In a small number of patients there is no appendix, either because it did not develop or because it has been digested or has atrophied as a result of previous inflammatory disease. In this case, what is the cause of the patient's symptoms? Carry out a search for disease of nearby organs (see below).

4 Confirm the diagnosis: the appendix, or more usually its tip, is swollen, congested, inflamed, even gangrenous, often with fibrin deposition, turbid fluid or frank pus.

> ? **DIFFICULTY**

> 1. If the appendix is not inflamed, examine its tip to exclude a neuroendocrine (carcinoid) tumour, which usually manifests as a yellowish swelling at the tip; such tumours are common, with low malignant potential, and appendicectomy may well be curative. Adenocarcinoma of the appendix, however, demands a right hemicolectomy.
> 2. Examine the caecum, since an ulcer, inflammation or cancer may present as appendicitis. Pass the distal 1.5 m of the ileum and its mesentery through your fingers to exclude mesenteric adenitis, Crohn's disease or Meckel's diverticulum. Palpate the posterior abdominal wall, ascending colon, liver edge and gallbladder fundus and the lower pole of the right kidney. Now feel below into the right rim of the pelvis, the bladder fundus, right iliac vessels and right inguinal region. In females examine the right ovary and fallopian tube, and attempt to feel the uterus and left ovary and tube.

> 3. Look for features of a distant cause such as bile-stained fluid tracking down from a perforated peptic ulcer, an inflamed gallbladder or gynaecological pathology. Be prepared to close a standard Lanz incision and make a fresh, well-placed incision, rather than struggle to deal with the problem by extending or stretching the incision in the right iliac fossa. The presence of free purulent fluid is an indication to embark on wider examination of the abdominal contents.

Action

1 Mobilize the appendix from base to tip by gently moving or peeling away adherent structures. Remember that the artery enters from the medial aspect. If the tip is adherent, improve the view. Do not dissect blindly. If necessary, extend the incision. Apply Babcock's tissue forceps to enclose, but not grasp, an uninflamed portion of the appendix, to hold it so you can view the mesentery against the light and identify the artery.

2 Pass one blade of the artery forceps through the mesoappendix and clamp the vessels (Fig. 7.4). If it is thickened, take the mesoappendix in two bites. Divide the mesoappendix distal to the clamp and ligate the vessel gently but firmly with 2/0 Vicryl or similar material, ignoring the slight back bleeding from the distal cut end.

3 Crush the base of the appendix with a haemostat then replace the clamp 0.5 cm distal to the crushed segment. Ligate the crushed segment with 2/0 Vicryl. Apply a haemostat to the ligature ends after trimming them.

4 Cut off the appendix just distal to the haemostat.

5 There is no need to invaginate the appendix stump by use of a purse-string suture, nor should the appendix stump be diathermized.

> ▶ **KEY POINT** Sterility

> ■ Stop! You have entered the bowel. Place the appendix, held by the Babcock's forceps, together with the knife, into a kidney dish for contaminated articles.

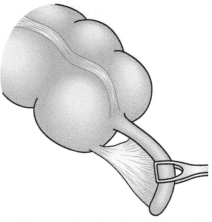

Fig. 7.4 Appendicectomy. Clamping the mesoappendix. The appendix is held up with tissue forceps.

1. If you cannot carry out the steps of the operation safely you must improve the exposure by extending the wound in the line of the skin incision laterally. Extension of the wound medially may encroach on the inferior epigastric vessels but once you enter the rectus sheath you can retract the rectus muscle medially.

2. If you cannot free the tip of the appendix, it is sometimes helpful to carry out retrograde appendicectomy. Crush, clamp and ligate the base of the appendix before dividing it. Now the base is free you will be better able to follow it to the tip.

3. If the appendix bursts in spite of gentle manipulations, remove it and look to see if a faecolith has escaped. Wash out any escaping material using saline lavage and suction. If there has been any contamination, consider inserting a drain into the superficial tissues, since the peritoneal cavity usually copes well with contamination provided the cause is removed.

4. If the base of the appendix is oedematous and fragile, do not attempt to crush it. If possible, carefully ligate it and divide it 5 mm distally. If it appears unsafe to insert a purse string, look for a piece of omentum or other peritoneum to draw over the stump and stitch it to a healthy piece of caecal wall.

5. If gangrene extends on to the caecal wall, first apply a non-crushing clamp gently across the bowel to limit contamination. Resect the gangrenous part to reveal healthy wall that can be closed with a suture line. If the hole cannot be closed, insert a large tube drain into the caecum and suture the edges of the bowel to the skin as a caecostomy. The stoma will close spontaneously in most cases when the tube is removed after 2 weeks.

6. If there is Crohn's disease and the appendix is not inflamed, do not carry out any procedure.

7. If you find an abscess, drain it but do not explore further or pursue a search for a buried appendix within the cavity. It will most probably be destroyed by the inflammatory reaction.

8. In the presence of purulent peritonitis, carry out appendicectomy. Now gently remove pus and debris and drain the wound. Instil copious saline lavage to cleanse the abdomen.

Closure

1. Pick up the edges of the peritoneum around the entire incision with fine haemostats to allow easy and safe suturing of the opening with continuous 2/0 Vicryl or similar material.

2. Insert interrupted stitches of the same material into the internal oblique muscle with just enough tension to appose but not strangulate the muscle fibres. Now close the external oblique aponeurosis with a continuous Vicryl stitch.

3. Apply povidone-iodine solution to the wound once the peritoneum is closed.

4. Appose the subcuticular tissues with fine sutures in an obese patient and close the skin with a continuous absorbable subcuticular suture or clips.

Postoperative

1. In the absence of general peritonitis, start oral fluids and a light diet as tolerated when the patient is fully awake.

2. If the appendix was perforated, and particularly in a high-risk patient, continue antibiotics for 5 days. These should be given intravenously until gut function returns.

3. Remove any drain after 2–3 days unless there is still profuse discharge.

4. Monitor the wound if pyrexia develops, and exclude chest and urinary infection.

Complications

1. Wound infection develops occasionally in patients with mild appendicitis but has a higher incidence in those who have had a gangrenous or perforated appendix removed. Anaerobic *Bacteroides* and aerobic coliform organisms are usually responsible. Examine the wound regularly and remove some of the skin suture or clips if there is evidence of infection, to allow any pus to drain. Check the results of any microbiological investigations taken at the time of surgery and tailor antibiotic therapy accordingly.

> **KEY POINT** Explain to the patient what was done
>
> ■ If you decided not to remove the appendix, ensure that you explain this to the patient. A future clinician, seeing a scar in the right iliac fossa, may wrongly assume that the appendix has been removed and attribute clinical features to other organs.

2. If pyrexia develops, always carry out a rectal examination. Pelvic infection produces localized heat, 'bogginess' and tenderness. Repeat the examination at intervals to detect if an abscess develops and 'points': be willing to aspirate it using a needle inserted through the vagina or rectum. If needle aspiration confirms the presence of an abscess, gently thrust closed, long-handled forceps into the cavity to drain it into the rectum. Ultrasound or radiological imaging may help if you are uncertain and may allow percutaneous drainage of a collection.

3. Reactive haemorrhage is infrequent, but occasionally the ligature falls off the appendicular artery. Return the patient to the operating theatre and re-open the wound to catch and re-ligate the artery.

4. Faecal fistula develops in two circumstances. Either the patient has unsuspected Crohn's disease or in florid appendicitis the appendicular stump or adjacent caecum has undergone necrosis. In the presence of necrosis do not over-optimistically rely on suturing the defect. Prefer to insert a large tube in the hole and suture the margins of the hole to the anterior abdominal wall where the tube emerges. The tube can be removed after 2 weeks and the fistula will heal spontaneously.

REFERENCES

1. Blomqvist PG, Andersson RE, Granath F, et al. Mortality after appendectomy in Sweden, 1987–1996. Ann Surg 2001;233: 455–60.
2. Andersson R, Lambe M, Bergstrom R. Fertility patterns after appendicectomy: historical cohort study. Br Med J 1999;318:963–7.
3. Paulson EK, Kalady MF, Pappas TN. Suspected appendicitis. N Engl J Med 2003;348:236–42.

LAPAROSCOPIC APPENDICECTOMY

Appraise

1. Most hospitals now have advanced laparoscopic equipment available and as a result the majority of appendicectomies are performed laparoscopically,[1] which has been shown to be as efficacious as open appendicectomy even for the treatment of complicated appendicitis.[2] Advantages claimed are decreased wound infection, reduced postoperative pain, better cosmesis and accelerated recovery, especially in obese individuals.[3] Laparoscopy also allows detailed pelvic and abdominal examination, which is particularly valuable in young women where preoperative diagnostic accuracy is low.

2. However, increased technical difficulty, longer operating time and increased risk of intra-abdominal abscess may offset these potential advantages.[1,4,5]

3. There are no absolute contraindications, and relative contraindications are the same as for other laparoscopic procedures.

> ### ▶ KEY POINTS Clinical diagnosis
>
> - In patients with equivocal symptoms and signs, repeated clinical examination is the mainstay of diagnosis.
> - Minimize negative laparotomy or laparoscopy rates.

Prepare

1. Obtain informed consent for both laparoscopic and open appendicectomy. Administer parenteral metronidazole and broad-spectrum antibiotics during anaesthetic induction.

2. Laparoscopic appendicectomy requires general anaesthesia with endotracheal intubation and muscle relaxation.

3. Place the patient supine. In females, the lithotomy position allows preoperative vaginal examination. You and your assistant stand on the patient's left side with the monitor on the right. The nurse also stands on the right, towards the foot end of the table.

4. Catheterize the urinary bladder to reduce risk of injury.

> ### ▶ KEY POINTS Examine the abdomen again
>
> - Re-examine the abdomen when the patient is anaesthetized.
> - The presence of a mass suggests likely technical difficulty but does not contraindicate a trial of laparoscopy.

Access

1. There is a great degree of variation between surgeons when deciding upon optimal port site configuration. Whichever configuration is used, it is essential to have a clear view of the right iliac fossa and for port site placement to allow adequate triangulation of the instruments on the appendix. Induce pneumoperitoneum, preferably using a Hasson's open technique at the umbilicus. Introduce a 10-mm port at the umbilicus. Set the insufflator pressure to 12 mmHg.

2. Use a 5-mm telescope if available. It can be used in all available ports and, therefore, allows a greater degree of flexibility when trying to obtain the best possible view. This flexibility is increased further if a 30° telescope is used. Insert the telescope through the umbilical port. Inspect the peritoneal cavity and confirm the diagnosis. To aid visualization of the structures in the right iliac fossa and pelvis, rotate the patient to the left side with some head-down tilt.

3. Introduce two 5-mm ports, one in the lower midline above the pubic symphysis, avoiding the bladder, and one in the left iliac fossa, lateral to the inferior epigastric artery. Always place ports under direct vision, to avoid inadvertently damaging bowel or vascular structures (Fig. 7.5).

Assess

1. Place the 5-mm telescope in the left iliac fossa port. With the help of atraumatic graspers in the other ports, examine all other pelvic and abdominal organs to exclude an ovarian cyst, ectopic pregnancy, pelvic inflammatory disease, cholecystitis, perforated peptic ulcer, Meckel's diverticulum, colonic diverticulitis and Crohn's disease. Your ability to examine abdominal contents is much greater using laparoscopy than at open surgery through a small incision.

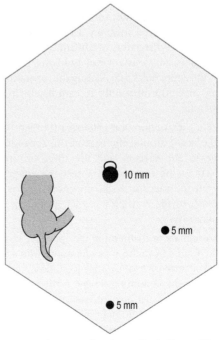

10 mm

5 mm

5 mm

Fig. 7.5 Laparoscopic appendicectomy. Port site positioning.

2 Identify the appendix which, in early appendicitis, may appear normal if mucosal inflammation has not yet extended to the peritoneum.

3 Plan to remove an apparently 'normal' appendix if you can find no other cause for the patient's pain.

Action

1 Your intention is to separate the appendix from its mesentery using diathermy dissection. The appendix mesentery is not removed. If this is a late presentation with advanced inflammation and oedema, this approach may not be possible. You may need to divide the appendix base and mesentery en masse, using a vascular stapler such as the EndoGIA Universal (Covidien).

2 Identify the appendix and aim to mobilize it fully before attempting to remove it. Break down inflammatory adhesions using blunt suction dissection. Occasionally, some lateral mobilization of the caecum may be necessary using scissor or hook diathermy dissection.

> ? DIFFICULTY

1. If you cannot find the appendix, insert the telescope in to one of the other ports to obtain a better view.
2. The appendix base is always found at the confluence of the three taenia coli on the caecum.

3 With the appendix tip elevated, identify the appendix base. The mesoappendix immediately adjacent to the appendix base is thin and usually only consists of a layer of peritoneum. Break down the peritoneum by carefully inserting a Petelin's forceps and opening the jaws, creating a small window in the mesoappendix. This window is a useful place to start separating the mesentery with a diathermy hook. Vessels close to the appendix are small and can be divided using diathermy alone, with minimal bleeding. If you cannot control an arterial spurter in this manner you may need to apply a clip through the 10-mm umbilical port. If dissection is difficult, insert a third port in the right flank. An assistant can hold the mesentery while you hold the appendix, so facilitating the separation. Continue dissecting until the appendix is completely free from the mesoappendix.

4 Introduce a Vicryl Endoloop (Ethicon) through the umbilical port and place it around the base of the appendix. Place two ties close to the caecum and the third tie approximately 1 cm distal to the first two. Transect the appendix, leaving two ties on the caecum. If the appendix base is friable and oedematous, divide it using a stapler, including some caecal wall if necessary.

5 Do not invaginate or diathermize the appendix stump. Remove any faecal residue from the appendix stump with a suction catheter, but avoid extensive saline irrigation unless there is gross contamination of the abdominal cavity. If there is contamination with pus and blood, perform extensive saline lavage of the right lower abdomen, pelvis and right subphrenic space until the irrigation fluid runs clear. In case of difficulty, leave a small-bore tube drain in the pelvis.

> ▶ KEY POINTS Technical considerations

- If you are applying a linear stapler, use a vascular rather than an intestinal cartridge for haemostasis.
- Experienced laparoscopic surgeons can reduce costs by tying knots extra-corporeally or intra-corporeally, rather than using endoloop or stapling devices.

6 The appendix base can usually be grasped and retrieved via the 10-mm umbilical port. If the appendix is very friable, use a retrieval bag to help prevent contamination.

> ▶ KEY POINTS Appendix normal?

- If the appendix looks normal and there is no other relevant pathology, remove the appendix as it may show early appendicitis on histology.
- This also eliminates appendicitis as a diagnosis if the patient has recurrent symptoms.

> ? DIFFICULTY

1. If the appendix is fixed or lying retrocaecally, place a port in the right upper quadrant of the abdomen to aid mobilization and dissection.
2. Be willing to move the telescope between ports to improve your view of the base of the caecum.
3. Do not hesitate to convert the procedure into an open operation if dissection is impossible, if bleeding is uncontrollable, and if you identify or suspect visceral damage.
4. If the appendix is perforated, as soon as possible apply an Endoloop below the perforation, so reducing contamination from leakage of bowel content into the peritoneal cavity. Cut this suture long so that it can be used for retraction. The appendix may be friable and disintegrate if held by forceps: place it in a retrieval bag to reduce contamination. Use liberal irrigation and suction to remove all purulent fluid from the pelvic, subhepatic and subphrenic spaces. Insert a small tube drain through one of the 5-mm ports, which can usually be removed on the next day.
5. If you are experienced you may be able to successfully manage an appendix abscess laparoscopically. When the appendix cannot be identified within an inflammatory mass, you may break down loculations, aspirate as much pus as possible and simply drain the area.
6. If you are in doubt, however, convert to open operation. In such cases, take special care to avoid inadvertently injuring the intestine, blood vessels or ureter.

Checklist

1 Inspect the pelvic, subphrenic and subhepatic spaces for any collection and use extensive saline irrigation if there is contamination.

2 Check the appendix stump to ensure that it is intact and safely closed.

3 Check for haemostasis and that any applied clips are well secured.

4 Ensure that there is no injury to the surrounding viscera.

Closure

1 Withdraw the ports under vision and try to allow all of the insufflation gas to escape.

2 Close the rectus sheath of the 10-mm incision site with a long-acting absorbable suture such as PDS. Close the skin with subcuticular absorbable sutures.

3 Infiltrate long-acting local anaesthetic at the port sites.

Postoperative

1 In the absence of general peritonitis allow oral fluids and food once the patient is fully awake.

2 Encourage the patient to get out of bed and walk on the day of operation. Most patients can be discharged on the first postoperative day and almost all by the second.

3 Continue metronidazole and a broad-spectrum antibiotic such as co-amoxiclav for 5 days if there was extensive sepsis or contamination, especially in high-risk patients. The antibiotics should be given parenterally until the patient is discharged.

4 If pyrexia develops, check the wounds and exclude chest and urinary infection.

Complications

1 *Bleeding* is one of the most common complications. Possible sources include the inferior epigastric artery, appendicular artery, retroperitoneal vessels or the staple line. You can injure the inferior epigastric artery when introducing the left iliac fossa port. Avoid this by placing the port well lateral to the rectus abdominus muscle. Attempt to identify and control the source of bleeding by re-laparoscopy if possible, before converting to open surgery.

2 *Perforation of the bowel* can occur either from puncture by the trocar, inadvertent electrosurgical injury or slippage of the appendix stump ligature. If you are an experienced laparoscopic surgeon you may close the perforation laparoscopically. Caecal perforation may be difficult to close laparoscopically, especially when it is inflamed and thick-walled. In these circumstances, convert to an open procedure.

3 Avoid *injury to the bladder* by catheterization and by introducing the suprapubic port under direct vision.

4 Postoperative *intra-abdominal and pelvic abscess* occurs in 3–5% of patients and can be detected or confirmed by ultrasound or computed tomography (CT). Perform percutaneous drainage under imaging guidance.

5 Significant *wound infection* is unusual. Examine the wound regularly and remove the superficial sutures or clips if there is evidence of infection.

6 There are several reports of *incomplete appendicectomy* leading to recurrent appendicitis. Avoid this problem by carefully identifying the appendix base during dissection.

7 *Incisional hernia* may develop through the trocar site, rarely complicated by a faecal fistula.

8 *Deep venous thrombosis* and *pulmonary embolus* can occur after appendicectomy, especially in the elderly. Reduce the risk by using low-molecular-weight heparin prophylaxis, anti-thromboembolic stockings and intermittent pneumatic calf compression devices intra-operatively.

REFERENCES

1. Ingraham AM, Cohen ME, Bilimoria KY, et al. Comparison of outcomes after laparoscopic versus open appendectomy for acute appendicitis at 222 ACS NSQIP hospitals. Surgery 2010;148(4):625–35.
2. Yau KK, Siu WT, Tang CN, et al. Laparoscopic versus open appendectomy for complicated appendicitis. J Am Coll Surg 2007;205(1):60–5.
3. Enochsson L, Hellberg A, Rudberg C, et al. Laparoscopic vs open appendectomy in overweight patients. Surg Endosc 2001;15(4):387–92.
4. Sauerland S, Lefering R, Holthausen U, et al. Laparoscopic vs conventional appendectomy: a meta-analysis of randomised controlled trials. Langenbecks Arch Surg 1998;383(3–4):289.
5. Ortega AE, Hunter JG, Peters JH, et al. A prospective randomized comparison of laparoscopic appendectomy with open appendectomy. Am J Surg 1995;169:208–12.

FURTHER READING

O'Reilly MJ, Reddick EJ, Miller WD, et al. Laparoscopic appendectomy. In: Zucker KA, editor. Surgical Laparoscopy. Update. St Louis; 1993. p. 301–26.
Richardson WS, Hunter JG. Complications in appendectomy. In: Ponsky JL, editor. Complications of Endoscopic and Laparoscopic Surgery. Prevention and Management. Philadelphia: Lippincott-Raven; 1997. p. 171–6.

APPENDIX MASS

Appraise

1 This is usually a late presentation of acute appendicitis.

2 It may result from the adherence of omentum and other viscera to the inflamed appendix. More usually the appendix has ruptured and an abscess has formed, its walls comprising the fibrin-lined omentum and adherent viscera.

3 Antibiotics are commonly given even when there are no clinical features of sepsis and the white cell count is not raised.

4 Provided the patient is well, with no features of sepsis, toxicity or peritonitis, expectant treatment without operation is the preferred management. Mark out the margins of the mass and regularly monitor progress. Provided the marked margins of the mass do not extend and features of toxaemia or peritonitis do not develop, wait for the mass to resolve.

5 Ultrasound scanning or computed tomography (CT) is valuable to confirm the diagnosis and determine whether an abscess is present, which can then be drained percutaneously.[1] If it extends into the pelvis it may be amenable to drainage transrectally under ultrasound guidance.

6 Perform open drainage only if worsening toxaemia or peritonitis develop, or if percutaneous drainage is not feasible or fails.

7 The subsequent management of patients with a resolved abscess remains controversial. Conventionally, the patient is re-admitted for interval appendicectomy after 1–2 months. However, at such operations one frequently finds no evidence of the appendix and, if no interval appendicectomy is undertaken, it is only rarely that recurrent appendicitis develops.[2]

Access

1. Define the mass when the patient is relaxed under anaesthesia.

2. Employ a standard Lanz incision. You may encounter oedema as you reach the deeper layers of the abdominal wall.

3. Alternatively, you may enter the abdomen and find the mass on the posterior wall.

Action

1. If you find on entering the abdomen that you are within the abscess cavity, do not rush to explore the wound. Take a specimen of the contents of the cavity for bacterial culture and to determine the antibiotic sensitivity of the contained organisms. Gently and thoroughly aspirate all pus and debris. Explore the cavity with your finger to decide whether it is safe to enlarge the opening without damaging viscera or disrupting the cavity wall.

2. If you gain an improved view you may see the appendix and be able to remove it safely. Sometimes the terminal part has separated and you will need to remove it piecemeal.

> ▶ KEY POINT The appendix looks normal

> ■ Do not misinterpret the presence of a short, apparently normal appendix. This is the stump left after the distal part has dropped off after a perforation and is lying in the abscess cavity. Look carefully for it and for a causative faecalith and remove both.

3. Sweep your finger round the cavity to identify any loose contents and remove them. Thoroughly aspirate any pus.

4. If you cannot find the appendix or if it is unsafe to open up the abscess cavity, insert a drain, closing the wound layers loosely around it.

5. If, when you open the abdomen, you enter the peritoneal cavity and find a mass lying on the posterior wall, pack it off from the remainder of the abdomen and gently explore it to determine if there is a plane of cleavage into the interior. Remember, inflamed tissues are friable; respond to the findings and be willing to stop if you encounter difficulty.

6. The mass or abscess may lie retrocaecally, retroileally, or within the pelvis. Be prepared to pack off the rest of the abdomen and mobilize the caecum by incising the peritoneum in the paracolic gutter so you can gently lift it off the mass. Now explore the mass to decide whether to enter it or leave it.

7. Whether you open the mass or leave it, insert a drain into the peritoneal cavity to provide a track for any pus.

REFERENCES

1. Brown CV, Abrishami M, Muller, et al. Appendix abscess: Immediate operation or percutaneous drainage? Am Surg 2003;69: 829–32.
2. Dixon MR, Haukoos JS, Park IU, et al. An assessment of the severity of recurrent appendicitis. Am J Surg 2003;186:718–22.

SUBPHRENIC AND SUBHEPATIC ABSCESS

Appraise

1. An abscess may form following major surgical procedures, operations performed in the presence of infection, or sometimes spontaneously following perforation of a viscus. It may result from a retained foreign body, necrotic tissue, inadequate drainage of blood or contaminated fluid, or an anastomotic leak. The abscess may develop above the liver (subphrenic), below the liver (subhepatic), along either paracolic gutter, between loops of bowel in the mid-abdomen or in the true pelvis.

2. Reserve the term 'subphrenic' for an abscess lying immediately below the diaphragm. On the right it lies above the right lobe of the liver, on the left it lies above the left lobe of the liver, gastric fundus and spleen (Fig. 7.6). Right subhepatic collections may be anterior (paraduodenal) or posterior (suprarenal, Fig. 7.7). Left subhepatic collections may lie anterior to the stomach and transverse colon or posteriorly in the lesser sac.

3. Suspect the diagnosis if the patient develops rigors, swinging pyrexia, toxicity and leucocytosis. In the presence of a subphrenic abscess the hemidiaphragm may be elevated, as demonstrated on a chest X-ray, and a reactive pleural effusion often develops above the diaphragm. You may see a fluid level with gas above if leakage from a viscus or anastomosis has developed, or in the presence of gas-forming organisms. Aspirate a specimen of pus for culture and determination of antibiotic sensitivity. CT or ultrasound scans are valuable means of confirming an abscess, and a radiolabelled white blood cell scan may reveal an occult abscess that is not detectable by other imaging methods.

4. The first-line method of dealing with subphrenic or subhepatic abscess should be percutaneous drainage. This is usually effective even for recurrent abscesses.[1] A needle is inserted under ultrasound or CT guidance to avoid damaging adjacent structures. A flexible guidewire is then passed through the needle, which is withdrawn. A bevel-tipped catheter is passed over the guidewire into the cavity and the guidewire is then withdrawn. This is the Seldinger technique. This technique may

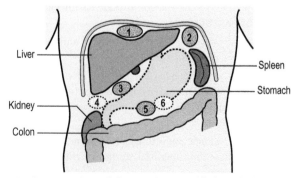

Fig. 7.6   Common sites of abscess above and below the liver: 1, right subphrenic; 2, left subphrenic; 3, right anterior subhepatic; 4, right posterior subhepatic (hepatorenal); 5, left anterior subhepatic; 6, left posterior subhepatic (lesser sac).

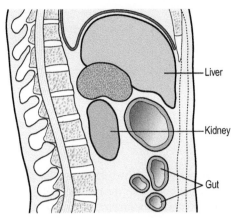

Fig. 7.7 Abscess in the hepatorenal pouch (right posterior subhepatic). This type of posterior collection may be drained by a posterior extra-peritoneal approach, through the bed of the 12th rib, or from an anterolateral direction.

not be successful in obtaining drainage of multiloculated abscesses but these may be successfully drained laparoscopically.[2] Send aspirated material for culture and to be tested for antibiotic sensitivity.

5 Open operation is now rarely necessary for large, loculated or recurrent abscesses and those containing necrotic or inspissated material.

6 The choice of approach depends on the site of the abscess. Ideally, an extrapleural, extra-peritoneal approach avoids the possibility of contaminating the peritoneal or pleural cavities. As a rule this is possible only for posterior collections, although a right anterior subphrenic abscess can sometimes be approached extra-peritoneally. Multiple or loculated abscess cavities usually demand a transperitoneal approach.

Prepare

Start antibiotic cover against the likely organisms before embarking on operation. Take advice from a clinical microbiologist, especially if you have managed to send a specimen of pus for study.

Action

Posterior approach

1 Place the patient in the full lateral position with the affected side uppermost. Identify the 12th rib and make a 10-cm transverse incision crossing its middle.

2 Cut down on to the rib, incise and elevate the periosteum so you can excise the rib. Incise the bed of the rib cephalad to the middle, to avoid entering the pleural cavity. Divide the origin of the diaphragm and displace the kidney forwards.

3 Feel for the lower edge of the liver and explore below it, using a needle and aspirating syringe to seek out pus. To drain a subphrenic abscess, separate the peritoneum from the undersurface of the diaphragm. When you find it, open the cavity, suck out the pus and debris. Explore it with your finger to avoid leaving necrotic or inspissated material. Now insert a drain.

Anterolateral approach

1 Place the patient supine but with the flank on the affected side elevated by placing a sandbag under the loin.

2 Make a lateral subcostal incision 1 cm below the costal margin and cut through all layers down to, but not including, the peritoneum.

3 Strip the peritoneum from under the diaphragm until you reach the abscess. Open it and drain it.

4 If you cannot find pus, carefully explore with a needle and finger through the peritoneum and be prepared to enter the peritoneal cavity.

Transperitoneal approach

1 Site the incision according to the site of the abscess derived from the preoperative ultrasound or CT scan.

2 If you are unsure of the site of the abscess or of the cause, carry out a complete exploration of the abdomen before entering the abscess cavity. This is to avoid the need to carry out an exploration after opening the abscess and risking general contamination. Explore the right and left subphrenic and sub-hepatic spaces, and enter the lesser sac through an avascular part of the hepatogastric omentum.

3 As soon as you encounter an abscess, pack off the area from the rest of the abdomen.

4 Now open the abscess, suck out the contents and drain the cavity through a separate stab wound in the abdominal wall.

REFERENCES

1. Gervais DA, Ho CH, O'Neill MJ, et al. Recurrent abdominal abscesses: incidence, results of repeated percutaneous drainage, and underlying causes in 956 drainages. AJR Am J Roentgenol 2004;182:463–6.
2. Lam SC, Kwok SP, Leong HT. Laparoscopic intracavitary drainage of subphrenic abscess. J Laparoendosc Adv Surg Tech A 1998;8:57–60.

FURTHER READING

Andersson RE. Meta-analysis of the clinical and laboratory diagnosis of appendicitis. Br J Surg 2004;91:28–37.

Cooper MJ. Manifestations of appendicitis. In: Williamson RCN, Cooper MJ, editors. Emergency Abdominal Surgery. Edinburgh: Churchill Livingstone; 1990. p. 221–32.

Engstrom L, Fenyo G. Appendicectomy: assessment of stump invagination versus simple ligature: a prospective, randomised trial. Br J Surg 1985;72:971–2.

Gillick J, Veayudham M, Puri P. Conservative management of appendix mass in children. Br J Surg 2001;88:1539–42.

Jones PF. Suspected acute appendicitis: trends in management over 30 years. Br J Surg 2001;88:1570–7.

Kirk RM. Basic Surgical Techniques. 5th ed. Edinburgh: Churchill Livingstone; 2002. p. 161–73.

Krukowski ZH, Irwin ST, Denholm S, et al. Preventing wound infection after appendicectomy: a review. Br J Surg 1988;75:1023–33.

Rao PM, Rhea JT, Rattner DW, et al. Introduction of appendiceal CT: impact on negative appendicectomy and appendiceal perforation rates. Ann Surg 1999;229:334–49.

Silen W. Cope's Early Diagnosis of the Acute Abdomen. Oxford: Oxford University Press; 2000.

Oesophagus

R. Mason

CONTENTS

ENDOSCOPY

Appraise

1 Endoscope every patient with dysphagia except when this is fully explained by the presence of neurological or neuromuscular disease.

2 Endoscope patients with suspected disease in the oesophagus producing pain on swallowing (odynophagia), heartburn not responding to simple medication or arising de novo in patients over 50 years, bleeding, or if accidental and iatrogenic damage are suspected.

Prepare

1 Ensure that the endoscope, the ancillary equipment and necessary spares are available, function correctly and are appropriately sterile. The endoscope must be thoroughly prepared between procedures according to the maker's instructions. Fibreoptic instruments, biopsy forceps and similar instruments are scrupulously cleaned using neutral detergent and usually disinfected with 2% alkaline glutaraldehyde. This is capable of eliminating all infective organisms, including HIV. Washing and sterilization are performed mechanically in an automatic machine to avoid exposure of endoscopy room staff to glutaraldehyde fumes.

2 Modern gastrointestinal endoscopes are slim, versatile, have remarkably flexible tips and can be passed with pharyngeal anaesthesia alone in most patients. They are safe, relatively comfortable for the patient and allow examination of the stomach and duodenum beyond. Use the end-viewing instrument routinely since it gives the best general view. Through it can be passed biopsy forceps, cytology brushes, snares, guidewires for dilators and needles for injection. Argon plasma coagulation or Nd-YAG laser may be applied through it for the palliation of inoperable neoplasms or for the treatment of Barrett's oesophagus. The technology of endoscopes is steadily improving and the rigid oesophagoscope is, to all intents and purposes, obsolete.

3 Obtain signed informed consent from the patient.

4 Remove dentures from the patient.

5 Except in an emergency, have the patient starved of food and fluids for at least 5 hours. In an emergency, especially in patients with upper gastrointestinal haemorrhage who cannot wait 5 hours for the stomach to empty, a crash general anaesthetic with cricoid pressure is the safest means of securing the airway and preventing aspiration.

6 Obtain a preliminary barium swallow X-ray if there is a suspected pharyngeal pouch.

7 Attach a pulse oximeter probe to the patient's finger if sedation is being used, and ensure that there are sufficient numbers of staff in the endoscopy room for safe care of a sedated patient.

8 Spray the pharynx with lidocaine solution just before passing the endoscope.

9 In anxious patients, or those in whom intervention (e.g. dilatation) is required, insert a small plastic cannula into a peripheral vein and through it inject slowly 1–2 mg of midazolam until the patient's eyelids just begin to droop. Remember that it takes 2 minutes for the full effect of midazolam to develop.

FIBREOPTIC ENDOSCOPY

1 Lay the patient on the left side with hips and knees flexed. Place a plastic hollow gag between the teeth. Ensure that the patient's head is in the midline and that the chin is lowered on to the chest.

2 Lubricate the previously checked end-viewing instrument with water-soluble jelly.

3 Pass the endoscope tip through the plastic gag, over the tongue to the posterior pharyngeal wall. Depress the tip control slightly so that the instrument tip passes down towards the cricopharyngeal sphincter. Do not overflex the tip or it will be directed anteriorly and enter the larynx. Visualize the larynx and pass the endoscope just behind it.

4 Ask the patient to swallow. Do not resist the slight extrusion of the endoscope as the larynx rises, but maintain gentle pressure so that it will advance as the larynx descends and the cricopharyngeal sphincter relaxes. Advance the endoscope under vision, insufflating air gently to open up the passage. Aspirate any fluid. Spray water across the lens if it becomes obscured. If no holdup is encountered, pass the tip through the stomach into the duodenum then withdraw it slowly, noting the features. Remove biopsy

specimens and take cytology brushings from any ulcers, tumours or other lesions.

5   If a stricture is encountered note its distance from the incisor teeth. Sometimes the instrument will pass through, allowing the length of the stricture to be determined. Always remove biopsy specimens and cytology brushings from within the stricture. If the stricture is benign in appearance, gentle dilatation to 12 mm can be attempted if the patient is symptomatic. Dilatation of malignant strictures is not indicated as any benefit is short-lasting and the risk of perforation is high (6–8%). Get biopsies and confirm the diagnosis prior to intervention. If nutritional support is required, fluoroscopic passage of a feeding nasogastric tube can be performed.

> **KEY POINT** Risk of perforation

■   Remember that malignant strictures are more easily perforated than benign strictures. This may influence the decision whether to dilate or not. Only dilate if this is important for treatment and then only to 12 mm (36 F).

Assess

1   Note the level of each feature. The cricopharyngeal sphincter is approximately 16 cm from the incisor teeth. The deviation around the aortic arch is 28–30 cm, the cardia lies at 40 cm and here the lining changes abruptly from the pale, bluish, stratified oesophageal epithelium to the florid, pinker, gastric columnar-cell epithelium.

2   Oesophagitis is usually from gastro-oesophageal reflux, but is not necessarily associated with hiatal hernia. Consult a colour chart that illustrates the grades of oesophagitis. Most commonly there are red streaking erosions just above the cardia. Oesophagitis may be seen above a benign stricture. Occasionally, in advanced achalasia, one may see a mild diffuse oesophagitis from contact with fermenting food residues. Thick white plaques indicate monilial infection, usually in association with oral involvement. Confirm the diagnosis by taking mucosal scrapings.

3   Sliding hiatal hernia produces a loculus of stomach above the constriction of the crura with a raised gastro-oesophageal mucosal junction. To determine the level of the hiatus, ask the patient to sniff, and note the level at which the crura momentarily narrow the lumen. Reflux and oesophagitis may be visible. A rolling hernia is visible only from within the stomach by inverting the tip of a flexible instrument to view the apparent fundic diverticulum. If the diagnosis is a possibility, confirm with a barium study.

4   Frank ulceration in the oesophagus is unusual, but may be due to severe reflux disease. In Barrett's oesophagus the lower gullet is lined with modified gastric mucosa and an ulcer may develop in the columnar-lined segment. In all cases of Barrett's take biopsies of the columnar segment from all four quadrants at 2-cm intervals. In patients with dysplasia even more biopsies are required for accurate assessment. Use 'jumbo' forceps. Ulcerating carcinomas may develop at any level. In most Western countries the majority of cancers comprise adenocarcinomas and these arise in the lower oesophagus in association with Barrett's oesophagus. Take multiple biopsies and cytological brushings from a number of areas of all ulcers.

5   Strictures from peptic oesophagitis or, rarely, ulceration in a Barrett's oesophagus develop at any time from birth onwards, but more frequently occur in middle or old age. Almost always there is a co-incidental hiatal hernia. If there is no hernia below the stricture, suspect cancer. Also suspect cancer if there is food residue above a stricture. Food residue may also be seen in achalasia and may be the only diagnostic clue. Take multiple biopsies and brushings for cytology. The cause of Schatzki's ring is unknown. It is usually asymptomatic, seen radiologically at the junction between gastric and oesophageal mucosa. Caustic strictures develop at the sites of hold-up of swallowed liquids at the cricopharyngeus, at the aortic arch crossing and at the cardia. Webs or strictures in the upper oesophagus are uncommon. However, it is not unusual to see a patch or ring of ectopic gastric mucosa in the upper oesophagus 1–2 cm below the cricopharyngeus, the so-called 'inlet patch'. Stricture may arise from external pressure, of which by far the most common cause is bronchogenic carcinoma.

> **KEY POINTS** Diagnostic appearances

■   Remember that it is possible to distinguish benign from malignant lesions from the gross appearances with a high degree of accuracy. Practise this skill, which is particularly useful for triggering speedy reinvestigation of suspicious lesions if biopsies are misleadingly negative.

■   Consult a good colour atlas or a CD-ROM. Become familiar with the appearances of early cancer of the oesophagus. Early diagnosis is the best means of improving cure rates.

6   Mega-oesophagus may be seen in achalasia of the cardia, but is now uncommon as most cases are diagnosed long before dilatation takes place. Mega-oesophagus may also be seen in the South American Chagas' disease and in some cases of advanced scleroderma.

7   Pulsion diverticula are related to abnormal oesophageal motility and are seen above the cricopharyngeus muscle (Zenker's diverticulum or pharyngeal pouch) and above segments of presumed spasm. Traction diverticula in the mid-oesophagus develop as a result of chronic inflammation of mediastinal glands, especially from tuberculosis.

8   Oesophageal varices are usually recognized just above the cardia as convoluted varicose veins, which may extend into the upper stomach.

DILATATION OF STRICTURES (Fig. 8.1)

1   Fragile strictures do not always require endoscopic dilatation if the diagnosis is not in doubt or has been confirmed by endoscopy. The safest oesophageal dilator is soft, solid food, provided that each bolus contains only aggregated small particles.

2   Record the distance of the stricture from the incisor teeth. If the stricture is short and appears benign, the best means for dilatation is by a through-the-channel balloon. These balloons have a fixed maximum diameter of 2 cm (60 F). Always check for perforation with endoscopy after dilatation. An alternative to these balloon dilatators are soft mercury-laden Maloney dilators. If problems occur inserting them through a tortuous stricture,

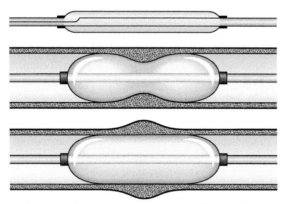

Fig. 8.1 Balloon dilatation. At the top is a balloon collapsed on its introductory catheter. There is a radio-opaque marker at each end of the balloon. In the middle drawing, the balloon is partly inflated within a stricture that has produced a waist. At the bottom, the waist has disappeared as the balloon is fully inflated.

balloon dilatation using a hydrophilic guidewire inserted under fluoroscopic control should be undertaken.

3 First outline the passage by getting the erect patient to swallow a thin contrast medium. Now introduce a fine, flexible guidewire through a nostril into the oesophagus and negotiate the tip through the stricture using a combination of rotating it and getting the patient to swallow a little water or more contrast medium to outline the passage. Now pass a well-lubricated catheter fitted with a deflated balloon over the guidewire and insinuate it through the stricture. The proximal and distal ends of the balloon have radio-opaque markers so that it can be placed accurately. Carefully inflate the balloon, watching it on the screen. A waist appears at the level of the stricture and as the pressure is gradually increased this disappears. If the patient is apprehensive or complains of discomfort, temporarily stop inflating the balloon.

4 Most strictures can be dilated at a single session, but do not persist unduly in the face of difficulty or discomfort. When the balloon is withdrawn, check to see if there is any blood on it. Now give the patient some contrast medium to swallow and carefully watch it pass through the stricture to ensure that there is no leak.

REMOVAL OF FOREIGN BODIES

Appraise

1 Swallowed articles impact at the sites of narrowing. Objects at the cricopharyngeus muscle are regurgitated but those that pass this point may impact at the crossing of the aortic arch or at the cardia. However, the normal oesophagus is extremely distensible and smooth objects usually pass into the stomach. The most frequent causes of impaction are pre-existing stricture or a sharp foreign body that penetrates the oesophageal wall.

2 Remember that many impacted foreign bodies are radiolucent. Sometimes they are demonstrable on X-rays by giving the patient a drink of water-soluble contrast medium.

3 Most foreign bodies may be removed using a variety of methods in conjunction with fibreoptic endoscopes and an overtube under local anaesthesia with sedation. If a foreign body cannot be removed with modern endoscopic instruments an operation

is probably required. Deeply and firmly impacted foreign bodies may require thoracotomy and oesophagotomy to remove them.

4 A smooth foreign body, or a food bolus, may be gently pushed into the stomach. As a rule it will pass through the gut but if it remains in the stomach removal is easier than from the oesophagus.

Action

1 There is a classic repertoire of methods to remove foreign bodies through the rigid oesophagoscope. The grasping forceps are strong and versatile, and can cope with open safety pins and coins. Version and extraction of an open safety pin with the point facing upwards is now part of the folklore of oesophageal surgery. However, the use of the rigid endoscope is not now to be encouraged. There are safer and better methods.

2 Ingenious methods have been used to remove foreign bodies using the end-viewing fibreoptic endoscope. The foreign body may be grasped with forceps or caught with a snare and withdrawn together with the instrument. An external flexible sheath may be pushed over the end of the endoscope tip into which a sharp foreign body can be drawn to protect the mucosa from injury. A variety of snares and grasping forceps should be kept available.

INJECTION OR BANDING OF VARICES

Appraise (see Chapter 17)

1 Recognize these as soft, collapsible, projecting columns in the lower oesophagus, sometimes continuing into the gastric cardia.

2 In patients with upper gastrointestinal bleeding who are found to have varices, do not assume that the bleeding is from the varices. A high proportion of such patients have another cause such as peptic ulcer, so always carry out a complete examination.

3 The varices thrombose when injected with ethanolamine oleate warmed to reduce its viscosity. An injection needle is passed down the biopsy channel and 2–5 ml is injected into each varix. The injections are repeated at intervals of 3–4 weeks until the varices are obliterated.

4 Banding of varices has a number of advantages, including better immediate control of active bleeding. A banding device that can fire several bands is loaded into and onto the endoscope. Always read the instructions on the device. Continuous design improvement is the norm and the device may have changed since you last used it. The varix is identified and then sucked into the banding cap on the end of the endoscope. When a 'red-out' is achieved the bander is fired and the suction released. The band should be seen clearly in the required position. Multiple varices can be ligated at a single session.

INTUBATION OF TUMOURS

Appraise

1 It is not necessary to intubate all strictures that cannot be resected. Malignant strictures that will be submitted to chemo-or radiotherapy may deteriorate temporarily and later expand, so it is worthwhile deferring intubation. Intubation of benign strictures

is not recommended unless in exceptional cases in very frail subjects with a limited life-expectancy. Intubation produces a rigid channel through which food must fall by gravity and which can easily become blocked, so reserve its use for patients with real need.

2 The development of expanding metal stents is a considerable advance and has replaced the rigid plastic tube. They provide a larger lumen for swallowing and do not require as much dilatation as semirigid stents such as the Nottingham tube. As a result insertion is safer. Expanding metal stents may be inserted at endoscopy, by radiological screening or by a combination of both methods. They are produced in both covered and uncovered formats.

Insertion of self-expanding metal stent (Fig. 8.2)

1 There are many different designs. Be familiar with the stent, its introducer and the method of deployment. Most expanding stents shorten as they expand and this must be taken into account during insertion. Some stents can be partially deployed and the position adjusted if it is not satisfactory. However, you may have to get it right first time, so be careful.

2 Such stents can be inserted under fluoroscopic or endoscopic control. Fluoroscopy has the advantage of outlining the length and position of the stricture accurately by using a radio-opaque

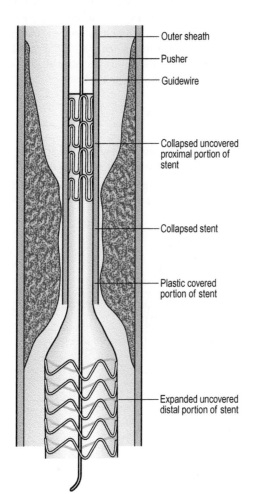

Outer sheath

Pusher

Guidewire

Collapsed uncovered proximal portion of stent

Collapsed stent

Plastic covered portion of stent

Expanded uncovered distal portion of stent

Fig. 8.2 Wall stent: self-expanding metal stent being deployed under fluoroscopic control.

contrast swallow prior to insertion. Dilatation up to 1 cm is usually required prior to stent deployment, as described above for dilatation of difficult strictures.

3 Pass the stent with its introducer over the guidewire and into the desired position. An endoscope may be passed alongside the guidewire so that deployment can be checked under vision.

4 Deploy the stent according to the manufacturer's instructions.

5 Correct stent deployment can be checked by endoscopy or contrast swallow. Some stents may be very slow to expand. Expansion may be hastened by dilatation with a through-the-scope balloon.

Aftercare

1 Make sure the patient does not have chest pain, air emphysema in the neck, or a raised temperature. Have a plain chest radiograph taken or perform a contrast swallow.

2 If there is evidence of a leak, confirm it and identify the site with X-rays using a water-soluble contrast medium. If an expanding stent is not sealing a leak consider inserting a second stent. Start the patient on broad-spectrum antibiotics and withhold food and fluids until the patient is entirely comfortable and a contrast swallow shows no leak.

3 Following stent insertion, warn the patient against swallowing unchewed food, particularly lumps of meat, fruit skins and stones, and to wash down the food with sips of water. Aerated drinks such as sodium bicarbonate solution (half a teaspoonful in half a glass of water half an hour before meals) or fresh pineapple juice help to wash away adherent mucus that may block the tube.

4 It is now extraordinarily uncommon to fail to intubate a tumour. If it cannot be done, a feeding gastrostomy or jejunostomy may be inserted after full discussion with the patient. This poses ethical and philosophical dilemmas, but these must be faced. However, always remember that the aim of palliation is to improve the quality of remaining life. If a particular therapy will not improve the quality of life in an individual patient, do not use it.

OESOPHAGEAL EXPOSURE

NECK (Fig. 8.3)

1 The cervical oesophagus may be approached from either side. Operations for the removal of pharyngeal pouch and cricopharyngeal myotomy, are usually carried out from the left side. For oesophageal anastomosis following resection, either side can be used. The right-sided approach minimizes risk of damage to the thoracic duct, although this is a rare complication for exposure of the oesophagus and usually occurs as a complication of biopsy of lymph nodes. The left recurrent laryngeal nerve is more likely to be injured during intrathoracic resection or be involved in the malignant process. It is better, therefore, to expose it to risk of injury rather than the right nerve.

2 The anaesthetized intubated patient lies supine on the operating table with the head turned to the opposite side from which the exploration will be made, resting on a ring with the neck extended. There is no need for complex head towelling, but drapes can be secured with skin staples.

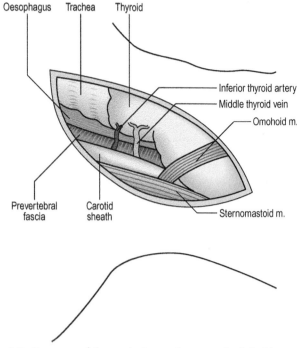

Fig. 8.3 Exposure of the cervical oesophagus on the left side. Sternomastoid muscle and the carotid sheath are drawn laterally. The space between these structures and the midline column of the pharynx and oesophagus, larynx, trachea and thyroid gland is crossed by the omohyoid muscle, middle thyroid vein and the inferior thyroid artery.

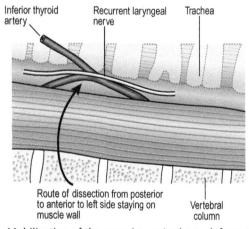

Fig. 8.4 Mobilization of the oesophagus in the neck from the left side preserving the recurrent laryngeal nerve.

3 Incise along the anterior border of sternomastoid muscle, through platysma muscle, cervical fascia, omohyoid muscle, ligating and dividing the middle thyroid vein to enter the space between the oesophagus, trachea and thyroid gland medially and the carotid sheath laterally. The inferior thyroid artery crosses the space; ligate and divide it laterally only if it interferes with the dissection.

4 Rotate the whole oesophageal-tracheal-thyroid column towards the opposite side, bringing into view the trachea-oesophageal groove, and display the posterior surface of the oesophagus and lower pharynx. Beware of inserting a Langenbeck's retractor into the trachea-oesophageal groove since it may well crush the recurrent laryngeal nerve.

5 Mobilize the posterior wall of the oesophagus with blunt dissection. Staying on the muscle wall of the oesophagus, come anteriorly and over the front, separating the trachea and recurrent laryngeal nerve anteriorly (Fig. 8.4). It is not necessary to mobilize the nerve and this prevents an ischaemic neuropraxia. Staying on the muscle wall, go round the oesophagus on the opposite side, retracting the oesophagus laterally. This exposes the prevertebral fascia on the opposite side. A curved forceps can then be placed around the oesophagus and a sling placed. With gentle traction on this, the oesophagus can be mobilized by finger dissection, staying on the oesophageal wall.

RIGHT POSTEROLATERAL THORACOTOMY (Fig. 8.5)

1 The anaesthetized patient, intubated with a double-lumen tube to allow exclusion of the right lung, lies on the left side. Carry out right posterolateral thoracotomy at the level of the fifth or sixth rib.

2 Ask the anaesthetist to collapse the right lung. Draw it downwards and forwards to reveal the mediastinal pleura. The oesophagus cannot be seen but the azygos vein can be seen arching over the lung root. Incise the mediastinal pleura, mobilize, doubly ligate and divide the azygos vein. This reveals the oesophagus running posterior to the trachea and lung root. The lower oesophagus is not visible between the left atrium and the vertebral column as it veers to the left. Expose it by dividing the pulmonary ligament until the inferior pulmonary vein is exposed. Then divide the mediastinal pleura anterior to the descending aorta. The upper stomach can be approached after dilating or incising the diaphragmatic crus to enlarge the hiatus.

LEFT THORACOTOMY (Fig. 8.6)

1 The lower thoracic oesophagus may be approached by left thoracotomy at the level of the seventh or eighth rib.

2 The left dome of diaphragm or the diaphragmatic crus may be incised to enter the upper abdomen.

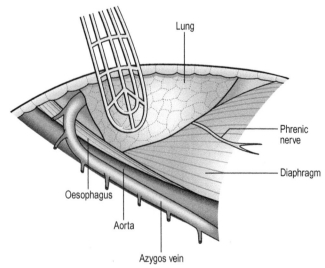

Fig. 8.5 Diagram of approach to the oesophagus through the right pleural space. The right lung is retracted anteriorly.

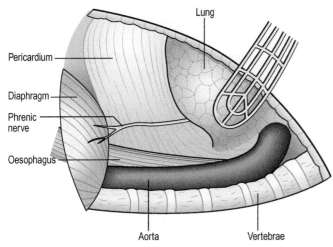

Fig. 8.6 Diagram of approach to the lower oesophagus through the left pleural space. The left lung is retracted anteriorly.

LEFT THORACOABDOMINAL APPROACH (Fig. 8.7)

1 The lower thoracic oesophagus and upper stomach are best approached using a combined thoracoabdominal approach.

2 Lay the anaesthetized intubated patient on the right side, left leg extended, right leg flexed at hip and knee, both arms flexed with forearms before the face. Allow the patient to lie back with the

shoulders at 30° from the vertical. Fix the patient's hips with an encircling band; support the left upper scapula against a padded post.

3 Prepare the skin and drape the area with sterile towels.

4 Start the incision 2.5 cm under the right costal margin in the mid-clavicular line, carry it obliquely upwards and to the left to cross the costal margin along the line of the seventh or eighth rib, extending to the posterior angle of the chosen rib and up behind the scapula. Deepen the incision to enter the thorax along the line of the rib, cutting and removing 1 cm of the costal margin. Incise the diaphragm peripherally parallel to the chest wall far enough in to enable the chest to be opened but not as far as the hiatus. This method spares the phrenic nerve.

5 In case of doubt make the abdominal or thoracic part of the incision first; assess the condition and now, if indicated, extend it fully.

6 After completing the procedure, close the diaphragm with strong absorbable material. Do not suture the costal margin but resect a wedge of cartilage to enable the ends to lie adjacent. Suture the abdomen in the usual manner. Close the chest after inserting an underwater-sealed drain.

ABDOMINAL APPROACH (Fig. 8.8)

1 The lower oesophagus is approachable through the abdomen and oesophageal hiatus.

2 The best access, especially in patients with a wide costal angle, is by a roof-top or bilateral subcostal incision. In those with a narrow costal angle an upper midline incision extending to the costal margin is preferable, opening the peritoneum just to the left of the falciform ligament. Ligate the ligamentum teres. Divide it and the falciform ligament.

3 Draw down the stomach while an assistant elevates the left lobe of the liver with a flat-bladed retractor. The lower oesophagus can be felt at the hiatus.

4 If necessary, cut the left triangular ligament and fold the left lobe of the liver to the right.

5 To display the lower thoracic oesophagus, transversely incise the peritoneum and fascia over the abdominal oesophagus for 5 cm, preserving the anterior vagal trunk. If greater exposure is

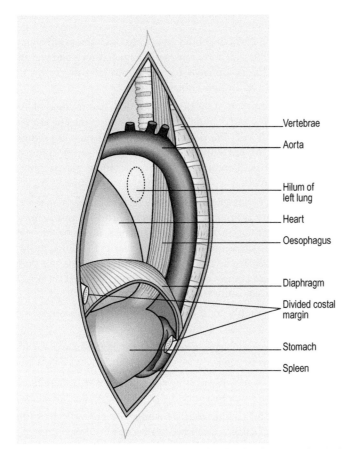

Fig. 8.7 Left thoracoabdominal approach. The diaphragm is divided circumferentially to enable the incision to open. It does not extend to the hiatus. The lung is elevated anteriorly.

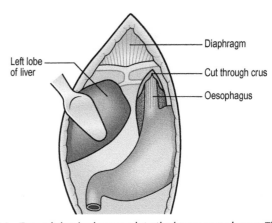

Fig. 8.8 Transabdominal approach to the lower oesophagus. The left lobe of the liver is folded to the right. If necessary, the diaphragmatic crus can be incised anteriorly.

necessary, insert a finger into the posterior mediastinum. Turn it forwards to separate the pericardium from the upper surface and incise the crus and diaphragm anteriorly for 5–7 cm. In patients of suitable build, the oesophagus can be viewed almost up to the carina of the trachea if the heart is gently elevated with a flat retractor. It is usually unnecessary to close the incision in the crus and diaphragm. The inferior phrenic vein will need to be oversewn.

TRANSHIATAL APPROACH (Fig. 8.9)

1 This encompasses both the abdominal and cervical approaches described above.

2 After division of the diaphragm anteriorly, dissect the fat pad off the back of the pericardium. It is common to take the pleura on the left side. Place an anterior resection retractor behind the heart and lift up and towards the head. Take care not to compress the left atrium. Dissect under direct vision to the carina using a harmonic scalpel, dividing the vagi.

3 Mobilize the oesophagus in the neck as described from the left side. After encircling the oesophagus, mobilize it with a finger into the upper mediastinum.

4 Place a tie around the oesophagus low down and produce a mucosal tube as described below. Open the anterior part of the mucosal tube and withdraw the nasogastric tube. Grasp the end of the nasogastric tube and place a tie into it to facilitate bringing it back to the conduit during the anastomosis.

5 Pass the wire of a varicose-vein stripper into the oesophagus and pass it into the stomach. Tighten the tie round the stripper wire distal to its insertion and divide the oesophagus. Place a medium head on the stripper. Gently pull the stripper distally, guiding the head into the posterior mediastinum avoiding damage to the adjacent structures. This will invert the oesophagus and deliver it to the abdomen. Vagal strands may prevent full delivery and need division under direct vision from below.

6 To guide the conduit to the neck for anastomosis use a chest drain to avoid rotation.

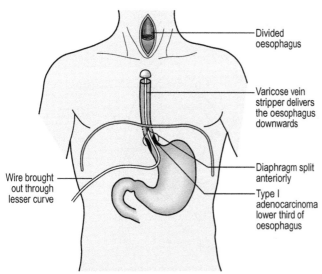

Fig. 8.9 The transhiatal approach, delivering the oesophagus with a varicose-vein stripper.

LAPAROSCOPIC APPROACH

1 Position the patient supine with the legs flat (for diagnostic or staging endoscopy) or with the legs apart in stirrups, as in rectal surgery (for major procedures, such as antireflux surgery).

2 Induce a pneumoperitoneum using a Veress needle or by an open technique.

3 Insert a 10-mm cannula in the midline approximately one-third of the distance between the umbilicus and the xiphisternum.

4 Liver retraction is best achieved by use of a Nathanson retractor inserted via a small 5-mm incision in the epigastrium. If not available, insert a 5- or 10-mm cannula, depending on what type of liver retractor is used, in the right subcostal region in the midclavicular line. Introduce a liver retractor and lift the left lobe of the liver upwards.

5 The number and position of additional cannulas depend on the procedure to be done and the preference of the operator. Commonly, additional cannulas are placed below the xiphisternum, in the left subcostal region in the midclavicular line and the anterior axillary line (the 'Liege' approach).

6 The oesophagus may then be approached as described in the previous section by dividing the peritoneum over the lower oesophagus. The precise approach to the oesophagus depends on the procedure to be done.

OPERATIVE CONSIDERATIONS

Appraise

1 Most other parts of the bowel are covered with serosa which rapidly forms fibrinous adhesions, sealing small defects and preventing leaks. The oesophagus has no serous coat except on the anterior wall of the abdominal segment.

2 A considerable part of the oesophageal wall is composed of longitudinal muscle. Longitudinally placed sutures thus have a tendency to cut out. The powerful longitudinal muscle produces shortening of the transected oesophagus when it contracts. Unless this is allowed for, the most carefully placed sutures may be torn out.

3 When the oesophagus is completely relaxed it has a remarkably large lumen. Commonly, the action of the circular muscle makes the diameter appear to be small. However, it can be stretched quite easily by insertion of a Foley catheter and inflating the balloon to facilitate the placement of sutures. If this is not done, closely spaced sutures may become widely separated on stretching, and leakage can easily occur between them.

4 The blood supply to the oesophagus is tenuous when it is mobilized, especially at the lower end.

5 The healthy oesophagus is easily damaged but disease may make it exceptionally fragile.

6 A diseased or partially obstructed oesophagus is contaminated. Prophylactic antibiotics must be given to cover the operation.

7 Although oral feeding may be stopped temporarily following oesophageal surgery, swallowed saliva must still pass through.

8 Intrathoracic oesophageal leakage produces posterior mediastinitis and if the pleura is damaged a pleural collection develops. The best hope for the patient's survival if major leakage occurs is rapid

clinical recognition with early re-operative repair and drainage. Minor leaks may be treated conservatively. Place chest drains in all opened chest cavities. Following transhiatal resection, even if the pleura is not opened a chest drain in the posterior mediastinum will prevent haematoma collection. A feeding jejunostomy should be placed at operation in all cases for postoperative nutrition and oral intake should not commence until the anastomosis is checked by contrast swallow at 5 days.

▶ KEY POINTS Technical considerations

- Never intubate the oesophagus unnecessarily. Never pass a rigid tube when a flexible one will suffice.
- Never carry out extensive oesophageal mobilization before forming an anastomosis.
- If the oesophagus retracts after division do not grab it with an instrument that may cause damage. Ask the anaesthetist to check the depth of anaesthesia – the longitudinal muscle of the oesophagus is one of the last to relax. The end of the oesophagus will often come easily back into view and stay sutures may be placed.
- Never leave the oesophagus sutured under tension. When joining it to another viscus, make sure there will be no traction, even when the oesophagus fully contracts.
- Never attempt an oesophageal anastomosis when access is poor. Improve the view or change tactics.
- Never perform an oesophageal anastomosis when tired. Take a short break if necessary.
- Never use small forceps to grasp the oesophagus. They cause damage. Use forceps with a large surface area and take a firm, but gentle grip. This is much kinder to tissue. Use grasping instruments as little as possible.

Anastomosis

1 The tenuous blood supply of the oesophagus makes it rarely possible to excise a segment, mobilize the cut ends and carry out an end-to-end union, except in neonates. Anastomosis is therefore usually to stomach, jejunum or colon.

2 Sutured anastomoses have been described using many different methods and materials. It is now recognized that single-layer anastomoses with continuous or interrupted sutures are best.

3 Circular stapling devices are often useful. Do not assume that perfection automatically follows their use. As with sutures, staplers give results commensurate with the care with which they are used. Which to choose? The stapling device saves a little time. It may allow an anastomosis to be accomplished where suturing is difficult high in the abdomen, under the aortic arch, or high in the thorax; but if it fails, suturing is usually impossible and a higher resection is necessary. The stapling gun has an inevitable crushing effect on the tissues. If a dilated and thickened oesophagus is to be joined to the cut end of bowel, the resulting tissue bulk cannot be accommodated in the staple gun. It is safer to use a sutured anastomosis. Hand suturing is usually preferable in the neck since there may be insufficient bowel accessible below the anastomosis for insertion of the gun.

Sutured anastomosis

1 Have you made sure that the oesophagus and conduit, which may be stomach, jejunum or colon, can be joined without tension and are not twisted? When the oesophagus contracts the powerful longitudinal muscle causes remarkable shortening. However, longitudinal muscle is of little value in retaining sutures, which easily cut out between the muscle fibres, so the strength of the anastomosis must depend upon the submucous coat and to some extent on the mucosa. To achieve this, when dividing the oesophagus first divide the muscle coat to produce a mucosal tube 1 cm long. Divide this in the middle with one cut, leaving the mucosa/submucosa pouting and associated with a little ooze. This is the layer that must be used for the anastomosis (Fig. 8.10).

2 Make sure the hole in the conduit matches the oesophageal lumen when it is slightly stretched. Place the oesophagus and conduit together as they will lie when joined. Avoid traction stitches as they can produce tears in the oesophageal walls. The ends should lie adjacent with no tension.

3 Suture material should be absorbable, such as polyglycolic acid, monofilament polyglyconate, polydioxanone or braided polyglactin 910 or braided lactomer 9–1. Use fine material such as 3/0.

4 The argument about continuous versus interrupted stitches continues. Good surgeons obtain good results with both methods. Continuous stitches, having fewer knots that weaken the thread, can, if inserted as an unlocked spiral, appose the tissues accurately without constricting them. Interrupted sutures tied without tension have the advantage that, if one cuts out, those on either side are not necessarily prejudiced. The choice is personal, often the result of following the tenets of an admired teacher. If you use interrupted stitches, those uniting the posterior walls are tied within the lumen, those uniting the anterior walls are tied on the outer walls.

5 For interrupted sutures, place three loose full-thickness sutures at the middle of the back wall and the angles 3 o'clock and 9 o'clock (Fig. 8.11). Insert further sutures, usually between two or three, again loosely. Make sure that there are no gaps and the sutures include the mucosal layer. When the back wall is complete, tie the sutures, leaving those at the angles long. Ask the anaesthetist to pass a nasogastric tube into the conduit and secure. The

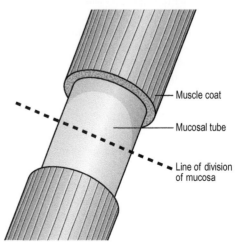

Fig. 8.10 The mucosal tube formed after division of oesophageal muscle.

Muscle coat
Mucosal tube
Line of division of mucosa

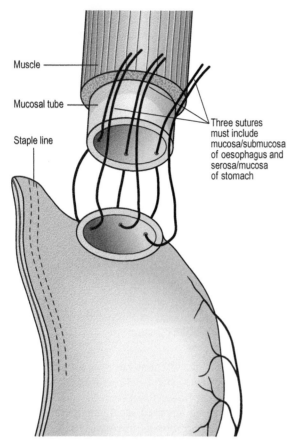

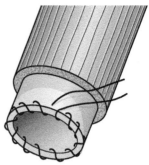

Fig. 8.12   Placement of the purse-string suture with 2/0 Prolene.

Fig. 8.11   Oesophageal anastomosis. The first three sutures are placed on the posterior wall to enable triangulation.

anterior layer of full-thickness sutures is now placed with knots on the outside. For continuous sutures it is best to use a double-ended monofilament suture and start at the middle of the back wall. Initial sutures can be placed loose and then tightened. Working from both sides, complete the back wall and introduce the nasogastric tube as before. Complete the anterior wall and tie the suture. Buttress sutures should be avoided; they narrow the lumen and can produce ischaemia.

6   As you draw stitches taut and tie them, remember that there will be some swelling of the tissues within the next few hours. If you have pulled the sutures too tight, they will cut through. Concentrate on placing each suture perfectly. Prefer to cut out and replace any that you are not satisfied with, rather than inserting extra 'bodging' stitches that may merely damage the blood supply. At the end, gently rotate the anastomosis to examine it, but remember that even more important is the integrity of the mucosal apposition.

Stapled anastomosis

1   Make sure that the oesophagus and bowel can be joined together without tension, are not twisted and that both ends have a good blood supply.

2   Transect the oesophagus, muscle first and the mucosa as described above. Insert a purse-string suture using 2/0 Prolene with an over-and-over suture encompassing the mucosal/submucosal layer (Fig. 8.12).

3   Assess the size of the oesophageal lumen by gently opening the jaws of an empty swab-holding forceps. Select the largest size of

stapler that easily fits the lumen. Do not attempt to force in a larger head as this will split the oesophageal wall. For a non-obstructed oesophagus a 25-mm head usually fits best.

> ▶ KEY POINT Do not split the oesophagus

- ■ A postoperative stricture is easy to dilate in contrast to a postoperative leak!

4   Open the circular stapling device to its maximum extent, separate the anvil from the spindle and then retract the stem by 'closing' the gun without the anvil. Introduce the anvil into the lower oesophagus. Tipping the anvil sideways may make introduction easier if it is a snug fit. Tighten and tie the previously inserted purse-string suture. Check that the purse string has drawn the oesophagus close to the stem. If there is a gap, insert a second purse string.

5   If the stomach is to be used, create a temporary anterior gastrotomy and insert the spindle of the stapler into the fundus at least 2 cm from any suture or staple line. 'Open' the instrument so that its sharp point comes through the stomach (Fig. 8.13). If the jejunum or colon are joined end-to-side, insert the stapler without the anvil head through the cut end; this will be closed later. Protrude the stem through the antimesenteric wall at a suitable point.

6   Attach the anvil on its spindle to the instrument and bring together the conduit and the oesophagus by closing the anvil down on to the cartridge. Check that there is no twisting and that nothing is interposed, nothing is protruding.

7   Release the safety catch.

8   Compress the handles fully and firmly: if using the Ethicon stapler a definite crunch will be felt. The gun has now been 'fired'.

9   Separate the jaws slightly. Gently rotate the device and draw it clear of the stapled anastomosis. Completely withdraw the instrument.

10   Remove the anvil head and check the toroidal ('doughnut'-shaped) oesophageal and viscus cuffs trimmed from the inside of the anastomosis. Make sure they are complete and then place them in fixative solution prior to histological examination.

11   Insert a finger through the anastomosis to check it. If an aspiration tube is to be passed, ask the anaesthetist to pass it now and guide it through the anastomosis with a finger.

12   Close the opening through which the instrument and finger were passed.

13   Carefully check that the anastomosis is complete all the way round and lies without tension.

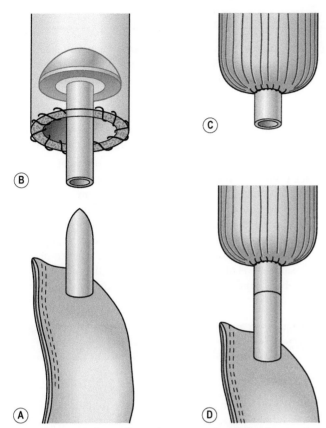

Fig. 8.13 A stapled oesophageal anastomosis: (A) the sharp point of the stapler shaft has been pushed through the stomach. (B) The anvil is inserted into the oesophagus. (C) The purse-string suture is tied around the shaft of the anvil (D). The two parts of the device are joined, the gun closed and actuated to produce an anastomosis.

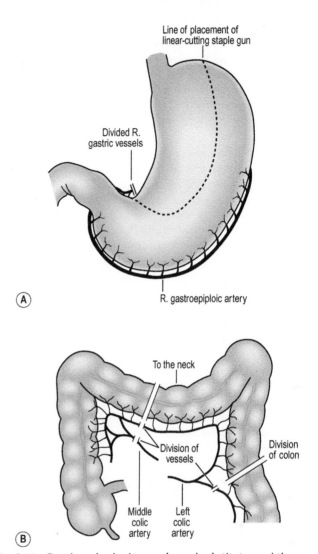

Fig. 8.14 Gastric and colonic oesophageal substitutes and the vascular pedicles on which they are based.

? DIFFICULTY

1. *The oesophagus splits when a large anvil is inserted.* Trim the split end and perform a sutured anastomosis. If the anastomosis is at the apex of the chest it may be necessary to perform a cervical incision for safe access to the oesophageal stump.
2. *A fragile oesophagus compressed normally within the jaws of the stapling machine is damaged.* The tenuous blood supply may be crushed between the staple carrier and the anvil. The longitudinal muscular wall may be traumatized. Abandon the anastomotic technique and perform a sutured anastomosis.
3. If the anastomosis is imperfect, reinforce the staple line with an encircling suture. Alternatively, abandon attempts to staple the viscera and rely on a carefully sutured anastomosis. Hoping for the best is a recipe for disaster in oesophageal surgery.

OESOPHAGEAL SUBSTITUTES (Fig. 8.14)

1. The alternatives are stomach, colon or jejunum. Jejunum is only applicable to anastomoses to the lower one-third of the oesophagus in most patients.

2. Both right and left colon can be used. Advocates exist for both, but the best is transverse and left colon based on the ascending branch of the left colic artery. The dogma that there is a vascular watershed at the splenic flexure is (usually) false, although the left colic artery may be stenosed or occluded in elderly, atherosclerotic patients, particularly those with aortic aneurysm. Provided there is a good marginal artery it is possible to mobilize a length of bowel, which will reach to the floor of the mouth. The right colon is bulky and more difficult to straighten. Either colon should be placed isoperistaltically.

3. The stomach is the favoured conduit due to its good vascular supply and adequate length. The conduit is based on the right gastroepiploic artery. The conduit should be a narrow tube 3–4 cm wide based on the greater curvature extending from the fundus to the lesser curve 3–4 cm proximal to the pylorus.

GASTRIC MOBILIZATION

Action

1. Identify the right gastroepiploic artery on the greater curvature of the stomach. Divide the greater omentum outside this arcade.

This is best achieved with a harmonic scalpel. Continue this mobilization proximally toward the pylorus taking care not to damage the vessel at its origin where it leaves the gastric wall. Continue dissection towards the fundus of the stomach dividing the left gastroepiploic and short gastric vessels and taking care not to damage the spleen. Dissection is continued to the left crus dividing small vessels to the stomach arising from the splenic artery.

2 The stomach is elevated to display the posterior gastric wall and left gastric pedicle. It is best to do a flush left gastric ligation removing all associated lymph nodes, including those on the common hepatic artery. Dissection is best achieved with bipolar scissors starting on the upper border of the pancreas. The left gastric vein is encountered first and ligated and divided. The left gastric artery is frequently 1 cm behind this and to the right. This should be double-ligated flush to the coeliac axis. The dissection is then continued to the crura which are cleaned of fat and lymphatics.

3 The right gastric artery is divided 3 cm from the pylorus and the gastric tube formed with a series of 'fires' of a TLC 100 linear cutting staple gun. This can be oversewn with a continuous running suture if required. The duodenum is Kocherized to complete mobilization. The gastric tube is usually fashioned in the abdomen and can be hitched to the oesophageal remnant to deliver to the chest or to a chest drain if it is to be delivered to the neck to avoid rotation. Except in cases of pyloric stenosis due to previous duodenal ulceration, there is no need to perform a pyloroplasty.

COLONIC MOBILIZATION

Action

1 Prefer the left colon. Mobilize it by dividing the peritoneum to the left from sigmoid to splenic flexure. Dissect the greater omentum from the colon. The colon can then be elevated and transilluminated to display the blood vessels. The marginal artery can be well visualized. Divide this distal to the ascending branch of the left colic and divide the colon with a linear cutting staple gun.

2 Continue the dissection of the vascular supply proximally, taking care with the middle colic artery which may divide just above its origin. Identify the proximal site of division of the colon and transect the colon with a linear cutting stapler and divide the marginal artery. If you doubt the viability then apply vascular clamps before dividing it.

3 Restore colonic continuity between proximal transverse and distal descending colon.

ROUTE OF RECONSTRUCTION

1 The best route for reconstruction is via the oesophageal bed in the posterior mediastinum. Alternatives include substernal and subcutaneous routes for neck anastomoses.

2 Use the substernal route with great caution if the colon is the conduit, since it is compressed at the root of the neck, resulting in venous congestion and conduit failure. If you employ this route you should resect the manubrium and first rib to prevent this.

LYMPHADENECTOMY

1 Controversy exists regarding the extent of lymphadenectomy in oesophageal cancer surgery. There is now no role for palliative resection leaving macroscopic disease. Remove all obviously involved nodes with the specimen.

2 As described above, perform coeliac lymphadenectomy as part of gastric mobilization. For transthoracic mobilization and anastomosis, take the para-oesophageal lymphatics with the specimen.

3 For operations through the right and left chest remove the subcarinal glands for accurate staging and, if approaching via the right chest, you can remove the thoracic duct. This involves dissecting along the azygos vein to the hiatus, taking all the tissue between the vein, vertebral column and aorta. The duct can be clearly seen in this tissue; double-ligate it at the lower end to prevent chylothorax. If you do not formally dissect it out, for safety place a suture at the level of T10 to encompass all the tissue between aorta, vertebral column and azygos vein after oesophageal mobilization.

TRAUMA, SPONTANEOUS AND POSTOPERATIVE LEAKS

Appraise

1 Swallowed foreign body, stab or missile wounds may immediately rupture the oesophagus, but crush injuries such as those sustained in road traffic accidents may cause necrosis with late rupture. Uncoordinated retching may tear the lower oesophagus, usually just above the hiatus, to the left side; this is Boerhaave's syndrome of 'spontaneous' or postemetic rupture. In some cases the tear is partial thickness, involving mainly mucosa, sometimes extending into the gastric cardia and presenting with acute haemorrhage. This is the Mallory-Weiss syndrome and it responds almost always to conservative management.

2 Iatrogenic rupture may follow endoscopy, dilatation of stricture or achalasia, removal of a foreign body, or follow an operation on the oesophagus including cardiomyotomy, vagotomy and resection or bypass.

3 The history of events, complaint of pain, collapse after injury or operation, presence of air emphysema in the neck and on plain radiographs demand radiological study with barium to determine the site, extent and localization of leakage. Barium gives much better imaging than water-soluble contrast and is perfectly safe. Modern water-soluble contrast media are relatively safe, but Gastrografin is hypertonic and should never be used. It is particularly dangerous if aspirated into the trachea. If these tests are negative and suspicion still exists perform endoscopy.

4 Late presentation may produce signs of cellulitis including mediastinitis, pleural effusion, empyema, peritonitis, abscess formation and fistula.

5 Following accidental or violent injury, assess the possibility of other injuries that must be dealt with.

6 Small cervical leaks following instrumental damage usually seal if the patient is fed parenterally for a few days.

7 Treat conservatively tears in the thoracic oesophagus that are: detected early, produced at endoscopy or instrumentation, associated with minimal contamination and are contained in the

mediastinum. Confirm that the mediastinal pleura is intact with X-rays, using barium. If the mediastinal pleura is breached or if the patient's condition deteriorates following initial conservative treatment, explore the leak. In general, postemetic rupture should be treated surgically as there is significant contamination of the mediastinum.

8 Intrathoracic leaks have a high mortality rate if not treated promptly. The worst results occur if the diagnosis is overlooked and the patient is fed.

9 If the oesophagus is split during dilatation of a carcinoma, immediate treatment is required: either resection or placement of a covered self-expanding metal stent. Remember that such tumours will present as advanced disease with limited life-expectancy.

CONSERVATIVE MANAGEMENT

1 Stop oral drinking or feeding.

2 Introduce a nasogastric tube into the stomach under X-ray screening.

3 Institute parenteral fluid replacement and feeding. For a minor leak in a fit patient, fluid and electrolyte replacement may suffice.

4 Administer broad-spectrum antibiotic cover and intravenous proton-pump inhibitors.

5 Do not place a self-expanding metal stent to seal the perforation other than in cases of established cancer. They will not seal the leak and inhibit healing.

6 If the general condition of the patient does not deteriorate, repeat the radiological examination after 7 days. Do not hurry to repeat the examination. This does more harm than good. If the leak is sealed, restart clear fluids orally, proceeding to all fluids, soft solids and full diet.

7 If the mediastinal pleura is breached so that contrast flows into the pleural space, or if the general condition of the patient deteriorates following initial conservative management, explore the leak without delay.

SURGICAL MANAGEMENT

Prepare

1 Resuscitate the patient with intravenous fluids and cross-match blood.

2 Start treatment with broad-spectrum antibiotic cover.

3 After induction of anaesthesia examine the perforation endoscopically to determine the length of mucosal tear. This is invariably longer than the muscle tear.

Access

1 Left thoracotomy gives good access to the lower oesophagus, right thoracotomy to the mid- and upper oesophagus.

2 If you suspect abdominal injuries use a left thoracoabdominal incision or be prepared to explore the abdomen subsequently.

3 If this is a postoperative leak, good drainage and placement of a T-tube into the hole may suffice (Fig. 8.15). If not, then resection;

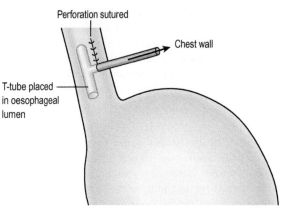

Fig. 8.15 Placement of a T-tube in a spontaneous oesophageal perforation.

you should perform proximal oesophagostomy and gastrostomy, with later reconstruction. Local debridement and re-anastomosis invariably fails.

4 Expose the oesophagus adequately to allow full assessment of the damage to the oesophagus and related structures.

Assess

1 Is there only a single site of damage? Can you identify healthy mucosa around the whole circumference? If not, extend the hole in the muscle until you can.

▶ KEY POINT Do not underestimate the size of a defect

■ Remember that the hole in the mucosa is often larger than the hole in the muscle wall.

2 Are the tissues healthy or ischaemic? Closing defects with unhealthy margins is doomed to failure.

3 Can the defect be repaired? Is there enough tissue for closure without tension?

4 Is there any foreign material? If so, remove it.

5 What is the condition of adjacent structures? Ensure that only healthy tissues remain.

6 If this is a postoperative leak, is the cause evident? What can be learned for future incorporation in your technique?

7 Take a specimen for culture of organisms and tests for antibiotic sensitivity.

Action

1 Remove any foreign material and excise dead or doubtful tissue.

2 Small tears of the cervical oesophagus need no sutures, but it is wise to drain the area. If the tear is large it may be sutured if good access can be obtained. Alternatively, insert a drainage tube through the tear to produce a controlled fistula. Tears of the 'cervical oesophagus' are usually tears of the lower pharynx or perforation of an unexpected pharyngeal pouch.

3 If the defect can be repaired with simple sutures, close it in a single layer using absorbable sutures in one or two layers. Reinforce this if possible with an intercostal muscle flap, a flap of diaphragm or pericardium. Lower oesophageal holes may be reinforced by wrapping with gastric fundus.

113

4 If the defect cannot be repaired, it may be possible to close it by mobilizing the gastric fundus and suturing the seromuscularis around the margins of the defect. Alternatively, insert a T-tube into the leak to produce a controlled fistula, or resect the oesophagus and perform cervical oesophagostomy and gastrostomy. Reconstruction may be delayed for weeks or months.

5 Facilitate enteral feeding below the leak by performing a jejunostomy.

6 In desperate circumstances isolate a severe leak by disconnecting the oesophagus above and below it, either as a temporary or a permanent measure. Transect the oesophagus in the neck leaving the lower cut end open and bring out the proximal end to the skin as a temporary cervical oesophagostomy. Transect the oesophagus below the leak using a 55-mm staple gun. The isolated segment of oesophagus will produce only a little mucus, which will drain by the open upper end. Never perform an oesophageal anastomosis in an unstable patient. Delayed reconstruction is safer.

Closure

1 Insert underwater-sealed drains to apex and base of the pleural cavity after thoracotomy. One of the drains should be sutured in place in the mediastinum close to the leak.

2 Insert closed suction drains into the neck or mediastinum and upper abdomen if the leak or site of trauma has been approached through the abdomen and hiatus.

3 If you decide to drain a leak, defunction the oesophagus and allow the hole to close spontaneously; place a soft drain close to the hole. If it lies at a distance from the hole, the drain will merely partially empty the large abscess cavity that will form.

Aftercare

1 Continue enteral or parenteral feeding, and antibiotics.

2 Remove chest drains when they cease to drain.

3 Monitor the patient's recovery clinically by progress charts and plain radiographs.

4 Check the repair and healing with a screened barium swallow on the seventh postoperative day. If there is no leak, oral feeding may be started, initially with clear fluids.

5 As drains cease to discharge, remove them. If fresh collections develop, drain them. Percutaneous drainage under computed tomographic (CT) guidance may be useful for secondary collections.

CORROSIVE BURNS

Appraise

1 Corrosives are swallowed accidentally or in suicide attempts during acute depression. Classically, the greatest damage occurs at the sites of hold-up above the cricoid sphincter, at the aortic crossing and above the cardia. The substance burns the mouth, pharynx and larynx; that which passes through the oesophagus into the stomach may remain there and cause ulceration, perforation and severe stricture at the gastric outlet.

2 A particular danger in children is the swallowing of small disc or 'button' batteries, which may release damaging caustic contents. These must be immediately and gently removed endoscopically.

It is important not to use instruments that might damage the capsule. Use a snare or dormia basket, but take care not to use excessive force.

3 The mucosa is damaged or destroyed, exposing the deeper layers to any remaining or subsequent passage of the corrosive. The wall then becomes friable and liable to rupture, especially if instrumentation is attempted. The oesophageal wall may become gangrenous and rupture spontaneously, resulting in septic mediastinitis.

4 If the oesophagus does not perforate, mucosal regeneration occurs during the next 10–14 days, but wound contraction and contracture often produce rapid and severe, sometimes long, strictures. There is a small long-term risk of carcinoma.

5 Initially exclude hoarseness, stridor and dyspnoea that suggest inhalation of the corrosive. Monitor the blood gases and carry out tracheostomy if the patient has, or develops, respiratory obstruction.

6 Exclude perforation of the oesophagus, which produces back and chest pain, and intra-abdominal perforation with pain, tenderness and guarding. Order plain X-rays of the chest and abdomen and, if necessary, chest and abdomen CT scan.

7 Do not perform a contrast swallow in the acute stage as it may be extremely painful. Early endoscopy is useful in judging the extent and severity of damage. It must be done gently with the minimum of air insufflation.

8 Start broad-spectrum antibiotic cover. Stop oral intake and institute intravenous fluid therapy with subsequent nutritional support.

9 If perforation has occurred or there is extensive necrosis, carry out emergency exploration with a view to oesophagectomy. Immediate reconstruction is not recommended and exteriorization of the surviving ends and later reconstruction with a suitable conduit is safest.

10 There is no role for steroids in this condition.

11 Do not allow the patient to swallow liquids until you, or another expert, have carried out a radiological or endoscopic examination to confirm that the passage is intact.

12 Anticipate the development of strictures. If they occur, start early treatment with balloon dilators. Do not overdilate the strictures but be prepared to repeat the procedure at gradually lengthening intervals.

13 Sometimes the strictures cannot be dilated, or they recur swiftly, demanding resection and anastomosis or bypass. Occasionally a broncho-oesophageal fistula develops, and this must be defunctioned, initially with a cervical oesophagostomy and gastrostomy. These stomata may be joined later using an isolated segment of colon.

GASTRO-OESOPHAGEAL REFLUX DISEASE

Appraise

1 The continence of the gastro-oesophageal junction is maintained by a combination of anatomical and physiological factors. Elegant anatomical studies have shown a gastro-oesophageal sphincter that corresponds to the high-pressure zone that can be measured by manometry. This area is still known as the lower oesophageal sphincter, although, in reality, it is more gastric than oesophageal.

The effect of the functioning sphincter is augmented by the muscle of the crura of the diaphragm and by having an intra-abdominal segment of oesophagus that is subject to a degree of external compression. The sphincter, including the diaphragm, is under integrated neurological control and relaxes during swallowing and belching. Stretch receptors in the upper stomach are responsible for relaxation of the sphincter during meals.

2 Gastro-oesophageal reflux disease (GORD) occurs when the function of the lower oesophageal sphincter is impaired. Oesophagitis is a complication of GORD that occurs when the lower oesophagus is exposed to irritant gastroduodenal contents long enough to overcome the normal mucosal protection mechanisms. Hiatal hernia has a variable association with GORD. In general, patients with the more severe stages of GORD with oesophagitis tend to have a hernia, but most GORD sufferers do not have a hernia and many of those with a hernia do not have GORD.

3 Careful clinical assessment remains paramount in making the diagnosis and determining its effects on the life of the patient. Endoscopy is valuable to monitor the state of the mucosa and to detect the complication of Barrett's oesophagus, which is a premalignant condition. Norman Barrett (1903–1979), surgeon at St Thomas' Hospital London, described the condition which was later shown to result from persistent acid reflux causing changes in the lower oesophageal mucosal cells, ulceration, strictures and eventual malignancy. If symptoms of reflux cannot be confirmed by endoscopy, 24-hour lower oesophageal pH recording is useful. Assessment of GORD and its complications by radiology is inaccurate and therefore plays little part.

4 The symptoms of reflux may be confused with many disorders causing dyspepsia. Always make an objective diagnosis if surgery is considered.

▶ **KEY POINTS** Discriminate

- Remember that early achalasia produces symptoms that can easily be confused with reflux. Manometry, carried out at the same time as pH recording, excludes achalasia and other motility disorders.
- Remember that in many patients with dyspepsia a hiatal hernia or gastro-oesophageal reflux can be demonstrated, but the symptoms may be due to other pathology.

---

5 Uncomplicated reflux can frequently be managed without surgical treatment. Many patients are overweight. The worst sufferers are sometimes those with good abdominal muscles, such as ex-sportsmen, who subsequently lay down fat that is not obvious, increasing intra-abdominal pressure. Sensible weight loss may cure the symptoms. Smoking, alcohol and fatty foods aggravate the symptoms and are best eschewed. Simple antacid or antacid/alginate preparations may help, but will have been tried long before the patient reaches a surgeon. H2-receptor antagonists will likewise often have been prescribed. Undoubtedly the most effective medication is a proton-pump inhibitor. Omeprazole, lansoprazole, pantoprazole and rabeprazole all have similar effects, although newer drugs such as esomeprazole have a longer duration of action and higher healing rates especially in grade 3 and grade 4 oesophagitis.

6 Consider operation if severe symptoms continue in spite of compliance with medical advice. Be wary of those who will not attempt to lose weight; they frequently put on more weight after operation. Of course, some patients cannot, for a variety of reasons, adhere to an effective regime. Warn the patient that the best reported results are about 85% excellent or good, and that 15% therefore still have symptoms. Be particularly wary of patients who continue to have dyspeptic pain during treatment with an adequate dose of a proton-pump inhibitor. The pain is highly likely to persist after surgery. If in doubt about the effectiveness of a given dose of proton-pump inhibitor, perform 24-hour monitoring of oesophageal and gastric pH to check that acidity is suppressed.

7 The best indication for surgery is persistent regurgitation (volume reflux). This responds poorly to medication and can be remarkably disabling. Beware of offering surgery to patients whose symptoms are well controlled on medical treatment.

8 Barrett's oesophagus is the result of reflux and seems to be increasing in incidence. The role of antireflux surgery in Barrett's oesophagus is still unknown. Patients with Barrett's require regular endoscopic surveillance. If persistently severe dysplasia or neoplasia develops then carry out oesophagectomy if the patient is fit enough to withstand it.

9 The most popular antireflux operation is the Nissen circumferential fundoplication. This can be performed by conventional open or laparoscopic surgery through the abdomen. The postoperative result may be marred by dysphagia, 'gas bloat' or change in bowel habit. The operation has been modified to avoid this, by making a short and loose ('floppy') fundic wrap or by performing a 270° wrap (Toupet). Other approaches such as the transthoracic Belsey are rarely used and will not be described further. There is a shift in opinion towards partial fundoplication, but good results may be obtained by either method if well done.

10 For complex cases in which there is fixed oesophageal shortening, the Collis procedure may be performed, in which a tube is formed from the upper part of the stomach. It is very rarely seen, however, and with proper mobilization the oesophagogastric junction can be brought below the hiatus in nearly all cases.

11 The vagi should never be divided deliberately as part of an antireflux operation since this risks producing postvagotomy symptoms. If the vagi are cut accidentally, as may well occur during revision operations, a pyloroplasty should not be performed. It is unnecessary and leads to additional side-effects.

12 Some patients with particularly difficult reflux problems complicating previous surgery may be helped by partial gastrectomy and Roux-en-Y reconstruction. However, this is not suitable for treatment of uncomplicated reflux and should not be undertaken lightly.

13 Finally, in extreme circumstances, if the cardia has been severely damaged by disease or surgery the only option may be to resect the oesophagus. Continuity may be restored by transposition of the stomach and anastomosis to the cervical or upper thoracic oesophagus, or by interposition of jejunum or colon.

14 Reflux may complicate cardiomyotomy, surgical damage to the hiatal mechanism and damage to, or resection of, the cardiac sphincter in the absence of hiatal hernia. The symptoms and effects may be disabling.

TRANSABDOMINAL FLOPPY NISSEN FUNDOPLICATION (Fig. 8.16)

Prepare

1 Do not operate upon an overweight patient until he or she has lost as much weight as possible.

2 Never operate before full investigation has confirmed the diagnosis and excluded other conditions of the upper gastrointestinal tract.

Access (Fig. 8.17)

1 Elevate the head end of the operating table.

2 Use an upper midline abdominal incision, opening the peritoneum to the left of the ligamentum teres and falciform ligament. An alternative is a bilateral Kocher's roof top incision.

3 If necessary, excise the xiphoid process.

4 Use an on-table mechanical retractor to lift the sternum and costal margin to flatten the diaphragm and give good access to the hiatal hernia.

5 Mobilize the left lobe of the liver and fold it to the right.

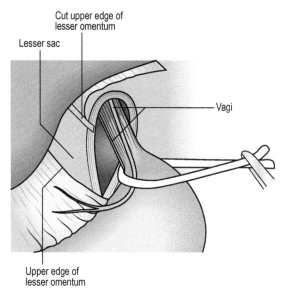

Fig. 8.17 Abdominal approach to the repair of hiatal hernia. The hernial sac has been excised to define the margins of the hiatus, and the upper edge of the lesser omentum has been detached from the diaphragm. Either an anterior or posterior repair may now be performed.

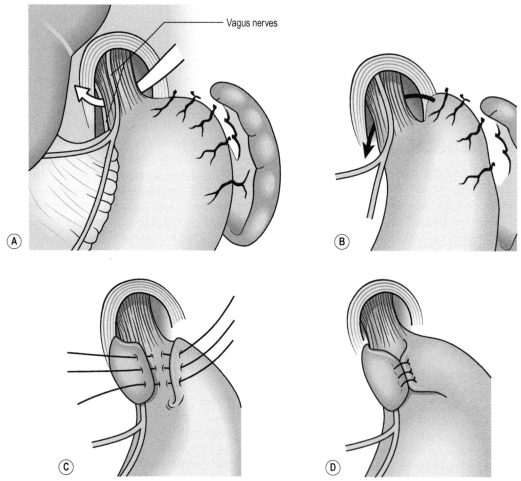

Fig. 8.16 Transabdominal Nissen fundoplication: (A) free the oesophagus in the hiatus, while preserving the vagi and branches; isolate, doubly ligate and divide the upper short gastric vessels; (B) gently fold the freed fundus behind the lower oesophagus to emerge on its right side; (C) insert three or four non-absorbable sutures to pick up the fold, the lower oesophagus and the anterior wall of the stomach to the left of the oesophagus; include the submucosa but not the mucosa; avoid piercing or damaging the vagi; (D) gently tie the sutures; you should be able to insert a finger beneath the cuff so formed.

Assess

1. Explore the abdomen.

2. Look for a sliding hiatal hernia. If the hernia reduces easily and does not tend to spring back into the chest it is safe to proceed with the Nissen operation. It is important to note that if the hernia appears fixed, careful dissection of the oesophagus into the chest may be required.

3. In rolling hernia the gastric fundus herniates alongside the gullet into the chest. The cardia may remain in the abdomen or slide into the chest.

Action

1. Resist the temptation to approach the oesophagus as the first manoeuvre. In open surgery it is much easier to perform a Nissen fundoplication if the fundus of the stomach is mobilized first.

2. Divide most of the short gastric vessels that tether the stomach to the spleen. This is best achieved using a harmonic scalpel. There is often a second layer of vessels entering the posterior aspect of the fundus directly from the splenic artery. Divide these also.

3. When the fundus has been mobilized, continue sharp dissection around the hiatus to expose the lower oesophagus and the crural margins. Identify the anterior and posterior vagal trunks and preserve them.

> **KEY POINTS** Dissect with care

- Do not use blunt dissection. This causes bleeding and may damage a friable oesophagus.
- Operate strictly under vision.

4. On the right side, divide the upper portion of the gastrohepatic omentum, to display the right margin of the hiatus. Leave the hepatic branches of the vagus nerve intact, together with an accessory hepatic artery.

5. Trim the sac, consisting of stretched peritoneum and phreno-oesophageal ligament, from the lower oesophagus.

Posterior repair

1. Ask the anaesthetist to pass a 50 F Maloney tapered mercury dilator into the stomach. This has a soft flexible tip and can be passed with safety.

2. Displace the gullet forwards and stitch the margins of the hiatus together behind it using 2–4 non-absorbable sutures. Leave a space between the hiatus and the stented oesophagus that will admit a finger. Take care not to overtighten the hiatus to avoid postoperative dysphagia.

3. Excise the fat pad that lies in front of the cardia. Take care not to damage the anterior vagus when doing this. There are some surprisingly large blood vessels in the pad that must be ligated.

4. Now gently fold the gastric fundus behind the lower oesophagus so that the greater curvature emerges above the lesser curvature. The posterior vagus nerve may be included in the wrap or the wrap may be placed between the posterior vagus and the oesophagus. Both methods have their advocates and are equally acceptable.

5. The fundus of the stomach should fold around the oesophagus with ease and should lie in place when released. If it tends to retract the fundus has not been adequately mobilized.

6. Insert a non-absorbable suture, such as braided polyamide, to pick up the upper anterior wall of the stomach on the left of the oesophagus, the lower oesophagus immediately above the cardia and the part of the stomach that has been folded behind and to the right of the oesophagus. Each stitch is deep enough to incorporate the submucosa but not to pierce the mucosa. Tighten the stitch so that the two folds of stomach are brought together in front of the oesophagus. Check that a finger can be passed easily between the wrap and the oesophagus which contains the 56 F dilator. The wrap must be really floppy to avoid postoperative dysphagia and gas bloat. Insert a second stitch 1 cm above the first one. The completed fundoplication must not be more than 1 cm long anteriorly. If it is too long, there will be an increased risk of dysphagia and gas bloat.

7. Resist the temptation to insert extra stitches and hitches. They do more harm than good.

8. Ask the anaesthetist to withdraw the mercury dilator but leave the nasogastric tube.

> **KEY POINTS** Avoid overtightening

- Remember, Nissen fundoplication is highly effective in controlling reflux, but it is easy to produce an overcompetent cardia.
- The wrap must be short and loose. It is impossible to make it too loose.

PARTIAL FUNDOPLICATION

1. In order to reduce the incidence of dysphagia and 'gas bloat', many surgeons favour partial fundoplication. There are various methods, which differ in detail, but the principle is the same.

2. The wrap encircles only 270° of the lower oesophagus. To carry this out, first have the anaesthetist pass a nasogastric tube into the stomach. Mobilize the upper half of the gastric greater curve by dividing at least half the short gastric vessels. Fold the gastric fundus loosely round the lower oesophagus. Insert stitches to produce a wrap not more than 3 cm long, around the lower oesophagus. Each of usually two or three stitches picks up gastric fundus on the right and the oesophagus. A second set of two or three stitches picks up the oesophagus and the left upper stomach, leaving the anterior 90° of oesophagus bare (Fig. 8.18).

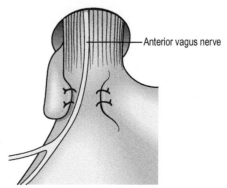

Anterior vagus nerve

Fig. 8.18 Partial fundoplication, leaving 90° of the oesophageal circumference bare.

3 In the Toupet operation the hiatus is not repaired. Instead, the completed fundoplication is stitched to the crura on both sides.

LAPAROSCOPIC FUNDOPLICATION

Appraise

The operation is exactly the same in principle as the 'floppy' Nissen. However, the technique is different because of the different access to the organs and because laparoscopic instruments have a different set of disadvantages from those encountered during a conventional approach.

Do not attempt laparoscopic fundoplication unless you are fully competent in the full range of laparoscopic skills and have been fully trained in the open approach. You must be able to convert to open surgery if difficulties are encountered.

? DIFFICULTY

1. If you cannot complete the procedure safely and effectively within a reasonable time, convert to open operation.
2. Safety is paramount.

Access

1 Place the patient supine with the legs in Lloyd-Davies stirrups as for a perineal operation.

2 Tilt the operating table 30° head up.

3 Have the anaesthetist pass a nasogastric tube to aspirate the stomach. Most surgeons now avoid the use of a 50 F Maloney dilator because of the risk of perforation.

4 Induce a pneumoperitoneum.

5 Place a mixture of 5- and 10-mm cannulas as shown in Figure 8.19.

6 Place a Nathanson retractor into the epigastric port to retract the left lobe of liver and expose the hiatus.

Action

1 First expose the distal oesophagus by dividing the gastrohepatic ligament from about the level of the left gastric artery to the hiatus (Fig. 8.20).

2 Divide the ligament with a harmonic scalpel taking care to identify any vascular structures in the ligament as they can bleed. You

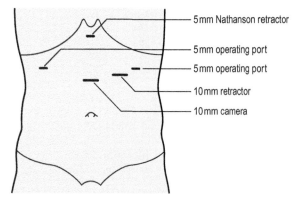

5 mm Nathanson retractor
5 mm operating port
5 mm operating port
10 mm retractor
10 mm camera

Fig. 8.19 Position of ports for laparoscopic Nissen fundoplication

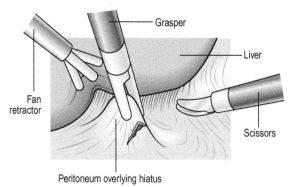

Grasper
Liver
Fan retractor
Scissors
Peritoneum overlying hiatus

Fig. 8.20 Division of gastrohepatic ligament.

now see the right crus of the diaphragm, even in obese patients, provided the liver and stomach are correctly retracted.

3 Now completely expose the crural structure, exposing the landmarks for safe posterior dissection of the oesophagus. Take your dissection over the top of the oesophagus and down the left crus dividing attachments between the angle of His, fundus and diaphragm. Again, a blood vessel is frequently encountered here. Use a harmonic scalpel for this (Fig. 8.21).

4 Take especial care to expose the most posterior aspect of the left crus in order to create the posterior window safely. When the crural muscular fibres are fully exposed, blunt dissection of the oesophagus can be safely accomplished from the lateral and anterior aspects.

5 If a hiatal hernial sac is present, deliver it during the exposure of the muscle fibres.

▶ KEY POINT Avoid damaging the oesophagus

■ Never grasp the oesophagus for retraction throughout the procedure.

---

6 Prepare to create a window posterior to the oesophagus. First ensure that the posterior left crus is completely dissected; it

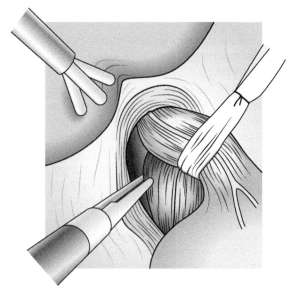

Fig. 8.21 Skeletonizing the hiatus to reveal the left crus.

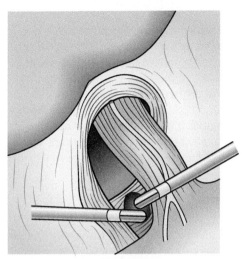

Fig. 8.22 Opening the posterior window with a chopsticks movement of two blunt forceps

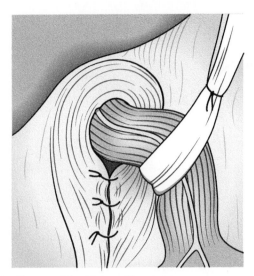

Fig. 8.23 Closure of the hiatus with sutures.

is 1 mm wide and has a firm consistency when you feel it with your right-handed blunt grasping forceps as they sweep inferiorly, following left lateral and anterior retraction of the oesophagus. In thinner patients the posterior crus presents as a visible ridge of tissue covered by para-oesophageal fat, provided retraction is correct. The left crus can also be identified by looking for the posterior vagus nerve as it curves over the structure.

7 You are at risk of gastric or oesophageal perforation if you dissect too inferiorly to the gastric wall, or too anteriorly to the gastro-oesophageal junction.

8 Create the window from the right side, elevating the oesophagus anteriorly with a blunt forcep, and with the other hand separate any strands posteriorly with a harmonic scalpel. Use a sweeping chopstick motion with two forceps to open a window, ensuring this is below the left crus seen from the right. It is easy to dissect into the chest above the crus in this situation (Fig. 8.22).

9 When the window is opened the spleen and post wall of the fundus may be seen. In fat individuals a curved forceps can help this dissection. Attempt to make the window behind the posterior vagus, keeping it next to the oesophagus.

? DIFFICULTY

1. Peri-oesophageal scarring, secondary to penetrating ulcers, and stricture formation are usually, but not always, predictable.
2. Do not dissect blindly. If you cannot confidently identify the posterior left crus and the posterior vagal branch, convert to open laparotomy.

10 In order to secure the wrap in the abdomen, you must close the hiatus by suturing the crura together. Use a 2/0 coated, braided polyester (Surgidac) on a curved needle. Take care to avoid injuring the posterior wall of the oesophagus when you place sutures in the left crus (Fig. 8.23).

? DIFFICULTY

1. Although posterior closure of the crura is easily accomplished in the case of small hernias, it may be difficult in a patient with a large para-oesophageal hiatal hernia. If necessary, carry out anterior repair with mesh reinforcement or suture the wrap to the right crus.
2. Fundoplication can be carried out to prevent reflux after widely mobilizing the oesophagus.

11 The right crus is thinner than the left so include its lateral peritoneal covering to prevent the stitch from tearing out. Two deeply placed stitches are usually sufficient, tied intracorporeally. It is important not to close the hiatus tightly as this will result in dysphagia.

If crural repair is difficult, suture the wrap with two non-absorbable sutures to the right crus to prevent wrap migration.

12 Greater curvature mobilization is currently a matter of debate and is usually not required. In some circumstances it allows the consistent formation of a loose wrap. Intend to divide the gastrosplenic ligament for 10 cm from the angle of His. Have the first assistant use an atraumatic, finely serrated 5-mm grasping forceps, in order to avoid tearing fatty tissue or the short gastric vessels. You hold the stomach so that the ligament is horizontal and under tension. Divide small amounts of tissue at a time, using harmonic scalpel scissors.

13 You are now ready to perform the fundoplication. Elevate the oesophagus and, under direct vision, insert the Babcock clamp through the window until you can see it on the left side of the oesophagus. Grasp the greater curve of the stomach approximately 5–7 cm from the angle of His and draw it to the right behind the oesophagus.

14 Avoid a spiral wrap, which can include the body of the stomach in the left limb of the wrap. Carefully choose the appropriate position for the left limb suture. Try to have the limbs in continuity so that traction on one limb moves the other (Fig. 8.24).

15 Place a full-thickness suture through the stomach but include only the muscular wall of the oesophagus to avoid the risk of

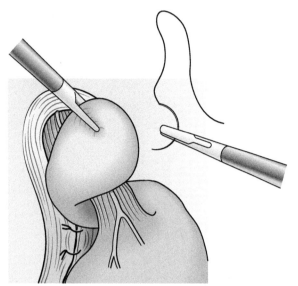

Fig. 8.24   The mobilized fundus is pulled behind the oesophagus and sutured.

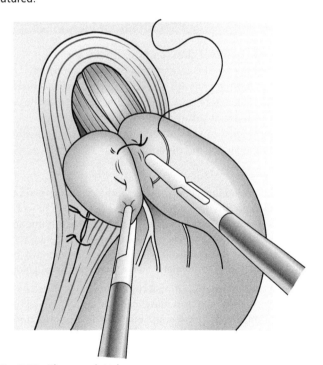

Fig. 8.25   The completed wrap.

postoperative oesophageal leakage. Incorporation of the oesophageal suture is important because it helps to secure the wrap. Sutures can be applied using either intra or extra-corporeal techniques. Perform a short 1–2 cm loose wrap with up to three sutures. There is no need to pass a bougie as these can damage the oesophagus and cause a perforation (Fig. 8.25).

? DIFFICULTY

1. Avoid the risk of perforation by refraining from applying excessive traction on the anterior stomach. If it does occur, repair it by inserting laparoscopic sutures, provided the extent of injury is clearly visible. If not, convert to open laparotomy.

2. Delayed greater curve perforation at the angle of His may follow excessive use of diathermy. Evade the possibility by using the most up-to-date ultrasonic dissector available for dissection in this area.
3. If injury to the oesophagus is suspected, endoscope the patient on the table and look for injury or inflate the oesophagus/stomach under water. Attempt laparoscopic closure of any perforation only if you are very experienced; otherwise, convert to open laparotomy.

Closure

Remove ports under direct vision. A nasogastric tube can be left in place for 12 hours until the patient demonstrates normal swallowing.

Postoperative

1 Order a postoperative Gastrografin swallow if you encountered any difficulties, but not routinely.
2 Encourage the patient to drink fluids after 6 hours. A sloppy diet can be taken within 12 hours.
3 Most patients can be discharged home within 24 hours with instructions to maintain the sloppy diet for the first 4 weeks.
4 Have the port-site sutures removed 1 week after the operation.

ROLLING HERNIA

Appraise

1 The gastric fundus may prolapse through the hiatus alongside the oesophagus alone, or alongside a sliding hiatal hernia of the cardia. The fundus may also prolapse through a congenital or acquired defect in the diaphragm near the hiatus.
2 Sometimes the rolling hernia becomes a volvulus of the stomach as the greater curvature increasingly prolapses through the hiatus.
3 Rolling hiatal hernias should always be repaired unless there is a contraindication to an operation. If the patient develops pain, vomiting from entrapment, obstruction or volvulus, operative repair should be performed as a matter of urgency.
4 Occasionally, a patient presents as an acute abdominal emergency, nearly always having had previous less severe attacks.

Access

Use an upper midline or roof top incision. These hernias can be reduced and repaired through the abdominal route.

Action

1 Identify the gastric fundus disappearing through the hiatus.
2 Reduce the hernia by gentle traction on the stomach. Do not use force or you will tear the gastric wall.
3 When you have completely reduced the stomach, it is very important to excise the sac, thus exposing the crura. This is best achieved by placing a Roberts forcep at the apex of the hiatus and, using long-handled diathermy, incising the peritoneum and carrying

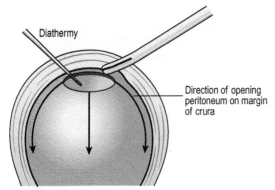

Fig. 8.26   Incising the peritoneum at the apex of a large rolling hiatal hernia.

it around the margin mobilizing the sac, which by gentle finger dissection can be mobilized from the chest (Fig. 8.26). The sac is then excised and the whole circumference of the oesophagus is carefully examined by rotating it.

4 In emergency operations for what is in these circumstances often a strangulated hernia, the gastric wall constricted in the crus may be gangrenous in places. Do not immediately get carried away with the desire to carry out a resection. The blood supply is usually intact proximal and distal to the constriction ring. If it is, invaginate the linear gangrenous ring with a running deep seromuscular stitch.

5 Carry out repair of the defect by uniting the crura posterior to the oesophagus, using four or five non-absorbable mattress sutures.

6 Some surgeons insert three or four non-absorbable sutures that fix the gastric fundus to the undersurface of the left diaphragm – a 'fundopexy' (Fig. 8.27).

7 Alternatively, a fundoplication may be performed. Although there is controversy about the need for an antireflux operation, in these circumstances it seems to do little harm, provides good fixation for the stomach and deals with concurrent reflux symptoms. A gastrostomy on the greater curve also fixes the stomach and acts as a vent.

LAPAROSCOPIC REPAIR

Appraise

Laparoscopic repair of a rolling hiatus hernia can be a challenging operation. Do not attempt it if you are an occasional operator for this condition.

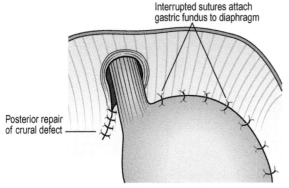

Fig. 8.27   Anterior fundopexy after reduction of gastric volvulus/rolling hiatal hernia. Interrupted non-absorbable sutures anchor the fundus and greater curve to the diaphragm and anterior abdominal wall.

Access

1 Place the patient supine with the legs elevated.
2 Insert five cannulas as for an antireflux operation.

Action

1 Elevate the left lobe of the liver and identify the hiatus and the herniated stomach.
2 Gently reduce the stomach into the abdomen.
3 The operation is greatly facilitated by early excision of the hernial sac. Divide the sac at the hiatal margin, pull down and excise the sac, taking care not to damage the vagi.
4 Repair the crura posterior to the oesophagus.
5 Some prefer to insert a mesh into the hiatus anteriorly to avoid suturing the crura under tension.
6 Fix the stomach in the abdomen with a fundoplication, if preferred.

SIMPLE LAPAROSCOPIC GASTROPEXY

Appraise

1 Many patients with rolling hiatal hernia are elderly, frail and unfit. They may be severely symptomatic, but not fit for major surgery.
2 If the hernia can be reduced and the stomach straightened out, the symptoms of a rolling hernia are relieved and the risk of gastric volvulus is avoided.
3 Simple laparoscopic gastropexy involves minimal surgical trauma and produces surprisingly good results.

Access

1 Place the patient supine with the legs elevated if it is safe to do so. Otherwise operate on the supine patient with the head of the table elevated.
2 Induce a pneumoperitoneum and place cannulas in the following positions: midline above the umbilicus one-third of the distance between umbilicus and xiphisternum; right subcostal, midclavicular; upper midline, below the left lobe of the liver so that the stomach can be sutured to this port site; left subcostal, midclavicular; left subcostal, anterior axillary.
3 Gently reduce the stomach into the abdomen.
4 Insert a non-absorbable suture through the upper midline port leaving the tail of the suture outside the abdomen. Gore-Tex is ideal for this purpose. Take a generous seromuscular bite of the upper stomach at a point that will maintain reduction of the stomach and allow it to be drawn up to the port site when the suture is tied. Bring the needle out of the port and leave the ends long and leave the needle in place.
5 Repeat the above manoeuvre with a suture passed through the left subcostal port.
6 When the sutures have been placed satisfactorily, remove the cannulas and deflate the abdomen.
7 Use the sutures to prolapse part of the stomach wall into the two port sites and stitch to the fascia of the abdominal wall.
8 Close the wounds.

ACHALASIA OF THE CARDIA

Appraise

1 Achalasia, in which the lower segment of the oesophagus fails to relax ahead of a peristaltic wave, is probably part of a generalized condition of neuromuscular origin associated with abnormal vagal motor input and myenteric ganglionic degeneration. The failure to relax is associated with a failure of peristalsis above.

2 As achalasia advances there is gradual dilatation of the oesophagus, ending below in a smooth, beak-like entrance into the stomach. Retention of contents within the oesophagus produces oesophagitis, and if the retained food is aspirated the patient may develop respiratory disorders, including pulmonary fibrosis. For these reasons do not delay effective treatment.

3 The diagnosis must be confirmed by oesophageal manometry. The aim should be to make the diagnosis at an early stage before the typical X-ray changes appear.

4 Achalasia can be treated using forceful dilatation of the lower oesophagus, or by surgical myotomy of the lower oesophageal sphincter. Injection of botulinum toxin also alleviates the symptoms, but has a relatively transient effect and is not recommended for routine use.

FORCEFUL DILATATION

1 This is carried out on the conscious patient under sedation with midazolam.

2 The procedure is undertaken using a plastic dilating balloon, which is specifically made for treating achalasia, is inelastic beyond a predetermined diameter and ruptures when it is overdistended. Increasing sizes of balloon may be used on successive days. The procedure must be performed under fluoroscopic control whether by an endoscopist or interventional radiologist. A radio-opaque, flexible, soft-tipped guidewire is passed through the cardia and the achalasia dilator is threaded over the guidewire until the radio-opaque markers at each end of the balloon lie above and below the cardia. The balloon is inflated under screening control until the waist, which initially appears at the level of the cardia, disappears. It is usual to start with a balloon of 2 cm in diameter and increase at increments of 0.5 cm until blood is seen on the balloon. It is advisable to check that there is no leakage by getting the patient to swallow contrast medium while screening the oesophagus.

3 This method requires significant expertise and should be carried out by skilled and experienced operators. Do not embark upon dilatation unless you, or others, are available with full surgical facilities in case the oesophagus is inadvertently ruptured.

4 If forceful dilatation has been successful for a reasonable period, such as a few months, it may be repeated. If a second dilatation fails to relieve the symptoms, cardiomyotomy should be advised.

LAPAROSCOPIC CARDIOMYOTOMY

Appraise

1 The aim of cardiomyotomy is to weaken the lower oesophageal sphincter sufficiently to allow food to pass, but not to allow gastro-oesophageal reflux. This may be achieved either by performing a limited myotomy with minimal disturbance of the hiatal anatomy or by a more extensive procedure together with an antireflux procedure. Limited myotomy seems the most logical option for most cases. However, if a revision procedure is required, more extensive dissection and an antireflux operation may well be needed.

2 The myotomy should not be carried more than 1 cm onto the stomach because the risk of gastro-oesophageal reflux is increased without improving oesophageal emptying. The proximal extent of the myotomy is not so critical, provided that the short, non-relaxing segment is divided. An oesophageal myotomy of 3–5 cm in length is sufficient.

3 Surgical access for cardiomyotomy may be thoracic or abdominal and there are strong proponents of both. Since myotomy is a limited technical manoeuvre, minimal access techniques are particularly appealing. Laparoscopic cardiomyotomy is probably the procedure of choice, provided expertise can be maintained by a sufficient volume of these uncommon cases.

Access

1 Place the patient supine with the legs elevated.

2 Induce a pneumoperitoneum.

3 Place 10-mm laparoscopic cannulas as follows: midline above the umbilicus one-third of the distance between umbilicus and xiphisternum; right subcostal, midclavicular; left subcostal, midclavicular; left subcostal, anterior axillary. Depending on the instruments that are available, 5-mm cannulas may be substituted for most of the above.

Action (Fig. 8.28)

1 Insert a Nathanson liver retractor through an incision in the epigastrium, deploy it under the left lobe of the liver and retract it upwards.

2 Identify the edge of the caudate lobe as it shows through the almost transparent lesser omentum. Divide the lesser omentum as far proximally as the diaphragm and distally to allow easy exposure of the hiatus. Look for the hepatic branch of the vagus nerve and an accessory hepatic artery, if present. Preserve these structures.

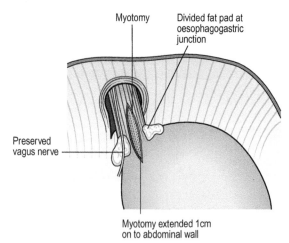

Fig. 8.28 Myotomy for achalasia. The defect can be covered with the gastric fundus to reduce reflux.

3 Identify the crural muscle on the right side of the hiatus. Divide the peritoneum at the edge of this muscle to open the hiatus. Extend the incision upwards and across the anterior aspect of the oesophagus. Do not take the incision downwards as in an antireflux operation. Disturb the hiatal anatomy as little as possible. It is only necessary to expose the anterior aspect of the oesophagus.

4 Identify the anterior vagus and preserve it.

5 Divide the pad of fat that lies anterior to the cardia. This is vascular and is perhaps the most difficult part of the operation.

6 Use curved, blunt-tipped dissecting scissors to make a small transverse incision through the muscle of the oesophagus, just above the cardia, until mucosa can be seen bulging through. This requires care and patience if the correct plane is to be entered and the mucosa kept intact. Wait until bleeding from the cut muscle subsides. Use a very gentle sucker technique to avoid injury to the mucosa.

7 When the mucosa has been exposed through the initial myotomy it is relatively simple to extend the myotomy proximally for 3–5 cm.

8 Extending the myotomy downwards onto the stomach is more difficult. Make repeated small longitudinal cuts under vision and inspect the mucosa at each stage.

9 Continue the myotomy 1 cm onto the stomach. The gastric mucosa has a different appearance to the oesophageal mucosa and can usually be recognized relatively easily.

10 Ask an experienced assistant to pass a gastroscope into the stomach. Use this to double-check that the myotomy is correctly sited and that the mucosa is intact. If there is any difficulty identifying the anatomical landmarks during the myotomy pass the gastroscope as a guide. It can be extremely useful.

11 If the mucosa is opened during the myotomy it may be repaired laparoscopically provided that the circumstances are ideal. Check the integrity of the repair with the gastroscope. If access to the site of injury is not ideal, or the area is obscured by blood, convert to an open procedure.

12 Close the wounds.

PHARYNGEAL POUCH

Appraise

1 This pulsion diverticulum of Zenker is a mucosal herniation between the transverse and oblique fibres of the inferior pharyngeal constrictor muscle, thought to result from incoordination or achalasia of the cricopharyngeal sphincter.

2 Recommend operation if the patient has dysphagia or regurgitation with the likelihood of aspiration pneumonia.

3 It is now usually treated by transoral stapling in which a linear cutting device both divides the cricopharyngeus and opens the diverticulum into the oesophagus (Fig. 8.29). Reserve operation for failures of this technique.

Access (Fig. 8.30)

1 The anaesthetized patient, with a cuffed endotracheal tube in place, lies supine with the head on a ring, turned to the right and neck extended. It is helpful to pass an oesophageal speculum and pass a tube or a small mercury dilator into the oesophagus.

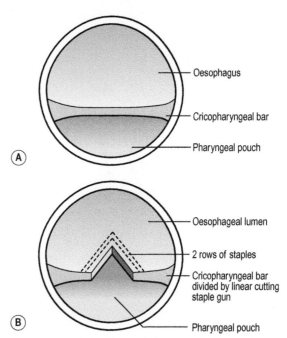

Fig. 8.29 Endoscopic treatment of pharyngeal pouch: (A) the special double-bladed speculum is introduced with the anterior blade in the oesophagus and the posterior blade in the pouch; (B) the bar of cricopharyngeus is divided with an endoscopic linear cutter staple gun.

2 After preparing the skin and towelling off the left side of the neck, make an incision along the anterior border of the left sternomastoid muscle from the greater horn of the hyoid bone to 5 cm above the sternoclavicular joint. Deepen the incision through the platysma muscle, ligating and dividing the external jugular vein if necessary, and then incise the deep fascia.

3 Identify the carotid sheath and retract it and the sternomastoid muscle posteriorly to view the groove between the carotid sheath laterally and the tracheo-oesophageal column medially.

4 Three structures cross the groove. Identify the belly of the omohyoid muscle and divide it. The middle thyroid vein may require double ligation and division but is usually lower. The inferior thyroid artery is lower and deeper than this dissection.

5 Rotate the thyroid gland, larynx, trachea and oesophagus to the right and gently separate the loose tissue in the groove to reach the prevertebral fascia. View the back of the lower pharynx and upper oesophagus to identify the pouch, which lies collapsed against the oesophagus. The neck of the sack lies at the level of the cricoid cartilage.

Action

1 Gently separate the sac from the oesophagus and elevate it from below until it is attached only by the neck. Avoid dissecting away from the sac and in particular keep away from the tracheo-oesophageal groove where the recurrent laryngeal nerve lies.

2 While the sac is still attached, identify the transverse fibres of the cricopharyngeus passing just distal to the neck of the pouch. Open the apex of the sac and insert a finger via the sac into the oesophagus. This enables easy identification of the cricopharyngeus, the fibres of which are divided with a scalpel, preserving mucosal integrity. Make absolutely sure that no horizontal muscle fibres remain.

123

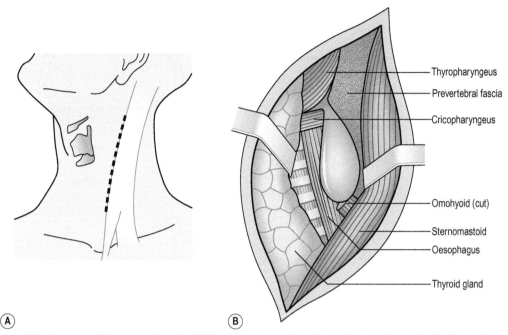

Fig. 8.30 Excision of pharyngeal pouch: (A) head rotated to the right and neck extended, with the incision indicated by a broken line; (B) the pouch and its relations.

3 The most important part of the operation is now completed.

4 A linear 55-mm staple gun is now placed across the neck of the sac to close it and the residual sac excised.

Closure

1 Insert a closed drainage system.

2 Repair the deep fascia and platysma, and close the skin.

Aftercare

1 Start oral fluids after 24 hours. Remove the drain after 2–3 days.

DIVERTICULA

Appraise

1 Traction diverticula result from fibrous adhesion, usually to a diseased, especially tuberculous, lymph node and subsequent contracture. They are rare and do not require specific treatment.

2 Pulsion diverticula result from motility disorders of the oesophagus. Apart from Zenker's diverticulum (pharyngeal pouch), most occur near the lower end of the oesophagus. These rarely require specific treatment. However, the associated motility disorder occasionally demands balloon dilatation or even surgical myotomy. If you need to perform myotomy, excise the diverticulum and close the mucosa. Make sure that the myotomy extends down to the cardia, otherwise there is a high risk of postoperative leakage.

FURTHER READING

Adam A, Ellul J, Watkinson AF, et al. A prospective randomised trial of laser therapy and stent placement. Radiology 1997;202:344–8.

Adam A, Mason RC, Owen WJ. Practical Management of Oesophageal Disease. Oxford: Isis Medical Media; 2000.

Agwunobi AO, Bancewicz J. Simple laparoscopic gastropexy as the initial treatment of paraoesophageal hiatal hernia. Br J Surg 1998;85:604–6.

Akiyama H. Surgery for Cancer of the Esophagus. Baltimore: Williams & Wilkins; 1990.

Anderson JR. Oesophageal injury: part I. The changing face of the management of instrumental perforations. Gullet 1990;10–5.

Bate CM, Keeling PWN, O'Morain C, et al. A comparison of omeprazole and cimetidine in reflux oesophagitis: symptomatic, endoscopic and histological evaluations. Gut 1990;31:968–70.

Coccia G, Bartolotti M, Mitchetti A, et al. Prospective clinical and manometric study comparing pneumatic dilatation and sublingual nifedipine in the treatment of oesophageal achalasia. Gut 1991;32:604–6.

De Meester TR, Wang CI, Wernly JA, et al. Technique, indications and clinical use of 24-hour oesophageal pH monitoring. J Thorac Cardiovasc Surg 1980;79:656–70.

Donahue PE, Bombeck CT. The modified Nissen fundoplication: reflux prevention without gas-bloat. Chirurgie et Gastroenterologie 1977;11:15–21.

Ellis Jr FH, Gibb SP, Crozier RE. Esophagomyotomy for achalasia of the oesophagus. Ann Surg 1980;192:157–61.

Fok M, Ah-Chong AK, Cheng SWK, et al. Comparison of a single layer continuous hand-sewn method and circular stapling in 580 oesophageal anastomoses. Br J Surg 1991;78:342–5.

Forshaw MJ, Gossage JA, Ockrim J, et al. Left thoracoabdominal oesophagogastrectomy: still a valid operation for carcinoma of the distal oesophagus and oesophagogastric junction. Dis Esophagus 2006;19:340–5.

Friedin N, Fisher MJ, Taylor W, et al. Sleep and nocturnal acid reflux in normal subjects and patients with reflux oesophagitis. Gut 1991;32:1275–9.

Gaudreault P, Parent M, McGuigan MA, et al. Predictability of esophageal injury from signs and symptoms. A study of caustic ingestion in 378 children. Pediatrics 1983;71:767.

Griffin SM, Raimes SA. Upper Gastrointestinal Surgery. 2nd ed. Philadelphia: Saunders; 2001.

Hallissey MT, Ratliff DA, Temple JG. Paraoesophageal hiatus hernia: surgery for all ages. Ann R Coll Surg Engl 1992;76:25.

Howard PJ, Mher I, Pryde A, et al. Systematic comparison of conventional oesophageal manometry with oesophageal motility while eating bread. Gut 1991;32:1264–9.

Hulscher JB, van Sandick JW, de Boer AG, et al. Extended transthoracic resection compared with limited transhiatal resection for adenocarcinoma of the oesophagus. N Engl J Med 2002;347:1662–9.

Jenkinson LR, Norris TL, Barlow AP, et al. Acid reflux and oesophagitis: day or night? Gullet 1990;1:36–44.

Khan AZ, Strauss D, Mason RC. Boerhaave's syndrome: Diagnosis and surgical management. Surgeon 2007;5:39.

Liu JF, Wang QZ, Hou J. Surgical treatment for cancer of the oesophagus and gastric cardia in Hebei China. Br J Surg 2004;91:90–8.

Lordick F, Srein HJ, Peschel C, et al. Neoadjuvant therapy for oesophago-gastric cancer. Br J Surg 2004;91:540–51.

Mason R. Palliation of malignant dysphagia, alternatives to surgery. Ann R Coll Surg Engl 1996;78:457–62.

McFarlane GA. Oesophageal injury: part II. The changing face of the management of ruptured oesophagus: Boerhaave's syndrome. Gullet 1990;1:16–23.

Nisson G, Wenner J, Larsson S, et al. Randomised clinical trial of laparoscopic versus open fundoplication for gastrooesophageal reflux. Br J Surg 2004;91:552–9.

Rohatgi A, Forshaw MJ, Sutcliffe RP, et al. Transhiatal oesophagectomy: techniques, tips and outcomes. Surgeon 2008;6:335–40.

Rokkas T, Sladden GE. Ambulatory pH recording in gastroesophageal reflux: relevance to the development of esophagitis. Am J Gastroenterol 1988;88:629–32.

Samuelson SL, Weiser HF, Bombeck CT, et al. A new concept in the surgical treatment of gastro-oesophageal reflux. Ann Surg 1983;197:254–9.

Temple DM, McNeese MC. Hazards of battery ingestion. Pediatrics 1983;71:100.

Thal AP. A unified approach to surgical problems of the esophagogastric junction. Ann Surg 1968;168:542–50.

Toussaint J, Gossuin A, Deruttere M, et al. Healing and prevention of relapse of reflux oesophagitis by cisapride. Gut 1991;32:1280–5.

Vaz F, Geoghegan J, Tanner A, et al. Conservative management of oesophageal perforation following pneumatic dilatation for achalasia. Gullet 1990;1:28–30.

Oesophageal cancer

H. Udagawa, H. Akiyama

INTRODUCTION

1 The epidemiology of squamous oesophageal carcinoma is the most varied of any tumour, so that in certain geographical regions there is a very high incidence and in other areas it is rare. Squamous cell carcinoma of the oesophagus often shows multicentric occurrence in association with head and neck tumours, suggesting that environmental factors are important. Many such factors have been postulated, including smoking, alcohol, dietary nitrosamines, fungal contamination, pickled vegetables, hot tea, gruel, the habit of chewing betel leaf and areca nut and deficiency of certain vitamins and trace elements. A number of benign diseases predispose to its development, including corrosive alkali burns, achalasia, the Paterson-Kelly-Plummer-Vinson syndrome and a history of irradiation. Studies have suggested a link between enzymatic polymorphism related to alcohol degradation (ALDH2) and the development of squamous cell carcinoma of the oesophagus. Genetic predispositions include the autosomal dominant condition tylosis (Greek: tylos = callus) which results in hyperkeratosis of the skin, papillomas and eventually squamous carcinoma of the oesophagus. On the other hand, Barrett's oesophagus is known to increase the risk of the development of adenocarcinoma: the incidence of adenocarcinoma of the lower oesophagus and gastric cardia is rapidly increasing in Western countries, although it is not clear if this increase is due to an increase in gastro-oesophageal reflux disease (GORD; gastro-oesophageal, hence GERD in the USA) and Barrett's oesophagus.

2 The oesophagus runs from the neck through the thorax and into the abdomen. Apart from the cervical region, the oesophagus is divided into upper, middle and lower thirds, although the abdominal segment is sometimes considered separately. Approximately half of all squamous carcinomas develop in the middle third of the thoracic oesophagus. A much larger number of adenocarcinomas develop in the lower third in Western countries.

3 The tumour spreads circumferentially and longitudinally within the mucosa (intraepithelial spread) and in the submucosa and muscle layer, either continuously or separate from the main tumour (intramural metastasis). It may invade the trachea, bronchi, lungs, thoracic duct, recurrent laryngeal nerves, pericardium and aorta. Spread to lymph nodes, both local and distant, is common: detailed Japanese studies have shown that even upper-third carcinomas may be associated with nodal metastases inside the abdomen, while lower-third tumours involve the supraclavicular nodes in a significant proportion of patients. Haematogenous spread is relatively late, and affects the liver, lungs and bones.

4 Because of its insidious development, many patients present with advanced disease, complaining of dysphagia, weight loss, substernal or back pain, aspiration pneumonia or hoarseness. Supraclavicular lymph nodes may be palpable on presentation. The prognosis at this stage is very poor.

5 In Japan, a large number of asymptomatic squamous cell carcinomas are detected through endoscopic examinations at the time of routine health checks, and many of them are treated with endoscopic mucosal resection (EMR) or endoscopic submucosal dissection (ESD). Such local treatment is highly curative as long as the tumour invasion is limited to the epithelium and lamina propria mucosae.

6 Contrast radiography typically demonstrates a long, irregular stricture. However, early lesions produce only slight or even no mucosal irregularities on contrast barium swallow films. The diagnosis is confirmed by endoscopy with biopsy. The technique of Lugol's iodine staining is useful as abnormal areas of mucosa (including carcinoma, oesophagitis, ectopic gastric mucosa and Barrett's epithelium) remains unstained. Newer technologies of image enhanced endoscopy such as narrow band imaging (NBI) and flexible spectral imaging colour enhancement (FICE) may make early detection easier. Biopsy specimens should be taken from all suspicious lesions, where there is an irregularity or a colour change. Take a number of biopsy specimens and record the levels at which they are taken. Do not take many biopsy specimens from one lesion, particularly when the lesion may be suitable for endoscopic resection, because biopsies often result in submucosal fibrosis and may make later intervention difficult.

7 If the cytological brushings and biopsy specimens are reported to be normal but you suspect carcinoma, repeat the examination and go on repeating it until you are absolutely sure that you are not missing a cancer. Cancers located in the hypopharynx, cervical and the thoracic inlet oesophagus are the most difficult to detect. They are very often overlooked by otolaryngologists, radiologists and endoscopists. Particular effort should be taken at endoscopy to observe the hypopharynx, including both piriform sinuses, at the beginning of the examination and the oesophageal inlet on removal of the scope to avoid misdiagnosis.

8 Other valuable imaging modalities are computed tomography (CT), endoscopic ultrasonography and magnetic resonance imaging: these provide information on tumour size, invasion of contiguous structures and extent of lymph node involvement.

Conventional endoscopic ultrasonography images the normal oesophageal wall as five to seven concentric layers; high-frequency ultrasound machines can visualize a nine-layered structure, allowing the depth of penetration to be estimated with greater accuracy. Ensure that CT scans include the upper abdomen and also the lower half of the neck, since enlarged lymph nodes that are not easily palpable may otherwise be missed. Conventional abdominal and cervical ultrasonography is also useful to detect abdominal and cervical nodal involvement, but remember that lymph node size is not diagnostic of metastasis: micrometastases are common and reactive hypertrophy of lymph nodes without metastasis is also frequent. FDG-PET is becoming routine for preoperative staging as it provides metabolic evidence of occult metastases, albeit with a significant incidence of both false negative and false positive results. Perform bronchoscopy with a flexible instrument in patients with middle- and upper-third advanced tumours to determine if there is invasion of the trachea or bronchi.

9 Preoperative staging should now be undertaken using the TNM classification of the International Union against Cancer (Table 9.1).

10 Carry out a careful assessment of the patient to exclude or confirm the presence of incidental disease, particularly that of the cardiovascular and respiratory systems.

11 Recent advances in the field of chemoradiotherapy (CRT) are rapidly changing the management of this disease. Although surgery remains the standard treatment for lesions where R0 resection is possible an increasing number of patients, particularly those with advanced disease, are treated with chemoradiation as the first mode of treatment.

12 As with many other fields of surgery, oesophagectomy has been influenced by the current trend towards minimally invasive surgery, and nowadays even Japanese-style extended radical oesophagectomy can be performed via Video-assisted thoracic surgery (VATS). Although the operation may not be truly minimally invasive because of the necessity for extended lymphadenectomy, the advantages of video-assisted surgery have been recognized.

Appraise

1 Because oesophageal carcinoma is so often advanced at the time of diagnosis, some surgeons feel that treatment should be palliative, thus depriving patients who might be cured of the opportunity to benefit from a radical approach. Our experience of over 25 years of extensive lymph node dissection proves that even patients with 'distant' lymph node metastases regarded as M1 in the TNM system still have a chance of being cured by surgery. With the recent advance of non-surgical treatments, some T4 tumours have also become candidates for radical operation after neoadjuvant therapy.

2 Except in a few areas, oesophageal carcinoma is not a common disease. Unless patients are referred to a specialist centre, the clinicians who see them have relatively little experience on which to base management decisions. It has also been shown that surgeons who regularly perform oesophageal operations achieve lower mortality rates and better results than occasional operators.

3 There is general agreement, at least among surgeons, that radical resection is indicated in otherwise fit patients with tumours at the loco-regional stage (TNM Stage I-III, excluding T4b). However, there are different opinions about what constitutes radical resection.

TABLE 9.1 TNM classification for oesophageal carcinoma (International Union against Cancer 2009)

T (primary tumour)

TX	Primary tumour cannot be assessed
T0	No evidence of primary tumour
Tis	Carcinoma in situ/high grade dysplasia
T1	Tumour invades lamina propria, muscularis mucosae or submucosa
T1a	Tumour invades lamina propria or muscularis mucosae
T1b	Tumour invades submucosa
T2	Tumour invades muscularis propria
T3	Tumour invades adventitia
T4	Tumour invades adjacent structures
T4a	Tumour invades pleura, pericardium, or diaphragm
T4b	Tumour invades other adjacent structures such as aorta, vertebral body, or trachea

N (regional lymph nodes)

Irrespective of the site of the primary tumour, those in the oesophageal drainage area including coeliac axis nodes and paraoesophageal nodes in the neck, but not supraclavicular nodes

NX	Regional lymph nodes cannot be assessed
N0	No regional node metastasis
N1	Metastasis in 1-2 regional lymph nodes
N2	Metastasis in 3-6 regional lymph nodes
N3	Metastasis in 7 or more regional lymph nodes

M (distant metastasis)

M0	No distant metastasis
M1	Distant metastasis

Other than the classical Stage grouping, new concept of Prognostic grouping has been introduced. The Prognostic grouping is different between squamous cell carcinoma and adenocarcinoma, although whether the new concept could be accepted widely is uncertain.

4 There is more disagreement about the treatment options for patients with advanced tumours that involve adjacent structures (T4, particularly T4b) or have more extensive nodal involvement (N3 or with M1 lymph node metastasis). Some surgeons still apply radical surgery with curative intent together with vigorous multimodality treatments to these diseases as long as R0 resection is possible. Even when only palliative treatment is indicated, resection or bypass surgery remains an important option for achieving the best palliation, especially with regard to dysphagia. Radiotherapy (including concurrent CRT), chemotherapy, stenting, laser therapy and laser-activated photodynamic therapy are all claimed to be beneficial alone or in combination. In recent reports, concurrent CRT has been shown to be more effective than single-modality treatments. A surgeon working alone is unable to

evaluate the various claims that are made. For this reason, work closely with your radiotherapy and oncology colleagues or refer your patients to a specialist centre.

5 Adequate resection of oesophageal carcinoma requires a tumour-free margin to avoid the development of recurrent malignant dysphagia. Because of the frequency of intraepithelial spread, intramural metastasis and multicentric tumours, precise preoperative diagnosis is of the utmost importance. Some surgeons send specimens from the upper and lower cut ends for frozen-section histology, but this does not entirely rule out the possibility of a 'skip' lesion remaining in the oesophageal remnant.

6 Do not make your decision without first discussing the possibilities and problems with the patient and, when appropriate, with the relatives. You must take into account the physical fitness and the psychological and philosophical attitudes of the patient. If you have obtained your patient's confidence, you will usually be entrusted with making the decision.

Prepare

1 Discuss the possibilities with the patient, since cooperation is essential to the success of major procedures.

2 Restore the dysphagic patient to a good nutritional state with soft oral foods and an elemental fluid diet, introducing a fine nasogastric tube into the stomach if necessary. Percutaneous endoscopic gastrostomy (PEG) is another option, particularly when neoadjuvant treatment requiring a longer time is planned. PEG is possible if a thin (transnasal) gastroscope can be introduced into the stomach, and it does not present an obstacle to future gastric pull-up. Parenteral intravenous alimentation is a useful option, although enteral feeding is more effective and preferred due to the concept of 'immuno-nutrition'.

3 Oral hygiene is very important to prevent postoperative pneumonia. Preoperative consultation by a dentist should be performed routinely, and the patient should be trained in vigorous self-oral care.

4 Preoperative consultation by an otolaryngologist is also important. It might reveal unexpected recurrent laryngeal nerve palsy and meso- or hypopharyngeal cancer, which often occurs synchronously. Coincidental hypopharyngeal cancer is, however, more often detected by careful endoscopy.

5 Although enteral feeding can be re-started on the first or second postoperative day, set up a central venous line before surgery commences to secure reliable blood access.

6 Achieve the best possible cardiorespiratory state with physiotherapy, blood replacement and correction of serum protein and electrolytes. Smoking should be stopped as early as possible. Order 2–3 units of cross-matched blood. Collecting 800 ml of the patient's own blood for autotransfusion is very useful to avoid allogenic blood transfusion. We also prepare cryoprecipitate from the patient's own blood to apply it to the operative field as fibrin glue.

7 Ensure that the oesophagus, stomach and colon are empty. If the colon may be used for reconstruction, commence 1 or 2 days of low residue diet and administer oral bowel preparation the day before surgery (see Chapter 13).

8 Commence intravenous prophylactic antibiotic cover prior to commencing surgery: second- or third-generation cephalosporins have been used routinely.

9 Institute prophylaxis against deep venous thrombosis. Application of pneumatic cuffs to the lower extremities during and for several days after operation is most effective. Start continuous intravenous administration of heparin (100-150 units/kg/day) from immediately after the operation until the patient is mobile.

10 Undertake urethral catheterization and monitor hourly urine output during and after the operation.

11 Administration of a small dose of a corticosteroid (methylprednisolone, 250 mg) 2 hours prior to surgery is recommended by some authors to prevent the release of cytokines, which may precipitate ALI (acute lung injury) or ARDS (adult respiratory distress syndrome).

RESECTION OF CARCINOMA OF THE LOWER OESOPHAGUS (LEFT THORACO-ABDOMINAL APPROACH)

Appraise

1 Our routine operation for carcinoma of the abdominal oesophagus and the cardia is resection of the lower thoracic oesophagus together with a cuff of the gastric cardia or entire stomach followed by jejunal interposition or Roux-en-Y reconstruction through the left thoracoabdominal approach (Fig. 9.1). Primary carcinoma of the lower thoracic oesophagus needs right thoracotomy for lymph node dissection.

2 You will nearly always find that the resection needs to go higher than you had planned. Technically, you can carry out anastomosis behind the carina through this approach. In doubtful cases, choose the right-sided approach, or bluntly dissect and resect the remaining upper thoracic oesophagus and then make an anastomosis in the neck between the cervical oesophagus and the gastric remnant or colon brought up either retrosternally or through the posterior mediastinum.

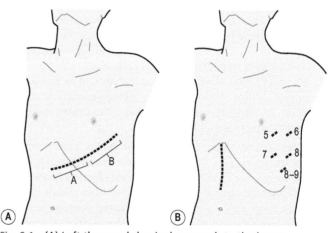

Fig. 9.1 (A) Left thoracoabdominal approach to the lower oesophagus. Dotted line A is for initial abdominal exploration. When the tumour is resectable, the incision is extended (Dotted line B). (B) The hand-assisted left thoracoscopic and abdominal approach to the lower oesophagus. The numbers on the chest wall indicate the levels of intercostal spaces for each port for thoracoscopic surgery.

3 The VATS procedure is a combination of upper median laparotomy and left thoracoscopic operation assisted by the operator's left hand inserted transhiatally (Fig. 9.1B). We call the conventional left thoraco-abdominal approach (LTA), and its VATS counterpart hand-assisted left thoracoscopic and abdominal approach (HLTA).

Access

1 Place the anaesthetized, intubated patient on the right side, with the left shoulder rotated back against a support attached to the operating table, or use a self-retaining mat.

2 Open the left upper abdomen obliquely along the line of the sixth or seventh intercostal space, starting in the midline halfway between the umbilicus and the tip of the xiphisternum and extending to the left costal margin. The sixth intercostal space is more suitable when the lesion has substantial extension in the thoracic oesophagus, and mediastinal lymph node dissection is planned. Palpate the liver and the pelvis to rule out distant spread. Determine the fixity of the cardia and feel for extensive lymph node involvement that would make resection useless. Laparoscopic assessment of the abdominal cavity may demonstrate peritoneal dissemination and avoid unnecessary laparotomy.

3 If resection seems feasible, cut across the costal margin and elongate the skin incision toward the posterior axillary line along the planned intercostal space. Open the chest, cutting along the lower attachment of the intercostal muscles. Even in elderly patients with fixed ribs, sufficient separation of the intercostal muscles from the rib will allow adequate access.

4 Cut the diaphragm radially 10–15 cm towards the right crus. Even in very advanced case with direct tumour invasion to the crural muscle, you can achieve a safe surgical margin with circular resection of the muscle around the hiatus. It is not necessary to transect the diaphragm completely from its periphery to the part around the hiatus. If necessary, circumferential resection of the diaphragm around the hiatus can be added.

5 Insert a self-retaining rib retractor and gently open it in stages.

6 Stop all bleeding meticulously.

7 Anchor the edge of the incised diaphragm to the edge of the skin incision so that the left lung will not prolapse and interfere with the operative field during the intra-abdominal procedure.

Assess

1 Determine the extent of spread to the gastric cardia and glands along the left gastric vessels and around the coeliac axis.

2 Even if the stomach and associated glands appear to be uninvolved remove the left gastric basin, including the root of the left gastric artery. If the cardia or upper stomach is widely involved, prefer total gastrectomy.

3 If radical resection is inappropriate because of the extended disease, be willing to carry out an adequate longitudinal resection in a fit patient with a resectable tumour. Treat unresectable lesions by bypass, taking the stomach, jejunum or colon well above the tumour and joining it to the oesophagus in the chest or the neck. In Britain, gastro-oesophageal anastomosis in the neck is associated with the name of Kenneth McKeown of Northallerton. For fixed, extensive, obstructing tumours in high-risk patients, dilatation and insertion of an expandable metallic stent is the treatment of choice. Tube jejunostomy is also recommended for supplementary nutrition.

Resect
Abdominal procedure

1 Open the lesser sac, dissecting the greater omentum from the transverse colon and severing the avascular portion of the gastric lesser omentum.

2 Ligate and divide each artery and vein of the stomach at the root according to the planned resection procedure.

3 Divide the stomach (for proximal gastrectomy) or the duodenal bulb (for total gastrectomy) with a linear stapling device.

▶ **KEY POINT** Distal pancreatectomy and splenectomy?

■ If the lymph nodes along the splenic artery are highly suspicious of metastasis or the tumour has directly invaded to the surface of the distal pancreas, distal pancreatectomy and splenectomy assures en bloc resection of the tumour.

4 Remove the anchoring stitch from the diaphragm and pass a tape through the hiatus. Pull the tape down to get good exposure of the left thoracic cavity.

Thoracic procedure

1 Gently free the lower lobe of the left lung, dividing the pulmonary ligament, taking care not to injure the pulmonary vein.

2 Elevate and pull forward the lower lobe of the lung to display the posterior mediastinum. Locate the lower thoracic aorta and incise the mediastinal pleura just anterior to it. Dissect the anterior surface of the aorta. Ligate and divide the proper oesophageal arteries, which are rather rarely found in the lower mediastinum.

3 Incise the mediastinal pleura just posterior to the pericardium. Gently mobilize the lower oesophagus, leaving the mediastinal adipose tissue on the oesophageal side and taking care not to accidentally injure the azygous vein and the thoracic duct on the left side. If necessary, excise the posterior pericardium and a portion of the right pleura.

4 Decide the level of oesophageal transection and do not mobilize too high above this point. Too-extensive mobilization (more than 5 cm) of the oesophagus may result in ischaemia of the oesophageal stump.

5 Gently grasp the oesophagus with Akiyama's oesophageal clamp or a right-angled vascular clamp and transect the oesophagus below it. Remove the specimen for histological examination. Immediate frozen section examination should be carried out if the upper margin is uncertain.

Unite (Fig. 9.2)

1 Plan the mesenteric incision line under transillumination to obtain the longest jejunal loop. The second or third jejunal artery is usually most suitable as a feeder. Cut the jejunum between two clamps and pull the distal end up retrocolically through the hiatus to the oesophageal stump.

2 Place a running purse-string suture in the oesophageal stump and insert the anvil of a 25 mm circular stapling device. Insert the circular stapler through the open jejunal end to construct an end-to-side (functionally end-to-end) oesophagojejunostomy. Close the

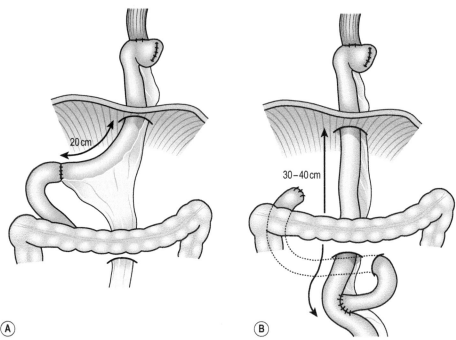

Fig. 9.2   Standard reconstructive methods after resection of lower oesophagus and stomach: (A) jejunal interposition; (B) Roux-en-Y reconstruction. (Modified with permission from Akiyama H 1990 Surgery for cancer of the esophagus. Williams & Wilkins, Baltimore.)

open jejunal stump using a linear stapling device. Add seromuscular sutures to bury the staple line. Insert a nasogastric tube though the anastomosis.

> ▶ KEY POINT   Confirmation of anastomosis
>
> ■ The easiest way to check the completeness of the anastomosis is to confirm the two 'donuts' of oesophageal and jejunal walls left in the circular stapler. If uncertainty remains, 'air-leak testing' is the next choice.

3 If the distal stomach is preserved, bury the line of staples on the gastric remnant with seromuscular stitches. Cut the elevated jejunum 20 cm below the hiatus, while preserving the feeding vessels. Make an anastomosis between the distal end of the jejunal segment and the anterior wall of the gastric remnant. Then form another end-to-end jejunojejunal anastomosis below the mesocolon to complete the reconstruction.

4 Following a total gastrectomy, Roux-en-Y reconstruction is a preferable choice.

> ▶ KEY POINT   Roux-en-Y reconstruction
>
> ■ If you create a Roux-en-Y anastomosis, unite the afferent jejunal segment from the ligament of Treitz, on the patient's left side of the elevated jejunum that has been anastomosed to the oesophagus. Otherwise, the afferent jejunal loop may prolapse to the left side through the space behind the raised segment of jejunum which may result in a complicated bowel torsion.

5 We routinely omit Heineke-Mikulicz pyloroplasty in spite of truncal vagotomy. Although this may result in early-stage gastric

stasis, patients have fewer episodes of bile regurgitation on long-term follow-up.

6 Make sure there is no tension on the anastomoses, and no twisting or kinking of the bowel.

Checklist

1 Make sure the intrathoracic anastomosis is perfectly fashioned and there is no evidence of tension or ischaemia. An intrathoracic leak is often fatal.

2 Has all the bleeding stopped?

3 Close all the defects of the mesentery and mesocolon in order to avoid internal herniation. Fix the organ that was elevated for reconstruction to the hiatus to prevent prolapse into the thoracic cavity. Do not tighten the hiatus unless it was widened during the tumour resection. If you perform hiatal narrowing, make sure that the hiatus is still loose afterwards.

> ? DIFFICULTY
>
> 1. There are wide variations in the extent of resection and the mode of reconstruction. It is most important to make sure that the anastomosis remains free from recurrence. Therefore, never skimp on tumour resection to facilitate anastomosis.
> 2. Has the tumour proved to be irresectable? A bypass operation usually preserves patency longer than oesophageal stenting and is functionally superior as long as it is done safely.
> 3. If the lesion is very extensive, abandon attempts to resect or bypass it.

4. If the respiratory function of the patient is too poor for left thoracotomy and the upper margin of the tumour is only 2 or 3 cm higher than the level of the hiatus, a transhiatal approach can be considered. Cut the central tendon of the diaphragm anterior to the hiatus so that you can achieve wide exposure of the lower posterior mediastinum. Take care not to place excessive compression on the heart when using this approach.

Closure

1 Insert an underwater-seal drain into the left pleural cavity through a separate stab incision near the costophrenic angle in the posterior axillary line.

2 Close the diaphragm using a continuous interlocking suture. The last 4–5 cm are closed with interrupted sutures from the abdominal side. Leave them unknotted until the incised intercostal space has been approximated with two thick, absorbable threads through both ribs.

3 Close the abdominal wound in your usual manner.

4 Close the chest wound, including the external oblique muscle and serratus anterior muscle above and below.

OPERATIONS FOR THORACIC OESOPHAGEAL CARCINOMA

INTRODUCTION

1 The two-stage operation of Ivor Lewis is the classic method for dealing with mid-oesophageal carcinoma. Many surgeons still employ this as their standard procedure for all oesophageal carcinomas. Newer and more radical techniques include the extensive (three-field) lymph node dissection popularized by Japanese surgeons.

2 VATS (video-assisted thoracic surgery) oesophagectomy is growing in popularity, as it offers advantages related to magnified view and variable view-point. It is also advantageous in surgical training because all the members of the team share the same view of the operative field and the instructor feels more confident when supervising a trainee performing a critical part of the operation.

3 It is not safe to embark on any of these advanced techniques, whether open or thoracoscopic, after simply reading a description. However, all the advanced techniques were developed as the result of step-by-step revision of older methods, enabling surgeons to make their operations more radical.

4 The more limited procedure of transhiatal oesophagectomy is still employed, combined with adjuvant therapy, and is claimed to be equally effective by its advocates.

IVOR LEWIS RESECTION FOR MID-OESOPHAGEAL CARCINOMA

Appraise

1 This operation is the source of other newer and more radical operations. Therefore, the essential points of the Ivor Lewis operation also apply to newer techniques. Only the general concept of the operation and a few specific points are presented here.

2 The first step is the abdominal operation, in which the whole stomach is mobilized for reconstruction leaving the right gastric and gastroepiploic vessels as feeding vessels. The second step is the thoracic operation, involving oesophageal resection and reconstruction using pulled-up stomach as an oesophageal substitute. An oesophagogastrostomy is made intrathoracically. This is performed with an end-to-end circular stapling device or side-to-side application of the linear stapling device and is rarely performed manually these days.

3 By careful positioning of the patient, it is possible for two surgical teams to work simultaneously, placing the upper part of the patient in the position for right thoracotomy, with the pelvis almost flat on the operating table. The position may thereafter be adjusted by tilting the table.

4 Carry out a full Kocher's mobilization of the head of pancreas and duodenal loop, because oesophageal reconstruction is usually done after closure of the abdominal incision.

RADICAL CURATIVE SURGERY: EXTENSIVE LYMPH NODE DISSECTION (AKIYAMA TECHNIQUE)

Appraise

1 Japanese surgeons have been performing extensive lymph node dissection for about 25 years, and more recently the technique has been adopted by surgeons in North America and Europe. The operative mortality is satisfactorily low and the 5-year survival rate exceeds 50% for those who undergo a curative (R0) resection. These good results are often attributed to differences in the type of tumour, population screening procedures, the general health and body habitus of the patients and stage migration due to extensive lymph node dissection itself (the Will Rogers phenomenon), but there is no good evidence that such factors play a part.

2 Achieving negative surgical margins for local control and extended lymphadenectomy for regional control are different but equally important targets of R0 resection. Skinner has advocated 'en bloc dissection' as a variation of such radical surgery. The essential concept of his operation is wide resection of tissues surrounding the oesophageal tumour, including mediastinal pleura, azygous vein, thoracic duct and pericardium for tumours with infiltrative growth beyond the adventitia. These days, such tumours are usually considered candidates for neoadjuvant chemoradiation.

3 The concept of extensive lymph node dissection was developed following investigation into the extent of lymphatic tumour spread, and made possible by careful attention to detail in planning and performing the operation. We do not take an inflexible attitude towards the extent of either oesophageal or lymph node excision, but try to match the operation to the site and extent of tumour growth and to the likelihood of invasion and spread to the lymph nodes.

4 Reliable preoperative assessment of the tumour by endoscopy, conventional ultrasound of the neck and abdomen, endoscopic ultrasound and CT is mandatory.

5 Although this preoperative assessment is helpful in detecting spread, it does not reveal micrometastases, so radical dissection must encompass what appears to be normal tissue.

6 Modern imaging techniques have made an initial abdominal exploration unnecessary in most patients. If uncertainty exists concerning resectability and curativity in the abdomen, start with the abdominal procedure. In such cases, the cervical and abdominal parts of the operation can be completed first (reconstruction-first approach). The order of mediastinal dissection and reconstruction is interchangeable so this is not a major problem.

7 Video-assisted radical oesophagectomy is now a standard procedure, particularly when the patient has no history of radio- or chemoradiotherapy. It is performed with the patient in a left lateral recumbent position similar to conventional open oesophagectomy. Because the essential operative technique of the two approaches is similar, details of the VATS procedure are appended to descriptions of the open procedure in the following paragraphs as necessary. Some surgeons prefer to perform VATS oesophagectomy in a prone position under positive pressure pneumothorax. Surgeons learning VATS oesophagectomy as part of a new team may find this approach easier, as it is almost 'solo-surgery' and no skilled assistant is necessary. However, for an experienced team the left lateral position has the advantage because the operation is performed within a view familiar to them.

THORACIC PROCEDURE

Access

1 Place the anaesthetized, intubated patient on the left side using a self-retaining mat.

2 Make a right anterolateral thoracotomy incision in the fourth intercostal space preserving the right latissimus dorsi muscle (Fig. 9.3).

3 Cut the intercostal muscles with electrocautery along the upper margin of the fifth rib from a point lateral to the internal mammary artery to a point lateral to the sympathetic trunk.

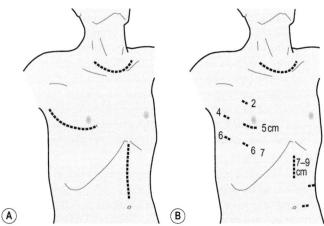

Fig. 9.3 (A) Skin incisions for the oesophagectomy with three-field lymphadenectomy. Thoracic incision is first made in left lateral recumbent position along the 4th intercostal space. The cervical and abdominal incisions are then made in supine position simultaneously by two teams. (B) Skin incisions for the video-assisted oesophagectomy with three-field lymphadenectomy. A minithoracotomy of 5 cm is placed along the 4th intercostal space. The numbers on the chest wall indicate the levels of intercostal spaces for each port for thoracoscopic surgery. A minilaparotomy of 7–9 cm and two port wounds are made for hand-assisted laparoscopic surgery. (Modified with permission from Akiyama H 1990 Surgery for cancer of the esophagus. Williams & Wilkins, Baltimore.)

4 Apply two self-retaining rib retractors in a crossed fashion to produce a square window for access to the right thoracic cavity.

▶ KEY POINTS Separating the ribs

■ We almost always divide the lower (usually 5th) costal cartilage near the sternocostal joint, and the upper (usually 4th) rib near the neck. These two cuts will prevent uncontrolled rib fracture or articular dislocation and reduce the incidence of chronic postoperative chest pain. The cut rib can be fixed at the time of wound closure using an absorbable hydroxyapatite intracostal implant.

■ When inserting the self-retaining rib retractor, open it gently and gradually.

■ When it becomes too tight, leave it for a few minutes and try again. In this way you improve the access without causing unnecessary rib fractures.

5 Free the lower lobe of the lung dividing the right pulmonary ligament.

6 For VATS oesophagectomy, a minithoracotomy of 5 cm in length is placed and four 11-mm ports are inserted, as shown in Figure 9.3B.

Assess

1 Rule out tumour implantation. Any suspicious nodules should be sent to the pathologist for frozen section diagnosis.

2 Check whether the main tumour is fixed to the surrounding organs. If direct invasion is suspected, carefully dissect the tumour from the organs around it. The trachea, left main bronchus, vertebra and descending aorta (those organs involved in T4b disease) are the most important to examine. Lung, pericardium, azygous vein, thoracic duct and diaphragm (organs involved in T4a disease) can easily be resected together with the oesophagus.

Action (Figs 9.4–6)

1 Incise the mediastinal pleura vertically over the right vagus nerve on the lateral tracheal wall. Elongate the pleural incision upward to the level of the subclavian artery. Identify the origin of the right recurrent laryngeal nerve and gently dissect it upward. The area behind this is the lower portion of the right recurrent laryngeal lymph node chain, which is a very frequent site of lymph node metastasis. It is possible to dissect this lymph node chain until the lower pole of the right thyroid lobe is encountered, but it is safer to leave the upper half untouched and dissect it from the neck (Figs 9.4, 5, 10). In VATS oesophagectomy a much higher portion of the right recurrent laryngeal lymph node chain can be reached safely under thoracoscopic vision.

2 Dissect the anterior and posterior ends of the azygous arch, ligate and divide it. Be sure that the right bronchial artery, which lies below the azygous arch, is not included (Fig. 9.5).

3 Identify the right bronchial artery, which is usually the main branch from the third right intercostal artery. Ligate and cut the (third) intercostal artery peripheral to the origin of the right

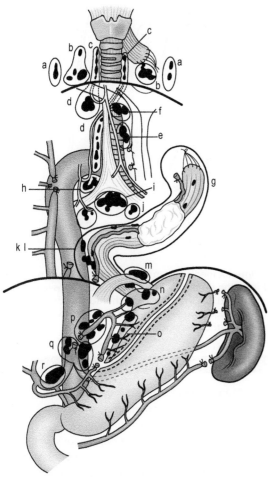

Fig. 9.4 Extent of resection and lymph node dissection of the standard radical oesophagectomy with extensive lymph node dissection for thoracic oesophageal carcinoma. Nodes to be dissected are in solid black. The mediastinal part is the lateral view. a, deep lateral cervical nodes; b, deep jugular nodes; c, cervical portion of recurrent nerve chain; d, thoracic portion of recurrent nerve chain; e, (right) pretracheal nodes; f, brachiocephalic artery nodes; g, upper thoracic para-oesophageal nodes; h, infra-aortic arch (left tracheobronchial) nodes; i, subcarinal nodes; j, main bronchus nodes; k, middle thoracic para-oesophageal nodes; l, lower thoracic para-oesophageal nodes; m, supradiaphragmatic nodes; n, right and left cardiac nodes; o, lesser curvature nodes; p, left gastric artery nodes; q, coeliac trunk nodes (including proximal splenic artery nodes); r, common hepatic artery nodes. Area k and l includes para-aortic nodes and thoracic duct nodes. (Modified with permission from Akiyama H 1990 Surgery for cancer of the esophagus. Williams & Wilkins, Baltimore.)

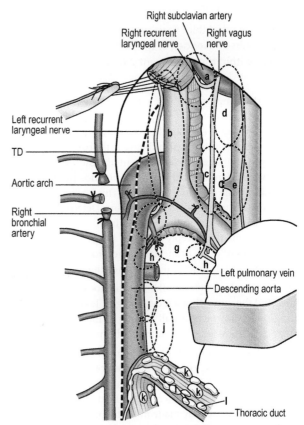

Fig. 9.5 Superior and middle mediastinum in the course of lymph node dissection viewed from the right side. Thoracic duct is resected with the oesophagus, and the third intercostal artery arising from its common trunk with the right bronchial artery is divided. Nodes indicated by dotted ellipsoids are to be dissected. Metastasis is rarely seen in the late stage in lower pretracheal nodes (e), so they are preserved to maintain tracheobronchial circulation when the tumour is located in the lower third of the oesophagus or the tumour is in the early stage. a, right recurrent nerve nodes; b, left recurrent nerve nodes; c, right tracheobronchial nodes; d, pretracheal nodes, upper one-third (brachiocephalic nodes); e, pretracheal nodes, lower two-thirds; f, left tracheobronchial nodes (subaortic arch nodes); g, subcarinal nodes; h, bilateral main bronchus nodes; i, para-aortic nodes; j, pulmonary ligament nodes; k, para-oesophageal nodes; l, thoracic duct nodes. The thick dotted line, TD, shows the running course of the thoracic duct before resection.

bronchial artery so that you can safely retract the mediastinum anteriorly without tension on the bronchial artery (Fig. 9.5).

4 Cut the thin membranous structure containing small sympathetic nerve branches behind the upper oesophagus, and dissect this plane to the left side leaving the thoracic duct and the adipose tissue around attached to the oesophagus. Cut the similar thin membranous structure on the left side, and you will observe the left lung translucently through the left mediastinal pleura. With anterior extension of the dissection along this plane, you will identify the pulsation of the left subclavian artery.

5 Identify the thoracic duct again in the middle and inferior mediastinum. It runs on the surface of the descending aorta anteriorly to the origin of the right intercostal bronchial artery. Dissect it

upward and downward for en bloc resection with the oesophagus, denuding the aortic surface. The thoracic duct runs over the vertebral bodies behind the oesophagus, lying between the azygous vein on its right and the aorta on its left in the middle and inferior mediastinum. Preserve the thoracic duct in T1 tumours or when the patient has liver cirrhosis.

▶ KEY POINTS Thoracic duct

■ If you are not able to preserve the thoracic duct without producing injury or stenosis, prefer to ligate it at its lower end in the thorax.

■ Beware, though, that ligation of the thoracic duct produces marked retroperitoneal oedema and a rapidly progressing decrease in the circulating plasma volume during the early postoperative period.

■ This augmented third space accumulation of extracellular fluid results in overload of the circulatory and respiratory organs within the subsequent 2 or 3 days.

6 Dissect the lymph nodes below the bilateral main bronchi and the carina, preserving the peripheral branches of the right bronchial artery and the bilateral pulmonary branches of the vagus nerves. First, identify the plane between the oesophagus and pericardium. Complete the circumferential dissection of the lower oesophagus identifying the bilateral inferior pulmonary veins. Then extend the dissection cephalad. This leads you to the anterior plane of the glands below the carina. Detach the nodes from the tracheobronchial wall beginning from the right end, toward the carina, and then deeply along the left main bronchus. Ligate the branches of other bronchial arteries from the anterior aspect of the subcarinal nodes if they are encountered (Fig. 9.5).

7 Dissect the plane between the membranous portion of the trachea and the upper thoracic oesophagus. Take care not to dissect too close to the tracheal wall in order to maintain the microvascular circulation and prevent tracheobronchial injury.

8 Anchor the upper thoracic oesophagus as high as possible using a tape, and retract the oesophagus posteriorly. Sharply dissect the soft tissue on the left lateral side of the trachea so that the fascia over the left subclavian artery is denuded. This dissection plane meets the space already made from the posterior side of the oesophagus in mobilizing the thoracic duct.

9 Identify the left recurrent laryngeal nerve in the soft tissue dissected from the left lateral side of the trachea. Dissect out the recurrent nerve using sharp dissection and perform en bloc dissection of the left paratracheal nodes (left recurrent laryngeal nerve chain nodes) remaining attached to the oesophagus.

▶ KEY POINTS Protect the recurrent laryngeal nerves

■ Golden rules for avoiding injury are:
■ gentle manipulation of the nerve
■ very slight traction to straighten it
■ close sharp dissection of the nerve without energy devices.

10 Transect the thoracic oesophagus at its upper end manually or with a linear stapling device. Divide and ligate the thoracic duct behind the upper thoracic oesophagus at its upper end in the thorax.

11 Dissect the nodes around the oesophagus, pulling the upper cut end of the oesophagus downwards past the arch of preserved right bronchial artery. Several proper oesophageal arteries that arise from the descending aorta need to be ligated and cut. Completely dissect the nodes in the posterior mediastinum so that the left lung can be observed through the thin left mediastinal pleura and the descending aorta is denuded widely to its left lateral margin (Fig. 9.5).

12 Ligate and cut the lower end of the thoracic duct. Dissect the soft tissues around the hiatus and visualize the crural muscles (Fig. 9.6).

13 In VATS oesophagectomy, you should complete the dissection described up to this point before you transect the oesophagus as traction on the oesophageal cut-end will not produce sufficient tension in the tissue to be dissected.

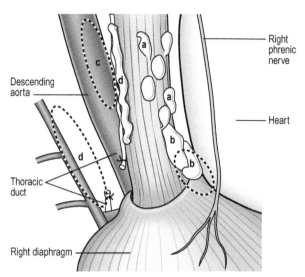

Fig. 9.6 Inferior mediastinum in the course of lymph node dissection viewed from the right side. The thoracic duct is resected with the oesophagus, and its lower end in the thoracic cavity is ligated and cut. a, para-oesophageal nodes; b, supradiaphragmatic nodes; c, para-aortic nodes; d, thoracic duct nodes.

▶ KEY POINTS Traction of the oesophagus

■ In VATS oesophagectomy, it is very important to achieve good traction on the oesophagus, which is easily achieved with your left hand in open surgery.
■ Apply additional tapes to the oesophagus whenever necessary. Secure the tape with an Endo-loop and hook the thread with the Endo-close device from any direction you need. Traction on this thread is very useful as long as the oesophagus is left uncut.

14 Go back to the superior mediastinum and dissect the pretracheal nodes if necessary. Also dissect the left tracheobronchial and subaortic arch nodes (Fig. 9.5).

15 Cover the fully mobilized oesophagus with nodes attached using a rubber sac in order to avoid possible scattering of tumour cells and loss of some nodes when the oesophagus is pulled out later from the thoracic cavity.

? DIFFICULTY

1. If you cannot find the right recurrent laryngeal nerve, search for it from the medial aspect. The left recurrent laryngeal nerve can be identified on the left lateral surface of the dissection plane when the soft tissue on the left side of the trachea is dissected en bloc. If you explore this soft tissue directly to identify the nerve, it may retract anteriorly behind the left posterior edge of the tracheal cartilage. There are a few mimicking sympathetic nerve branches running parallel to the left recurrent laryngeal nerve. If there are two or more candidates, follow them downwards: only the true left recurrent laryngeal nerve arises from the left vagus trunk and runs around the lower surface of the aortic arch. Do not cut any suspicious

structure until you are quite sure that you have found the correct one.

2. The right bronchial artery can be sacrificed when it is too thin to preserve or too close to the tumour. However, it is safer to preserve it if you plan extensive lymph node dissection in the superior mediastinum. If you have sacrificed the right bronchial artery, you should avoid too-extensive dissection of the subaortic arch space so as not to sacrifice the left bronchial arteries.

3. A frequent variation in the anatomy of the thoracic duct is a persistent left thoracic duct. The most frequent pattern is a confluence of the bilateral thoracic ducts dorsally above the aortic arch. If you cannot identify this confluence, the left thoracic duct would be left unligated resulting in a postoperative chylothorax, which cannot be controlled by the approach to the right lower mediastinum.

4. Transection can be performed at the lower end of the thoracic oesophagus when the upper margin of the tumour is so high that simple transection at the upper end cannot obtain a safe surgical margin (discussed under the cervical procedure).

Checklist

1 Has all the bleeding stopped? Most bleeding points are on the dissected oesophagus, which has to be left in the thorax for a while.

2 Are the lower end of the thoracic duct and its small branches completely ligated? An unligated small branch can cause postoperative chylothorax.

3 If the left mediastinal pleura is opened, suck out all the fluid that has accumulated in the left pleural cavity during the thoracic operation.

4 If pulmonary injury occurred during the thoracic operation, repair it meticulously with manual suturing, ligation, linear stapling and fibrin glue. Newer synthetic sheets of absorbable fibres are very effective in controlling difficult air leaks and persistent bleeding.

Closure

1 Insert an underwater-seal drain into the right pleural cavity through a separate stab incision in the sixth or seventh intercostal space in the posterior axillary line. The lowest port site can be utilized in VATS.

2 Approximate the incised intercostal space with two thick, absorbable sutures through both ribs.

3 Close the chest wound, including the pectoralis and serratus anterior muscles above and below.

ABDOMINAL AND CERVICAL PROCEDURES

Access

1 Move the patient to a supine position with the neck extended.

2 Make an upper median laparotomy incision for the abdominal operation and a collar incision for the cervical operation. These two operations are started simultaneously by two separate teams.

Assess: abdominal procedure

1 Determine the extent of spread to the lymph nodes along the left gastric vessels and around the coeliac axis.

2 Also check for para-aortic lymph node involvement. Peritoneal dissemination, which occurs when tumour seeds from the main lesion or massively metastatic lymph nodes, should also be excluded. Such advanced tumour growth should be suspected as a result of preoperative assessment, and a 'reconstruction-first' method should be employed.

Action: abdominal procedure

1 The basic manoeuvres applied around the root of the left gastric artery are very similar to the Japanese D2 dissection for gastric cancer. We routinely dissect the nodes on the common hepatic artery, the root of splenic artery and the nodes around the coeliac axis (Fig. 9.7).

2 After complete mobilization of the stomach by dividing the left gastroepiploic, short gastric, posterior gastric and left gastric vessels, while dissecting the nodes mentioned above, cut the phreno-oesophageal ligament and carefully pull out the oesophagus from the thorax with lymph nodes attached. Cover the oesophagus with a towel.

3 Find the highest point by the 'pinching up' technique (Fig. 9.8). Design the resection line for the stomach by connecting the points where the vessels from the left gastric artery enter the gastric wall so that the pericardiac nodes and the nodes in the left gastric basin are all removed. Resection is done along this line with two or three applications of a linear stapling device. The suture line is covered with interrupted seromuscular stitches.

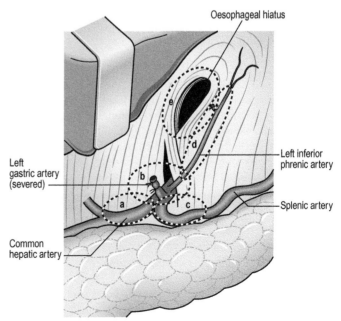

Fig. 9.7 Upper abdomen in the course of lymph node dissection. a, common hepatic artery nodes; b, coeliac nodes; c, proximal splenic artery nodes; d, inferior phrenic artery nodes; e, hiatal nodes.

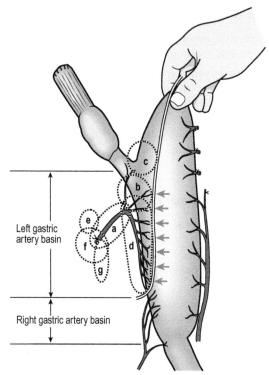

Fig. 9.8 'Pinching-up' technique to select the 'highest point'. Resection is done along the line connecting the points (short arrows) where the vessels of the left gastric area enter the gastric wall. Take care not to injure the right gastric vessels by traction. Nodes indicated by a–g are dissected. a, left gastric artery nodes; b, right paracardiac nodes; c, left paracardiac nodes; d, left lesser curvature nodes; e, proximal splenic artery nodes; f, coeliac nodes; g, common hepatic artery nodes.

▶ KEY POINT Gastric circulation

■ Take care to avoid injuring the right gastric vessels. They are very fragile, are easily torn, and bleed when pulled downwards. Although they are safely sacrificed in most cases, try not to injure them to preserve better circulation of the gastric remnant.

Technical point

Hand-assisted laparoscopic surgery (HALS) can also be applied to oesophageal operations. The smaller laparotomy wound, about 7 cm in length, reduces postoperative pain. Although a standard lymph node dissection can be performed using HALS, we do not recommend this procedure in patients with obvious, large abdominal lymph node metastases for fear of tumour implantation.

? DIFFICULTY

1. When another abnormality of the stomach has been detected preoperatively, such as an ulcer scar or early gastric cancer, try to include such lesions in the resected portion.
2. Mark the lesion preoperatively using endoscopic clips, or make a longitudinal incision in the gastric wall near the lesser curvature to observe the lesion directly and perform intraoperative mucosal resection.

3. If time allows, small neoplastic lesions should be resected preoperatively using the ESD technique, which allows a definitive pathological diagnosis and makes subsequent decision-making more logical.
4. If the stomach is not suitable for oesophageal reconstruction, ileocolon is the next best choice.

Action: cervical procedure

1 Mobilize the bilateral sternomastoid muscles widely. Separate the clavicular part from the sternal part, and place tapes around each muscle. Supraclavicular dissection can be achieved by pulling these tapes laterally and medially without cutting the muscle head (Fig. 9.9).

2 The area to be cleared extends from the cervical oesophagus laterally to the lateral supraclavicular nerve and from the level near the laryngeal promontory down to the subclavian vein and apical pleura (Fig. 9.9). More than 90% of cervical lymph node metastases arising from tumours of the thoracic oesophagus are located within the triangle defined by the bilateral omohyoid muscles and subclavian veins.

3 First, dissected out lymph nodes lateral to the common carotid arteries. Clear away the areolar tissue and lymph nodes from the posterior surface of the platysma, to the anterior, middle and posterior scalene muscles, the thyrocervical trunk and its three branches. Identify and preserve the phrenic and vagus nerves. Sacrifice the omohyoid muscle.

4 Draw up the cut end of the thoracic duct into the neck on the left side and ligate and cut its entry into the junction of the internal jugular and subclavian veins.

5 Now dissect out the lymph nodes along the carefully preserved recurrent laryngeal nerves. They may be very small, but are liable to contain micrometastases. Make sure that the paratracheal

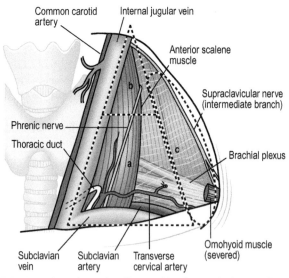

Fig. 9.9 Lymph nodes to be dissected in the cervical procedure except the paratracheal nodes. The thoracic duct is preserved. a, supraclavicular fossa nodes; b, deep jugular nodes; c, lateral cervical nodes.

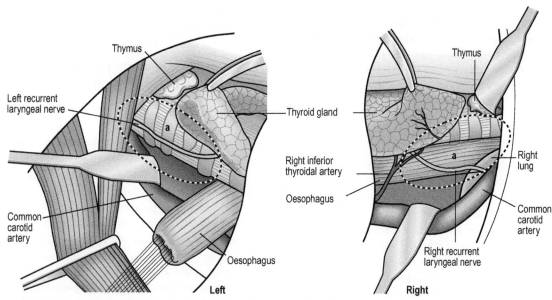

Fig. 9.10 Completion of lymph node dissection in bilateral cervical paratracheal area. a, cervical recurrent nerve nodes (paratracheal and para-oesophageal nodes).

dissection plane of the thoracic operation and the cervical operation are completely continuous on both sides (Fig. 9.10).

> **KEY POINTS** Recurrent laryngeal nerves and thoracic duct

- Be aware that metastatic nodes tend to be located posterior to the recurrent laryngeal nerve on the right, and anterior to the nerve on the left. Performing left paratracheal dissection is easier when the upper oesophageal stump is pulled out to the left with the left recurrent laryngeal nerve lying in front, and the left strap muscles are transected at their lower end.
- When you preserve the thoracic duct in the intrathoracic procedure, you must identify its entry to the left cervical venous angle. Make sure that it is not injured or stenosed in the neck. If it has been injured, ligate it at its lower end through the abdominal wound where it lies behind the right crural muscle.

RECONSTRUCTION

Appraise

As is well known, there are three possible routes for oesophageal reconstruction: subcutaneous, retrosternal and posterior mediastinal. There are pros and cons for each route. You should select one of them by considering all the relevant possibilities. Our standard procedure for advanced thoracic oesophageal carcinoma using the retrosternal route is presented here.

Action

1 Dissect the cervical oesophagus from the surrounding tissue to obtain enough length for anastomosis. Transect the left sterno-hyoid and sternothyroid muscles with electrocautery near their heads. Then bluntly open the retrosternal space behind the sternal incisura with a finger.

2 In the abdominal operating field, close the oesophageal hiatus with three interrupted sutures. Place the gastric remnant with the suture line on the dorsal side of the patient. Fix two tapes of different colours on each side near the tip with suture-ligatures.

3 Make a retrosternal tunnel using blunt finger dissection and a long, delicately curved, flat, flexible intestinal retractor with a hole at the tip. Ligate the two coloured tapes on the same side of the retractor through the hole at the tip.

4 Then pass the retractor through the retrosternal tunnel again and catch the two tapes in the neck. Bring the tip of the gastric remnant up to the neck by pushing from the abdominal side and gently pulling on the tapes in the neck. Take care to avoid rotation of the gastric remnant in the tunnel, using the coloured tapes as a guide.

5 Oesophagogastrostomy is performed manually in two layers or with Gambee's technique using 5/0 absorbable monofilament thread. Pass a nasogastric tube for decompression.

6 Place an enteral feeding tube: either a classical Witzel-type jejunostomy or a direct epigastric gastrostomy when the reconstruction route is retrosternal. Alternatively, duodenostomy using a feeding tube through the hepatic falciform ligament is a good choice because it does not increase the risk of postoperative bowel obstruction.

> ? **DIFFICULTY**

1. When the upper margin of the main tumour is high, there are multiple lesions or intramural metastasis is suspected near the cervical oesophagus, the upper margin of the oesophagectomy should be determined using the cervical operating field:
   - The oesophagus should have been divided at a lower level in the thorax. Pull out the thoracic oesophagus to

the left cervical area with nodes attached, and cover it with a towel. Then dissect the cervical oesophagus from the surrounding tissue to as high a level as possible. Cut up the cricopharyngeal part of the inferior pharyngeal constrictor muscle on the left posterolateral side for better exposure and, more importantly, to facilitate postoperative swallowing function.

■ Incise the oesophagus longitudinally on the contralateral side of the suspected lesion. The lumen can be opened easily when you cut the wall over a nasogastric tube.

■ Wipe the mucosal surface gently with a dry soft cotton ball, and then spread Lugol's solution evenly over the mucosa with a cotton ball. All the unstained mucosa should be included in the resected segment. Remember that submucosal spread cannot be ruled out by this technique and should be excluded by pathological examination of frozen sections.

2. If the gastric remnant is too short for cervical anastomosis, add Kocher's mobilization. If this is not enough, cut the peritoneum over the hepatoduodenal ligament transversely near the duodenum and carefully divide the restraining strands of lesser omentum that prevent the lesser curve from straightening. The gastric remnant can be stretched further if it has been made narrower, but the circulation is uncertain.

▶ KEY POINT Preventing gastric prolapse

■ If you choose the posterior mediastinal route for reconstruction, slightly pull down the elevated stomach and fix it to the crural muscles after completing the cervical anastomosis. This prevents the gastric remnant from prolapsing into the right thoracic cavity.

Check

Has all the bleeding in the neck and the abdomen stopped? The supraclavicular fossa is a very frequent site of postoperative re-bleeding. Most frequently, re-bleeding is from the cut end of a small branch of the transverse cervical artery, the posterior surface of the sternomastoid muscle, or a small branch of the inferior thyroid artery.

Closure

1 Insert a pair of silicone cylinder drains 5 mm in diameter with multiple holes or longitudinal grooves, through small incisions on the anterior chest surface. Pass them into the dissected supraclavicular fossae through the two heads of sternomastoid muscle on both sides and connect them to the closed low-pressure suction bag.

2 Close the cervical collar incision in the same airtight manner as after a thyroid operation.

3 Close the abdominal wound in your usual manner except that, when the retrosternal route has been chosen for reconstruction,

the peritoneal incision line is not sutured at the most cephalic 10 cm so that the elevated stomach is not constricted.

RESECTION OF THE THORACIC OESOPHAGUS WITHOUT THORACOTOMY

Appraise

1 Palliative resection of the oesophagus may be achieved by combined transhiatal abdominal and cervical approaches.

2 We believe that this procedure should be restricted to high-risk patients in whom standard thoracotomy is impossible, or you will deprive some patients with potentially curable disease of the chance to undergo a more radical resection.

3 Transhiatal oesophagectomy also offers a convenient means of providing a gastric conduit following pharyngolaryngectomy. Although a free jejunal graft with microvascular anastomosis is the current standard, the transhiatal procedure is preferable in patients with vascular disease who are unsuitable for microvascular surgery or those with thoracic oesophageal involvement. It may also be of value in patients with widespread or multiple superficial mucosal cancers for which EMR or ESD are impractical, although superficial mucosal cancers are now conventionally treated with chemoradiation therapy. The technique can also occasionally be employed for adenocarcinoma of the cardia and lower oesophagus, intractable benign stricture, incapacitating motility disorders and irrevocable damage following trauma.

4 Take into account all the advantages and disadvantages before you perform this procedure on oesophageal malignant disease. There are many other options for palliation including bypass surgery, indwelling expandable metallic stents, palliative (chemo-) radiation and simple feeding gastrostomy or enterostomy.

5 Do not embark upon this technique unless you have an intimate knowledge of the mediastinal anatomy and are competent to carry out a formal thoracotomy if necessary. Clumsy and ignorant blunt dissection can lead to calamitous bleeding or tearing of the fragile posterior membrane of the trachea or bronchi, with disastrous results.

6 Orringer and colleagues have claimed that this approach, together with CRT, is an acceptable alternative to other methods of radical oesophagectomy. However, we can see no prognostic benefit in this approach compared with the results obtained by oesophagectomy with extensive lymphadenectomy.

Access

1 Place the anaesthetized, intubated patient supine, with the head turned moderately to the right, and insert a small folded sheet beneath the scapulae to extend the neck.

2 Approach the abdomen through an upper midline incision.

3 Video mediastinoscopy from the hiatus is useful.

4 Make a neck incision along the lower anterior border of the left sternomastoid muscle. Cut platysma, dissect the medial border of sternomastoid muscle and cut the omohyoid muscle and the middle thyroid vein. This gives you entry to the space between the common carotid artery and the left lateral surface of the trachea and the thyroid gland.

Assess

1 Explore the abdomen to assess the intra-abdominal spread and operability. Do not commit yourself to resection until you are sure that the procedure is feasible and you can achieve it safely.

2 Do not forget that this procedure is limited in radicality for thoracic oesophageal cancer with submucosal or deeper infiltration. If the tumour is located low enough to obtain a safe surgical upper margin by resecting the lower thoracic oesophagus through a widened oesophageal hiatus, palliative resection of the main lesion together with proximal or total gastrectomy followed by jejunal interposition or Roux-en-Y reconstruction is a reasonable alternative with the same limited radicality. If the tumour is too advanced or the patient is unfit, consider inserting a stent to relieve dysphagia. In the absence of dysphagia, do not feel under pressure to 'do something'. Be prepared to simply close the abdomen.

Action

Abdominal procedure

1 If resection is feasible, mobilize the left lobe of the liver and fold it to the right (Fig. 9.11).

2 Incise the peritoneum and the transversalis fascia over the front of the oesophageal hiatus. Insert a finger into the posterior mediastinum and separate the pericardium from the upper surface of the diaphragm. Incise the central tendon of diaphragm forwards for 7–8 cm from the hiatus, while ligating and dividing the inferior phrenic vessels.

3 Assess the extent of the tumour in the lower oesophagus.

4 Mobilize the lower oesophagus keeping well clear of the tumour and excising a cuff of diaphragmatic crus, posterior pericardium, mediastinal pleura and posterior connective tissue as necessary. The oesophagus can be mobilized under vision almost up to the level of the tracheal carina. Carefully avoid excessive compression of the heart, which might cause hypotension,

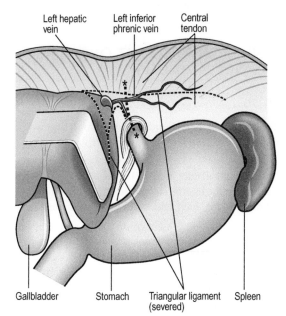

Left hepatic vein   Left inferior phrenic vein   Central tendon

Gallbladder   Stomach   Triangular ligament (severed)   Spleen

Fig. 9.11 Incisional line (∗—∗) of the diaphragm for widening of the hiatus.

tachyarrhythmia and even cardiac arrest in patients with cardiovascular risk factors.

5 Now proceed close to the oesophagus, carefully separating it from the back of the trachea. Hook the branches of the vagus nerves within the flexed index and middle fingers, and cut them using long scissors within the protection of the fingers.

Cervical procedure

1 Access is increased, if necessary, by transecting the strap muscles on the left. Median sternotomy or excision of the medial clavicle, a portion of the first rib and a half of the manubrium sterni on one side will very efficiently widen the operative field, but it is usually not necessary unless a bulky tumour, primary or metastatic, interferes with the access.

2 Expose the left lateral surface of the cervical oesophagus behind the trachea. The longitudinal fat pad along the posterior margin of the tracheal cartilage contains the left recurrent laryngeal nerve. Sharply dissect this fat pad from the oesophagus and enter the space between the membranous portion of the trachea and the anterior surface of the oesophagus. Widen this space upward and downward. Dissect the posterior surface of the cervical oesophagus from the prevertebral fascia. Place a tape around the oesophagus just on its right lateral surface to avoid injury to the right recurrent laryngeal nerve. Care should also be taken not to compress the left recurrent laryngeal nerve on the left lateral tracheal surface.

3 Continue freeing the oesophagus downwards into the superior mediastinum. Final mobilization is best achieved by inserting the index finger of one hand through the neck and passing the other hand up from the abdomen through the posterior mediastinum.

Resect

1 Remove the nasogastric tube.

2 Apply a ligature (or a linear stapling device) around the cervical oesophagus as low as possible.

3 Transect the oesophagus above the ligature, sterilize the tip and allow the lower ligated cut end to retract into the mediastinum. Connect a tape to the oesophageal stump to guide pulling up the oesophageal substitute later.

4 In the abdomen, transect the upper part of the stomach in the same manner described for extended lymph node dissection (Fig. 9.8) to prevent early recurrence around the elevated stomach. Cover the suture line with seromuscular stitches.

5 Remove the specimen for histology.

6 Insert a basal or apical underwater-seal drain whenever the pleural cavity has been breached.

Unite

1 If the gastric remnant can be used as the conduit, mobilize it as previously described. Ensure that the tip of the gastric remnant will reach the neck by laying it on the chest wall. Bring up the gastric remnant to the neck through one of the three possible routes (usually posterior mediastinal) and unite it to the cervical oesophagus.

2 The alternatives have already been discussed under 'Assess'.

OESOPHAGEAL BYPASS

1 Resection may not be possible, or may be contraindicated because the tumour is too extensive. Bypass is preferable to stenting in patients with a prognosis of months rather than weeks. Bypass does not preclude radiotherapy as the conduit lies some distance from the field of irradiation.

2 The mobilized stomach may be raised above the unresected tumour when the left thoracoabdominal operation or the Ivor Lewis operation is planned. The anastomosis above the tumour can be fashioned after transection of the oesophagus and closure of the cut lower end or, if there is no fistula, it can be made in the lateral wall of the oesophagus without transection. If possible, leave the lower oesophagus in continuity with the stomach. Sometimes it is necessary to divide the lower oesophagus to free the stomach, so that it can be joined well above the tumour.

3 Kirschner's operation (total bypass of the thoracic oesophagus with stomach) is preferable when bypassing unresectable middle-third lesions. Mobilize the stomach through the abdomen. You can transect the oesophagus at the cardia and use the whole stomach, but our preference is to prepare the stomach as described for extensive lymph node dissection (Fig. 9.8), but without the 'pinching up' technique so as not to pull up the stomach with metastatic lymph nodes. The bypass route can be retrosternal or subcutaneous. For the subcutaneous route elevate the skin at the upper end of the wound. Use long-handled scissors to create a track 7–10-cm wide in the subcutaneous tissue over the sternum and manubrium with a combination of blunt and sharp dissection. Mobilize the cervical oesophagus through an incision in the side of the neck (we prefer the left side) in the same manner as that described for resection of the thoracic oesophagus without thoracotomy (P.139), and use this incision to complete the subcutaneous track into the neck. Grasp the oesophagus with a clamp as low as possible in the mobilized cervical oesophagus. Transect the oesophagus above the grasped level, close the lower cut end, and allow it to retract into the superior mediastinum. Gently manoeuvre the stomach through the subcutaneous track by a combination of pushing and traction. Avoid tension and twisting of the organ. Now anastomose the upper cut end of the oesophagus to the upper surface of the drawn-up stomach.

4 It is often said that it is safe to leave the oesophagus in situ after closing both ends of a segment containing an unresectable tumour. However, this holds true only for a limited period: internal or external (tube) drainage is necessary when continuity of the oesophagus and the lower gastrointestinal tract cannot be maintained unless there is a large fistula with the tracheobronchial tree. This can be achieved by simply inserting a drainage tube from the lower cut end, or anastomosing the lower end to a Roux loop of jejunum. We prefer tube oesophagojejunostomy with Witzel jejunostomy on the anal side (Fig. 9.12).

5 Oesophageal bypass can be accomplished using a long jejunal pedicle taken up subcutaneously or retrosternally to the neck, but mobilization of such a long segment of jejunum is difficult. A segment of colon (see below) taken out of circuit is usually more easily fashioned into a conduit between the cervical oesophagus and the distal stomach.

6 When the tumour is too high to get enough length of cervical oesophagus for anastomosis, often with impending higher airway

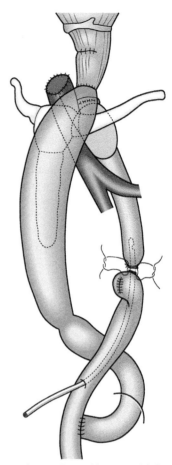

Fig. 9.12 Diagram of oesophageal bypass with laryngectomy. Drainage of the isolated oesophagus is accomplished by a simple technique of tube oesophagojejunostomy. Two sites of purse-string sutures around a thin drainage tube are approximated with a few additional stitches. (Modified from Udagawa H. Esophageal bypass with laryngectomy: a method of palliation for nonresectable upper esophageal carcinoma. Diseases of the Esophagus 1991; 4: 63–70.)

obstruction or recurrent laryngeal nerve palsy, oesophageal bypass with laryngectomy (Fig. 9.12) is a possible means of palliation.

COLONIC REPLACEMENT OR BYPASS OF THE OESOPHAGUS

Appraise

1 The colon usually has a good marginal blood supply (Fig. 9.13) and it makes an excellent oesophageal replacement.

2 An antiperistaltic loop can be created by swinging up the mobilized left colon after dividing the left colic vessels, so that it is supplied through the middle colic vessels. Because it does not always function well, this method should be the last alternative.

3 An isoperistaltic loop of right colon can be swung up, based on the middle colic vessels, after dividing the right colic and ileocolic vessels. The bulky caecum is brought to the neck after closing the terminal ileum and carrying out appendecectomy. The caecal bulk soon diminishes.

4 Our preference is to use an ileocolic segment including 15–20 cm of terminal ileum with the caecum and ascending colon for reconstruction or bypass. There are several advantages in this

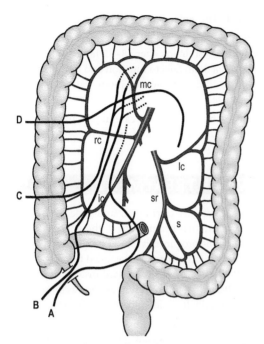

Fig. 9.13 Cutting lines for oesophageal reconstruction or bypass with isoperistaltic colonic segment. Additional separation of the vasculature along the dashed lines is possible unless it spoils the circulation of the segment. We routinely begin with A, shifting step by step to B, C and D according to the circulatory state of the tip and the length of the segment. ic, ileocolic, rc, right mc, middle colic; lc, left colic; S, sigmoidal; Sr, superior rectal artery.

procedure: the right colic vessels can often be preserved, the bulky colon tends to remain in the thorax and preservation of the ileocaecal valve provides an antireflux mechanism. Perfusion of the ileum should be carefully examined because the vascular arcade between the ileocolic and the right colic vessels is poor in some patients.

5 If the tip of the elevated colon shows poor arterial circulation or bad venous return and microvascular expertise is available, addition of an arterial or venous anastomosis of the sacrificed colonic vessels to a suitable cervical vessel (usually called 'supercharge' and 'superdrainage') can save this difficult situation.

Prepare

The colon must be prepared beforehand by feeding the patient with a low residue or liquid diet for 1–2 days preoperatively and administering oral bowel preparation the day before surgery. Prophylactic oral antibiotics are unnecessary.

Action

1 Carefully study the anatomy of the marginal vessels.

2 Any bypass route for a colonic segment, particularly when the right colon is used, should be designed to be wider than for gastric pull-up.

3 Mobilize the caecum, ascending colon and right transverse colon on its primitive mesentery. Check for vascular continuity by inspecting the mobilized mesocolon against a light. In case of doubt, gently apply bulldog clips to the blood vessels at the intended sites of division and an intestinal clamp on the terminal

ileum for several minutes, and then check the colour and circulation. Do not commit yourself to colonic bypass with an ischaemic or congested segment of colon. Remember, the venous drainage is as important as the arterial supply.

4 Doubly ligate and divide the ileocaecal vessels near their origin from the superior mesenteric vessels. Do not divide the right colic vessels at this stage, because it is often unnecessary. Then divide the ileum at the point about 20 cm (depending on the pattern of mesenteric vasculature) proximal to the ileocaecal valve with a linear stapling device. Apply seromuscular stitches to the distal cut end of the terminal ileum. Check the length of the ileocolic segment placing it on the anterior chest wall. The right colic vessels can be divided if greater length is required. Swing the mobilized ileocolon upwards and gently push and pull it along the prepared track. Carefully avoid violent traction on the root of the draining vein when you are pulling up any colonic segment. Anastomose the terminal ileum to the cervical oesophagus in an end-to-side fashion.

5 Meticulously divide the marginal vessels for 3 cm at a suitable point on the transverse colon for distal anastomosis whilst avoiding injury to the vascular arcade. Divide the transverse colon at the centre of the devascularized segment. Anastomose the proximal cut end of the colon to a suitable organ (i.e. distal stomach, duodenal bulb or side of the jejunal loop brought up antecolically), depending on the situation. Then anastomose the proximal cut end of the terminal ileum to the distal cut end of the transverse colon.

▶ **KEY POINTS Small-bowel complications**

■ Ischaemic contraction of the bowel may be observed when the ileocolic vessels are divided in patients with poor vascular arcade between the right colic and ileocolic vessels. This usually resolves: if you observe palpable or visible pulsation of the ileocolic trunk after 10–20 minutes it is a reliable sign that the arterial perfusion to the ileocolic arterial basin is sufficient. If you are not sure, remove the ligature from the ileocolic artery: if there is good backflow, you can safely continue the procedure. If there is not, it is safer to cut off the ileocolic arterial basin or to consider cervical microvascular anastomosis.

■ Only the antimesenteric wall of the ileum is necessary for the oesophagoileostomy in the neck. Furthermore, the real distance via the retrosternal tunnel is shorter than the distance you can measure on the body surface. This means that the length of the mesentery required for ileocolic pull-up is not as long as one may imagine. Therefore avoid unnecessary division of right colic vessels by precisely estimating which vessels must be divided.

■ If you carry out end-to-side colonojejunostomy, as mentioned for Roux-en-Y reconstruction, place the afferent loop on the patient's left side, that is the same side as the ligament of Treitz. If you do not, the anastomosis may undergo torsion when the fluid accumulates in the afferent loop, possibly causing bowel obstruction.

■ When you try to pull up the bulky colon via the posterior mediastinal route, the tracheal bifurcation very often becomes an obstacle. When the ileocolon is used, the bulky caecum may be stuck below the carina and only ileum may be brought up behind the trachea. In such case, put the bowel segment to be brought-up in a plastic bag. Fix the bag firmly only at the tip. Apply a small amount of sterilized glycerin over the bag as lubricant. When the tip of the bag reaches the neck, gently pull out the plastic bag to the neck from the mediastinum. In this way, the bulky part easily passes the narrowness caused by the bifurcation.

6 Close the mesenteric window to prevent internal herniation. Close the diaphragm or anterior abdominal wall slackly around the colon so that it is not constricted. Ensure that the bowel and blood vessels are not twisted and are not under tension before closing the incisions.

7 Belsey has described the use of an isoperistaltic loop of transverse colon based on the left colic vessels. If necessary, the left branch or even the right branch of the middle colic artery can be divided.

Checklist

1 Ensure that bleeding and oozing from the many raw surfaces has been controlled before closing the wounds.

2 Have all the anastomoses been performed satisfactorily? Leakage of an anastomosis including colon is often fatal. If you have even a slight doubt, refashion the anastomosis.

AFTERCARE (Common to all procedures described)

1 Following major oesophageal surgery, the patient should remain in the intensive care unit for at least 24 hours, so that cardiorespiratory, renal and cerebral functions can be monitored with early correction of any abnormalities. After extensive radical oesophagectomy, it takes much longer for pulmonary function to be restored, so it is advisable to keep the patient in intensive care for 3–4 days. Some patients benefit from initial mechanical ventilation via an endotracheal tube. Arrange for regular chest X-rays to ensure full pulmonary expansion. Order chest physiotherapy and aspiration of bronchial secretions either orally, through the endotracheal tube or using a flexible bronchoscope.

2 Order adequate regular analgesics, and continue antibiotics and prophylaxis for venous thrombosis.

3 Aspirate the visceral tube regularly but, as bowel function recovers, the tube may be used for feeding if its position has been checked radiographically. After 7 days, screen the patient following a swallow of water-soluble contrast to exclude anastomotic leakage. Withdraw the tube and start oral feeding, progressing to solids over a day or two. Then stop parenteral feeding. If a feeding enterostomy was created, start by giving small volumes of dilute fluid on the first postoperative day, gradually increasing to larger volumes of full-strength feeds until oral feeding is established. The enterostomy catheter can be left for several months for supplementary feeding.

4 Remove the chest drains after 48–72 hours unless fluid is being produced. If a drain fails to function and intrapleural fluid or air persists, do not hesitate to insert further suitably placed underwater-sealed drains.

5 Study the pathologist's report carefully. Is adjuvant radiotherapy or chemotherapy justified and required?

ADJUVANT TREATMENT

1 Although squamous carcinoma, and indeed adenocarcinoma, responds to external beam therapy, the effect of such adjuvant treatment on the prognosis is questionable. Most controlled trials of preoperative radiotherapy have failed to show any prognostic benefit. Radiotherapy has been used instead of surgery in some series and Pearson reported results as good as those obtained with surgery, especially for mid- and upper oesophageal tumours.

2 Brachytherapy (intracavity irradiation with caesium-137 or iridium-192) offers certain advantages, notably that the radiation is concentrated on the tumour. A guidewire is inserted endoscopically or under fluoroscopy and an external applicator tube is passed over the guidewire to straddle the tumour. Pellets of caesium or iridium, stored in a safe source, are then pneumatically transferred into the applicator and are transferred back at the end of treatment. This is an effective way to increase the local control rate of radiotherapy. However, care should be taken as local tissue damage may lead to perforation if the tube positioning was not appropriate.

3 Endoscopic Nd-YAG laser therapy is valuable for palliation of dysphagia but it often has to be repeated to alleviate symptoms and to maintain patency.

4 Photodynamic therapy involves giving sensitizing drugs, usually haematoporphyrin derivatives or phthalylcyanates, which are retained by tumour cells. When exposed to certain light wavelengths, these agents produce cytotoxic substances such as oxygen free radicals. The light is usually delivered via optical fibre, but there is little tissue penetration, so the activity is mainly confined to the surface of lesions.

5 Chemotherapy has been tried alone or in a variety of combinations. Cisplatin has been combined with 5-fluorouracil, and this combination (FP) is still regarded as the standard regimen. Many other drugs such as Adriamycin, etoposide, vindecine and recently paclitaxel, docetaxel and irinotecan have also been tried usually in combination with diamminedichloroplatinum or FP. Postoperative chemotherapy had been thought to lack scientific evidence in survival benefit, but a Japanese multicentric phase III trial with FP successfully showed significant prolongation of disease-free survival. More recently, the same Japanese group (JCOG) reported the superiority of two courses of preoperative chemotherapy with FP over the same chemotherapy given postoperatively. Consequently, neoadjuvant chemotherapy + surgery is currently regarded as standard in Japan.

6 The concept of neoadjuvant treatment was proposed in 1981. Since then, a variety of preoperative treatments have been tried. Among them, concurrent CRT (chemoradiotherapy) has attracted wide attention and most of the trials of neoadjuvant

CRT yielded positive results. It is often claimed that neoadjuvant CRT does not increase the risk of a subsequent operation, but this claim remains controversial.

7 Chemoradiotherapy may also be used as a definitive treatment not only in non-resectable advanced tumours but also in earlier stage tumours to preserve the oesophagus. Recent trials suggest that, following a good response to chemoradiation therapy, the addition of surgery results in better local control but no survival benefit. However, the presence or absence of residual tumour after definitive CRT is very difficult to diagnose and its late adverse effects are not fully understood. Salvage operations for recurrent tumour after definitive CRT are not easy and the postoperative quality of life is often poor.

8 The many treatment options for oesophageal cancer now allow individualization of treatment, combining two, three or more modalities. Research is currently geared to rationalizing this individualization, applying techniques of molecular biology and genetics. More experimental treatments such as adoptive immunotherapy and gene therapy are also being tried in several centres.

▶ KEY POINTS Decision-making and patient consent

- Informed consent is a first priority in modern society.
- Because many different modes of therapy are available and effective against oesophageal cancer, you need to give patients the best information possible. You must, therefore, be fully aware of the vast field of oncology.
- With the easy availability of information technology you can remain aware of the very latest knowledge in the field.
- Remember that 'evidence-based medicine' is based on a notional average patient. You must take into account all the unique factors for each individual and offer the treatment option that you decide is the best for your patient.

FURTHER READING

Ajani JA. Resectable esophageal cancer: surgery as primary therapy is not the answer, but then, what is and why? J Clin Oncol 2010;28(15):e243–4.

Akiyama H. Surgery for carcinoma of the esophagus. In: Current problems in surgery. Chicago: Year Book Publishers; 1980.

Akiyama H. Surgery for cancer of the esophagus. Baltimore: Williams & Wilkins; 1990.

Akiyama H, Udagawa H. Total gastrectomy and Roux-en-Y reconstruction. In: Pearson FG, Cooper JD, Deslauriers J, et al., editors. Esophageal surgery. 2nd ed New York: Churchill Livingstone; 2002. p. 871–9.

Akiyama H, Tsurumaru M, Ono Y, et al. Transoral esophagectomy. Surg, Gynecology Obstet 1991;173:399–400.

Akiyama H, Tsurumaru M, Udagawa H, et al. Esophageal cancer. In: Current problems in surgery. St Louis: Mosby; 1997.

Allum WH, Stenning SP, Bancewicz J, et al. Long-term results of a randomized trial of surgery with or without preoperative chemotherapy in esophageal cancer. J Clin Oncol 2009;27:5062–7.

Ando N, Iizuka T, Ide H, et al. Surgery plus chemotherapy compared with surgery alone for localized squamous cell carcinoma of the thoracic esophagus: a Japan Clinical Oncology Group Study—JCOG9204. J Clin Oncol 2003;21:4592–6.

Ando N, Kato H, Igaki H, et al. A randomized trial comparing postoperative adjuvant chemotherapy with cisplatin and 5-fluorouracil versus preoperative chemotherapy for localized advanced squamous cell carcinoma of the thoracic esophagus (JCOG9907). Ann Surg Oncol 2012;19(1):68–74.

Bedenne L, Michel P, Bouche O, et al. Chemoradiation followed by surgery compared with chemoradiation alone in squamous cancer of the esophagus: FFCD 9102. J Clin Oncol 2007;25:1160–8.

Boonstra JJ, Koppert LB, Wijnhoven BP, et al. Chemotherapy followed by surgery in patients with carcinoma of the distal esophagus and celiac lymph node involvement. J Surg Oncol. 2009;100(5):407–13.

Cooper JS, Guo MD, Herskovic A, et al. Chemoradiotherapy of locally advanced esophageal cancer: long-term follow-up of a prospective randomized trial (RTOG 85-01). Radiation Therapy Oncology Group. JAMA 1999;281:1623–7.

Cuschieri A. Invited introduction. Treatment of carcinoma of the oesophagus. Ann R Coll Surg Engl 1991;73:1–3.

D'Journo XB, Doddoli C, Michelet P, et al. Transthoracic esophagectomy for adenocarcinoma of the oesophagus: standard versus extended two-field mediastinal lymphadenectomy? Eur J Cardiothorac Surg 2005;27 (4):697–704.

Dimick JB, Pronovost PJ, Cowan JA, Lipsett PA. Surgical volume and quality of care for esophageal resection: do high-volume hospitals have fewer complications? Ann Thorac Surg 2003;75:337–41.

Earlam R. An MRC prospective randomized trial of radiotherapy versus surgery for operable squamous cell carcinoma of the oesophagus. Ann R Coll Surg Engl 1991;73:8–12.

Fujita H, Kakegawa T, Yamana H, et al. Mortality and morbidity rates, postoperative course, quality of life, and prognosis after extended radical lymphadenectomy for esophageal cancer Comparison of three-field lymphadenectomy with two-field lymphadenectomy. Ann Surg 1995;222:654–62.

Gebski V, Burmeister B, Smithers BM, et al. Survival benefits from neoadjuvant chemoradiotherapy or chemotherapy in oesophageal carcinoma: a meta-analysis. Lancet Oncol 2007;8:226–34.

Ilson DH, Bains M, Ginsberg RJ, et al. Neoadjuvant therapy of esophageal cancer. Surg Oncol Clin N Am 1997;6:723–40.

Ishikura S, Nihei K, Ohtsu A, et al. Long-term toxicity after definitive chemoradiotherapy for squamous cell carcinoma of the thoracic esophagus. J Clin Oncol 2003;21:2697–702.

Isono K, Sato H, Nakayama K. Results of a nationwide study on the three-field lymph node dissection of esophageal cancer. Oncology 1991;48:411–20.

Jamieson GG. Surgery of the oesophagus. Edinburgh: Churchill Livingstone; 1988.

Japan Esophageal Society. Japanese classification of esophageal cancer, tenth edition: part I. Esophagus 2009;6:1–25.

Japan Esophageal Society. Japanese classification of esophageal cancer, tenth edition: part II and III. Esophagus 2009;6:71–94.

Kelsen DP, Winter KA, Gunderson LL, et al. Long-term results of RTOG trial 8911 (USA Intergroup 113): a random assignment trial comparison of chemotherapy followed by surgery compared with surgery alone for esophageal cancer. J Clin Oncol 2007;25:3719–25.

Khoury GA. Squamous cell carcinoma of the oesophagus: 10 years on. Ann R Coll Surg Engl 1991;73:4–7.

Kitagawa Y, Fujii H, Mukai M, et al. Intraoperative lymphatic mapping and sentinel lymph node sampling in esophageal and gastric cancer. Surg Oncol Clin N Am 2002;11:293–304.

Kodama M, Kakegawa T. Treatment of superficial cancer of the esophagus: a summary of responses to a questionnaire on superficial cancer of the esophagus in Japan. Surgery 1998;123:432–9.

Krasna MJ, Tepper J. The role of multimodality therapy for esophageal cancer. Chest Surg Clin N Am 2000;10:591–603.

Mathisen DJ. Ivor Lewis procedure. In: Pearson FG, Deslauriers J, Ginsberg RJ, et al., editors. Esophageal surgery. New York: Churchill Livingstone; 1995. p. 669–76.

Matthews HR, Powell DJ, McConkey CC. Effect of surgical experience on the results of resection for oesophageal carcinoma. Br J Surg 1986;73:621–3.

Minsky BD, Pajak TF, Ginsberg RJ, et al. INT 0123 (Radiation Therapy Oncology Group 94-05) phase III trial of combined-modality therapy for esophageal cancer: high-dose versus standard-dose radiation therapy. J Clin Oncol 2002;20:1167–74.

Murata Y, Suzuki S, Ohta M, et al. Small ultrasonic probes for determination of the depth of superficial esophageal cancer. Gastrointest Endosc 1996;44:23–8.

Orringer MB. Transhiatal esophagectomy without thoracotomy. In: Pearson FG, Deslauriers J, Ginsberg RJ, et al., editors. Esophageal surgery. New York: Churchill Livingstone; 1995. p. 683–701.

Osugi H, Takemura M, Higashino M, et al. Learning curve of video-assisted thoracoscopic esophagectomy and extended lymphadenectomy for squamous cell cancer of the thoracic esophagus and results. Surg Endosc 2003;17:515–9.

Palanivelu C, Prakash A, Senthilkumar R, et al. Minimally invasive esophagectomy: thoracoscopic mobilization of the esophagus and mediastinal lymphadenectomy in prone position–experience of 130 patients. J Am Coll Surg 2006;203:7–16.

Raijman I, Siddique I, Ajani J, et al. Palliation of malignant dysphagia and fistulae with coated expandable metal stents: experience with 101 patients. Gastrointest Endosc 1998;48:172–9.

Rice TW, Blackstone EH, Rusch VW. A cancer staging primer: esophagus and esophagogastric junction. J Thorac Cardiovasc Surg 2010;139:527–9.

Rizk NP, Ishwaran H, Rice TW, et al. Optimum lymphadenectomy for esophageal cancer. Ann Surg 2010;251:46–50.

Rutgeerts P, Vantrappen G, Broeckaert L, et al. Palliative Nd:YAG laser therapy for cancer of the esophagus and gastroesophageal junction: impact on the quality of remaining life. Gastrointest Endosc 1988;34:87.

Shimada H, Okazumi S, Matsubara H, et al., Effect of steroid therapy on postoperative course and survival of patients with thoracic esophageal carcinoma. Esophagus 2004;1:89–94.

Skinner DB. En bloc resection for neoplasms of the esophagus and cardia. J Thorac Cardiovasc Surg 1983;85:59–71.

Sobin LH, Gospodarowicz MK, Witteind Ch, editors. International Union Against Cancer. TNM classification of malignant tumors. 7th edn. Wiley; 2009. p. 66–72.

Stahl M, Walz MK, Stuschke M, et al. Phase III comparison of preoperative chemotherapy compared with chemoradiotherapy in patients with locally advanced adenocarcinoma of the esophagogastric junction. J Clin Oncol 2009;27:851–6.

Tepper J, Krasna MJ, Niedzwiecki D, et al. Phase III trial of trimodality therapy with cisplatin, fluorouracil, radiotherapy, and surgery compared with surgery alone for esophageal cancer: CALGB 9781. J Clin Oncol 2008;26:1086–892.

Thomas RJ, Abbott M, Bhathal PS, et al. High-dose photoirradiation of esophageal cancer. Ann Surg 1987;206:193.

Udagawa H. Esophageal bypass with laryngectomy: a method of palliation for nonresectable upper esophageal carcinoma. Dis Esophagus 1991;4:63–70.

Udagawa H, Akiyama H. Surgical treatment of esophageal cancer: Tokyo experience of the three-field technique. Dis Esophagus 2001;14:110–4.

Udagawa H, Ueno M, Shinohara H, et al. The importance of grouping of lymph node stations and rationale of three-field lymphoadenectomy for thoracic esophageal cancer. J Surg Oncol 2012;106(6):742–7.

Udagawa H, Ueno M, Kinoshita Y. Rationale for video-assisted radical esophagectomy. General Thoracic and Cardiovascular Surgery 2009;57:127–31.

Urschel JD, Vasan H. A meta-analysis of randomized controlled trials that compared neoadjuvant chemoradiation and surgery to surgery alone for resectable esophageal cancer. Am J Surg 2003;185:538–43.

Urschel JD, Ashiku S, Thurer R, et al. Salvage or planned esophagectomy after chemoradiation therapy for locally advanced esophageal cancer: a review. Dis Esophagus 2003;16:60–5.

Yokoyama A, Omori T. Genetic polymorphisms of alcohol and aldehyde dehydrogenases and risk for esophageal and head and neck cancers. Jpn J Clin Oncol 2003;33(3):111–21.

Yokoyama A, Hirota T, Omori T, et al. Development of squamous neoplasia in esophageal iodine-unstained lesions and the alcohol and aldehyde dehydrogenase genotypes of Japanese alcoholic men. Int J Cancer 2012;130(12):2949–60.

Stomach and duodenum

M.C. Winslet, K.I. Dawas

ENDOSCOPY

Appraise

1 Consider endoscopy when there is a likelihood that tissue biopsy is required. Radiology contrast studies complement endoscopy.

2 Endoscopy is mandatory in the investigation of gastrointestinal bleeding. It is also extremely useful in delineating anatomy, particularly in cases where there has been previous surgery.

3 Endoscopy is also a useful adjunct intra-operatively. It allows for intra-luminal examination if required when the diagnosis remains unclear.

4 The therapeutic capabilities of an endoscope should not be underestimated. Benign strictures can be dilated (bougie or balloon); malignant strictures cored out using Nd-YAG laser; polyps snared and removed; stones removed from the biliary tree; and stents inserted into the oesophagus, pylorus and biliary tree.

5 Percutaneous endoscopic gastrostomies are commonly performed for patients who are unable to swallow adequate volumes of nutrition. In addition, percutaneous endoscopic jejunostomies and nasojejunal feeding tubes are placed with the aid of endoscopy.

Prepare

1 Familiarize yourself with the endoscopes available in your hospitals. Ensure you are able to set up the scope and the stack independently in case you need to do so out of hours without experienced assistance (Fig. 10.1). Make sure that the instrument, light source, suction apparatus, biopsy forceps and air insufflation pump all work satisfactorily and that the instrument has been sterilized according to the manufacturer's recommendations. Sterilization of instruments during an endoscopy list demands careful organization to guard against transmission of micro-organisms such as *Salmonella* spp, *Pseudomonas aeruginosa* and *Mycobacterium* as well as hepatitis B virus (HBV) and human immunodeficiency virus (HIV). Thorough cleaning is followed by immersion in 2% alkaline activated glutaraldehyde or 10% succine dialdehyde for a minimum of 4 minutes. Since these substances are toxic, irritant and may cause allergic reactions, the endoscopes must be washed thoroughly afterwards.

2 End-viewing endoscopes are most commonly used and are very versatile but side-viewing scopes are used to cannulate the ampulla of Vater.

3 Obtain written, informed consent from the patient, highlighting the indications for the procedure and the potential complications.

4 The patient takes no food or fluids for 6 hours. In an emergency, attempt endoscopy even if the patient has had a recent meal, but there is a higher risk of aspiration. It is prudent to have an anaesthetist in attendance.

5 Don protective gloves and spectacles before starting the procedure.

6 Try to minimize the use and the dose of sedative (midazolam). For simple diagnostic endoscopy, it is often sufficient to use a local anaesthetic throat spray. Monitor all patients using a pulse oximeter and administer oxygen if necessary. Elderly or infirm patients given analgesics and sedatives are at risk of hypoxia, especially during prolonged procedures.

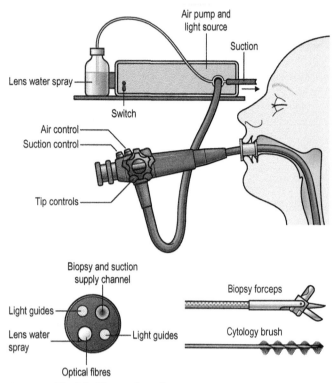

Fig. 10.1 Flexible fibreoptic endoscopy.

7 Ensure that the patient has no dentures. Insert a plastic mouthpiece between the patient's teeth or gums through which the instrument will slide easily. Smear the endoscope shaft with water-soluble lubricant. Secretion and mucus are less likely to adhere to the lens if it is smeared with silicone liquid and lightly polished to leave a thin film.

8 The patient may be laid on the left side, with no pillow but with the head steadied by an assistant who maintains neck flexion, discouraging the patient from extending his neck which tends to make the instrument pass into the larynx. The patient's pronated left hand lies on the right chest, the right hand grasps the edge of the bed. Both knees and hips are flexed. Alternatively, the patient may lie supine but with the head of the bed raised.

Access

1 Slightly flex the tip of the instrument. Pass it through the mouthpiece, over the tongue, keeping the flexed tip strictly in the midline pointing towards the cricopharyngeal sphincter. As the tip reaches the sphincter there is a hold-up. Ask the patient to swallow. The tip will be slightly extruded, and do not resist this, but suddenly the obstruction disappears as the sphincter relaxes and the instrument can be smoothly passed into the stomach after unflexing the tip.

▶ **KEY POINTS Be cautious**

■ Do not use force.
■ Never advance the endoscope blindly.

2 Watch the screen and concentrate on safely passing the instrument through the oesophagus and stomach and into the duodenum, noting incidentally if there is any abnormality. Insufflate the minimum

of air to open up the passage. Hold and adjust the tip controls with the left thumb and index finger. Hold the shaft of the endoscope with the right hand close to the patient's mouth, advancing, withdrawing and rotating it as necessary. When the gastric angulus is passed, flex the tip to identify the pylorus. Advance the tip, keeping the pylorus in the centre of the field until the tip slips through.

3 The side-viewing endoscope has a rounded tip which makes it easier to negotiate the pharynx. If there is any doubt about the free passage, always examine the patient first with an end-viewing endoscope. Become familiar with the tip control and angle of view before passing it. When it has passed into the stomach, rotate it to bring into view the relatively smooth, straight lesser curve which ends at the arch of the angulus, below which can be seen the pylorus in the distance. Angle the instrument up towards the roof of the antrum while advancing the instrument. The view of the pylorus is lost momentarily as the tip slips through into the duodenum. Paradoxically, if the shaft is slightly withdrawn, the instrument is straightened and the tip advances further into the duodenum. Rotate the shaft to bring the medial duodenal wall into view and, as the instrument enters the second part of the duodenum, the ampulla of Vater is usually seen as a nipple, often with a hooded mucosal fold above it.

Assess

1 Withdraw the end-viewing instrument in a spiral fashion to bring into view the whole circumference of the duodenum and stomach. Withdraw the side-viewing endoscope whilst rotating it 180° either side to view the whole circumference. Do not overinflate the stomach and duodenum with air. In the duodenum and distal stomach, keep the endoscope still and watch the peristaltic waves form and pass distally, to estimate the suppleness of the walls and exclude rigidity from infiltration or disease. With the tip of the end-viewing instrument lying in the body of the stomach, flex it fully while gently advancing the shaft to bring the fundus and cardia into view (the 'J' manoeuvre). Flex the side-viewing instrument to produce the same view. From just above the cardia the end-viewing instrument displays the pinchcock action of the diaphragmatic crura at each inspiration. If gastric mucosa is seen above this, there is a sliding hiatal hernia. The gastric mucosa is pink and shiny; at the crenated transition to the thinner and more opaque oesophageal squamous mucosa, the colour becomes paler and sometimes slightly bluish. Islands of pink gastric mucosa may be seen above the line of transition.

2 If the view disappears, withdraw the instrument and insufflate a little air. If the lens is obscured, clean it with the water jet or wipe it against the mucosa to free it of adherent mucus.

3 Look out for inflammation in duodenitis, gastritis and oesophagitis. As a rule, the mucosa appears florid and reddened, but endoscopy is uncertain and biopsy specimens should be taken when in doubt. In atrophic gastritis the distal mucosa is thinned and translucent so that submucosal vessels are visible through it. In gastric atrophy, associated with pernicious anaemia, the fundic mucosa is particularly affected, being flat and featureless. Menetrier's hypertrophic gastritis results in strikingly florid mucosal folds, as may the fundic mucosa in the Zollinger-Ellison syndrome.

4 Peptic ulcers usually display a basal slough, but adherent mucosa may simulate a crater. Healed ulcers typically appear flat and white, with radiating mucosal folds. Diverticula, seen usually high on the gastric lesser curve, have healthy mucosa entering the mouth of the diverticulum. Mallory-Weiss tears show a ragged, often bleeding edge in the mucosa at the cardia.

> ### ▶ KEY POINT Cellular diagnosis
>
> ■ Never fail to remove cytology brushings and biopsy specimens for examination.

5 Tumours are typically elevated and malignant ulcers have raised, everted edges. Gastric polyps may be single or multiple, and can be mucosal or submucosal, such as leiomyomas and leiomyosarcomas, which frequently have healthy mucosa overlying them. Lymphomas – sometimes with mucosal hypertrophy, sharply differentiated from normal mucosa – may reveal no histological abnormality on biopsy, since they tend to spread in the submucosa. They may produce multiple shallow ulcers, or ulcers with raised edges. By the time tumours become obvious they are usually well advanced and the best time to recognize them is in the early pre-invasive stage. Any slight irregularity of the mucosa is suspicious, whether it is a localized depression, plateau, cobblestone irregularity or ulcer, especially if this is an unusual site for a peptic ulcer. In cases of reflux, peptic ulcer disease or dyspepsia remove a sample to be tested for *Helicobacter Pylori* (Clotest).

6 Oesophageal varices, seen in portal venous hypertension, appear as tortuous, sometimes bluish, projections into the lumen of the lower oesophagus and may continue into the gastric fundus or are occasionally visible only in the upper stomach. Do not assume in patients who have gastrointestinal bleeding that visible varices are necessarily the site of bleeding.

7 Pyloric stenosis may prevent the passage of the instrument into the duodenum and it is sometimes impossible to assess whether the obstruction is from benign duodenal ulceration, a mucosal diaphragm in the distal stomach or neoplastic infiltration.

8 Previous gastric surgery distorts the anatomy and preliminary radiological examination is helpful. A stoma or pyloroplasty allows bile to reflux into the stomach. The mucosa around a stoma is often florid. Stomal ulcers usually develop just distal to the anastomosis and the instrument can be passed through it to view them. Recurrent gastric and duodenal ulcers are usually easy to see but remember that carcinoma occurs more frequently following previous gastric surgery for peptic ulceration.

9 Bleeding from the upper gastrointestinal tract can often be localized at endoscopy. If possible use an instrument with a wide-bore channel through which efficient suction can be applied. If necessary, rotate the patient to bring the site of bleeding uppermost, so that it is not hidden at the bottom of a pool of blood and other gastroduodenal contents. If the source of bleeding cannot be found, remember that the examination can be repeated. If an operation is to be performed, repeat endoscopy can be carried out just prior to surgery.

10 Always ensure that endoscopy can be repeated during an operation for upper gastrointestinal bleeding. It is sometimes invaluable in locating the bleeding site while avoiding extensive gastrotomy or gastroduodenotomy.

Action

1 Remove biopsy specimens under vision from any suspicious sites, including tumours, the edges of ulcers, irregularities of the mucosa and suspected inflammation. Take specimens from different places, preferably from each quadrant of the edge of an ulcer and not from the sloughy base. If lymphoma is a possibility, take multiple deep biopsies, since the disease often spreads in the submucosa. Place the specimens in carefully labelled separate pots containing formal saline fixative for histological examination.

2 Polypoid lesions can be caught in a snare for removal and histological examination. If the polyp has a broad base ensure that this is completely caught and, if bleeding is likely, coagulate the base with the diathermy before it is removed.

3 Foreign bodies can be grasped with forceps, snared or caught in a modified Dormia basket for withdrawal. An external tube may be slid over and pushed beyond the endoscope tip, enclosing a sharp foreign body as it is withdrawn to protect the mucosa from damage.

4 Bleeding oesophageal varices can be injected under direct vision using sclerosant solution injected through a long needle passed down the biopsy channel (see Chapter 17). Bleeding ulcers may be coagulated by spraying on thrombogenic substances or using the diathermy point. Argon gas laser or a solid state Nd-YAG laser may be used to coagulate the bleeding vessel by energy release at the point of contact. Since laser light is absorbed by blood clot this must first be gently washed away with a fine water jet. The depth of laser penetration is crucial: too superficial and the effect is lost, too deep and the resulting necrosis penetrates the wall. For this reason, laser coagulation must be performed by a skilled, experienced operator.

5 *Endoscopic retrograde cholangiopancreatography* (ERCP). A cannula can be passed through a special side-viewing endoscope for insertion in the bile and pancreatic ducts to obtain radiographic pictures following the injection of radio-opaque medium. The ampulla and lower bile duct can be slit with a diathermy wire, and stones can be removed with a modified Dormia basket. A stricture can be dilated from below followed by the insertion of a prosthetic indwelling plastic tube to maintain a passage. These techniques require special training and equipment.

6 Oesophageal dilatation can be carried out with bougies, balloons or by Nd-YAG laser destruction of tissue. The lumen may be held open by inserting a stent (see Chapter 8).

7 Endoscopic ultrasound is a novel diagnostic tool which is most helpful in oesophageal tumour staging but also useful in some gastric pathologies. It also allows for advanced therapeutic manoeuvres such as endoscopic resections of mucosal lesions.

Postoperative

1 Lay a heavily sedated patient in the recovery position (on the left side, slightly face-down), under the care of a trained nurse who will watch him until he recovers fully. If he has any respiratory obstruction this must be overcome; chest physiotherapy will help him to cough up his retained secretions. Do not allow any fluids or foods to be given until the patient is fully recovered and until the effect of pharyngeal anaesthesia has worn off.

2 Carefully clean and check the instrument.

PERIOPERATIVE CARE

Preoperative

1 Patients are assessed before an operation and routine check of blood count, blood urea, serum electrolytes and chest X-ray for those who have pre-existing disease, those who smoke or those over 40 years of age is performed. If there is suspicion of cardiac disease, arrange an electrocardiogram (ECG).

2 Explain the intended operation to the patient and obtain informed, signed consent. Detail the risks as well as the benefits.

3 Institute prophylaxis against deep venous thrombosis according to agreed protocol dependent on procedure risk classification.

4 The patient receives no food for 6 hours and water for only 2 hours before operation. If there is evidence of gastric retention, then the stomach should be emptied the day before operation by passing a nasogastric tube for aspiration. Such patients should have an intravenous infusion set up to ensure that they are not dehydrated or electrolytically depleted.

5 Ask the anaesthetist to pass a nasogastric tube as soon as anaesthesia is induced.

6 For straightforward elective operations, some surgeons would not give prophylactic antibiotics, but for emergency surgery such as perforated or bleeding ulcer or surgery for carcinoma or pyloric stenosis give a bactericidal antibiotic, such as a first- or second-generation cephalosporin, before the operation starts and continue it if there is contamination.

Action

1 Although the contents of the healthy stomach are virtually sterile, this is not so in the presence of disease and especially if there is any gastric stasis, as in pyloric stenosis, carcinoma of the stomach and re-operative gastric surgery.

2 Adopt a routine of performing as much dissection as possible before opening the stomach, then isolate the area using added towels of distinctive colour. Keep within the isolated area during the part of the operation that requires the gut to be opened and use a limited number of instruments that are kept separate. Sometimes, in spite of careful preoperative preparation and aspiration of the indwelling nasogastric tube, the stomach is distended with content. In this case, after isolating the area, make an incision into it that will just allow the sucker tube to be inserted and empty it before proceeding; otherwise, the area is likely to be flooded with foul, retained gastric content. Following this, apply non-crushing clamps to occlude the lumen to prevent further efflux. When the stomach or bowel is closed, discard the special towels and the instruments and change into fresh, sterile gloves to continue the operation.

3 The stomach is well supplied with blood and tolerates extensive mobilization without risk to its blood supply. However, this rich blood supply can lead to bleeding from the suture line so consider a haemostatic over-and-over stitch as opposed to a Connell type of stitch, unless the blood vessels are first picked up individually and tied or coagulated.

4 The duodenum is fragile and does not tolerate tension or vigorous mobilization. However, the Kocher manoeuvre often renders it mobile and prevents tension (see Fig. 10.3). Rather than anastomose it under tension, be prepared to close it and perform gastroenterostomy if this is possible.

Aftercare

1 Have the patient's condition monitored carefully until he recovers from the anaesthetic. In particular, note his colour, respiration, pulse rate and blood pressure. The blood pressure is taken every 15 minutes for the first 3 hours and then half-hourly until it is stable. Have the wound checked regularly to ensure that there is no bleeding.

2 See that the urinary output is checked hourly. Following major operations, an indwelling catheter is necessary so that urinary output can be monitored and when an epidural analgesic has been used. It can be removed as soon as the patient has recovered and is active.

3 Order nasogastric tube drainage to be recorded every hour. It may be gently aspirated every 4 hours if there is a high output. If gastric aspirate is recorded as nil, suspect that the tube is either in the wrong place or blocked. Remove the tube when the amount aspirated is less than the oral intake and the aspirate is clear, provided the patient is comfortable, with a soft abdomen. Try to remove the nasogastric tube early in patients with respiratory problems, if necessary restricting oral fluid intake. It is very difficult to cough with a tube irritating the pharynx.

4 Order intravenous fluids, remembering that sodium retention is frequent following operations and that, provided the patient started in fluid and electrolyte balance, only lost electrolytes need be replaced. Provided also that renal function is good, then, if sufficient fluid is given, small imbalances will be compensated. Since enteral feeding is safer and cheaper than parenteral feeding, consider placing a feeding jejunostomy tube or inserting a fine nasoenteric feeding tube at the time of operation in such patients.

5 On the morning after operation, allow 30 ml of water each hour, increasing incrementally to liberal fluid intake on the third day, after which normal intake can be resumed and intravenous fluid replacement stopped. Following many operations, especially when the stomach and duodenum have not been opened, this regime may be speeded up so that the morning after operation the nasogastric tube can be removed and oral fluid intake allowed in increasing amounts, depending on the patient's tolerance and general condition. Withhold oral fluids following gastric operations with oesophageal anastomosis but allow the patient to have sips as this is no different to swallowing one's saliva. It is not possible to prevent a little fluid and saliva from being swallowed, but as a rule wait for 4–5 days after operation. It is reasonable to check the intactness and adequacy of the anastomosis radiologically using a water-soluble contrast medium such as Gastrografin before commencing oral fluids and proceeding gradually to full diet. Others do not rely on this test and will start oral intake as long as there are no clinical markers of a leak, such as fever or rising inflammatory markers.

6 Encourage the patient to sit out of bed the morning following operation and have him walking a little during the next day or two, depending upon his general condition. The help of a cheerful physiotherapist in encouraging the patient to cough up retained sputum and move freely is of enormous value in preventing stasis. The use of epidural anaesthesia greatly facilitates such early mobilization.

ACCESS IN THE UPPER ABDOMEN

Do not attempt difficult manoeuvres in the upper abdomen unless there is an adequate view. As a rule, routine exposures are satisfactory, but in occasional patients the view is severely restricted.

GASTRIC CARDIA

1 Tilt the whole patient in a reverse Trendelenberg position (head up).

2 Use an upper midline incision, opening the peritoneum to one or other side of the falciform ligament. Start the incision at or alongside the xiphoid process and carry it vertically down for 20 cm, skirting the umbilicus.

3 Transverse (rooftop) and oblique incisions are also used but may be restricting in patients with a narrow costal margin. They may also be combined with vertical incisions to form a flap. A rooftop (or inverted 'V') incision offers good access since the apex of the 'V' can be folded down and sutured to the lower abdominal wall.

4 Carefully place retractors and ensure that the operating theatre light is correctly focused and aimed. To gain access under the diaphragm, use a retractor that elevates the lower sternum and costal margin, attached to a frame fixed to the operating table.

5 Mobilize the left lobe of the liver if this interferes with the view. Insert the fully pronated left hand with the index and middle fingers passing on each side of the left triangular ligament to draw down the lobe. Cut the ligament from its free edge towards the right with long-handled scissors, avoiding damage to the subphrenic vessels and left hepatic veins. Fold the lobe to the right, cover it with a gauze pack and have it held out of the way with a large curved retractor. Remember to replace it carefully at the end of the operation.

6 Carry the whole depth of the incision right up to the xiphisternum or into the angle between it and the costal margin. Do not hesitate to excise the xiphisternum using bone-cutting forceps, after dissecting off the two diaphragmatic muscle slips from its under-surface (Fig. 10.2).

7 If access is still inadequate, particularly for oesophageal anastomosis, consider performing thoracotomy.

8 If using a rooftop incision, make the incision at least an inch below the costal margin to facilitate closure at the end. Make the incision long enough so that you can fold the apex of the V downwards and suture it in the midline below the umbilicus if that helps with exposure.

KOCHER'S DUODENAL MOBILIZATION

Appraise

1 This manoeuvre (Fig. 10.3) raises the head of the pancreas contained within the duodenal loop into its embryological midline position, restrained by the structures in the free edge of the lesser omentum above, the superior mesenteric vessels below, and the body and tail of the pancreas to the left.

2 The head and neck of the pancreas can be examined from behind and palpated between fingers and thumb. The lower end of the common bile duct can be palpated and sometimes seen, although it is usually buried within the pancreatic head. The

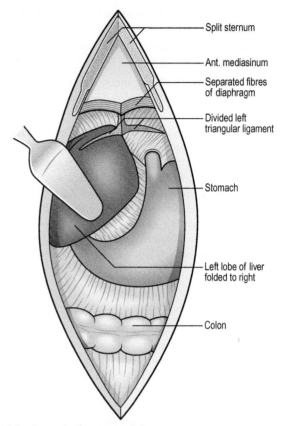

Fig. 10.2 Access in the upper abdomen.

Labels: Split sternum; Ant. mediasinum; Separated fibres of diaphragm; Divided left triangular ligament; Stomach; Left lobe of liver folded to right; Colon

duodenum and especially the ampullary region can be palpated. Duodenotomy allows inspection of the interior of the duodenum. If the incision is placed at the level of the ampulla this can be seen and palpated for tumours or stones. Biopsy, excision of ampullary neoplasms, sphincterotomy, sphincteroplasty, and

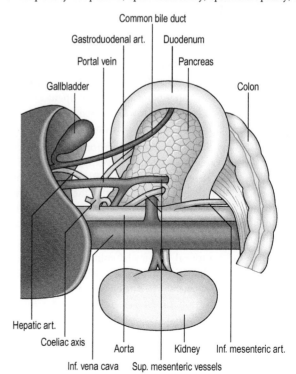

Fig. 10.3 Kocher's duodenal mobilization, as seen from the right side of the patient.

Labels: Common bile duct; Gastroduodenal art.; Duodenum; Portal vein; Pancreas; Gallbladder; Colon; Hepatic art.; Coeliac axis; Aorta; Kidney; Inf. mesenteric art.; Inf. vena cava; Sup. mesenteric vessels

cannulation or instrumentation of the bile and pancreatic ducts can be carried out under vision.

3 Mobilization is essential for excision of the pancreatic head and duodenal loop in Whipple's pancreatoduodenectomy.

4 Elevation of the duodenal loop and pancreatic head reveals the inferior vena cava when performing portocaval anastomosis or major hepatic resections.

5 The manoeuvre is particularly valuable in gastroduodenal operations. Pyloroplasty can be performed easily and the extremities of the gastroduodenal incision can be brought together without tension. In gastrectomy, the proximal duodenum is easily dissected and can be closed or united to the stomach with ease. Full mobilization may be a useful step when the stomach is drawn up for gastro-oesophageal or gastropharyngeal anastomosis. However, it is usually the porta hepatis and its connection to the first part of the duodenum that limits further mobilization.

Action

1 If incomplete mobilization is sufficient, as for palpating the lower end of the bile duct or the pancreatic head or for the purpose of carrying out pyloroplasty and gastrectomy by the Polya method, then it may be sufficient to elevate only the superior part of the duodenal loop and pancreatic head. Insinuate a finger into the aditus to the lesser sac and then divide the floor of the foramen downwards, to separate the upper duodenum and pancreas from the inferior vena cava. Extend the mobilization by continuing the division with scissors or diathermy blade, downwards, just outside the convexity of the duodenal loop.

2 For full mobilization, have your assistants draw the hepatic flexure of the colon downwards, the right edge of the wound outwards and the duodenal loop to the left.

3 Incise the peritoneum and underlying fascia of Toldt for 5 cm, placing the incision 1 cm from and parallel to the convex border of the second part of the duodenum.

4 Insinuate your fingers beneath the descending duodenum and pancreatic head. A natural plane of cleavage opens up between the embryological layers which were present when the duodenum was freely suspended in the peritoneal cavity.

5 Having defined the plane, cut the peritoneum and fascia upwards, just outside the duodenal convexity, into the mouth of the aditus to the lesser sac, meanwhile lifting the proximal duodenum forward with a finger, so protecting the inferior vena cava from damage. The dissection is easy and can be carried out by splitting with the finger except in the presence of severe scarring, as from severe duodenal ulceration.

6 Continue the peritoneal and fascial split below, taking care to avoid damaging the right colic vessels, which must be pushed downwards with the hepatic flexure of the colon and mesocolon, to release the junction of the second and third parts of the duodenum.

7 Continue the separation of the pancreas and duodenum across the aorta where it is tethered below by the superior mesenteric artery and its pancreatic branches. The structures in the free edge of the lesser omentum restrain it superiorly.

8 When the appropriate procedure is completed, carefully check the pancreatic head, duodenal loop and the bed from which the structures have been mobilized, before laying them back in place.

EXAMINATION OF THE STOMACH AND DUODENUM

1 Did you make a firm diagnosis before operation? Mucosal lesions within hollow organs are best assessed from within the lumen by radiology and endoscopy, not by examination of the exterior at operation.

2 Look at the exposed stomach. Is it distended as may be seen in pyloric obstruction? Is the musculature hypertrophied as seen in longstanding partial obstruction? The serous surface may be inflamed and oedematous, or scarred and puckered with petechiae overlying an ulcer. It may be covered with miliary tubercles in tuberculous peritonitis, or metastatic deposits of tumour. The thickened rigid appearance of 'leather-bottle' stomach may be accompanied by serosal extension, giving an appearance resembling crystallized sugar adherent to the serosa.

3 Feel for the lower oesophagus and diaphragmatic crura. Sometimes there is an obvious invagination of the gastric cardia through the diaphragmatic hiatus. If the normal anatomy can be restored by applying traction to the lesser curve of the stomach, this is a sliding hiatal hernia. If the cardia cannot be drawn down, there is a fixed hiatal hernia which may be primary or may be secondary to disease in the posterior mediastinum. There may be a gap between the crura into which the fingers can be inserted but the stomach remains fixed within the abdomen. Gently grasp the gastric cardia between finger and thumb and see if it can be slid through the hiatus into the chest. Record an asymptomatic hiatal hernia discovered incidentally when carrying out another procedure but do not repair it. Palpate the fundus of the stomach. If it disappears through the hiatus into the posterior mediastinum, this is a rolling hernia which may cause obstructive symptoms. If the patient has complained of this then consider repairing it, depending upon the severity of the symptoms, the extent of herniation, the fitness of the patient and the severity of the proposed operation.

4 Examine the body and lesser curve of the stomach for evidence of ulcers and ulcer scars. Ulcers and healed scars are often palpable and visible, and former ulcers can sometimes be detected by pinching the stomach along the lesser curve. Normal mucosa can be felt to slip away from your fingers but it may be tethered at the site of a healed ulcer. The stomach can be palpated most readily by making holes through avascular parts of the lesser and gastrocolic omenta so that fingers can be passed behind to feel the two layers of gastric wall against the thumb placed anteriorly (Fig. 10.4). The scar of an undetected posterior gastric ulcer may be adherent to the pancreas, but there are normally flimsy adhesions across the lesser sac between the stomach and pancreas. A pre- or intra-operative endoscopy may be very helpful in confirming mucosal pathology site or anatomical abnormalities. If this is not possible, carry out gastrotomy, preferably in the middle of the anterior wall of the stomach at the level of the suspected ulcer or other lesion and evaginate the lesion through the gastrotomy for visual assessment, biopsy or excision. Alternatively, it can be opened along the greater curvature in order to neither compromise any subsequent resection nor endanger the lesser curve's integrity if you decide to perform ulcer

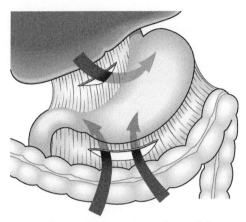

Fig. 10.4 Approaches to the posterior surfaces of the stomach and duodenal bulb, through the gastrohepatic and gastrocolic omenta.

excision. The gastrotomy may then be closed, either because no further action is necessary or prior to carrying out gastrectomy if a hitherto unsuspected chronic gastric ulcer is causing the patient's symptoms. In poor-risk patients, gastric ulcer may be treated by ulcer excision. Vagotomy is now seldom used when most patients with benign ulcers can be treated successfully with antibiotics and proton-pump inhibitors.

5 Look and feel for neoplasms. These will in nearly all cases have been diagnosed and thoroughly staged by the TNM system before operation. Staging is by computed tomographic (CT) scanning, endoluminal ultrasound and, often, laparoscopy. Carcinoma is most frequently seen, although lymphoma, reticulum-cell sarcoma, leiomyoma, leiomyosarcoma and gastrointestinal stromal tumours (GIST) are not rare, and adenomatous polyps may be felt. Carcinoma may produce a tumour within the stomach or be felt as an ulcer with raised margins. Remember that early gastric cancers may be impalpable.

> **KEY POINT** Biopsy all gastric ulcers

■ Regard all gastric ulcers as malignant until proved, by biopsy, to be benign.

An apparently benign ulcer may have developed malignant characteristics. Extensive submucosal infiltration produces the rigid 'leather-bottle' stomach (linitis plastica), often with penetration of the serosa producing a crystallized sugar appearance with beaded irregular blood vessels. If carcinoma is suspected, proven or unexpectedly encountered, do not touch it but examine the prerectal pouch, the ovaries in the female, the remainder of the peritoneal cavity, the root of the mesentery and the liver to assess the degree of spread before palpating the primary tumour, so that malignant cells are not carried around on the gloves. Feel the local glands along the greater and lesser curves, and through holes in the avascular portions in the lesser and gastrocolic omenta assess the degree of posterior infiltration into the pancreas and the involvement of glands around the coeliac axis and along the superior border of the pancreas. When, in some cases, the diagnosis remains in doubt, gastrotomy should be performed, with the removal of a specimen for frozen-section histology, and then closed. On the basis of the report and the operative assessment, decide on the immediate action. If a

distal carcinoma appears to be totally resectable, carry out a radical distal gastrectomy. An apparently curable proximal carcinoma is ideally treated by radical total gastrectomy. This may be carried out through a left thoracoabdominal incision and the abdominal incision can be extended to the left after the patient has been turned onto the right side, has had the skin prepared and fresh sterile towels have been applied. This approach is very useful for Siewert type II or III tumours of the gastro-oesophageal junction. Alternatively, for Siewert type I, II and small type III tumours, an Ivor Lewis right thoracoabdominal approach gives good access and permits adequate proximal clearance of the tumour. Early tumours of the cardia may also be excised using a proximal gastrectomy. This procedure is associated with intractable symptoms of biliary reflux, which may be reduced by the use of a jejunal interposition graft in place of the excised proximal stomach (Merendino Procedure). Midgastric tumours can sometimes be adequately excised by abdominal total gastrectomy. Carry out palliative resection or exclusion gastrectomy if inoperable distal carcinoma threatens to cause obstruction or is the source of recurrent bleeding or anaemia. A defunctioning gastroenterostomy offers palliative relief, although patients often experience prolonged delayed gastric emptying.

Completely excise adenomas since histology may reveal malignant changes. Sometimes they are multiple and gastrectomy may be more appropriate. Benign tumours such as angioma and lipoma require merely local removal. Leiomyoma or GIST cannot be differentiated at operation, or even by frozen-section histology, from leiomyosarcoma. Excise it with a healthy margin and await definitive histological analysis. Leiomyoblastoma is less frequently seen and is usually benign. Lymphoma may be primary gastric or nodal in type. Primary gastric lymphoma is associated with only regional lymphadenopathy. In nodal lymphoma there may be splenic and hepatic involvement. It may be difficult to diagnose before operation and frozen-section histology at the time of operation may be valuable in case of doubt.

6 Examine the pyloroduodenal region. The pyloric ring can be picked up between the index finger and thumb of both hands, but the mucosal ring may be smaller than the muscular ring. To check this, invaginate the anterior antral wall through the pylorus on an index finger and invaginate the anterior duodenal wall back into the stomach in a similar manner. If there is obstruction, look again at the stomach. Is it dilated? Is the muscular wall hypertrophied? Look and feel for a duodenal ulcer, remembering that the majority of ulcers lie in the bulb, although they may be in the postbulbar region or further distally, especially in the Zollinger-Ellison syndrome. Sometimes an ulcer crater can be palpated, sometimes there is gross and incontrovertible scarring and narrowing, together with pseudo-diverticulum formation but there may be minimal scarring, a few petechial haemorrhages – which could be iatrogenic – or there may be nothing abnormal to see or feel. Of course the diagnosis should have been made endoscopically before operation, but occasionally endoscopy has failed because the tip of the instrument could not negotiate the narrow or distorted pyloroduodenal canal. If doubt remains, could a small endoscope be passed and the tip guided through manually to allow the interior to be viewed? Alternatively, create a small prepyloric gastrotomy and examine the interior with a finger, or by placing small retractors within the pyloroduodenal canal. A mucosal diaphragm that is soft and easily stretched can be dilated, or conventionally treated by pyloroplasty.

7. Diverticula of the stomach are most frequently found on the upper lesser curve, sometimes produced by traction from a leiomyoma. If no primary lesion is present, leave an asymptomatic diverticulum alone. Pseudodiverticula of the duodenum develop when chronic duodenal ulcer causes distortion. The most frequent duodenal diverticulum is not seen unless it is sought for, since it lies close to the ampulla, protruding into the pancreas, which must be mobilized by Kocher's manoeuvre to approach from posteriorly. It rarely causes symptoms and should normally be left alone.

SUTURING AND STAPLING THE STOMACH AND DUODENUM

SUTURES

1. There is a wide choice of sutures. As with all sutures, they are severely weakened by crushing, abrasion and rough handling, especially when drawing them through the tissues and tying knots.

   Braided polyglycolic acid and monofilament polyglyconate retain their tensile strength reliably for longer than catgut. Polydioxanone also retains its tensile strength for longer than catgut and, because it degrades by hydrolysis, there is relatively little inflammatory response during absorption. Braided polyglactin 910 has good handling qualities with slow absorption. For use in the gastrointestinal tract 3/0 or 4/0 has adequate strength.

   Some surgeons still insert a serosal layer. Non-absorbable 3/0 or 4/0 braided polyamide may be used, but slowly absorbing synthetics are probably better.

2. Innumerable papers have been written about the best ways of suturing stomach and intestine. Should we use interrupted or continuous, one layer or two, simple through-and-through or complex stitches, including or excluding the mucosa, inverted or edge-to-edge? It is obvious from listening to, and reading the papers of, the various advocates that all the methods are successful. There is but a single common factor and that is the care with which sutures are inserted and tied. If you bring together the edges of stomach or bowel that have a good blood supply, are not under tension and are apposed carefully with sutures that do not strangulate the included tissue, they will heal. Many of us continue to use the methods we learned whilst training, because they have demonstrably worked, even though we accept that they may no longer be in vogue. The one layer that must always be included in the stitches, as shown by Halsted, is the submucosa.

   Since all the methods work provided they are employed carefully, it seems logical to employ a single-layer edge-to-edge apposition, allowing each component of the gut wall to join directly to the same component on the opposite edge. Preference for interrupted or continuous stitching is constantly argued. Interrupted stitches have the advantage that, if one cuts out, others remain, and, if they are tied too tightly, the intervening tissue that is not enclosed will survive and unite. Continuous unlocked stitches produce a spiral that does not strangulate the tissues yet allows the tension to be evenly distributed; they withstand much greater distraction of the edges than do interrupted stitches.

LIGATURES

- As with sutures, ligatures are applied using the finest possible materials, although silk and linen are still popular because of their excellent handling properties. Metal clips are convenient to seal blood vessels but they easily catch in swabs and can be dragged off. One instrument applies two clips side by side and cuts between them, for dividing vascular tissue. Unless they offer advantages in saving time, prefer to tie ligatures, which is more versatile.

- Absorbable synthetic clips have also become more commonly used.

STAPLES

- The development of reliable instruments for joining bowel has potentially great value in gastroduodenal surgery. However, they are not as versatile as sutures. If you are a trainee, by all means learn to use stapling instruments but more importantly take every opportunity to master the accurate placement of sutures.

- There are two overriding indications for using stapling instruments. The first is when the difficulties of suturing, perhaps because of inadequate access that cannot be improved, make stapling safer. The second is when speed is essential, perhaps during a major operation.

GASTROTOMY AND GASTRODUODENOTOMY

Appraise

1. Gastric, gastroduodenal and duodenal incision allows the interior of the bowel to be examined to confirm, biopsy or treat a suspected lesion such as an ulcer, tumour or source of bleeding.

2. Gastrotomy allows access from below to the lower oesophagus. Strictures are often dilated more safely from below than from above.

Access

1. As a rule, open the stomach on the anterior wall midway between the greater and lesser curves.

2. For the purpose of diagnosis, start with a small incision, 3–4 cm long, the proximal end of which is 5–6 cm from the pylorus. This incision ensures that the intact pylorus or mucosal diaphragm can be examined and it may be unnecessary to destroy the pyloric muscular ring. The incision can be extended proximally or, if it becomes necessary, distally through the pyloric ring onto the anterior wall of the duodenal bulb.

3. To view the interior, first aspirate all the contents. Retractors may be placed to hold open the stomach so that it can be examined by adjusting the theatre light to shine through the opening. The stomach can be manoeuvred manually to bring different parts of the interior into view. Frequently the gastric wall can be evaginated through the incision so that it can be examined and any lesion excised or biopsied. If the pylorus is not too narrow, small retractors may be placed in to allow the duodenal bulb to be viewed, and, if it is wide, an unscarred duodenal bulbar wall may be evaginated through it on a finger. If there is difficulty in viewing the duodenum to exclude or confirm disease, a per-oral endoscope may be introduced through it. Sometimes, when fibreoptic endoscopy is ineffective before operation, perhaps resulting from inability to evacuate the gastric contents, the stomach may be emptied and endoscopy can then be performed. The gastrotomy can be temporarily occluded with a clamp to allow the stomach to be inflated but as a rule the stomach can be held open to allow endoscopy to be accomplished without the need for inflation.

Closure

1. Close a gastrotomy in one or two layers, leaving a longitudinal suture line.

2. It is conventional practice to close a gastroduodenotomy as a Heineke-Mikulicz pyloroplasty. This may be accomplished using a single edge-to-edge row of sutures, a two-layer invaginating suture or with a row of staples. However, this destroys the pyloric metering function and it may be preferable to carefully close the incision to create a longitudinal scar, bringing the edges together without invagination in a single layer, taking care to appose the pyloric edges perfectly. Cover the suture line with a layer of omentum as an extra precaution.

3. Use ingenuity to incorporate the gastrotomy in plans for other procedures. A distal gastrotomy may be incorporated in a gastroenterostomy. The proximal part of a long gastroduodenotomy may be closed longitudinally and the distal part converted into a pyloroplasty if necessary. If gastrectomy is intended, temporarily close the gastrotomy with stitches or staples to keep soiling to a minimum.

PYLOROMYOTOMY

Appraise

1. Pyloromyotomy for infantile pyloric stenosis is described in Chapter 34.

2. Adult hypertrophic pyloric stenosis is rarely discovered as a cause of gastric retention. It is not known whether or not this represents undiagnosed infantile pyloric stenosis.

3. Pyloromyotomy is sometimes carried out following oesophagectomy with oesophagogastric anastomosis, in the hope of preventing gastric retention. Failure of the stomach to empty in the absence of pyloric stenosis results from gastric atony following the inevitable gastric vagotomy. Many surgeons employ a pyloroplasty to compensate for this postvagotomy gastric atony.

Assess

Endoscopy should have been performed before operation, but, if this was not possible, pick up the pylorus and feel the thickness of the muscular ring. Assess the size of the mucosal channel by attempting to invaginate the anterior antral wall and the anterior duodenal wall through the pylorus on the tip of an index finger.

ACTION

1. Grasp the pylorus between finger and thumb of the left hand to steady it (Fig. 10.5).

2. Incise the seromuscularis along the middle of the anterior antral wall from 1 cm proximal to the thickened segment and carefully extend it distally across the pylorus onto the anterior duodenal wall for 1 cm. The duodenal wall at the fornix is very thin, so take care not to incise into the lumen.

3. Deepen the incision through the thickened muscle of the distal antrum until the mucosa bulges into the split. Make sure all the muscle fibres are divided. The final split may be accomplished by grasping the wall on each side of the split with dry gauze swabs and separating the edges, to allow mucosa to bulge freely along the whole of the incision.

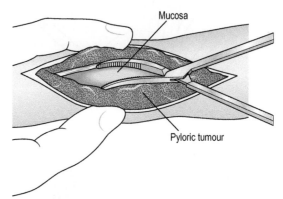

Fig. 10.5 Pyloromyotomy.

4. Carry the split distally to the pylorus and carefully divide all the circular muscle fibres here, again taking care to expose but not damage the mucosa of the first part of the duodenal bulb. Lift the muscle fibres free of the mucosa with closed fine non-toothed dissecting forceps, allow the forceps blades to open and then cut the fibres between them.

Check

1. Make sure all the fibres have been cut.

2. Gather some gastric air into the segment with the pyloromyotomy, to distend the mucosa so that it bulges into the split. Watch carefully for any leaks. It is no disaster to find a leak and carefully close it with fine stitches: it may be disastrous to miss a leak.

OPERATIVE GASTROSTOMY

Appraise

1. Gastrostomy offers a valuable method of feeding patients who are unable to swallow because of oesophageal obstruction, bulbar palsy and other causes. Patients with mechanical obstruction who will have reconstructive surgery utilizing the stomach as a conduit should not normally have a temporary gastrostomy since this will interfere with subsequent reconstructive surgery. They are better served by a jejunostomy.

2. Gastrostomy offers a means of providing gastric aspiration without nasogastric intubation, valuable in patients who have respiratory difficulties and those who cannot tolerate the presence of the tube in their pharynx, during the postoperative recovery period from gastric operations.

3. As a rule gastrostomy is placed endoscopically (Percutaneous Endoscopic Gastrostomy – PEG) and is intended as a temporary measure. When all else fails, do not hesitate to offer it after discussion with the patient.

4. Operative gastrostomy is often unnecessary following the advent of percutaneous endoscopic gastrostomy. If necessary, a number of operative techniques have been described. Stamm's gastrostomy (Fig. 10.6) is almost universally used now and is described below. The tube passes through the abdominal wall and enters the stomach through a small stab wound. The hole is prevented from leaking by invaginating it using a series of purse-string sutures so that it resembles a non-spill inkwell. Witzel's gastrostomy is similar, but leakage is prevented by laying the emerging tube along

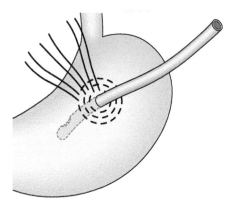

Fig. 10.6   Stamm gastrostomy.

the stomach wall and covering it by suturing over it ridges of gastric wall so that it lies in a tunnel. The Depage-Janeway gastrostomy employs a flap of stomach formed into a tube which is brought to the skin surface to create a permanent conduit.

PERCUTANEOUS ENDOSCOPIC GASTROSTOMY

Appraise

1. The commonest application is for intragastric or enteral nutritional support in the presence of, for example, bulbar palsy. Another indication is to enable prolonged gastric aspiration to be performed, especially in those who cannot tolerate nasogastric intubation.

2. Do not attempt this method if the patient has an impassable oesophageal stricture, or previous upper abdominal surgery that produces adhesions preventing expansion of the stomach to contact the anterior abdominal wall, or a partial gastrectomy. Gross ascites or sepsis makes the procedure dangerous so a surgical gastrostomy or jejunostomy is preferred. Portal venous hypertension, coagulopathy/gastric ulcer or tumour at the elective site of gastrostomy is also a contraindication. Gross obesity may make the procedure difficult.

3. There is a choice of methods, and some excellent commercially produced kits are available with tubes 9F or 15F in size. A popular, simple pull-through technique is described below.

Prepare

1. Administer intravenous sedation according to protocol.

2. Lie patients who can tolerate it supine. Alternatively, pass the endoscope with the patient lying on the left side and then roll the patient into the supine position.

3. Give a single intravenous injection of a broad-spectrum antibiotic.

Action

1. Pass an end-viewing endoscope into the stomach. In the presence of an oesophageal stricture it may be necessary to dilate it using bougies or a balloon, and then introduce a paediatric endoscope. Pass the tip into the distal stomach.

2. Inspect the stomach and duodenum to exclude any condition that would contraindicate gastrostomy.

3. Gently inflate the stomach to distend it.

4. Have the abdomen exposed and the room lights dimmed.

5. Turn the endoscope tip towards the anterior abdominal wall. The light should be visible through the gastric and abdominal walls.

6. Have the abdominal operator indent the anterior abdominal wall with a finger placed where the endoscope light is seen most brightly. The indentation should be visible from within the stomach.

7. Pass a polypectomy snare through the biopsy channel of the endoscope (Fig. 10.7A).

8. If you are the abdominal operator, prepare the skin, infiltrate the chosen puncture spot with local anaesthesia into the skin and abdominal wall (and most often into the gastric lumen under direct vision), then make an incision in the skin sufficiently large to allow the passage of the gastrostomy tube.

9. Pass a needle carrying a smooth, closely fitting plastic cannula through the abdominal wall into the stomach. This catheter is usually in the PEG kit but a standard intravenous catheter may be employed.

10. If you are the endoscopist, manoeuvre the loop of the snare over the cannula (Fig. 10.7B). The needle is withdrawn by the abdominal operator and either a flexible wire or a strong thread is passed through the cannula into the stomach.

11. Withdraw the snare from the end of the cannula under vision, in order to grasp the thread or wire that protrudes from the end of the cannula into the stomach (Fig. 10.7C). While the abdominal operator holds the other end of the thread or wire, withdraw the endoscope, snare and trapped thread or wire out through the mouth.

12. Attach the emerging thread or wire to the tapered end of the gastrostomy tube (Fig. 10.7D). The bulbous or inflatable end of the gastrostomy tube will remain in the stomach, pulling it against the abdominal wall.

13. Apply lubricant to the gastrostomy tube.

14. Draw upon the thread or wire emerging from the abdominal cannula while guiding the tapered tip of the gastrostomy tube through the patient's mouth and into the oesophagus and stomach. Eventually the tapered tip is drawn against the cannula tip, extruding it. As you continue to pull, the tapered end of the gastrostomy tube will emerge through the gastric and abdominal walls (Fig. 10.7E).

15. Re-pass the endoscope into the stomach and observe the enlarged end ('bumper') of the gastrostomy tube as it is drawn up against the gastric wall. In some tubes the end is shaped so that it expands automatically; in others, a balloon is expanded by distending it with air or fluid through a side channel. Make sure that the tension on the gastrostomy tube is not sufficient to cause gastric mucosal blanching.

16. Withdraw the endoscope.

17. Cut off the tapered end of the gastrostomy tube and ensure that the expanded end is inflated if it is of this type, and seal the side-tube inflation channel.

18. The tube must be fixed to hold the stomach against the abdominal wall. Most kits contain a fixation base that fits over and holds the gastrostomy tube, having an expanded flat surface that lies against the abdominal wall (Fig. 10.7F).

Aftercare

1. Feeding with suitable varied fluids can usually start within 24 hours.

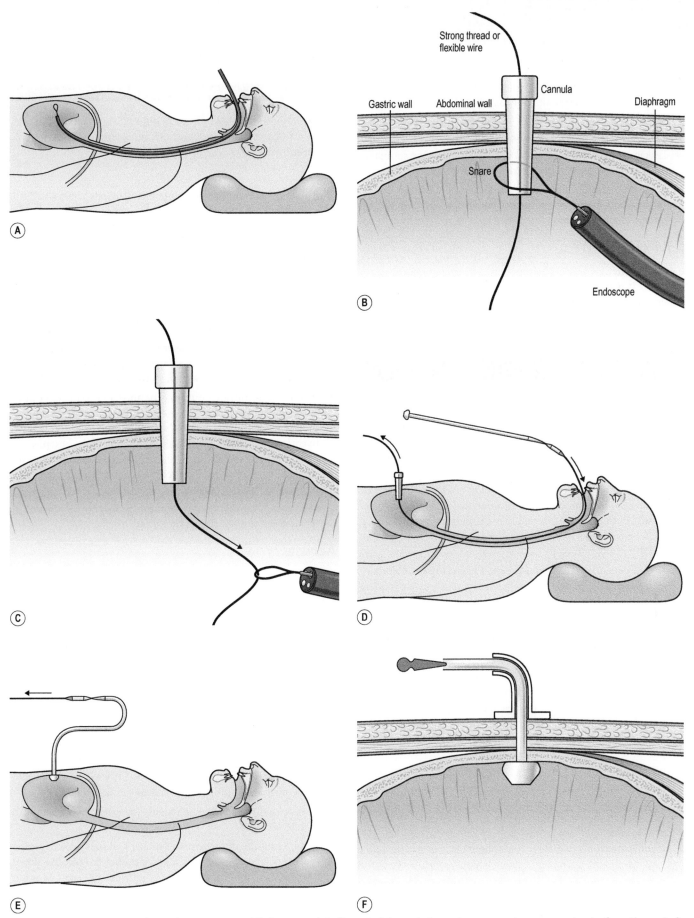

Fig. 10.7 Percutaneous endoscopic gastrostomy: (A) the stomach is distended through the endoscope; a wire snare protrudes from the end of the endoscope; (B) strong thread or wire passed into the stomach; (C) thread or wire snared for withdrawal through the mouth; (D) the tapered end of the gastrostomy tube is fixed to the strong thread or flexible wire; (E) the gastrostomy tube has been pulled through the pharynx, oesophagus and stomach; the bulbous or inflatable end is about to be drawn against the anterior gastric wall; (F) the gastrostomy tube in position.

2 Monitor the patient to ensure that there is no chest infection, since reflux and aspiration pneumonia is a well-recognized complication.

3 Check the gastrostomy site since infection is frequent.

4 Leakage around the gastrostomy catheter may develop spontaneously or in the presence of gastric outlet obstruction.

5 Some gastrostomy tubes can be removed by deflating the expanded end and drawing them through the abdominal wall. Others require endoscopic withdrawal.

JEJUNOSTOMY

It is possible to pass a longer, narrower tube through the gastrostomy tube after it is in place. This can be advanced through the pylorus, either spontaneously, under radiographic control, or endoscopically, into the duodenum and jejunum. In this way a jejunostomy is created for distal enteral feeding.

PERFORATED PEPTIC ULCER

Appraise

1 Record the patient's age, blood pressure and the presence or absence of serious associated disease such as cardiac, respiratory or renal failure. Fully resuscitate the patient before performing the operation.

2 Perforation of other viscera such as colon or gallbladder may be confused with gastroduodenal perforations. A laparoscopic approach may aid diagnosis and may be adequate for treatment. A CT scan is vital in making a clear diagnosis as long as the patient is stable enough to go through the scanner.

3 Not all patients who have a perforated peptic ulcer should have an operation. Patients seen within 8 hours, in whom a confident diagnosis is made, and who are haemodynamically stable, may be treated conservatively. Ensure that the tip of an 18F nasogastric tube is accurately placed in the most dependent part of the stomach. A disadvantage is that peritoneal toilet cannot be performed. Proceed to operation at once if the patient develops pyrexia, tachycardia, pain, distension or increasing intra-peritoneal gas on X-rays. A few patients develop intra-peritoneal abscesses if there has been significant leakage and soiling. Nasogastric suction, parenteral feeding, systemic antibiotics and chest physiotherapy are instituted, and operation is resorted to only if the patient fails to improve or deteriorates.

4 Perforated gastric ulcer carries a higher mortality than perforated duodenal ulcer, because the patients are, on average, older and generally less 'fit'. Most gastric ulcer perforations are successfully managed by simple suture after excising a specimen from the edge for histology. Sometimes they are difficult to close and demand gastrectomy. If there is doubt about the nature of the ulcer, treat it as though it is benign, remove a biopsy specimen from the edge and, if malignancy is demonstrated histologically, carry out the appropriate operation later as an elective procedure. If the ulcer cannot be sutured but is of doubtful origin and frozen-section histology is equivocal or cannot be arranged, then carry out gastrectomy as for a benign ulcer and be prepared to re-operate to carry out an elective radical procedure later. The added risks of performing a radical operation are not justified without confirming the diagnosis.

5 Bleeding associated with perforation demands control of both complications. A bleeding perforated gastric ulcer is conventionally controlled by distal gastrectomy, including the ulcer. Bleeding is rarely a complication of anterior perforating duodenal ulcer but if there is a co-existent bleeding posterior duodenal ulcer, the anterior perforation can be incorporated into a gastroduodenotomy. Insert non-absorbable stitches into the base of the posterior ulcer to control the bleeding and then close the gastroduodenotomy as a pyloroplasty. If unable to close the duodenotomy due to friable tissue then perform a distal gastrectomy, close the duodenal stump over a Foley catheter balloon (exteriorized as a controlled fistula) and place a large surgical drain next to the stump. These patients need long-term proton-pump inhibitors.

6 Perforated gastric carcinoma may be amenable to the same operation as would be carried out electively. If not, consider suturing it or plugging the defect with omentum and re-operating electively later after the patient has been brought to the best possible condition. Sometimes inadequate resection is forced upon the surgeon. If so, consider whether this can be corrected later by a more adequate operation.

7 Laparoscopy may be used to confirm the diagnosis, followed by repair using sutures, staples or a plug.

Access

If a laparoscopic approach is used four ports are needed, one of which is for retraction of the liver, with two operating ports (for suturing) and a central camera port. If a laparotomy is chosen, use a midline incision from the xiphisternum to the umbilicus, 10–12 cm long.

Assess

1 Remove all instruments from the field with the exception of a retractor for your assistant and the sucker tube for yourself.

2 Aspirate any free fluid after collecting a specimen for laboratory examination. Gastric juice is usually bile-stained.

3 Examine the duodenal bulb and the stomach, especially along the lesser curve. If necessary, open the lesser sac of omentum through the lesser or gastrocolic omenta to view the posterior gastric wall.

4 Remember that multiple perforations can occur.

5 Always locally excise or remove a biopsy specimen from the edge of a gastric ulcer.

6 If you cannot find the perforation after a diligent search, explore the whole abdomen, if necessary extending the incision downwards. Examine in particular the gallbladder and sigmoid colon. If you are still puzzled, consider the possibility of Boerhaave's syndrome (spontaneous rupture of distal spontaneous oesophagus).

7 If you are a surgeon in training and find yourself in difficulty either because of failure to discover the cause, or indecision about the best course of action, or because the required procedure is beyond your capabilities, do not hesitate to contact your chief for advice and assistance.

- Your function at this emergency operation is to perform the simplest procedure that will correct the catastrophe.
- If you do more than this, will you be able to justify it to yourself and others if the patient succumbs?

Simple closure

1 Place two or three parallel sutures of 3/0 synthetic absorbable material through all coats, passing in 1 cm proximal to the ulcer edge and emerging 1 cm distal to the ulcer (Fig. 10.8). Do not pick up the opposite wall as this will obstruct the lumen. When all the sutures are in place, mobilize a tongue of omentum, place it over the perforation and tie the sutures just tightly enough to hold it in place.

2 Insert further sutures to reinforce the obturating action of the omentum and ensure the defect is adequately sealed.

3 Even when closure seems secure, do not hesitate to suture omentum over it.

4 Aspirate any free fluid from above and below the liver, from within the lesser sac, the right paracolic gutter and from the pelvis.

Checklist

1 Re-examine the closure of the perforation.

2 Aspirate in the collection areas once more.

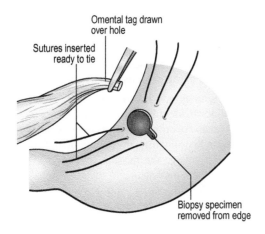

Omental tag drawn over hole

Sutures inserted ready to tie

Biopsy specimen removed from edge

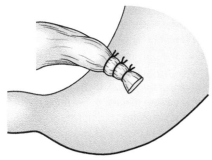

Fig. 10.8 **Suture of a perforated peptic ulcer.**

Drain?

1 If the perforation was sutured without delay, if the closure is secure and peritoneal toilet was adequate, drainage is unnecessary.

2 Make sure the insertion of a drain does not replace careful technique.

ELECTIVE SURGERY FOR PEPTIC ULCER

Appraise

1 Medical treatment has become the mainstay with potent antacids, atropine-like drugs, liquorice extracts, mucosal-coating substances, histamine H_2-receptor-blocking drugs and proton-pump inhibitors. The elimination of *Helicobacter pylori*, using so-called triple therapy of a proton-pump inhibitor combined with two antibiotics such as clarithromycin and metronidazole, reduces the relapse rate. Most patients can be controlled with these powerful and safe agents and the only people who may require operation are the minority who cannot be controlled medically, who cannot or will not take the required treatment, or who develop complications of the ulcer.

2 The operation in vogue in the 1960s and 1970s was proximal gastric vagotomy, known also as highly selective vagotomy. Some centres report high rates of recurrence after long-term follow-up but variations in recurrence rates probably reflect variations in completeness of parietal cell denervation and are thus dependent on the skill of the surgeon. An adjunctive operation to overcome gastric retention is unnecessary if there is no evidence of impending pyloroduodenal stenosis resulting from the chronic ulcer scarring. If there is, some surgeons dilate the canal through a prepyloric gastrotomy using Hegar-type dilators or a finger, or by invaginating the anterior duodenal and gastric antral walls through the stenosed canal on an index finger tip – a manoeuvre introduced by Jaboulay. If the stenosis is confined to the bulb, a longitudinal incision can be made through it without impinging on the pyloric ring, closing it as a transverse suture line after the manner of a pyloroplasty; hence it is termed a duodenoplasty. A few surgeons still prefer truncal vagotomy combined with pyloroplasty, gastroenterostomy or distal gastrectomy to improve gastric emptying.

3 Gastric ulcer was treated more aggressively by surgeons in the past than was duodenal ulcer. Many surgeons adopt a fixed policy of carrying out endoscopy and biopsy to confirm that the ulcer is benign, then give the patient a 6–8-week course of medical treatment followed by a further check endoscopy. If the ulcer is healed, operation is deferred. If the ulcer is not healed, or if it soon recurs, then surgical treatment is recommended. This more aggressive treatment stems partly from anxiety about the possibility of early malignancy or impending change and partly from the pragmatic knowledge that chronic gastric ulcers are less likely than chronic duodenal ulcers to become quiescent.

Gastric ulcers sometimes develop in patients taking non-steroidal anti-inflammatory drugs (NSAIDs). Misoprostol, a prostaglandin analogue, appears to reduce this tendency.

The operation of choice for gastric ulcers is a Polya partial gastrectomy, including the ulcer in the specimen.

4 Postbulbar duodenal ulcers are quite frequently seen in certain countries, especially southern India, but are relatively uncommon in Western countries. They are often severe and stenosing so that operation may be recommended for fear of incipient

obstruction. Proximal gastric vagotomy is effective if the lumen is still widely patent; if it is not then add gastroenterostomy, thus retaining the vagal supply to the gallbladder, pancreas and small intestine.

5 Zollinger-Ellison syndrome associated with hypergastrinaemia, usually from G-cell hyperplasia or gastrin-secreting tumour in the pancreas, generally produces peptic ulcers in usual sites. If an ulcer lies in an unusual site, or if there are multiple ulcers and especially if the ulcer is in the upper jejunum, suspect the Zollinger-Ellison syndrome (vide infra).

6 Oesophageal peptic ulceration occurs when gastric acid refluxes into the oesophagus where the squamous mucosa is unresistant to acid attack. This develops most frequently as a result of hiatal hernia but can occur in the absence of herniation of the stomach into the chest. A less frequent cause of peptic ulcer in the oesophagus is the condition of Barrett's oesophagus. This appears to be acquired, although it used to be called 'congenitally short oesophagus'. There is intestinal metaplasis in the distal oesophagus and the oesophagogastric mucosal junction moves progressively upwards; an ulcer sometimes develops just above the junction. There is a greatly increased risk of developing adenocarcinoma of the distal oesophagus (see Chapter 9).

VAGOTOMY

The various types of vagotomy are now seldom used in the elective treatment of peptic ulceration, because of the success of medical treatment with antibiotics and potent antacids. Proximal gastric, or highly selective, vagotomy is preferable to truncal vagotomy and 'drainage' because side-effects such as dumping and diarrhoea are fewer in incidence and less in severity.

> ### ▶ KEY POINT 'Blind' vagotomy
>
> ■ Never embark on elective vagotomy without confirming the diagnosis of peptic ulcer.

TRUNCAL VAGOTOMY

Appraise

1 Per-hiatal truncal vagotomy was formerly indicated for the management of uncomplicated duodenal ulcer when the full range of medical treatment had been tried and failed to control the symptoms. It is normally accompanied by pyloroplasty or gastroenterostomy to improve the rate of gastric emptying, so-called drainage procedures. Pyloroplasty (vide infra) is simple to perform unless the patient is very obese with a deep abdomen and with a fixed, very scarred pylorus. Anterior juxatapyloric gastroenterostomy is convenient if pyloroplasty is difficult to perform, and has the advantage that it is not irrevocable.

2 Truncal vagotomy may be used when controlling gastroduodenal bleeding from peptic ulcer. At such operations the main task is to stop the bleeding, but the secondary task is to prevent bleeding from recurrent or persistent ulcer.

3 In the surgical management of recurrent peptic ulcer truncal vagotomy is best combined with partial gastrectomy.

4 Truncal vagotomy combined with a 'drainage' operation is sometimes advocated for the definitive management of a perforated duodenal ulcer. The improvement in medical management of uncomplicated duodenal ulcer has rendered this approach obsolete.

5 Truncal vagotomy and a drainage operation is often effective treatment for chronic gastric ulcer in an unfit patient, but gastrectomy including the ulcer is preferred treatment whenever possible.

Access

1 Use a midline incision 20 cm long, skirting the umbilicus.

2 Mobilize the left lobe of the liver, folding it to the right, to obtain a good view.

3 In an obese patient with a high diaphragm try the effect of tilting the patient 25–30° head-up.

4 Insert a retractor fixed to the table, to elevate the sternum.

Assess

1 Explore the whole abdomen. Remember that patients with proven peptic ulceration may have incidental conditions such as gallstones or colonic carcinoma which might help to explain their symptoms.

2 Examine the stomach and duodenum and note the effects of the ulcer in distorting the duodenum and fixing it, so that you may make a decision about the easiest and safest adjunctive operation.

> ### ▶ KEY POINTS Favour simple and safe procedures
>
> ■ There is little difference between the results of the various operations.
> ■ Do not perform a difficult procedure regardless of other considerations.

Action

1 Make sure there is a nasogastric tube in place, as a guide to the line of the gullet at the oesophageal hiatus.

2 While an assistant grasps the lower anterior wall of the stomach and draws it down, identify the hiatus by feeling for the nasogastric tube. Open the peritoneum transversely, avoiding the inferior phrenic vessels. Beneath this is the phreno-oesophageal ligament. Open this and enlarge the incision to 3–4 cm. You can now pass the closed scissors anterior to the gullet into the posterior mediastinum. If you cannot, you have not yet opened the phreno-oesophageal ligament. Thorough mobilization of the distal oesophagus is the key to the achievement of complete vagotomy.

3 Look out for the anterior vagal trunk lying in front of the oesophagus (Fig. 10.9) and separate it upwards for 5 cm and downwards to where it gives off the hepatic and gastric body branches, continuing as the anterior nerve of Latarjet. Transect it where it breaks up below, crushing the distal stump to occlude the small vessels running with it. Place a curved Moynihan clamp across it as high as possible and transect it just below the clamp, then remove the clamp. This is a 'vagectomy' and ensures that the whole trunk is removed but does not guarantee that vagotomy is complete, since fine branches may come off higher up and bypass the 'vagectomy'.

4 Encircle the lower gullet with the right forefinger and thumb. There is a 'mesentery' behind the gullet in which lies the posterior

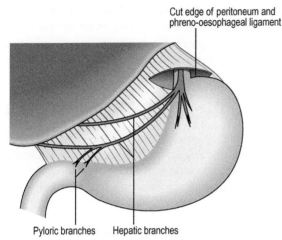

Fig. 10.9 Truncal vagotomy. Exposure of the anterior nerve; the distribution of the nerve is indicated.

vagal trunk (Fig. 10.10). Pass the middle finger to the left of the gullet and push this 'mesentery' to the right so that the nerve trunk can be identified. Separate the oesophagus from the vagus and burst through the mesentery behind the vagus. As the trunk is traced down, part of it passes backwards to the coeliac plexus (Fig. 10.11), part continues downwards as the posterior nerve of Latarjet and branches leave to reach the body of the stomach. Crush and cut the nerve below and again as high as possible to remove a segment of nerve to insure against leaving a separate branch intact.

5 Search for missed, separate branches around the whole circumference of the oesophageal wall. They feel like tight threads and should be divided. Make sure that there is no damage to the oesophagus and that all the bleeding is controlled.

6 Repair the horizontal defect in the hiatus using non-absorbable sutures.

7 Carry out the selected adjunctive procedure of pyloroplasty, gastroenterostomy or gastrectomy.

1. Access can be very difficult in obese patients. Do not proceed if you do not have an adequate view. Tilt the patient head-up, remove the xiphoid process, mobilize the left lobe of the liver and fold it to the right. If the view is still restricted, do not hesitate to split the sternum in the midline. The only danger is of embarking on vagotomy without being able to see properly and control what is done.

2. The assistant's hand drawing down the stomach may be in the way. Make a hole in an avascular part of the upper lesser omentum, pass curved forceps behind the fundus of the stomach and push them through the gastrophrenic ligament near the angle of His. Draw a rubber tube through the hole as a sling to exert traction without distorting or obscuring the cardia.

3. *Damage to the oesophagus?* Repair the hole carefully, using all-coats sutures followed by a muscle coat stitch. Leave a nasogastric tube in the stomach.

4. *Cannot find the vagi?* Clumsy opening of the phreno-oesophageal ligament may lead to inadvertent anterior vagotomy. Carefully open the peritoneum and phreno-oesophageal ligament until the oesophagus can be seen encircled above by the diaphragmatic crus. The cut anterior trunk will be seen lying on the oesophagus. Alternatively, you will see that the anterior trunk has been displaced to one side.

5. The posterior vagal trunk does not always lie close to the oesophagus. If it cannot be felt, carefully display the oesophagus emerging through the crus. The vagal trunk may be seen lying against the muscle of the crus. If you are a surgeon in training and cannot find the vagi, call for advice and assistance. Otherwise remember that more than half of patients treated surgically by gastroenterostomy will be cured of their symptoms. An experienced surgeon may carry out polya gastrectomy in appropriate circumstances.

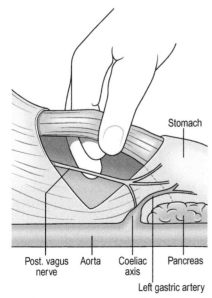

Fig. 10.10 Truncal vagotomy. Exposure of the posterior nerve as seen from the right side of the patient. While the gullet is encircled by the right thumb and forefinger, the right middle finger pushes the 'mesentery' containing the dorsal nerve to the right.

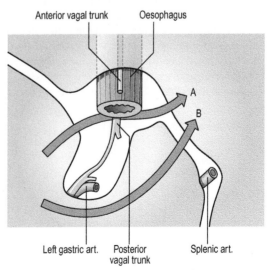

Fig. 10.11 Diagram of peritoneal reflections from the posterior abdominal wall. The posterior vagal trunk is gathered along path A but not along path B.

PROXIMAL GASTRIC VAGOTOMY

Appraise

- This operation is otherwise known as highly selective vagotomy.
- Proximal gastric vagotomy aims to denervate only the acid-secreting proximal part of the stomach, leaving the alkali-secreting antrum, with its muscular pumping action, still innervated. Thus gastric acid secretion is reduced but gastric emptying is usually unimpaired. The addition of a drainage operation can be dispensed with in most patients in the absence of pyloroduodenal stenosis.

Access

Use an upper midline incision, skirting the umbilicus, 20 cm long.

Action

1 Make a hole through an avascular area in the mid-portion of the gastrocolic omentum. While the stomach is lifted forwards, carefully and completely separate the flimsy attachments of the stomach to the pancreas, watching out for, and preserving, the fold of peritoneum that contains the left gastric vessels. Separate the stomach from the posterior wall right up to the roof of the lesser sac. Occasionally you will be surprised to find the scar of an unsuspected posterior gastric ulcer.

2 Pass the right index finger through the hole in the gastrocolic omentum and grasp the gastric antrum to draw it down, so stretching the lesser curve of the stomach. In all but the most obese patients the taut anterior nerve of Latarjet can be seen running parallel to the lesser curve, separating into branches which form a 'crow's foot' pattern as they cross the curvature at the angulus, accompanied by blood vessels from the descending branch of the left gastric artery (Fig. 10.12). The posterior nerve cannot usually be seen from the front but can be displayed by looking through the hole in the gastrocolic omentum after turning the stomach forwards and upwards.

3 Carefully make a hole through the lesser omentum close to the gastric wall, just to the left of the 'crow's foot' of nerves, while protecting the posterior structures from damage with the right index finger passed through the defect in the gastrocolic omentum. Pass one end of a tape through the hole in the lesser omentum, drawing it out through the hole in the gastrocolic omentum. The tape now encircles the stomach at the level of the angulus, marking the lower limit of dissection. Clip the ends of the tape together so

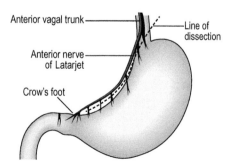

Fig. 10.12 Proximal gastric vagotomy. The anterior nerve of Latarjet, showing line of separation by dissection. The posterior nerve runs parallel to the anterior nerve.

they may be used to exert gentle downward traction on the stomach by an assistant to tauten and define the nerves of Latarjet.

4 Make a second, higher hole in the lesser curve close to the stomach just above the next visible vessels. Double-clamp, divide and ligate the vessels and accompanying nerve filaments.

> ### KEY POINTS Take care!
>
> - The length of tissue available for double-clamping between the nerve of Latarjet and the lesser curve is short.
> - If you place the haemostats well apart you risk damaging the lesser curve, or the nerve of Latarjet or both.

5 A better method is to pass double ligatures with an aneurysm needle or with Lahey's fine curved forceps, tie them carefully and divide the tissue between them. It is possible to use haemostatic clips instead of ligatures. One instrument applies two clips side by side and cuts between them: there is not usually sufficient tissue but it may be carefully used where the vessel and nerve length is adequate. If you do use haemostatic clips, take care that you do not inadvertently brush them off, thus tearing the delicate blood vessels.

6 Proceed upwards step by step, dividing the vessels and nerves that cross the lesser curve, carefully preserving the nerves of Latarjet as they are separated from the stomach. Higher up on the stomach, the vessels and nerves do not tend to penetrate at the lesser curve but cross it to enter on the posterior or anterior wall. Take advantage of this extra length by carrying the dissection onto the anterior and posterior walls. The separation of the anterior and posterior nerves of Latarjet from the stomach now proceeds independently onto the anterior and posterior gastric walls.

7 As the anterior and posterior layers of lesser omentum separate, slide non-toothed forceps under avascular sections and cut between the opened blades. Small vessels may be sealed with low-power diathermy applied for the minimum time through fine forceps applied well away from the main nerves and from the gastric musculature.

8 At the level of the main left gastric artery and vein quite large vessels must be ligated and divided on the anterior and posterior walls, together with their accompanying nerve filaments. Above these, the lowest portion of the oesophagus can be separated from the nerves of Latarjet without dividing any large vessels.

9 As the dissection reaches the cardia, the main trunks of the nerve are separated from the gullet, the nerves of Latarjet being the inferior prolongations of them. At this point temporarily stop the dissection.

10 Draw down the gastric fundus while an assistant retracts the left costal margin. Identify the angle of His between the fundus and the left edge of the lower gullet. Carefully incise the peritoneum in the angle, without damaging the stomach or oesophagus. Open up the hole gently with the right index finger and pass the right thumb through the upper part of the defect in the lesser omentum, behind the fundus of the stomach. Thumb and finger are prevented from meeting by the peritoneum of the roof of the lesser sac, which can now be broken through.

11 At the level of the cardia separate, doubly ligate and divide the peritoneum, phreno-oesophageal ligament and nerve fibres

across the anterior aspect of the lower oesophagus, leaving the muscle coat denuded but intact.

12 Divide loose tissue and nerve fibres around the posterior aspect of the lower oesophagus, rotating it to improve the view. A troublesome fragile vein is encountered, running posteriorly from the cardia, often in a crescentic peritoneal fold. Tie it, seal it with diathermy current or apply a haemostatic clip. Do not encroach more than 2 cm on the greater curve aspect of the gastric fundus or you will damage the short gastric vessels and the spleen.

? DIFFICULTY

1. *Bleeding into the lesser omentum?* A vessel retracts out of the ligature and continues to bleed between the layers of the omentum to form a large, spreading swelling. Do not try to grab it with large artery forceps. The ooze does not emerge directly from the vessel but trickles through the haematoma. Gently close the blades of a Rampley swab holder over the area and leave them for 5 minutes, timed by the clock. Remove the forceps. If bleeding does not recur during the remainder of the operation it is safe to leave the vessel. If oozing recurs or you are in doubt, gently dissect between the layers, identify the vessel and ligate it.
2. *Thick, fatty omentum?* Do not attempt to ligate it as a single layer. If you bunch it, subsequent traction on the stomach stretches the base of the bunch, and the ligature is forced off. If you are lucky, bleeding starts now. If you are unlucky, it will start later and you will miss it. Safeguard against this by picking up vessels with the minimum extraneous tissue. If necessary, perform the dissection in three separate layers, along the anterior leaf of lesser omentum, the lesser curve and the posterior leaf.
3. The operation can be difficult in an obese patient, in spite of taking steps to obtain a good view. Consider if truncal vagotomy would be easier, combined with a drainage operation. If you decide to proceed with proximal gastric vagotomy, concentrate on each step, not anticipating the difficulties of the next step. Remarkably, the dissection usually becomes easier as the stomach is mobilized.

---

13 Clear the whole circumference of the lower 5–7 cm of the oesophagus of nerve fibres. Do not damage the longitudinal muscle coat. Catch any small veins that have retracted into the muscle coat using fine sutures if necessary (Fig. 10.13).

Checklist

1 Examine the lesser omentum, lesser curve of stomach, lower oesophagus and upper lesser sac for signs of damage or bleeding. Have the short gastric vessels or spleen been damaged?

2 Re-examine the lower oesophagus for the presence of persistent vagal fibres and for signs of damage to the muscular coat. Re-examine the incisura angularis, where vagal fibres to the parietal cell mass may also have escaped detection. Finally, look again at the gastric lesser curve to ensure there is no damage. Ensure that 5–6 cm of distal stomach remains innervated.

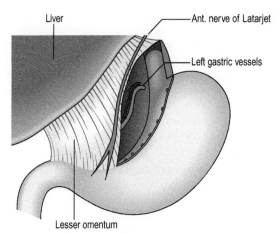

Fig. 10.13 Proximal gastric vagotomy. The nerves of Latarjet have been separated from the lesser curvature of the stomach.

PYLOROPLASTY

Appraise

1 Re-formation of the pylorus has the effect of increasing the size of the lumen and also destroys the pyloric sphincteric metering function. It can be used to overcome stricture of the pylorus and also to improve gastric emptying following truncal vagotomy. Following proximal gastric vagotomy, the distal stomach or 'antral mill' remains innervated so that gastric emptying is not usually prejudiced and pyloroplasty is not required.

2 Pyloroplasty is simple to perform in most circumstances and has enjoyed great popularity as an adjunctive operation with truncal vagotomy for duodenal ulcer. It may be difficult to perform if the duodenum is very scarred and adherent to the pancreas and the structures in the free edge of the lesser omentum if the abdomen is obese and deep.

3 It is probable that many postvagotomy symptoms are attributable to the drainage procedure and not to the vagotomy. Many such patients are improved if the drainage procedure is reversed. Although the pylorus can be anatomically restored to normal, the long-term results are not impressive.

4 Inevitably a number of methods of performing pyloroplasty have been described. The Heineke-Mikulicz method is the simplest, but some surgeons favour the Finney pyloroplasty.

5 The use of pyloroplasty or pyloromyotomy to facilitate gastric emptying following transection of the cardia for oesophagectomy is controversial. Some surgeons perform it only if there is evidence of stenosis (see Chapter 9). In the event of delayed gastric emptying they give metoclopramide 5–10 mg intravenously, and balloon dilatation of the pylorus under radiological control; they reserve re-operation for patients in whom these methods fail. The experience of other surgeons gives less cause for optimism so they routinely perform pyloroplasty or pyloromyotomy to circumvent gastric delay.

HEINEKE-MIKULICZ PYLOROPLASTY

Access

Gently mobilize the pyloroduodenal region by Kocher's manoeuvre and place a large pack behind the upper duodenal loop to bring it forwards in the wound.

Action

1. Make a longitudinal incision through all coats starting on the anterior wall of the duodenal bulb, carried through the pylorus and on to the anterior gastric antral wall (Fig. 10.14). Centre the incision, 4–5 cm long, on the narrowest part of the pyloroduodenal canal. If there is an active anterior ulcer, encircle it so that a lozenge-shaped segment of anterior pyloroduodenal wall is excised, containing the ulcer. This 'pylorectomy' was described by Judd.

2. Aspirate the contents and inspect the interior of the distal stomach and proximal duodenum. Sometimes there is a mucosal diaphragm with no evidence of ulcer in patients with typical features of pyloric stenosis in whom an endoscope would not pass. If a diaphragm is suspected, start the incision on the anterior antral wall 3–4 cm proximal to the pylorus and inspect the interior before cutting through the pyloric ring. Make sure there is not a second narrow duodenal segment distal to the pyloroplasty, as may develop in postbulbar duodenal ulceration.

3. Gently apply tissue forceps to the middle of the upper and lower cut edges and draw them apart, allowing the proximal and distal limits of the incision to come together, transforming the longitudinal cut into a transverse slit.

4. Close the incision, starting from the upper tissue forceps and ending at the lower forceps. Three methods are possible. The traditional technique is to insert an invaginating continuous all-coats layer reinforced with a second seromuscular layer of sutures. However, the invaginated edges may cause a temporary

holdup and many surgeons therefore employ a single layer of all-coats sutures placed closely together, uniting the walls edge-to-edge without invagination. In the last few years stapling devices have gained popularity. Place a single straight stapler along the edges as they are held in their new position, with the opposed edges everted. Close and activate the stapler. Cut off the excess tissue with a scalpel blade held in contact with the upper surface of the stapler, which is then removed. Insert a reinforcing layer of seromuscular stitches if desired.

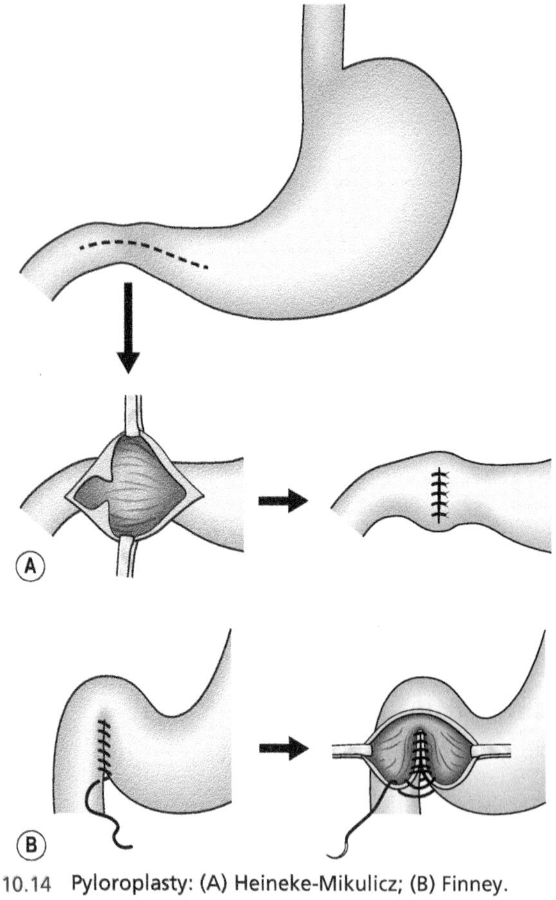

FINNEY PYLOROPLASTY

Appraise

Advocates claim that this produces a wider lumen than the Heineke-Mikulicz pyloroplasty. Of course the lumen size depends to some extent on the length of the incision. The Finney technique merely represents a generously fashioned Heineke-Mikulicz pyloroplasty with the inferior 'dog ear' pushed in.

Action

1. Gently mobilize the duodenal loop by Kocher's manoeuvre so the descending duodenum can be laid alongside the greater curve part of the gastric antrum.

2. Unite the adjacent gastric and duodenal walls with a seromuscular stitch, from above downwards, closing the angle below the pylorus.

3. Incise the full thickness of the stomach, pylorus and duodenum along an inverted horseshoe-shaped line which runs from the gastric antrum 4–5 cm proximal to the pyloric ring, through the pylorus, curving through the duodenal bulb and down the descending duodenum.

4. Starting at the pylorus, unite with an all-coats stitch the adjacent walls of the stomach and duodenum. Continue the stitches round the lower limits of the incisions to unite the right duodenal cut edge to the left gastric cut edge, using an invaginating stitch.

5. Continue the seromuscular stitch to cover the anterior all-coats suture line.

DUODENOPLASTY

Appraise

1. The advent of proximal gastric vagotomy removed the need to perform an adjunctive drainage operation in the majority of patients with duodenal ulcer since in modern times most patients with incipient pyloric stenosis are operated upon before it becomes severe.

2. Even if pyloroplasty is necessary there are advantages in performing proximal gastric vagotomy. If truncal vagotomy is performed, gallbladder dilatation results and there is an increased risk of gallstones; loss of vagal supply to the pancreas reduces its exocrine secretion and there is a significantly increased risk of severe diarrhoea. In some patients, stenosis is distal to the pylorus and can be overcome without damaging the sphincteric mechanism. This is particularly true when the patient has postbulbar duodenal ulceration. Proximal gastric vagotomy can then be justified.

Fig. 10.14 Pyloroplasty: (A) Heineke-Mikulicz; (B) Finney.

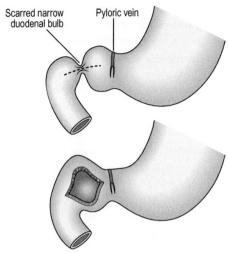

Fig. 10.15   Duodenoplasty.

Action

1. Mobilize the pyloroduodenal region by Kocher's manoeuvre and confirm that the pyloric ring itself is widely patent by invaginating the anterior antral wall through it on an index finger. The site of stenosis should have been determined before operation but this is not always easy to assess.

2. Make a longitudinal incision through the anterior duodenal wall, stopping short of the pyloric ring (Fig. 10.15). This needs to be only about 1.5–2 cm long. If the ulcer and stenosis are postbulbar remember that the distortion may draw the ampulla out of its normal place, exposing it to inadvertent damage.

3. Gently apply tissue forceps to the middle of each cut edge and separate them to produce a transverse slit.

4. Close the slit transversely. Insert a single layer of closely applied stitches, bringing the edges together without inversion.

GASTRODUODENOSTOMY

Appraise

- This resembles the Finney pyloroplasty but does not include division of the pyloric ring.

- It is an alternative method to pyloroplasty or gastroenterostomy for overcoming pyloric obstruction and may be appropriate if the descending duodenum has been opened. It is seldom used.

Action

1. Mobilize the descending duodenum by Kocher's manoeuvre and join the descending duodenum to the anterior wall of the distal stomach with a running seromuscular stitch.

2. Incise the descending duodenum and anterior gastric walls for 5 cm, parallel and close to each side of the seromuscular stitch. Aspirate the contents and inspect the interior (Fig. 10.16).

3. Join the adjacent gastric and duodenal walls with a continuous all-coats stitch, carrying this round on to the anterior walls as an invaginating stitch to encircle the anastomosis.

4. Continue the seromuscular stitch onto the anterior wall to bury the all-coats stitch and complete the two-layer anastomosis.

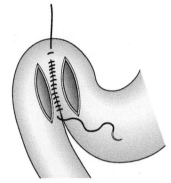

Fig. 10.16   Incisions for gastroduodenostomy.

5. The anastomosis can be accomplished using a stapling device that will insert four linear rows of staples and incise in the same line between the inner rows of staples. Bring the stomach and duodenum together with a posterior seromuscular stitch. Make a stab hole in the stomach and the duodenum at the lower limit of the intended anastomosis. Insert the separated limbs of the stapler, one into each hole, with the points towards the pylorus. Lock the limbs together so they lie just anterior to the seromuscular stitch line with no extraneous tissues intervening. Fire the stapler to insert the rows of staples and cut between the middle rows. Unlock the stapler, withdraw the limbs, inspect the completeness of the union and pick up the extremities of the staple lines through the stab wounds, which are now united, with tissue forceps. Separate the tissue forceps to draw the defect into an everted slit. Close the defect with sutures or a linear stapler. Check the integrity of the anastomosis and if desired continue the seromuscular stitch from the posterior suture line to bury the anterior staple line.

GASTROENTEROSTOMY

Appraise

1. Gastroenterostomy was originally applied to the relief of pyloric obstruction from distal gastric carcinoma. It offers an important method of relief when gastrectomy cannot be carried out because the tumour is locally too extensive or has already metastasized. Always place the gastroenterostomy as high on the stomach as possible to guard against the stoma becoming obstructed by advancing tumour growth. However, always prefer an exclusion gastrectomy if this is possible because high gastroenterostomy often fails to drain the stomach and may provoke bilious vomiting.

2. Gastroenterostomy was used for the relief of benign pyloric stenosis from duodenal ulceration, but in the absence of stenosis it diverts some of the acid away from the ulcer, which usually heals. A proportion of patients eventually develop an ulcer at the stoma, although this may be delayed for many years. An advantage is that if the patient subsequently has postprandial symptoms from the drainage operation, it can be taken down quite simply provided that the pyloroduodenal canal is adequate. Gastroenterostomy for duodenal ulcer is placed as close to the pylorus as possible.

3. Gastroenterostomy may be used as a bypass in the presence of duodenal ileus or fistula. For many years surgeons argued about the merits of different techniques for gastroenterostomy. As a

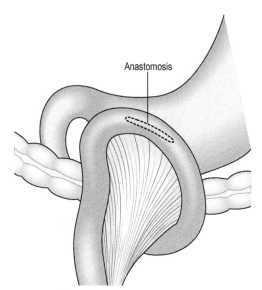

Fig. 10.17   Juxtapyloric anterior gastroenterostomy.

general rule, surgeons now use only anterior juxtapyloric gastro-enterostomy for benign disease (Fig. 10.17); this will be described in detail with a note on the previously very popular posterior gastroenterostomy.

Access

Use a midline incision 15 cm long.

Assess

1 Explore the abdomen.
2 If the patient proves to have extensive and inoperable carcinoma with no evidence of impending distal obstruction, carry out limited exploration only, but take a biopsy specimen.

Action

Suture technique

1 Pick up a longitudinal fold of anterior gastric wall and grasp it with one of Lane's twin clamps. Choose a fold as close to the pylorus as possible if this is for benign pyloric obstruction or accompanies vagotomy for ulcer. Choose a fold as high as possible if this is to bypass an unresectable distal gastric carcinoma.

2 Lift up the greater omentum and transverse colon to identify the duodenojejunal junction. Draw the first loop of jejunum up over the colon and greater omentum to the stomach, with the short but not taut afferent loop against the proximal part of the clamped gastric fold and the efferent loop against the distal end of the fold. Place the second twin clamp along the apposed bowel, avoiding the mesentery, to occlude the lumen but not the blood supply. Lock the clamps together.

3 Unite the adjacent gastric and jejunal walls with a running sero-muscular stitch on an eyeless needle. Leave the ends long so that the stitch can be continued to encircle the anastomosis.

4 Open the stomach and jejunum parallel to the seromuscular stitch and 0.5 cm from it on each side, for 4–6 cm if this is for benign disease and for as long as possible if it is to bypass malignant obstruction.

5 Apply fresh drapes to isolate the area and keep separate instruments during the next part of the operation when the potentially infected interior of the bowel will be exposed.

6 Unite the adjacent gastric and jejunal walls with a running all-coats stitch. Carry the stitch round the corner on to the anterior wall to complete the anastomosis. As the anterior gastric and jejunal walls are brought together, invert the edges. A Connell mattress stitch may be used as an alternative to the simple over-and-over stitch but take care that the blood vessels are picked up and tied along the edges since the Connell stitch is not haemostatic.

7 Remove the twin clamps, discard and replace the soiled towels, instruments and gloves.

8 Carry the seromuscular stitch round the end onto the anterior wall and complete it to encircle the anastomosis, burying the all-coats stitch.

Checklist

1 Examine the anastomosis and make sure it is patent.
2 Make sure there is no tension on the loop of jejunum. Draw the transverse colon and greater omentum to the right so there is no weight of bowel to drag on the anastomosis.

? DIFFICULTY

1. The duodenum may be bound down in patients with severe duodenal ulcer. It is then difficult to make a juxtapyloric anastomosis. Make a more proximal, safe and easy anastomosis.
2. It may be difficult to draw down sufficient proximal stomach to make a high anastomosis as a palliative bypass operation for obstructing distal carcinoma. Do not hesitate to enlarge the incision and abandon clamps if they are difficult to apply.

Staple technique

1 The anastomosis can be fashioned using a linear-cutter stapling device. Draw the jejunum up to the stomach and attach it along the proposed line of the anastomosis with a seromuscular stitch at each end. Make stab wounds in the stomach and the jejunum close to the stitch uniting the afferent jejunal loop to the proximal stomach.

2 Insert a sucker to empty the gastric and jejunal contents.

3 Separate the two halves of the stapler and insert one blade into each of the stab wounds, pointing towards the distally placed stitch. Lock the blades together, taking care not to include extraneous tissue.

4 Fire the device to insert four parallel rows of staples and cut between the central rows, forming an anastomosis between stomach and jejunum. Unlock the blades and withdraw them.

5 Inspect the anastomosis all round from within and without, inserting sutures to reinforce doubtful areas. Pick up the ends of the staple lines on each side of the defect and draw them apart to create a linear slit. Apply a linear stapling device along the everted edges of the defect to seal the edges. Remove the device and examine the anastomosis to ensure it is perfect, inserting further stitches if necessary. Alternatively, close the defect with sutures.

Checklist

1 Is the anastomosis intact and patent?

2 Ensure that there is no tension on the loop of jejunum. Draw the transverse colon and greater omentum to the right so there is no weight of bowel to drag on the anastomosis.

Technical points

■ Suture material and stitches vary from surgeon to surgeon. We have described a sutured anastomosis using two layers of continuous absorbable stitches. A single all-coats stitch is also quite adequate. Many surgeons insert interrupted non-absorbable stitches such as silk on the outer, seromuscular layer. It is not the suture material or method but the care with which they are inserted that determines whether the patient will recover without complications.

■ The use of non-crushing clamps is argued about by surgeons. Certainly many successful surgeons use them routinely when they can be conveniently applied to prevent the leakage of bowel content into the wound, and to hold the stomach and bowel perfectly apposed while the anastomosis is fashioned. If you use clamps, apply them to the bowel only and not across the mesentery. Apply them sufficiently firmly to occlude the arteries as well as the veins, otherwise the bowel becomes congested and oedematous.

POSTERIOR GASTROENTEROSTOMY

1 This method was used with success for many years. From time to time it offers a convenient way of fashioning the anastomosis for benign disease. It cannot be used conveniently for high gastroenterostomy to relieve malignant distal gastric obstruction.

2 Hold up the greater omentum and transverse colon in order to inspect the mesocolon. Identify the middle colic vessels and make a conveniently placed vertical hole through the mesocolon to one or other side of them, 5–7 cm long.

3 Identify the posterior wall of the stomach through the hole and draw it down. Select a dependent and distal part of the stomach.

4 Apply the twin clamps to the protruding part of the stomach and to the first loop of jejunum beyond the ligament of Treitz. Lock the clamps and carry out the anastomosis.

5 Suture the margins of the cut mesocolon to the stomach to prevent small bowel loops from slipping through into the lesser sac and becoming obstructed.

BILLROTH I PARTIAL GASTRECTOMY

Appraise

■ Billroth I gastrectomy was first used to resect a distal gastric carcinoma in Frau Heller on 29 January 1881, by Theodore Billroth (1829–1894) of Vienna. The size of the anastomosis between the proximal gastric stump and the duodenum is restricted to the diameter of the duodenal lumen and if the cancer recurs there is a risk of anastomotic obstruction. In Billroth II or polya gastrectomy the whole width of the cut end of the proximal gastric stump can be used for the anastomosis, which is at less risk of obstruction, and this technique has replaced the Billroth I operation.

■ In its developed form the lesser curve of the proximal gastric stump is excised with closure to form a new lesser curve to match the duodenal lumen: thus a proximal gastric ulcer can be included in the tongue of excised lesser curve. However, effective non-surgical treatment of gastric ulcers reduces the need for operation and, if it is needed, polya gastrectomy is suitable.

POLYA PARTIAL GASTRECTOMY

Appraise

■ At an emergency operation for bleeding peptic ulcer the most certain procedure is excision of the ulcer-bearing area. If the ulcer is duodenal then polya gastrectomy with closure of the duodenum gives good results if the main end-point is prevention of re-bleeding. However, the operative mortality is twice that following vagotomy with under-running of the bleeding vessel, and the side-effects and late sequelae may be more severe. Consequently, the most frequently performed procedure is vagotomy with pylorotomy following under-running of the ulcer with non-absorbable stitches. Erosive bleeding rarely demands operation but multiple haemorrhages can be dealt with only by excision of the affected gastric wall by gastrectomy. Fortunately such bleeding is usually from the distal stomach.

■ The most frequent indication for gastrectomy is distal gastric carcinoma. Polya gastrectomy allows the creation of a stoma the full width of the stomach, which is thus unlikely to become obstructed if the tumour recurs. Since the duodenum is closed, this isolates it from distal spread as may occur if gastroduodenal anastomosis is used. The preferred method of resecting distal gastric carcinoma is by radical subtotal gastrectomy with Polya or Roux-en-Y reconstruction.

Access

Make a midline incision that skirts the umbilicus, extending downwards from the xiphoid process for 20 cm. Ligate and divide the ligamentum teres and divide the falciform ligament.

Assess

1 Explore the whole abdomen. If the operation is for carcinoma, start in the pelvis and lower abdomen, para-aortic region and root of the mesentery, proceeding to the liver before touching the stomach in order to avoid carrying malignant cells around the peritoneal cavity.

2 Carefully examine the stomach and duodenum to confirm the diagnosis and assess the strategy of the operation. If necessary, open the lesser omentum or gastrocolic omentum to examine the posterior wall of the stomach and contents of the lesser sac, including the glands around the coeliac axis and along the superior border of the pancreas.

Resect

Benign disease

1 Make a hole in an avascular area of the gastrocolic omentum to the left of the gastroepiploic vascular arch. Identify the posterior gastric wall and separate it from the pancreas and transverse mesocolon.

2 Clamp in sections, ligate and divide the gastrocolic omentum, extending on the left up to and including the main left gastro-epiploic vessels and the first one or two short gastric vessels. Avoid damaging the spleen directly or by exerting heavy traction on the stomach. To the right, divide and ligate the main right gastroepiploic vessels as they lie near the inferior border of the pylorus. The separation of this vascular tissue can be accomplished rapidly using ultrasonic (e.g. Harmonic Scalpel, Ethicon Endosurgery) or tissue response generator (Ligasure, Covidien) dissection.

> ▶ KEY POINT Inadvertent vascular damage

> ■ Identify to avoid damaging the middle colic vessels, which lie within 1 cm of the right gastroepiploic vessels.

3 Clamp, divide and ligate the right gastric vessels after identifying and isolating them as they run to the left in the lesser omentum just above the duodenal bulb and pylorus. Divide the lesser omentum proximally, if possible preserving an accessory hepatic artery if one is present.

4 Free the first 1–2 cm of duodenum after applying fine artery forceps on the small vessels posteriorly, dividing and ligating them with fine ligatures. Divide with a linear stapler or Payr's clamp across the duodenum just beyond the pylorus. Place a second clamp just proximal to this to occlude the stomach. If there is insufficient room for this, apply a non-crushing clamp across the distal stomach. Transect the duodenum just above the distal Payr clamp, ensuring that no gastric mucosa remains attached to the duodenum. Cover the cut distal stomach with a swab.

5 Dissect the duodenum free for 2–3 cm so that it can be safely closed, applying fine forceps and ligatures to the vessels, keeping close to the duodenal wall.

> ▶ KEY POINTS Distorted anatomy?

> ■ The common bile duct lies near the posterior and superior parts of the proximal duodenum and may be drawn out of its normal relationship by scar tissue.
> ■ The gastroduodenal artery runs close to the medial wall of the duodenum.

6 Close the duodenal stump, as a rule using a linear stapling device. This places a double row of staples across the duodenum. Apply it just distal to the pylorus in place of the Payr's crushing clamp and place a proximal clamp across the distal stomach. Activate the stapling device to staple and seal the duodenum and transect this with a scalpel applied closely to the upper edge of the stapler. Alternatively, close the distal stomach and duodenal stump with GIA staplers. It is wise to invaginate and reinforce the everted staple line with a layer of sutures.

7 Alternatively, close the duodenal stump with sutures. First use a running over-and-over spiral stitch that encircles the clamp and the enclosed crushed duodenum. Gently ease out the clamp, tightening the stitches seriatim as it is withdrawn. Tie the stitch. Insert a second invaginating seromuscular suture to cover the first stitch line or insert a purse-string suture and invaginate the first suture line as it is tightened and tied. If possible, insert a third stitch that picks up and draws together the ligated right gastric and right gastroepiploic vessel stumps, the anterior duodenal wall and the peritoneum over the head of the pancreas.

8 Exert a little tension on the left gastric vessels by elevating the pyloric end of the stomach. Identify the artery by feeling for the pulsations. Isolate the vessels from the lesser curve of the stomach, doubly clamp, divide and ligate them.

9 Select the line for the transection of the stomach (Fig. 10.18). When Polya gastrectomy was the standard operation for duodenal ulcer, a two-thirds gastrectomy was usually carried out.

10 Ask the anaesthetist to withdraw the nasogastric tube until the tip lies above the line of transection.

Malignant disease

1 Radical subtotal gastrectomy is described later, but non-radical partial gastrectomy is appropriate in frail patients and in those who have a resectable carcinoma but already have metastatic deposits in the liver or elsewhere which make radical resection impossible.

2 It may not be possible to be sure that the distal resection is clear of tumour but always ensure that the proximal line of resection is well clear of growth. Aim at a minimum of 5 cm apparently tumour-free margin. If the resection line cuts through tumour, the anastomotic line may break down during recovery from the operation. If it does not do so, recurrent tumour at the anastomosis may soon obstruct the lumen.

3 It is useless to carry the line of resection widely beyond the stomach, so adopt the same technique as for resection for benign disease.

4 Plan to provide a full-width gastroenterostomy to guard against recurrent tumour causing obstruction.

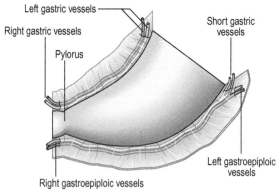

Fig. 10.18 Polya partial gastrectomy. The removed specimen.

Unite

Staples

1. The gastroenterostomy can be accomplished using stapling devices. Place a long straight stapling device across the stomach at the proposed line of section and cut off the distal gastric specimen with a scalpel run along the distal edge of the stapler. Remove the stapler.

2. Bring up a proximal loop of jejunum and suture it to the posterior wall of the stomach 5 cm above the staple line, placing a seromuscular stitch at each end, with the afferent loop to the lesser curve, the efferent loop to the greater curve. Make a stab wound in the greater curve aspect of the posterior wall of the stomach 2 cm proximal to the staple line and a matching stab wound in the jejunum at the origin of the efferent loop.

3. Insert the two limbs of the stapler separately into the holes, with the tips pointing to the lesser curve. Ensure that there is no interposed tissue, lock the two limbs together and fire the instrument. Four lines of staples will have united stomach to jejunum and the knife will have cut a stoma between the centre rows of staples. Unlock and withdraw the stapler.

4. Carefully check that the staple lines are perfect. Place tissue forceps at the ends of the inner and outer staple lines and separate the forceps to create an everted linear defect in the anastomosis. Place a short straight stapler across the everted lips of the defect, tighten and actuate it. Cut off the excess tissue, remove the stapler and check the line of closure carefully, if necessary reinforcing the whole anastomosis all round with sutures.

Sutured

1. Place one of the twin gastroenterostomy clamps across the stomach 2 cm above the proposed line of transection, from greater to lesser curve. Place a long non-crushing clamp across the stomach 3 cm distal to the twin clamp and parallel to it. The stomach will be transected just above this clamp.

2. Fold the distal part of the stomach upwards. Reach down and identify the duodenojejunal junction. Draw up to the stomach the first loop of jejunum, with afferent loop to lesser curve with no slack but not tight. The efferent loop is placed at the greater curve. Place the second of the twin clamps across this loop of bowel, occluding only the lumen and not the mesentery. Marry and lock the clamps together.

3. Run a continuous seromuscular stitch to unite the adjacent gastric and jejunal walls.

4. Incise the full width of the posterior gastric wall 0.5 cm above the clamp, taking care at this time to leave the anterior wall intact. Make a parallel incision in the jejunum, 0.5 cm from the seromuscular suture line. Join the adjacent gastric and jejunal edges with an all-coats stitch.

5. Now cut through the anterior wall of the stomach 1 cm distal to the clamp and remove the specimen of distal stomach. Continue the all-coats stitch round on to the anterior wall and along it to completely encircle the anastomosis.

6. Remove the clamps, discard and replace the towels, gloves and instruments. Complete the seromuscular suture line onto the anterior wall to encircle the anastomosis.

Valved anastomosis

1. When performing gastrectomy for benign disease it is conventional to close the lesser curve half of the stomach and form a small stoma between the greater curve half of the stomach and the jejunum. This is referred to as a valved anastomosis (Fig. 10.19).

2. A different technique is used after uniting the stomach and jejunum in the twin clamps and with the posterior seromuscular stitch. Have the distal stomach held vertically and place halfway across it from the lesser curve, and 1 cm distal to the twin clamp, a short Payr's crushing clamp. Cut halfway across the stomach just distal to the Payr clamp, transecting the lesser curve half of the stomach. Oversew the clamp and contained crushed stomach edge with a running loose spiral stitch. Release and gently withdraw the clamp as the sutures are tightened seriatim. This manoeuvre leaves just the greater curve half of the stomach to be united to a matched hole made in the jejunum. The anastomosis is accomplished in a similar manner to the creation of a full-width stoma.

3. After the gloves, towels and instruments have been replaced, continue the posterior seromuscular stitch round and along the anterior wall to encircle the stoma and closed lesser curve.

Technical points

1. The inside of the stomach and bowel are colonized with microorganisms. While fashioning anastomoses, isolate the interior of the bowel from the peritoneal cavity and wound edges by using separate towels, instruments and gloves. When the bowel is repaired, discard and replace them with sterile gloves, towels and instruments.

2. Retrocolic anastomosis may be fashioned following gastrectomy but it does not confer any benefits over the antecolic anastomosis.

3. Some surgeons avoid the use of clamps during the fashioning of gastric anastomoses. There is, however, no evidence that clamps damage the bowel.

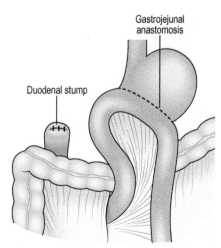

Fig. 10.19 Polya partial gastrectomy. The antecolic valved gastrojejunal anastomosis, with afferent loop joined to lesser curve, is complete. The duodenal stump is closed.

1. It may be difficult and hazardous to dissect out and close the duodenum in the presence of extensive scarring and distortion from chronic severe duodenal ulceration. There are alternative techniques available. If you are committed to closing the duodenum then an alternative is to transect the gastric antrum, dissect out and excise the antral mucosa and close the cut edge of duodenal mucosa, leaving raw antral seromuscularis. Now close this using a series of internal purse-string sutures.

2. If you have committed yourself to dissecting out and closing the duodenum and now find yourself in difficulty, carefully stick close to the duodenal wall. If you encounter a large ulcer crater, this cannot be mobilized to help close the duodenum. There are three choices. The best choice is to carefully pinch off the duodenum just at the distal ulcer edge and carefully mobilize a sufficient cuff of duodenum beyond to close safely, leaving the ulcer crater undisturbed. The second choice is to leave the duodenum attached to the ulcer and mobilize the anterolateral duodenal wall so that it can be sewn down to the distal fibrotic edge of the ulcer crater, thus closing off the duodenum. If neither of these is possible, nor can be safely accomplished, then do not try to close the duodenum. Sew in a large tube and bring this to the surface of the abdomen. Leave it attached to a closed drainage system for 10 days and, if the patient is well, gradually withdraw it. The duodenal fistula will heal spontaneously provided there is no distal obstruction or adynamic ileus. Even if it does not do so, the track is so well established that there will be no intra-abdominal complications.

3. *Is it difficult to mobilize the proximal stomach?* The spleen may be adherent to the diaphragm and the costal margin may be narrow in an obese patient. Make sure the stomach is not adherent posteriorly through adhesions or a previously unsuspected gastric ulcer; if it is, pinch off the ulcer and, if necessary, temporarily close the defect with sutures, and include the ulcer in the gastrectomy specimen.

4. In time of difficulty make sure that the light, the exposure and the assistance are all optimal.

5. *Bleeding?* Avoid panic measures. Control severe bleeding with local pressure while preparing to pick up the bleeding point accurately with artery forceps. Do not tie blood vessels together with large pieces of omentum or mesentery. The blood vessel may retract and quietly bleed into the closed mesentery. If the splenic capsule is torn, try to preserve the spleen by suture repair or packing with Surgicel. Splenectomy is undesirable because of the thrombotic, infective and immunological complications (but see Chapter 18).

6. *Damage to the common bile duct?* Correct it now, or call upon a more experienced person to do so. Ensure that you have available radiography to help in elucidating the damage. Repair the injured duct as you would at a routine biliary operation and plan to leave a 'T-tube' drain in the common duct to drain the biliary tract. Immediate and perfect repair of the bile duct injuries ensures minimal disability; missed or imperfectly repaired injuries seriously threaten the patient's life or well-being.

Checklist

1. Examine the anastomosis. See that it is perfectly fashioned and intact. If necessary insert extra sutures. Ensure that you can invaginate the gastric and jejunal walls through the stoma.

2. Check each of the main vascular ligatures. Re-tie them if they are insecure.

3. Check the spleen. Aspirate all the blood from under the left cupola of the diaphragm and re-check it just before closing the abdomen to ensure that there has been no further collection of blood.

4. Make sure the duodenal stump is safely closed. Should you leave a drain down to it? If so, does this replace careful technique and should you therefore re-close the duodenum or reinforce the closure?

5. Examine the colon to ensure there is no damage to it, or the mesocolon or middle colic vessels. Draw the greater omentum, transverse colon and mesocolon through to the right so there is no weight of colon resting on the anastomosis.

6. Aspirate any blood from under the right cupola of the diaphragm, from under the liver and in the right prerenal pouch. Finally, aspirate any blood that has collected in the pelvis.

GASTRODUODENAL BLEEDING

Appraise

1. Bleeding is the most life-threatening complication of peptic ulcer. Its management is best carried out by experienced clinicians, endoscopists and surgeons acting as a team. Dedicated units achieve much better survival than those undertaking it as part of a general service.

2. Erosive bleeding sometimes complicates bleeding elsewhere, sepsis, burns, head injury and major trauma. Drugs such as steroids and NSAIDs can cause erosive bleeding or be associated with ulcer bleeding. Alcohol causes acute gastritis with bleeding from this or, following retching, from Mallory-Weiss tears around the cardia. For this reason take a careful history, asking specific questions about drugs.

3. Assess the patient's general condition so that you can carry out appropriate resuscitation. Check the haemoglobin and haematocrit, and exclude clotting deficiencies if suspected. In appropriate circumstances have blood cross-matched. Routinely give intravenous omeprazole or an equivalent proton-pump inhibitor.

4 Do not make a once-and-for-all assessment but carefully monitor the patient thereafter. Remember that mortality is highest among the over-60s, those with massive haemorrhage and shock, and those with serious associated disease.

> ### ▶ KEY POINT Decision making
>
> ■ Remember that more than 80% of gastrointestinal bleeding stops spontaneously, but also remember that you do not know which 80%.

5 Carry out endoscopy as soon as possible to determine the cause, site, state and number of lesions. Look for continuing bleeding and the presence of visible vessels which indicate that the bleeding is likely to continue or recur. Even if you cannot identify the source you can usually exonerate particular areas, for example excluding oesophageal varices.

6 If you are expert in their use, have available instruments to control bleeding through the endoscope. These include the Nd-YAG laser, heater probes and diathermy, together with needles for injecting adrenaline (epinephrine), ethanol or polidocanol through the biopsy channel. Other methods that are under trial include application or injection of cryoprecipitate or thrombin to induce clotting, the adhesive trifluoroisopropylcyanoacrylate to seal the vessel, and endoscopic clipping or suturing of vessels. Combinations of these methods are proving effective. Haemostatic substances can be injected in association with local application of heat. They should be the first line of treatment in most patients. They may be repeated if re-bleeding occurs.

7 For this reason, if you are inexperienced or do not have the equipment available, call in an expert or be willing to transfer the patient rather than operate precipitately. Surgery produces its own immediate and long-term complications. Inexpert and ineffective surgery is disastrous.

8 The origin of obscure recurrent upper gastrointestinal bleeding can sometimes be elucidated by injecting radioisotope-labelled red cells into the circulation with gamma-camera monitoring of leakage into the gut. Most surgeons would now opt for angiography carried out during bleeding episodes. In appropriate circumstances the radiologist may be able to embolize the feeding vessel.

9 Relative indications for operation when other methods of control have failed remain:
- Continuing bleeding which fails to respond to other measures
- Bleeding that recurs
- Patient more than 60 years old
- Gastric ulcer bleeding
- Patients with cardiovascular disease, who do not withstand hypotension well. This makes it dangerous to defer operation if bleeding is serious and not controllable.

> ### ▶ KEY POINTS Intra-operative endoscopy
>
> ■ Always have an endoscope available in the operating theatre, even when the diagnosis seems certain.
> ■ When the patient is anaesthetized, be willing, in case of doubt, to perform endoscopy

10 Although exploratory laparotomy allows access to the abdomen, the exterior of the gut is exposed, not the interior where the cause lies. Do not embark on surgery for upper gastrointestinal bleeding alone if there is someone more experienced available. Eschew the temptation to carry out 'blind' gastrectomy if you cannot identify the cause of bleeding. This merely confuses the problem while risking the possible complications.

Access

Make a generous upper abdominal midline incision skirting the umbilicus, 20–25 cm long. Ligate and divide the ligamentum teres and incise the falciform ligament.

Assess

1 As the abdomen is opened, blood which appears bluish through the bowel wall may be seen in the small or large bowel. Dilated and congested veins on the viscera with a stiff cirrhotic liver make portal venous hypertension obvious. Scarring and oedema of the stomach or duodenum may indicate the site of bleeding.

> ### ▶ KEY POINT Multiple sites
>
> ■ Do not assume there is a single cause.

2 Remember that, in Britain, most upper gastrointestinal bleeds requiring emergency surgery are from peptic ulceration or erosions, but also remember that there are sometimes multiple causes and the detection of a possible site does not exclude the possibility of other causes. Therefore carry out a thorough check of the lower oesophagus, stomach and duodenum, remembering that there may be an unsuspected lesion in the small or large bowel.

3 If no cause is detected and there is no site of active bleeding, do not hesitate to repeat the endoscopy yourself or ask an experienced colleague to do so. It may be valuable first to have a large-bore gastric tube passed so that the stomach can be washed out if it contains blood or retained food.

4 Alternatively, but often less satisfactorily, perform gastrotomy or gastroduodenotomy. Make an incision through the anterior gastric wall midway between the greater and lesser curves in the distal stomach, carrying this through the pylorus into the anterior duodenal wall for 2–3 cm if necessary. Aspirate the gastric contents. Insert large-bladed retractors for your assistants, have the light adjusted to shine into the stomach and carefully examine the interior of the stomach and if necessary the duodenal bulb, seeking the cause of bleeding. Sometimes the gastric wall can be evaginated through the gastric wound to allow close inspection. If the pylorus has not been incised it is often possible to insert thin-bladed retractors through it to view the duodenal bulb, or a flexible cystoscope may be passed, offering excellent views of the bulb.

5 Do not carry out a procedure unless the cause is found. Make a thorough examination of the whole gastrointestinal tract including structures that could produce bleeding into it, such as the biliary tract. If there is no active bleeding and no cause is found, close the abdomen and determine to repeat the endoscopy at the first sign of re-bleeding, followed if necessary by other methods of detection and isolation of bleeding sites.

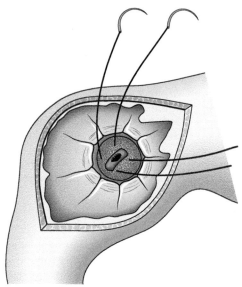

Fig. 10.20   Suture-ligature of gastroduodenal artery in the base of posterior duodenal ulcer, using 2/0 silk.

Action

1 Bleeding duodenal ulcer is preferably treated at present by pyloroplasty or duodenotomy, and suture of the bleeding vessels. Vagotomy is now usually omitted in favour of postoperative medical treatment of the ulcer. Create a gastroduodenotomy of the size that would usually be made for a pyloroplasty. Aspirate blood and clot from the ulcer base and isolate the site of bleeding. This is usually from the gastroduodenal artery. Carefully insert stitches of 2/0 non-absorbable material on a round-bodied small curved needle placed transversely to pick up the artery (Fig. 10.20).

> ### ▶ KEY POINTS Crucial aims
>
> ■ Make sure you have completely controlled the bleeding.
> ■ Insert the sutures carefully because the common bile duct lies close by.

2 Close the gastroduodenotomy either as a pyloroplasty or longitudinally as it was made.

3 The florid duodenal ulcers that were formerly seen are less common now but occasionally the duodenal ulcer is so large, the walls so thickened and distorted that pyloroplasty will not be successful. One possibility is to close the gastroduodenotomy longitudinally, and if necessary create a gastrojejunostomy. Alternatively, perform Polya gastrectomy, although this should rarely be necessary. The difficulty will be in freeing and closing the duodenum. If the duodenum has already been opened to perform pyloroplasty before the problem is appreciated, first control the bleeding with 2/0 non-absorbable sutures. Now decide whether to dissect the duodenum distal to the ulcer sufficiently to allow it to be closed. This is feasible only if the ulcer is close to the pylorus. If it lies distally, you will endanger the ampullary region. Nissen's manoeuvre may succeed: suture the anterior cut duodenal

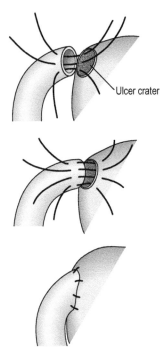

Fig. 10.21   Nissen's manoeuvre for closure of duodenal stump. The cut anterior duodenal edge is first sutured to the distal ulcer edge. The anterior duodenal wall is then sutured to the proximal ulcer edge.

edge to the distal ulcer edge and, if there is sufficient free anterior duodenal wall, suture it over the ulcer to the proximal ulcer edge (see Fig. 10.21).

4 If the difficulty of performing pyloroplasty is appreciated early, perform Polya gastrectomy, preserving as much of the anterior duodenal wall as possible, provided the ulcer base can be exposed and the bleeding controlled with sutures. This allows the closure of the duodenum to be carried out securely.

5 Control of the bleeding may be difficult in the presence of a large ulcer and the base may be exposed most easily by 'pinching off' the duodenum from the ulcer edge to leave the base free. Control the bleeding. The problem of closing the duodenum can now be tackled calmly, either accomplishing it in the post-ulcer segment, or closing the hole created by the ulcer defect.

6 If all else fails, insert a large catheter into the duodenal defect and close the duodenum around it. Bring the catheter to the surface of the abdomen to create a controlled fistula. This can be removed after 10–14 days and always closes without complication unless there is distal obstruction.

7 The surgical treatment of erosive gastritis is often unsatisfactory and most surgeons are conservative whenever possible. If bleeding is uncontrollably severe, then perform high or even total gastrectomy. Roux-en-Y reconstruction is then usually appropriate.

8 Gastric carcinoma or sarcoma are rare causes of severe gastrointestinal bleeding and should have been diagnosed before surgery was contemplated. Ideally, the operation to be performed is the one that would be selected at an elective operation. However, as a life-saving operation, be prepared to carry out a limited resection. In suitable patients it is reasonable to plan re-operation after 2–3 weeks to carry out radical resection.

RECURRENT PEPTIC ULCER

Appraise

1. The effectiveness of modern drugs has drastically reduced the indications for peptic ulcer surgery and therefore the risk of recurrent ulcer. In consequence, many surgeons are inexperienced in dealing with the challenging problems encountered in this field. Do not hesitate to refer patients with recurrent ulcer to someone who has specialized experience.

2. Test the basal, pentagastrin-stimulated and insulin-stimulated gastric acid secretion. High basal secretion suggests the possibility of a Zollinger-Ellison tumour. In all cases estimate the serum gastrin level and exclude hyperparathyroidism (see Chapter 21). A positive insulin test may suggest incomplete vagotomy if that was the original operation.

3. An episode proton-pump of recurrent ulcer does not necessarily demand re-operation. Try the effect of H2-receptor-blocking drugs in high dosage or proton-pump inhibitors (PPI), or PPI with antibiotics. The ulcer may heal and not recur.

4. If the recurrent ulcer is associated with high basal gastric acid output, carefully explore the pancreas and duodenum to exclude the presence of a Zollinger-Ellison tumour.

5. Recurrent gastric ulcer is rare following Billroth I gastrectomy but, if it does develop, carry out a higher gastrectomy, excising the ulcer. The anastomosis may once again be gastroduodenal, but Polya gastrectomy is highly effective in preventing recurrence. Recurrent ulcer following proximal gastric or truncal vagotomy with excision of the ulcer or a 'drainage procedure' is best treated by partial gastrectomy.

6. Recurrent ulcers may develop following conversion surgery to relieve dumping, bile vomiting or diarrhoea. Combine vagotomy and partial gastrectomy.

Action

1. Truncal vagotomy demands expert knowledge of the area. If the trunks were missed previously, search carefully not only around the lower oesophagus but also within the whole of the oesophageal hiatus. The posterior trunk may lie posteriorly on the right crus of the diaphragm. Remember that missed trunks may have been displaced at the first operation.

2. Partial gastrectomy is not necessarily more difficult than at a primary operation but great care is necessary to mobilize the stomach or remnant.

3. Do not leave a complicated anatomical result but prefer to take down anastomoses, leaving the anatomy simple. Blind and redundant loops of bowel endanger the patient's long-term well-being.

REVISION SURGERY FOLLOWING PEPTIC ULCER SURGERY

Appraise

1. It is surprising how infrequently patients having gastric surgery for cancer develop disabling chronic symptoms compared with those having surgery for peptic ulcer.

2. If you are an inexperienced and occasional gastric surgeon do not embark on revision surgery for the relief of sequelae following operations for peptic ulcer. Resist the desire to 'do something'. Very few of the many papers written on revision operations are objective or have sufficient numbers, or sufficient follow-up. Many of the patients improve with time following reassurance, and almost all of them can be improved by adherence to simple rules such as avoiding large meals and food that they have learned is likely to be upsetting, by taking small meals separate from fluids and resting after meals, and by avoiding food and drinks containing excessive sugar. In any case, it is wise to wait at least 2 years from the primary operation before contemplating a revision operation.

3. Bilious vomiting following the creation of a gastroenterostomy stoma is most likely to respond to anatomical revision. Indeed, disabling bilious vomiting is the only symptom for which a mechanical conversion can be offered with reasonable confidence. It is thought that the afferent loop is functionally or mechanically obstructed and distends with bile, pancreatic juice and duodenal secretions discharging intermittently into the stomach. The gastric lining is irritated and the patient may vomit or regurgitate some of the bile-stained fluid. At endoscopy, the region of the stoma reveals florid gastritis. If bilious vomiting follows gastroenterostomy plus truncal vagotomy, the anastomosis can often be simply disconnected provided the pyloroduodenal canal has an adequate lumen. If it follows Polya gastrectomy, conversion to a Roux-en-Y anastomosis (see Fig. 10.22) with drainage of the duodenal loop into the efferent limb at least 50 cm from the stomach diverts bile away from the stomach.

4. An alternative is a Roux-19 conversion in which the afferent loop is divided and the ends are anastomosed into the efferent loop at

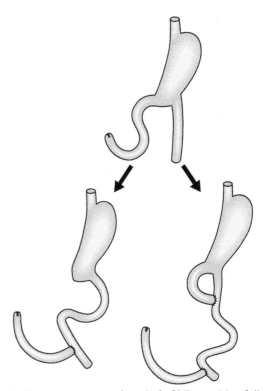

Fig. 10.22 Conversion surgery for relief of bile vomiting following polya partial gastrectomy. Lower left is the Roux-Y operation. Lower right is the Tanner Roux-19 operation.

least 50 cm apart; this procedure can be carried out without mobilizing the stomach. These operations increase the risk of stomal ulceration and, if the original operation was for duodenal ulcer, it is wise to perform truncal vagotomy.

5 Occasionally, bilious vomiting complicates Billroth I gastrectomy. The anastomosis can be disconnected, the duodenum closed and the stomach connected to a Roux-Y loop of jejunum.

6 Dumping syndrome is named from the probability that it develops because of the destruction of pyloric metering of gastric contents into the small bowel. Thus food and fluid may be rapidly deposited into the jejunum, causing overdistension and discomfort, usually within 30 minutes of the meal. This is called 'early' dumping. Rapid absorption of fluid may produce circulatory disturbances, while hyperosmolar solutions attract fluid into the lumen, depleting the circulating fluid volume and at the same time overfilling the jejunal lumen. Rapid absorption of sugars may evoke hyperglycaemia stimulating insulin release, followed by rapid fall in blood glucose and the symptoms of hypoglycaemia, usually 2–4 hours after meals. This is called 'late' dumping. Proximal gastric vagotomy without drainage for duodenal ulcer greatly reduces the incidence and severity of dumping, since the metering function of the antrum and pylorus is left intact.

7 Following Polya partial gastrectomy, dumping may be diminished by conversion to a Billroth I anastomosis or by conversion to a Roux-en-Y, adding truncal vagotomy if the first operation was for duodenal ulcer, to protect from recurrent ulceration. Neither of these procedures is totally satisfactory in every patient. Elaborations have been recommended, usually in the form of interposed antiperistaltic or isoperistaltic jejunal segments between the gastric remnant and the duodenum or efferent loop of small bowel. As a trainee surgeon, do not attempt to perform these complicated and often ineffective operations.

8 Severe dumping infrequently complicates Billroth I gastrectomy. It is sometimes improved by interposing an isolated isoperistaltic or antiperistaltic loop of jejunum between the gastric remnant and the duodenum.

9 Dumping following vagotomy is usual only when accompanied by an adjunctive procedure to improve gastric emptying. Gastroenterostomy can be taken down if the pyloroduodenal canal is adequate and the results are usually good. Pyloroplasty can be revised so that the pylorus is restored to anatomical normality but reports are varied on the success of the procedure. Probably it does little to improve the patient's symptoms in the long term.

10 Gastric retention produces a postprandial bloating sensation and regurgitation or vomiting of gastric contents, often with eructation. It was notorious in a proportion of patients treated by truncal vagotomy alone for the cure of duodenal ulcer and was relieved or prevented by the addition of gastrectomy, gastroenterostomy or pyloroplasty. As a rule, improvement occurs with time even when there is no drainage operation. Some patients appear to develop complete gastric atony following vagotomy, including proximal gastric vagotomy, whether or not a drainage operation has been added; this also tends to improve slowly with time. If a drainage operation was not used originally, then perform gastroenterostomy.

11 Occasionally, gastric retention develops from stomal obstruction associated with adhesions trapping the efferent bowel, intussusception of the afferent loop into the stomach or prolapse of hypertrophic gastric mucosal folds into the stoma, and from stenosis following recurrent ulcer. The diagnosis is made by contrast radiography and endoscopy. Treatment is surgical relief of the obstruction, or bypass. In the case of stenosis from recurrent ulcer, truncal vagotomy and gastrectomy are usually necessary.

12 In postgastrectomy patients who swallow indigestible food without first chewing it, the bolus of food may impact in the bowel, usually in the terminal ileum. Surgical relief is necessary: the bolus can usually be broken up without opening the bowel. If it cannot be broken up, 'milk' it proximally and open the bowel to extract the bolus. Then repair the incision in the bowel. Subsequently adjure the patient to avoid eating unchewed meat, fruit and other foods.

13 Diarrhoea may complicate peptic ulcer surgery. Make sure that the patient does not have some unrelated cause. An occult tendency to coeliac disease, colitis or irritable bowel disease may become manifest following peptic ulcer surgery. Dumping of food and fluid, especially hyperosmolar fluid, provokes intestinal hurry and diarrhoea as well as dumping syndrome and these symptoms can be controlled with simple dietary advice. Nearly all patients following gastrectomy have a tendency to steatorrhoea, although this may not be clinically evident. In most patients diarrhoea can be controlled using codeine phosphate. A rare cause of diarrhoea is inadvertent gastroileostomy instead of gastrojejunostomy; this requires surgical correction.

14 A few patients have crippling, uncontrollable diarrhoea following truncal vagotomy and drainage for peptic ulcer. Diarrhoea is associated with dumping and can usually be alleviated by controlling the dumping. A 10–12-cm length of jejunum may be taken out of circuit, reversed and inserted 100 cm beyond the ligament of Treitz; alternatively, reverse an 8-cm loop of ileum 40 cm proximal to the ileocaecal valve. The results have been disappointing in the long term.

15 Surgery for peptic ulcer is thought to predispose to gastric carcinoma. The cause is probably excessive bile reflux onto the gastric mucosa following Polya gastrectomy or gastroenterostomy with vagotomy. The detergent bile breaks the protective mucosal barrier, which may provide access to the mucosa for ingested carcinogens. A diet poor in vitamins and antioxidants, together with hypoacidity in the stomach, may be other predisposing factors. Do not assume that all symptoms, especially those developing late or with a changed pattern from previous symptoms, are 'post peptic ulcer surgery syndrome'. Carry out endoscopy and remove numerous biopsies, especially near the stoma. The reassurance that serious disease has been excluded often leads to an improvement in the symptoms. Successful resection is possible in some patients with stump carcinoma.

GASTRIC CARCINOMA

Appraise

1 At present, the best hope of cure is radical resection. Gastric carcinoma is usually resistant to radiation therapy, but responds to chemotherapy.

2 Unfortunately, most tumours present late. In Japan, a high proportion of early cancers are detected by screening or open-access endoscopy and are successfully treated by surgery. Early gastric

cancer is defined as a cancer that is confined to the mucosa or submucosa, with or without spread to the lymph nodes. In the UK, not even those at higher-than-normal risk are routinely and regularly screened. They include those with a family history of the disease, pernicious anaemia and gastric atrophy, hypergammaglobulinaemia, atrophic gastritis, intestinal metaplasia, dysplasia, polyps and previous gastric surgery. Blood group A confers a higher than normal risk. Early gastric cancer is often asymptomatic, yet even patients presenting with dyspepsia are not routinely endoscoped.

3 Lauren of Finland described in 1965 two types of gastric carcinoma. The first is intestinal in type, developing in areas of intestinal metaplasia and tending to be localized. The reduction in gastric cancer that is seen in many Western countries stems from a reduced incidence of this type. The second type is diffuse and tends to spread rapidly within the stomach, often in the submucosa, causing the rigidity that gives it the name 'linitis plastica'. It also spreads widely outside the stomach and carries a gloomy prognosis. Nevertheless, gastric cancer should be primarily regarded as a locoregional disease which is potentially curable by classical oncological surgery that removes the primary tumour and its draining lymph nodes.

4 Although most gastric carcinomas are sited distally, a tendency for a higher proportion to develop proximally has been noticed in recent years; the reason is unknown.

5 Endoscopy with cytology and biopsy is the best method of screening and diagnosis. It is valuable in detecting early gastric cancer (Fig. 10.23).

6 Improvements in imaging have facilitated preoperative staging. Barium meal X-ray is often now deprecated if endoscopic diagnosis has been made, but in expert hands it can sometimes give valuable information. For example, gastric rigidity and lack of peristalsis suggest extensive submucosal spread. Chest X-ray may reveal enlarged mediastinal nodes or pulmonary metastases. The preferred imaging modality is CT scanning, which demonstrates spread into adjacent organs, the liver and lymph nodes but does not pick up very early lesions. Endoluminal ultrasound is a valuable means of assessing infiltration and local nodal involvement. Laparoscopy is useful for determining tumour spread in the peritoneal cavity and assessing any fixation of the tumour to surrounding organs.

7 The ability to determine the extent of the tumour before operation saves many patients from fruitless exploratory laparotomy, although the preoperative, perioperative and postoperative staging may prove to be different. The combined TNM (tumour, nodes, metastases) staging of the International Union against (contra) Cancer (IUCC) in 1987 modified the staging to reflect the realization that the depth of invasion is more important than the topographical distribution.

8 Careful studies, carried out mainly in Japan, have demonstrated the sequential spread of cancer from various sites in the stomach to the lymph nodes. Local nodes within 3 cm of the primary tumour are designated N_1, the next nodes to be affected are N_2, the third tier is N_3 and distant spread is N_4 (Fig. 10.24, Table 10.1). If the tumour has not spread into unresectable local structures, or been metastasized by the blood stream, curative resection can be attempted. En bloc resection of the tumour with the N_1 nodes is designated a D_1 resection, with the N_1 and N_2 nodes a D_2

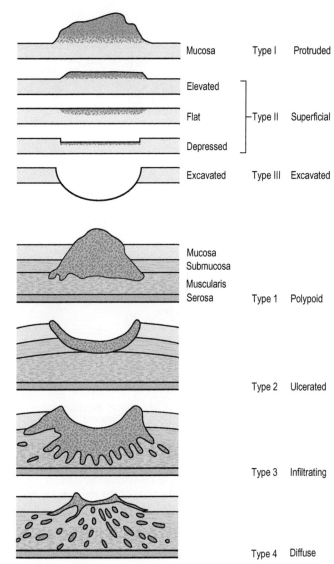

Fig. 10.23 Early and invasive gastric cancer. The upper types I-III are superficial carcinoma confined to the mucosa, described by the *Japanese Society of Gastroenterological Endoscopy*. The lower types 1–4 show advanced carcinoma described by Borrmann.

resection. D_2 resection is the standard procedure. On occasion a D_3 resection may be performed, incorporating the N_3 nodes.

9 Other structures may be removed in continuity with the stomach, including the parietes, the spleen, transverse colon or pancreas. The aim is to achieve circumferential resection margins that are clear of tumour: if you succeed in this endeavour, there is a 20–90% chance of cure, depending on the stage (90% in early gastric cancer, 20% in stage IIIb). Overall, 5-year survival in Britain is now about 40% after potentially curative D_2 resection.

10 Radical subtotal gastrectomy carried out through the abdomen is the standard operation for localized distal tumours. For diffuse distal growths and those in the body of the stomach a radical total gastrectomy is required. This is sometimes performed through a left thoracoabdominal incision but can often be performed satisfactorily through the abdomen. For lesions at the gastro-oesophageal junction (Siewert type I and II), a radical oesophagogastrectomy is usually required and this must be performed through a left or right thoracoabdominal approach. However,

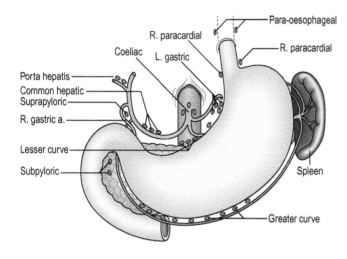

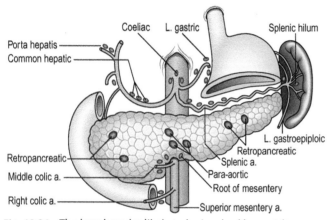

Fig. 10.24 The lymph nodes likely to be involved by gastric carcinoma. In the lower diagram the body of the stomach has been removed to display the deeply placed nodes.

Siewert type II and III tumours (truly junctional and ones encroaching the proximal 3 cm of stomach, respectively) may be tackled by performing a total or extended gastrectomy. An extended gastrectomy needs a left thoracoabdominal approach.

11 Palliative distal gastrectomy is occasionally helpful if gastric outlet obstruction is not relieved by a stent or a gastroenterostomy.

12 When resection is impracticable, try to relieve existing or impending obstruction. Distal obstruction can usually be bypassed using a proximal gastrojejunostomy. For a proximal obstruction consider dilating a stricture with bougies or inflatable balloons followed by the insertion of a stent. If a large tumour bulges into and blocks the lumen, reduce it using radiotherapy or endoscopically delivered Nd-YAG laser beam vaporization.

D₂ RADICAL ABDOMINAL SUBTOTAL GASTRECTOMY

Appraise

■ Radical resection for localized carcinoma of the distal stomach will be described. It resembles radical total gastrectomy except that a fringe of proximal stomach is retained; its size is determined by the extent of proximal spread of the tumour since the resection margin should be 5 cm clear of detectable tumour. Preservation of the proximal stomach allows gastrojejunostomy to be accomplished through the abdomen. It is carried out on patients who have no evident involvement of the peritoneum distant from the tumour or of N3 and N4 nodes. Any local invasion of contiguous structures must be resectable with the stomach, such as proximal duodenum, a segment of small bowel, transverse colon, pancreas or spleen.

■ Ensure that the resection margin is well clear of growth, because a resection that does not protect the patient against stomal recurrence and obstruction is not worth carrying out. If there are extensive metastases, palliative resection is probably inappropriate. Bypass existing or impending pyloric obstruction with proximal gastroenterostomy.

TABLE 10.1 The successive tiers of lymph nodes affected by adenocarcinoma at different sites within the stomach				
	N₁	**N₂**	**N₃**	**N₄**
Distal primary carcinoma	Lesser curve Greater curve Suprapyloric Subpyloric	Right paracardial Left gastric Common hepatic Coeliac axis	Hepatoduodenal ligament	Middle colic artery
Middle third carcinoma	Right paracardial Lesser curve Greater curve Suprapyloric	Splenic artery Splenic hilum Left paracardial Left gastric	Posterior aspect of pancreas	Para-aortic
Subpyloric	Common hepatic	Para-oesophageal Coeliac axis		
Upper-third carcinoma	Left paracardial Right paracardial Lesser curve Greater curve	Suprapyloric Subpyloric Common hepatic Left gastric Splenic artery Splenic hilum Coeliac axis	Diaphragmatic Root of mesentery	

Access

1 Make a long vertical midline incision skirting the umbilicus.

2 If necessary excise the xiphoid process. Be prepared to mobilize the left lobe of liver and fold it to the right.

Assess

1 Do not immediately palpate the stomach. Note any ascites and peritoneal deposits. Start your complete exploration from the pelvis and work towards the stomach in order not to disperse malignant cells. Exclude pelvic deposits and, in the female, ovarian seedlings. Examine the greater omentum for deposits and then raise it to feel the para-aortic nodes and those around the root of the mesentery, and the right colic and middle colic arteries. Examine the full length of the small and then large intestine, seeking peritoneal deposits on the bowel wall, the mesentery and the parietal peritoneum. Look for incidental disease. Throughout the examination confirm pulsation in the arteries, noting atheromatous rigidity, aneurysms and venous or lymphatic obstruction.

2 Now draw the omentum caudally to examine the upper compartment. Feel both lobes of the liver and adjacent diaphragm, gallbladder and free edge of the lesser omentum, the spleen, kidneys and adrenal glands. Starting at the oesophageal hiatus and working distally, look and feel for tumour involvement, fixity, glands and also incidental disease. Systematically move distally, avoiding handling or squeezing the tumour if possible.

3 Palpate the duodenum and feel the head of the pancreas between finger and thumb. Now palpate the body and tail of the pancreas through the lesser omentum and transverse mesocolon, then the region of the coeliac axis just above the neck of the pancreas. This part of the examination cannot be exact and must be repeated as the dissection allows. If you are seriously in doubt whether to proceed, incise the lesser omentum in an avascular area near the liver and examine the coeliac axis and emerging arteries and assess the spread across the lesser sac. If you are doubtful about involvement of the head of the pancreas, perform Kocher's manoeuvre in order to palpate it adequately. None of these manoeuvres commits you to proceed with radical resection if you discover unsuspected spread.

> ▶ **KEY POINTS** Avoid too early commitment to resection
>
> ■ If you are still in doubt, plan to mobilize the stomach without dividing any vital structures until you have ensured that resection is appropriate and achievable.
> ■ This may entail a change in the order of the procedure, approaching the suspect area from a different aspect.

Resect

1 Lift the great omentum and dissect it from the transverse colon. There is a bloodless plane of fusion between the folded omentum, which was part of the dorsal mesogastrium, and the anterior leaf of mesocolon. Gently peel off the omentum, taking care not to damage the anterior leaf of mesocolon or the middle colic and marginal vessels. Continue on to the pancreas until you reach its upper border. Take care to avoid damaging the pancreas or its blood vessels. It is easy to get lost during this manoeuvre and

end up posterior to the pancreas. Therefore, remain vigilant and lift the peritoneum off the anterior surface of the pancreas, which will lead to the coeliac axis and its branches. This manoeuvre is often referred to as a 'bursectomy'.

2 At the left extremity of the greater omentum the left gastroepiploic vessels pass forwards in the gastrosplenic omentum from the hilum of the spleen. Carefully dissect out the lymph nodes at the origin of the left gastroepiploic artery, then doubly ligate and divide the artery and vein. An ultrasonic dissector is useful for this.

3 At the right extremity of the greater omentum the right gastroepiploic vessels pass forwards from the gastroduodenal vessels. Carefully isolate them and the subpyloric lymph nodes before doubly ligating and dividing them at their origins.

4 Now draw the distal stomach caudally to put on stretch the free edge of the lesser omentum. Carefully make a transverse incision in the anterior leaf above the pylorus to reveal the right gastric vessels and the suprapyloric lymph nodes. Dissect the nodes and doubly ligate and divide the right gastric blood vessels.

5 Gently burst through an avascular area of the lesser omentum close to the liver and extend this towards the cardia, keeping close to the liver. Look for and divide between ligatures the accessory hepatic artery crossing from the left gastric artery.

6 Perform Kocher's mobilization of the duodenum so that the first part can be dissected from the head of the pancreas. The blood vessels are short and fragile. In order to avoid damaging the pancreas, apply fine haemostasis forceps on the vessels a few millimetres from the duodenal wall, divide the vessels between the tips of the forceps and the duodenal wall, then pick up the short duodenal cut ends to ligate them.

7 Mobilize 5–6 cm of duodenum beyond the pylorus.

> ▶ **KEY POINT** Keep in the correct tissue plane
>
> ■ Do not wander from the duodenal wall; you risk damaging the bile duct and pancreas.

8 Use a GIA or similar mechanical stapler to transect the duodenum.

9 From the site of ligature of the right gastric artery, strip the peritoneum, connective tissue and lymph nodes from the hepatic artery, proximally along the upper border of the pancreas, to the coeliac artery en-bloc.

10 Have the distal stomach elevated by an assistant, to tauten the left gastric vessels in their peritoneal fold. In the free edge of the fold lies the left gastric vein; identify, doubly ligate and divide this first. Now extend the dissection of the hepatic artery to the coeliac artery, in order to dissect all the glands from this area, including those around the origin of the splenic artery and look out for the left adrenal gland. Elevate the gland mass into the column of tissue around the now cleaned origin of the left gastric artery. Doubly ligate and divide the left gastric artery. We always place two ties on the proximal cut stump or transfix it with an arterial suture.

11 Have the stomach drawn caudally and to the patient's left, to place the cardia on stretch. Complete the division of the lesser omentum until the right side of the cardia is reached; now gently

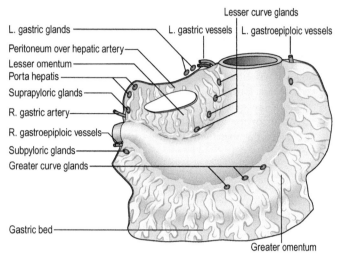

Fig. 10.25 Radical subtotal gastrectomy; the removed specimen.

Labels (figure): L. gastric glands; Peritoneum over hepatic artery; Lesser omentum; Porta hepatis; Suprapyloric glands; R. gastric artery; R. gastroepiploic vessels; Subpyloric glands; Greater curve glands; Gastric bed; Lesser curve glands; L. gastric vessels; L. gastroepiploic vessels; Greater omentum

clean the upper lesser omentum, connective tissue and right cardiac lymph nodes from the gastric lesser curve down to the selected site of transection. The nerves of Latarjet will be transected during this manoeuvre.

12 Turn the distal stomach cranially again, to examine the upper posterior wall, ensuring that it is free of adhesions; there is often a vein, arching backwards in a peritoneal fold from the posterior gastric fundus, which bleeds annoyingly if it is torn.

13 Transect the stomach with a mechanical stapling device. When the stomach is transected it appears as in Figure 10.25.

Technical

1 Remember that the more extensive the operation the greater the morbidity and mortality. Do not deprive a fit patient of the chance for cure by being too conservative. However, do not place a patient at risk unnecessarily with a radical resection if the N_3 nodes (porta hepatis, root of mesentery, para-oesophageal and retropancreatic) and N4 nodes (middle colic and para-aortic) are already involved. If in doubt, take biopsies of these nodes and obtain frozen-section histology.

2 Remember the two principles of cancer surgery enunciated by the great surgeons, William Halsted and Keiichi Maruyama: whenever possible, dissect the lymph nodes en bloc with the primary tumour so that you do not transect the intervening lymphatics, and obtain clear circumferential resection margins.

3 An argument could be made for less extensive nodal dissection for early gastric cancer. However, in a fit patient, perform D_2 resection, because 10–30% of UK patients with early gastric cancer have nodal metastases.

4 The D_2 resection may be selectively extended to encompass N_3 nodes (a $D_{2/3}$ resection):
  ■ Tumour cells may travel retrogradely towards the hilum of the liver. Routinely remove these nodes when radically excising distal gastric carcinoma, in continuity with the dissection of the common hepatic artery. Make a careful incision across the upper free edge of the lesser omentum over the hepatic arteries, which can be found by palpation between a finger placed in the upper aditus to the lesser sac, and a thumb

placed anteriorly. Carefully strip down the connective tissue and glands from the hilum of the liver to the point of right gastric artery ligation and beyond, along the common hepatic artery to the coeliac axis. Take care not to damage the common bile duct; the portal vein is less at risk since it lies posteriorly.

■ After Kocher's manoeuvre has been performed to dissect off the duodenal bulb, carefully seek and excise retropancreatic (N3) nodes from the posterior aspect of the pancreatic head. Of course, these cannot be removed in continuity with the main specimen. During this manoeuvre also look for and remove nodes at the root of the mesentery (N_3 nodes) and close to the aorta (N_4 nodes). Always have isolated nodes placed separately in labelled pots for histology and prognostication.

■ If the distal carcinoma extends proximally into the body of the stomach it is wise to excise the nodes along the upper and lower borders of the pancreas (N_2 nodes for carcinoma in the body of the stomach). When the omentum has been stripped as far as the pancreas, gently dissect the mesocolon caudally to display the lower border of pancreas. Seek and remove any glands that lie around the emerging superior mesenteric vessels and the inferior mesenteric vein.

■ Having stripped the greater omentum as far as the pancreas, peel the continuation of posterior parietal peritoneum, in a cephalad direction, from the upper part of the body and tail of the pancreas to reveal the serpentine splenic artery. Carefully dissect from it the connective tissue and lymph nodes proximally along its whole length from its origin at the coeliac artery.

■ Some surgeons remove the spleen and body and tail of the pancreas in order to remove the supra- and infrapancreatic nodes together with retropancreatic nodes around the splenic vein. To achieve this, draw the spleen forwards and to the right to display and divide the left leaf of the lienorenal ligament. Gently mobilize the spleen and tail and body of pancreas forwards with the splenic artery and vein. Doubly ligate and divide the splenic vein just distal to the entry of the inferior mesenteric vein. Carefully dissect the lymph nodes from the splenic artery, starting at the coeliac artery and working distally until you reach the level at which the splenic vein was divided. Now doubly ligate and divide the splenic artery, leaving the dissected nodes attached to the distal segment. Transect the body of the pancreas, carefully preserving the inferior mesenteric vein junction with the splenic vein. If possible, isolate and separately ligate the cut pancreatic duct. Oversew the proximal cut end of the pancreas with fine non-absorbable sutures. Since the splenic artery no longer supplies the proximal stomach through the short gastric vessels, the proximal stomach will receive its blood supply only from the oesophagus, so perform a near-total gastrectomy, leaving but a fringe of stomach.

▶ KEY POINTS Cost–benefit decision

■ Addition of splenopancreatectomy to D_2 subtotal gastrectomy triples the operative mortality, from approximately 4% to 10–15%. Spleen and pancreas so removed are usually uninvolved.

- Do not, therefore, routinely perform splenectomy or pancreatectomy in standard D2 subtotal gastrectomy, but assiduously try to clear suprapancreatic lymph nodes.
- However, direct posterior invasion of the pancreas may force you to carry out splenopancreatectomy en bloc with stomach.

Unite

1. Fashion a Roux-en-Y loop. Draw up the alimentary limb and ensure it measures at least 50 cm to the jejunojejunal anastomosis to minimize the risk of biliary reflux.

2. The anastomosis can be made using a combined linear stapling and cutting device. In this case transect the stomach with a double line of staples applied with a long linear stapler and transect it below the line of staples. Bring up the selected jejunal end then make stab wounds through the gastric and jejunal walls close to the uniting stitch at the greater curve end of the proposed anastomosis and pass in the separate blades of the combined linear stapler and cutter, one into the stomach, one into the jejunum, lying parallel to each other and pointing to the gastric lesser curve.

3. Lock the two blades together after ensuring that there is no intervening tissue. Actuate the stapler to insert four parallel rows of staples uniting the stomach and jejunum and cutting between the middle rows to form a stoma. Unlock and remove the stapler. Inspect the interior to ensure the anastomosis is perfect.

4. Pick up the incomplete ends of the staple lines with tissue forceps and separate them to leave a longitudinal defect. Close this with an absorbable continuous suture or a short straight stapling device, being careful not to narrow the new anastomosis. Thus you end up with a side stomach to side jejunum anastomosis.

5. Alternatively, draw up a loop of proximal jejunum in exactly the same manner as following Polya gastrectomy for benign disease. The disadvantage of this method is the biliary reflux which can cause discomfort and ulceration at the gastroenterostomy.

ABDOMINAL TOTAL GASTRECTOMY

Resect

1. Complete the gastric mobilization by dividing the lesser omentum right up to the diaphragm and dividing the gastrophrenic ligament close to the diaphragm. Posteriorly, there is a vein arching backwards from the upper stomach that must be ligated or occluded with haemostatic clips and divided. Splenectomy and distal pancreatectomy are not always necessary.

2. The stomach is now attached only to the oesophagus. Gently free this in the hiatus. Transect the anterior and posterior vagal trunks and decide on the level of transection. Divide the oesophagus once you have secured the oesophagus to prevent retraction. Prevent retraction of the oesophagus into the chest by placing a 2/0 PDS suture through the full thickness of the oesophagus about 5 cm proximal to the line of transection or by application of a Satinsky clamp.

3. If a nasojejunal tube is to be used, have it drawn up into the lower oesophagus. It can be pulled down when making a sutured

anastomosis when the posterior all-coats suture is in place and pushed on into the jejunum. If a stapled anastomosis is made, have the anaesthetist push it on with a twisting motion when the stapler is withdrawn.

Unite

1. Oesophagojejunostomy is preferably performed using a Roux-en-Y jejunal loop (see Chapter 11). Transect the jejunum close to the ligament of Treitz and divide sufficient primary vascular arcades to allow the distal portion to be taken up to the oesophagus. Transect the bowel beyond the duodenojejunal junction and join the cut proximal end into the side of the Roux loop 50 cm downstream. If a sutured oesophagojejunal anastomosis is used, close the end of the jejunum in two layers, or staple it. The loop should be led up to the oesophagus posterior to the transverse mesocolon. Make sure it lies without tension or twisting. Insert a posterior running suture line of Lembert stitches joining the posterior wall of the oesophagus to the posterior wall of the Roux loop about 5 cm from the closed end. Now transect the oesophagus below the suture line and remove the specimen.

2. Create a hole in the antimesenteric border of the jejunum exactly matching the oesophageal lumen. Insert a stitch through all coats of the oesophagus and jejunum at each end so they can be slightly stretched. Carefully insert a circular all-coats stitch to produce perfect union. Now carry the posterior Lembert stitch onto the anterior wall to encircle the anastomosis, trying to draw up the jejunal wall to cover the inner all-coats stitch.

3. Discard and replace the soiled towels, instruments and gloves.

4. End-to-end Roux loop anastomosis is rarely possible if the oesophagus is sufficiently dilated so that its lumen matches that of the cut end of the jejunum and if the jejunum can be laid straight with not too much tendency to curve at its free end. A two-layer anastomosis is usually fashioned, but one-layer anastomosis is probably equally satisfactory.

5. The oesophagojejunal anastomosis may be accomplished using one of the circular stapling devices. Just after the oesophagus is completely transected, an encircling all-coats purse-string suture is inserted. Introduce a size-testing head so that the correct size of stapler can be used (usually 25 mm). An end-to-side Roux anastomosis does not require a separate stab since the instrument, without the anvil, can be passed in through the cut end of bowel, which will be closed with a linear stapler or in two layers after it is withdrawn. In an end-to-end anastomosis the anvil remains in place but well separated from the staple cartridge, and a purse-string suture is used to draw in the jejunal end over the cartridge.

6. Now feed the anvil head into the cut end of the oesophagus, tighten and tie the purse-string suture and close the anvil head onto the cartridge after ensuring there is no extraneous tissue trapped and that the oesophagus and jejunum lie without tension or twist. Release the safety catch and actuate the gun. Open it, remove it, check the intactness of the anastomosis and of the doughnut-shaped rings on the spindle. Close the portal of entry of the device in two layers.

7. In case of doubt about the integrity of the anastomosis, retain the closed stapler and use it to rotate the anastomosis while inserting reinforcing sutures around the circumference of the stoma. Only now release and remove the stapler.

Check

1. Stop all bleeding.
2. Ensure that the anastomoses are perfect, the bowel is a good colour, untwisted and not stretched and the mesentery lies free.
3. Check all the other structures that have been disturbed. The hiatus does not need to be repaired if total gastrectomy has been carried out. The liver must be replaced if the left lobe was folded to the right. Repair the transverse mesocolon if there is a hole through which small bowel may prolapse.

Closure

1. Drain the cut end of the pancreas and leave the drain in situ for 6–10 days to form a track. Pancreatic fistula is common and very dangerous if it cannot freely drain externally.
2. Close the abdomen in routine fashion.

Postoperative

1. Manage a patient following subtotal gastrectomy in the same manner as following gastrectomy for benign disease.
2. Following transabdominal total gastrectomy manage the patient in a similar manner to one who has had thoracoabdominal total gastrectomy (vide infra).

RADICAL THORACOABDOMINAL TOTAL GASTRECTOMY

Appraise

1. Never embark upon this operation without first obtaining a tissue diagnosis with endoscopic biopsy or cytology or frozen-section histology at operation. Never embark upon it without making every effort by preoperative and operative assessment to exclude metastatic tumour.
2. As a rule, this is a radical operation undertaken for carcinoma of the gastro-oesophageal junction, proximal stomach or cardia with encroachment into the distal oesophagus.
3. Accomplish it through a left thoracoabdominal incision. It can be carried out through an upper midline abdominal incision only if the tumour does not extend proximally beyond the gastro-oesophageal junction and where there is a 5-cm length of intra-abdominal oesophagus.

> ▶ KEY POINT Insure against anastomotic recurrence
>
> ■ It is tragic for the patient to undergo a major resection only to rapidly develop malignant stenosis at the anastomosis.

4. Sarcoma of the stomach is best treated by radical gastrectomy but even if it extends beyond the scope of the operation total gastrectomy may be justified to reduce the bulk of the tumour. Radiotherapy and chemotherapy may then be more effective, with a reduced risk of hollow viscus perforation.
5. Non-radical total gastrectomy through the abdomen was conventionally carried out on patients with Zollinger-Ellison syndrome, whether or not a gastrin-secreting tumour had been totally excised. It is now reserved for the minority of patients whose ulcer cannot be controlled medically or by extirpation of the tumour.
6. This major resection must sometimes be offered to patients who are elderly, have other conditions that prejudice recovery and are also malnourished. Ensure that the nutritional state is restored by oral feeding with high-calorie, high-protein and vitamin-rich diet, nasoenteric feeding or, if necessary, intravenous feeding through a centrally placed venous catheter. Organize preoperative chest physiotherapy and check all other body systems to anticipate and prevent complications. It is recommended that the patient have a double lumen endotracheal tube to allow for deflation of the left lung. Make sure that the patient has an indwelling urinary catheter in place during and after the operation to allow the urinary output to be monitored.

Access

1. The anaesthetized, intubated patient lies on the right side (Fig. 10.26), tilted backwards 30°, right hip and knee flexed, left leg straight and separated from the right leg by a pillow. The pelvis is fixed by a wide strip of adhesive tape to prevent it from rolling backwards; a fixed post, covered with sponge, supports the left scapula posteriorly to maintain its position. The arms are brought in front of the face in the 'hornpipe' position.
2. Stand on the patient's right.
3. Open the abdomen obliquely from the midline to the costal margin in the line of the left seventh or eighth rib.

Assess

1. Note any free fluid. Feel the pelvic peritoneum for deposits, then the para-aortic and middle colic nodes, then the liver.
2. Examine the stomach and its related nodes, in particular the coeliac nodes by making a hole in an avascular part of the lesser omentum near the liver. Note if the tumour is fixed to adjacent structures such as the liver, pancreas, colon or abdominal wall and if partial resection of these allows radical resection to be accomplished. Decide if radical resection is feasible.

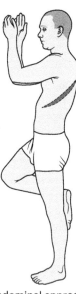

Fig. 10.26 Left thoracoabdominal approach to total gastrectomy, as seen from above the patient. The shaded section shows the extent of the incision.

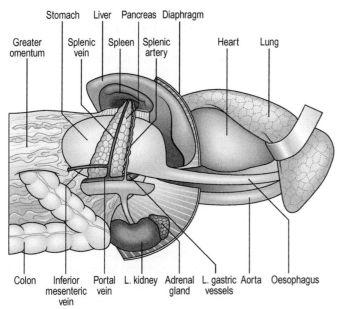

Stomach Liver Pancreas Diaphragm

Greater   Splenic Spleen Splenic   Heart   Lung
omentum   vein   artery

Colon   Inferior   Portal L. kidney Adrenal L. gastric Aorta Oesophagus
         mesenteric vein   gland   vessels
         vein

Fig. 10.27 Through a left thoracoabdominal incision the diaphragm has been incised. The spleen, splenic vessels and body and tail of the pancreas have been elevated, together with the greater curve of the stomach.

Resect

1 Extend the incision along the seventh or eighth rib as far as the lateral border of the sacrospinalis muscle. Open the chest by resecting the costal margin and then incise along the upper border of the rib. Isolate and divide the intercostal nerve posteriorly to prevent postoperative girdle pain.

2 Incise the diaphragm circumferentially about 3 cm from the chest wall to allow easy reconstruction at the end. It may be necessary to resect the crural part en bloc with the growth.

3 Mobilize the spleen forwards (Fig. 10.27) after incising the lienorenal ligament, lifting up the tail and body of the pancreas. When the inferior mesenteric vein is encountered, doubly ligate and divide the splenic vein distal to it and separate the proximal pancreas from the right part of the splenic vein, ligating any small vessels joining the two structures.

4 Lift up the greater omentum and separate its whole length from the transverse colon in the bloodless plane just above the colon, so that the omentum can be stripped upwards as an intact leaf from the mesocolon. Avoid damaging the mesocolon or its contained blood vessels.

5 Carry out Kocher's manoeuvre. Carefully identify and dissect out the lymph nodes on the posterior surface of the pancreatic head, para-aortic area, origin of the superior mesenteric artery, and also the origins of the middle colic and right colic arteries. Pot these separately in formalin for histology.

6 Rotate the spleen, tail of pancreas, omentum and greater curve of stomach over to the right. At the pyloric end the right gastroepiploic vessels are taut and at the cardiac end of the stomach the left gastric vessels are tensed. Dissect out the right gastroepiploic vein on the pancreas and doubly clamp, divide and ligate it. Dissect out the origin of the right gastroepiploic artery. Clamp, divide and ligate it, dissecting out the lymph nodes with the vessels. Above the pylorus, identify the right gastric vessels, trace the arteries up to their origin

from the hepatic artery and doubly clamp, divide and ligate them, dissecting out the lymph nodes with the vessels. Mobilize the duodenum for at least 5 cm beyond the pylorus. There are small vessels connecting it to the pancreas; clamp these close to the duodenum, divide them between the clamps and the duodenum, pick up the vessels on the duodenal wall and ligate them.

7 Isolate the area with distinctive coloured towels. Transect the duodenum 3–5 cm beyond the pylorus using a linear stapler or between thin crushing clamps such as Lang Stevenson's. Close the distal cut end with a loose running over-and-over absorbable stitch. Insert a second layer of invaginating stitches to bury the first layer. Alternatively, close the duodenum with a straight stapling device, with or without a row of reinforcing invaginating stitches.

8 Fold the distal stomach to the left. Expose the porta hepatis and incise the peritoneum over the hepatic artery, recognized by palpation. Strip the peritoneum, connective tissue and lymph nodes from the hepatic artery back to the coeliac artery. Continue the peritoneal incision in the porta hepatis to the left, keeping close to the liver, to detach the lesser omentum up to the diaphragm.

9 Have the distal stomach drawn upwards to place the left gastric vessels on stretch within their peritoneal fold. Continue the dissection of peritoneum, connective tissue and nodes along the hepatic artery to clear the coeliac axis and origins of the splenic and left gastric arteries. Dissect in continuity any glands from the aorta above the coeliac axis. Isolate, doubly clamp, divide and ligate the left gastric vein on the posterior abdominal wall. Doubly clamp, divide and ligate the left gastric artery at its origin.

10 If a distal pancreatectomy is required, then just below and to the right of the coeliac axis gently separate the neck of the pancreas from the splenic vein lying behind it and transect the pancreas here, picking up and ligating the small vessels above and below. Identify the main duct and separately ligate it. Close the raw proximal cut end of the pancreas with a running absorbable stitch or with interrupted sutures.

11 The coeliac axis has been cleared of connective tissue and nodes. Now sweep off the tissue on the left-hand side to reveal the cleaned origin of the splenic artery. Doubly clamp, divide and ligate the splenic artery at its origin. Separate the splenic vein from the posterior surface of the pancreas as far as the ligature placed distal to the entrance of the inferior mesenteric vein. The distal splenic artery with its associated glands is now freed, together with the body and tail of the pancreas and spleen.

12 The distal stomach is free. Decide whether or not to excise a cuff of diaphragmatic crura in continuity with the upper stomach and lower oesophagus. In any case, continue up the dissection of the upper stomach and lower oesophagus, keeping well away from them so the loose connective tissue, paracardial glands and lymphatics will be incorporated in the specimen.

13 Have the left lung deflated and retracted or the lower lobe held forwards with a lung retractor. Incise the pleura over the lower oesophagus. Mobilize the oesophagus above the diaphragm and dissect downwards, stripping all the surrounding connective tissue, lymphatics and lymph nodes with it and from the aorta lying posteriorly and the pericardium medially.

14 Extend the radial cut in the diaphragm to the crura. Now, preferably dissect on either side to leave a cuff of crus still attached to the free oesophagus. If the tumour is well away, it is permissible

179

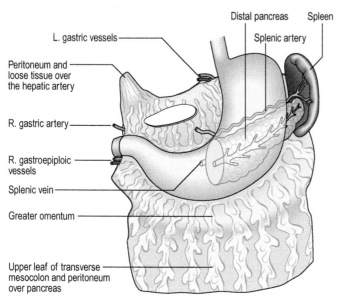

L. gastric vessels

Peritoneum and
loose tissue over
the hepatic artery

R. gastric artery

R. gastroepiploic
vessels

Splenic vein

Greater omentum

Upper leaf of transverse
mesocolon and peritoneum
over pancreas

Distal pancreas   Spleen

Splenic artery

Fig. 10.28   Radical total gastrectomy. The resected specimen.

to split through the crus and dissect out all the loose tissue with the oesophagus.

15 The specimen is now attached only by the oesophagus and vagal trunks. Divide the vagi. Decide the level of oesophageal transection to be 5–10 cm clear of detectable tumour. In case of doubt, obtain frozen-section histological confirmation that the resection margin is free from tumour. Reconstruction will be easy if the oesophagus is cut at the level of the lower edge of the left pulmonary vein. Do not stint on the resection, however. It is tragic to succeed in extirpating all the peripheral growth only to have the patient develop recurrence at the stoma. If necessary, the oesophagus can be freed and united on the outside of the arch but this is usually too high for the jejunal limb to reach, or freed up to the neck and united to a conduit there. Transect the oesophagus cleanly (Fig. 10.28). If a nasogastric tube was in place, have it first withdrawn to just above the line of transection.

16 Scrupulously ensure total haemostasis now. It will be impossible to examine the area when the reconstructive conduit is in place.

Unite

1 Pick up the proximal jejunum. Carefully examine the vascular pattern. Hold up the loops and view them against a light. Create a Roux loop that will easily reach the retracted oesophagus. Draw the loop through a hole in an avascular portion of the posterior part of the mesocolon, subsequently suturing the margins of the mesocolon carefully to the loop and its mesentery to prevent other loops of bowel from herniating through.

2 The anastomosis may be end-to-end but the jejunum usually sits most comfortably with the oesophagus joined end-to-side. If this is a sutured anastomosis, close the end of the jejunum with a purse-string suture or a linear stapler, reinforced with an invaginating seromuscular stitch. Make a hole in the antimesenteric border of the jejunum to match the lumen of the oesophagus. Place stay sutures through all coats of oesophagus and jejunum at each end and have these drawn apart to slightly stretch the anastomotic lines. Now carefully insert an all-coats stitch uniting

the adjacent oesophageal and jejunum walls, placing the sutures 2 mm apart, with 2–3-mm bites. The stitches may be continuous or interrupted, absorbable, braided or monofilament plastic thread. The material and method are less important than the perfection of every stitch (Fig. 10.29).

3 Many surgeons employ a single suture layer. Alternatively, a second layer may be inserted of continuous or interrupted stitches which pick up the muscularis and submucosa of the oesophagus close to the anastomosis and the seromuscularis of the jejunum 5 mm below the anastomosis so that as it is gently tightened it draws a cuff of bowel up and over the all-coats suture line. The anastomosis can be rotated to allow the stitch to be inserted around the whole circumference.

4 Now discard and replace the soiled towels, instruments and gloves.

5 The anastomosis can be fashioned using circular staplers. Choose a suitable cartridge size (usually 25 mm) by inserting a test head into the oesophagus. Do not unite the jejunal end. When turned over the cartridge head with a purse-string suture, it would prove too bulky in conjunction with the thick-walled oesophageal end also drawn into the gap between anvil and cartridge by a purse-string suture.

6 Apply the stapler safety catch and remove the anvil from the spindle. Introduce the spindle and cartridge through the open end of the jejunum, cut down upon the spindle end 5–7 cm from the jejunal end, on the antimesenteric border, and advance the spike through the jejunum. Replace the anvil. Introduce a purse-string suture of monofilament plastic suture around the cut oesophageal end. Introduce the anvil into the oesophagus and tighten the purse-string suture, cutting off the spare thread. Close the anvil onto the cartridge with the intact purse-stringed oesophagus and jejunal wall separating them and with no extraneous tissue caught. Release the safety catch and actuate the stapler. Separate the anvil from the cartridge and gently withdraw the instrument.

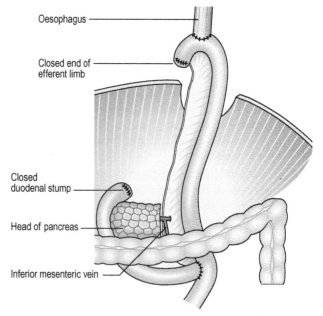

Oesophagus

Closed end of
efferent limb

Closed
duodenal stump

Head of pancreas

Inferior mesenteric vein

Fig. 10.29   Radical total gastrectomy. The oesophagojejunal anastomosis is complete, using a Roux loop of jejunum taken behind the mesocolon. The duodenal bulb is closed, and duodenal loop is joined end-to-side to the jejunum.

7 Confirm that there are two intact toroidal fragments ('doughnuts') of oesophagus and jejunum on the spindle. Check the suture line. If necessary, reinforce it partially or completely with sutures.

8 Now close the cut jejunal end using a short straight stapler. If the oesophagus is very thick, dissect back the muscular coat as a cuff which is not included in the stapler. After 'firing' and withdrawing the stapler, unite the oesophageal muscle to the jejunum with a continuous ring of sutures. The technique is simplified using the stapling device in which the anvil, together with the spindle, can be separated from the cartridge.

9 Manoeuvre the nasogastric tube through the anastomosis and if possible down to or beyond the duodenojejunal anastomosis if it is intended to use it for feeding.

Technical points

1 Radical and potentially curative resection may be accomplished if the tumour has invaded the diaphragm provided it is possible to excise part of this en bloc with the tumour. If the body or tail of the pancreas is invaded posteriorly, this part of the gland will have been removed as a routine together with the spleen. The transverse colon can be resected en bloc with the stomach. If the tumour spreads distally into the duodenum or into the head of the pancreas then pancreatoduodenectomy would be necessary and this is very rarely feasible.

2 It is important to stretch the anastomosis slightly when uniting it with sutures, since the oesophagus contracts down to a narrow tube and sutures placed close together become widely separated when a bolus of food stretches it, allowing leakage to occur.

3 If the oesophagus retracts under the aortic arch gently free it until it can be brought onto the outside of the arch and complete the anastomosis there. With care this can be accomplished perfectly but occasionally it is worth creating a second, higher thoracotomy. If anastomosis cannot be safely performed, do not persist. Dissect up the oesophagus to the neck and complete it safely there, using a suitable conduit such as a segment of colon.

4 A jejunostomy may be created (see Chapter 11) to allow early feeding if the patient was severely undernourished or if slow recovery is possible. Alternatively, the nasal tube may be passed into the upper jejunum for feeding purposes. In patients who find the tube intolerable, the upper end can be brought out in the neck as a pharyngostomy.

Checklist

1 Check that you have completed the D_2 glandular clearance (see Table 10.1).

2 In the chest, make sure the anastomosis is perfectly executed, that it lies without tension and is not twisted. Ensure that the lung is undamaged and that it can be re-expanded by the anaesthetist if he has deliberately collapsed it.

3 Check all the main ligatures. Re-examine the closed neck of pancreas and duodenal stump closure. Check that there is no continuing oozing from the raw surfaces.

4 Check the jejuno-jejunal anastomosis, ensure that the Roux loop passes upwards without twisting, and that its blood supply is not prejudiced. Re-examine the passage of the jejunum through the mesocolon and ensure that the blood supply to the colon is not damaged.

Closure

1 Insert a left basal chest drain and connect it to an underwater seal. Insert an abdominal drain to the distal cut pancreas.

2 Close the cut diaphragm using mattress sutures of non-absorbable material. Even if a cuff of crura has been removed it will close without tension. Do not tighten the new hiatus to constrict the jejunal loop. Do not suture the bowel to the diaphragm but allow it to lie freely.

3 Close the chest in layers.

4 Close the abdomen.

Postoperative

1 Nurse the patient in a high dependency unit for the first 24 hours.

2 Institute physiotherapy for the chest. Remove the underwater drain after 48 hours if the output is less than 100 ml per day and the drain to the pancreas after 6–10 days. Order daily chest X-rays until the chest is clear. If fluid collects in the base of the left pleural cavity, aspirate it.

3 Give jejunostomy feeds preferably, or parenteral feeds. Some surgeons arrange a contrast swallow after 4–5 days to examine the anastomosis radiologically, but there is little evidence that this changes outcomes: it may be preferable to arrange such studies only if there is a clinical need. Start oral fluid intake at day 3 or 4 and at this stage remove the nasogastric tube if it is not draining much.

PALLIATIVE OPERATIONS FOR GASTRIC CARCINOMA

Appraise

■ Palliative resection for carcinoma implies apparently complete removal of the primary tumour where there is metastatic growth outside the scope of a radical resection. If residual tumour remains at the gastric resection margin the anastomosis may not heal, so that the patient develops leakage and peritonitis, or soon develops stomal obstruction from recurrent tumour, or tumour is disseminated widely during the procedure. As cytotoxic chemotherapy improves, palliative resection may be of greater value since some agents are more effective if the tumour bulk is reduced.

■ If resection is precluded, the patient can still be relieved of impending or existing obstruction in many cases.

PROXIMAL GASTRECTOMY OR MERENDINO PROCEDURE (PROXIMAL GASTRECTOMY AND JEJUNAL INTERPOSITION)

Appraise

■ Fit patients with early (T1) cancer of the cardia or upper body of the stomach where a lymphadenectomy is not required are suitable candidates for this procedure.

■ Ensure that staging is accurate (including endoscopic ultrasound).

■ This is not a lesser procedure for patients thought to be unfit for a total gastrectomy.

Action

1. Access is through an upper midline or a roof top incision.

2. Examine the stomach and its related nodes. If there is a suspicion the tumour stage is greater than T1 or that there is nodal involvement then a D2 total gastrectomy should be performed.

3. After performing a thorough inspection to exclude metastases as with previously described resections, start by mobilizing the proximal stomach. Open a window in the gastrocolic ligament and use a device such an ultrasonic dissector to coagulate and divide the left gastroepiploic and short gastric arteries. You must preserve the right gastroepiploic artery as this will be the main supply to the stomach remnant.

4. Once at the diaphragm, divide the peritoneum over the crura and clear the abdominal part of the oesophagus.

5. Ask your assistant to lift the stomach anteriorly to stretch the left gastric vessels and double ligate then divide these as described previously.

6. Divide the lesser omentum at the edge of the liver from the level of the left gastric vessels to the diaphragm.

7. If performing a proximal gastrectomy (Fig. 10.30), proceed to the oesophago-jejunal anastomosis as described below. (Unite, point 3)

8. If performing a Merendino Procedure you will need a 15 cm length of jejunum to interpose between the oesophagus and the distal stomach. Divide the jejunum about 20 cm from the DJ flexure and then 15 cm beyond that using a linear stapler, preserving a cone of mesentery with the blood supply to this length. Create a window in the transverse mesocolon to allow the jejunum through.

Unite

1. Once you have satisfied yourself that the jejunal loop will sit comfortably between the oesophagus and distal stomach apply a stay suture through the wall of the oesophagus at least 2 cm from the gastro-oeosphageal junction and then divide the distal oesophagus. Allow at least 2 cm clearance from the tumour in both directions.

2. Using a linear stapler, divide the stomach and remove the specimen.

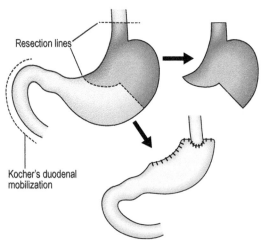

Resection lines

Kocher's duodenal mobilization

Fig. 10.30   Upper partial gastrectomy.

3. Perform either a handsewn or stapled oesophago-jejunal anastomosis. If stapled, use a circular device as described earlier for total gastrectomy.

4. The jejuno-gastric anastomosis is easily hand sewn using two layers of a continuous absorbable suture.

5. Use a linear stapler to perform the side-to-side jejuno-jejunal anastomosis and close the enterotomy with a continuous absorbable suture.

6. Finally, check the transverse mesocolon and mesenteric windows will not allow any internal herniation and close these if necessary.

Postoperative

1. Close the incision in the routine fashion.

2. Ensure good analgesia, early mobilization and chest physiotherapy.

3. Introduce nutrition as you would for a total gastrectomy.

> ▶ **KEY POINTS** Guard against mesenteric tension or twisting
>
> ■ Ensure against twisting the jejunal graft when you pass it through the transverse mesocolon.
> ■ Once the jejunal ends are connected to each other the jejunal graft and its mesentery should not be under any tension.

PALLIATIVE PARTIAL GASTRECTOMY

Appraise

For distal gastric carcinomas associated with metastases outside the scope of radical surgery, distal gastrectomy may still offer good palliation. However, the proximal cut edge should be well clear of growth or the stoma will either leak or subsequently obstruct from recurrent growth. However, if the tumour is very extensive it may be more damaging to perform gastrectomy than to leave the patient alone.

Action

1. Perform the gastrectomy in the same manner as for benign disease. Make sure that the line of proximal section is at least 5–7 cm above detectable disease.

2. Close the duodenal stump; bring up a proximal loop of jejunum and create a full-width stoma to guard as far as possible against stomal obstruction if the carcinoma recurs. Alternatively use a Roux-en-Y reconstruction.

GASTROENTEROSTOMY

Appraise

■ If a distal growth is extensive and cannot be resected or if there are gross metastases, relieve existing or impending obstruction in the pyloric region by creating a proximal gastroenterostomy.

■ Bypass may offer as good palliation and disturb the patient less than a resection that cuts through tumour.

Action

1 The procedure may be performed either laparoscopically or at open surgery.

2 Reach below the transverse mesocolon and draw up the proximal jejunum, selecting the first loop that will reach easily to the upper stomach.

3 If a laparoscopic approach is used, select a long laparoscopic linear stapler. Put a stay suture through the jejunal loop and ask an assistant to hold the suture. This will aid you, once you have made the enterotomy and gastrotomy, to place the ends of the stapler into each opening. Close the remaining defect either with another linear stapler or using an absorbable suture.

4 The same principle applies to the open approach. Create a high, wide stoma between the upper anterior gastric wall and the jejunum. Use twin gastroenterostomy clamps only if they facilitate the procedure.

CARDIAC OBSTRUCTION

Appraise

1 An inoperable proximal carcinoma that obstructs the cardia offers a challenge. If nothing is done the patient will starve to death.

2 An oesophagus narrowed by a tumour can be opened using laser, gently dilated and a stent placed either endoscopically or under radiological control.

3 Occasionally, it is valuable to insinuate a nasogastric tube through into the stomach for feeding purposes before trying the effect of radiation therapy. In some patients this may result in dramatic shrinkage of the tumour and relief of the obstruction.

4 Many surgeons deprecate the use of a feeding gastrostomy in patients with terminal disease.

GASTRIC LYMPHOMA

- Most lymphomas are generalized nodal disease, affecting the stomach secondarily. Primary gastric lymphoma is a non-Hodgkin's B-cell lymphoma characterized by the absence of peripheral node enlargement, mediastinal gland enlargement on chest X-ray, or liver and spleen enlargement. In addition, there is no bone marrow evidence of leukaemia. Some tumours that appear to be neoplastic run a benign course and are labelled pseudolymphomas. They may represent reactive hyperplasia.

- Both symptomatically and at endoscopy, primary gastric lymphoma often resembles adenocarcinoma. There may be a mass, a plaque, sessile or pedunculated polyps, or infiltration resembling linitis plastica. Ulcers are irregular and dendritic, sometimes with raised edges, sometimes multiple. The rugae tend to be hypertrophic. The condition can be multicentric. Since the lesions are essentially in the submucosa, the best diagnostic method is deep biopsy.

- Staging is by clinical, endoscopic, ultrasound and CT scanning.

- The best method of treatment is a combination of chemotherapy and radiotherapy.

BENIGN AND NON-EPITHELIAL TUMOURS

- Polyps may be regenerative, hyperplastic or adenomatous. Employ endoscopic biopsy, snare and diathermy to establish the diagnosis.

- Leiomyomas and leiomyosarcomas are difficult to distinguish histologically. Excise lesions with a clear margin of healthy gastric wall. For larger and doubtful lesions carry out an appropriate gastric resection.

- Fibrosarcoma, angiosarcoma, Kaposi's sarcoma and haemangiopericytoma are rare in the stomach.

GASTROINTESTINAL STROMAL TUMOURS

- These are tumours of mesenchymal origin and are recognized by the presence of proteins expressed in gastrointestinal stromal tumours (GISTs) called DOG-1 (discovered on GIST-1) and CD117.

- Histopathological diagnosis often needs EUS directed biopsy as the tumour is submucosal.

- Surgery is the mainstay of therapy for non-metastatic GISTs. These tumours rarely spread to lymph nodes and a local resection is all that is required. It is important not to burst the tumour during the resection as this increases the risk of early recurrence. A laparoscopic approach is often employed but tumours in the posterior wall of the stomach are difficult to reach and open access may be better.

- Tyrosine kinase inhibitors play a role in the management of large and metastatic GISTs.

- The risk of recurrence of GISTs is dependent on three variables: location in the GI tract, size and mitotic rate.

ZOLLINGER-ELLISON SYNDROME

Appraise

1 The classic syndrome consists of severe and sometimes intractable peptic ulcer developing as a rule in expected sites but sometimes distally in the duodenum and proximal jejunum, associated with gastric acid hypersecretion of marked degree.

2 Exclude it in all patients developing recurrence following surgical treatment of duodenal ulcer. The ulcers may be multiple. There may be diarrhoea, usually attributed to irritability of the bowel from contact with its high acid content. The syndrome is caused by a gastrin-secreting tumour of the pancreatic islets which may be benign or malignant, or there may be hyperplasia without tumour formation (see Chapter 16). The serum gastrin is raised and appears to act as a trophic hormone acting on gastric parietal cells which undergo hyperplasia. The gastric fundic mucosa appears hypertrophied and extends almost to the pylorus, hypersecreting acid in response to the hypergastrinaemia at basal rates approaching maximal acid output. Zollinger-Ellison syndrome is part of a multiple endocrine neoplastic (MEN) syndrome in a quarter of cases, the parathyroid glands being particularly frequently

involved. The features of hypergastrinaemia are reproduced in the absence of a pancreatic tumour when the antrum is congenitally duplicated and when it is sequestered in an alkaline medium.

3 Suspect the diagnosis when duodenal ulcer does not respond as expected to medical treatment; or is multiple; or ulcers occur in the stomach, distal duodenum and upper jejunum or in unexpected areas of the stomach such as the greater curvature. The suspicion is confirmed when very high basal levels of acid output are measured and maximal pentagastrin stimulation has little or no added effect. Serum gastrin is raised. In case of doubt, carry out calcium stimulation test (5 mg/kg/hour infused for 3 hours) or a secretin challenge (4 units/kg intravenously). These cause a sharp release of gastrin from tumours. Search for other endocrine abnormalities, particularly of the parathyroid glands.

4 Total gastrectomy was previously advocated but should now be reserved only for those who fail to respond to adequate treatment with H_2-receptor-blocking drugs, omeprazole or somatostatin analogues.

5 After employing scanning techniques to exclude metastases, and angiography to try to localize the tumour, plan to explore the abdomen and carefully examine the pancreas, duodenum, stomach, liver and remainder of the abdomen, searching for single or multiple tumours and metastasis. Debulking of metastases is worthwhile. If a solitary tumour is found in the head of the pancreas in the absence of metastases, enucleate it. If a tumour is found in the body or tail of the pancreas, excise the body and tail. If no tumour is found in the pancreas, duodenum or elsewhere, excise the body and tail of the pancreas for histological exclusion of hyperplasia.

FURTHER READING

Akiyama H. Thoracoabdominal approach for carcinoma of the cardia of the stomach. Am J Surg 1979;137:345–9.

Allum WH, Griffin SM, Watson A, et al., the Association of Upper Gastrointestinal Surgeons of Great Britain and Ireland, the British Society of Gastroenterology, and the British Association of Surgical Oncology. Guidelines for the management of oesophageal and gastric cancer. Gut 2002;50(Suppl V):v1–v23.

Barkun A. *Helicobacter pylori* eradication prevents ulcer recurrence after simple closure of duodenal ulcer perforation. Evidence-Based Gastroenterology 2001;2:6–8.

Bell GD, McCloy RF, Charlton JE, et al. Recommendations for standards of sedation and patient monitoring during gastrointestinal endoscopy. Gut 1991;32:823–7.

Higham J, Kang J-Y, Majeed A. Recent trends in admissions and mortality due to peptic ulcer in England: increasing frequency of haemorrhage among older subjects. Gut 2002;50:460–4.

Imamura H, Kurokawa Y, Kawada J, et al. Influence of bursectomy on operative morbidity and mortality after radical gastrectomy for gastric cancer: results of a randomized controlled trial. World J Surg 2011;35 (3):625–30.

Kodera Y, Fujiwara M, Ohashi N, et al. Laparoscopic surgery for gastric cancer: a collective review with meta-analysis of randomized trials. J Am Coll Surg 2010;211(5):677–86.

McCulloch P. The role of surgery in patients with advanced gastric cancer. Best Pract Res Clin Gastroenterology 2006;20(4):767–87.

Rabine JC, Barnett JL. Management of the patient with gastroparesis. J Clin Gastroenterol 2001;32:11–8.

Sasako M. Principles of treatment of curable gastric cancer. J Clin Oncol 2003;21(Suppl. 23):2745–55.

So JBY, Yam A, Cheah WK, et al. Risk factors related to operative mortality and morbidity in patients undergoing emergency gastrectomy. Br J Surg 2000;87:1702–7.

Thorban S, Bottcher K, Etter M, et al. Prognostic factors in stump carcinoma. Ann Surg 2000;231:188–94.

Small bowel and operations for obesity

D.E. Whitelaw, V. Sujendran

CONTENTS

▶ KEY POINTS What is normal?

- Take every opportunity to see and feel normal bowel.
- You can determine what is abnormal only by knowing the limits of normality.
- You can determine the limits of normality by taking every opportunity to examine normal bowel.

Abnormalities

1   *Diverticula.* These are common. Meckel's diverticulum, which arises from the distal ileum, is considered below. Acquired diverticula may affect the duodenum, jejunum and to a lesser extent the ileum, and are frequently multiple. Do not remove incidental diverticula unless they are inflamed, bleeding or appear diseased.

2   *Inflammation.* Crohn's disease may affect any part of the alimentary tract but especially the terminal ileum. Affected segments of bowel are inflamed, thickened and narrowed, and often covered with fibrinous exudate. The mesentery is thickened and the mesenteric fat often extends over the serosa of the bowel towards the anti-mesenteric border (fat wrapping). Adjacent lymph nodes are often enlarged. Look for evidence of disease elsewhere in the small and large bowel. Segmental resection is often required for chronic Crohn's enteritis. Tuberculous and Yersinial infection can produce similar changes of ileitis; if in doubt remove a lymph node for bacteriological and histological examination. Coeliac disease predominantly affects the jejunum. The diagnosis is indicated by dilatation of subserous and mesenteric lymphatics, thinning and pigmentation of the bowel wall and splenic atrophy. Severe refractory coeliac disease may cause ulcerative jejunitis and predispose to small bowel lymphoma.[1] Full-thickness biopsy is usually required to make this diagnosis (see below). Small-bowel ulcers and strictures may occur spontaneously, follow radiotherapy or transient strangulation in an external hernia or after the ingestion of potassium tablets.

3   *Infarction.* The viability of the small bowel must be carefully checked after reduction of a strangulated hernia or untwisting of a volvulus in adhesional obstruction. Any frankly necrotic or perforated loops should be excised. If you are in doubt about the viability of a dusky segment, return it to the abdomen and wait for 5 minutes (timed by the clock). The return of a shiny, pink appearance, pulsation of the mesenteric vessels and peristalsis across the affected segment indicate viability. If doubt persists, resect.

EXAMINATION OF THE SMALL BOWEL

Normal appearance

1   The duodenum [From Greek: *duodekadaktulon* = 12 fingers (breadth)] is 25 cm long. Apart from the proximal 2–3 cm, it is retroperitoneal. The remaining small bowel, which has a mesentery, is variable in total length (about 3–5 m) and difficult to measure with accuracy in vivo. It is arbitrarily divided into a proximal 40%, the jejunum (Latin: *jejunus* = hungry, empty), and a distal 60%, the ileum (Greek: *eilios* = twisted). On palpation the jejunal wall is thicker than that of the ileum, so that the examining fingers gain the impression of a double layer, rather like feeling a shirt through the sleeve of a jacket.

2   Examine the duodenal loop. Locate the duodenojejunal flexure by displacing the transverse colon upwards and tracing the coils of jejunum proximally to the ligament of Treitz. Pick up the small bowel at the duodenojejunal flexure and feed it through your fingers down to the ileocaecal valve. Note the diameter and contents of the bowel and the thickness and colour of its wall.

3   Examine the small-bowel mesentery throughout. Its thickness varies with the patient's adiposity. In a thin patient mesenteric lymph nodes can often be seen: determine whether the nodes are enlarged or inflamed.

4 *Tumours.* Serosal deposits occur in carcinomatosis peritonei and may cause kinking and obstruction of the small bowel, requiring side-to-side bypass (see below). Primary neoplasms are less common. Benign tumours such as adenoma, leiomyoma, lipoma and Peutz-Jeghers hamartomas can cause intussusception. Carcinoid tumours favour the ileum, but may be multiple and metastasizing; they are hard with a yellowish cut surface. Other malignant tumours comprise adenocarcinoma, lymphoma and leiomyosarcoma in that order of prevalence. Primary neoplasms should be resected or, if unresectable, bypassed and biopsied.

Biopsy

1 Duodenal lesions can be biopsied endoscopically under direct vision.

2 The small intestine can be examined using flexible endoscopy or capsule endoscopy. Capsule endoscopy is now widely used clinically, complementing other enteroscopic techniques.[1] It employs a capsule containing a digital camera with a radio transmitter, an external receiving antenna and a computer workstation for review of images. The technique is increasingly used for the diagnosis of obscure gastrointestinal bleeding, iron-deficiency anaemia and Crohn's disease.[2,3] Biopsy of any identified abnormalities, on the other hand, requires small bowel enteroscopy.

3 Operative biopsy of the small intestine is seldom indicated. It is usually possible to excise the segment of bowel in question, and intestinal biopsy should be avoided in Crohn's disease. If a full-thickness biopsy is required, however, the incision should be closed in two layers in the same fashion as an intestinal anastomosis.

4 Mesenteric lymph nodes can be biopsied with relative ease, either laparoscopically or at open surgery. Where possible, select a node close to the bowel wall and avoid dissecting deep into the root of the mesentery. Carefully incise the peritoneum and dissect out the entire node, using diathermy to coagulate small blood vessels.

REFERENCES

1. Rubio-Tapia A, Murray JA. Classification and management of refractory coeliac disease. Gut 2010;59(4):547–57.
2. Liao Z, Gao R, Xu C, et al. 2010 Indications and detection, completion, and retention rates of small-bowel capsule endoscopy: a systematic review. Gastrointest Endosc 2010;71(2):280–6.
3. Maieron A, Hubner D, Blaha B, et al. Multicenter retrospective evaluation of capsule endoscopy in clinical routine. Endoscopy 2004;36:864–8.

INTESTINAL ANASTOMOSIS

General principles

1 Several hundred intestinal anastomoses are carried out each week in Britain, and the vast majority heal rapidly by primary intention.

2 Remember that most of the intestinal tract is contaminated with bacteria. Take appropriate precautions against disseminating faecal organisms before dividing and re-suturing the bowel; clamps are usually indicated to prevent spillage of faeces or small bowel contents.

3 Ensure that the bowel ends are pink and bleeding freely, and leave the mesentery attached to the bowel right up to the point of intestinal transection. If either cut end is bruised or dusky, it is usually sensible to sacrifice a few more centimetres of intestine, even if, in the case of the large bowel, this requires further mobilization.

4 Tension usually results from inadequate mobilization, especially of the colon. Though readily avoidable, twisting of the mesentery can also render an anastomosis ischaemic. Repair mesenteric/mesocolic defects after completing an intestinal anastomosis to prevent postoperative internal herniation, but take care not to compromise the vessels supplying the bowel ends.

5 Distended loops of bowel are heavy and difficult to handle. Moreover, healing is impaired because the bowel wall is somewhat ischaemic. Distended small bowel may be decompressed by milking contents upwards into the reach of the nasogastric tube or by enterotomy and insertion of a sucker (see below). Gaseous distension of the large bowel can be relieved by introducing a needle obliquely through its wall.

▶ KEY POINT A safe small-bowel anastomosis

■ The key to a successful anastomosis is the accurate union of two viable bowel ends with complete avoidance of tension.

Hand-suturing techniques

1 Traditionally, bowel is united in two layers, using absorbable suture material such as polyglactin 910 (Vicryl) for the inner, all-coats layers and an outer stitch, named after its inventor in 1826, the Parisian surgeon Antoine Lembert (1802–1851), to join the seromuscular layers. More recently, one-layered anastomoses have gained popularity and have proved safe. They are used in colorectal, small bowel and bilio-enteric anastomoses and in oesophago-jejunostomy.

2 Surgeons have long disputed the best suture material, the best type of stitch and the best methods of fashioning a suture line. These technical points are less important than the principle stated above: to achieve accurate and tension-free coaptation of two healthy mucosal surfaces. Nevertheless, each surgeon develops his own variations of technique which he believes to be the most appropriate. As an assistant, therefore, follow the method of your present chief and aim to experience a number of methods before you select one for yourself.

3 Surgical trainees are often uncertain whether to use continuous or interrupted sutures in a given situation. A continuous (running) stitch is undoubtedly quicker and it achieves good haemostasis. It can be used for straightforward gastric, enteric and colonic anastomoses.

4 Interrupted sutures allow greater precision and may be more convenient than a continuous stitch when there is marked disparity in the size of the bowel ends to be united or the anastomosis is technically difficult. In inaccessible situations, such as a colorectal anastomosis deep in the pelvis or hepaticojejunostomy, it may be wise to insert the entire posterior row of interrupted sutures before trying any individual stitch.

5 Many surgeons routinely use two layers of continuous absorbable sutures for gastric and intestinal anastomoses. If impaired

healing is anticipated, as in Crohn's disease, an inner layer of continuous Vicryl and an outer layer of interrupted 2/0 polyester (Ethibond) or similar non-absorbable suture may provide additional security. Non-absorbable sutures are often also used when joining small bowel to the oesophagus, pancreas or rectum.

6 Whichever type of suture and suture material you employ, take care to achieve the correct degree of tension when pulling through and tying the stitch. Insert each stitch separately and invert the bowel edges as the suture is tightened. Once the bowel edge is inverted, prevent the suture material from slipping by getting your assistant to 'follow', keeping the tension on the suture already placed. Alternatively, follow for yourself, using the taut suture as a means of steadying the bowel against the thrust of the needle. The objective is a snug, watertight anastomosis. Excessive tension risks strangulating the bowel incorporated in the stitch and perhaps causing subsequent leakage.

7 Do not place the sutures so close to the edge of the bowel that they might tear out or so deep that they turn in an enormous cuff of tissue and narrow the bowel: usually 3–5 mm is about the correct depth of 'bite'. Be sure that the all-coats suture does in fact incorporate all coats of the bowel wall. The best way to master these important technical points is to assist at, and then perform under supervision, a number of intestinal anastomoses.

8 The seromuscular stitch unites the adjacent bowel walls outside the all-coats stitch. Sometimes the posterior seromuscular layer is inserted before opening the gut, as in side-to-side anastomoses (Fig. 11.1). After the all-coats stitches have been inserted, carry the seromuscular sutures round the ends of the anastomosis and across the front wall, ultimately encircling the anastomosis so that the all-coats stitches can no longer be seen. For end-to-end anastomoses in small and large intestine it may be simpler to complete the all-coats layer before placing any Lembert sutures. Thereafter, the seromuscular layer can be inserted all the way round by rotating the bowel.

9 There are many ways of inserting the all-coats stitch; two popular methods are described here:

■ *Continuous over-and-over suture.* Approximate the two edges of cut bowel. Starting at one end, insert a corner stitch from outside to in, then over the adjacent edges of bowel and out through the other corner. Tie the suture and clip the short end. Pass the stitch back through the nearest bowel wall, over the contiguous cut edges and back through the full thickness of both walls. Continue over-and-over stitches to the opposite corner (Fig. 11.2A). After the last stitch is inserted right into the

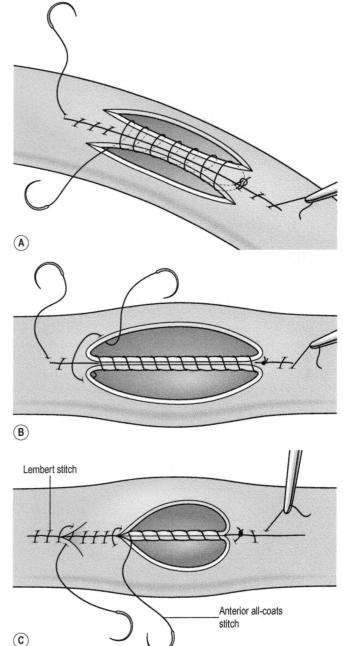

Lembert stitch

Anterior all-coats stitch

Fig. 11.2 Continuous over-and-over stitch. (A) The all-coats stitch is being inserted in a continuous over-and-over fashion. Care is taken to include mucosa and muscularis in each bite. (B) The all-coats stitch is continued round the corner. A single loop-on-the-mucosa stitch starts the return over-and-over stitch. (C) The anterior all-coats stitch is continued then the anterior seromuscular stitch completes the anastomosis.

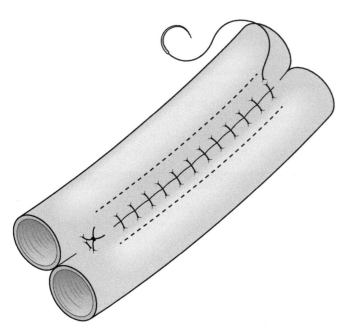

Fig. 11.1 A continuous layer of posterior seromuscular sutures has been inserted before fashioning a side-to-side anastomosis. The dotted lines indicate the lines of incision of the bowel.

corner, take it back through the nearest corner leaving a loop on the mucosa so that the stitch emerges from the outer wall of the bowel (Fig. 11.2B). Now sew the front walls together by passing the stitch over and over, from out to in and then from in to out (Fig. 11.2C). Continue until the anastomosis has been encircled and the edges inverted, then tie off the ends of suture material. This over-and-over stitch is haemostatic.

■ Continuous *over-and-over plus Connell suture*. Commence in the middle of the posterior wall by placing a stitch between the adjacent cut edges of bowel and tying it on the luminal surface. Now continue towards one corner with over-and-over stitches. At the corner the needle passes from in to out on the nearside cut surface, then crosses to the far edge and is passed in and out to leave a loop on the mucosa (Fig. 11.3). The needle returns to the near edge and another loop-on-the-mucosa stitch (named after the American surgeon Gregory Connell born 1875, who popularized it) is inserted. These Connell stitches turn the corner neatly. Once you are round the corner, leave this stitch and return to the middle of the posterior wall. Use a new length of suture material, unless there is a needle at each end of the original length. Insert and tie a stitch close to the site of the original knot, and proceed towards the opposite corner, using Connell sutures to negotiate the corner again. Once round the corner, return to over-and-over stitches. Tie the ends of suture material together where they meet in the middle of the anterior wall.

Mechanical stapling techniques

1 Stapling devices can be used to carry out most types of gastrointestinal anastomoses. Disposable and angled instruments are available for use in particular circumstances, and the metal staples come in different lengths to accommodate the different tissue thicknesses encountered. For end-to-end anastomosis (e.g. colorectal, oesophagojejunal) a circular stapling gun (Fig. 11.4A) is introduced into the intestinal lumen downstream, brought out through the distal cut end of bowel and then insinuated into the proximal cut end.

Choose the largest anvil that will fit comfortably into the proximal lumen. Tightly snug the proximal and distal gut around

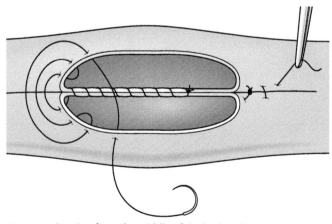

Fig. 11.3 Starting from the middle of the back wall, an over-and-over stitch has been inserted as far as the corner. Two or three Connell stitches are placed to turn the corner, followed by an anterior over-and-over stitch. A separate suture is used to fashion the other half of the anastomosis.

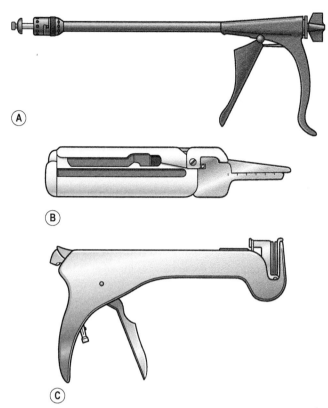

Fig. 11.4 Auto Suture instruments used for gastrointestinal anastomosis: (A) model EEA is for end-to-side anastomosis; (B) model GIA is for side-to-side anastomosis; (C) model TA30 is for closing off the end of the bowel.

the central rod using a polypropylene purse-string suture, and then approximate the anvil to the cartridge by closing the instrument. When the gun is fired, a circular double row of titanium staples is inserted and at the same time a complete 5-mm rim of each bowel end (the 'doughnut') is resected. Withdraw the machine and check the 'doughnuts' to confirm that they are complete and that the anastomosis is perfect.

2 For side-to-side anastomoses a different instrument called a linear stapler/cutter is used. It resembles a pair of scissors (Fig. 11.4B). One 'blade' is inserted into each of the two intestinal segments to be united, and the blades are closed. Firing the gun advances a knife, which divides the adjacent surfaces of bowel between three parallel rows of staples.

The resulting opening can then either be sutured or stapled closed using a further staple cartridge.

> ### ▶ KEY POINTS Stapled anastomosis
>
> ■ Using a mechanical stapler does not guarantee a perfect result. It is just as important to prepare healthy bowel ends and avoid tension as it is in hand-sewn anastomoses.
> ■ Stapling devices require less fine manual dexterity than suturing, so as a trainee take every opportunity to practice perfect stitching.

3 Stapling devices reduce the time involved in creating an anastomosis and are used extensively in laparoscopic bariatric and oesophago-gastric surgery.

Types of anastomosis

End-to-end anastomosis

1. This is the simplest way of restoring intestinal continuity after partial enterectomy where there is little or no size disparity. After removal of the resected specimen, clean and approximate the bowel ends. The anastomosis is usually created in one layer, using interrupted absorbable sutures (e.g. 2/0 or 3/0 Vicryl).

    Interrupted sero-muscular suture. Insert three stay sutures from out to in and in to out evenly spaced around the bowel circumference. Clip the ends and get your assistant to hold the clips to exert traction on the cut edges of bowel. This causes the bowel lumen to adopt a triangular appearance (Fig. 11.5). Between two of the stay sutures, held taught, insert a row of sutures 2–3 mm apart, taking serosa and muscularis only and tying the knots on the serosal surface.

2. Now rotate the anastomosis using the stays and place a further row of sutures between the next adjacent stay sutures. Finally turn the anastomosis over and suture the third side of the triangle. All knots should lie uniformly on the outside of the anastomosis.

Oblique anastomosis

1. When the ends of bowel are disproportionate in size, they may be matched by incising the antimesenteric border of the narrow bowel longitudinally (Fig. 11.6A).

2. This manoeuvre is useful in joining obstructed bowel to collapsed bowel or ileum to colon. In neonates with congenital intestinal atresia, the lumen of the distal bowel is particularly narrow and this type of 'end-to-back' anastomosis is necessitated. When two segments of narrow intestine must be united, they may both be opened along their antimesenteric borders, which are then joined back-to-back (Fig. 11.6B). The mesenteries are now on opposite sides of the anastomosis and cannot always be neatly approximated.

End-to-side anastomosis

1. This is most commonly used when creating a Roux-en-Y anastomosis. Approximate the cut end to the side of bowel to which it

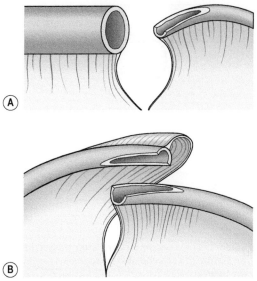

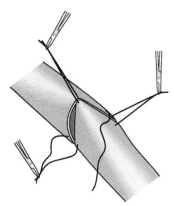

Fig. 11.5 **End-to-end anastomosis using interrupted sutures.** Two of the three corner stitches are held taught and interrupted sero-muscular sutures are placed between them with the knots on the outside. The anastomosis is turned over and the process repeated for all three sides. The stay sutures are then tied.

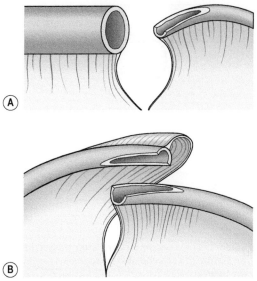

Fig. 11.6 **End-to-end intestinal anastomosis:** (A) and (B) two layers of stitches being inserted.

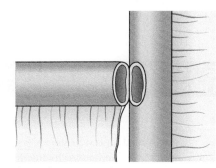

Fig. 11.7 **End-to-side anastomosis.**

will be joined and insert a posterior seromuscular suture (Fig. 11.7).

2. Incise the antimesenteric border of the side of bowel to accommodate the cut end. Insert the all-coats stitch as before, remove the clamps and complete the seromuscular stitch. Lastly, join the cut edge of mesentery to the side of the intact mesentery.

Side-to-side anastomosis

1. This can be used to joint two loops of bowel without resection, or to unite intestine to stomach, bile duct, etc. (Fig. 11.8).

2. It may also be employed as an alternative to end-to-end anastomosis after intestinal resection, in which case the cut ends of bowel should first be closed and invaginated. The advantages of the side-to-side anastomosis are that the segments of bowel to be united have no interruption to their blood supply at all and that the incisions can be made exactly congruous. The disadvantages are that there are more suture lines involved and that there may be some degree of stasis and bacterial overgrowth.

3. Lay the segments to be joined side by side in contact for 8–10 cm and insert a posterior seromuscular stitch. Incise the antimesenteric borders for about 5 cm and insert an all-coats stitch. Remove

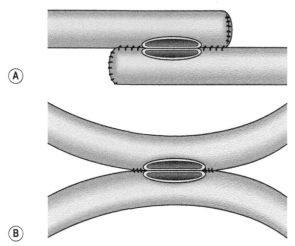

Fig. 11.8 Side-to-side anastomoses: (A) after transection of the bowel, with closure of each end; (B) two segments are joined without dividing the bowel.

the clamps and complete the anterior seromuscular layer of stitches. When side-to-side anastomosis follows bowel resection, suture the cut edge of mesentery to the adjacent intact mesentery on each side of the anastomosis.

ENTERECTOMY (SMALL-BOWEL RESECTION)

Appraise

1 Resection is often indicated for congenital lesions of the small bowel such as atresia and duplication; traumatic perforation; critical ischaemia from mesenteric trauma, strangulation or arteriosclerosis; Crohn's disease or other cause of stricture; tumours of the bowel or its mesentery. Resection is sometimes indicated for fistula, diverticulitis, intussusception and a symptomatic blind loop. Small portions of the duodenum and ileum are removed during partial gastrectomy and right hemicolectomy respectively.

2 There are several reasons for being conservative in the management of Crohn's disease: the indolent nature of the disease, its relapsing course and its strong tendency (>50%) to recur anywhere in the intestinal tract, but especially at and just proximal to the anastomosis. Despite many advances in the treatment of Crohn's disease, the course of the disease in any given patient remains unpredictable. A multivariate analysis has shown that the only independent predictors of earlier postoperative recurrence after initial operation are an initial presentation with peritonitis secondary to perforation, and a longer preoperative disease duration.[1]

> ▶ KEY POINT Avoid unnecessary intestinal resection in Crohn's disease
>
> ■ Do not resect for Crohn's ileitis discovered incidentally during laparotomy for suspected appendicitis.

3 On the other hand, most patients with chronic Crohn's enteritis eventually require resection of the affected segment because of subacute obstruction, fistula or abscess. Bypass is obsolete: although it may achieve remission of active disease in the defunctioned segment, bacterial overgrowth of the blind loop may aggravate diarrhoea and there is a long-term risk of carcinoma. For short stenotic areas of bowel strictureplasty (see below) is an alternative to resection.

4 When operating for radiation enteropathy, establish the extent both of the original cancer and of the radiation damage. Where possible, avoid bypass or exclusion procedures: the defunctioned bowel may still give rise to problems such as bleeding and fistula. Wide resection is the optimal approach, ensuring that at least one side of the subsequent anastomosis employs healthy, non-irradiated, bowel.

Prepare

1 In the presence of an obstructing lesion, ensure that the patient is adequately resuscitated before operation with nasogastric intubation and intravenous rehydration.

2 Healthy ileum has a resident bacterial flora, and in the presence of obstruction the entire small bowel may be colonized. It is sensible to employ appropriate prophylactic antibiotic cover, such as a cephalosporin plus metronidazole given preoperatively in a single injection, in all operations likely to involve intestinal resection.

3 Nutritional status may be impaired in some patients requiring small-bowel resection, for example those with Crohn's disease, cancer, radiation enteropathy or enterocutaneous fistula. In the absence or obstruction or fistula, supplemental enteric feeds may reverse the nutritional defect, but some patients require a period of preoperative parenteral nutrition.

Access

1 Employ a midline incision that skirts the umbilicus and can be extended in either direction as necessary.

2 Remember that the small bowel quite often adheres to the back of a previous laparotomy incision, so take particular care during abdominal re-entry. An accidental perforation is unlikely to be located in a segment of bowel you intended to remove.

Assess

1 Expose and examine the entire small bowel. Continue by examining the stomach, large bowel and remaining abdominal viscera.

2 If a loop of small bowel has been strangulated in an external hernia, release the obstruction and check the viability of the bowel after allowing a period of 5 minutes for possible recovery in doubtful cases.

3 Do not gratuitously sacrifice healthy bowel, particularly terminal ileum which has specialized transport functions. Except when operating for primary malignant tumours it is quite unnecessary to excise a deep wedge of mesentery, which might increase the extent of small bowel requiring removal. In Crohn's disease do not remove more than a few centimetres of gut on either side of the affected segment, but include any fistulas or sinuses. It is more than likely that further resection will be required in future, and microscopic inflammation of the bowel at the resection margin does not appear to increase subsequent anastomotic recurrence.

Formal right hemicolectomy is unnecessary for Crohn's disease of the terminal ileum; undertake a limited ileocaecal resection.

4   Sometimes a partial resection of small bowel can be performed, leaving the mesentery intact. Appropriate conditions include Richter's hernia, Meckel's diverticulum and small benign tumours arising on the antimesenteric border.

Action

1   Isolate the diseased loop of bowel from the other abdominal contents by means of large, moist packs or a special towel.

2   Hold up the bowel and examine the mesentery against the light. Note the vascular pattern.

Standard resection

1   Determine the proximal and distal sites for dividing the bowel, and select the line of vascular section in between; keep close to the bowel wall (Fig. 11.9) except when resecting a neoplasm (Fig. 11.10). Incise the peritoneum along this line on each aspect of the mesentery.

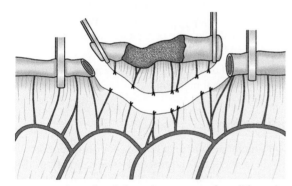

Fig. 11.9   Resection of an ischaemic segment of small bowel including a shallow wedge of mesentery. The narrower bowel end has been cut obliquely to match the wider end.

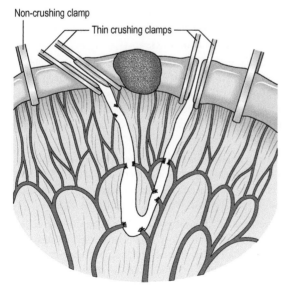

Non-crushing clamp

Thin crushing clamps

Fig. 11.10   Resection of a small-bowel tumour. A deeper wedge of mesentery is included than in operations for benign disease (see Fig. 11.9). As before, the narrower segment of bowel (on the left) is transected obliquely, removing more of the mesenteric border with the specimen.

This manoeuvre is most easily accomplished by inserting one blade of a pair of fine, curved scissors beneath the peritoneum and cutting superficially to expose the mesenteric vessels.

2   Using small artery forceps, create a small mesenteric window right next to the bowel wall at each point chosen for intestinal transection. Starting at one end, insinuate a curved artery forceps through this window and back through the mesentery, denuded of peritoneum, 1–2 cm away, thus isolating a small leash of mesentery with its contained vessels. Divide the vessels between artery forceps, ligating the mesentery beneath each pair of forceps using 2/0 or 3/0 Vicryl ties, according to the thickness of the mesentery. Proceeding in this manner, divide the mesentery right up to the bowel wall at the further end of the line of peritoneal incision. Take care in placing and tying each ligature: if the knot slips, there can be troublesome haemorrhage.

3   Apply four intestinal clamps (Fig. 11.9). The first two clamps are crushing clamps (Payr's, Lang Stevenson's or Pringle's). They should be applied obliquely at the points of intended intestinal transection, so that slightly more of the antimesenteric border is resected than of the mesenteric border; the obliquity reduces the risk of a tight anastomosis. Now apply a non-crushing clamp about 5 cm outside each crushing clamp, having milked the intervening bowel free of contents.

4   Place a clean gauze swab beneath the clamps at each end to catch spills, and divide the bowel with a knife flush against the outer aspect of each crushing clamp. Place the specimen and the soiled knife in a separate dish, which is then removed.

5   Cleanse each bowel end, using small swabs or pledgets of gauze soaked in 10% povidone-iodine. Then remove the protective gauze swab and proceed to intestinal anastomosis. In an attempt to limit contamination, some surgeons divide the intestine between two pairs of light crushing clamps (i.e. six clamps in all) and insert the posterior seromuscular layer of sutures before removing the outer clamps and excising the narrow rim of crushed tissue (Fig. 11.10).

6   Perform a single-layer, end-to-end anastomosis, as described in the previous section.

Partial resection

1   A diverticulum on the antimesenteric border may be locally excised. Clamp and cut it off at the neck, then close the defect in two layers as a transverse linear slit. Try to avoid narrowing the intestinal lumen during this procedure.

2   A diamond-shaped area of the antimesenteric border may be included in the resection of a localized tumour or wide-mouthed Meckel's diverticulum. Apply two light crushing clamps (Lang Stevenson's or Pringle's) across the antimesenteric border, meeting in a 'V' (Fig. 11.11). Incise the bowel flush with the outer aspect of each clamp, and close the wall in two layers, leaving a transverse suture line.

3   A similar defect results if the antimesenteric lesion is excised through a longitudinal ellipse. Approximate the ends of the ellipse, pull apart the sides and close transversely as before.

Checklist

1   Take a last look at the anastomosis. Check that the bowel is pink, that haemostasis is secure and that all mesenteric defects are closed.

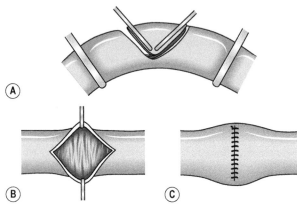

Fig. 11.11 Partial resection of small bowel: (A) a wedge of antimesenteric bowel is removed; (B) the defect is opened out transversely; (C) closure across the long axis of the bowel prevents narrowing.

> ▶ KEY POINTS Swabs

- It is easy to lose a swab among the coils of small intestine.
- Check the entire abdominal cavity and make sure that the swab count is correct.

2 Remove any ends of suture material that might provoke subsequent adhesions.

3 Replace the intestine and the greater omentum in their normal anatomical position.

4 Aspirate any blood or fluid from the peritoneal cavity using a pool sucker.

5 Drains are usually unnecessary following small bowel anastomoses.

? DIFFICULTY

1. *Is the bowel obstructed?* Decompress obstructed jejunum by milking the contents upwards until they can be aspirated through the nasogastric tube. The obstructed ileum may be decompressed prior to performing an anastomosis if the obstructed segment is being resected. If no bowel is being resected or anastomosed, do not open the bowel to attempt decompression,

2. In the presence of obstruction there may be marked disparity between the diameters of the bowel ends. In practice, moderate incongruities can be overcome by adjusting the size of suture bites while suturing proximal to distal bowel. The diameter of the distal bowel can be increased by transecting it more obliquely, sparing the mesenteric border, and by opening it along the antimesenteric border. If there is gross disparity, consider a side-to-side sutured or stapled anastomosis.

3. Resection and anastomosis can usually be completed outside the abdomen. Sometimes this is not possible, in which case you may not be able to apply all the clamps described above. Try to retain the non-crushing clamps placed at a distance from the anastomosis, if possible around all or most of the circumference.

4. *A haematoma develops in the mesentery or in the submucosa at the point of intestinal transection.* Compression of the area with a swab usually stops the bleeding. If the bleeding is not fully controlled, incise the peritoneum, find the bleeding point, pick it up with fine artery forceps and ligate it. Check the colour of the bowel to confirm that the blood supply is not prejudiced.

5. *One or other intestinal end becomes dusky during the anastomosis.* Allow time to be certain the anastomosis is ischaemic. Non-viable bowel will not heal; so if you are in any doubt excise a few more centimetres and start again.

Aftercare

1 Anticipate a period of postoperative paralytic ileus during which maintain the patient on intravenous fluids. Leave the nasogastric tube on free drainage, aspirated regularly for the first 24 hours. Allow water 30 ml/hour by mouth. The tube can usually be removed when the volume of aspirate drops below the volume of fluid taken by mouth.

2 If restoration of oral feeding is delayed for more than a few days, consider parenteral nutrition.

Complications

1 Good surgical technique in limiting contamination from bowel contents reduces the incidence of wound infection. If it does develop, remove sufficient sutures to allow the pus to drain, irrigate the wound, obtain bacteriological cultures and, if cellulitis is present, institute appropriate antibiotic therapy. Once the infection is controlled, the wound usually heals without the need for secondary suture.

2 As with any abdominal operation there is a risk of chest infection resulting from atelectasis. Institute vigorous physiotherapy to avert the need for antibiotics.

3 Occasionally a collection of infected material develops within the abdominal cavity. Abscess sites may be subphrenic, subhepatic, pelvic or adjacent to the anastomosis. The patient develops fever and leukocytosis; localize the collection with ultrasound or CT scans and radiologically place a percutaneous drain.

4 A leaking anastomosis often presents with pain, fever, tachycardia and erythema of the wound or drain site before intestinal contents begin to discharge. The management of an established small-bowel fistula is described later in this chapter.

5 It is occasionally necessary to undertake massive resection of the small bowel, for example when volvulus complicates an obstruction. Repeated enterectomies in Crohn's disease can similarly remove a substantial percentage of the small intestine. Increased frequency of bowel actions may follow loss of a third to a half of the small bowel, and more extensive resections produce short-bowel syndrome.[2] During the initial phase of recovery and adaptation, anticipate and replace losses of fluid and electrolytes, notably potassium. Give codeine or loperamide to control

diarrhoea. The body compensates better for proximal than distal enterectomy. After an extensive ileal resection regular injections of vitamin B_{12} may be needed indefinitely; cholestyramine may diminish the irritative diarrhoea that results from bile-acid malabsorption. A proton pump inhibitor is indicated to reduce gastric acid hypersecretion. Parenteral nutrition will be required in severe short-bowel syndrome.

REFERENCES

1. Bernell O, Lapidus A, Hellers G. Risk factors for surgery and postoperative recurrence in Crohn's disease. Ann Surg 2000;231:38–45.
2. Bristol JB, Williamson RCN. Postoperative adaptation of the small intestine. World J Surg 1985;9:825–32.

ENTERIC BYPASS

Appraise

1 Small-bowel loops may become obstructed as a result of carcinomatosis peritonei or particularly dense adhesions, sometimes deep in the pelvis. Irradiated small bowel may fistulate into other organs, such as the bladder or vagina. In these unfavourable circumstances it is often better just to bypass the affected segment of intestine (Fig. 11.12) rather than embark on a difficult and hazardous disentanglement. In radiation enteritis choose overtly normal bowel for the anastomosis, otherwise healing is likely to be impaired.

2 Resection is almost always a better option than bypass in Crohn's disease of the small bowel. For unresectable carcinoma of the caecum, however, side-to-side bypass is indicated between the terminal ileum and the transverse colon.

Action

Bypass of an unresectable lesion

1 A midline incision is usually appropriate. Aim to anastomose healthy bowel on either side of the diseased segment. Side-to-side anastomosis avoids the risk of closed-loop obstruction developing in a sequestered loop of bowel.

2 Occasionally, if there are multiple sites of actual or imminent obstruction, two or more side-to-side anastomoses between adjacent loops may cause less of a short circuit than one enormous bypass.

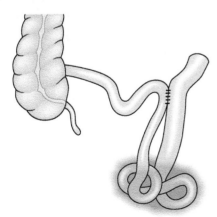

Fig. 11.12 Bypass procedure for small-bowel obstruction resulting from irresectable pelvic cancer. A side-to-side anastomosis is fashioned between a (proximal) distended loop of bowel and a (distal) collapsed loop.

3 Approximate a distended loop of proximal intestine to a collapsed loop of distal small bowel (Fig. 11.12) or transverse colon. Pack off the remaining viscera. Consider decompression of the obstructed loops.

4 Carry out a two-layer, side-to-side anastomosis, as previously described. Do not prolong the operation unnecessarily if the patient has advanced disease. A stapled side-to-side anastomosis is appropriate and quick in this situation.

Aftercare and complications

The principles of management are as for enterectomy. Short-bowel syndrome is inevitable after subtotal (about 90%) jejunoileal bypass, although adaptation can still be anticipated.

STRICTUREPLASTY

Appraise

1 This technique is virtually confined to patients with Crohn's disease causing one or more strictures in the small intestine.[1,2] It can avoid the need for resection and may therefore be appropriate for patients with disease at several sites or those with recurrent disease and a limited length of residual small bowel.

2 Florid inflammatory change or bowel containing several strictures within a relatively short segment is better treated by local resection. Sometimes you may combine one or more strictureplasties with resection to reduce the total length of bowel excised.

Assess

The tightness of the stricture(s) can be assessed by making a small enterotomy and passing a balloon catheter. Moderate strictures of 20–25 mm diameter may be treated by balloon dilatation, but tight strictures of less than 20 mm diameter require either strictureplasty or resection.

Action

1 Carry a longitudinal full-thickness incision across the stenotic area and for 1 cm into the 'normal' bowel on either side.

2 Close the bowel transversely, using either one or two layers of 3/0 Vicryl sutures. Test that the anastomosis is airtight and watertight.

3 This modification of the Heineke-Mikulicz pyloroplasty is suitable for short stenoses. For long stenoses, a modification of the Finney pyloroplasty can be performed, but local resection may be a simpler alternative.

Complications

1 Wound infections are uncommon.

2 Anastomotic leakage may occur, particularly if tight strictures distal to the strictureplasty are not treated.

3 Several studies have reported excellent symptomatic improvement following strictureplasty. Perioperative complication rates are comparable to standard surgical resection, with low rates of recurrent stricture.

4 It is of concern that small bowel adenocarcinoma has been reported at the site of a previous strictureplasty, so bear this possibility in mind if there is a sudden clinical deterioration.[3]

REFERENCES

1. Froehlich F, Juillerat P, Mottet C, et al. Obstructive fibrostenotic Crohn's disease. Digestion 2005;71(1):29–30.
2. Felley C, Vader JP, Juillerat P, et al. Appropriate therapy for fistulizing and fibrostenotic Crohn's disease: Results of a multidisciplinary expert panel. Journal of Crohns & Colitis 2009;3(4):250–6.
3. Jaskowiak NT, Michelassi F. Adenocarcinoma at a strictureplasty site in Crohn's disease: report of a case. Dis Colon Rectum 2001;44:284–7.

THE ROUX LOOP

Appraise

1 A defunctioned segment of jejunum provides a convenient conduit for connecting various upper abdominal organs to the remaining small bowel. The technique was originally described by the Swiss surgeon Cesar Roux in 1907 for oesophageal bypass.

> **KEY POINT** The versatile Roux loop

■ The method has proved invaluable in gastric, biliary and pancreatic surgery.[1] It can be used to bypass or replace the stomach or the distal bile duct and to drain the pancreatic duct or a pseudocyst.

2 Roux-en-Y anastomosis has two advantages over an intact loop: it can stretch further and it is empty of intestinal contents, thus preventing contamination of the organ to be drained, such as the bile duct. Active peristalsis down the loop encourages this drainage.[2]

3 Probably the commonest indications for Roux-en-Y anastomosis are biliary drainage in unresectable carcinoma of the pancreatic head and reconstruction after total gastrectomy (Fig. 11.13) or oesophagogastrectomy.

4 Isolated jejunal loops may be interposed between the stomach and duodenum in an isoperistaltic or antiperistaltic direction

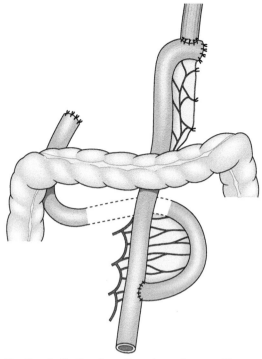

Fig. 11.13 One indication for a Roux loop: Roux-en-Y anastomosis between the oesophagus and jejunum after total gastrectomy.

for different facets of the postgastrectomy syndrome. A reversed loop can be used further downstream in certain cases of intractable diarrhoea (Fig. 11.14).

Action

1 Select a loop of proximal small bowel, beginning 10–15 cm distal to the ligament of Treitz. Hold up the jejunum and transilluminate its mesentery to display the precise blood supply, which varies from patient to patient. The number of vessels requiring division depends on the length of conduit required.

2 Starting at the point chosen for intestinal transection, incise the peritoneal leaves of the mesentery in a vertical direction

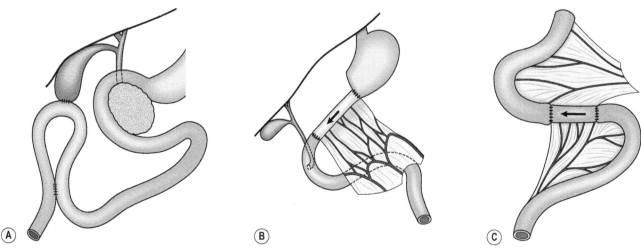

Fig. 11.14 Other types of enteric loop: (A) intact loop used to drain the distended gallbladder in a case of irresectable pancreatic cancer; side-to-side anastomosis below the cholecystojejunostomy may divert food away from the biliary tree; (B) isoperistaltic 20-cm jejunal loop interposed between the stomach remnant and the duodenum to treat reflux alkaline gastritis after partial gastrectomy; (C) reversed 10-cm loop inserted 1-m distal to the ligament of Treitz to treat severe postoperative diarrhoea.

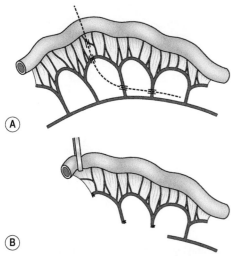

Fig. 11.15 Creation of a long Roux loop: (A) three arcade vessels have been divided; (B) the bowel is transected at a point previously selected and the loop is mobilized.

(Fig. 11.15). Divide at least one vascular arcade and the smaller branches that lie between the arcade vessels and the bowel. In laparoscopic cases, a harmonic scalpel may be used to divide the mesentery. Now divide the bowel between clamps.

3 If a longer loop is required, sacrifice two or three main jejunal vessels, preserving an intact blood supply to the extremity of the bowel via the arcades (Fig. 11.15). Individual ligation of the arteries and veins is recommended, using 3/0 vicryl sutures. Check the viability of the bowel at the tip of the loop, and sacrifice the end if it is dusky.

4 Straighten out the efferent limb and take it up by the shortest route for anastomosis to the oesophagus, stomach, bile duct, common hepatic duct or pancreatic duct. It is usually easier to close the end of the limb and fashion a new subterminal opening of the correct diameter. Make a window in the base of the transverse mesocolon, to the right of the duodenojejunal flexure, for passage of the Roux loop. At the end of the operation suture the margins of this defect to the Roux loop to prevent internal herniation.

5 Restore intestinal continuity by uniting the short afferent limb to the base of the long efferent limb, using a sutured end-to-side or stapled side-to-side anastomosis. Ensure that the efferent limb is at least 40 cm long and that the afferent loop is joined to its left-hand side.

REFERENCES

1. Allison PR, da Silva LT. The Roux loop. Br J Surg 1953;41:173–80.
2. Kirk RM. Roux-en-Y. World J Surg 1985;9:938–44.

ENTEROTOMY

APPRAISE

1 Enterotomy is sometimes needed to extract a foreign body, for example in gallstone ileus or bolus obstruction. After partial gastrectomy, the absence of the antropyloric mill means that whole orange segments or pith, for example, are inadequately broken up and may impact further down the gut. Benign mucosal or submucosal tumours may be explored and removed through an enterotomy incision.

2 Traumatic enterotomy can result from blunt or penetrating abdominal injuries. After a closed injury there is typically a rosette of exposed mucosa on the antimesenteric border of the upper jejunum. After knife or gunshot injuries, look for entry and exit wounds: holes in the small bowel nearly always come in multiples of two.

3 Occasionally, operative enteroscopy may be indicated for unexplained bleeding localized to the small bowel. A paediatric colonoscope or gastroscope can be introduced through a mid-enterotomy and threaded up and down the gut.

Action

Extraction enterotomy

1 It may be possible to knead a foreign body, especially a bolus of food, onwards into the caecum. If so, it will pass spontaneously per rectum. Do not persist with this manoeuvre if it is difficult.

2 Before opening the bowel, pack off the area carefully. Try and manipulate an impacted foreign body upwards for a few centimetres, away from the inflamed segment in which it was lodged.

3 Apply non-crushing clamps across the intestine on either side of the enterotomy site. Open the bowel longitudinally over the foreign body or tumour and gently extract or resect the lesion. Close the bowel transversely in two layers to prevent stenosis.

4 In gallstone ileus examine the right upper quadrant of the abdomen. It is rarely, if ever, appropriate to proceed to cholecystectomy and closure of the biliary-enteric fistula. Examine the rest of the small bowel to exclude a second gallstone.

Traumatic enterotomy

1 Excise devitalized tissue and close the intestinal wound(s) in two layers. Explore an associated haematoma in the mesentery and ligate any bleeding points. Check the viability of the bowel thereafter, and if in doubt resect the damaged segment with end-to-end anastomosis.

2 Examine the other abdominal viscera for concomitant injuries (see Chapter 3).

ENTEROSTOMY

Appraise

1 A feeding jejunostomy permits enteral nutrition in patients who are unable to take sufficient food by mouth.[1] Prefer feeding by the enteral route to parenteral nutrition if practicable. Before considering surgical jejunostomy, it may be possible to pass a fine-bore naso-gastric feeding tube through a malignant stricture under endoscopic control.

2 A feeding tube should be placed as high as possible in the jejunum. Even so, troublesome diarrhoea often occurs when feeding is commenced. Some surgeons use a feeding jejunostomy routinely after major oesophagogastric resections. Others reserve it for postoperative complications such as fistula, or serious upper gastrointestinal conditions such as corrosive oesophagogastritis or pancreatic abscess.

3 The ideal feeding jejunostomy is easily inserted, if necessary under local anaesthesia and seals off immediately it is removed. It

neither obstructs the bowel nor permits the escape of intestinal contents. It can be placed at laparotomy or laparoscopy via an enterotomy.

4 A terminal ileostomy replaces the anus after total colectomy for malignancy, ulcerative proctocolitis or Crohn's colitis. The ileostomy may be temporary, if subsequent ileorectal anastomosis is planned or permanent after panproctocolectomy. Improvements in stoma care make ileostomy less of a burden to patients, many of whom are young. It is desirable and usually possible to select and mark the site for ileostomy preoperatively. Choose a point just below waist level and 5 cm to the right of the midline, unless there is a previous scar in this region. It is important to create a spout that will discharge its irritative contents well clear of the skin.

5 Defunctioning loop ileostomy is used to defunction the distal colon after low anterior resection. In comparison with transverse colostomy, it produces predictable volumes of relatively inoffensive faecal effluent and is truly a defunctioning stoma to which an appliance can easily be attached. As a result it has become the temporary stoma of choice. Split ileostomy, with separated stomas, completely defunctions the distal bowel and has been advocated in selected cases of colitis. Split enterostomy has also been advocated to protect a lower enteric anastomosis created in the presence of peritonitis. The distal cut end is either exteriorized as a mucous fistula or oversewn and fixed to the parietal peritoneum to facilitate later retrieval. Kock's continent ileostomy is now rarely employed: it consists of an ileal reservoir discharging by a short conduit to a flush stoma; a nipple valve is created to preserve continence, and the patient empties the reservoir regularly with a soft catheter. Lastly, a 'wet' ileostomy together with an ileal conduit provides one of the commoner methods for achieving urinary diversion.

Action

Feeding jejunostomy

1 Expose the upper jejunum, either laparoscopically or through a small left upper quadrant transverse incision. Trace the bowel proximally to the duodenojejunal flexure. Select a loop 10–20 cm distal to this point, so that it will easily reach the anterior abdominal wall.

2 Insert a Vicryl purse-string suture on the antimesenteric border of the bowel. Make a tiny enterotomy in the centre of the purse-string and introduce a 9Fr feeding jejunostomy tube into the lumen of the bowel (Fig. 11.16). Tighten the purse-string snugly around the tube.

3 To exclude the enterotomy from the peritoneal cavity, suture the bowel to the parietal peritoneum at four points around the entry site of the tube.

Terminal ileostomy

▶ KEY POINT A durable ileostomy

■ Permanent ileostomies are prone to complications such as retraction, prolapse and parastomal hernia that require operative correction. Take extra care when fashioning an ileostomy to reduce the incidence of these problems.

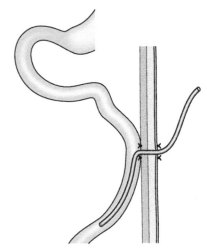

Fig. 11.16 Feeding jejunostomy. The 9Fr Feeding jejunostomy tube is brought out through the abdominal wall and the jejunum is stitched to the peritoneum around the tube.

1 Excise a circular disc of skin and subcutaneous fat, 3 cm in diameter, at the site chosen and marked preoperatively. Make a transverse incision in the exposed anterior rectus sheath, split the fibres of the rectus muscle and open the posterior sheath and peritoneum. The defect should comfortably accommodate two fingers.

2 The terminal ileum will previously have been clamped and transected. Now exteriorize 6–8 cm of bowel, with its mesentery intact, through the circular opening in the abdominal wall, leaving its end securely clamped. Make sure that the mesentery is neither twisted nor tight and that the tip of the ileum remains pink.

3 Some surgeons close the lateral space between the ileostomy and the abdominal wall, using a continuous Vicryl suture (Fig. 11.17). Others tunnel the ileum extraperitoneally. We prefer transperitoneal ileostomy, leaving the lateral space widely open.

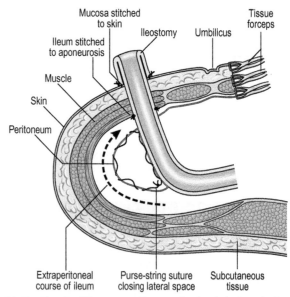

Fig. 11.17 Terminal ileostomy. Two methods of closing the lateral space are shown: a purse-string suture or taking the ileum along an extraperitoneal track. Alternatively, the lateral space can be left widely open. Tissue forceps on each layer of the wound edge prevent retraction of the layers while the ileostomy is being fashioned.

4 After closing the main abdominal incision, remove the clamp and trim the crushed portion of ileum. Now suture the edge of the ileum directly to the skin, using Vicryl mounted on a taper-cutting needle. After inserting three or four evenly spaced sutures, the bowel begins to evert spontaneously; if not, use Babcock's forceps to encourage eversion. Complete the circumferential sutures, producing a spout, which should project about 3 cm from the abdominal wall.

5 Carefully clean and dry the skin around the ileostomy and apply an ileostomy bag at once.

Loop ileostomy

1 Excise a disc of skin and fat and deliver a loop of ileum onto the abdominal wall.

2 Open the bowel, not at the apex of the loop as for a loop colostomy but close to skin level.

3 Suture the mucosa of the distal bowel to the skin. Use Babcock's forceps to evert the mucosa of the proximal bowel before suture.

4 The completed loop ileostomy looks very like a standard end ileostomy. Attach a suitable appliance, with flange and clip-on bag, to the skin over the stoma.

Aftercare

1 *Feeding jejunostomy.* Keep the tube patent by introducing 10 ml of water hourly initially. Feed may start at 30 ml per hour on the first postoperative day and be built up incrementally. Consult the dietician about the patient's individual nutritional needs. Give codeine or loperamide to control diarrhoea. When oral feeding is resumed spigot the tube for 24–48 hours before removal.

2 *Ileostomy.* Increase oral fluids when the stoma commences to discharge. The effluent will be very loose at first, but will gradually thicken as the ileum adapts. Give bulking agents or antidiarrhoeal drugs as needed. Consult the stomatherapist directly, if he or she has not already seen the patient before operation. Make sure that the patient is competent and confident at managing the stoma before he leaves hospital.

REFERENCE_

1. Niv E, Fireman Z, Vaisman N. Post-pyloric feeding. World J Gastroenterology 2009;15(11):1281–8.

MISCELLANEOUS CONDITIONS
MECKEL'S DIVERTICULUM

1 Potential complications include bleeding, infection, peptic ulceration, perforation, intestinal obstruction or fistulation to the umbilicus. Usually this remnant of the vitello-intestinal duct gives no trouble at all throughout the patient's life.

2 Incidental Meckel's diverticulectomy has now been abandoned. A retrospective analysis[1] found that the probabilities of producing surgical morbidity and mortality in the adult population were far higher when resecting incidental diverticula.

► KEY POINT Removal of Meckel's diverticulum

■ Do not carry out incidental Meckel's diverticulectomy.

3 The first step in diverticulectomy is to divide the small vessel that crosses the ileum to supply it. Depending on the size of its mouth, the diverticulum can simply be transected across the neck using a linear stapler or excised with a portion of the antimesenteric border of the bowel. Local resection of the ileum with end-to-end anastomosis may be preferable in a complicated case.

INTUSSUSCEPTION

In infants

1 Ileocolic intussusception usually presents in a child of a few months old with abdominal colic and rectal passage of blood and mucus. Besides confirming the diagnosis, barium enema may reduce the intussusception totally or subtotally. On examination under anaesthetic, if not before, a mass can be felt in the central or upper abdomen with an 'empty' right iliac fossa.

2 Open the abdomen through a right Lanz incision and find the sausage-shaped mass. Starting at the apex, squeeze the intussusceptum back along the intussuscipiens as though extracting toothpaste from the bottom of the tube. Do not remove the bowel from the abdominal cavity during this manoeuvre.

3 The final portion of the intussusception is the most difficult to reduce. Deliver the affected segment from the abdomen and gently compress it with a moist swab, before resuming the squeeze. Make certain that reduction is complete before replacing the bowel. No fixation is required, except in the rare event of a recurrent intussusception.

4 If the bowel is clearly gangrenous or the intussusception cannot be reduced, proceed to resection. Usually an end-to-end ileo-ileostomy can be performed.

In adults

1 Intussusception is rare and is nearly always associated with an underlying lesion in the bowel wall such as a benign tumour, metastatic deposit or Meckel's diverticulum.

2 Reduce the intussusception as far as possible then proceed to local resection of the affected segment of bowel with end-to-end anastomosis.

INTESTINAL ISCHAEMIA

1 The small intestine is supplied by the superior mesenteric (midgut) vessels. Thrombosis may occur on arteriosclerotic plaques at the origin of the superior mesenteric artery, especially if the patient is shocked. The superior mesenteric artery is an uncommon site for peripheral embolism in patients with cardiac arrhythmia or a recent myocardial infarction. Venous gangrene may result if the superior mesenteric or portal veins suddenly undergo thrombosis, for example in extreme dehydration or disseminated intravascular coagulation. Lastly, non-occlusive mesenteric infarction may occur secondary to microcirculatory damage in critically ill patients. Although the diagnosis may be difficult to make, suspect it if unexplained lactic acidosis develops in a postoperative or critically ill patient.

2 Patients with severe mesenteric vascular insufficiency are extremely ill with evidence of peritonitis and shock. Early operation is needed to prevent death.[2] At laparotomy, the bowel appears ischaemic or frankly infarcted without evidence of strangulation.

3 Examine the whole intestinal tract and feel for pulsation in all accessible gut arteries. Examine the aorta and its main divisions to determine the extent of atherosclerosis. If the main intestinal vessels and their arcades are patent, the circulation is probably occluded at capillary level.

4 Resect obviously necrotic bowel. Recovery is unlikely if the entire midgut is infarcted following occlusion of the superior mesenteric artery. If an extensive segment is affected, be as conservative as possible to avoid severe short-bowel syndrome. Multiple patches of ischaemia can be oversewn or locally resected.

5 Early cases of arterial embolus or acute in-situ thrombosis may be amenable to revascularization. It is much easier to mobilize the caecum and identify the ileocolic artery than to expose the origin of the superior mesenteric artery itself. Control the vessel with tapes and perform a longitudinal arteriotomy. Pass a Fogarty catheter proximally into the superior mesenteric artery and aorta to dislodge the clot, and try to establish free flow. Rapid injection of heparin saline up the vessel may achieve the same effect. If the bowel regains its normal colour, close the arteriotomy with a venous patch. Otherwise consider side-to-side anastomosis between the ileocolic and right common iliac arteries.

6 Following direct arterial surgery, or in any case in which bowel of doubtful viability has been left in the abdomen, plan to repeat the laparotomy after 24 hours. Further resection of bowel may be clearly indicated at this time.

> ### KEY POINT Mesenteric ischaemia: urgency of management
>
> ■ Regardless of aetiology, recovery in patients with mesenteric ischaemia is dependent upon rapid diagnosis and surgical treatment. Conservative management is rarely successful; more often laparotomy is required and can be life-saving.

SMALL-BOWEL FISTULA

1 The spontaneous discharge of bowel contents onto the abdominal wall is a rare event. The vast majority of external fistulas arise either from a leaking anastomosis or from operative injury to the intestine. Impaired healing, radiation enteritis, multiple adhesions, diffuse carcinoma and Crohn's disease predispose to fistula formation.

2 Do not rush to re-operate once there is an established small-bowel fistula. Correct fluid and electrolyte depletion. Switch to total parenteral nutrition which will reduce the amount of fistula discharge. There is some evidence that Octreotide 150 μg tds may reduce the time for fistulae to heal.[3] Consult a stomatherapist on how best to protect the wound and abdominal wall from the effluent, using adhesive seals and collecting bags as appropriate.

3 Obtain an early fistulogram to delineate the leak. A side hole may well close if there is no distal obstruction, but a complete anastomotic dehiscence is almost certain to require re-operation once the patient's general condition allows.

4 If the patient is toxic, early drainage of an associated abscess may improve the patient's general health and sometimes allow the fistula to heal. If you encounter a complete dehiscence at this time, it is probably better to exteriorize the bowel ends rather than attempt

a repeat anastomosis under unpromising circumstances. This advice may not be appropriate for a high jejunal fistula, however.

5 Do not ordinarily undertake a definitive operation to close a small-bowel fistula if you are an inexperienced surgeon. As a rule resect the damaged portion of bowel. Take care to divide any adhesions that could partially obstruct the distal gut and lead to recurrence of the fistula. Continue nutritional support during the postoperative healing phase.

REFERENCES

1. Peoples J. Incidental Meckel's diverticulectomy in adults. Surgery 1995;118:649–52
2. Herbert GS, Steele SR. Acute and chronic mesenteric ischemia. Surg Clin North Am 2007;87(5):1115–34.
3. Lloyd DA, Gave SM, Windsor AC. Nutrition and management of enterocutaneous fistula. Br J Surg 2006;93(9):1045–55.

LAPAROSCOPIC APPROACH TO THE SMALL BOWEL

Appraise

1 Diagnostic laparoscopy can be performed with minimal morbidity and can prevent additional complications arising from laparotomy such as wound infection and respiratory complications. In addition to this diagnostic role, laparoscopic surgical techniques can now be applied to most of the therapeutic procedures that were traditionally performed at open surgery and laparoscopic treatment of small bowel complication of Crohn's disease is now well-established.[1]

> ### KEY POINT Laparoscopy: risk of small-bowel injury
>
> ■ In patients in whom previous laparotomy has been carried out or in those with distended loops of bowel, an open method of initial port placement is the only safe way to avoid inadvertent puncture of the small bowel.

2 Diagnostic laparoscopy is useful in patients with peritonitis or possible small-bowel ischaemia; any subsequent therapeutic procedures being carried out either laparoscopically or via open laparotomy. The small bowel can be examined in detail via the laparoscope. Use a standard infra-umbilical port and a 30°-angled endoscope. Identify the ligament of Treitz initially. Thereafter, by alternately using two atraumatic graspers, expose the entire length of the small bowel to the caecum, dividing any intervening adhesions with laparoscopic scissors. Inspect both the serosal surface and the mesentery.

3 A clinical diagnosis of small-bowel ischaemia is notoriously difficult to make. Laparoscopic examination of the bowel is helpful in determining whether bowel is viable or not. If you are in doubt about the viability of the bowel, make a small incision in order to deliver the suspect segment for closer inspection. Diagnostic laparoscopy is safe and can be performed with minimal morbidity and mortality. It is particularly useful in critically ill patients in whom you wish to avoid unnecessary laparotomy.

4 Small-bowel resection can be performed entirely laparoscopically or with laparoscopic assistance. Determine the segment for resection, dissect the mesentery and divide it using the

harmonic scalpel. Perform the subsequent anastomosis intraperitoneally using three firings of a laparoscopic linear stapling device or by standard extracorporeal anastomosis after delivering the bowel to the exterior through a small abdominal incision.

5 Laparoscopic creation of stomas such as loop ileostomy, loop sigmoid colostomy and end colostomy can all be carried out relatively easily. Studies have reported a high success rate in excess of 95%, and a low morbidity rate.

6 Laparoscopic management of acute small-bowel obstruction is theoretically attractive, but may be difficult. Adhesions and distended loops of bowel make establishing pneumoperitoneum hazardous, so an open pneumoperitoneum technique is mandatory and port placement should be under direct vision. If obstruction is due to a single adhesion, this can readily be identified and divided. If adhesions are more extensive, adhesiolysis and relief of obstruction is more difficult. The procedure demands painstaking care, whether performed by the open or the laparoscopic route. Several studies have shown however, that laparoscopy is both effective and safe in patients with small-bowel obstruction. One study in particular[2] reported that laparoscopy was effective in a high proportion of patients and that hospital stay was reduced. However, a recent Cochrane systematic review found no randomized or prospective controlled trials comparing laparoscopic with open surgery for small bowel obstruction.[3]

REFERENCES

1. Dasari BV, McKay D, Gardiner K. Laparoscopic versus open surgery for small bowel Crohn's disease. Cochrane Database Syst Rev 2011;1: CD006956.
2. Wullstein C, Gross E. Laparoscopic compared with conventional treatment of acute adhesive small bowel obstruction. Br J Surg 2003;90:1147–51.
3. Cirocchi R, Abraha I, Farinella E, et al. Laparoscopic versus open surgery in small bowel obstruction. Cochrane Database Syst Rev 2010;2: CD007511.

FURTHER READING

Irwin ST, Krukowski ZH, Matheson NA. Single layer anastomosis in the upper gastrointestinal tract. Br J Surg 1990;77:643–4.
Mackey WC, Dineen P. A fifty year experience with Meckel's diverticulum. Surg Gynecol Obstet 1983;156:56–64.
Michelassi F. Strictureplasty for Crohn's disease: techniques and long-term results. World J Surg 1998;22:359–63.
Ottinger L. Mesenteric ischaemia. In: Williamson RCN, Cooper MJ, editors. Emergency abdominal surgery. Edinburgh: Churchill Livingstone; 1990. p. 242–57.
Studley JGN, Williamson RCN. Malignant tumours of the small bowel. In: Taylor TV, Watson A, Williamson RCN, editors. Upper digestive surgery. Oesophagus, stomach and small intestine. London: Saunders; 1999. p. 949–62.
Thomas WEG. Complications of small bowel diverticula. In: Williamson RCN, Cooper MJ, editors. Emergency abdominal surgery. Edinburgh: Churchill Livingstone; 1990. p. 191–208.
Williams NS, Nasmyth DG, Jones D, et al. De-functioning stomas: a prospective controlled trial comparing loop ileostomy with loop transverse colostomy. Br J Surg 1986;73:566–70.

OPERATIONS FOR OBESITY

Appraise

1 Obesity is becoming more prevalent worldwide, leading to an increasing incidence of related co-morbidities such as type II diabetes, obstructive sleep apnoea, coronary artery disease and stroke. To date, surgery is the only reliable way to produce significant and sustained weight loss and reverse weight-related illnesses.

2 Surgical treatment of obesity can produce significant weight loss and resolve diabetes, hypertension, hypercholesterolaemia and decrease the incidence of malignancy. Furthermore it can improve quality of life and lead to a reduction in medical costs for the health service over the long term.

3 Current UK recommendations allow bariatric surgery for any adult whose body mass index (BMI) is greater than 35 kg/m^2 if they have weight-related co-morbidity or a BMI of greater than 40 kg/m^2 if they do not.

4 Operations for obesity were originally carried out at laparotomy, but since the late 1990s laparoscopy has become the established method. Open operation is reserved for patients requiring complex revision surgery or for those whose weight precludes pneumoperitoneum.

5 The most commonly performed bariatric surgical procedures are the laparoscopic adjustable gastric band, laparoscopic sleeve gastrectomy and laparoscopic Roux-en-Y gastric bypass. Other less commonly performed procedures include laparoscopic duodenal switch, open biliopancreatic diversion and vertical banded gastroplasty (Fig. 11.18). We shall discuss the first three of these procedures in detail.

6 Assess patients requiring bariatric (Greek barys = heavy + iatros = physician) surgery within a multidisciplinary team (MDT) before embarking on operation. We recommend involvement of a bariatric surgeon, endocrine physician, psychologist, dietician, bariatric anaesthetist and specialist nurse.

7 Obtain a detailed history to establish the severity of co-morbidities, eating habits and psychological triggers. Only then can you enter into a detailed discussion on which operation is most suitable for the patient. This is influenced by the patient's weight and BMI, eating habits and the presence of co-morbidities such as diabetes, which responds particularly well to gastric bypass.

8 The decision on choice of procedure ultimately lies with the patient. There are no absolute contraindications to any of the procedures in any patient:
   ■ Adjustable gastric band is perceived as the least radical operation, and is wholly reversible so is often favoured by patients with a BMI between 30 and 40 and by younger patients. Because the typical weight loss achieved with gastric banding is of the order of 40–50% of *excess* weight, patients with an extremely high BMI having gastric bands have little prospect of achieving a final BMI <30 despite a successful operation, and the higher the initial BMI the more marked is this effect. We recommend that patients with a BMI >55 consider an alternative to a gastric band.
   ■ Gastric bypass is perceived as very radical and is irreversible.
   ■ Sleeve gastrectomy lies between the two other operations. With both this procedure and gastric bypass weight loss of the order of 60–70% of *excess* weight is achievable; thus even patients with a high BMI can achieve a significantly lower final BMI.

9 Co-morbidity influences the choice of procedure. The presence of type II diabetes is a clear indication for gastric bypass as resolution of diabetes occurs in approximately 80% of patients and is independent of weight loss. In addition, sleep apnoea, which *is* dependent on weight loss, is best improved by choosing a

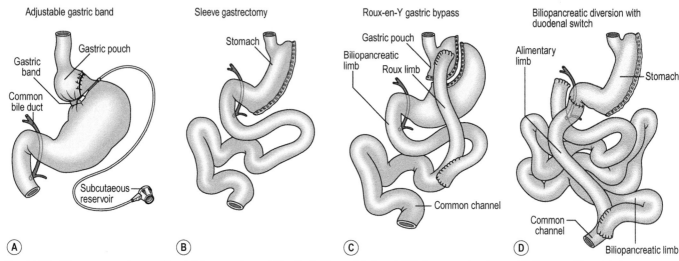

Fig. 11.18 The common types of bariatric procedures: (A) adjustable gastric band; (B) sleeve gastrectomy; (C) Roux-en-Y gastric bypass; (D) biliopancreatic diversion with duodenal switch. (Modified with permission from The New England Journal of Medicine Copyright 2007 Massachusetts Medical Society).

procedure which maximizes this. The presence of gastro-oesophageal reflux-disease (GORD) is a relative contraindication to sleeve gastrectomy where symptoms may be exacerbated by removing the fundus of the stomach. Gastric bypass may be impossible in patients with extensive previous abdominal surgery involving the small bowel.

10 Take possible surgical risks into account when planning the operation. Patients with poor cardiovascular reserve who are unlikely to survive re-operation for anastomotic leakage might benefit from gastric banding since the risk of early reoperation is negligible. Also, gastric banding can be abandoned safely and rapidly at any point during the operation if the patient's condition deteriorates. In contrast, during gastric bypass, once the gastric pouch is created you must complete the operation.

Prepare

1 Equip the surgical unit with an operating table capable of withstanding patient's excess weight, specialist equipment for moving the anaesthetized patient from table to bed and the necessary laparoscopic stapling devices for the operation proposed. Ensure that the wards are equipped with beds and furniture capable of accommodating larger patients.

2 Fully control any diabetes prior to operation.

3 Commence patients with severe obstructive sleep apnoea on home continuous positive airway pressure (CPAP) for at least 6 weeks prior to surgery.

4 Restrict carbohydrate diet for 2–3 weeks prior to surgery to reduce the size of the liver. Otherwise the enlarged liver will prejudice surgical exposure of the stomach.

5 Order perioperative prophylaxis with low-molecular-weight heparin and pneumatic calf compression to minimize the risk of deep vein thrombosis (DVT).

▶ KEY POINT Is surgery right for the patient?

■ Do not proceed straight to surgery without thorough prior assessment by the multi-disciplinary team

LAPAROSCOPIC ADJUSTABLE GASTRIC BAND

This is a purely restrictive operation, which involves placing a silicon band around the upper stomach, just below the gastro-oesophageal junction. On the inside surface of the band is a balloon which can be inflated with saline to tighten the band. Following surgery the band can be adjusted via a filling port which lies on the abdominal wall beneath the skin.

▶ KEY POINT Become familiar with the band closure before surgery

■ There are a number of different adjustable gastric bands available, each with its own particular closing mechanism. Ensure that the company representative demonstrates the closing mechanism to you on a specimen band prior to attempting the manoeuvre laparoscopically.

Access

1 Has the anaesthetist available a calibration tube? This has an expandable balloon at its tip, which can be passed to lie at the upper extremity of the stomach and inflated. The gastric band can be placed directly below it.

2 Position the patient on a split leg bariatric table, with exaggerated reversed Trendelenburg (head up) attitude. Separate the legs and stand between them.

3 Create a pneumoperitoneum using a Veress needle in the midline between the umbilicus and xiphisternum. Once pneumoperitoneum is established, place a 12-mm optical port at the same spot. Now place the remainder of the ports and liver retractor under direct vision (Fig. 11.19).

Assess

1 Assess the size and texture of the left lobe of liver and exclude the presence of a large hiatus hernia.

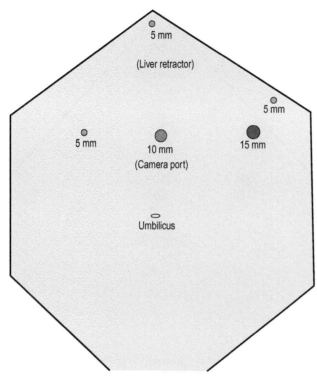

Fig. 11.19 Port positions for Laparoscopic gastric band insertion.

2 Gently elevate the left lobe of liver using the Nathanson liver retractor and clamp it in position to make the gastro-oesophageal junction easily visible.

> ▶ KEY POINTS Use the Veress needle safely

- It is easy to puncture the liver inadvertently with the Veress needle.
- Pay close attention to the insufflation pressure gauge and end tidal carbon dioxide level to prevent CO_2 embolism.

Action

1 Starting from the angle of His (Wilhelm His 1831–1904, Swiss anatomist), gently free the fundus of the stomach from the left crus of diaphragm using the diathermy hook.

2 Identify the pars flaccida window in the gastro-hepatic omentum and open it gently using the diathermy hook. Incise the peritoneum at the junction between the posterior wall of stomach and the right crus of diaphragm. Through the space which opens here, pass a disposable 'Goldfinger' probe behind the stomach to emerge at the angle of His. Angle this so that the tip is clearly visible (Fig. 11.20).

> ? DIFFICULTY

- If you are uncertain whether the Goldfinger probe has passed posterior to the stomach, ask the anaesthetist to place the calibration tube into the stomach. It is then easy to confirm that the Goldfinger is in the correct place by elevating it and lifting the tube forwards.

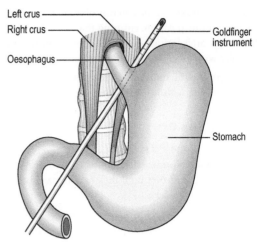

Fig. 11.20 Position of Goldfinger dissector prior to insertion of laparoscopic gastric band.

- If the Goldfinger does not readily appear at the angle of His, gently dissect both at the angle of His and between the right crus and stomach to clearly identify the correct route.

> ▶ KEY POINT Prepare the gastric band

- Prior to inserting the adjustable gastric band fill the balloon with sterile water and remove the dead-space air.

3 Pass the adjustable gastric band into the abdomen via the 15-mm port and hook it onto the tip of the Goldfinger instrument. Now straighten and retract this, pulling the gastric band from left to right behind the stomach into its correct position. Close the band around the stomach, below the 20-ml calibration balloon placed in the uppermost part of the stomach. Take care not to damage the balloon with the atraumatic graspers.

4 Once the band is in position, place three interrupted non-absorbable sutures between the fundus of the stomach and gastric pouch to completely cover the antero-lateral surface of the band. We use 2/0 polyester (Ethibond) sutures for this purpose (Fig. 11.21).

5 Bring the end of the band tubing out of the abdomen via the 15-mm port and connect it to the filling port. Create a small

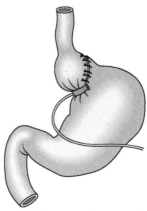

Fig. 11.21 Appearance of laparoscopic gastric band in position at completion of operation.

pocket on the surface of the anterior oblique muscle and fix the filling port in this position, ensuring that the rubber diaphragm of the filling port is facing outwards. Close the muscle around the filling tube with a non-absorbable suture.

6 Close Scarpa's fascia and the skin incisions with absorbable sutures and seal the wounds with skin glue.

Postoperative care

1 Gastric bands may be inserted as a day-case procedure. Oral fluid can be introduced immediately. Patients then progress though pureed food and soft diet until they can manage solid food, in approximately 6–8 weeks.

2 Discharge patients home on daily self-injected low-molecular-weight heparin for 2 weeks as prophylaxis against DVT.

3 Perform the first band inflation 6 weeks after surgery.

4 Long-term successful weight loss following laparoscopic gastric band placement requires a dedicated specialist nurse and dietician to monitor progress and provide close dietary support.

Complications

1 More than 20% of patients may have poor weight loss or regain significant weight after a period of time.

2 Long-term complications such as pouch dilatation, band slippage and band erosion occur rarely but often require removal of the band.

3 A slipped band causing complete obstruction of the gastric pouch is a surgical emergency. Recognize it early if a patient has persistent dysphagia despite deflation of the band. Urgently remove the band surgically to prevent ischaemic necrosis of the gastric wall.

LAPAROSCOPIC SLEEVE GASTRECTOMY

This is a restrictive operation in which the fundus of the stomach is resected using a linear stapling device leaving a narrow stomach tube between the gastro-oesophageal junction and the distal antrum.

Access

Position the patient similar to that for laparoscopic gastric banding. Ports positions are shown in Figure 11.22.

Assess

Is the left lobe of liver small enough to allow the operation to take place?

Action

1 Using a harmonic scalpel or Ligasure haemostatic device, start the dissection on the greater curve of stomach approximately one-third of the way from pylorus to the angle of His. Open a window into the lesser sac through the gastro-colic omentum, staying close to the greater curve of stomach. Proceed towards the angle of His achieving control of all the short gastric vessels. Where the tissue is thick, at the gastro-splenic ligament, begin by dividing the anterior leaflet before continuing with the posterior one. Continue dissection until the entire fundus of stomach is mobile, all the way to the angle of His.

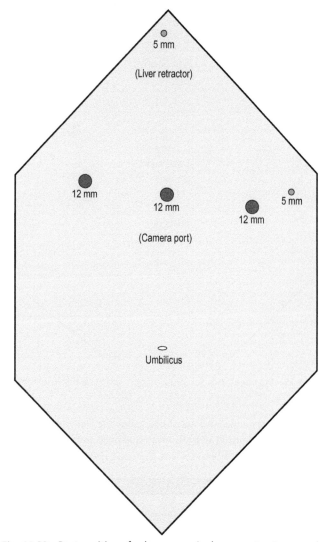

Fig. 11.22 Port positions for laparoscopic sleeve gastrectomy and laparoscopic gastric bypass.

■ *The stomach appears fused to the splenic hilum.* By gentle retraction on the stomach it is always possible to develop a safe plane between the two organs without the need to use the haemostatic device on the splenic tissue.

2 Return to the starting point of the dissection and separate the gastro-colic omentum from the gastric wall, this time proceeding toward the pylorus (the patient's right). Stop the dissection approximately 4 cm proximal to the pylorus. The entire greater curve of stomach should now be freely mobile.

3 Advance a 12.7-mm diameter calibration tube from the mouth along the lesser curve of the stomach until it passes through the pylorus. Using a 60-mm linear stapler, starting 4 cm proximal to the pylorus, staple the greater curve snugly to the calibration tube using green (4.1 mm), cartridges. We favour reinforcing each staple line with Peri-strips® which minimize bleeding from the staple line. Continue the staple line snug to the tube all the way to the angle of His (Fig. 11.23).

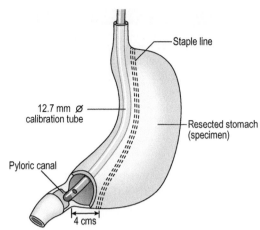

Fig. 11.23   Dissection for laparoscopic sleeve gastrectomy.

> ▶ KEY POINTS Ensure staple placement is precise

- When stapling, ensure both anterior and posterior walls of stomach are stretched laterally to avoid forming a baggy stomach tube.
- Make sure the narrow stomach along the lesser curve does not twist during stapling so that the staple line lies laterally along its entire length.

4 Inspect the staple line carefully and clamp the pylorus with an atraumatic grasper. Using the calibration tube, fill the stomach with methylene blue dye until the stomach tube appears tense. Inspect the staple line for blue dye while slowly withdrawing the tube.

5 Remove the resected stomach in a bag through a 12-mm port site and send it for histological examination.

6 The port sites do not routinely require deep closure. Close the skin with absorbable sutures and skin-glue.

Postoperative

1 Patients can drink water immediately after surgery and free fluids the following day. Provided there is no tachycardia or significant abdominal pain, allow them to go home on the first postoperative day. Instruct patients to follow a 6-week dietary regime identical to that following gastric banding.

2 Discharge patients home on low-molecular-weight heparin for 2 weeks with daily gastric acid suppression therapy for 3 months.

> ▶ KEY POINT

- Specific vitamin and mineral supplementation is not required, although we recommend a daily multivitamin tablet.

Complications

1 Patients frequently feel severe nausea in the first 24–48 hours after surgery. Manage this by anti-emetics. It always settles spontaneously.

2 Leakage from the gastric staple line occurs in 1–2% of patients. This presents with sudden acute abdominal pain and warrants immediate return to the operating theatre. It is extremely unlikely to occur more than 2 weeks postoperatively.

3 If the patient develops increasing pain with a falling haemoglobin, suspect bleeding from the omentum or spleen. This is usually easy to control by re-laparoscopy and washout of the blood.

LAPAROSCOPIC ROUX-EN-Y GASTRIC BYPASS

Access

Position the patient as per laparoscopic gastric banding. Position ports as in Figure 11.22.

Assess

Check that there are no adhesions which would prevent mobilization of the small intestine. Often the omentum is firmly stuck in a previously undetected para-umbilical hernia. If so, reduce it completely. If the defect is large enough to allow small bowel to enter, repair it at the end of the procedure.

Action

1 Carefully dissect to open up the angle of His. Inflate a 20-cc calibrating balloon in the stomach and retract it until it is stopped by the elastic resistance of the diaphragmatic crura. Start the dissection of the lesser curve just inferior to the balloon. Using the harmonic scalpel, dissect close to the lesser curve posteriorly until the space opens into the lesser sac behind the stomach. After removing the calibration tube, staple horizontally across the medial part of the stomach at this level using the 45-mm linear stapler with blue (3.5 mm staples). Lift the stomach upwards to view the posterior surface of the gastro-oesophageal junction and bluntly dissect to produce a passage through to the left crus of the diaphragm. Using two further cartridges staple vertically upwards towards the left crus to separate the small rectangular pouch of stomach from the main body of the stomach. Open the lower left corner of this pouch with the diathermy hook to produce a passage into the lumen of the pouch.

2 Grasp the greater omentum using atraumatic forceps and lift it superiorly until the transverse colon is suspended horizontally. Starting close to the transverse colon, bisect the omentum vertically until it forms a right and left leaf. Close to the colon extend the dissection to the left and to the right, close to the colonic wall, taking care not to damage the colon. This omental dissection provides a tension-free passage for the jejunum up to the gastric pouch.

3 Lift the colon upwards to expose the mesocolon. Identify the duodeno-jejunal flexure and carefully grasp the proximal jejunum. Draw up a loop of jejunum anterior to the colon until it reaches the pouch without tension. Create a small hole in the anti-mesenteric border of the jejunum and pass the stapling device superiorly into the jejunum. Grasp the pouch on each side of its opening and without force, pass the passive (anvil) blade of the stapler into the pouch until the tissue abuts the angle of the stapler. Fire the stapler (and then ask the anaesthetist to

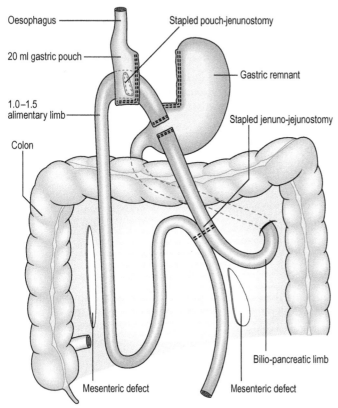

Fig. 11.24 Configuration of laparoscopic gastric bypass at completion of operation.

advance the tube until the tip is visible within the pouch. Suture the resultant defect closed with a continuous, absorbable 2/0 mattress suture (Fig. 11.24).

■ *The jejunum appears too short to reach the gastric pouch.* This indicates an inadequate omental dissection. Extend the dissection between the transverse colon and omentum further to the patient's left to create a more direct route for the jejunum to the gastric pouch.

4 Measure 100–150 cm distally along the jejunum from the anastomosis and place a stay suture between the measured jejunum and jejunum midway between the DJF and anastomosis. Using the diathermy hook create adjacent enterotomies close to the stay suture and pass the stapler with a white (2.5 mm) staple cartridge superiorly to join the two bowel lumens. Insert a second straight stapler pointing downwards and fire it, to enlarge the anastomosis lumen. Follow this with a transverse staple firing to close the enterotomy. Insufflate the tube with methylene blue dye under pressure to check both anastomoses for leaks and then divide the short length of jejunum between them with a further white (2.5 mm) staple cartridge.

5 Close the two mesenteric defects created by the anastomoses with a purse string suture of non-absorbable 2/0 Ethibond.

▶ KEY POINT

■ Handle the small intestine very gently. It is vital to avoid creating multiple serosal tears to the jejunum whilst manipulating the stapling devices and constructing the anastomoses. As a rule, repair all serosal tears with seromuscular interrupted sutures.

Postoperative

1 Water may be sipped on the first postoperative day with free fluids reintroduced on the second day.

2 If observations are stable patients may be discharged home 2 days after surgery.

3 Patients require prophylactic low-molecular-weight heparin for 2 weeks after discharge and acid suppression therapy for 3 months. The postoperative dietary regime is identical to laparoscopic gastric band insertion, but all patients require vitamin B12 injections 3 monthly and lifelong regular iron, calcium, vitamin D and multivitamin supplements.

Complications

1 If the patient complains of severe pain or develops tachycardia with increased inflammatory markers, consider imaging with CT and oral contrast to assess the anastomosis and exclude significant bleeding. Anastomotic leaks and significant bleeding usually occur within 48 hours of surgery: if you suspect it carry out immediate re-laparoscopy:

■ Anastomotic stenosis and internal herniation are extremely rare, but suspect them in any patient who re-presents with abdominal symptoms more than 3 months following surgery.

■ Make sure the narrow stomach along the lesser curve does not twist during stapling so that the staple line lies laterally along its entire length.

FURTHER READING

Buchwald H, Avidor Y, Braunwald E, et al. A systematic review and meta-analysis. JAMA 2004;292:1724–37.

Frachetti KJ, Goldfine AB. Bariatric surgery for diabetes management. Current Opinion in Endocrinology, Diabetes and Obesity 2009;16:119–24.

O'Brien PE, Sawyer SM, Laurie C, et al. Laparoscopic adjustable gastric banding in severely obese adolescents: a randomized trial. JAMA 2010;303(6):519–26.

Sjöström L, Gummesson A, Sjöström CD, et al. Effects of bariatric surgery on cancer incidence in obese patients in Sweden (Swedish Obese Subjects Study): a prospective, controlled intervention trial. Lancet Oncol 2009;10:653–62.

Sjöström L, Narbro K, Sjöström CD, et al. Effects of bariatric surgery on mortality in Swedish obese subjects. N Engl J Med 2007;357:741–52.

Tice JA, Karliner L, Walsh J, et al. Gastric banding or bypass? A systematic review comparing the two most popular bariatric procedures. Am J Med 2008;121:885–93.

12

Colonoscopy

R.J. Leicester

CONTENTS

DESCRIPTION OF OPERATION

Appraise

1 Colonoscopy has revolutionized the diagnosis and treatment of colonic disease, allowing accurate mucosal visualization, biopsy and therapeutic polypectomy. Technological advances in instrumentation allow rapid and safe examination of the whole colon, provided the endoscopist has been adequately trained in the technique.

2 Use diagnostic colonoscopy to evaluate an abnormal or equivocal barium enema or CT cologram, particularly where diverticular disease or colonic spasm may often obscure a small mucosal lesion. Colonoscopy should be the first-line investigation for unexplained rectal bleeding or iron deficiency anaemia and is the investigation of choice for all patients with a positive faecal occult blood test. Colonoscopy is the most accurate diagnostic tool for differential diagnosis and assessment of extent in inflammatory bowel disease, but should be avoided in acute disease, where technetium-labelled white cell scanning, if available, is a safer alternative.

3 Therapeutic colonoscopy has changed the management of colorectal polyps, facilitating removal of all pedunculated and most sessile adenomatous lesions, particularly with the advent of endoscopic mucosal resection (EMR) and endoscopic submucosal dissection (ESD), thus providing an opportunity for colorectal cancer prevention. Diathermy coagulation or laser therapy of vascular abnormalities such as angiodysplasia may pre-empt laparotomy in acute colonic haemorrhage or cure anaemia due to chronic blood loss.

4 Relief of obstruction in colorectal cancer, either as an initial procedure prior to surgical resection or as long-term palliation, may be achieved using either laser vaporization or stent insertion.

5 Perform surveillance colonoscopy with chromoscopy and biopsy of abnormal areas of mucosa in all individuals with a 10 year history of ulcerative or Crohn's colitis. Further surveillance should be according to current BSG or NICE guidelines, which outline high-risk factors for dysplasia, concomitant family history and primary biliary cirrhosis with recommended intervals between surveillance colonoscopies. Surgery is indicated only in those with definite dysplasia or carcinoma, thus avoiding colectomy in over 80% of cases.

6 Following polypectomy or curative resection for colorectal cancer, carry out regular follow-up colonoscopy, according to the risk factors as outlined in the current BSG guidelines.

7 Commence screening of patients with familial polyposis coli from age 15 years (if gene-positive) and continue approximately 2-yearly until the age of 40 years. Hereditary non-polyposis coli families should undergo 1–2-yearly surveillance, commencing at least 10 years younger than the index case. If facilities exist, then screen subjects with a strong family history of colorectal cancer (i.e. one first-degree relative with onset before 40 years of age, or more than one first-degree relative of any age) in the hope of reducing the incidence of colorectal cancer by removing adenomatous lesions.

8 Emergency colonoscopy is rarely helpful in cases of acute, severe rectal bleeding. Anorectal and upper gastrointestinal causes should be excluded by rigid proctosigmoidoscopy and gastroscopy. Bleeding usually ceases in up to 90% of patients, allowing colonoscopy within 4 to 6 weeks after bowel preparation. In those cases where haemorrhage continues, angiography with embolization of a bleeding point may be helpful. However, if a diagnosis has not been reached and emergency laparotomy becomes necessary, you may perform colonoscopy under general anaesthetic with the peritoneal cavity exposed, following on-table lavage with saline or water introduced via a Foley catheter through a caecostomy.

Prepare

1 Accurate, rapid examination depends upon effective bowel preparation. Advise patients to discontinue any iron preparation or stool-bulking agents 1 week prior to endoscopy and change to a low-residue diet for at least 2 days. Twenty-four hours before examination restrict oral intake to clear fluids such as coffee or tea without milk, concentrated meat extract and glucose drinks. Give a purgative such as sodium picosulphate or 'low volume' polyethylene glycol preparation 12–18 hours before colonoscopy and repeat it 4 to 6 hours before examination. Alternatively, give 'high volume' balanced electrolyte solution combined with polyethylene glycol, which have been shown to produce rapid preparation without the need for dietary restriction. Administration of metoclopramide 10 mg prior to ingestion of the 3–4 L of solution enhances gastric emptying and reduces nausea and vomiting.

Any patients with evidence of renal impairment should undergo renal function testing prior to administration of bowel preparation and if necessary be referred to a renal physician for advice.

2 Written, informed consent for the procedure should be obtained from all patients prior to bowel preparation and arrival for the

procedure. The nature, purpose and risks of the procedure, together with alternatives, should be explained, including the implications of sedation. Give reassurance about the examination to allay fears, allowing minimal levels of sedation to be used.

3 Colonoscopy is usually performed under intravenous sedation with the addition of an analgesic. Do not give excessive sedation or analgesia as this may result in circulatory or respiratory depression. Additionally, it will dull appreciation of severe pain which should occur only when a poor technique is used, causing dangerous overstretching of the bowel. For similar reasons do not perform colonoscopy under general anaesthesia, apart from as an intra-operative procedure in cases of acute colonic haemorrhage. Elderly patients in particular can suffer significant hypotension following pethidine, and this, combined with the synergistic effect of opiates and benzodiazepines, can also cause significant falls in oxygen saturation. In order to avoid these complications, use only small doses of analgesic and hypnotic such as intravenous pethidine 25 mg or fentanyl 50 ug plus midazolam 2–3 mg. Monitor all patients by pulse oximetry, during and after the procedure, and give added inspired oxygen in all cases. Always have available antidotes to benzodiazepines (flumazenil) and opiates (naloxone), together with full cardiorespiratory resuscitation equipment and staff trained to use it in case of emergency. Occasionally an antispasmodic, either intravenous hyoscine butylbromide (Buscopan) or intraluminal peppermint oil suspension may be employed.

4 As a rule, commence examination of the patient in the left lateral position or, alternatively, supine. Use a tipping trolley in case of cardiorespiratory problems. Have available at least two trained assistants: one to observe the patient's vital signs and the other to assist with the accessories for biopsy or snare polypectomy.

5 Check all equipment prior to intubation. The colonoscope must have been adequately cleaned and disinfected. The light source, endoscope angulation controls, air/CO_2 insufflation, lens washing and suction facilities must be in full working order. If using a variable stiffness colonoscope ensure that the dial is at '0'. Check the diathermy equipment for correct, safe operation. Ensure that all accessories, such as biopsy forceps polypectomy snares and injection needles, are available in the room.

Access

1 Modern colonoscopes are sophisticated precision instruments designed to enhance intubation of the colon in the most efficient manner. As well as a wide-angled lens to allow a greater field of vision and high definition video chip camera, graduated torque characteristics assist variability in the stiffness of the instrument. In addition, some colonoscopes have an ability to vary the stiffness of the insertion shaft.

2 During intubation, the instrument may be pushed forward or pulled back. Change of direction may be achieved by angulation of the distal end, up/down or left/right. Change of direction may also be achieved by up/down deflection, combined with rotation or torque. Keeping the distal section of the instrument as straight as possible and restoring this to a neutral position as soon as possible after angulation around an acute bend helps to prevent loop formation. Avoid maximum up/down and left/right angulation, as this results in a J-shape and rotation of the end of the instrument rather than change of direction. Advancement may also be

achieved by the straightening of a loop using torque and withdrawal or by suction, causing a concertina effect of the bowel over the endoscope.

3 Colonoscopy is made easier if the anatomy of the colon is properly understood. The rectum is fixed in a retroperitoneal position and consists of alternating mucosal folds forming the valves of Houston. The sigmoid colon is freely mobile on its mesentery and of variable length and configuration. The descending colon and splenic flexure are relatively fixed by their peritoneal attachments. At the splenic flexure, the direction of the colon is forwards and downwards to the transverse colon which, like the sigmoid, is of variable length and freely mobile on the transverse mesocolon. The bowel becomes fixed again at the hepatic flexure and the direction passes forwards and downwards into the ascending colon and caecum, which are usually fixed by peritoneal attachments, though less consistently than the descending colon. It is the mobile and variable-length sigmoid and transverse colon that cause the most difficulty through looping of the instrument.

4 The aim of colonoscopy is to achieve intubation from the anus to caecum with the minimum possible length of instrument. Characteristically, the colonoscope, when straight and without loop formation, should be in a roughly U-shaped configuration with 70–80 cm of instrument inserted to the caecal pole (Fig. 12.1). Significantly greater insertion length indicates the presence of a loop.

> **KEY POINTS** Achieving successful colonoscopy

- Avoid creating loops by minimal air/CO_2 insufflation, minimal tip angulation, using torque to steer, particularly in the left colon, and early position change of the patient whenever acute angles in the colon are encountered.
- Recognize loop formation early by lack of one-to-one advancement of the instrument tip compared with shaft insertion, paradoxical movement of the tip or patient pain.
- If loop formation occurs, provided there is little or no patient discomfort, try 'pushing through' the loop. Otherwise reduce the loop, using a logical approach of first pulling back with clockwise torque. If this fails to reduce the loop pull back with anti-clockwise torque. If still not resolved then change patient position and repeat the above steps if necessary.
- Successful loop resolution requires at least 90° and often 180° of torque. Luminal view should be maintained by

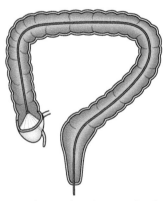

Fig. 12.1 Colonoscope inserted to the caecal pole.

adjustment of the up/down and left/right angulation controls as torque is applied. Continue pulling back until one-to-one withdrawal occurs and then reinsert whilst maintaining the torque and steering with the angulation controls, to avoid re-looping.

- If a loop continues to reform after successful resolution, first try changing patient position, followed if necessary by abdominal compression by an assistant or application of the stiffener in colonoscopes having this facility.

- Successful colonoscopy depends on the application of any one or more of these techniques as visual appearances and feedback of longitudinal and rotational forces on the colonoscope are detected by you via the instrument shaft and control wheels. By using a tactile approach, assessing the forces on the instrument, you can often prevent unnecessary looping before it occurs.

5 Liberally lubricate the anus and perianal area with lubricating gel. Carry out a thorough digital examination then introduce the instrument along the forefinger of the right hand. Repeated lubrication is required to prevent friction at the anus, one of the commonest causes of failure to advance the endoscope. Control of the instrument is best achieved by rotation of the up/down and left/right angulation control wheels, using your left thumb. Place your index finger to allow it to operate the air/water and suction valves. Manipulation of the colonoscope shaft is performed with the right hand (Fig. 12.2).

6 On entering the rectum, aspirate excess fluid and adjust the tip of the instrument, using torque, until it is in the centre of the lumen. During intubation, insufflate only the minimum amount of air to allow adequate visualization of the lumen. Excessive air leads to distal distension and accentuation of angles in the bowel. At the rectosigmoid junction the lumen passes upwards and to the right. Intubation at this point can be achieved by upward deflection of the tip and clockwise rotation of the shaft. In patients with a relatively short sigmoid colon, continuation of the clockwise rotation with advancement often leads to passage as far as the descending sigmoid junction. Intubation of the rectosigmoid can often be the most uncomfortable part of the procedure for the patient; if excess angulation is required to view the lumen then change the patient position to supine or right lateral to decrease the rectosigmoid angle and allow intubation with minimal tip angulation. In many patients, particularly those with diverticular disease or those who have undergone pelvic surgery, the configuration is variable and there may be a number of acute angles. In these cases, achieve advancement by a combination of, position change, torque and adjustments to the left/right wheel. Aim to take the shortest possible route through the bowel, keeping the instrument tip in the centre of the lumen and keeping to the inside of each bend.

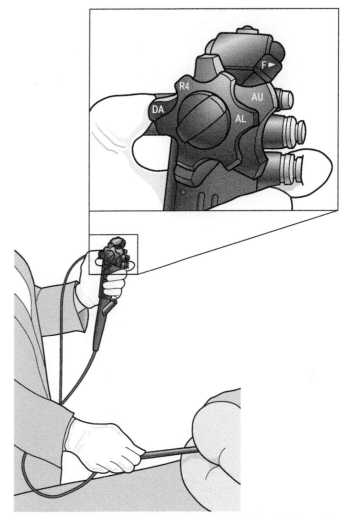

Fig. 12.2 The right hand, which should be gloved, manipulates the colonoscope shaft.

in patients with diverticular disease, as advancement of the instrument into a diverticulum is potentially hazardous.

3. Clues as to the position of the lumen can be obtained from the arcuate folds and the light reflex caused by the instrument. As a general rule, steer towards the concavity of the folds and away from the bright light reflex (Fig. 12.3).

4. Position change will often allow a better luminal view and advancement with minimal angulation (Fig. 12.4).

7 Looping of the colonoscope may occur in the sigmoid colon, indicated by a lack of one-to-one advancement of the instrument tip compared with the shaft, which may also cause the patient some discomfort. Straighten the loop by applying rotational torque to the shaft, in the direction that produces the least resistance, while at the same time withdrawing the instrument. Once one-to-one withdrawal has been achieved, re-advance the instrument while maintaining the same torque, preventing reformation of the loop. In the sigmoid colon, the torque usually needs to be applied in a clockwise direction. The effect of this is to fold the sigmoid loop over and achieve a relatively straight sigmoid colon (Fig. 12.5).

? DIFFICULTY

1. If at any time the luminal view is lost, withdraw the instrument until the view is regained.
2. Pushing against the colon wall tends to create loops and may also lead to perforation. This is particularly important

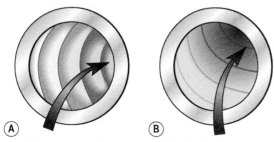

Fig. 12.3 Steer towards the concavity of the folds (A) and away from the bright light reflex (B).

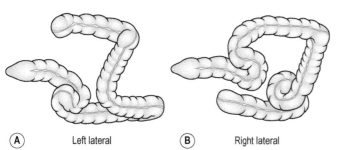

(A) Left lateral   (B) Right lateral

Fig. 12.4 Effect of changing position from left lateral to right lateral.

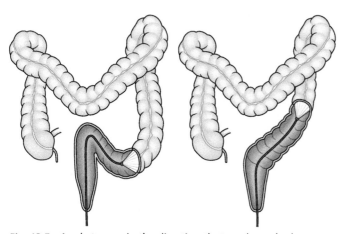

Fig. 12.5 Apply torque in the direction that produces the least resistance while withdrawing the instrument, to straighten the sigmoid colon so that the colonoscope can advance into the descending colon.

On reaching the descending colon, often recognizable by its long, straight appearance, straighten the tip of the instrument and advance it by insertion, maintaining the torque applied to keep the sigmoid colon in a straight configuration. The splenic flexure may be recognized by a bluish discoloration produced by the spleen adjacent to the colon wall, or a gate-like appearance at the entrance to the transverse colon.

8 Although there are variations between patients, the transverse colon is usually found by rotating the tip to the left and downwards. In many patients, the splenic flexure is acutely angled, resulting in sigmoid looping as advancement is attempted. Changing the position of the patient to the right lateral allows the transverse

colon to drop away from the flexure thus decreasing the angle. Once the characteristic triangular lumen of the transverse colon is recognized, straighten the tip and advance the instrument with a combination of intermittent suction and insertion. This has the effect of making the bowel concertina over the colonoscope and shortening the effective length. The transverse colon usually has at least one acute angle at its centre point, but may have more, particularly if postoperative adhesions are present. On reaching such an angle, angle the tip around the bend and, while maintaining a luminal view, apply torque and withdrawal as for the sigmoid loop, again in the direction of least resistance. In order to prevent possible trauma to the colon, always maintain a luminal view and do not hook the end of the instrument into the bowel wall. The effect of this manoeuvre is to straighten the transverse colon (Fig. 12.6).

As soon as one-to-one advancement is achieved, straighten the tip and advance the instrument, again using intermittent suction. If this manoeuvre does not result in easy one-to-one advancement, position change to supine or right lateral can be helpful. The tip of the instrument should then pass rapidly to the hepatic flexure, which may be recognizable by a bluish hue of the right lobe of the liver visible through the colonic wall. However, this is an unreliable landmark as the left lobe of the liver can give the same appearance in the mid-transverse colon. Occasionally, during the process of straightening the transverse colon, the sigmoid loop may re-form. It is useful at this stage, having re-straightened the sigmoid loop, either to employ an assistant to hold the sigmoid or transverse loop in its straightened configuration or increase the stiffness of the insertion shaft if using a variable stiffness colonoscope. In the case of the sigmoid colon, abdominal compression is performed using the flat of the hand to exert pressure downwards and towards the left iliac crest (Fig. 12.7A). For recurrent transverse looping, the colon is splinted by the assistant's hand pushing upwards from just above the umbilicus (Fig. 12.7B).

9 At the hepatic flexure, entrance to the caecum is usually found by angulation down and rotation to the left. The caecum often has a pool of fluid at its pole and the ileocaecal valve is visible as a shelf-like protrusion, with a lip-like centre. Advancement to the caecal pole can usually be achieved by a combination of suction and gentle advancement. If a transverse loop has re-formed, then

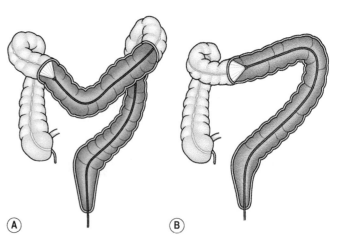

(A)   (B)

Fig. 12.6 Negotiating the transverse colon. Always maintain a luminal view.

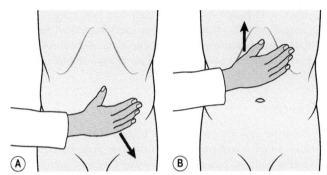

Fig. 12.7 (A) Have the colon held in the straightened configuration by an assistant's hand placed on the abdominal wall. (B) For recurrent transverse colon looping, have the assistant's hand push upwards from just below the umbilicus.

straighten the loop and re-advance, using assistant compression, or, providing the patient does not experience excessive discomfort and there is no resistance to intubation, a transverse loop can be deliberately formed and then, following angulation of the tip into the upper ascending colon, straightening of the scope by withdrawal combined with torque achieves advancement to the caecal pole. An alternative solution is to ask the patient to move back into the left lateral position, which will often result in a less-acute angle to be negotiated.

10 The only reliable landmarks in colonoscopy are seen on entering the caecum. Typically, there is a triradiate fold at the caecal pole, representing the convergence of the taeniae coli, at the centre of which may be seen the base of the appendix. Palpation of the abdomen, laterally in the right iliac fossa, produces indentation of the caecal wall, and the light of the colonoscope may also be visible through the abdominal wall. However, all of these appearances may be mimicked by a deep transverse loop, and the ileocaecal valve or terminal ileum is the only reliable sign that the caecum has been reached. The appearance of the ileocaecal valve may vary, but its usual appearance is of a lip-like structure. Intubation of the valve shows an obvious change in the mucosal pattern, from the shiny mucosa of the colon with visible blood vessels to the rather granular appearance of the distal ileum, often with visible lymphoid patches, and a characteristic advancing peristaltic movement.

Assess

1 Whilst much of the examination is carried out during intubation, perform a thorough inspection of the colon during withdrawal of the instrument. By using a combination of up/down deflection and rotation to create a figure-of-eight motion, it is possible to examine the colonic mucosa completely, particularly behind the circular muscle folds. A proper examination during withdrawal should take at least 6 minutes to avoid missing any mucosal lesions.

2 Keep your right hand on the shaft of the colonoscope, approximately 15–20 cm from the anus, since straightening of a loop often leads to rapid distal progression of the instrument. This requires rapid re-insertion to avoid overlooking any area of the mucosa. During extubation, insufflate more air/CO_2 in order to straighten the haustral folds. As each segment of colon is

examined, suck out the air in order to prevent undue discomfort and possible vasovagal attacks due to over-distension. At this stage, if spasm becomes a problem then inject intravenous hyoscine butylbromide or instil peppermint oil suspension into the colon via the biopsy channel to relieve the spasm and allow adequate visualization.

3 The normal appearance of the colon is a shiny mucosal surface, with a clearly visible vascular pattern. Loss of vascular pattern is the earliest sign of inflammatory bowel disease, followed by granular, friable mucosa and frank ulceration as the disease intensifies. Chronic disease may be manifest by pseudopolyps and stricture formation. The presence of 'skip lesions' separated by areas of normal mucosa, aphthous ulceration and deep fissuring ('cobblestone mucosa') is characteristic of Crohn's disease. The commonest types of polyp to be encountered are either adenomatous or hyperplastic. High definition endoscopes combined with either chromoscopy or narrow band imaging will allow classification of most polyps; however, in cases of doubt, or operator inexperience, remove these for histological assessment. Biopsy polypoid or plaque-like areas in cases of established ulcerative colitis to exclude dysplastic or neoplastic change.

Action

1 During colonoscopy, take biopsies or perform polypectomy. Introduce endoscopic accessories only when there is a clear luminal view, to avoid the risk of perforation. The most convenient biopsy forceps are those of the spiked variety, which remove adequate-sized samples of tissue and will not slide off the mucosa when attempting biopsy at a tangent. Hot biopsy, traditionally used for small sessile polyps, is potentially dangerous, carrying a high risk of perforation or delayed bleeding, and often produces inadequate material for accurate histology, whilst showing no evidence of decreasing polyp recurrence. Mount biopsy specimens carefully according to the preference of the histopathologist. Clearly label containers. Preferably, use a diagram of the colon on the histology request form, with specimens appropriately labelled to allow accurate identification of biopsy sites. In the case of strictures, use brush cytology when adequate biopsies cannot be obtained.

2 Perform coagulation of areas of angiodysplasia only if there are signs of ulceration or recent bleeding. Using coagulation forceps pick up the edge of the lesion, tenting it away from the colonic wall and drawing it over the centre of the lesion before applying the current. Alternatively, use argon plasma coagulation or laser vaporization.

3 Prior to snare polypectomy, make sure that you are familiar with the diathermy equipment and manufacturer's guidance. Diathermy power is delivered in different modes: coagulation, cut, a blend of coagulation and cut, or sequential cut and coagulation. The way in which the power is delivered affects both the mode of application of current and tightening of the snare. Always mark the snare in the fully closed position, allowing assessment of the amount of tissue enclosed in the snare: this avoids the risk of over-enthusiastic tightening or 'cheese-wiring' of the polyp with the risk of subsequent haemorrhage. Make sure that injection needles with adrenalin solution, together with endoscopic clips and endoloops are readily available in order to deal with any bleeding. Ensure that the colonoscope is as straight as

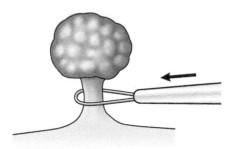

Fig. 12.8   When snaring a polyp, gradually close the snare while advancing the covering tube up to the stalk.

possible and the instrument tip is rotated to position the biopsy channel in line with the polyp. After introducing the snare, open it and manoeuvre it over the polyp. Adjust its position around the polyp stalk. Gradually close the snare while advancing the covering tube up to the stalk (Fig. 12.8). Do not apply diathermy current until the snare is closed around the polyp stalk, or the colonic wall beyond the polyp could be burned. Apply coagulation diathermy in the manner recommended by the diathermy manufacturer whilst slowly closing the snare.

> **KEY POINT** Take care with diathermy coagulation

- For safe diathermy coagulation of a polyp, look for blanching of the stalk; as this occurs, gradually draw the wire through.

On separation of the polyp head, observe the remaining stalk for bleeding. If haemorrhage does occur, replace the snare over the stalk, tighten it and leave it in place for 2–3 minutes. Do not apply further diathermy, but if necessary inject the stalk with a 1:10 000 adrenaline (epinephrine) solution using an endoscopic injection needle, and apply endoscopic clips or an endoloop.

4 Retrieve polyps for histological examination by either lassoing them with the snare or capturing them in a polyp retrieval basket. Alternatively, they may be sucked on to the end of the endoscope and withdrawn en masse by extubation. Small polyps (≤5 mm) may be sucked through the biopsy channel and retrieved into a polyp trap inserted into the suction line. Snares may be used not only for pedunculated polyps but also for sessile lesions. Submucosal injection of saline to raise the polyp from the muscularis mucosae not only facilitates placement of the snare, but reduces the risk of perforation and makes dealing with any bleeding vessels much easier. This technique allows snare polypectomy of lesions up to 2 cm in size. Larger lesions should be removed by endoscopic mucosal resection or submucosal dissection, usually in specialist centres that have expertise in these techniques. Piecemeal polypectomy should be avoided as it makes histopathological assessment of completeness of excision and staging impossible. If the polyp does not completely raise after the injection and there is central tethering, malignancy should be suspected and a biopsy taken. When large polyps are removed, the mucosa adjacent to the polypectomy site (distal to the site in the right colon, proximal in the left colon) should be marked by raising a bleb of submucosal saline injection, followed by injection of Indian ink into the bleb in at least three quadrants circumferentially. This allows easy identification of the site at follow-up colonoscopy, or marking of the site for subsequent laparoscopic or open resection if the polyp exhibits malignant change.

Aftercare

1 Have the patient observed by a trained nurse during recovery from sedation and ensure continuation of pulse oximetry monitoring until the patient is fully awake. Excessive insufflation of air during intubation may lead to nausea and vomiting, which is potentially dangerous in the sedated patient. Once fully awake, allow patients to go home provided they are accompanied by a responsible adult. Advise patients against driving or operating machinery for a period of 24 hours after sedation.

2 Ensure that the colonoscope is cleaned and disinfected following the procedure in accordance with the appropriate guidelines for decontamination of flexible endoscopes, and all equipment is checked for correct operation.

Complications

1 Apart from the effects of sedation, complications of diagnostic colonoscopy include perforation and haemorrhage, occurring in 0.1% to 0.3% of cases, with approximately 10 times this rate following polypectomy. However, these rates are quoted from a number of colonoscopic series, some very early in the evolution of colonoscopy, when instrument design was less advanced and endoscopists were learning the techniques. Nevertheless, complications still occur, particularly when the colonoscopist is inexperienced, so remember that patient pain is an important warning sign of dangerous overstretching of the bowel. This must not be masked by heavy sedation or analgesia. Similarly, never perform routine colonoscopy under general anaesthesia.

2 Many of the reported cases of postpolypectomy perforation and haemorrhage occur late (up to 72 hours post-procedure), usually because excessive diathermy current has been used, causing transmural burns or secondary haemorrhage. Advise patients to be seen by an experienced clinician if pain or bleeding occurs at any time following the procedure.

FURTHER READING

American Society for Gastrointestinal Endoscopy, Standards of Practice Committee. Complications of colonoscopy. Oak Brook, IL: ASGE. Available at http://www.asge.org/WorkArea/downloadasset.aspx?id=3342&LangType=1033; accessed 2003.

British Society of Gastroenterology. Guidelines for colorectal cancer screening and surveillance in moderate and high risk groups (update from 2002). London: BSG. Available at http://www.bsg.org.uk/clinical-guidelines/endoscopy/guidelines-for-colorectal-cancer-screening-and-surveillance-in-moderate-and-high-risk-groups-update-from-2002.html; accessed 2010.

British Society of Gastroenterology. Guidelines on decontamination of equipment for gastrointestinal endoscopy. London: BSG. Available at www.bsg.org.uk/pdf_word_docs/decontamination_2008.pdf; accessed 2008.

British Society of Gastroenterology. Guidance for obtaining a valid consent for elective endoscopic procedures. London: BSG. Available at http://www.bsg.org.uk/clinical-guidelines/endoscopy/guidance-for-obtaining-a-valid-consent-for-elective-endoscopic-procedures.html; accessed 2008.

British Society of Gastroenterology. Guidelines on safety and sedation during endoscopic procedures. London: BSG. Available at http://www.bsg.org.uk/clinical-guidelines/endoscopy/guidelines-on-safety-and-sedation-during-endoscopic-procedures.html; accessed 2003 and 2006.

Cotton PB, Williams CB, Hawes RH, Saunders BP. Practical Gastrointestinal Endoscopy: The Fundamentals. 6th ed. London: Wiley-Blackwell; 2008.

National Institute for Clinical Excellence. Colonoscopic surveillance for prevention of colorectal cancer in people with ulcerative colitis, Crohn's disease or adenomas. London: NICE. Available at http:// guidance.nice.org.uk/nicemedia/live/13415/53592/53592.pdf; accessed March 2011.

Riley SA. Colonoscopic polypectomy and endoscopic mucosal resection: A practical guide. London: BSG. Available at http://www.bsg.org.uk/pdf_word_docs/polypectomy_08.pdf; accessed 2008.

Wada Y, Kashida H, Kudo SE, et al. Diagnostic accuracy of pit pattern and vascular pattern analyses in colorectal lesions. Dig Endosc 2010;22 (3):192–9.

Waye JD, Rex DK, Williams CB. Colonoscopy: Principles and Practice. 2nd ed. London: Wiley-Blackwell; 2009.

13

Colon

R. Novell, M.K.W. Li, O. Ogunbiyi, H.Y.S. Cheung

PREOPERATIVE ASSESSMENT OF THE LARGE BOWEL

1 Obtain a full history and examine the abdomen, anus and rectum in every patient before undertaking surgery. Carry out further investigations as necessary:

- *Rigid sigmoidoscopy.* Although increasingly superseded by flexible sigmoidoscopy, this remains a useful investigation in outpatients presenting with bowel symptoms as it allows for prompt identification and biopsy of rectal pathology such as carcinoma, proctitis or solitary rectal ulcer.
- *Flexible sigmoidoscopy.* This can be undertaken as an outpatient procedure without sedation after bowel preparation with phosphate enemas. 60-cm scopes are available and easier to control but if you are experienced choose either a 90-cm scope or full-length colonoscope as they allow examination of the entire left colon in all patients.
- *Colonoscopy* (see Chapter 12). This is the investigation of choice for the large bowel, although not without risks, especially in the elderly or during therapeutic procedures. Biopsies can be obtained from tumours and inflammatory bowel disease and pedunculated polyps can be removed by colonoscopic snaring. More advanced procedures, such as endoscopic submucosal

resection and stenting, are available in many centres. The risk of perforation is approximately 1:800; removal of large polyps also carries a significant risk of bleeding although this can usually be controlled endoscopically.

- *CT colography (virtual colonoscopy).* With the advent of spiral computed tomography (CT), the technique of CT colography or virtual colonoscopy has achieved diagnostic sensitivity equivalent to optical colonoscopy. Advantages over colonoscopy are a reduced risk of perforation, the ability to image the bowel proximal to strictures and the detection of other intra-abdominal and pelvic pathology. A significant abnormality on virtual colonoscopy usually demands confirmation by optical colonoscopy and biopsy.
- *Barium enema.* Double-contrast barium enema is less sensitive than colonoscopy but is still widely used in hospitals where access to endoscopy and CT is limited.
- *Contrast-enhanced CT scan.* The investigation of choice in the acute abdomen, bowel obstruction and acute diverticulitis. A CT of the chest, abdomen and pelvis is now routinely used in staging colorectal cancer.
- *MRI.* The 'Gold Standard' investigation in preoperative staging for rectal cancer and increasingly employed in imaging inflammatory bowel disease due to the absence of radiation risks.
- *Other examinations.* **Stool microscopy** and culture are essential to differentiate bacterial and parasitic infection from inflammatory bowel disease. Order an **erect chest/abdominal X-ray** in suspected bowel obstruction or perforation. Serial abdominal films are also important in acute fulminant colitis to detect the onset of toxic megacolon. **Ultrasound scans** are of value in diagnosing abdominal masses, intra-abdominal collections and possible metastases. Ultrasonography is more readily available than CT scanning, but diagnostic accuracy is operator-dependent. Employ **angiography** in the management of severe gastrointestinal haemorrhage: this can be combined with therapeutic embolization of the bleeding vessel.

ELECTIVE OPERATIONS

CARCINOMA

▶ KEY POINTS Precautions

- Plan elective surgery carefully.
- Always obtain informed consent for removal of any organs which preoperative investigations indicate may be affected by the disease process.

- Always have X-rays and results of other investigations available for review in the operating theatre.
- Ensure you have the right equipment and assistance available. Endoscopy equipment should be available to allow examination of the bowel lumen if necessary during the procedure.
- Re-examine the abdomen and rectum when the patient is anaesthetized and relaxed.

Assess

1 Perform a full laparotomy or laparoscopy, particularly if preoperative CT scanning has not been performed.

2 Examine the whole of the colon from the appendix to the rectum. Synchronous carcinomas occur in 4% of patients; adenomatous polyps cannot usually be palpated.

3 Avoid handling the carcinoma. Cover it with a swab soaked in 10% aqueous povidone-iodine solution.

4 Feel for enlarged lymph nodes in the mesentery and para-aortic region. Look and feel for liver and peritoneal metastases.

5 Assess the resectability and curability of the tumour.

6 If you discover unexpected liver metastases in the presence of a potentially resectable tumour do not biopsy them, as this may result in trans-peritoneal spread of tumour. In selected patients with solitary or localized liver metastases it may be appropriate to perform a synchronous metastasectomy if you have the relevant expertise. For multiple liver metastases the increased morbidity outweighs any benefit. Proceed with the planned bowel resection and refer the patient to a specialist liver centre for further assessment.

? DIFFICULTY

1. If a tumour is potentially resectable but fixed to another viscus such as bladder, uterus, a loop of bowel, duodenum, stomach, gallbladder, liver, kidney or to the abdominal wall, the prognosis is not adversely affected if it can be resected en bloc with part or all of the adjacent structure.
2. Resection of the primary tumour provides better palliation than a bypass procedure even in the presence of peritoneal metastases, but adopt a less radical approach.

7 Curative resection should incorporate complete mesocolic excision (analogous to total mesorectal excision, vide infra). Excise the colon, segmental blood supply and associated lymph nodes en bloc within an intact mesocolic fascial envelope. If you fail to dissect in this plane you increase the risk of dissemination of tumour cells, resulting in local recurrence.

8 Treat carcinoma of the right colon by right hemicolectomy, taking the ileocolic pedicle at its origin from the superior mesenteric vessels (Fig. 13.1). For tumours of the hepatic flexure perform an extended resection, dividing the right branch of the middle colic pedicle at its origin (Fig. 13.2). If metastases are present perform a less radical resection without wide mesenteric

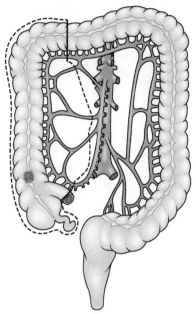

Fig. 13.1   Radical right hemicolectomy. The ileocolic artery and vein are divided at their origins from the superior mesenteric vessels. The right branch of the middle colic artery is divided.

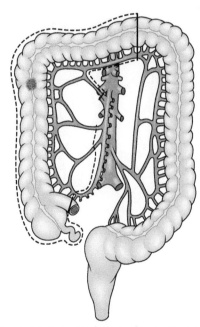

Fig. 13.2   Extended right hemicolectomy for carcinoma of the hepatic flexure.

clearance. Treat carcinoma of the transverse colon by extended right hemicolectomy or transverse colectomy (Fig. 13.3), mobilizing the hepatic and/or splenic flexure as required.

9 Treat carcinoma of the splenic flexure with left hemicolectomy, dividing the left colic pedicle at its origin (Fig. 13.4). If distal diverticular disease is present, perform an extended left hemicolectomy and swing the transverse and right colon down the right side of the abdomen to anastomose it to the rectum (Fig. 13.5). Alternatively, perform a subtotal colectomy and ileorectal anastomosis.

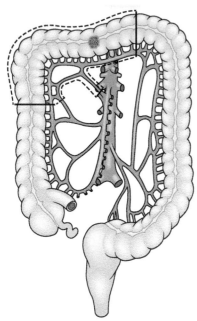

Fig. 13.3   Transverse colectomy.

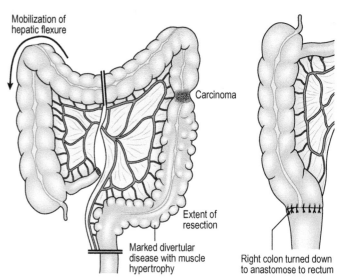

Fig. 13.5   Management of carcinoma of the splenic flexure or distal transverse colon with sigmoid diverticulosis.

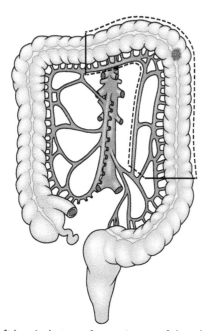

Fig. 13.4   Left hemicolectomy for carcinoma of the splenic flexure.

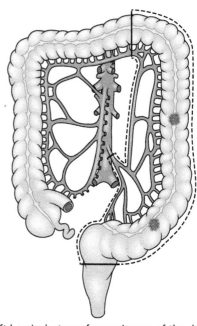

Fig. 13.6   Left hemicolectomy for carcinoma of the descending and sigmoid colon.

10 Treat carcinoma of the descending or sigmoid colon by left hemicolectomy, dividing the inferior mesenteric artery at its origin from the aorta and the inferior mesenteric vein at the same level (Fig. 13.6).

11 The surgical management of rectal carcinoma has undergone radical evolution over the last 20 years. Most cases of carcinoma of the rectum are now treated by restorative anterior resection using either a sutured, stapled or per-anal anastomosis. Abdominoperineal excision of the rectum and anus is required in around 20% of cases when it is impossible to obtain adequate distal clearance of the tumour. Carefully dissect in the pelvis to remove the mesorectum without breaching the fascial plane in which it is contained. Preserve the hypogastric nerve plexus if it is uninvolved with tumour, thereby reducing the incidence of erectile dysfunction and urinary complications. In expert hands total mesorectal excision (TME) results in very low local recurrence rates with an acceptable incidence of complications.

12 For high rectal carcinoma (tumours situated above the peritoneal reflection) with metastases, perform an anterior resection and primary anastomosis if you are able to perform this without the need for a defunctioning colostomy. These patients often have a limited survival and may never have the colostomy closed. For rectal carcinoma with unresectable local extension into the pelvic side wall, a Hartmann's operation provides the best palliation.

DIVERTICULAR DISEASE

1 Diverticular disease is common and elderly patients having abdominal surgery are often found to have diverticula, most

commonly in the sigmoid colon. Although diverticular disease may be pancolonic, symptoms usually result from muscle hypertrophy causing thickening and shortening of the sigmoid colon.

2 Indications for elective resection are rarely absolute. Consider surgery in patients in good general health who have severe episodes of left iliac fossa and suprapubic pain with marked diverticular disease on a barium enema or CT scan and who are unresponsive to dietary change and antispasmodic drugs. More definite indications for surgical treatment include:
- Younger male patients (less than 50 years of age) with symptomatic disease, since statistically over 80% eventually come to surgery, many with complications
- Patients with urinary symptoms associated with their attacks or with pneumaturia, indicating a colovesical fistula. Female patients who have undergone hysterectomy may also present with offensive vaginal discharge secondary to a colovaginal fistula
- Patients with recurrent attacks of acute diverticitis presenting with fever, and tenderness in the left iliac fossa or mass or evidence of a pericolic abscess on CT scan
- Patients with recurrent lower gastrointestinal bleeding: surgery is not mandatory following a single episode of bleeding.

3 Colectomy for diverticular disease is frequently more challenging than similar operations for cancer. Even elective resections may be associated with pericolic inflammation, oedema and pericolic abscess formation in the mesentery.

> ### ▶ KEY POINT Avoid operation
>
> - Avoid operation in patients with few diverticula and irritable bowel symptoms. They are unlikely to benefit from resection and may develop greater urgency.

4 It is unnecessary to remove all the proximal diverticula. Resect the hypertrophied section of bowel (usually the sigmoid colon), with anastomosis between the descending colon and the upper third of the rectum at or below the sacral promontory.

5 The elective treatment of choice is primary resection and anastomosis. If there is acute inflammation at the time of surgery or the anastomosis is difficult, perform a temporary defunctioning ileostomy.

ULCERATIVE COLITIS

1 Offer elective surgery to patients with persistent bloody diarrhoea, anaemia, weight loss and general ill-health who do not respond to treatment with corticosteroids and immune modulators such as azothiaprine. The majority of these patients have pancolitis (Greek: pan = all, total). Patients with distal disease involving the rectosigmoid or left hemicolon can usually be managed medically. Try to operate on patients during a remission.

2 Active colitis of 10 or more years' duration may result in epithelial dysplasia with eventual progression to carcinoma, even in the absence of any symptoms. These patients require yearly surveillance with colonoscopy and mucosal biopsy. Advise operation if they develop severe dysplasia. Advise colectomy on any patient with total colitis and a stricture on barium enema or

colonoscopy. Steroid therapy is not a contraindication to surgery, but steroid cover is required during and after the operation.

3 In longstanding total colitis, the colon is thickened, shortened and featureless in appearance. The macroscopic appearances may vary with parts of the colon appearing more actively inflamed with thickening, oedema and marked hyperaemia. The paracolic and mesenteric nodes may be enlarged.

4 The simplest operation is a proctocolectomy with a conventional end (Brooke) ileostomy, which removes all the inflamed bowel and potential cancer risk in one procedure.

5 Consider alternative procedures:
- If you are inexperienced in pelvic surgery, carry out a colectomy and ileostomy, retaining the whole rectum, and refer the patient to a specialist centre for subsequent reconstruction. This is also the procedure of choice in the urgent or emergency situation.
- In patients wishing to avoid a permanent ileostomy, perform a restorative proctocolectomy, preserving the anal canal and sphincters, and create an ileo-anal reservoir.
- In older or obese patients who wish to avoid a stoma but in whom the risks and uncertainties of pouch surgery do not seem justified, consider performing a colectomy and ileorectal (or if possible ileosigmoid) anastomosis. To achieve the best functional results, operate early in the course of the disease when the rectum is still distensible and there is no dysplasia present in rectal biopsies.
- The Kock reservoir is a continent ileostomy designed to spare patients the need to wear a stoma appliance. It is prone to complications and poor function and is, as a result, now rarely performed.

CROHN'S DISEASE

1 This can affect any part of the gastrointestinal tract from the mouth to the anus and is primarily treated medically.

2 Resort to surgery if medical treatment fails to control the disease, or for complications such as stricture causing obstructive symptoms, abscess or fistula formation.

> ### ▶ KEY POINT Operate on clinical grounds, not merely on investigation results
>
> - Surgery is not curative, so treat the patient and their symptoms, not the X-ray.

3 All or part of the colon may be involved in Crohn's disease. At laparotomy or laparoscopy carefully exclude disease in the stomach, duodenum and small bowel. Measure and record the sites and extent of disease and the length of residual small bowel following resection: patients with Crohn's disease may require multiple operations and may develop short bowel syndrome if surgery is not carefully planned.

4 Crohn's disease of the terminal ileum or ileocaecal region should be treated by ileocaecal resection, removing only the diseased segment: there is no advantage to removing macroscopically normal bowel. If there is a chronic abscess cavity in the right iliac fossa, position the anastomosis in the upper abdomen away from the inflamed tissues.

5 For extensive colitis unresponsive to medical treatment, perform a colectomy and ileorectal anastomosis or a total proctocolectomy and ileostomy. Stenosing or fistulating disease involving only the rectum may require abdominoperineal excision with an end colostomy.

6 Segmental colonic resection is appropriate for localized segmental involvement of the colon, or to treat internal fistula between the terminal ileum and the transverse or sigmoid colon.

POLYPS AND POLYPOSIS

1 Rectal polyps found at rigid sigmoidoscopy should be biopsied. If the polyp proves to be an adenoma, arrange a colonoscopy to find and remove any proximal polyps. Sessile villous adenomas usually occur in the rectum and can be removed by endoanal local excision. Transanal endoscopic microsurgery (TEMS) and endoscopic laser ablation (useful in the frail and elderly) are available in specialist centres.

2 If large colonic polyps are present in a patient undergoing surgery for carcinoma, extend the resection to include them or consider subtotal colectomy and ileorectal anastomosis.

3 Circumferential villous adenomas of the rectum are at high risk of malignant change and are difficult to resect peranally. Perform anterior resection with colo-anal anastomosis or a modified Soave procedure, particularly for tumours extending more than 10 cm from the anus.

4 Surgery is mandatory in familial adenomatous polyposis (FAP) to avoid inevitable malignant change. Options include colectomy and ileorectal anastomosis or proctocolectomy and ileoanal pouch reconstruction. Following ileorectal anastomosis the rectum still carries the potential for malignant change. Inspect sigmoidoscopically every 6–12 months with fulguration of polyps over 5 mm in diameter.

URGENT OPERATIONS

1 Urgent operations on the colon or rectum are required for obstruction, perforation, acute fulminant colitis and, less frequently, life-threatening acute haemorrhage.

2 Stabilize the patient's condition prior to surgery by replacing blood, fluid and electrolyte losses. Give broad-spectrum antibiotics (co-amoxiclav or a cephalosporin with metronidazole) to counteract sepsis.

3 Major abdominal sepsis, perforation or torrential haemorrhage demand operation as soon as the patient's condition allows. Patients with colonic obstruction or inflammatory bowel disease rarely require immediate surgery and frequently benefit from appropriate investigation and resuscitation.

> **KEY POINT** Operate under the best conditions

- Whenever possible avoid operating in haste at night, when you are tired, the patient is ill-prepared and the assistance and equipment are inadequate.

OBSTRUCTION

1 Establish the site of obstruction with a CT scan or water-soluble contrast enema.

2 If the patient is unfit for surgery, a stenosing tumour may be suitable for radiological stenting to open up the bowel lumen, allowing the patient's condition to be optimized for subsequent elective surgery. Stenting is less successful for benign strictures due to diverticulitis, Crohn's disease or external compression and carries a higher morbidity: a defunctioning proximal stoma provides better palliation in patients who are unfit for major surgery.

3 Urgent resection should be as radical as would be achieved electively, provided the patient's condition permits this. If metastases are present, undertake a less radical resection if possible, as this will give better palliation.

> ▶ KEY POINTS Do not lose sight of your objective

- You are operating in an emergency to relieve a life-threatening condition.
- Do not undertake unnecessary procedures which may prejudice the patient's recovery.

4 Perform a right hemicolectomy for carcinoma of the right colon causing acute intestinal obstruction. It is rare to find a proximal tumour that is not resectable. Avoid a bypass operation if possible as this may relieve the obstruction but it will not stop bleeding from the tumour and consequent anaemia, nor will it palliate pain or complications resulting from invasion of other structures.

5 Historically, left-sided obstruction was treated by a three-stage procedure with an initial proximal stoma to relieve the obstruction, subsequent resection and anastomosis and, when the anastomosis was healed, closure of the stoma. Obstructing carcinoma of the sigmoid or descending colon is now usually treated by a one-stage colectomy with ileosigmoid or ileorectal anastomosis (Fig. 13.7). If a left-sided tumour is unresectable, create a proximal defunctioning colostomy.

6 Treat carcinoma of the rectosigmoid junction or rectum by resection and primary anastomosis with or without a defunctioning ileostomy. Alternatively, perform a Hartmann's procedure (vide infra).

7 Acute obstruction due to diverticular disease is often complicated by paracolic abscess formation, and is most commonly treated by

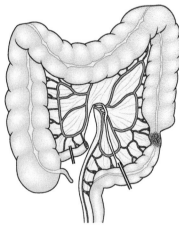

Fig. 13.7 Ileosigmoid anastomosis for obstructing carcinoma of the sigmoid colon.

Hartmann's procedure. However, if the infection is localized and can be completely excised then primary resection and anastomosis, with or without a defunctioning ileostomy, may be appropriate.

PERFORATION

1. Perforation of a carcinoma or diverticular disease requires resection and anastomosis with a covering stoma; if major faecal contamination is present, perform a Hartmann's procedure.

2. If CT scanning demonstrates a localized perforation and pericolic abscess, drain it percutaneously. Operate if initially localized abdominal signs become more generalized or if the infection fails to settle despite adequate conservative therapy. Generalized purulent peritonitis secondary to diverticulitis may be managed by laparoscopic peritoneal lavage and drainage, provided there is no evidence of a free perforation. In patients with more extensive contamination and a free perforation, resection and primary anastomosis is possible in selected cases, but do not perform this in the presence of faecal peritonitis.

3. Primary anastomosis is increasingly popular because:
   - Patients require one operation rather than two
   - Following Hartmann's procedure many patients are left with a permanent stoma, because they are unwilling or unfit to have further surgery
   - Reversal of Hartmann's procedure can be challenging, particularly if attempted too early.

4. Always aim to resect the perforated segment of bowel, even in an acutely ill patient, to minimize the risk of persistent contamination. Also, it is difficult at operation to decide whether a lesion is a perforated carcinoma or diverticular phlegmon: up to 25% of patients with a preoperative diagnosis of perforated diverticulitis will prove to have malignancy. If carcinoma is suspected perform a radical resection: examination of the resected specimen in theatre may help to confirm the diagnosis.

ACUTE INFLAMMATORY OR ISCHAEMIC BOWEL DISEASE

1. Treat acute fulminant colitis, with or without toxic megacolon, by colectomy and ileostomy. Do not excise the rectum. It is usually safe to close the rectal stump but if it is very inflamed or friable you may need to bring it out as a mucous fistula. Alternatively, close the stump directly under the wound so that if it breaks down it will not contaminate the peritoneal cavity.

2. In ischaemic colitis, excise the segment of acutely ischaemic colon and create a proximal (and if necessary a distal) colostomy. Do not remove the rectum or distal sigmoid colon as these usually recover sufficiently for an anastomosis to be carried out later.

ACUTE MASSIVE HAEMORRHAGE

1. If possible, determine the site of bleeding by sigmoidoscopy, colonoscopy, upper gastrointestinal endoscopy and angiography. In patients with episodes of haemorrhage and diverticular disease do not assume causation: 50% have another cause for the bleeding.

2. It is usually possible to arrest life-threatening bleeding by interventional radiology and embolization, which carries a much lower morbidity and mortality than emergency colectomy.

Surgery may still be required if the embolized segment becomes ischaemic, but at least you will be sure which part to remove.

PRINCIPLES OF COLECTOMY

Appraise

1. Morbidity and mortality following colonic surgery are higher than following small bowel resection. Infection is more common, resulting in abscess formation with potentiation of collagenase activity which predisposes to anastomotic dehiscence.

2. In addition, the colonic blood supply is more tenuous and tissue perfusion may be suboptimal postoperatively, resulting in ischaemia to the anastomosis. If available, we recommend goal-directed intra-operative fluid replacement using peroperative transoesophageal Doppler monitoring.

Prepare

1. Enhanced recovery protocols ('fast track surgery') have demonstrated reduction in both morbidity and length of stay following elective colorectal resections. They typically include:
   - Avoidance of mechanical bowel preparation (vide infra)
   - Preoperative carbohydrate loading to prevent the development of a catabolic state and insulin resistance
   - The use of minimally invasive surgery or small incisions
   - Goal-directed fluid replacement (vide supra)
   - Prevention of intra-operative hypothermia
   - Avoidance of opiates by the use of epidural anaesthesia, transversus abdominis plane (TAPP) blocks or wound catheters to infuse local anaesthetics
   - Avoidance or early removal of nasogastric tubes, drains and urinary catheters
   - Early enteral feeding
   - Early mobilization.

2. There is no evidence to support the routine use of bowel preparation before elective colonic operations and good evidence that the resulting fluid and electrolyte imbalances delay postoperative recovery. Some surgeons nonetheless prefer to prepare the left colon, but there is no need to clear the bowel prior to right hemicolectomy. Always prepare the bowel prior to low anterior resection with a loop ileostomy, as this will otherwise leave a long segment of faecally loaded colon between the covering stoma and the anastomosis. Sodium picosulfate and magnesium citrate (Picolax™, Citrafleet™), sodium phosphate (Fleet™) and polyethylene glycol (Kleanprep™, Moviprep™) are all suitable. Encourage adequate oral fluids during bowel preparation: intravenous fluids may be required in elderly patients. Patients likely to have a transanal stapled anastomosis should have an enema prior to surgery to avoid the problem of a rectum loaded with stool.

3. Give preoperative prophylactic antibiotics at induction of anaesthesia: a cephalosporin or a broad-spectrum penicillin plus betalactamase inhibitor (co-amoxiclav) plus metronidazole are suitable. Give a second dose of antibiotics if the duration of operation is more than 2 hours or if there is significant intraoperative contamination. There is no evidence that routine use of more than one dose of prophylactic antibiotics reduces the risk of infection, unless gross faecal contamination is present, when antibiotics should be continued for several days postoperatively.

4 Catheterize the patient after induction of anaesthesia and monitor urinary output during and after surgery.

> **KEY POINTS** Complete the World Health Organization (WHO) preoperative checklist

- Is this the right patient, accompanied by the completed consent form? Has the abdomen been marked for potential stoma sites?
- Is the patient correctly positioned on the operating table? Do you have adequate assistance and all the necessary equipment?
- Are the imaging results available? Has blood been cross-matched?

Action

1 Clamp the segment of bowel to be resected with Parker-Kerr clamps or use a cross-stapling technique. Do not clamp the ends to be sutured: apply non-crushing clamps 5 cm away from the bowel end to avoid contamination while constructing the anastomosis.

2 A good blood supply is crucial to anastomotic healing. Ensure that both limbs of the anastomosis are pink and well perfused: visible or palpable pulsation in the mesenteric vessels is an added reassurance, as is pulsatile flow on dividing the marginal artery whilst preparing the bowel for anastomosis.

3 Divide the colon at right-angles to the mesentery. If there is disparity in size between the ends, particularly when carrying out a right hemicolectomy or an ileorectal anastomosis, make a slit in the antimesenteric border of the ileum until the two ends approximate in size. Alternatively, carry out a stapled side-to-side anastomosis. When anastomosing a long proximal limb of mobilized colon to the rectum check that it is not twisted through 360°. Clean the ends of the bowel to be sutured with swabs moistened in aqueous 10% povidone-iodine solution.

4 Suture the bowel using a single-layer seromuscular suture such as 3/0 PDS (polydioxanone sulphate) using either an interrupted or continuous technique. Invert the edges to ensure no mucosa protrudes from the suture line. Where the two bowel limbs are sufficiently mobile and well perfused a side-to-side stapled anastomosis is a quick and reliable technique, although significantly more expensive. This technique is ideally suited to small bowel and right colonic resections, but should be used with caution in the left colon where the blood supply is more tenuous.

5 Colorectal anastomosis is most easily accomplished using a circular stapling device such as the CEEA stapler, using a 28-or 31-mm diameter device. We particularly recommend it for anastomosis low in the pelvis where suturing may be technically difficult.

6 Prevent contamination of the operative field by placing a non-crushing clamp across the bowel 10 cm from the end before this is swabbed out and cleaned. Isolate the anastomosis from the peritoneum and wound edges while it is being constructed, using disposable drapes or abdominal packs soaked in 10% aqueous povidone-iodine solution. On completion of the anastomosis, discard any soiled packs and instruments and change gloves before closing the abdomen.

7 Intra-peritoneal drains are of no proven value and may actually increase the risk of anastomotic leakage. Some surgeons prefer to drain the pelvic cavity following low anterior resection or abdominoperineal excision.

LAPAROSCOPIC COLECTOMY

1 The indications for laparoscopic colectomy are essentially the same as for open surgery. The laparoscopic approach is associated with some short-term benefits when compared with open surgery, notably faster recovery and reduced postoperative pain and wound infection. Data from randomized trials have demonstrated oncological outcomes comparable to open surgery.

2 Like other advanced laparoscopic procedures, laparoscopic colectomy is associated with a steep learning curve, requiring around 30 resections to achieve competence. Mobile lesions in the right colon or rectosigmoid junction are ideal for the novice. Lesions in the upper sigmoid or descending colon which necessitate splenic flexure mobilization and mid or low rectal tumours, which require pelvic dissection, require considerably more skill and experience.

3 Patient-related factors such as obesity and previous abdominal operations can make laparoscopic surgery more difficult, although conversely laparoscopic colectomy may result in greater short-term benefits in these patients. Patients with compromised cardiopulmonary function require special attention as they tolerate prolonged pneumoperitoneum poorly: close liaison with an experienced anaesthetist is recommended. Patients with locally advanced disease (tumours with fixation to surrounding structures or contiguous organ involvement) should be selected with extreme caution. Such tumours often preclude a pure laparoscopic approach (although you may employ a 'hand-assisted' laparoscopic approach with the use of hand-access devices) and are better managed through a conventional laparotomy incision.

4 As abdominal organs cannot be palpated during laparoscopy, preoperative colonoscopy and imaging studies are important both for tumour localization and disease staging. If preoperative colonoscopy is incomplete, either barium enema examination or CT virtual colonoscopy should be considered for proximal colonic evaluation; the latter also facilitates better patient selection by providing information on tumour staging.

5 'Tattoo' small mucosal lesions during endoscopic examination to facilitate identification at subsequent laparoscopy. Alternatively, carry out perioperative colonoscopy, preferably with CO_2 insufflation, during surgery.

6 Laparoscopic colectomy is never a single surgeon operation. Always use a dedicated team of at least two experienced surgeons and one camera assistant. Experienced anaesthetists, nurses and technicians who are familiar with the procedures, laparoscopic instruments and ancillary technology also form an integral part of the team. The operating theatre should accommodate staff and equipment in an unencumbered fashion. If possible, carry out laparoscopic colectomy in an integrated endo-laparoscopic operating suite where all equipment, including the optical system, energy source and monitors, is placed on ceiling-mounted platforms. Back-up equipment and facilities are essential.

7 Recommended instruments for laparoscopic colectomy:
- A 30° telescope

- Three to four atraumatic forceps for handling of bowel and fine tissues
- Two grasping forceps for holding sutures or cotton tapes
- Ultrasonic dissection device, 5 or 10 mm in size; or Ligasure™ device (Tyco Healthcare Group LP, Boulder, U.S.A.), 5 or 10 mm in size
- Laparoscopic bipolar coagulating forceps (Gyrus Medical Limited, Cardiff, U.K.), 5 mm in size
- Endoscopic clip applicators and clips
- Endo-staplers of various sizes, used for bowel transection (blue, gold or green cartridge) and vascular division (white cartridge)
- Circular staplers for trans-rectal bowel anastomosis
- A sterile plastic zip-lock bag, used as a parietal protector during specimen retrieval.

> ▶ KEY POINTS Identifying the pathology

- Identification of pathology at the time of laparoscopic colectomy may be difficult or impossible when there is no serosal involvement unless a hand-assisted device is used.
- Accurate delineation of the lesion is aided by preoperative endoscopic tattooing of the normal colonic wall around the lesion, or by perioperative colonoscopy with CO_2 insufflation.

RIGHT HEMICOLECTOMY

Appraise

1 Perform this operation for carcinoma of the caecum and ascending colon, benign tumours of the right colon, perforated caecal diverticulum, midgut neuroendocrine tumours and carcinoma of the appendix. Small, low-grade neuroendocrine tumours of the tip of the appendix (appendiceal carcinoid) found incidentally at appendicectomy do not require subsequent hemicolectomy.

2 In benign disease of the terminal ileum, particularly Crohn's disease, resect the diseased ileum together with the caecum and 2–3 cm of the right colon. If ileocaecal Crohn's disease is associated with abscess formation in the right iliac fossa, place the anastomosis in the upper abdomen away from the abscess cavity to reduce the risk of postoperative fistula formation.

3 Do not site a small bowel anastomosis close to the ileocaecal valve, as this may predispose to anastomotic leakage. It is preferable to remove the caecum and a small part of the ascending colon to achieve an ileocolic anastomosis.

4 In patients with distal colonic obstruction the caecum may be ischaemic: include any non-viable bowel in the resection, either by means of an extended right hemicolectomy or subtotal colectomy with ileorectal anastomosis.

Action

Resect

1 Make a midline incision centred on the umbilicus or a transverse incision extending laterally from the umbilicus. Handle the tumour as little as possible. If the serosa is infiltrated by carcinoma, cover it with a swab soaked in aqueous 10% povidone-iodine solution.

2 Draw the caecum and ascending colon medially. Divide the parietal peritoneum in the lateral paracolic gutter from the caecum to the hepatic flexure. If the carcinoma infiltrates the lateral abdominal wall do not attempt to dissect it off, but excise a disc of peritoneum and underlying muscle en-bloc with the specimen.

3 Dissect the plane between the right colon and posterior abdominal wall, identifying and preserving the right gonadal vessels, ureter and duodenum.

4 Mobilize the hepatic flexure and posterior attachments of the terminal ileum so that the whole of the right colon can be lifted medially and out of the abdomen.

> ▶ KEY POINTS Anatomy

- You are elevating the bowel on its embryological mesentery consisting of blood vessels, lymphatics and nerves contained in an envelope of adipose tissue (the mesocolon).
- Maintain meticulous dissection in the mesocolic plane between the mesocolon and posterior abdominal wall to avoid breaching the primary tumour or any mesenteric nodal metastases.

5 Clamp and divide the ileocolic artery and vein close to their origin from the superior mesenteric vessels, being careful not to tent the superior mesenteric trunk up and thereby inadvertently damage it. Divide the right colic vessels (if present) and the right branch of the middle colic vessels close to their origin.

6 The extent of the resection depends on the size and site of the tumour but normally extends from terminal ileum to the mid-transverse colon. In operations for carcinoma of the right colon it is not necessary to resect more than a few centimetres of terminal ileum.

7 Remove the right half of the greater omentum with the specimen. If the tumour is situated near the hepatic flexure remove the adjacent gastroepiploic vascular arcade to ensure adequate clearance.

8 Place a Parker-Kerr clamp or cross-stapler across the ileum and transverse colon at the site of division. If the patient is obstructed place towels around the bowel at the time of division as described above.

9 Divide the bowel proximally and distally and remove the specimen.

10 Hold the ends of the ileum and colon to be anastomosed in Babcock's forceps and clean them with mounted swabs soaked in aqueous 10% povidone-iodine solution.

Unite

1 Construct a functional end-to-end anastomosis using a linear cutting stapling device. Alternatively, suture the terminal ileum end-to-end to the transverse colon, if necessary widening the ileum with a Cheatle antimesenteric slit, described by the English surgeon Sir George Cheatle, 1865–1951 (Fig. 13.8). Mark the anastomosis with radio-opaque clips if desired.

2 Appose the cut edges of the mesentery with a 2/0 polyglactin 910 (Vicryl) or 3/0 PDS suture.

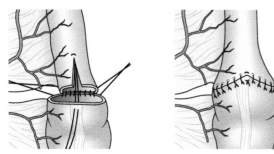

Fig. 13.8 Cheatle slit on antimesenteric aspect of the ileum to accommodate the discrepancy in size.

3 Return the anastomosed bowel to the right paracolic gutter, covering it with the remaining omentum.

Technical points

1 Resections for benign conditions such as Crohn's disease or caecal diverticulum should be conservative. Divide the vessels in the middle of the mesentery rather than at their origin.

2 If a carcinoma is locally invasive but can be excised radically, include abdominal wall or involved organs in the resection as required.

3 For carcinoma of the transverse colon you may need to mobilize the splenic flexure. This is best achieved by entering the lesser sac of the peritoneum through the gastrocolic omentum. Divide the middle colic vessels close to their origin and anastomose the terminal ileum to distal transverse colon, if adequately perfused, or else the descending or sigmoid colon.

4 If multiple metastases are present, a limited segmental resection provides better palliation than a bypass procedure.

Checklist

1 Make sure the anastomosis is viable and not under tension.

2 Examine the raw surfaces, particularly in the right paracolic gutter, for bleeding. Lavage the operative field with warm isotonic saline and remove any blood which may have collected above the right lobe of the liver and in the pelvis. Do not add antiseptics or antibiotics to the fluid as these irritate the peritoneum and promote adhesion formation.

LAPAROSCOPIC RIGHT HEMICOLECTOMY

Access

1 Stand on the left side of the patient. The monitor is placed next to the patient's right shoulder (Fig. 13.9).

2 Establish pneumoperitoneum via a 10–11-mm subumbilical incision using an open technique. Place further ports as shown in Figure 13.10.

3 Place the patient in steep head-down position and rolled to the left so that the small bowel falls away from the pelvis, the caecum and terminal ileum. Re-position the patient into the head-up position as the operation field moves to the hepatic flexure and transverse colon.

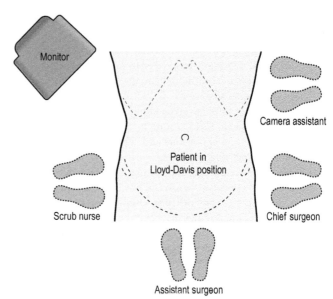

Fig. 13.9 Position of operating team for laparoscopic right hemicolectomy.

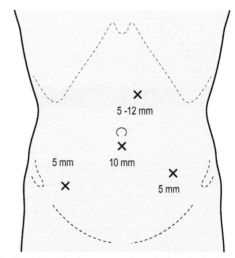

Fig. 13.10 Port sites for laparoscopic right hemicolectomy.

▶ KEY POINTS Principles of laparoscopic colonic resection

■ Identification of lesion
■ Assess suitability for laparoscopic resection: if not appropriate convert to open or hand-assisted laparoscopic approach
■ Mobilization
■ Pedicle division
■ Resection
■ Restore continuity.

Action

1 We describe the medial-first approach here. Identify first the ileocolic vessels near the third part of duodenum. Have the assistant surgeon hold up the caecum, putting the vascular pedicle on stretch. Divide the pedicle between endo-clips close to the

duodenum (i.e. 'high' ligation). Take care to avoid inadvertent injury to the superior mesenteric artery and vein.

2 Continue the mesenteric division upwards above the second part of duodenum. Display the right colic vessels by gently lifting the mesentery upwards; avoid excessive traction, which may tear the right colic vein. Once identified, the right colic vessels, usually shorter and smaller than the ileocolic pedicle, are controlled and divided.

3 Blunt dissection (e.g. with the use of the closed jaws of a 10-mm Ligasure™) is then carried out laterally in the plane between the colonic mesentery and the retroperitoneum. The right ureter and gonadal vessels are identified beneath the retroperitoneal fascia. Perform dissection as far lateral as possible, till the lateral abdominal wall is reached. Lateral to the second part of duodenum, carry out similar blunt dissection to separate the ascending colon and its mesentery from Gerota's fascia. Always keep the plane of dissection anterior to the duodenum at all times and do not Kocherise the duodenum. Perform blunt dissection as far upwards as possible; the inferior border of the liver is sometimes visible through the fascial covering at the end of dissection. The medial dissection is now complete.

4 Start the lateral dissection by incising the fascia inferio-lateral to the ileocaecal junction. Have the assistant surgeon pull the caecum cranially and medially to provide the necessary countertraction. Follow the 'white line' of Toldt's fascia and mobilize, in this order, the terminal ileum, caecum and ascending colon. The right ureter and gonadal vessels are identified once again under the retroperitoneal fascia.

5 Next, place the table in head-up position to keep the small bowel away from the upper abdomen. Starting at proximal to mid transverse colon, incise the greater omentum close to the colon and enter the lesser sac, caution being taken not to damage the colonic wall or transverse mesocolon. When the lesser sac is entered the posterior wall of the stomach should be clearly visible. Follow the upper border of the transverse colon and continue the division of the greater omentum and fascia towards the hepatic flexure. Have the assistant retract the hepatic flexure medially and caudally to provide countertraction. Divide the final fascial attachments near the hepatic flexure. The duodenum is again identified underneath the colon. The intra-corporeal stage of the operation is now complete.

6 Finally, pneumoperitoneum is abolished for extra-corporeal resection and anastomosis. The 5–12-mm epigastrium port is extended and shielded with a plastic bag or wound protector. The tumour is delivered and excised through this protected wound. Ileo-transverse anastomosis is performed using either a hand-sewn or stapled technique.

LEFT HEMICOLECTOMY

Appraise

1 Undertake left hemicolectomy for tumours of the left and sigmoid colon, sigmoid volvulus and diverticular disease.

2 If the operation is for an obstructing neoplasm, carry out an extended colectomy with an ileosigmoid or ileorectal anastomosis. Alternatively, carry out a resection with on-table decompression or irrigation of the obstructed proximal colon and primary anastomosis. Try to avoid Hartmann's procedure as patients are often unfit or reluctant to undergo a further reversal operation.

3 In diverticular disease, resect the sigmoid colon and as much of the rectum and descending colon as is necessary, whilst avoiding potential tension on the anastomosis. Isolated diverticula in the descending and transverse colon can safely be left, providing the bowel wall is not thickened. Anastomose the proximal bowel to the rectum at or below the sacral promontory.

4 Mobilization of the splenic flexure and the left half of the transverse colon is required for tumours of the descending colon, but may not be necessary for a tumour in the mid or lower sigmoid colon.

Prepare

1 Place the patient in the lithotomy Trendelenburg (Lloyd-Davies) position (Fig. 13.11).

2 Pass a catheter to empty the bladder and to monitor urine output during and after the operation.

Access

1 Stand on the patient's right side.

2 Make a midline incision downwards from the umbilicus. If mobilization of the splenic flexure is required, the incision will need to be extended upwards.

Assess

1 If the operation is for a carcinoma, palpate the liver for occult metastases, examine the colon and entire small bowel, look for enlarged mesenteric and para-aortic nodes and examine the peritoneal cavity and pelvis for metastases.

2 Assess the mobility of the carcinoma; if the serosal surface is involved, cover it with a swab soaked in 10% aqueous povidone-iodine solution.

3 If you are performing colectomy for a benign condition, assess the diseased colon to decide the extent of resection.

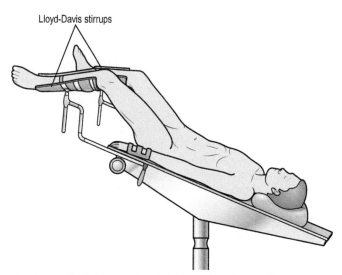

Lloyd-Davis stirrups

Fig. 13.11 The lithotomy Trendelenburg (Lloyd-Davies) position for operations involving the left side of the colon or the rectum. This allows access to the rectum for on-table endoscopy or transanal stapled anastomosis.

- Start with an incision of sufficient length to assess the anatomy and pathology, but do not hesitate to extend it to achieve a safe and radical excision. Remember – incisions can always be made bigger, but never smaller.
- Always perform a radical resection of a carcinoma where possible. Do not stray out of the mesocolic plane during your dissection. Tie the inferior mesenteric artery at its origin from the aorta and the inferior mesenteric vein below the inferior border of the pancreas.
- If the patient is very elderly and unfit or the blood supply to the colon is tenuous because of severe atheroma, undertake a less radical procedure, retaining the inferior mesenteric trunk and ligating the segmental left colonic and sigmoid branches as appropriate.
- If the operation is for a benign condition, or a palliative resection for carcinoma, undertake a conservative resection and ligate and divide the vessels close to the bowel wall.

Resect

1 Divide the congenital adhesions that bind the sigmoid colon to the abdominal wall in the left iliac fossa and then divide the lateral peritoneum in the paracolic gutter, following the 'white line', which represents the conjunction of posterior and visceral peritoneum.

2 If required, mobilize the splenic flexure by dividing the phreno-colic ligament. Avoid damaging the spleen and the tail of the pancreas. If the carcinoma is distal, preserve the greater omentum by dividing the adhesions between the omentum and the colon proximally to the middle of the transverse colon and entering the lesser sac. If the tumour is situated near the flexure, divide the left side of the gastroepiploic vascular arcade and excise the lesser and greater omentum with the specimen.

3 Elevate the left colon on its mesentery and separate it from the duodeno-jejunal flexure, left ureter and gonadal vessels using blunt dissection.

4 Incise the peritoneum medial to the colon and separate the inferior mesenteric artery from the sacrum by gentle blunt dissection. Create a window in the mesentery and trace the artery proximally. Clamp, ligate and divide the artery close to its origin. Identify the inferior mesenteric vein lying laterally and clamp, ligate and divide it below the lower border of the pancreas.

5 Divide the mesentery and marginal vessels at the chosen proximal and distal resection sites.

6 Place a non-crushing right-angled clamp across the rectosigmoid junction and irrigate the rectum with 10% povidone-iodine solution via a catheter passed through the anus until it is clean. This cytotoxic washout removes any viable tumour cells that may otherwise implant in the anastomotic line.

1. If the carcinoma involves the abdominal wall, excise the area with the tumour and repair the defect at the end of the procedure. Be prepared to resect a loop of small bowel or excise part of the bladder fundus en bloc if they are attached to the tumour. Likewise, a hysterectomy may be necessary if the tumour invades the uterus. Involvement of the ureter usually occurs as it crosses the iliac vessels at the pelvic brim: you may be able to resect this portion and reimplant the proximal end into the bladder using a psoas hitch and/or a Boari flap.

2. Do not hesitate to involve another specialist if you are not experienced enough to deal with an unfamiliar area or technique.

3. If the tumour is situated in the left half of the transverse colon or at the splenic flexure, excise most of the transverse colon and unite the hepatic flexure to the descending or sigmoid colon. Alternatively, perform an extended right hemicolectomy with an ileocolic anastomosis.

7 Prepare the proximal colon for division by placing a non-crushing clamp across the bowel proximal to the intended site of division. Cross-staple or use a Parker-Kerr clamp just distal to the intended site of division. Divide the colon, hold the proximal end in Babcock's forceps and swab the bowel lumen with aqueous 10% povidone-iodine solution.

8 Divide the rectosigmoid below the right-angled clamp and remove the specimen comprising the left hemicolon, inferior mesenteric pedicle and the whole of the mesentery. Do not divide the sigmoid higher than 10 cm above the rectosigmoid junction or you will leave an ischaemic segment distally.

Unite

1 Anastomose the bowel ends with a single layer of seromuscular inverting 2/0 polyglactin 910 (Vicryl) or 3/0 PDS sutures.

- Beware when using the CEEA stapler with a long distal stump. Select the 28-mm diameter stapler and take care when advancing it around the rectal valves or you may tear the rectum. If it will not advance to the top of the rectum, resect a further segment of rectum or anastomose the colon end-to-side to the rectum.

LAPAROSCOPIC LEFT HEMICOLECTOMY

Access

1 Stand on the right side of the patient, facing the monitor at the table end. A second monitor is positioned as shown for the assistant (Fig. 13.12).

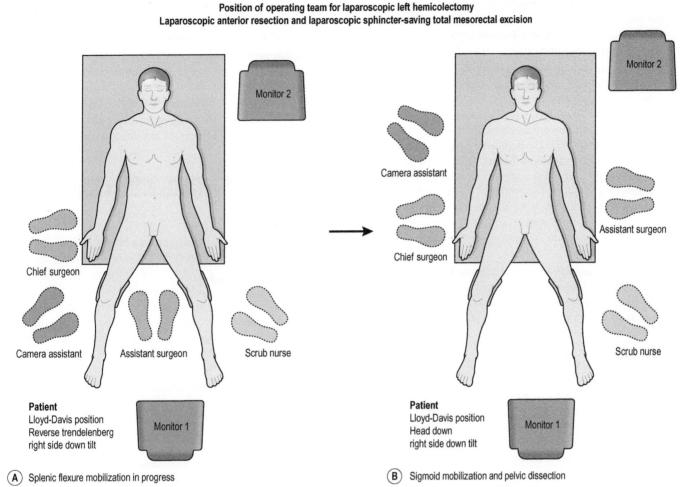

Position of operating team for laparoscopic left hemicolectomy
Laparoscopic anterior resection and laparoscopic sphincter-saving total mesorectal excision

Monitor 2

Chief surgeon

Camera assistant   Assistant surgeon   Scrub nurse

Patient
Lloyd-Davis position
Reverse trendelenberg
right side down tilt

Monitor 1

(A) Splenic flexure mobilization in progress

Monitor 2

Camera assistant

Assistant surgeon

Chief surgeon

Scrub nurse

Patient
Lloyd-Davis position
Head down
right side down tilt

Monitor 1

(B) Sigmoid mobilization and pelvic dissection

Fig. 13.12 Position of operating team for laparoscopic left hemicolectomy, laparoscopic anterior resection and laparoscopic sphincter-saving total mesorectal excision. (A) Position of the operating team for laparoscopic splenic flexure mobilization using monitor 2. (B) Position of the operating team during laparoscopic sigmoid mobilization and pelvic dissection using monitor 1.

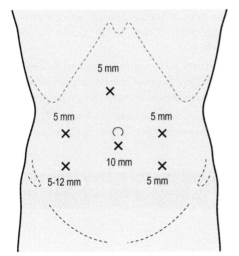

5 mm

5 mm   5 mm

10 mm

5-12 mm   5 mm

Fig. 13.13 Port sites for laparoscopic left hemicolectomy, laparoscopic anterior resection and laparoscopic sphincter-saving total mesorectal excision.

2 Place the ports as shown in Figure 13.13.

3 Put the patient in a steep head-down position with the table rotated to the right, a position that allows the small bowel to fall away from the left lower quadrant and the pelvis.

Action

1 Splenic flexure mobilization is carried out first, once the tumour is judged to be resectable: the medial-to-lateral approach is described here. The small bowel is kept in the right side of the abdomen by tilting the operating table to the right (right side down position). The inferior mesenteric vein (IMV) is identified lateral to the duodeno-jejunal flexure, and is controlled and divided with the Ligasure™. Using the same device, blunt dissection is carried out in the avascular plane between the descending colon mesentery and the retroperitoneal fascia. Continue this dissection laterally towards the splenic flexure as far as possible until Gerota's fascia is exposed. The inferior border of the pancreas should be clearly evident: avoid dissecting deep to the pancreas. After completion of the medial dissection, start the lateral dissection at the mid-transverse colon. The greater omentum is peeled off the colon by incising the fascia just above the bowel, caution being taken to avoid damage to either colon or mesocolon. The posterior wall of the stomach should be clearly seen once the lesser sac is entered. By keeping close to the colon at all times, further dissection along the upper and lateral border will allow complete mobilization of the splenic flexure. Identify the pancreas once more and divide the attachment of the transverse mesocolon to its inferior border, taking care to avoid injury to

223

the middle colic vessels. Sufficient mobilization is achieved when the splenic flexure can be swung to the midline. A head-up (reverse Trendelenburg) tilt helps improve exposure during the final stage of lateral dissection.

2   Debate continues as to whether a lateral or medial-first approach should be used for sigmoid colon mobilization and vascular control. The lateral-first approach is easier for the novice as it is the same as for open surgery and is described here.

The lateral peritoneal attachment of the sigmoid (Toldt's fascia) is first divided. This is continued upwards to the previously dissected area near the splenic flexure. Following this, a window is created in the sigmoid mesentery at the rectosigmoid junction. A cotton tape 15–20 cm long is then passed through the window and tied around the bowel. By grasping the tape and moving it to and fro, the assistant surgeon can provide the necessary countertraction and exposure for subsequent mesenteric division and colon mobilization.

3   Identify the left gonadal vessels and ureter under the retroperitoneal fascia in the left lateral peritoneal space. Now incise the retroperitoneal fascia medial to the ureter (beware of the iliac vein which lies deep to the ureter), and enter the presacral space in a plane anterior to the left presacral hypogastric nerve, which is located 1–2 cm lateral to the midline at the level of the sacral promontory. The lateral dissection is now complete.

4   Swing the sigmoid colon to the left side and incise the retroperitoneal fascia at the base of the sigmoid mesentery, starting at the level of the sacral promontory. Take care to avoid damage to the underlying right hypogastric nerve and right ureter. If adequate lateral dissection has been performed, a generous retromesenteric window is easily made at the base of the mesosigmoid, which should by now look paper-thin. Visualize the left ureter through this retromesenteric window. Continue to divide the mesosigmoid cranially, anterior to the aorta, until you encounter the inferior mesenteric artery (IMA). Divide the IMA using a linear endo-stapler (white cartridge), clips or the Ligasure™ device: do not use the latter option in patients with extensive atherosclerosis and calcification as haemostasis may be suboptimal.

5   The medial mesenteric division is continued further cranially to join the previous window from the divided IMV. Divide the remaining posterior fascial attachments between the mesentery and the retroperitoneum. Following this, the whole left-side colon should be freely mobile. At a trial descent, the splenic flexure should reach the pelvis easily without tension. Divide the mesentery at the rectosigmoid with the Ligasure™, and after performing cytocidal lavage, transect the rectum with a linear endo-stapler (blue or green cartridge) at a level distal to the sacral promontory.

6   Abolish pneumoperitoneum, deliver the specimen and excise it via a 5–6 cm Pfannestiel incision protected with a sterile plastic bag. Use a muscle-splitting incision which is less painful than a muscle-cutting incision and results in fewer postoperative hernias. Check again that the colon is long enough to allow for a tension-free anastomosis low down in the pelvis, reaching the symphysis pubis extra-corporeally without tension. Secure the anvil of a circular stapler in the colonic stump with a purse-string suture. Replace the colon in the abdomen, and close the retrieval wound. Re-establish pneumoperitoneum and reposition the small bowel. Insert the circular stapler transanally and perform intra-corporeal anastomosis as for open surgery. Inspect the tissue doughnuts for completeness.

7   You may perform perioperative colonoscopy following construction of the anastomosis to carry out air-testing for leaks and inspect the anastomosis for staple line bleeding; confirm that the colonic mucosa is adequately perfused at the same time.

8   If the proximal or distal doughnuts are incomplete or the air-leak test is positive, drain the pelvis and create a covering stoma.

CARCINOMA OF THE RECTUM

Appraise

1   Confirm the diagnosis in all patients with sigmoidoscopy and biopsy, and evaluate the proximal colon with colonoscopy or CT colography.

2   If possible, perform magnetic resonance imaging in lower and middle third tumours to assess T and N stage and potential involvement of the circumferential resection margin (CRM). If MRI is not available, perform an examination under anaesthetic to assess the fixity of low tumours. Exclude distant metastases with CT chest, abdomen and pelvis.

3   Short-course preoperative radiotherapy has been shown to reduce the risk of local recurrence following resection of rectal cancer, but this benefit must be weighed against poorer functional results following low anterior resection, impaired healing of the perineal wound following abdominoperineal resection and an increased risk of late malignancy. Consider radiotherapy in lower third tumours, particularly those sited anteriorly, fixed or tethered tumours and lesions staged T_3 or T_4 and those with a threatened CRM on MRI scanning. Long-course chemoradiotherapy is used to 'downstage' locally advanced, fixed rectal cancers. It may result in complete clinical and radiological resolution of the tumour: if so, a 'wait-and-watch' policy may be appropriate. The management of low rectal cancers is summarized in Figure 13.14.

4   If the patient presents as an emergency with obstructive symptoms or pain, perform a trephine colostomy (see below) and then undertake a full assessment and appropriate neoadjuvant treatment.

5   A few patients with small early carcinomas (T_1 or T_2 assessed by transrectal ultrasound) are suitable for a peranal local excision.

ANTERIOR RESECTION OF THE RECTUM

Prepare

1   Place the anaesthetized patient in the lithotomy Trendelenburg (Lloyd-Davies) position.

2   Insert an indwelling Foley catheter into the bladder.

Access

1   Stand on the patient's right.

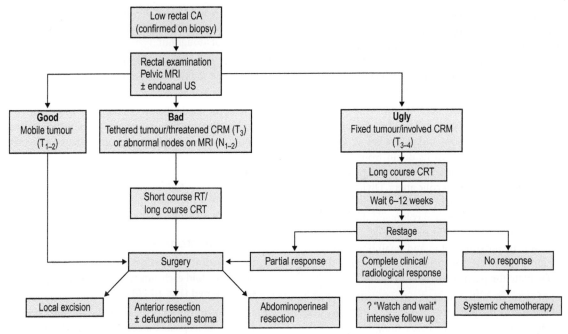

Fig. 13.14 **Management of low rectal cancer: the Good, the Bad and the Ugly.**

2 Make a midline incision downwards from the umbilicus to the symphysis pubis. If mobilization of the splenic flexure is required, the incision will need to be extended upwards.

Assess

1 Proceed as described above under left hemicolectomy. Note the relation of the tumour to the peritoneal reflection and decide whether it is mobile, adherent to other organs or fixed within the pelvis.

? DIFFICULTY

1. A large rectal carcinoma lying within a small male pelvis may seem daunting. Take your time and deepen the dissection in the mesorectal plane in a circumferential manner. As you mobilize the rectum, dissection will become progressively easier.
2. Do not compromise the success of radical resection by breaching the mesorectal plane of dissection.

Action

1 Mobilize the left side of the colon by dividing the congenital adhesions as described for left hemicolectomy. Assess the length of colon required to achieve a tension-free anastomosis: if the planned proximal resection margin will reach to the pubic symphysis, it will reach to the pelvic floor.

2 If necessary, mobilize the splenic flexure and the left half of the transverse colon, preserving the omentum unless there are metastases present in it. Avoid damage to the spleen (Fig. 13.15).

3 Mobilize the left colon by pulling it to the right on its mesentery. Identify the left ureter and gonadal vessels and sweep them away from the mesocolon.

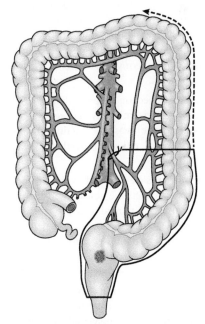

Fig. 13.15 Anterior resection of the rectum: the inferior mesenteric artery has been ligated and divided on the aorta and the inferior mesenteric vein at the upper border of the pancreas. The splenic flexure may be mobilized as shown.

▶ KEY POINTS Anatomy

- You are mobilizing the left colon onto its embryological mesentery.
- Make sure you do not breach the mesocolic envelope containing potentially involved lymph nodes: dissect in the correct plane which lies between the mesocolon and the posterior abdominal wall.

4 To enter the mesorectal plane lift the sigmoid loop vertically. Divide the peritoneum on the right side to expose the inferior mesenteric artery and follow it proximally to its origin and distally into the loose areolar tissue of the mesorectal plane. Push away the tissue containing the pelvic nerve plexus which lies deep to the vessels: both branches of the plexus should be visible as they divide around the rectum at the level of the sacral promontory.

5 Make a similar incision in the peritoneum of the left side to produce a window with artery above and nerves below. Clamp, divide and ligate the artery close to its origin from the aorta. If the patient is old and atherosclerotic, divide the pedicle further from the aorta, preserving the left colic artery. Divide the inferior mesenteric vein below the lower border of the pancreas. Select a suitable area to transect the proximal colon and divide the mesentery up to this point. Transect the bowel using a linear cutting stapler and pack the proximal colon and small bowel out of the way in the upper abdomen. The specimen can now be pulled anteriorly to facilitate the pelvic dissection.

6 The extent of rectal mobilization depends upon the level of the tumour. If it is below the peritoneal reflection, mobilize the rectum and mesorectum down to the pelvic floor.

7 Move to the left of the patient. Pull the rectum forwards to dissect the plane between presacral fascia and mesorectum from the sacral promontory to the tip of the coccyx. This is facilitated by an assistant using a St Mark's lipped retractor to pull the rectum forwards whilst the operating surgeon carries out sharp dissection with scissors or diathermy. Take care to visualize and preserve the presacral nerves.

8 As the posterior dissection deepens, divide the peritoneum over each side of the pelvis, mid-way between the rectum and pelvic side-wall, uniting the incisions anteriorly in the midline 1 cm above the peritoneal reflection, overlying the seminal vesicles anterolaterally.

9 Hold the seminal vesicles forwards with a St Mark's lipped retractor and dissect between the vesicles and the rectum to expose the rectovesical fascia, named after the Parisian anatomist and surgeon Charles Denonvilliers (1808–1872). Incise this and dissect distally in the male to the lower border of the prostate. In the female, dissect distally between the rectum and vagina as far down as necessary to achieve adequate mobilization of the tumour.

10 While retracting the rectum first to one side and then the other side of the pelvis, continue dissecting in the avascular plane between the mesorectum and pelvic side wall. If available, employ the Ligasure™ device or harmonic scalpel as a useful aid to bloodless dissection. Do not clamp and ligate the so-called 'lateral ligaments' as this may tent up and damage the third sacral nerve root, resulting in loss of sexual function in the male.

11 Lift the rectum and tumour out of the pelvis and select a suitable site for division of the rectum, if possible leaving a 5-cm clearance below the carcinoma. For lower third tumours this degree of clearance is not possible in a restorative procedure. Provided you have performed a total mesorectal excision, a 1 to 2-cm distal margin of rectum is sufficient to achieve a curative resection. For lesions of the upper rectum divide the mesorectum perpendicularly to the rectal wall at the level of resection using the Ligasure™, or divide it between mounted ligatures. Avoid oblique dissection, which may breach mesorectal tumour deposits. Apply a transverse stapler or right-angled clamp to the rectum

at the site selected for division. Remember, if you are performing a stapled anastomosis an extra 8 mm of rectal wall is excised in the distal 'doughnut'.

12 Irrigate the rectum through the anus with aqueous 10% povidone-iodine solution. If only a small cuff of sphincter and rectum remains, swab it out with the same solution.

13 Divide the rectum below the stapler or clamp with a long-handled scalpel. Remove the specimen containing the rectal carcinoma, the complete mesorectal envelope and inferior mesenteric pedicle.

Unite

Staple or suture the anastomosis, depending upon the level of anastomosis, ease of access to the pelvis and the obesity of the patient.

Sutured anastomosis

1 Insert vertical mattress sutures into the posterior layer but do not tie them. Hold each suture with artery forceps until they have all been inserted (Fig. 13.16).

2 Have the sutures all held taut while you push down the proximal colon until its posterior edge is in contact with the rectum. This is the 'parachute' technique. Tie the sutures with the knots within the lumen. Hold the two most lateral sutures and cut the others. Suture the anterior layer using interrupted seromuscular inverting sutures, again inserting them all before tying them.

3 Radio-opaque clips may be used to mark the anastomosis if desired.

Stapled anastomosis

1 Low colorectal anastomosis is more easily accomplished using the CEEA circular stapling device. Carry out the operation exactly as described above but close the rectal stump using a cross stapler. Insert a 2/0 Prolene™ purse-string suture into the end of the proximal colon. Holding the bowel edges with Babcock's forceps, insert the anvil of a 28-mm or 31-mm stapling gun and tie the purse-string suture as tightly as possible.

2 Introduce the body of the CEEA gun through the anus and open it, guiding the spike of the gun through the posterior aspect of the stapled rectal stump in the middle and just behind the staple line. Remove the spike if it is detachable and connect the anvil to the cartridge (Fig. 13.17).

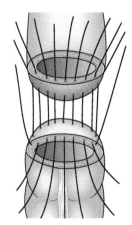

Fig. 13.16 Anterior resection of the rectum with one-layer sutured anastomosis showing the insertion of sutures in preparation for the descending colon to be 'railroaded' down to the rectum.

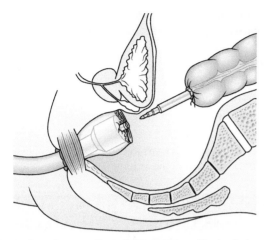

Fig. 13.17 Anterior resection of the rectum with stapled anastomosis showing insertion of the circular stapling device, inserted transanally through the stapled rectal stump, connecting to the anvil which is tied into the sigmoid colon.

3 Have the assistant operating the gun approximate the anvil to the cartridge while you ensure that the vaginal vault and any loops of small bowel are not trapped in the closing stapler. Fire the staple gun to construct the anastomosis. Open the gun two full turns to separate the anvil from the cartridge and rotate it 360° clockwise and again anti-clockwise to ensure the anastomosis is free before gently extracting it from the anus.

4 Check the integrity of the stapled anastomosis:
   ■ Examine the 'doughnuts' of colon and rectum removed from the gun. They should be complete. Identify the distal doughnut and send it for histological examination.
   ■ Perform a digital rectal examination to exclude any palpable abnormality.
   ■ Fill the pelvis with saline and place a non-crushing clamp on the distal colon. Gently insufflate air into the rectum through a sigmoidoscope or bladder syringe: if no bubbles appear and the doughnuts are complete, the anastomosis is satisfactory.

Checklist

1 Wash out the paracolic gutter with warm isotonic saline and make sure there is no bleeding, particularly in the region of the splenic flexure and spleen.

2 Check that the anastomosis is not under tension and that the proximal colon is viable.

3 Some surgeons prefer to drain the pelvis to prevent an infected pelvic haematoma, using a suction drain inserted through a stab wound in the left iliac fossa. Meticulous haemostasis is preferable.

4 Replace the small bowel and cover it with the omentum before closing the abdomen.

LAPAROSCOPIC ANTERIOR RESECTION

Assess

1 The position of the patient, surgical team and laparoscopic ports are similar to those for laparoscopic left hemicolectomy (see Figs 13.12, 13.13). If splenic flexure mobilization is not required, omit the 5-mm right upper quadrant port.

2 Throughout the procedure place the patient in a 20° Trendelenburg position with a right-side-down tilt, a position that helps to clear the small bowel off the lower abdomen and pelvis.

ACTION

1 In a female patient, hitch up the uterus by passing sutures (OO Prolene on a straight needle) underneath the two fallopian tubes near the uterine cornu and tying them to the lower anterior abdominal wall. The stitch should pass through the skin and be tied over a piece of gauze as a reminder to the surgeon to replace the uterus at the end of operation.

2 Splenic flexure mobilization is rarely required for 'high' anterior resection, as long as the sigmoid colon is healthy and can be brought down to the pelvis for a tension-free anastomosis after mobilization. When the sigmoid colon is diseased, as from severe diverticular disease or previous radiotherapy, or becomes ischaemic following high ligation of the IMA (as occasionally arises in elderly patients with extensive atherosclerosis), it is preferable to use the descending colon for anastomosis. In this case proceed to splenic flexure mobilization as previously described.

3 Carry out sigmoid mobilization and vascular control as previously described for laparoscopic left hemicolectomy.

4 Retract the rectum upwards and forwards, and identify the loose areolar plane between the mesorectum and the presacral fascia, with the hypogastric nerves lying on it. Continue dissection of the presacral space posteriorly and laterally, using a combination of sharp and blunt dissection in a similar manner to open surgery. Slowly divide the posterior mesorectum 5 cm distal to the tumour, using an ultrasonic dissector or Ligasure,™ until you expose the rectal tube. Have the assistant pull the rectum in a cephalad direction. Following cytocidal lavage through the anus transect the rectum with a linear endo-stapler (blue or gold cartridge). Two to three firings are sometimes required, and an angulating stapler works better in the lower pelvis. Perform a trial descent to confirm that there is a sufficient length of colon for anastomosis.

5 Undertake laparoscopic total mesorectal excision (TME) for cancers in the mid and low rectum. After initial posterior and lateral dissection, pull the rectum in a cephalad direction to expose the rectovesical or rectouterine pouch. Then incise the anterior peritoneal refection. Proceed with the anterior dissection as in open surgery, in male patients between the rectum and Denonvillier's fascia covering the seminal vesicles and in females between the rectum and upper vagina. Have the assistant insert a finger into the vagina, retracting it upward, to help with dissecting the rectovaginal plane. Facilitate the posterior dissection distally by turning the 30° laparoscope 180° upwards. Continue the dissection laterally until the whole rectum is mobilized distally down to the pelvic floor. After cytocidal lavage divide the rectum with an endo-stapler just above the pelvic floor. A smaller size stapler (30 mm) works better in the restricted space of the true pelvis but several firings may be required. A blue cartridge gives the best haemostasis, but in patients who have received neoadjuvant radiotherapy the tissues are thicker and more oedematous and it may be preferable to use a greater staple height (gold or green

cartridge). After rectal transection perform a trial descent as described above.

6 Specimen retrieval and intra-corporeal anastomosis are performed as described for laparoscopic left hemicolectomy. In low anterior resection be extremely cautious to avoid inadvertent stapling of the levator muscles or adjacent structures. In female patients, the assistant surgeon lifts the vagina upwards with a finger while closing the circular stapler; this manoeuvre helps to exclude the vaginal vault from the anvil and prevent an unintentional rectovaginal fistula.

7 Either a side-to-end anastomosis (L-pouch) or a colonic J pouch can be constructed to improve subsequent bowel function. For colonic J pouch, fashion a 5-cm long pouch with a 60-mm linear cutter, using either the descending or the proximal sigmoid colon. Secure the detachable anvil of a circular stapler into the apex of the pouch with an O Prolene string suture. Put the pouch back into the peritoneal cavity, and close the incision in layers.

8 We recommend a covering stoma following TME to guard against the relatively high rate of anastomotic leakage, which is 20% or more. Either loop ileostomy or transverse loop colostomy is suitable, but loop ileostomy is easier to create and close subsequently. Identify a point in the terminal ileum about 20 cm from the ileocaecal valve for the formation of a loop ileostomy. Mark the antimesenteric border lightly with bipolar cautery at two different points to differentiate the proximal and distal limbs. Tie a cotton tape around this segment via a mesenteric window, and retract the ileal segment by grasping the cotton tape, taking care to ensure that the ileum is not twisted during extraction. Since the patient has been in a right-side down position, make sure no small bowel loops are trapped in the lateral space. Abolish the pneumoperitoneum and raise a covering ileostomy over the premarked stoma site. If desired, drain the presacral space via the left lower quadrant 5-mm port.

Aftercare

1 A nasogastric tube is occasionally required to deflate the stomach for better exposure of the transverse colon and splenic flexure. Remove it at the end of the operation before the reversal of anaesthesia.

2 Whilst postoperative feeding can be started as early as the day of operation, it is usually more sensible to start oral intake on the first postoperative day if there is no evidence of nausea or abdominal distension.

HARTMANN'S OPERATION

This was first described by the French surgeon Henri Hartmann in 1921, for cancer of the rectum, as a safer alternative to the then more commonly performed operation of abdominoperineal excision.

Appraise

1 After carrying out an anterior resection of the rectum or rectosigmoid it may be inadvisable to proceed with an anastomosis if:
   ■ The procedure is palliative and the anastomosis demands the addition of a defunctioning colostomy, or there is residual carcinoma in the lateral pelvic wall

■ The operation is an emergency for obstruction or perforation and sepsis, or faecal soiling or poor bowel perfusion is evident.

Action

1 Close the distal rectum, ideally with a cross-stapler. If the rectum is divided low down in the pelvis and the end is difficult to suture or staple, leave it open and insert a drain through the anus into the pelvis.

2 Bring out an end colostomy as described below under abdominoperineal excision of the rectum.

ABDOMINOPERINEAL EXCISION OF THE RECTUM

Prepare

1 Ask the stomatherapist to mark the ideal position for the stoma on the skin of the left iliac fossa: this will depend on the patient's body habitus and should be assessed lying, sitting and standing to ensure that the stoma appliance stays in place.

2 This operation may be carried out using a synchronous combined approach with two teams of surgeons, but is better performed by one experienced surgical team carrying out the abdominal and perineal parts sequentially.

3 Do not give the patient preoperative bowel preparation; it is difficult to construct a perfect end colostomy in the presence of liquid stool.

4 Place the patient in the lithotomy Trendelenburg position. Rest the sacrum on a pad to allow the coccyx to overhang the end of the table.

5 Insert a urinary catheter.

6 Strap up the scrotum so that it is clear of the perineal operative field.

7 Perform a digital rectal examination to determine the distance of the carcinoma from the anal verge and its fixity to pelvic structures.

8 Close the anus with a strong non-absorbable purse-string suture such as 0 silk: encircle the anus twice before tying the purse-string to prevent faecal leakage.

ABDOMINAL OPERATION

Access

1 Stand on the patient's right side.

2 Open the abdomen through a lower midline incision extending from the umbilicus to the symphysis pubis.

Assess

1 Proceed as described above under left hemicolectomy.

Action

1 Suture the lower cut edge of the peritoneum and bladder to the skin.

2 Place the small bowel on the right side of the abdomen and cover it with a pack.

3 Divide the lateral attachments of the sigmoid and descending colon.

4 Lift the colon upwards and to the right, identify the left ureter and gonadal vessels and sweep them away from the vascular pedicle.

5 Enter the mesorectal plane and preserve the pelvic nerve plexus as described for anterior resection of the rectum. Divide the inferior mesorectal artery at its origin from the aorta, and the inferior mesenteric vein at the same level.

6 Select a suitable site in the sigmoid colon for transection of the bowel, taking into account the patient's body habitus and the pre-operative skin marking. If the colon easily reaches the symphysis pubis there should be sufficient length to allow construction of the stoma without tension and risk of subsequent retraction. Divide the mesocolon, ligating and dividing the marginal vessels to this point. Divide the colon using a Parker-Kerr clamp on the rectal side and non-crushing clamp on the colonic side or, ideally, divide the colon with a linear cutting stapler. This maintains sterility and the staple line can be excised from the colonic end when the wound is closed and the colostomy is constructed.

7 Construct a trephine in the left iliac fossa at the previously marked site for the colostomy. Remove a disc of skin 2 cm in diameter together with the underlying subcutaneous fat. Divide the rectus sheath, separating rather than cutting the underlying muscle fibres and incise the peritoneum.

8 Move to the patient's left side and continue the mesorectal dissection posteriorly, laterally and anteriorly as for anterior resection of the rectum. Define the course of both ureters in the pelvis and be careful to preserve them. Continue the dissection as far as required, usually down to the pelvic floor and the tip of the coccyx posteriorly. For tumours adjacent to or involving the levator ani muscles a wider 'extralevator' abdominoperineal excision (ELAPE) will be required, and you should halt the abdominal dissection before the tumour is reached.

▶ KEY POINTS Anatomy

■ Take care to stay in the correct mesorectal plane: if you stray into the mesorectum you risk disseminating cancer cells and condemning the patient to a painful and debilitating local recurrence.
■ Identify and preserve the presacral sympathetic nerves.

9 When the perineal dissection is completed withdraw the specimen through the perineal wound. Irrigate the pelvic cavity with aqueous 10% povidone-iodine solution.

10 Deliver the proximal colon through the trephine incision.

11 Ensure that you have achieved complete pelvic haemostasis.

12 It is not necessary to close the pelvic peritoneum. Attempts to approximate it under tension may result in subsequent dehiscence and herniation of the small bowel, resulting in a closed loop obstruction.

13 Close the abdominal wound.

14 Trim the staple line from the colostomy to leave 1 cm projecting above the skin. Suture the edge of the colon to the edge of the skin wound with interrupted polyglactin 910 sutures on a cutting needle.

PERINEAL OPERATION

In the male

1 Opinion is divided on the optimal positioning of the patient. Many surgeons advocate the prone jack-knife position, which gives superior views of the anterior dissection, particularly for wide 'extralevator' excision. If you select this option construct the colostomy, close the abdomen and turn the patient prone before commencing the perineal dissection.

2 Make an elliptical incision around the closed anus (Fig. 13.18) and deepen the incision to expose the fat of the ischiorectal fossae and the coccyx. Insert a Norfolk and Norwich self-retaining retractor.

3 Begin the dissection posteriorly. Lift the anus forward, palpate the tip of the coccyx, and divide the anococcygeal raphe (Fig. 13.19). In extralevator excision the coccyx is excised: flex the coccyx to open the coccygeal joints and divide across it with a scalpel or reticulating bone saw to separate the distal portion. Coagulate any bleeding from the middle sacral vessels.

4 For small, mobile tumours the pelvic floor can be preserved by dissection in the intersphincteric plane, separating the levator

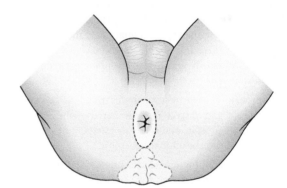

Fig. 13.18 Abdominoperineal excision of the rectum: perineal skin incision.

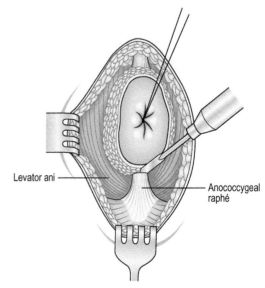

Levator ani

Anococcygeal raphé

Fig. 13.19 Abdominoperineal excision of the rectum: posterior dissection.

muscles and puborectalis sling from the adjacent rectal fascia (see 'Elective total proctocolectomy' below). For extralavator excision extend the dissection outside the external sphincter, dividing the levator muscles laterally at their origin. Ligate or coagulate the inferior haemorrhoidal and pudendal vessels. If available, the Ligasure dissector is a great aid to bloodless dissection throughout the perineal operation.

5 Separate the mesorectum from the anterior aspect of the presacral fascia to enter the plane of the abdominal operation.

6 When the posterior and lateral dissection is complete, begin the anterior dissection. Retract the rectum posteriorly and make a transverse incision anteriorly to expose the superficial and deep transverse perineal muscles.

> ▶ KEY POINT Anatomy
>
> ■ Great care must be taken to avoid injury to the urethra: keep the plane of dissection behind the transverse perineal muscles.

7 Divide the pubococcygeus and puborecto-urethralis muscles on either side of the rectum (Fig. 13.20). Then divide the underlying fascia, which is the lateral continuation of the fascia of Denonvilliers and Waldeyer, to expose the rectal wall. Palpate the prostate gland anteriorly and define the plane between the rectum and prostate.

8 Divide the fibres of the rectourethralis muscle to expose the prostatic capsule and dissect rostrally between the visceral pelvic fascia and the prostate and seminal vesicles until your dissection meets that of the abdominal operation.

9 Divide any remaining lateral attachments and draw the rectum and sigmoid colon through the perineal incision.

10 Flatten the operating table, irrigate the pelvis with warm isotonic saline and secure pelvic haemostasis using diathermy or 2/0 polyglactin 910 sutures. Place a suction drain into the pelvis through a stab wound anterolateral to the perineal wound (being careful to avoid the scrotum and the femoral vessels) and secure it to the skin.

11 Close the pelvic floor and subcutaneous tissue in two layers using interrupted 0 polyglactin 910 sutures. Close the skin with interrupted 3/0 Ethilon on a cutting needle.

12 If a wide extralavator excision has been performed primary closure of the perineal wound is likely to fail, particularly following preoperative radiotherapy. Reconstructive options include omentoplasty, biological meshes or a local flap (VRAM, Gracilis or Inferior Gluteal Artery Perforator). The VRAM flap gives superior results compared to omentoplasty, with no increase in morbidity or postoperative stay, but adds an additional 2 hours to the procedure: it is best planned preoperatively as a joint procedure with a plastic surgeon. Early reports suggest that biological meshes may be equally effective but they are expensive and this currently limits their use in many hospitals.

In the female

1 For bulky, fixed tumours situated anteriorly it may be necessary to remove the posterior vaginal wall. Make your incision from the posterior angle of the labia around the anus to the coccyx.

2 The posterior part of the dissection is as in the male. Carry the anterior incision upwards through the posteriolateral wall of the vagina as far as the posterior fornix. Make a transverse incision to join the two lateral incisions and deepen it to expose the rectal wall.

3 It may be difficult to reconstruct the vagina, particularly following preoperative radiotherapy. Oversew the cut edge of the vagina with a continuous 2/0 synthetic absorbable suture to secure haemostasis.

4 Close the subcutaneous tissue in two layers using interrupted 0 polyglactin 910 sutures. Close the skin with interrupted 3/0 Ethilon on a cutting needle.

> ? DIFFICULTY
>
> 1. Do not attempt to close the pelvic peritoneum under tension, particularly following preoperative radiotherapy.
> 2. If pelvic haemorrhage cannot be controlled, pack the pelvis with gauze Caesar roll inserted via the perineal wound. Remove the pack under GA at 48–72 hours and inspect the pelvis: most cases are due to venous haemorrhage and will have ceased. Any arterial bleeding should be controlled by under-running the vessel with a 2/0 Vicryl suture.

TRANSVERSE COLOSTOMY

Appraise

> ▶ KEY POINT Carefully assess the options
>
> ■ Transverse colostomy can be difficult to manage and is prone to prolapse. Colonic stenting, if available, may be a better option in the frail elderly patient.

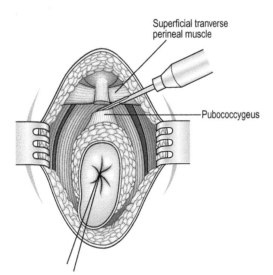

Superficial transverse perineal muscle

Pubococcygeus

Fig. 13.20 Abdominoperineal excision of the rectum: anterior dissection.

1 Carry out a transverse colostomy in patients presenting with distal obstruction who are unfit to undergo resection (or if you are too inexperienced to do this), or to defunction a distal anastomosis instead of a loop ileostomy. A transverse colostomy may be easier to manage than an ileostomy as the effluent is more formed, and can if necessary be performed under local anaesthetic in a severely ill patient.

2 Site the stoma in the right upper quadrant of the abdomen, midway between the umbilicus and the costal margin: you should position the colostomy as far to the right of the transverse colon as possible to minimize the risk of prolapse.

Access

If you are using a trephine technique, make a transverse incision 5 cm long centred on the upper right rectus muscle between the umbilicus and the costal margin so that an appliance can be fitted without encroaching upon either. Divide the anterior and posterior rectus sheath, and split the rectus muscle. Through this, locate the transverse colon, which is recognized by the presence of attached omentum and the lack of appendices epiploicae.

Assess

If you are undertaking the operation through a laparotomy to relieve a distal obstruction, inspect the obstructing mass in the distal colon. It is, in practice, impossible to distinguish with absolute certainty between carcinoma and a diverticular phlegmon. Palpate the remainder of the colon and the liver and examine the peritoneal cavity for metastases.

Action

1 Draw the loop of proximal transverse colon out of the abdomen so that it lies in the wound without tension.

2 Open the colon longitudinally for 4 cm along one of the taenia coli, turn back the edges of the colotomy and suture the whole thickness of the colon to the edge of the skin incision with interrupted 2/0 Vicryl sutures mounted on a cutting needle. Take generous bites of the bowel wall and smaller bites of skin.

3 Insert a finger into each loop of the colostomy to make sure it is not too narrow and that the finger passes into the underlying colon.

Aftercare

Fix a suitable disposable appliance over the loop colostomy. The use of a rod or bridge passed under the loop through a window in the mesocolon is archaic and unnecessary. The stoma will not retract if fashioned without tension and the bridge makes it more difficult to fit the stoma appliance securely.

Closure

1 Do not close the colostomy until at least 6 weeks after it has been formed: 3 months is better. This period allows resolution of the acute healing phase and makes the operation easier and therefore safer.

2 Before closure ensure that any distal anastomosis is soundly healed and patent by sigmoidoscopy, Gastrografin enema or CT scan. Bowel preparation is unnecessary.

3 Circumcise the mucocutaneous junction using a cutting diathermy or scalpel and pick up the bowel using Babcock's forceps.

4 Deepen the incision to expose the colon and the anterior rectus sheath. Dissect the colonic loop from the abdominal wall until the peritoneum is entered and the whole loop can easily be drawn out of the abdominal cavity.

5 Close the colostomy transversely using a single layer of seromuscular sutures. Alternatively, if the two limbs are sufficiently mobile, a functional end-to-end stapled anastomosis may be constructed.

6 Replace the colon in the peritoneal cavity and place the omentum over it.

7 Close the abdominal wound in one layer with interrupted 1 PDS sutures. Close the skin.

SIGMOID COLOSTOMY

Appraise

1 It is usually possible to raise a sigmoid colostomy without recourse to laparotomy, unless the sigmoid is bound down by adhesions from previous diverticulitis. Laparoscopy is helpful in mobilizing the sigmoid and, more importantly, confirming the proximal and distal ends, and is the preferred option in suitable patients.

2 Use the trephine technique to construct a loop colostomy for patients with advanced rectal carcinoma who are too frail for resection, have extensive metastatic disease precluding radical surgery, or to defunction the bowel prior to chemoradiotherapy to downstage the tumour. It may also be used when the patient requires a permanent end colostomy for incontinence and in some cases of prolapse and solitary rectal ulcer when no other definitive operation is possible, but the proximal and distal ends must be correctly identified (vide infra).

Action

1 Place the patient in the lithotomy Trendelenburg (Lloyd-Davies) position.

2 Make a 5-cm transverse incision through the rectus sheath in the left iliac fossa at the site marked for the colostomy.

3 Find the sigmoid colon (identified by the absence of omentum and the presence of appendices epiploicae) and make sure the mesentery is not twisted.

4 Using an assistant to retract the wound laterally, locate the 'white line' marking the lateral peritoneal attachment of the sigmoid and incise it. Using a finger, gently sweep the parietal tissues posteriorly, mobilizing the sigmoid loop.

5 Take great care to identify the correct orientation of the colon, particularly when constructing an end stoma, to ensure that the proximal end is delivered as the stoma. If you have not confirmed this with a laparoscope, introduce a sigmoidoscope into the rectum, insufflate air and confirm that it distends the distal limb.

6 When constructing an end stoma, divide the loop of sigmoid across, together with 5 cm of mesentery, and examine the bowel lumen with a finger to confirm its orientation. Close the distal end with 2/0 polyglactin 910 sutures or a transverse stapler and return it to the peritoneal cavity. Fashion the colostomy from the proximal end using interrupted 2/0 Vicryl sutures.

7 If a loop stoma is required, proceed as described above for Transverse colostomy.

> ### ▶ KEY POINTS Anatomy

> - ■ It is disastrous to bring out the wrong end of the bowel when constructing an end stoma using the trephine technique.
> - ■ Laparoscopic-assisted colostomy (or laparotomy) allows you to confirm the correct end.
> - ■ If in doubt perform a flexible sigmoidoscopy on table, or create a loop colostomy.

COLECTOMY FOR INFLAMMATORY BOWEL DISEASE

Appraise

1 Acute fulminant colitis, with or without toxic megacolon, usually occurs in idiopathic ulcerative colitis but may occur in Crohn's disease. It is also increasingly seen in acute *Clostridium difficile* colitis.

2 The operation of choice is colectomy and ileostomy. Emergency proctocolectomy is technically demanding, carries a higher mortality and morbidity, and removes the option of later restorative surgery.

3 Manage these patients jointly with an experienced senior gastroenterologist: the first line treatment is high-dose intravenous corticosteroids.

4 Surgical treatment is usually indicated if:
- ■ The patient's condition does not improve within 72 hours and he or she still has more than 6–8 bowel actions containing blood each day
- ■ There is a fever of 38 °C or more and a tachycardia in excess of 100 beats/min
- ■ The C reactive protein is significantly elevated and rising.

5 Carry out daily plain X-ray of the abdomen: if this demonstrates toxic dilatation or evidence of perforation, proceed to emergency surgery.

6 Beware of being lulled into a false sense of security by a lack of abdominal tenderness: high-dose steroids mask clinical signs and the patient's condition may be more critical than is apparent.

Prepare

1 Continue steroid therapy with 100 mg of hydrocortisone 6-hourly. Commence full antibiotic cover with Augmentin, gentamicin or a cephalosporin and metronidazole.

2 Mark the ileostomy site.

3 Place the patient in a supine position and catheterize the bladder.

Access

1 Make an ileostomy trephine 2 cm in diameter at the previously marked site. If the patient is very sick and this has not been done, site it in the mid-inguinal line just below the umbilicus.

2 Open the abdomen through a midline incision.

Assess

1 The colon is hyperaemic, thickened and oedematous. Do not handle it excessively and do not pull away adherent omentum or lateral pelvic wall adhesions as these may be the site of sealed perforations.

2 Note any free gas, denoting that perforation has occurred. If there is a perforation, try and close it with a purse-string suture before proceeding. Note any free fluid and obtain a swab for culture and antibiotic sensitivity.

3 Examine the small bowel for skip lesions and the small bowel mesentery for enlarged lymph nodes which might denote Crohn's disease.

Action

1 Ensure that there is good access. Gently dissect the colon from its lateral attachments, starting at the caecum and mobilizing it completely round to the rectum, taking care to avoid too much traction. Try to preserve the omentum as it will prevent adhesions between the small bowel and laparotomy wound, which cause small bowel obstruction in around 25% of patients. If it proves difficult to dissect it from the transverse colon, remove the omentum with the colon as further attempts to dissect it away may lead to a perforation. If the colon is fixed to the lateral abdominal wall, remove a disc of peritoneum with the colon rather than risk opening a sealed perforation.

2 Transilluminate the mesentery and divide the vessels at a suitable place near to the bowel. Take care to preserve the terminal ileal arcades, which may provide the blood supply for a subsequent ileal pouch.

3 Mobilize the terminal ileum and transect it using a linear cutting stapler 1–2 cm proximal to the ileocaecal valve.

4 Divide the lower sigmoid colon between Parker-Kerr clamps, or using a linear cutting stapler. If the distal bowel is too friable to close, it can be brought out through the lower end of the wound as a mucous fistula. Do not divide the colon close to the sacral promontory in the mistaken belief that all of the inflamed colon must be resected.

5 Bring the ileum through the ileostomy trephine hole and trim the staple line prior to constructing the ileostomy with polyglactin 910. It is not necessary to suture the mesentery to the abdominal wall.

6 Secure haemostasis and close the abdomen. When constructing a mucous fistula bring the sigmoid colon into the lower aspect of the abdominal wound and suture it to the skin with polyglactin 910. Alternatively, close the colon with sutures or staples and leave it under the closed skin incision.

- In any operation for inflammatory bowel disease or familial adenomatous polyposis, never carry out a proctocolectomy without considering whether a sphincter-saving operation would potentially be more appropriate.
- If there is any doubt in your mind, leave the rectum intact.

ELECTIVE COLECTOMY AND ILEORECTAL ANASTOMOSIS

Appraise

1. Elective colectomy and ileorectal anastomosis may be indicated for ulcerative colitis, Crohn's disease or familial adenomatous polyposis.
2. In ulcerative colitis there must be no associated carcinoma or severe dysplasia. The rectum must be compliant enough to act as a reservoir and the anal sphincter function normal.
3. In Crohn's disease the rectum must be relatively free of disease with good anal sphincter function and no evidence of severe perianal disease such as fistulae.
4. In familial adenomatous polyposis there must be no carcinoma in the rectum. If there are confluent rectal polyps a proctocolectomy, with or without ileoanal reservoir, is preferable.
5. Never assume a patient with multiple polyps has familial adenomatous polyposis until several have been biopsied and proved to be adenomas.
6. Order an upper gastrointestinal endoscopy to exclude duodenal adenomas in patients with familial adenomatous polyposis.

Access

1. Place the patient in the lithotomy Trendelenburg position with the legs supported on Lloyd-Davies stirrups. Insert a Foley catheter into the bladder.
2. Open the abdomen through a midline incision.

Assess

1. Palpate the liver and examine the whole of the gastrointestinal tract including the stomach and duodenum. Carefully examine the small bowel for skip lesions in Crohn's disease.
2. Examine the colon carefully to make sure there is no carcinoma. An ileorectal anastomosis is still possible in the presence of a carcinoma, provided it is not in the rectum, but perform a radical colonic resection as described above.

Action

1. Mobilize the colon completely as previously described, starting at the caecum and working around to the rectosigmoid junction. Preserve the omentum by separating it from the transverse mesocolon.
2. Divide the mesenteric vessels at a suitable place in the mid-part of the mesocolon. Preserve the superior rectal artery and vein and avoid damaging the presacral nerves.

3. Place a Lloyd-Davies right-angled clamp across the rectosigmoid junction and irrigate the rectum through the anus with 10% povidone-iodine.
4. Place a Parker-Kerr clamp at right-angles across the terminal ileum close to the ileocaecal valve. Wrap a gauze swab soaked in povidone-iodine around the ileum at the site of division, protect the abdominal contents with packs and divide the ileum close to the proximal side of the clamp.
5. Divide the rectosigmoid below the Lloyd-Davies clamp with a long-handled scalpel and remove the specimen. Hold up the rectum with Babcock's forceps.
6. The ileal lumen is usually narrower than that of the rectosigmoid. Widen the ileum with a longitudinal cut along the antimesenteric border to facilitate anastomosis.
7. Construct an anastomosis using a single layer of seromuscular inverting sutures according to your preferred technique. Alternatively, cross-staple the rectosigmoid with a transverse stapler and construct the anastomosis using a 28-mm CEEA gun. Do not force the stapling gun when advancing it through the upper rectum or it may tear the rectal wall.
8. Return the bowel to the abdomen in an anatomical position and cover it with the omentum.
9. Close the abdomen.

Technical

1. If the colectomy and ileorectal anastomosis is carried out for polyposis, excise or fulgurate any rectal polyps adjacent to the transaction line before constructing the anastomosis.

ELECTIVE TOTAL PROCTOCOLECTOMY

Appraise

1. The rectum may be excised as part of the proctocolectomy or as a secondary procedure following previous subtotal colectomy and ileostomy.
2. Either excise the rectum conservatively using a close rectal dissection to conserve the pelvic floor and protect the pelvic autonomic nerves, or ensure that similar care is taken as for total mesorectal excision of the rectum for cancer to ensure preservation of these structures.
3. Mark the ileostomy preoperatively. Place it in the right iliac fossa through the right rectus muscle, as described above.

Access

1. Place the patient in the lithotomy Trendelenburg position.
2. Catheterize the bladder.
3. Open the abdomen through a midline incision.

Action

1. Carry out the colectomy and ileostomy as previously described. If the patient has previously had a colectomy and a mucous fistula, mobilize the mucous fistula when the wound is reopened and staple or oversew the lumen of the sigmoid colon.

2 Mobilize the rectum with peritoneal incisions on both sides close to the rectal wall, joined anteriorly just above the peritoneal reflection. Preserve the superior rectal artery together with the presacral fat and nerves. Clamp, divide and ligate the individual sigmoid and rectal arteries close to the rectal wall with fine ligatures. Alternatively, excise the mesorectum as for anterior resection of the rectum but do not breach the presacral fascia or damage the presacral nerves.

3 Dissect posteriorly as far as the coccyx to meet the upward dissection of the perineal operation.

4 Dissect anteriorly between the rectum and the vagina in the female. In the male, retract the seminal vesicles anteriorly with a lipped St Mark's retractor. Divide Denonvilliers' fascia transversely and dissect down between the rectum and prostate.

5 Approach the lateral dissection as for anterior resection, dividing this tissue using diathermy and sharp dissection as far down as the pelvic floor. It is not necessary to ligate and divide the so-called lateral ligaments.

Perineal operation

1 Place a strong purse-string suture around the anus close to the anal margin, aiming to remove a minimum of perianal skin.

2 Make a circumferential incision and deepen it to expose the intersphincteric plane between the pale fibres of the internal sphincter and the darker voluntary muscle fibres of the external sphincter. A Norfolk and Norwich self-retaining retractor or alternatively a Lone Star retractor is extremely useful for this dissection.

3 Deepen the dissection bilaterally, separating the internal sphincter from the puborectalis and levator muscles to establish a plane into the pelvis and then dissect posteriorly up to the puborectalis sling.

4 Deepen the anterior part of the dissection behind the superficial and deep transverse perineal muscles and then continue the dissection upwards, in the female between the vagina and the rectal wall. In the male, the external sphincter decussates in the midline to merge with the fibres of the rectourethralis muscle. Cut the strap-like rectourethralis to expose the posterior aspect of the prostate gland and divide the visceral pelvic fascia laterally on each side where it is condensed on to the lateral lobe of the prostate. The seminal vesicles are then visualized in the upper part of the wound. The use of the Ligasure or harmonic scalpel greatly aids haemostasis during the perineal dissection.

5 Divide Waldeyer's fascia posteriorly to meet the abdominal dissection. Divide any remaining lateral attachments and remove the specimen through the perineum, leaving a small wound with the external sphincter and the whole of the levator muscles intact.

Closure

1 Place a suction drain into the pelvis through a stab wound anterolateral to the perineal wound (being careful to avoid the scrotum and the femoral vessels) and secure it to the skin.

2 Approximate the puborectalis and levator muscles using interrupted 0 polyglactin 910 sutures.

3 Close the subcutaneous tissue in two layers using interrupted 2/0 polyglactin 910 sutures. Close the skin with interrupted 3/0 Ethilon on a cutting needle.

RESTORATIVE PROCTOCOLECTOMY

This is now the procedure of choice in patients with ulcerative colitis or familial adenomatous polyposis who wish to avoid a permanent conventional ileostomy and are not suitable for an ileorectal anastomosis.

1 Divide the anorectal junction at the level of the puborectalis sling, preserving the internal and external sphincters.

2 Construct a pelvic reservoir and create an anastomosis to the anal canal. The most frequently employed configuration is the stapled 'J' pouch. This is constructed from a 40-cm loop of terminal ileum using multiple firings of a linear cutting stapler to produce a pouch 20 cm in length (Fig. 13.21A). Some surgeons prefer the sutured 'W' pouch, which is technically more complex to construct, but has a greater capacity and compliance. The functional results and long-term success rates are similar for both types. The ileoanal anastomosis is usually constructed using a 25-mm diameter CEEA circular stapler, the anastomosis lying 1–2 cm above the dentate line (Fig. 13.21B). Ensure that you do not leave a cuff of residual rectum below the anastomosis as this will result in persistent inflammation, bleeding and urgency ('cuffitis'), which may result in failure of the pouch.

3 We advise you to defunction the pouch-anal anastomosis with a loop ileostomy.

4 An alternative is the Kock continent ileostomy, which consists of a reservoir constructed from 45 cm of terminal ileum with an intussuscepted nipple valve in the efferent ileum. The reservoir is continent and emptied by catheterization, so no external appliance is necessary. It is prone to complications and poor function and is now rarely performed.

SOAVE OPERATION

Appraise

1 This operation was devised by the Italian surgeon of that name in 1964 for the treatment of Hirschsprung's disease. It is rarely performed for this indication in adults, having been supplanted by Duhamel's procedure (described by the Parisian surgeon in 1956). Hirschsprung's disease is very rarely encountered in a typical colorectal practice and will not be considered further. The Soave operation is, however, a useful procedure in patients undergoing revision of a failed pelvic anastomosis and in the treatment of large villous tumours, radiation proctitis, rectovaginal and rectoprostatic fistulas and haemangiomas of the rectum.

Access

1 Place the patient in the lithotomy Trendelenburg position. Drain the bladder with an indwelling catheter.

2 Open the abdomen through a midline incision.

Action (Fig. 13.22)

1 Mobilize the sigmoid, descending colon and splenic flexure as required. Transect the rectum to leave a 10-cm long stump and resect any diseased bowel above this.

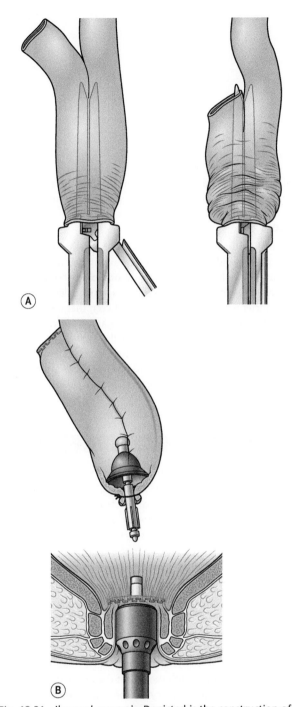

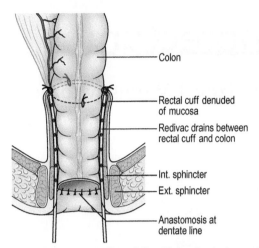

Fig. 13.22   Soave operation. The mobilized left colon is drawn through the retained rectum, which has been denuded of mucosa, and sutured to the dentate line. Suction drains are inserted through the perianal skin to drain the potential space between the rectum and colon.

5 Place two suction drains in the intersphincteric plane to drain the space between the colon and the rectal cuff.

6 Close the abdomen.

FURTHER READING

Chung CC, Ha JPY, Tsang WWC, Li MKW. Laparoscopic-assisted total mesorectal excision and colonic J pouch reconstruction in the treatment of rectal cancer. Surg Endosc 2001;15:1098–101.

Chung CC, Ng DCK, Tsang WWW, et al. Hand-assisted laparoscopic versus open right colectomy: a randomized controlled trial. Ann Surg 2007;246:728–33.

COST Study Group. A comparison of laparoscopically assisted andopen colectomy for colon cancer. N Engl J Med 2004;350:2050–9.

Guillou PJ, Quirke P, Thorpe H, et al. Short-term endpoints of conventional versus laparoscopic-assisted surgery in patients with colorectal cancer (MRC CLASICC trial): multicentre randomized controlled trial. Lancet 2005;365:1718–26.

Hohenberger W, Weber K, Matzel K, et al. Standardised surgery for colonic cancer: complete mesocolic excision and central ligation – technical notes and outcome. Colorectal Dis 2009;11:354–65.

Keighley MRB, Williams NS. Surgery of the Anus, Rectum and Colon. 2nd ed. London: Saunders; 1999.

Leung KL, Kwok SPY, Lam SCW, et al. Laparoscopic resection of rectosigmoid carcinoma: prospective randomised trial. Lancet 2004;363:1187–93.

Nicholls RJ, Dozois RR. Surgery of the Colon and Rectum. Edinburgh: Churchill Livingstone; 1997.

Novell JR, Lewis AAM. Peroperative observation of marginal artery bleeding: a predictor of anastomotic leakage. Br J Surg 1990;77:137–8.

Phillips RKS. Colorectal Surgery: A Companion to Specialist Surgical Practice. London: Saunders; 1998.

Shihab OC, Moran BJ, Heald RJ, et al. MRI staging of low rectal cancer. Eur Radiol 2009;19:643–50.

Soni N. Focus on enhanced recovery. Curr Anaesth Crit Care 2010;21(3): 105–106.

Veldkamp R, Kuhry E, Hop WC, et al. Survival after laparoscopic surgery versus open surgery for colon cancer: long-term outcome of a randomized clinical trial. Lancet Oncol 2009;10:44–52.

Walter CJ, Collin J, Dumville JC, et al. Enhanced recovery in colorectal resections: a systematic review and meta-analysis. Colorectal Dis 2009;11:344–53.

West NP, Anderin C, Smith KJE, et al. Multicentre experience with extralevator abdominoperineal excision for low rectal cancer. Br J Surg 2010;97:588–99.

Fig. 13.21   Ileoanal reservoir. Depicted is the construction of a 'J' configuration reservoir (A), stapled to the anal canal 1–2 cm above the dentate line (B).

2 Working both from above and through the anus with a self-retaining retractor, inject a solution of 1:200 000 adrenaline (epinephrine) in saline under the mucosa to lift it clear of the underlying circular muscle.

3 Denude the mucosa from the whole of the rectum down to the dentate line.

4 Bring down normal colon through this muscular tube and suture it with polyglactin 910 sutures to the dentate line, making certain that the anal sutures include part of the internal sphincter muscle. Approximate the upper end of the rectal cuff to the descending colon using interrupted absorbable sutures.

14

Anorectum

C.J. Vaizey, J. Warusavitarne

CONTENTS

INTRODUCTION

The anus is a very precise mechanism – it is able to distinguish gaseous, liquid and solid matter with greater sensitivity than the fingers. The controlling sphincter muscles are finely balanced to prevent leakage and urgency and allow us to retain continence. Meticulous attention to detail and carefully supervised postoperative care are necessary to ensure preservation of these extra-ordinary and vital functions. It is also essential to have a sound understanding of the anatomy of the area in order to make a precise diagnosis and perform effective treatment.

Wherever possible, perform a full rectal examination, including inspection, palpation, sigmoidoscopy and proctoscopy, before carrying out any procedure. Where appropriate, serious underlying diseases such as neoplasms or inflammatory bowel disease should be excluded with colonoscopy or computed tomography (CT) pneumocolonography.

Most operations can be performed with the patient in the lithotomy position. The prone (Latin: *pronus* = bent forward) jack-knife position has the advantage of superior visibility and superior access for your assistant.

ANATOMY

The anal canal extends from the anorectal junction to the anal margin and is approximately 3–4 cm long in men and 2–3 cm long in women. The lining epithelium is characterized by the anal valves midway along the anal canal. This line of the anal valves is often referred to as the 'dentate line' (Fig. 14.1): it does not represent the point of fusion between the embryonic hindgut and the proctoderm, which occurs at a higher level, between the anal valves and the anorectal junction. In this zone, sometimes called the transitional zone, there is a mixture of columnar and squamous epithelium.

Sphincters

The anal canal is surrounded by two sphincter muscles. The internal sphincter is the expanded distal portion of the circular muscle of the large intestine. It is only about 2 mm thick, composed of smooth muscle and is grey/white in colour. The external sphincter lies outside the internal sphincter with a palpable gutter between them. It is usually nearly 1 cm thick, composed of striated muscle and is brown in colour.

There is usually a pigment change in the skin over the outer margin of the external anal sphincter muscle, with lighter skin outside and darker skin over the muscle and towards the anal canal. This demarcation is useful when siting the skin incision to operate on the external anal sphincter.

? DIFFICULTY

1. Identification and differentiation of the internal and external sphincters can be difficult. Electrical stimulation, using an electrical stimulator or electrocautery, causes twitching of the external sphincter but the internal sphincter does not respond in this way. Superiorly it is contiguous with the puborectalis and levator ani muscles, forming one continuous striated muscle sheet (Fig. 14.1). The external sphincter is supplied by the pudendal nerve entering the muscle from its outer aspect posterolaterally, and the levator ani from branches of the fourth sacral nerve on its superior aspect.
2. The levator ani and puborectalis muscles are responsible for holding the anal canal in its correct position in relationship to the bony pelvis; this is with the top of the anal canal on the line joining the tip of the coccyx to the inferior aspect of the symphysis pubis. They also maintain the correct angle between the rectum and anal canal at less than 90° (Fig. 14.2).

Spaces

There are three important spaces around the anal canal: the intersphincteric space, the ischiorectal fossa and the supralevator space (Fig. 14.1). These spaces are important in the spread of sepsis and in certain operations:

- The *intersphincteric space* lies between the two sphincters and contains the terminal fibres of the longitudinal muscle of the large intestine. It also contains the anal intermuscular glands, approximately 12 in number, arranged around the anal canal. The ducts of these glands pass through the internal sphincter and open into the anal crypts.

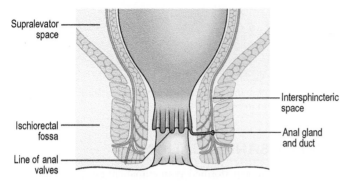

Fig. 14.1 Diagram to show the essential anatomy of the anal canal.

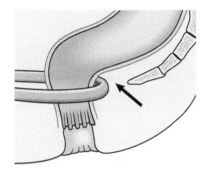

Fig. 14.2 Sagittal diagram to show the relationship of the distal rectum to the anal canal. The anorectal angle is just less than a right-angle in most people.

■ The *ischiorectal fossa* lies lateral to the external sphincter and contains fat. Abscesses may occur in this site as the result of horizontal spread of infection across the external sphincter.

■ The *supralevator space* lies between the levator ani and the rectum. It is also important in the spread of infection.

Prepare

1 Familiarize yourself with the small range of essential instruments for examination of the patient, such as the proctoscope and the rigid sigmoidoscope. In awake patients with anal sphincter spasm, use a small paediatric sigmoidoscope.

2 Operating proctoscopes of the Eisenhammer, Parks and Sims type are essential for operations on and within the anal canal.

3 Use a pair of fine scissors, fine forceps (toothed and non-toothed), a light needle-holder, Emett's forceps and a small no. 15 scalpel blade for intra-anal work. Alternatively, diathermy dissection creates a virtually bloodless field.

4 For fistula surgery have a set of Lockhart-Mummery fistula probes (Fig. 14.3), together with a set of Anel's lacrimal probes.

5 Most patients require no preparation, or two glycerine suppositories, to ensure that the rectum is empty before anal surgery. If for any reason the bowels need to be confined postoperatively, carry out a full bowel preparation to empty the whole large intestine.

6 Minor operations can be performed under local infiltration anaesthesia; larger procedures demand regional or general anaesthesia.

7 For outpatient procedures use the left lateral position, or alternatively the knee-elbow position. For anal operations most British surgeons favour the lithotomy position, although the prone jack-knife position (Fig. 14.4) can also be used.

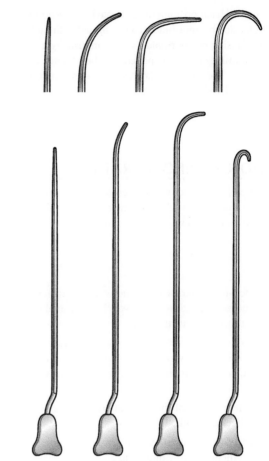

Fig. 14.3 A set of four Lockhart-Mummery fistula probes.

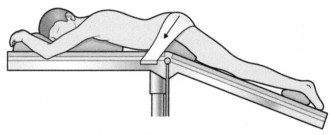

Fig. 14.4 The jack-knife position.

8 If you prefer to shave the area before starting an anal operation, carry it out in the operating theatre immediately beforehand, where there is good illumination.

HAEMORRHOIDS

Appraise

▶ KEY POINT Primary, secondary or incidental?

■ Have you excluded pelvic tumours, large-bowel carcinoma and inflammatory bowel disease?

1 Haemorrhoids usually do not need treatment if the symptoms are minimal and you have excluded a primary cause.

2 Small internal haemorrhoids can be treated by injection sclerotherapy. Prolapsing haemorrhoids may be ligated with rubber-bands. Large prolapsing haemorrhoids, which are usually accompanied by a significant external component, are best treated by haemorrhoidectomy. The advent of day-case diathermy haemorrhoidectomy has rendered surgical treatment simpler and more available than in the past.

3 As a rule avoid treating haemorrhoids if the patient also has Crohn's disease.

INJECTION SCLEROTHERAPY

This is an outpatient procedure and does not require any anaesthesia. It is most conveniently carried out following a full rectal examination if no further investigation is required. Leave the patient in the left lateral position.

Action

1 Pass the full-length proctoscope and withdraw it slowly to identify the anorectal junction – the area where the anal canal begins to close around the instrument.

2 Place a ball of cotton wool into the lower rectum with Emett's forceps to keep the walls apart. Since you will not usually remove it, warn the patient that it will pass out with the next motion.

3 Identify the position of the right anterior, left lateral and right posterior haemorrhoids.

4 Fill a 10-ml Gabriel pattern syringe with 5% phenol in arachis oil with 0.5% menthol (oily phenol BP).

5 Through the full-length proctoscope, insert the needle into the submucosa at the anorectal junction at the identified positions of the haemorrhoids in turn. Inject 3–5 ml of 5%phenol in arachis oil into the submucosa at each site, to produce a swelling with a pearly appearance of the mucosa in which the vessels are clearly seen. Move the needle slightly during injection to avoid giving an intravascular injection.

6 Delay removing the needle for a few seconds following the injection, to lessen the escape of the solution. If necessary, press on the injection site with cotton wool to minimize leakage.

7 Warn the patient to avoid attempts at defecation for 24 hours.

> ► **KEY POINTS** Injection sclerotherapy caution

- Avoid injecting the solution too superficially. This produces a watery bleb, which may ulcerate and subsequently cause haemorrhage.
- Avoid injecting the solution too deeply. This produces an oleogranuloma with subsequent features of an extrarectal swelling. Too deep anterior injection in male patients causes perineal pain and sometimes haematuria from prostatitis. This is a serious problem. Halt the injection immediately.
- If you suspect that the needle has entered the urinary tract, administer antibiotics. Do not hesitate to admit the patient, since septicaemia is common and may be severe.

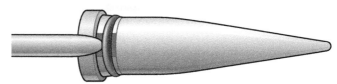

Fig. 14.5   A simple instrument with which to perform elastic-band ligation of haemorrhoids.

RUBBER-BAND LIGATION

1 This can also be performed as an outpatient procedure and does not require anaesthesia.

2 There are several different designs of band applicator (Fig. 14.5); the suction bander is relatively expensive, but is convenient and easy to use.

3 There are two conceptually different strategies:
- Band, or inject, above the haemorrhoid in order to 'hitch' it back into its normal place. Grasp the redundant mucosa proximal to the haemorrhoid and band that.
- Try to destroy the haemorrhoid itself.

4 Enquire about anticoagulants pre-procedure. Banding should not be performed if the patient is on Warfarin or Clopidigrel and some surgeons prefer to stop Aspirin as well.

NOTE: the bands are usually marked as being latex-free.

Action

1 Load one band onto the end of the sucker and one onto the applicator before applying your gloves.

2 Pass the full-length proctoscope and withdraw it slowly to identify the anorectal junction. Position the end of the proctoscope midway between the anorectal junction and the dentate line.

3 The haemorrhoids will fall into view and then the end of the suction device can be applied. Cover the hole on the device to activate the suction and then wait for a few seconds.

4 The band can then be deployed.

5 Any number of haemorrhoids can be banded on each occasion; however, the view is often obscured once two bands have been applied. Repeat banding where necessary but delay it for 6–8 weeks.

Aftercare

1 Advise the patient to take a mild analgesic and sit in a hot bath if the procedure causes discomfort.

> ? DIFFICULTY

1. If the procedure produces severe pain it may be because you applied the band too low onto the sensitive epithelium of the lower anal canal.
2. Try the effect of analgesics.
3. If they do not control the pain, remove the bands – this can be difficult in the outpatient setting and can require a light anaesthetic and the use of an operating proctoscope.

2 Pain developing slowly in 1–2 days may be from ischaemia. Analgesics relieve the pain. Give metronidazole tablets 200–400 mg three times daily, which may help reduce inflammation.

3 Advise the patient that the haemorrhoid and the band should drop off after 5–10 days and may be accompanied by a small amount of bleeding.

4 Warn the patient that secondary haemorrhage occurs in approximately 2% any time up to 3 weeks after the application. Tell the patient to report to hospital if this is severe, since it may require transfusion and operative control of the bleeding.

> ▶ KEY POINT Monitor temperature

- If the patient develops severe fever, admit the patient for treatment with intravenous antibiotics.

HAEMORRHOIDECTOMY

Appraise

1 There are several methods of performing a haemorrhoidectomy. We shall describe the diathermy technique, which has evolved out of the ligation and excision technique of Milligan and Morgan.

2 Haemorrhoidectomy should be a curative procedure. Perform it carefully and thoroughly.

Prepare

1 Start lactulose, a non-absorbed disaccharide which produces an osmotic bowel action, 30 ml twice daily 2 days preoperatively. This reduces postoperative pain.

2 Give oral metronidazole 400 mg t.d.s. for 5 days, which also significantly reduces postoperative pain.

3 Place the anaesthetized patient in the lithotomy position with some head-down tilt. Avoid caudal anaesthetic as it may provoke retention of urine.

Assess

1 Plan the operation by inserting the Eisenhammer retractor and establish which haemorrhoids need to be removed; also estimate the state and size of the skin bridges (Fig. 14.6).

2 Determine whether:
- A three-quadrant haemorrhoidectomy will be sufficient
- There is one additional haemorrhoid that needs removal, or the situation is more complex than this.

3 If there is one additional haemorrhoid you may:
- Leave it and be prepared to return on another occasion if it proves troublesome
- Fillet it out by undermining the skin bridge
- Another technique is to divide the skin bridge above the dentate line, reflect it out of the anus, and trim the

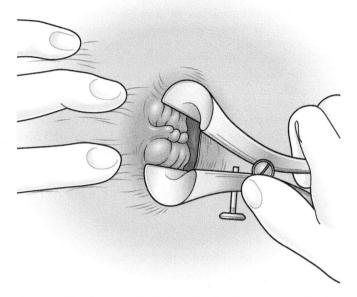

Fig. 14.6 Plan the operation by inserting the Eisenhammer retractor, establish the site and size of the haemorrhoids and identify the skin bridges to preserve them.

haemorrhoid with the back of a pair of scissors. Now excise any redundant mucosa and stitch the trimmed flap back into position with 2/0 synthetic absorbable sutures of Vicryl (Fig. 14.7).

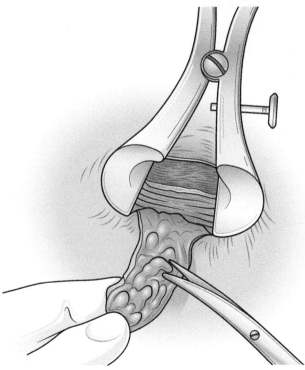

Fig. 14.7 In the event that there is an additional haemorrhoid, over and above the usual three, divide the skin bridge above the dentate line, reflect it out of the anus, trim the haemorrhoid with the back of a pair of scissors, excise redundant mucosa and stitch the trimmed flap back into position with 2/0 Vicryl.

4 The haemorrhoids may be even more extensive and may be circumferential. In this case:
- Perform a standard three-quadrant haemorrhoidectomy and return on another occasion to deal with any residual haemorrhoids
- If you are experienced in the technique, consider performing the circumferential Whitehead haemorrhoidectomy described in 1882 by the English surgeon Walter Whitehead (1840–1914). He described the excision of a tubular segment of the anal canal, with mucosal-cutaneous re-anastomosis. Use polyglactin 910 (Vicryl). Difficulties include the Whitehead deformity – mucosal ectropion (Greek: *ek* = out + *trepein* = to turn) – and late stenosis.

Action

1 Inject bupivacaine (Marcaine) 0.25% with adrenaline (epinephrine) 1:200 000 into each skin bridge and into the external component of each haemorrhoid to be excised.

2 Wait, and gently massage away excess fluid from the injection with a moistened gauze.

3 Commence with the left lateral haemorrhoid. Place the Eisenhammer retractor in the anal canal and open it sufficiently to put the internal sphincter under tension. This demonstrates the plane of the dissection (Fig. 14.8).

4 Grasp the external component and excise it with electrocautery, using cutting diathermy on skin and coagulating diathermy for all other dissection (Fig. 14.9).

> **KEY POINT** Avoid diathermy burns

- When using cutting diathermy on skin, do not linger in one area or the skin develops indolent burn marks.

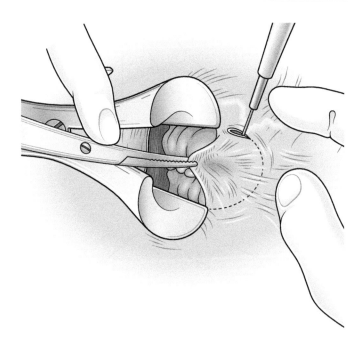

Fig. 14.8 Commence with the left lateral haemorrhoid. With the Eisenhammer in the anal canal, the internal sphincter is put on stretch allowing easy identification.

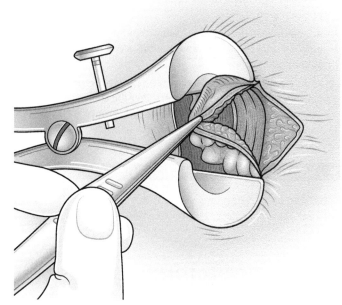

Fig. 14.9 Using electrocautery dissection, excise the external skin component and then continue the dissection up the anal canal separating haemorrhoid from anal sphincter.

5 Now extend the haemorrhoidal dissection up the anal canal, separating the haemorrhoid from the underlying internal sphincter.

6 Narrow the pedicle as you dissect up towards the apex, otherwise you risk encroaching on the skin bridge.

7 When you have encompassed the internal component of the haemorrhoid, simply transect the pedicle with diathermy.

8 Repeat the procedure on the right anterior haemorrhoid and then the right posterior haemorrhoid.

9 Ensure complete haemostasis and check each wound and apex.

> **KEY POINT** Haemostasis

- Remember that bleeding comes from what remains inside the patient, not from what has been removed.

10 Inspect the skin bridges and perform any further procedure as necessary and as earlier decided in the 'Assess' section (Fig. 14.10).

11 Do not apply any anal canal dressing.

12 Insert a diclofenac (Voltarol) suppository into the anus.

Aftercare

1 Allow the patient home after recovery from the anaesthetic.

2 Warn that there is likely to be an early increase in pain 3–5 days postoperatively.

3 Pain can usually be satisfactorily controlled with non-steroidal anti-inflammatory drugs (NSAIDs).

4 Manage the bowels with lactulose 30 ml orally twice daily until defecation is comfortable.

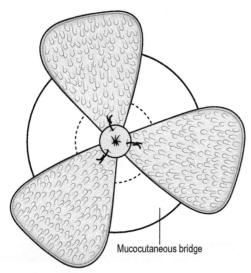

Fig. 14.10 Haemorrhoidectomy: it is essential to preserve three mucocutaneous bridges.

5 Some surgeons advocate a reversible chemical sphincterotomy with locally applied 0.2% glyceryl trinitrate (GTN) applied three times daily.

6 Review the patient in the outpatient clinic within 10–12 days.

OTHER PROCEDURES

Closed haemorrhoidectomy

The principle is a limited removal of anoderm with immediate suturing. Randomized trials have failed to show any advantage.

Stapled haemorrhoidectomy

Linear staples impinging on skin or the rectum are painful. Circular stapling above the dentate line, originally advocated by Longo, has had a variable reception from surgeons across the world. A major advantage over conventional haemorrhoidectomy is a reduction in short-term postoperative pain. However there can be major complications, including fistula formation, and tenesmus and faecal urgency are more common. Symptom control and safety are similar for the two treatments but the re-treatment rate for recurrent prolapse at 1 year is higher following a stapled operation when compared to conventional haemorrhoidectomy.

HALO procedure

This ligation procedure employs Doppler-guided haemorrhoid artery ligation. At best it is a more accurate alternative to haemorrhoidal banding and may reduce the need for conventional haemorrhoid surgery in patients who fail rubber-band ligation treatment. It does not address the external component of haemorrhoids, which are commonly the major presenting feature.

FISSURE

Appraise

1 Most ulcers at the anal margin are simple fissures in ano, possibly associated with a sentinel skin tag and/or hypertrophied anal papilla or anal polyp.

2 Exclude excoriation in association with pruritus ani, Crohn's disease, primary chancre of syphilis, herpes simplex, leukaemia and tumours.

3 Treat superficial fissures with 2% diltiazem ointment (Anoheal™) or 0.4% glyceryl trinitrate cream (Rectogesic™) twice a day. GTN can cause headaches; diltiazem occasionally causes local irritation.

4 Botulinum toxin injection is an alternative therapy, especially useful in patients who are non-compliant in regularly applying creams. Doses of botulinum toxin type A (Botox) may range from 2.5 to 50 units and reports have included injections into the internal and external anal sphincter either directly into the fissure or at sites removed from it. Dysport is an alternative preparation which requires roughly three times the number of units used with Botox. However, studies suggest that the two formulations are not bioequivalent, whatever the dose relationship.

5 Reserve operation for failures, which are more common when there is a sentinel tag, an anal polyp, exposure of the internal sphincter or undermining of the edges (Fig. 14.11).

6 Anal dilatation is no longer an acceptable treatment as it causes unpredictable stretching of the internal and external sphincters and lower rectum, producing an unacceptable risk of incontinence.

7 The standard procedure is a lateral (partial internal) sphincterotomy.

The position statement for the Association of Coloproctology of Great Britain and Ireland includes an algorithm on the treatment of fissures. Only resistant high-pressure fissures should be treated with lateral sphincterotomy, resistant low-pressure fissure may heal with the use of an anal advancement flap.

LATERAL SPHINCTEROTOMY

Appraise

1 This is very successful, curing more than 95% of patients. It was introduced by Eisenhammer in 1951.

2 To avoid exacerbating the pain, avoid preoperative preparation.

3 The operation can be carried out as a 'day-case' procedure.

4 Warn the patient of a 1 in 20 chance of permanent flatus incontinence and a 1 in 200 chance of faecal leakage.

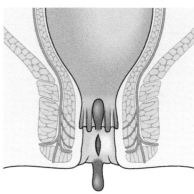

Fig. 14.11 A fissure with a sentinel skin tag, an anal polyp and undermining of the edges of the ulcer.

Action

1. Place the patient in the lithotomy position, with general or regional anaesthesia.

2. Pass an Eisenhammer bivalve operating proctoscope. Examine the fissure to exclude induration suggestive of an underlying intersphincteric abscess.

3. Remove hypertrophied anal papillae or a fibrous anal polyp, sending them for histopathological examination. Remove a sentinel skin tag.

4. Rotate the operating proctoscope to demonstrate the left lateral aspect of the anal canal. Palpate the lower border of the internal sphincter muscle. If desired, you may replace the Eisenhammer retractor with a Parks' retractor which permits outward traction, making the internal sphincter more obvious.

5. Make a small incision 1 cm long in line with the lower border of the internal sphincter. Insert scissors into the submucosa, gently separating the epithelial lining of the anal canal from the internal sphincter, and also into the intersphincteric space to separate the internal and external sphincters.

6. If you make a hole in the mucosa open it completely to avoid the risk of sepsis.

7. Clamp the isolated area of the internal sphincter with artery forceps for 30 seconds. This markedly reduces haemorrhage.

8. With one blade of the scissors on each side of it, divide the internal sphincter muscle up to the level of the top of the fissure (Fig. 14.12).

> ▶ KEY POINTS Limit the sphincteric division
>
> ■ Do not extend the division of the internal sphincter above the upper limit of the fissure.
> ■ Never extend it above the line of the anal valves.

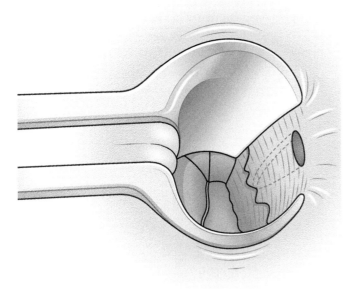

Fig. 14.12 Lateral partial internal sphincterotomy.

9. Press on the area for 2–3 minutes to stop the bleeding. The wounds do not normally need to be closed.

10. Do not apply a dressing unless there is excessive bleeding that will be controlled by pressure from it. The dressing exacerbates postoperative pain.

11. Apply a perineal pad and pants.

Aftercare

1. Prescribe a bulk laxative such as sterculia (Normacol™) 10 ml once or twice a day.

2. Bruising under the perianal skin signifies a haematoma, but it requires no treatment.

ANAL ABSCESS AND FISTULA

Appraise

1. Most abscesses and fistulas in the anal region arise from a primary infection in the anal intersphincteric glands. Furthermore, they represent different phases of the same disease process. An acute-phase abscess develops when free drainage of pus is prevented by closure of either the internal or external opening of the fistula (or both).

2. Other causes of sepsis in the perianal region include pilonidal infection, hidradenitis suppurativa, Crohn's disease, tuberculosis and intrapelvic sepsis draining downwards across the levator ani.

3. Once established, an intersphincteric abscess may spread vertically downwards to form a perianal abscess or upwards to form either an intermuscular abscess or supralevator abscess, depending upon which side of the longitudinal muscle spread occurs (Fig. 14.13A). Horizontal spread medially across the internal sphincter may result in drainage into the anal canal, but spread laterally across the external sphincter may produce an ischiorectal abscess (Fig. 14.13B). Finally, circumferential spread of infection may occur from one intersphincteric space to the other, from one ischiorectal fossa to the other and from one supralevator space to the other (Fig. 14.13C).

4. Once an abscess has formed surgical drainage must be instituted; antibiotics have no part to play in the primary management. As the tissues are inflamed and oedematous, do the minimum to promote resolution of the infection. More tissue can be divided later to resolve the condition. Send a specimen of pus to the laboratory for culture. The presence of intestinal organisms suggests the presence of a fistula.

5. Avoid preoperative preparation of the bowel as it causes unnecessary pain.

6. Place the anaesthetized patient in the lithotomy position and shave the operation area.

PERIANAL ABSCESS

1. Recognize the abscess as a swelling at the anal margin.

2. Make a radial incision and excise overhanging edges. Allow pus to drain and send a sample to the laboratory.

3. Gently examine the wound to see if there is a fistula.

4. Insert a gauze dressing soaked in normal saline solution and surrounded by Surgicel. Do not pack the wound tightly.

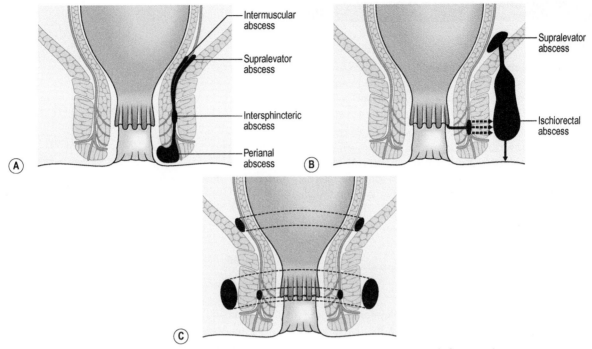

Fig. 14.13 Spread of intersphincteric abscess. (A) Vertical spread upwards and downwards from a primary intersphincteric abscess. (B) Horizontal spread from infection medially across the internal sphincter into the ischiorectal fossa, upwards into the supralevator space. (C) Circumferential spread.

INTERMUSCULAR ABSCESS

1. Recognize the abscess as an indurated swelling, sometimes mobile within the lower rectal wall.

2. As this is an upward extension of an intersphincteric abscess, manage it similarly, but the upper limit of division of the internal sphincter and/or circular muscle of the rectum is higher.

3. Control bleeding from the divided edges of the rectal wall.

4. Insert a gauze dressing soaked in normal saline to the upper limit of the wound. Do not pack the wound tightly.

SUPRALEVATOR ABSCESS

1. This is recognizable as a fixed indurated swelling palpable above the anorectal junction.

2. Drainage of a supralevator abscess extends upwards to a similar level as an intermuscular abscess, except that the whole rectal wall needs to be divided.

3. Insert a gauze dressing soaked in normal saline, surrounded by Surgicel, into the anal canal to the upper limit of the wound. Do not pack the wound tightly.

ISCHIORECTAL ABSCESS

1. Recognize this as a brawny inflamed swelling in the ischiorectal fossa.

2. An ischiorectal abscess often spreads circumferentially from one side to the other, so carefully examine the patient under anaesthesia to determine if this has occurred. Recognize the abscess by feeling the induration inferior to the levator ani muscle.

3. For the same reason, employ a circumanal incision to establish drainage. Excise the skin edges to create an adequate opening and send a specimen of pus to the laboratory.

▶ **KEY POINTS** Gentleness

- Be very careful when exploring the cavity with your finger. You may spread infection, damage the levator ani or injure the rectum itself.
- Never use a probe.

---

4. Gently insert a gauze dressing soaked in normal saline surrounded by Surgicel to the upper limit of the wound. Do not pack the wound tightly.

Postoperative

1. Remove the dressing on the second postoperative day while the patient lies in the bath, having been given an intramuscular injection of pethidine 100 mg or papaveretum 7–15 mg.

2. Initiate a routine of twice-daily baths, irrigation of the wound and the insertion of a tuck-in gauze dressing soaked in physiological saline or 1:40 sodium hypochlorite solution.

3. If the patient has evidence of persistent local or systemic sepsis, administer systemic antibiotics guided by the culture report. Metronidazole is effective against anaerobic organisms.

4. Assess the patient for the possible presence of a fistula detected at the time of abscess drainage, or a history of recurrent abscesses, or palpable induration of the perianal area, anal canal and lower rectum, or the presence of gut organism in the pus. If so, plan to re-examine the patient under anaesthesia and carry out the appropriate treatment.

FISTULA

Appraise

1 A fistula is an abnormal communication between two epithelial-lined surfaces. Therefore, in the context of fistula in ano, there should be an external opening on the perianal skin, an internal opening into the anal canal and a track between the two.

2 There may be no external opening, or it may be healed over. Likewise, there may be no internal opening as the sepsis arises in the area of the intersphincteric gland, which is the primary site of infection. It may not drain across the internal sphincter into the anal canal. Finally, the track may follow a very complicated path.

3 The presence of infection is characterized by the physical sign of induration, detected by palpation with a lubricated, covered finger.

SUPERFICIAL FISTULA

Assess

1 Place the anaesthetized patient in the lithotomy position. Always perform sigmoidoscopy, looking especially for inflammatory bowel disease.

2 Palpate the perianal skin, anal canal and lower rectum to detect induration. This is confined to the distal anal canal and localized to one area, as superficial fistulas are really fissures covered with skin and lower anal canal epithelium (Fig. 14.14).

Action

1 Insert a bivalve operating proctoscope and pass a fine probe along the track.

2 Lay open the fistula using a no. 15 bladed knife or electrocautery.

3 Curette the granulation tissue and send a specimen for histopathology.

4 If there is no induration deep to the internal sphincter, fashion the external skin wound so that it becomes pear-shaped and perform a lateral sphincterotomy (see above).

5 Insert a gauze dressing soaked in normal saline solution and surrounded by Surgicel to the upper limit of the wound.

INTERSPHINCTERIC FISTULA

1 An intersphincteric fistula results when the sepsis is inside the striated muscle of the pelvic floor and the anal canal (Fig. 14.15).

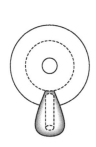
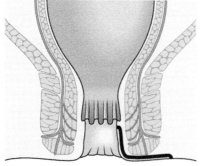

Fig. 14.14 A diagram to show a superficial fistula and the pear-shaped wound required to treat it.

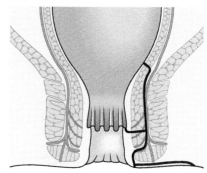

Fig. 14.15 Intersphincteric fistula. Note how the track may extend upwards into the rectum above the level of puborectalis and subcutaneously some distance from the anus.

Assess

1 Have the anaesthetized patient in the lithotomy position. Perform sigmoidoscopy in all cases, especially looking for inflammatory bowel disease.

2 Palpate carefully for induration. There is often a long subcutaneous perianal track leading to the external opening. You can feel induration in the wall of the anal canal between a finger in the anal canal and the thumb externally. If there is an upward extension, you feel induration in the rectal wall. Although the internal opening into the rectum may be above the anorectal ring, laying it open is not difficult, as the striated muscle will not be divided. Remember that there may not be an internal opening.

Action

1 Insert a bivalve operating proctoscope and pass a fistula probe, such as Lockhart-Mummery's, or Anel's lacrimal probe, along the track. This runs parallel to the long axis of the anal canal.

▶ KEY POINT Gentle manipulation

■ Never force a probe or you may create false passages.

2 If there is a long subcutaneous track, the probe is directed from the external opening towards the anus. Lay it open and remove the granulation tissue with a curette. The upward extension between the sphincters becomes apparent as granulation tissue exudes from the opening.

3 Divide the internal sphincter as high as the tip of the probe. Again remove granulation tissue by curettage. If no granulation tissue protrudes from a residual part of the track, and palpation reveals no more induration, do nothing more.

4 If necessary, totally divide the internal sphincter and the muscle of the lower rectum completely, to lay open the fistula.

5 Create an adequate external wound to allow drainage.

6 Insert a gauze dressing soaked in normal saline solution surrounded by Surgicel. Do not pack the wound tightly.

7 Apply a perineal pad and pants.

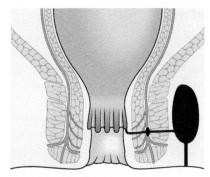

Fig. 14.16 Trans-sphincteric fistula.

TRANS-SPHINCTERIC FISTULA

1 In a trans-sphincteric fistula, the primary track passes across the external sphincter from the intersphincteric space to the ischio-rectal fossa. The infection may also have drained across the internal sphincter into the anal canal, where you find the internal opening of the fistula, which is usually at the level of the anal valves (Fig. 14.16).

Assess

1 Have the anaesthetized patient in the lithotomy position with the buttocks well down over the end of the table. Invariably perform sigmoidoscopy, especially looking for inflammatory bowel disease.

2 Palpate carefully for induration. The external opening(s) are usually laterally placed and indurated, but there is not usually any induration extending towards the anus subcutaneously in a trans-sphincteric fistula. You may palpate induration within the wall of the anal canal, the site of the primary anal gland infection. Induration is also detected under the levator ani muscles and is often circumferential. Palpate between a finger in the lower rectum, and thumb on the perianal skin, for a large area of induration. This is especially obvious if circumferential spread has not occurred and the contralateral side is normal.

> ▶ KEY POINTS Complex presentations
>
> ■ Remember that there may be no internal opening – the infection has not crossed the internal sphincter.
> ■ If there is an internal opening at the level of the anal valves, the level at which the primary track crosses the external sphincter may not be the same – it may be lower or higher (Fig. 14.17).
> ■ Infection can spread vertically in the intersphincteric space and open into the rectum, in addition to spreading across the external sphincter.
> ■ Circumferential spread of infection and other secondary tracks may also develop.

Action

1 Pass a bivalve operating proctoscope in order to try and identify the internal opening.

2 Pass a Lockhart-Mummery probe into the external opening. It may extend several centimetres and can be felt very close to a finger in the rectum. Do not force the probe, and do not pass it into the rectum, as this is never the site of the internal opening.

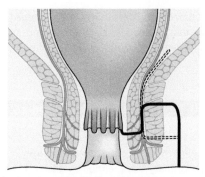

Fig. 14.17 The level at which the primary track crosses the external sphincter is not necessarily at the same level as the internal opening into the anal canal. It may be higher or lower; furthermore, there may be an upward intersphincteric extension.

3 If there is spread of infection towards the midline posteriorly, direct the probe previously inserted into the external opening, posteriorly towards the coccyx. With a scalpel (no. 10 blade) in the groove of the probe divide the tissue between the skin and the probe; divide skin and fat only, you should not divide any muscle. Apply tissue-holding forceps to the skin edges and secure any major bleeding points. Alternatively, perform the laying open with electrocautery.

4 Curette away granulation tissue, sending some for histopathological examination, and look for a forward extension from the site of the external opening. Lay it open.

5 Seek any extension of the sepsis to the opposite side by palpation, probing and looking for granulation tissue pouting from an opening in the previously curetted track. Use a no. 10 bladed knife or electrocautery to divide skin and fat to lay open any further tracks.

6 Insert the bivalve proctoscope again and re-identify the internal opening. It may or may not be possible to pass a probe either through the internal opening into the previously opened tracks or from the previously opened tracks into the anal canal.

7 Divide the anal canal epithelium and the internal sphincter to the level of the internal opening, if present, with a no. 15 bladed knife or electrocautery, thus opening up the intersphincteric space. If there is no internal opening, open the intersphincteric space in a similar way, to the level of the anal valves. Curette any granulation tissue.

8 Now identify the primary track across the external sphincter. If it is at or below the line of the anal valves, divide the muscle. If it is higher, as it often is, it may be possible to divide the muscle, but determining this requires considerable experience. It is often safer to drain the track by inserting a seton: use a length of fine silicone tubing (1 mm diameter) or no. 1 braided suture material. Mono-filaments such as nylon are often uncomfortable for the patient because of the sharp ends beyond the knot.

> ? DIFFICULTY
>
> 1. Accurate definition of a complex fistula can be difficult. Do not be tempted to risk causing incontinence by dividing the external sphincter.
> 2. Insert a loose seton (Latin: seta = bristle; a ligature threaded through the track), and order a magnetic resonance imaging (MRI) scan to clarify the situation; you can then plan effective and safe definitive treatment.

9 Once all the septic areas have been drained, fashion the wound so that drainage can continue and the wound can heal from its depths. You almost certainly need to trim the skin and fat.

> ▶ **KEY POINTS** The phases of the procedure
>
> ■ Drain the secondary tracks.
> ■ Drain the intersphincteric abscess of origin.
> ■ Drain the primary track, either by dividing the muscle or by inserting a seton.

10 Insert gauze dressings soaked in normal saline surrounded by Surgicel into the wounds and the anal canal. Do not pack the dressings tightly.

11 Apply a perineal pad and pants.

SUPRASPHINCTERIC FISTULA

■ In a suprasphincteric fistula, the primary track crosses the striated muscle above all the muscles of continence (Fig. 14.18). As this is a variant of a 'high' trans-sphincteric fistula, manage it on similar principles.

■ This is a very rare form of fistula. When possible refer the patient to a surgeon specializing in this field.

EXTRASPHINCTERIC FISTULA

1 An extrasphincteric fistula arising from an upward extension of infection from the ischiorectal fossa is also unusual and may result from the injudicious use of a probe during operation.

2 Create a defunctioning loop colostomy as a preliminary to closing the opening in the rectum and treat the fistula along the lines indicated above.

3 Manage a fistula arising from pelvic sepsis (for example from acute appendicitis, Crohn's disease or diverticular disease and not, therefore, of anal gland origin) by treating the primary disease (see Chapters 11, 13).

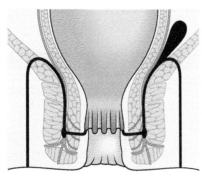

Fig. 14.18 Suprasphincteric fistula. There may be an associated supralevator abscess.

Postoperative

1 Remove the dressing on the second or third postoperative day after giving an intramuscular injection of pethidine 100 mg or papaveretum 7–15 mg. Carry out the first dressing in the operating theatre under general anaesthesia if the wound is very extensive.

2 Initiate a routine of twice-daily baths, irrigation of the wound and insertion of gauze soaked in physiological saline.

3 Inspect the wound at regular intervals until healing is complete.

4 Encourage the bowel movements to coincide with these dressing times by giving laxatives. If they do not coincide, arrange bath-irrigation-dressing routines as necessary.

5 If there is voluminous discharge of pus, review the wound in the operating theatre under general anaesthesia after 10–14 days. In patients with large wounds, this may need to be repeated. Lay open any residual tracks and curette away the granulation tissue.

6 Administer antimicrobial agents such as ciprofloxacin or metronidazole for up to 28 days, to assist in the elimination of the sepsis. A pus swab may further guide the choice of antibiotic.

7 A seton does not complicate the postoperative routine. Allow the wound to heal around it; this may take 3 months. Then, under general anaesthesia, remove the seton and curette its track free of granulation tissue. Spontaneous healing occurs in approximately 40% of patients. If healing does not occur, lay open the residual track. The advantage of this staged division of the external sphincter is that healing occurs around the 'scaffolding' of the external sphincter. When it is subsequently divided – and this is not always necessary – its ends separate only slightly. This produces a better functional result than if it were divided at the outset.

Complications

1 Failure to heal may result from inadequate drainage of the intersphincteric abscess, of secondary tracks, or of the primary track. Give the nurses clear instructions and advice about the dressings. Inadequate postoperative dressings allow bridging of the wound edges and pocketing of pus. If there is excessive growth of granulation tissue, cauterize it with silver nitrate or curette it away under general anaesthetic.

> ▶ **KEY POINTS** Slow healing?
>
> ■ Is the patient malnourished or suffering from zinc deficiency?
> ■ If hairs are growing into the wound, shave the area.
> ■ Have you missed a specific cause for the fistula, such as Crohn's disease?

2 Secondary haemorrhage may occur from any potentially septic, open wound healing by second intention.

3 Anal incontinence of varying degrees may follow division of the sphincter muscles. If the entire sphincter complex has inadvertently been divided, consider repairing it once the sepsis has been eradicated and healing has occurred.

4 Successful fistula surgery depends upon accurate definition of the pathological anatomy, drainage of the intersphincteric abscess of origin, the primary and secondary tracks, and excellent postoperative wound care.

OTHER PROCEDURES

■ A loose seton can be very acceptable to the patient even in the long term, provided that the seton is discrete and comfortable. The use of rubber sloops tied with several silk knots and left dangling between the buttocks will cause irritation and soreness. A neat 1 Ethibond thread, with only two knots, secured with 3/0 Ethibond to anchor the 'whiskers' can be completely comfortable, especially with the knots turned into the track.

■ A tight seton is designed to cut through the fistula track slowly, in the hope of reducing the separation of muscle ends. Apply it firmly but not tightly. Replace it at monthly intervals.

■ Specialist colorectal surgeons may create advancement flaps to avoid sphincter division and employ an intersphincteric approach and core-out fistulectomy. The technique is employed particularly in high trans-sphincteric fistulae, especially when situated anteriorly in women, who have a short anal canal, and is successful in around 50% of cases.

■ The use of fibrin glues injected into the track and bioprosthetic plugs sutured to the track is appealing in that there is no sphincter destruction and continence is maintained. However, initial enthusiasm over the short-term external opening healing rates has been tempered by a lack of evidence of healing of the track on MRI scanning and high recurrence rates.

PILONIDAL DISEASE

A simple pilonidal sinus detected as a chance finding during routine examination probably does not require treatment. Operate only if it is painful or infected, producing a pilonidal abscess.

Prepare

Place the anaesthetized patient in the left lateral position with the right buttock strapped to hold it up. Elastic adhesive strapping is adequate and adheres better if the skin has been sprayed with compound tincture of benzoin. Carefully shave the area.

Action

1 Determine the extent of sepsis by palpation for induration and by using probes.
2 Completely excise the skin of the septic area.
3 Curette away the granulation tissue and embedded hairs.
4 Check with a probe in the base of the wound to detect any side tracks, and look for any residual granulation tissue that may be pouting from a side track.
5 Fashion the wound so that there are no overhanging edges.
6 Secure haemostasis.
7 Dress the wound with gauze soaked in physiological saline solution and apply pressure to it.

Postoperative

1 Initiate a twice-daily routine of bath, irrigation and dressing.
2 Keep the wound edges shaved.
3 Cauterize any excess granulation tissue with silver nitrate.
4 Complications include haemorrhage, delayed healing and recurrence. If necessary, repeat the operative procedure.

OTHER PROCEDURES

1 Lay open a simple pilonidal sinus and marsupialize (Latin: *marsupium* = pouch; create a pouch with an open mouth) the wound. This keeps the wound open until the interior has filled up.
2 In Bascom's operation each pit is excised with a no. 11 bladed knife. Drain the cavity through a laterally placed incision.
3 Various rotation flaps can be used, all having the objective of avoiding a midline suture line.

HIDRADENITIS SUPPURATIVA

Appraise

1 Hidradenitis (Greek: *hidros* = sweat + *aden* = gland + *itis* = inflammation) suppurativa (Latin: = pus-forming) is a septic process that involves the apocrine (Greek: *apo* = off + *krinein* = to separate; the secretion is a breakdown product of the cell) sweat glands. It occurs in the perineum as well as the axillae.
2 Recurrent abscess formation often results from inadequate drainage. There is no communication with the anal canal and the infection is superficial. Occasionally, hidradenitis occurs in association with Crohn's disease and lithium therapy.
3 Combine surgical treatment of acute abscesses with continuing dermatological input as topical or systemic antimicrobial agents, retinoids, hormonal therapy and immunosuppressive medications may also help to control the disease.

Action

1 Drain the pus from each abscess. They are often multiple and may intercommunicate.
2 Curette away all the granulation tissue.
3 Remove all overhanging skin.
4 Allow the defect to heal by second intention.
5 In very severe cases it may be necessary to excise and graft an area most affected in order to prevent multiple recurrences.

ANAL MANIFESTATIONS OF CROHN'S DISEASE

Appraise

1 These occur in approximately 50% of patients affected with Crohn's disease.
2 The perianal area has a bluish discoloration and there may be oedematous skin tags. Ulceration, which can be extensive, may involve the perianal skin, anal margin and anal canal. Sepsis may occur in the form of either an abscess or a fistula (Fig. 14.19).

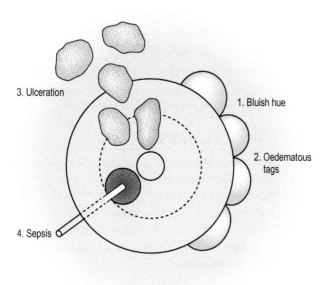

3. Ulceration

1. Bluish hue

2. Oedematous tags

4. Sepsis

Fig. 14.19　Diagram to show the anal manifestations of Crohn's disease.

Action

1　Remove a small biopsy specimen of a skin tag, or granulation tissue together with a rectal mucosal biopsy for histopathological examination.

2　Drain any abscess in the usual way, taking care not to divide any muscle.

3　For long-term seton drainage of fistulas, again prefer a soft suture material such as No. 1 Ethibond. By using 3/0 Ethibond a secure knot can be tied without the need for too many 'throws' that would create a bulky knot. Again turn the knot so that it lies within the track, leaving only a smooth loop of suture on the outside.

4　Fully investigate the patient.

CONDYLOMATA ACUMINATA

Appraise

1　Condylomata acuminata (genital warts) result from human papillomavirus (HPV) infection of the squamous epithelium. Papilliferous lesions may develop on the perianal skin, within the anal canal and on the genitalia. Exclude other forms of sexually transmitted disease and attempt to trace contacts.

2　Treat scattered lesions by applying 25% podophyllin in compound benzoin tincture. Treat more extensive lesions by operation using the technique of scissor excision.

Action

1　Have the anaesthetized patient placed in the lithotomy or prone jack-knife positions.

2　Infiltrate a solution of 1:300 000 adrenaline (epinephrine) in normal saline under the epithelium bearing the perianal lesions to reduce bleeding during excision of the warts and to separate the individual lesions, thus preserving the maximum amount of normal skin.

3　Hold the warts with fine-toothed forceps and remove them with pointed scissors.

4　Remove intra-anal canal warts in the same way after inserting a bivalve operating proctoscope. There is often a confluent ring of lesions in the upper anal canal. Totally remove these and then join the mucosa of the lower rectum to that of the anal canal at the dentate line with sutures (Fig. 14.20). In addition to achieving mucosal apposition, this mucosal anastomosis is haemostatic.

5　Send the excised lesions, particularly the intra-anal ones, for histopathological examination.

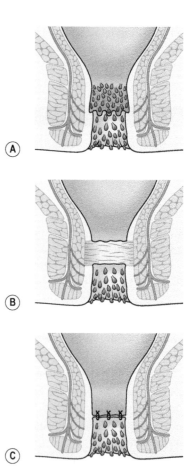

(A)

(B)

(C)

Fig. 14.20　(A) Confluent intra-anal canal warts above the dentate line. (B) The warts, together with all the mucosa, are removed, leaving a section of muscle denuded of mucosa. (C) The lower rectal mucosa is attached to the dentate line by interrupted absorbable sutures.

Postoperative

1 No special measures are needed.

2 Carry out regular examinations to detect further wart formation, which usually occurs within the first 3 months. Treat scattered lesions with podophyllin. More extensive recurrences require further inpatient treatment.

ANAL TUMOURS

Tumours in this region may be divided into two groups, although opinions differ as to the anatomical level of division.

For the purposes of this chapter anal canal tumours arise from the dentate line and above. Anal margin tumours arise below the dentate line.

ANAL MARGIN TUMOURS

Appraise

1 These may be benign or malignant. Condylomata acuminata, keratoacanthoma, apocrine gland tumours, premalignant Bowen's disease and Paget's disease are benign.

2 Excise condylomata acuminata (warts) with scissors as above.

3 Totally excise other tumours. If the defect is not too large allow the wound to heal by second intention. Close large defects with split skin grafts.

4 Histopathological information is essential in deciding whether or not any further treatment is required.

5 Malignant tumours of the anal margin are mainly squamous cell carcinomas, although basal cell carcinoma can occur. Induration suggests malignancy. Small microinvasive carcinomas can be adequately treated by wide local excision, but more advanced cancers require a combination of radiotherapy and chemotherapy (see below).

ANAL CANAL TUMOURS

Appraise

1 These are almost always malignant and include squamous cell carcinoma, basaloid carcinoma, adenocarcinoma and malignant melanoma.

2 Examine the tumour under anaesthesia and remove a biopsy specimen.

3 There is virtually no indication for local excision in infiltrative squamous carcinoma of the anal canal, which may be treated conservatively in the majority of cases by primary radiotherapy with chemotherapy. Reserve surgery for residual tumour, complications of therapy or subsequent tumour recurrence.

4 If surgery is indicated after failed combined modality therapy, then this usually requires abdominoperineal excision of the rectum and anal canal (see Chapter 13), widely excising the perianal skin, ischiorectal fossa fat and the levator ani muscles near the lateral pelvic wall. Ensure that you have positive histology after radiochemotherapy of a squamous carcinoma prior to performing an abdominoperineal resection.

RECTAL ADENOMAS

Appraise

1 Adenomas of the rectum may be classified on a histopathological basis into tubular, tubulovillous and villous. From the clinical viewpoint these three types of adenoma are similar in their behaviour as there is no invasion of neoplastic cells across the muscularis mucosae. A more useful classification is according to their clinical appearance; for example, are they pedunculated or sessile?

2 Are there any other neoplastic lesions – benign or malignant – in the large intestine? In patients with lesions more than 2 cm in diameter, there is an incidence of further tumours of 25% (benign 18%, malignant 7%). Order a colonoscopy.

> **KEY POINT** Familial disease?
>
> ■ Multiple small adenomatous polyps in the rectum suggest the diagnosis of familial adenomatous polyposis.

3 Is the lesion totally benign or does it have malignant areas? There is a 50% chance of malignant areas in patients with lesions larger than 2 cm in diameter.

4 Be sure to remove the whole lesion by performing a total excision biopsy, which is diagnostic as well as therapeutic if the lesion proves to be totally benign. Do not perform an incision biopsy as it is not representative of the whole lesion and makes subsequent submucosal excision difficult.

Action

1 Totally remove lesions less than 5 mm across by twisting with a pair of Patterson biopsy forceps.

2 Employ diathermy snare excision for those that are pedunculated.

3 Submucosally excise those that are sessile, non-circumferential and confined to the lower two-thirds of the rectum (see below).

4 Those in the lower third of the rectum that are circumferential may be suitably excised by a modified Soave operation (see below).

5 Employ anterior resection for sessile non-circumferential tumours with the lower border in the upper third of the rectum, and circumferential tumours with the lower border in the upper two-thirds of the rectum.

SUBMUCOSAL EXCISION OF SESSILE ADENOMA

Appraise

1 Undertake this technique only if there are no malignant lesions at a higher level.

2 Undertake this technique provided the tumour does not feel indurated on palpation with the finger or the end of the sigmoidoscope, suggesting malignant change.

Prepare

1. Order full bowel preparation.
2. Place the patient in the lithotomy position or the jack-knife position, which is especially suitable for anterior lesions.

Action

1. Insert a bivalve operating proctoscope and ensure that illumination is adequate. You may find it advisable to wear a headlamp.
2. Inject 1:300 000 adrenaline (epinephrine) in physiological saline into the submucosa under the tumour.

> ▶ KEY POINT Cause for suspicion
>
> ■ Benign tumours are entirely mucosal; therefore, if you find it difficult to create artificial oedema in the submucosa, suspect malignant invasion (Fig. 14.21).

3. With sharp scissors or electrocautery incise the mucosa approximately 1 cm from the edge of the tumour and then dissect it free of the circular muscle of the rectum, which appears as white fibres in the distended submucosal layer (Fig. 14.22).
4. Seal bleeding points with diathermy.
5. Allow the wound to heal spontaneously without suturing it. Close any defect you inadvertently created in the muscle with sutures.
6. Pin the specimen to a cork board before fixing it, so that the pathologist can determine whether or not there is any malignant invasion, by taking serial sections (Fig. 14.23).

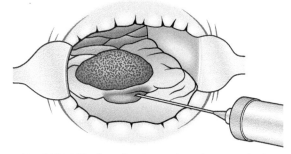

Fig. 14.21　1:300 000 adrenaline (epinephrine) in normal saline is injected into the submucosa to elevate the mucosa and the tumour within it. This will prove difficult if there has been a previous incision biopsy, or malignancy is present.

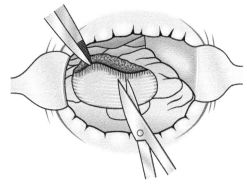

Fig. 14.22　The mucosa is dissected from the underlying circular muscle (white fibres).

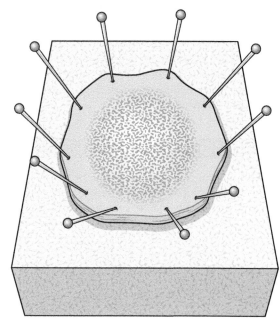

Fig. 14.23　The specimen with a margin of normal mucosa is pinned to a cork board prior to fixing to assist the histopathologist.

Postoperative

1. No special measures need be adopted other than to ensure that constipation does not occur.
2. Haemorrhage is a rare complication.
3. Study the histopathological report. If there are malignant foci, decide whether or not to proceed to a more radical procedure.
4. Follow-up the patient to detect any recurrence and metachronous (sequential but separated by appreciable intervals) lesions.
5. Stenosis of the rectum may develop if excision was performed for too large a lesion.

MODIFIED SOAVE OPERATION

1. Reserve this operation for large circumferential lesions with their lower border in the lower third of the rectum and extending into the upper third.
2. In principle the entire tumour is excised submucosally by a combined abdominal and peranal approach. The rectal muscular tube is relined with descending colon, anastomosed through the anus to the level of the dentate line (Fig. 14.24) as described in Chapter 13.
3. Circumferential lesions extending over only a few centimetres can be treated by submucosal excision, with plication of the muscle tube to allow mucosal anastomosis.
4. This is an unusual operation best reserved for performance in a specialist centre.

OTHER PROCEDURES

Both transanal endoscopic microsurgery (TEMS) and extended endoscopic mucosal resection (EMR) can be used to cure superficial mucosal tumours of the gastrointestinal tract, regardless of their size, as long as the tumours are localized and without metastases. They are both very specialist techniques.

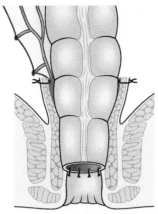

Fig. 14.24 Modified Soave operation. The mucosa has been removed from the distal rectum by both the abdominal and perineal surgeon. The descending colon is now passed into the muscle tube and sutured at the dentate line.

TEMS is a minimally invasive surgical technique that allows the surgeon to operate on lesions in the mid and upper rectum with an operating microscope inserted into the anus. An operating proctoscope (a 2 inch wide tube) is placed through the anus and positioned over the lesion. The rectum is filled with carbon dioxide gas so there is room to work. A special microscope is used to look at the area directly and with a video camera. Long instruments are then used to grasp, cut and suture.

The application of conventional EMR with snaring was somewhat limited by the size of the tumour. The Japanese introduced extended EMR or endoscopic submucosal dissection (ESD) with a new endoscopic resection technique using sodium hyaluronate and a needle knife resection for en bloc resection of large but superficial gastric neoplasms in 1998. This has been extended to other areas of the gastrointestinal track including the colon and rectum.

Recent non-randomized studies suggest that EMR is equally effective in removing large rectal adenomas when compared to TEM. Current clinical practice mainly depends on local expertise in TEM or EMR.

RECTAL PROLAPSE

Appraise

1 The symptom of prolapse (i.e. tissue slipping through the anus) may result from causes other than complete rectal prolapse. Distinguish haemorrhoids, anal polyps, mucosal prolapse and rectal adenomas. An internally intussuscepted rectum lies in the lower third of the rectum (the first phase of prolapse), whereas a complete prolapse passes through the anal sphincter and keeps it open: sphincter function is inhibited in both cases.

2 Treatment consists of control of the prolapse, re-education of the bowel habit and improvement, if necessary, of sphincter function.

3 First control the prolapse. Many operations have been described to achieve control: in the UK complete rectal prolapse is usually treated either by abdominal rectopexy or by perineal mucosal sleeve resection (Delorme's procedure, see below).

4 An open abdominal rectopexy is currently rarely performed, but follows the same steps as the laparoscopic operation described below.

5 Abdominal rectopexy is associated with unpredictable postoperative constipation, which in some patients can be severe. There are claims that concomitant sigmoid resection (resection rectopexy, also known as the Frykman-Goldberg operation) reduces this risk.

6 After rectopexy only a few patients have sphincter dysfunction severe enough to produce significant incontinence. Pelvic floor physiotherapy, faradism and electrical stimulators give little long-term benefit. The problem results from pelvic floor neurogenic myopathy producing a shortened anal canal with widening of the anorectal angle. Postanal pelvic floor repair reduces the anorectal angle and lengthens the anal canal, restoring satisfactory continence in some patients.

7 All abdominal pelvic dissection in male patients has the potential to cause either erectile or ejaculatory dysfunction. Because of this it is essential that this complication be mentioned and recorded when obtaining informed consent.

8 The laparoscopic ventral rectopexy is a newer technique which is particularly beneficial in the presence of a rectocele and enterocele as it bolsters the rectovaginal septum. Proponents of the operation suggest it should be the treatment of choice for all patients with rectal prolapse.

LAPAROSCOPIC ABDOMINAL RECTOPEXY

Prepare

1 No bowel preparation is usually required but can be used at the discretion of the clinician.

2 Order metronidazole 500 mg intravenously and Augmentin 1.2 g intravenously at induction of anaesthesia.

3 The patient should be catheterized.

4 Place the anaesthetized patient in the Lloyd-Davies (lithotomy Trendelenburg) position.

Action

1 Make a subumbilical 12-mm incision and enter the peritoneal cavity using the Hasson technique. Place a Hasson trocar in the peritoneal cavity. The camera and stack should be on the patient's left side. The bed should be tilted to the head down and left lateral position to allow the small bowel to migrate to the upper abdomen. Measures should be taken to avoid the patient slipping off the table.

2 Achieve CO_2 pneumoperitoneum to 12–15 mm Hg.

3 Place a 12-mm trocar under direct vision in the right iliac fossa. Insert another 5-mm trocar a hand's breadth above this trocar. Insert a 3rd 5-mm trocar in the left lateral region.

4 If the small bowel cannot be adequately moved out of the pelvis the ileal attachments to the lateral abdominal wall should be divided to allow the bowel to move cephalad. Starting at the level of the sacral promontory, incise the peritoneum on the medial side beside (but not damaging) the superior haemorrhoidal artery using an energy device such as the harmonic scalpel. Prior to making this incision, use a non-traumatic bowel grasping forceps to retract the rectum superiorly (assistant through the left sided port) and cephalad (surgeons left handed grasper pulling the rectosigmoid cephalad). The incision will result in gas entering the plane

of dissection, enabling good visualization of the plane. The ureters lie laterally on both sides, but always check their position. The presacral nerves lie just behind the superior haemorrhoidal artery; take care to preserve them. Extend the dissection in the lateral direction till the left ureter is identified. As the dissection progresses ensure the bow created by the superior haemorrhoidal artery is placed on tension with the left handed grasper. Now extend the peritoneal incision to the bottom of the prerectal pouch, then across the midline between the rectum and vagina or bladder, so that the rectum may be separated from them.

5   Enter the postrectal space and open it up by dissection, holding the rectum forward with your left handed grasper. Exert adequate tension on the rectum to display the areolar tissue. Seal any vessels with the energy device.

6   Now that the anterior and posterior dissection of the rectum is complete its only attachments are the two lateral ligaments. It is arguable whether or not these should be divided.

7   Achieve perfect haemostasis.

8   Using a 3/0 ethibond suture and two needle holders inserted through the right sided port, place a stitch between the upper parts of the lateral ligaments on the right side and the vertebral disc just distal to the sacral promontory; avoiding the median sacral artery. These will suspend the rectum while scarring fixes it in place. Two to three such sutures will ensure the rectum stays attached to the promontory. If the surgeon is not skilled in intracorporeal knot tying, a knot pusher can be used after suture placement.

9   Observe whether the sigmoid loop is redundant. If it is, and particularly if there is a background history of constipation, perform sigmoid resection with end-to-end anastomosis. Otherwise it is not worth resecting the sigmoid colon (Fig. 14.25). To remove the specimen and create the purse-string suture for anvil placement a 3–4-cm left iliac fossa incision can be made.

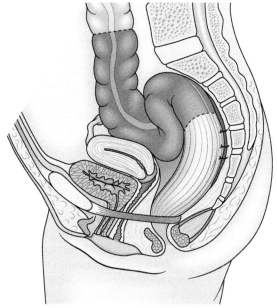

Fig. 14.25   Abdominal rectopexy can be done with or without sigmoid resection and is now usually achieved simply with a series of non-absorbable sutures rather than as previously with sponge or mesh.

10   A drain is not usually necessary, but if there is a persistent collection of blood and fluid in the pelvis insert a tube drain for 24 hours.

11   Close the laparoscopic port sites.

Postoperative

1   The patient can be commenced on an enhanced recovery programme. If no resection is performed start a normal diet as soon as the patient is able to tolerate it. If a resection is performed, start with free fluids till the patient passes flatus.

2   Remove the catheter on the first postoperative day.

3   Avoid constipation. Give a mild osmotic laxative to initiate bowel movement. Subsequently use suppositories such as glycerine and bisacodyl.

Complications

1   Haemorrhage may lead to a pelvic haematoma.

2   Postoperative constipation is unpredictable and can be troublesome.

MUCOSAL SLEEVE RESECTION (DELORME PROCEDURE)

The functional results of this procedure (Fig. 14.26) are good and it is particularly useful if the prolapse is small or incomplete and in high-risk patients who are unsuitable for abdominal surgery.

Prepare

1   Order a full bowel preparation.

2   The patient is given general or regional anaesthesia and lies in the lithotomy position.

Action

1   Reproduce the prolapse and infiltrate the submucosal plane with saline containing 1:300 000 adrenaline (epinephrine) to facilitate the dissection and to limit bleeding.

2   Make a circumferential incision through the mucosa 1 cm proximal to the dentate line. Identify the white annular fibres of the rectal wall lying deep to the submucosa.

3   Develop the submucosal plane circumferentially using either scissor dissection or electrocautery until you reach the apex of the prolapse.

4   Continue the dissection back up inside the prolapsed rectum until close to the level of the anus. Unless you do this, only half of the prolapse will have been treated.

5   Re-approximate the mucosal edges using interrupted 2/0 polyglactin 910 (Vicryl) sutures, which are also used to plicate the denuded rectal wall. Ensure that each suture takes several bites of the rectal wall in order to obliterate any potential dead space beneath the mucosa.

6   The plicated rectal wall returns to the pelvis and lies above the sphincter, preventing further prolapse.

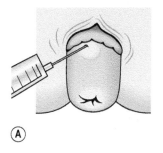 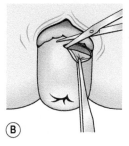 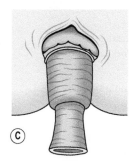 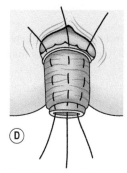 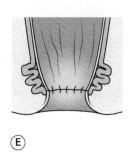

Fig. 14.26 Delorme Prodedure. (A) Infiltration with adrenaline-saline solution. (B) Beginning the mucosal sleeve dissection. (C) Completion of the mucosal sleeve dissection. (D) Insertion of muscle plication sutures. (E) The completed procedure.

Postoperative

1. Avoid constipation by using an osmotic laxative.
2. Complications can include haemorrhage, anastomotic breakdown and stricture formation.

FAECAL INCONTINENCE

Appraise

1. Determine the cause of faecal incontinence. If the anal sphincter is normal consider causes such as faecal impaction or irritable bowel syndrome. If the anal sphincter is abnormal consider the possibility of a congenital abnormality, complete rectal prolapse (see above), a lower motor neurone lesion, disruption of the sphincter ring due to trauma (including surgical and obstetric trauma) or muscle atrophy.
2. Operative treatment may be employed for the correction of some congenital abnormalities, complete rectal prolapse and simple disruption of the external sphincter (sphincter repair). Severe incontinence may need to be treated with the implantation of an artificial bowel sphincter. Sacral nerve stimulation is an alternative approach which is gaining in popularity.
3. Disruption of the sphincter ring may be suggested by a history of trauma – accidental, obstetric or surgical – and diagnosed by detecting a defect in the sphincter ring using endoanal ultrasound.

INJECTION OF BULKING AGENTS

1. The use of polytetrafluoroethylene (Teflon or polytef) was first reported in the context of a weakened or defective internal anal sphincter muscle by Shafik in 1993.
2. Injection of PTQ (silicone based) implants is now licensed in the UK. Reports on the use of other substances in faecal incontinence have been limited. Most substances have limited, if any, durability whether injected submucosally, intramuscularly or into the intersphincteris space.
3. The use of radiofrequency ablation has been employed as an alternative in the USA, but is not currently in use in the UK. It uses circumferential treatments to produce scarring of the anal canal.

Prepare

1. The patient should be put onto laxatives 2 days pre-injection, to continue for a week after injection.
2. An enema can be given preprocedure.
3. If the procedure is to be performed under local anaesthesia, a local anaesthetic cream can be used prior to injection of the anaesthetic agent.
4. Antibiotics are given intravenously at the time of the first injection and continued orally for a week after.

Action

1. There is little agreement on the optimal injection methodology.
2. The patient may be in the prone jack-knife, lithotomy or left lateral position.
3. Injections are sometimes given circumferentially in all patients and sometimes only into a specific site in those with a single internal anal sphincter defect.
4. Trans-sphincteric injection may reduce infection when compared to direct anal canal injection.
5. The site of the injection may be guided by the index finger to avoid any dispersal of product; however, some centres prefer to use a retractor or ultrasound guidance.

OVERLAPPING SPHINCTER REPAIR

A colostomy is necessary only in complex cases, such as patients with Crohn's disease, rectovaginal fistula or where the injury is very extensive (e.g. a cloacal defect extending into the vagina).

Prepare

1. Order a full bowel preparation.
2. The patient is given a general anaesthetic and placed in the supine position if construction of a loop sigmoid colostomy is required (see Chapter 13). Then place the patient in the lithotomy position for the sphincter repair.
3. Pass a urinary catheter.

Action

1. Make an incision following the slight pigment change seen around the anus. Centre it on the point of injury and extend it through 180° (Fig. 14.27).

2. Dissect out into ischiorectal fat. This means that the anal sphincter now lies between the depths of the wound and the anal canal (Fig. 14.28).

3. For an anterior, usually obstetric, injury mobilize the anus from the vagina. It helps to place two fingers in the vagina and two Allis forceps on the anal margin of the wound. The plane lies fractionally posterior to any large veins (because these will be paravaginal veins) (Fig. 14.29).

4. Split the muscle scar down its length and develop the plain between the anal mucosa and the muscle on either side.

5. After sufficient mobilization you can achieve a muscle overlap of about 2 cm, extending the length of the anal canal. Suture with 2/0 polydioxanone (PDS) (Fig. 14.30).

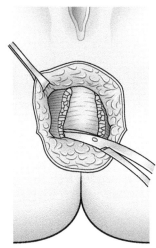

Fig. 14.29   Next, dissect close to the anal mucosa. This leaves a bulk of tissue between the lateral ischiorectal plane and the perianal plane that will contain the divided ends of internal and external sphincter.

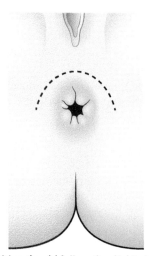

Fig. 14.27   The incision should follow the slight pigment change seen around the anus. It should be centred on the point of injury and will usually extend 180°.

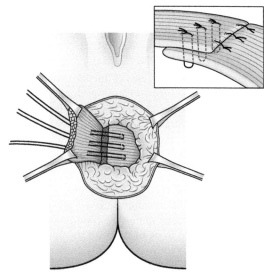

Fig. 14.30   After sufficient mobilization a muscle overlap of about 2 cm can be achieved, extending the length of the anal canal. Suture with 2/0 polydioxanone (PDS).

6. When possible, close the wound. Otherwise leave it open to heal by second intention (Fig. 14.31).

Postoperative

1. The patient can eat and drink normally and does not need confinement of the bowels.

SACRAL NERVE STIMULATION

1. This is performed in two stages: a temporary testing phase and a permanent implant for those patients who are found to gain benefit during the testing phase.

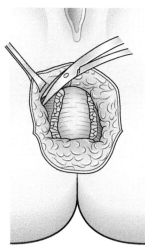

Fig. 14.28   Dissect out laterally into ischiorectal fat. This means that the anal sphincter now lies between the depths of the wound and the anal canal.

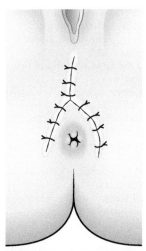

Fig. 14.31 When possible, close the wound. It may help to close it in an inverted 'Y' fashion allowing reconstruction of the perineal body and lengthening the distance between the posterior fourchette and the anal canal. Otherwise leave it open to heal by second intention.

2 There is no need for any bowel preparation.

3 The patient is given a general anaesthetic without muscle relaxants and lies in the prone jack-knife position. The anus and the big toes should be visible.

TEMPORARY TEST WIRE INSERTION

Action

1 Mark out the bony landmarks for the position of the S3 foramina. They are typically 1 cm cephalad to the crest of the sacrum and 1 cm lateral to the midline.

2 Insert the 20 G, 3.5-inch (9-cm) spinal insulated needles (Medtronic 041828–004) into S3 on either side, and find the best response to stimulation using an external, hand-held neuro-stimulator (Medtronic Model 3625 Screener). The current used for stimulation usually ranges from 0.5 to 2 mA at a rate of 20 Hz and a pulse width of 200 seconds.

3 Response to the stimulus is assessed clinically, looking for deepening and flattening of the buttock groove from lifting and dropping of the pelvic floor (known as a 'bellows' action) and a flexion of the big toe.

4 If the response if suboptimal it may be necessary to insert the needles into S2 or S4. Stimulation at the level of S2 usually causes a clamp-like contraction of the anal sphincter with rotation of the leg, ankle flexion and calf contraction. S4 is associated with a 'bellows' action and a pulling sensation on the perineum but not with any toe movement.

5 Using the foramen of maximal response, thread a temporary percutaneous stimulator test lead (Medtronic 3057) down through the needle and re-test the adequacy of the stimulation with the external stimulator and the wire. If a good response is still obtained slide the needle out over the wire, being very careful not to dislodge the wire. Secure the wire.

Postoperative

1 When the patient is awake and co-operative, attach the wire to the external stimulator (Medtronic Model 3625 Screener).

2 The stimulus employed for the 3-week temporary test phase is that which is the maximum comfortably tolerated by the patient, and usually ranges between 0.5 and 3 mA at 15 pulses/second with a pulse width of 210 microseconds.

THE PERMANENT IMPLANT

The decision to proceed to permanent implantation is based on the patient's and the doctor's subjective assessment of a significant improvement and on a 50% quantitative improvement in episodes of faecal incontinence, either frequency or amount lost.

Action

1 The initial steps taken to find the correct foramen during the test are repeated. The permanent electrode (Medtronic 3093) is then inserted instead of the wire and this self-secures with barbs. This is then tunnelled subcutaneously out to the permanent stimulator which is implanted in the buttock.

2 The stimulator is left turned off until the patient is awake and responsive.

Postoperative

The stimulator is externally programmed using telemetry. The current required for stimulation is usually between 0.5 and 2 volts at a frequency of 15 pulses/second and a pulse width of 210 microseconds.

ARTIFICIAL BOWEL SPHINCTER (THE ACTICON)

The operation to implant the Acticon is relatively simple. However, infection is a major hazard and preoperative preparation should be meticulous.

Prepare

1 Order a full bowel preparation.

2 Irrigate the rectum and vagina with Betadine wash-outs.

3 Get the patient to shower in antiseptic.

4 Swab the patient for MRSA (methicillin-resistant *Staphylococcus aureus*).

5 Plan to use adequate antibiotic cover in the perioperative period.

Action

1 Make an incision similar to that for an anterior overlapping repair arcing around the front of the anus.

2 A tunnel is then created around the outside of the anal sphincters to accommodate the hydraulic cuff. Sizers can be used to assess the size of the cuff to be implanted. All parts of the sphincter are carefully primed with radio-opaque fluid, with the exclusion of all air bubbles prior to implantation.

3 A further 'bikini-line' incision a few centimetres long is then made on the side chosen for implantation of the pump (this depends on whether the patient is right- or left-handed).

4 The connector tube from the cuff is tunnelled up to the abdominal incision; the pump and the preperitoneal reservoir are

implanted through the same incision. The pump sits in the labia majorum in women and in the scrotum in men. All three major components are connected by fully implanted silicone tubing.

5. The pump is squeezed to achieve cuff deflation via a temporary transfer of fluid into the balloon. A push-button device on the pump locks the pump closed until healing has occurred at about 6 weeks.

Postoperative

1. Continence is restored by re-activating the pump with a sharp squeeze in the clinic setting at about 6 weeks.

2. Time must be spent with the patient to ensure his full understanding of the pump mechanism or he may not be able to pass stools on discharge.

FURTHER READING

Beck DE, Wexner SD. Fundamentals of Anorectal Surgery. 2nd ed. Philadelphia: Saunders; 1998.

Fielding LP, Goldberg SM. Rob and Smith's Operative Surgery. 5th ed. Oxford: Butterworth-Heinemann; 1993.

Goldberg SM, Gordon PH, Nivatvongs S. Essentials of Anorectal Surgery. Philadelphia: Lippincott; 1980.

Goligher JC. Surgery of the Anus, Rectum and Colon. 5th ed. London: Baillière Tindall; 1984.

Henry MM, Swash M. Coloproctology and the Pelvic Floor. 2nd ed. Oxford: Butterworth-Heinemann; 1992.

Keighley MRB, Williams NS. Surgery of the Anus, Rectum and Colon. 2nd ed. London: Saunders; 1999.

Martin M-C, Givel J-C. Surgery of Anorectal Diseases. Berlin: Springer-Verlag; 1990.

Nicholls RJ, Dozois RR. Surgery of the Colon and Rectum. Edinburgh: Churchill Livingstone; 1997.

Phillips RKS. Colorectal Surgery: A Companion to Specialist Surgical Practice. London: Saunders; 1998.

Sir Alan Parks Symposium Proceedings. Ann R Coll Surg Engl 1983; (Supplement).

Thomson JPS, Nicholls RJ, Williams CB. Colorectal Disease. London: Heinemann Medical Books; 1981.

Todd IP, Fielding LP. Rob and Smith's Operative Surgery: Alimentary Tract and Abdominal 3. Colon, rectum and anus. 4th ed. London: Butterworths; 1983.

15

Biliary tract

B.R. Davidson, A.B. Cresswell

CONTENTS

INTRODUCTION

Gallstones are common and represent the most frequent indication for biliary tract surgery. Around 12% of males and 24% of females will develop stones in the gall bladder and of these around 2–4% per year will become symptomatic.

Whilst symptomatic stones are generally accepted as a clear indication for surgical intervention (assuming the patient is otherwise fit), there is no clear evidence of benefit for cholecystectomy for asymptomatic stones.

Obstructive jaundice and biliary pancreatitis are amongst the most serious complications of gallstone disease and some stones present de novo with these complications.

Cholecystectomy is by far the commonest intervention and accounts for around 50,000 procedures a year in the UK. The laparoscopic approach is now firmly established as the technique of choice. However, some surgeons support an open or 'mini-open' technique.

Though laparoscopic cholecystectomy has become established as a 'routine' operation and is often performed as a day case, the importance of good surgical technique should not be underestimated. This operation results in an average of 23 claims for negligence per year to the UK NHS Litigation Authority, with a the majority being for bile duct injury and resulting in compensation payments of up to £350,000 per case.

Cholecystectomy has traditionally been performed as an elective procedure wherever possible, with acute episodes of inflammation being treated with antibiotics and allowed to settle for 2–3 months prior to an interval operation. There has, however, been a more recent vogue for the removal of the gallbladder during an index admission with acute symptoms. This approach undoubtedly leads to a more challenging operation in the face of acute inflammation, but has not been shown to be associated with higher rate of bile duct injury or conversion to open operation in the published reviews. There is, however, clear health economic evidence that performing cholecystectomy at the time of index presentation results in a shorter overall hospital stay (due to avoidance of recurrent admissions whilst on a waiting list) and lower total costs. The timing of acute cholecystectomy remains contentious, with traditional dogma suggesting that it must be performed within 5 days of the onset of symptoms. It has been the authors' experience that absolute duration of symptoms is less important than clinical signs and previous history of symptoms in predicting success with a laparoscopic approach in the acute setting.

The advent of endoscopic retrograde cholangiopancreatography (ERCP) combined with endoscopic sphincterotomy and balloon trawl has reduced the frequency with which surgical exploration of the bile duct and treatment of the sphincter of Oddi is undertaken; however, these techniques remain an important part of the surgical armamentarium and can be undertaken by both laparoscopic and open approaches.

Further interventions on the biliary tree for benign indications are uncommon, but include biliary tract reconstruction and excision of choledochal cysts. Such procedures should be confined to specialist centres and require meticulous technique with careful follow-up.

CHOLECYSTECTOMY

Appraise

1. The majority of patients with typical biliary pain undergoing surgery for documented gallstones may expect an excellent response to their operation in terms of symptom resolution and postoperative side-effects.

2. Asymptomatic gallstones are common and it is vital to obtain a careful corroborating history before ascribing vague upper abdominal symptoms to stones seen on imaging.

3. In patients where symptoms are not typical, there should be a warning that the operation may not provide complete relief and a thorough search for an alternative diagnosis should be undertaken prior to surgery.

4. The aim of the operation is to remove the gallbladder with division of the cystic duct, which connects the gallbladder to the main biliary tree and the cystic artery, which is the major blood supply to the gallbladder and usually a branch of the right hepatic artery.

5. Significant variation exists in both biliary and hepatic arterial anatomy and, although the majority of these variations will have little impact on a safely performed cholecystectomy, full advantage should be taken of any preoperative imaging that may be available and careful note made of any anatomical anomalies identified on ultrasound scans, magnetic resonance cholangiograms (MRCP) or ERCPs where available.

Prepare

1 The majority of patients can be treated laparoscopically. Fitness for surgery should be considered on the basis that an open operation may be required. The cardiovascular effects of a pneumoperitoneum should be borne in mind.

2 Patients should be booked to appropriate lists based on any underlying medical co-morbidity and clues as to the likely severity of their disease process, such as a long history of severe and constant pain and ultrasound findings of a very thick-walled gallbladder with surrounding oedema or empyema.

3 Informed consent should be obtained with mention of specific risks such as bleeding, infection, injury to surrounding blood vessels, bowel or the main bile duct, to include bile leak. General complications of surgery such as venous thromboembolism (VTE), acute coronary events, pulmonary and cerebrovascular events and anaesthetic complications should also be discussed. In general terms' any complications that occur relatively frequently (>1 in 1000) should be outlined, along with other rarer, but very significant risks.

4 Ensure that a sample of blood has been obtained for group and save of serum and review the preoperative blood results – specifically, the liver function tests.

5 If it is planned to undertake the operation laparoscopically, the patient should be warned of the possibility of conversion to open surgery depending on intra-operative findings or events.

6 Instigate adequate VTE prophylaxis, according to local protocol, which may include the use of pre- or perioperative prophylactic heparin therapy, compression stockings or pneumatic compression devices.

7 A meta-analysis has shown no benefit to the routine use of antibiotic prophylaxis in the prevention of wound infection and septic complications, but they should be considered if the biliary tree is considered to be infected.

8 The operation is conducted under general anaesthesia and care should be taken to ensure that a radiolucent operating table is used, as regardless of whether an intra-operative cholangiogram is performed routinely or selectively, it may be essential in the case of intra-operative difficulties.

LAPAROSCOPIC TECHNIQUE

Action

1 The patient is positioned supine, and following the application of a warming device, antiseptic skin preparation should be applied from an area extending from the nipples to the symphisis pubis, with the drapes positioned such that the full costal margin and the lower border of the sternum are within the sterile operative field.

2 The convention is for the operating surgeon to stand on the patient's left hand side with an assistant to their left and the scrub nurse with instruments on the patient's right. Some surgeons prefer to place the patient in a Lloyd-Davies position and to operate from between the legs and a few will stand on the right side of the table.

3 The monitor is placed at the surgeon's eye level at the patient's right shoulder (Fig. 15.1).

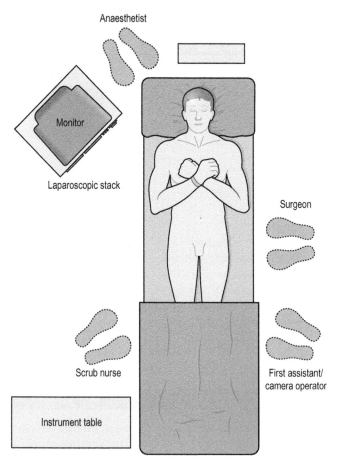

Fig. 15.1 The authors' favoured operating room set-up for laparoscopic cholecystectomy.

4 The pneumoperitoneum may be safely established by either an open cut-down or through the use of a Veress needle. Although numerous safe techniques exist for an open approach, the authors favour a 1-cm vertical supraumbilical incision with sharp scissor dissection down to the linea alba. A stay suture is then placed either side of the midline and the sheath and peritoneum incised to enter the peritoneal cavity whilst maintaining upward traction on the fascial stay stitches. A blunt trocar is then used to insert a 10- or 11-mm cannula to be used as the optical port. An operating pressure of 12 mmHg is favoured.

5 If a Veress needle technique is preferred, this is introduced through a similarly sited skin incision and gentle upward traction applied by grasping the surrounding skin of the abdominal wall until two distinct clicks of the needle are felt as it passes through first the abdominal wall fascia and then the peritoneum. Correct positioning can be confirmed by either placing a drop of saline at the injection port of the needle with the valve closed – the fluid should be 'sucked' into the needle when the valve is opened and the abdominal wall lifted – or, alternatively, the insufflation machine can be attached and should show a high flow rate and low intra-abdominal pressure. Following insufflation of at least 3 L of gas and with an intra-abdominal pressure of 12 mmHg, the needle is removed and an armed, sharp trocar used to introduce the first port, again whilst maintaining traction on the upper abdominal wall. You must be certain of correct positioning of the Veress needle and of an adequate peritoneum prior to the blind

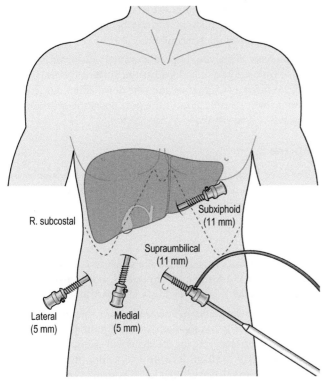

Fig. 15.2 The standard port positions for a laparoscopic cholecystectomy – the supraumbilical port is used for the laparoscope and may need to be placed more cranially in the larger patient.

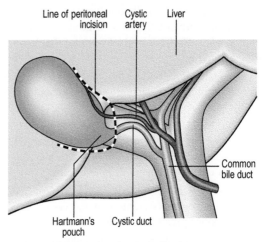

Fig. 15.3 The initial peritoneal incision for laparoscopic cholecystectomy should free Hartmann's pouch and cross Calot's triangle. Extending the initial incision a little way along the medial and lateral borders of the gallbladder with the liver will increase mobility of Hartmann's pouch and facilitate the dissection of Calot's triangle.

insertion of a sharp port and if in any doubt, should consider reverting to an open introduction technique.

6 Following insertion of the optical port, the laparoscope should be introduced and a full inspection of the abdominal contents performed to identify concomitant pathology outside of the vicinity of the gallbladder.

7 Tilt the operating table head-up and to the patient's left in order to facilitate an optimal view.

8 A standard four-port laparoscopic cholecystectomy requires the introduction of three further ports which should be introduced under direct vision and usually consist of a further 11-mm port in the epigastrium, one 5-mm port in the right upper quadrant and a further 5-mm port in the right lower quadrant (Fig. 15.2). A three-port cholecystectomy has also been described whereby all retraction is supplied by the surgeon's left hand instrument and there is no dedicated fundal retractor. There has been no evidence that the elimination of the fourth port alters outcome in terms of postoperative pain or complications – nor have there been any studies addressing safety of the three-port technique.

9 Divide any omental or visceral adhesions to expose the fundus of the gallbladder, which is then grasped with a suitably robust, ratcheted instrument inserted through the RLQ port and retracted cranially to expose Hartmann's pouch and Calot's triangle (the area between the cystic duct, common hepatic duct and liver).

10 If the view is obscured by distended duodenum or stomach then the anaesthetist should be asked to aspirate via a nasogastric tube.

11 Apply traction to Hartmann's pouch using a suitable instrument (Johann or dolphin grasper) in your left hand and use an instrument for dissection in the right hand – usually a diathermy

hook, scissors, curved dissecting forceps or a combination of the above.

12 Make a peritoneal incision at the medial aspect of the lower border of Hartmann's pouch and continue to divide the peritoneum around the base of the gallbladder and extended a little way up each of the medial and lateral borders with the liver (Fig. 15.3). This will increase mobility and facilitate the dissection of Calot's triangle.

13 Carefully dissect Calot's triangle to expose the cystic duct and artery (with the artery usually, but not always, lying between the cystic duct and liver plate and usually related to a cystic lymph node). Following isolation of these structures, about 1/3 of the proximal gallbladder should be dissected from the liver in order to be sure of the correct identity of the cystic structures – the so-called critical view of safety (Fig. 15.4).

14 Only when you are absolutely satisfied that the structures are the cystic artery and duct may they be secured and divided. Mechanical clips are the commonest technique used (either metal

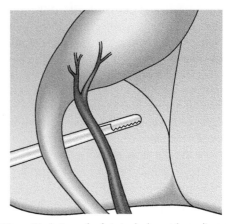

Fig. 15.4 The critical view of safety includes a 'clean dissection' of the cystic artery and duct with separation of the proximal 1/3 of the gallbladder wall from the liver bed. This ensures that the structures isolated are indeed the cystic structures and that they do not re-enter the liver.

or polypropylene) and usually the structures are clipped twice proximally and once distally before division with scissors, ensuring that a safe cuff of tissue is left beyond the proximal clips (at least 3 mm).

15 Now grasp Hartmann's pouch with your left hand and retract it cranially to facilitate dissection of the gallbladder from the liver bed in the layer of the cystic plate.

16 Care should be taken not to stray too deeply towards the liver substance as the middle hepatic vein can lie quite superficially within the gallbladder bed and will be the source of significant and difficult-to-control haemorrhage if injured.

17 A small blood vessel or occasionally a bile duct (of Lushka) may be encountered during dissection of the cystic plate – these should be clipped proximally if they are to be divided.

18 The final dissection of the fundus of the gallbladder from the liver bed is facilitated by conversion to caudal traction with the fundal grasper. However, the cystic structures and the gallbladder bed should be checked for haemostasis and bile leaks prior to division of the final gallbladder attachments, as retraction is more difficult when the gallbladder has been completely detached.

19 Retrieve the gallbladder in an impermeable extraction bag to minimize the risk of port site infection and to protect the wound in the infrequent case of an incidental carcinoma. Extraction is best performed through the umbilical port, as this fascial incision is usually the largest and the simplest to extend and subsequently close.

20 Make a final inspection of the operative field to exclude bleeding and bile leaks and remove each port under direct vision, again to check haemostasis.

21 Close the 11-mm fascial defects using an 0 absorbable suture. The 5-mm ports are not often closed routinely, though some surgeons would advocate doing so to avoid the infrequent hernias encountered through these port sites.

22 Close the skin according to your own preference and instil local anaesthetic into each of the wounds, based on the safe maximum dose for the individual patient.

> **? DIFFICULTY**
>
> 1. If you cannot extract the gallbladder from the port site then open a portion of the gallbladder wall that you have been able to deliver between clips and use the laparoscopic sucker to aspirate bile from the portion of the organ that is lodged inside the abdomen, taking care not to spill bile outside of the bag and onto the wound.
> 2. If the gallbladder still cannot be removed – pass some Rampley's sponge holding forceps through the hole in the gallbladder and extract some stones, or let the organ pass back into the abdomen (keeping hold of the retrieval bag) and extend the skin and fascial incisions.

OPEN TECHNIQUE

Appraise

1 The majority of cholecystectomies are now performed laparoscopically, with the open procedure usually reserved for cases where laparoscopic progress is impossible or when the gallbladder is being removed in conjunction with another procedure that is being performed via an open technique.

2 The presence of previous upper abdominal incisions is not an absolute contraindication to laparoscopic surgery. It is usually possible to insert a laparoscope and take down adhesions (perhaps with a slight modification of the port positioning) in order to proceed to a laparoscopic cholecystectomy.

Prepare

1 The same preoperative steps are required as for the laparoscopic procedure. In addition, antibiotic prophylaxis against wound infection is usually given in all cases.

Action

1 The surgeon usually stands on the patient's right side with the first assistant and scrub nurse opposite. A second assistant is very useful, if available, and should stand to the surgeon's left.

2 Make a transverse subcostal incision on the right hand side and deepen this using monopolar diathermy through the fat layer, down to the fascia overlying the rectus and external oblique muscles. Usually a 6–10-cm incision will suffice, though this may need to be extended according to the patient's build and the degree of inflammation of the gallbladder.

3 Incise the fascia in the same oblique line and stay at least 3–4 cm beneath the costal margin to allow closure of the wound without having to stray too close to the periosteum of the ribs.

4 Some surgeons will pass a swab or tape beneath the rectus muscle prior to division, but it is perfectly safe to simply divide the muscle using diathermy until the posterior fascial layer is reached. Any large vessels encountered within the muscle can be grasped with forceps and diathermized or ligated as required.

5 Grasp the posterior layer of fascia with two clips and incise between them, then extend the full length of the wound with a hand inside the abdominal cavity to protect any underlying bowel.

6 Following an inspection of the abdominal contents, place a folded swab above the right dome of the liver in order to bring the gallbladder and hilum into the operative field.

7 Divide any omental or visceral adhesions to allow the colon and small bowel to be retracted caudally beneath a further folded pack and use a deep retractor such as a 'Kelly' held in the assistant's left hand to maintain a clear view of the gallbladder neck and the hepatic hilum.

8 A 'Rampley's' sponge holding forceps on the fundus of the gallbladder and retracted towards the right shoulder by a second assistant is often useful to display Calot's triangle.

9 Cholecystectomy may commence with either dissection of the structures in Calot's triangle, as with the laparoscopic operation, or by a fundus-first dissection of the gallbladder from the liver bed. It is the authors' preference to first identify and divide the cystic artery and duct and to divide the tissue within Calot's triangle prior to detaching the gallbladder, as this helps guide the final stage of mobilization of the gallbladder from the liver.

10 Transfix the cystic duct and artery proximally and ligate them distally prior to division. An absorbable suture is adequate and the authors' preference is for 3/0 vicryl.

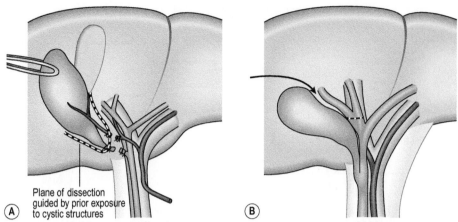

(A) Plane of dissection guided by prior exposure to cystic structures

(B)

Fig. 15.5 The correct line of dissection on reaching Hartmann's pouch is made far more obvious by isolating the structures in Calot's triangle as the initial manoeuvre during an open cholecystectomy. The cystic plate is continuous with the hilar plate and a fundus-first dissection of the gallbladder will lead directly to the right portal structures.

11 Dissection should follow the same plane within the cystic plate as with the laparoscopic operation and as the cystic plate is continuous with the hilar plate it is necessary to direct dissection over the cystic structures on reaching Calot's triangle, as continuing along the cystic plate will lead to the right hilar structures. Determining the correct plane to follow at this stage of the dissection is made very much easier if Calot's triangle has been dissected in the first instance (Fig. 15.5).

12 Following removal of the gallbladder, check the cystic plate for bile leaks and bleeding by applying a clean white swab.

13 Unless the gallbladder was perforated during removal, routine lavage or drainage is not required. If bile or stones were spilt, then a careful wash should be performed and all stones retrieved.

14 A drain will not be necessary unless you have any doubts about the integrity of your closure of the cystic duct stump.

15 You may close the wound using either a heavy permanent or an absorbable suture, either in two layers or by mass closure, according to preference. A 'fat stitch' is not usually necessary and skin can be closed, again according to preference.

SINGLE INCISION LAPAROSCOPIC SURGERY TECHNIQUE

1 There is a growing interest in single incision laparoscopic surgery (SILS) and some centres offer SILS cholecystectomy.

2 This technique is undoubtedly more challenging and is limited by poor separation of the longitudinal axis of the instruments from the optical axis of the endoscope and by a severely restricted operating angle between the instruments. Careful patient selection is key and the technique is feasible for the more straightforward cases.

3 The advantages of SILS surgery over conventional laparoscopic surgery are yet to be proven and the technique is still far from mainstream. It is mentioned here for the sake of completeness, but should not be attempted without a firm grounding in the laparoscopic technique and specific SILS training.

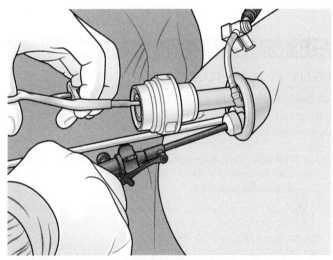

Fig. 15.6 A single incision laparoscopic surgery (SILS) port will allow passage of several instruments and a laparoscope through a large 'mother' port. Each sub-port has its own independent gas seal; however, the manipulation angles between instruments are very limited. Several brands of SILS port are available and there are subtle differences between the brands.

Action

1 Insert a special SILS port, via an open incision through the umbilicus, which allows passage of a number of standard instruments and a 10-mm laparoscope (Fig. 15.6).

2 The technique for the operation is the same as for the laparoscopic procedure; however, manipulation angles for the instruments are restricted and high-quality camera work is essential.

3 Some lateral retraction of the gallbladder can be achieved by passing a suture on a straight needle through the anterior abdominal wall in the left upper quadrant, passing the suture through Hartmann's pouch and out through the abdominal wall in the right upper quadrant. Ligaclips are then placed on the suture on either side of Hartmann's pouch and

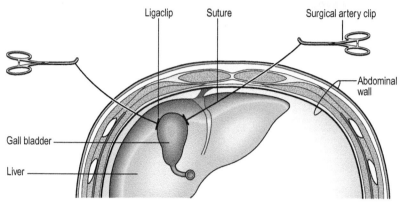

Fig. 15.7   A suture passed through the abdominal wall and through the fundus of the gallbladder can be used to provide some lateral retraction of the gallbladder. A ligaclip should be applied to the suture on either side of the gallbladder to provide countertension for retraction.

external traction on either end of the suture will provide some lateral retraction of the gallbladder to facilitate dissection (Fig. 15.7).

THE DIFFICULT GALLBLADDER

PATIENT HABITUS

All surgical techniques are more challenging in patients with a high body mass index. Cholecystectomy in obese patients is usually easier laparoscopically than by open surgery:

1. Initial port access may be difficult, especially with the open technique and a larger skin incision may be required in order to reach the abdominal wall fascia.

2. It is helpful to grasp the base of the umbilicus with a 'Littlewood's' forceps and to retract this upwards in order to minimize the distance between the skin and the fascia.

3. In particularly challenging cases a 'visiport', which allows insertion of the first port through the various layers under direct vision, may be useful.

   It may be necessary to use longer ports and instruments and particular care should be taken in ensuring that the patient is secure on the operating table prior to tilting the table.

4. Fatty change in the liver may severely restrict the ability to retract the gallbladder due to stiffness and bulk of the liver and the liver substance itself becomes far more friable. Some of these difficulties can be overcome by placing the fundal retractor around a third of the way between the fundus and Hartmann's pouch, rather than on the very tip of the gallbladder.

5. In severe cases, there has been a suggestion that the fatty infiltration of the liver can be minimized for the procedure by a 2-week ultra-low-calorie and ultra-low-fat diet prior to surgery. For this, the patient should be allowed 2 pints of skimmed milk daily along with a balanced multi-vitamin supplement, unlimited water based drinks and a stock-cube to maintain electrolyte balance. Substantial improvements in the bulk of the liver can be obtained by this diet, but it must be stressed to the patient that it is only safe for a very limited period of time preoperatively.

ANATOMY

1. Biliary and hepatic arterial anatomy is extremely variable, although the majority of variations will have no impact on laparoscopic cholecystectomy.

2. It is crucial to begin dissection around Hartmann's pouch and not to stray too far down the cystic duct – identifying the cystic duct/CBD junction is not helpful and may lead to unnecessary injury.

3. The cystic artery should similarly be dissected at its junction with the gallbladder in order to avoid injury to the right hepatic artery.

4. It is essential that the critical view of safety is obtained, that the cystic duct and artery have been positively identified and that no other structures are present in Calot's triangle prior to clipping or dividing any structures.

5. A right posterior sectional duct that joins the cystic duct is not too uncommon and is easily injured or mistaken for a duct of Lushka (Fig. 15.8).

6. Any doubts about the anatomy that has been displayed should prompt you to either perform a laparoscopic cholangiogram to confirm ductal anatomy or to convert to an open procedure.

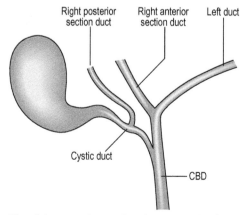

Fig. 15.8   The right posterior section duct may arise from the cystic duct or directly from the common bile duct (CBD) and can traverse Calot's triangle – where it can easily be damaged. The critical view of safety should be widely exposed and both the cystic duct and artery positively identified prior to clipping or dividing any structures.

PATHOLOGY

1. Severe inflammation can make cholecystectomy extremely challenging and is sometimes difficult to predict from preoperative ultrasound scanning.

2. Dense omental adhesions to the body of the gallbladder may also involve the colon or the duodenum and care should be taken to identify these viscera during dissection.

3. Fistulae between these hollow organs and the gallbladder occur occasionally and an open procedure is usually required to facilitate safe dissection and closure of fistulae if present.

4. A severely inflamed Hartmann's pouch that is filling Calot's triangle and adherent to the hilar structures is one of the commonest causes of misidentification of the cystic duct/CBD and, classically, a tubular structure that appears to be funnelling into the gallbladder actually turns out to be the CBD adherent to Hartmann's pouch (Fig. 15.9). Injury in these circumstances can be avoided by completing the dissection of Calot's triangle to provide the critical view of safety prior to dividing the duct. If this view cannot be obtained, then conversion to open or a subtotal cholecystectomy may be required.

5. If a Mirizzi's syndrome exists (obstructive jaundice due to compression from a stone in the cystic duct or Hartmann's pouch) the inflamed gallbladder is usually densely adherent to the main bile duct). Have a low threshold for subtotal cholecystectomy or enlist specialist HPB assistance if available.

6. In the case of a very badly inflamed gallbladder in the acute setting, it may be wise to abandon the procedure following initial laparoscopy to allow the inflammation to settle down, and perform an interval cholecystectomy in 6 to 8 weeks. If the patient is acutely unwell – consider either a surgical or percutaneous cholecystostomy as a temporising measure.

CONVERSION

1. Have a generally low threshold to convert a difficult laparoscopic cholecystectomy if inflammation is severe, in the event of intraoperative complications or if the anatomy cannot be adequately visualized. Be under no illusions, however, that the open procedure will be any easier and ensure that your incision, lighting and assistance are adequate.

2. A common cause of bile duct injury following conversion is fundus first dissection of the gall bladder, especially when Calot's triangle has been obliterated. In such circumstances, the cystic plate will lead directly onto the right hilar structures and care must be taken to avoid injury. Have a low threshold for subtotal cholecystectomy in such circumstances.

SUBTOTAL CHOLECYSTECTOMY

This technique is invaluable when it proves difficult to identify and mobilize the cystic duct and can be performed as a laparoscopic or open operation:

1. Start by aspirating the fluid from the gallbladder as this may well be infected (A Veress needle attached to a 50-ml syringe with a Leuer lock is useful). Send the fluid for culture. Then open the gallbladder at the fundus using diathermy.

2. Remove all the stones and stop any bleeding from the gallbladder wall.

3. Place a finger inside the gallbladder and palpate the cystic duct orifice or Hartmann's pouch, if performed as an open operation, or identify these structures visually if laparoscopic.

4. Incise longitudinally along the inferior border of the gallbladder to a level just above the cystic duct orifice and then extend the incision circumferentially across the gallbladder.

5. If possible, dissect the posterior wall of the gallbladder from the liver and simply amputate the gallbladder at the level of Hartmann's pouch.

6. If bleeding is encountered in dissecting the cystic plate, then simply carry the circumferential incisions upwards when reaching the junction between the gallbladder and liver and leave the posterior gallbladder wall on the liver.

7. The cystic duct orifice within Hartmann's pouch should be closed using a purse-string stitch and if the posterior wall of the gallbladder is left behind – destroy its mucosa with diathermy.

8. A closed non-suction tube drain should be left at the cystic duct stump and can be removed after 48 hours in the absence of bile (Fig. 15.10).

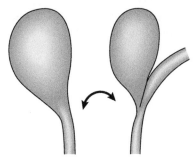

Fig. 15.9 Hartmann's pouch and the cystic duct may become inflamed and adherent to the main bile duct. In such circumstances a tubular structure may be dissected which seems to funnel out into the gallbladder. Full dissection of Calot's triangle with lateral traction and inspection will identify this situation and avoids one of the commonest reasons for iatrogenic bile duct injury.

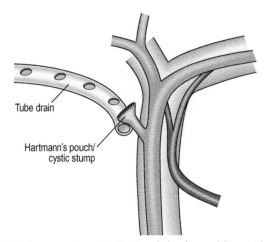

Tube drain

Hartmann's pouch/ cystic stump

Fig. 15.10 In cases where Calot's triangle has been obliterated by inflammation a subtotal cholecystectomy with removal of all gallstones is a safer option. Following closure of Hartmann's pouch/cystic duct stump, a non-suction tube drain should be placed adjacent to the closure.

ENTERIC FISTULAE

1 If a fistula to the colon or duodenum is discovered, this should be detached by blunt finger dissection.

2 Debride and close the fistula in one or two layers using an absorbable suture and leave a drain at the site of the closure.

3 If a sizable defect exists, it is occasionally necessary to perform a segmental colonic resection with primary anastomosis or a duodenoplasty.

DUCTAL CALCULI

1 Up to 10% of patients with symptomatic gallstones will have occult ductal calculi.

2 If a stone is identified incidentally during cholecystectomy it may be either removed by surgical exploration of the common bile duct or by postoperative ERCP, depending on the surgeon's experience and the availability of ERCP services. Duct exploration is a high-risk procedure in frail and elderly patients.

3 Be mindful of any previous surgery or anatomical considerations that would preclude subsequent ERCP, as surgical removal of the ductal stone is mandated in these patients (e.g. previous gastric surgery, which prevents endoscopic access to the ampulla, or the presence of a large duodenal diverticulum).

4 If a postoperative ERCP is planned then a more secure method of securing the cystic duct stump than clips alone is wise as intraductal pressure may be high postoperatively, which would increase the risk of a stump blow out and bile leak. Acceptable techniques would include the use of locking clips, suture ligation, pre-tied endoloops or stapling devices.

INTRA-OPERATIVE COMPLICATIONS

HAEMORRHAGE

1 Small amounts of blood can look very significant when viewed laparoscopically. Care should be taken to cauterize all small vessels, as bleeding during the dissection will obscure the view of vital structures.

2 If bleeding is encountered apply pressure and wait rather than rushing to cauterize or clip a vessel that has not been clearly identified.

3 If there is a significant bleed discuss the likely source and the management plan with your anaesthetist so that blood can be available if transfusion is required.

4 Torrential bleeding can be encountered by injury to the right hepatic artery, portal vein or middle hepatic vein branches.

5 Arterial bleeding is the easiest to deal with as it is usually possible to identify the precise source of the bleeding and to control this with pressure or a grasper in order to repair the laceration with sutures. This can be performed laparoscopically if you are sufficiently experienced or may require conversion to an open approach.

6 Although the right hepatic artery can be ligated without serious consequence this is best avoided wherever possible and a careful suture repair with fine non-absorbable sutures is a far better option. Place a bulldog clip proximally and distally to the injury if bleeding is brisk and you cannot see to perform the repair.

7 Portal venous bleeding is more difficult to control and a significant injury usually mandates conversion to open surgery. Control the bleeding by gentle pressure and dissect and sling the vessel proximally and distally if possible. If necessary, apply a Pringle clamp across the hilar structures at the free edge of the lesser omentum; although this will not prevent back-bleeding from the vein, it can allow better visualization.

8 The extent of the injury must be carefully defined and the venotomy closed by fine non-absorbable sutures (e.g. 5/0 Prolene).

9 Avoid blind stitching in the hilum of the liver. Repair is very much preferable to ligation of the vein, so control the situation with pressure and enlist the help of an HPB or vascular surgeon if necessary.

10 The middle hepatic vein or branches can run very superficially in the gallbladder fossa. Avoid straying into the liver substance during dissection of the gallbladder from its bed. A hole in the gallbladder is far preferable to a hole in the vein. If heavy bleeding is encountered in this area, control it initially by pressure and consider whether you need to convert to open surgery.

11 It is usually necessary to complete the removal of the gallbladder prior to attempting a repair, in order to gain adequate access.

12 With gentle pressure applied to the bleeding point, take a deep bite either side of the injury and with tension on the suture, take a second bite to complete a 'figure of 8 stitch'. The suture needs to be tied gently to avoid tearing through the parenchyma and a relatively loose stitch will effectively control the bleeding.

13 If you think that you have made a significant sized hole in the middle vein, warn the anaesthetist as air embolism is possible, which could lead to circulatory disturbance and/or a drop in oxygen saturation, and suture the injury as soon as possible.

14 On occasion, following both laparoscopic and open cholecystectomy, a significant degree of ooze can be encountered from the gallbladder bed. Use diathermy set to spray to control the area and then press with a damp swab for 4 minutes (timed by the clock).

15 If the ooze continues, consider whether there is a focal area that needs to be stitched, or try a topical haemostatic product, combined with further pressure.

16 In all cases, ensure that haemostasis is secured before closing the patient as significant blood loss can occur from an oozing gallbladder bed.

BILE LEAK

1 Spillage of bile during mobilization and dissection of the gallbladder due to either a retraction or diathermy injury is relatively common but is usually avoidable with careful technique.

2 If this happens, start by emptying the gallbladder by suction and retrieving any stones that have been spilt. These can act as a nidus for infection if left and may present even years later.

3 If possible, close any holes in the gallbladder using clips, pre-tied loops or by suturing to prevent further stone loss.

4 Biliary injury during cholecystectomy is an unusual but important complication.

5 Occasionally clips on the cystic duct may become loose. If this is noticed intra-operatively then reclip, perhaps using a locking clip, or apply a pre-tied loop to the cystic duct stump.

6 If a bile leak is encountered following gallbladder removal carry out a careful inspection of the operative field. If there is no leakage from the cystic duct stump then an intra-operative cholangiogram should be performed.

7 Apart from cystic stump leaks, the commonest significant injury is damage to (usually transection of) the right posterior sectional duct. It is important that this duct is clearly identified on the cholangiogram as it can occasionally drain into the cystic duct itself.

8 Injury to the main biliary tract should be managed in a specialist setting and may require a biliary reconstruction.

9 If you identify such an injury or cannot locate the source of a bile leak then place a large closed non-suction drain in the region of the porta hepatis and arrange transfer to an HPB centre for further assessment.

VISCERAL INJURY

1 The most commonly injured viscera are the transverse colon and the duodenum.

2 Beware diathermy injury to these structures and if a burn is caused, even if it is not full thickness, it should be oversewn, even if this requires conversion to open surgery.

3 Full-thickness injuries can usually be closed primarily in one or two layers, though some debridement of devitalized tissue may be required.

4 Maintain a low threshold for conversion to open repair in such circumstances.

INTRA-OPERATIVE IMAGING OF THE BILIARY TRACT

Appraise

1 The ability to image the biliary tract during cholecystectomy should be regarded as a core skill.

2 Some surgeons routinely image the bile duct, others use the technique selectively.

3 There is no definite evidence that routine imaging prevents bile duct injury; however, the technique is mandatory if there is the suspicion of injury to the bile duct or if the biliary anatomy cannot be clearly identified.

4 In the elective setting, the presence of small stones or sludge on dividing the cystic duct stump should prompt cholangiography to exclude stones in the common bile duct.

5 The choice of technique depends on local expertise and availability of equipment. Cholangiography is the most commonly employed technique, though endoscopic ultrasound and choledochoscopy are also practised.

CHOLANGIOGRAPHY

1 Care should be taken at the start of every cholecystectomy to position the patient's upper abdomen over a radiolucent portion of the operating table and to obtain consent for cholangiography.

2 Following dissection of the structures in Calot's triangle, place a clip on the cystic duct at its origin from Hartmann's pouch – this is to prevent spillage of bile or small stones.

3 With the gallbladder retracted laterally make a small transverse incision in the cystic duct with fine scissors – this should be sufficient to allow passage of the cholangiogram catheter and is usually around 50% of the calibre of a normal-sized cystic duct.

4 Some bleeding may be expected from the edge of the duct and this does not need intervention unless it is very heavy.

5 Ensure that the catheter is connected to a syringe of diluted contrast (50/50 mix of contrast and saline) and a syringe of plain saline via a three-way tap.

6 The catheter should be flushed to exclude any air bubbles which may later be mistaken for ductal stones and initially opened to the saline-containing syringe.

7 The authors prefer to use Olsen-Reddick Cholangiogram Forceps to introduce the catheter as this allows easy insertion and securing of the catheter in the cystic duct with the instrument's in-built clamp (Fig. 15.11).

8 Regardless of the equipment you use, make fine adjustments with the gallbladder retraction and have your assistant continuously flush the catheter gently to facilitate insertion.

9 Following clipping or clamping of the catheter in position ensure that the saline flushes freely into the bile duct.

10 Return the table to a flat position and then slowly remove the fundal retracting grasper and allow the gallbladder to rest in its usual position.

11 Check again that the saline is flushing freely, without significant leakage prior to opening the three-way tap to the contrast syringe.

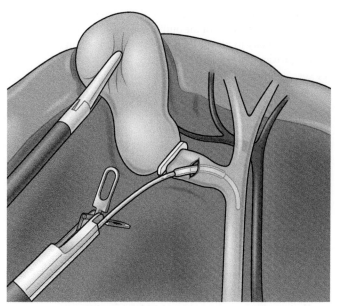

Fig. 15.11 The authors favour the Olsen-Reddick cholangiogram forceps, which allow easy placement of the catheter within the cystic duct, which can be secured without the need for additional clips.

12 After covering the patient's abdomen with a sterile drape move the C-arm of the image intensifier into position with the radiation source placed around 20–30 cm above the patient's abdomen.

13 Take care not to disturb the cholangiogram catheter whilst positioning the C-arm.

14 Make sure that all operating theatre personnel are covered by protective lead aprons or screens. Place a pair of scissors on the skin surface on the RUQ of the abdomen with the tip pointing upwards and roughly in the position of the junction between the cystic duct and the bile duct. Use the scissors to confirm the orientation and positioning of the radiographic image following a brief burst of screening.

15 The position of the lumbar spine and the right lower ribs also helps to identify the appropriate area of the abdomen prior to contrast injection.

16 When you are happy with the positioning, remove the scissors and screen continuously while you inject contrast. You should see the biliary tree outlined in its entirety, without any filling defects.

17 First concentrate on the lower end of the CBD and its insertion into the duodenum. You should look for free flow of contrast into the duodenum without any filling defects. If contrast does not flow freely to outline the duodenal mucosa, it may be due to a small stone or ampullary spasm: the administration of 20 mg of intravenous buscopan may be helpful.

18 Next direct your attention to the upper duct and follow this along its course into the liver. You should again note the free flow of contrast and absence of filling defects.

19 You should check the calibre of the bile ducts and ensure that they taper smoothly along their length with no extravasation of contrast.

20 Finally, check that you have seen all of the second order branches with the liver, especially the right posterior section duct. As a minimum, you must see the right main duct branching into its anterior and posterior sections and the left duct giving rise to the medial and lateral branches (Fig. 15.12).

21 Although the majority of stones will be seen distally you should check that the whole of the outlined ducts are clear. Occasionally it is necessary to tilt the table slightly head-down in order to see the proximal ducts.

22 When you are happy that the cholangiogram is complete, remove the C-arm and ensure that the images have been stored.

23 Reinsert the laparoscope and retract the gallbladder fundus to display the cystic duct. Remove the catheter under direct vision.

24 Clip the cystic duct distal to the incision, divide the duct and complete the cholecystectomy.

LAPAROSCOPIC ULTRASOUND

Appraise

1 Some centres favour the use of laparoscopic ultrasound over cholangiography.

2 The perceived advantages are that the procedure is less invasive, does not require the use of contrast and can be performed without an incision in the biliary tract.

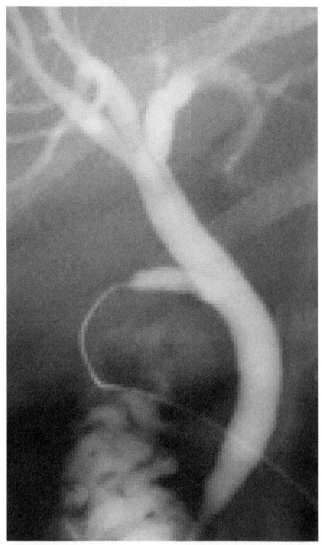

Fig. 15.12 A complete cholangiogram should demonstrate flow into the duodenum and second-order divisions of the intrahepatic ducts – namely the left main and right anterior and posterior sectional ducts. Check for filling defects which may represent retained stones and also for the continuity of the vital anatomy.

3 The use of ultrasound is limited by the availability of the equipment and expertise; however, it has been shown to be as sensitive and specific as cholangiography for the determination of biliary anatomy and the detection of ductal calculi.

Action

1 A flexible linear probe is inserted (usually through the epigastric port) and the entire biliary tree from the intra-pancreatic portion of the bile duct to the second order divisions of the intrahepatic ducts may be visualized.

2 The procedure is difficult in the presence of large volumes of intra-peritoneal fat, dense adhesions and a markedly fatty liver; however, adequate views can usually be obtained with careful retraction of the gallbladder. The technique has the added advantage of being able to identify the location of both the ductal and vascular structures prior to dissection in cases of severe inflammation.

LAPAROSCOPIC CHOLEDOCHOSCOPY

This technique will be fully outlined in the section on bile duct exploration and is not commonly used for the routine inspection of the biliary tree at elective cholecystectomy.

SURGICAL EXPLORATION OF THE COMMON BILE DUCT

Appraise

1. Operative exploration of the bile duct has become far less common with the advent of ERCP. Despite this, there remains a role for single-stage management of gallbladder and ductal stones, retrieval of incidental stones detected on routine intra-operative ductal imaging and for those patients in whom endoscopic clearance has either failed or is technically impossible.

2. Several choices for technique are available and procedures can be performed both laparoscopically or open and via the cystic duct or common bile duct.

3. The choice of technique depends partly on the availability of surgical expertise, equipment and preference.

4. Although the majority of common bile duct stones can be removed laparoscopically, the same relative contraindications to laparoscopic cholecystectomy (such as significant cirrhosis or adhesions in the upper abdomen) apply to laparoscopic duct exploration.

5. Large stones that are impacted in the duct can be difficult to dislodge without the benefit of bimanual palpation.

6. A non-dilated bile duct (<8–10 mm) is a contraindication to direct laparoscopic exploration due to the high risk of stricture formation following closure of the choledochotomy. Such cases are better served by trans-cystic or endoscopic retrieval.

7. Relative contraindications to trans-cystic stone retrieval include numerous and large ductal stones, a narrow cystic duct and a low cystic duct insertion.

The authors' favoured technique is described – other methods are available.

Prepare

1. The same general preparations as for cholecystectomy are required.

2. In addition, the necessary supplemental equipment should be available and checked, specifically: cholangiogram catheters, balloon dilators, soft-tipped guidewires, balloon catheters, choledochoscope and lithotripsy basket.

Action

Laparoscopic duct exploration

Trans-cystic

1. Following dissection of the structures at Calot's triangle, make a 50% cystic dochotomy. The duct should then be 'milked' by gently squeezing it proximally to distally to dislodge any small stones or sludge. Now perform a cholangiogram.

2. Make a note of the size, number and location of the ductal stones and evaluate the calibre, length, insertion level and configuration of the cystic duct.

3. Move the fundal retractor a little way proximally along the body of the gallbladder in order to allow use of the RUQ operating port for the insertion of instruments to explore the duct.

4. It is sometimes difficult to maintain adequate exposure and it may be necessary to insert a further 5-mm port in the RUQ between the fundal retractor and working port.

5. Depending on the calibre of the duct and size of the stones, insert a balloon dilator into the cystic duct and gently dilate this to facilitate removal of the stones (Fig. 15.13).

6. Under X-ray screening, pass a lithotripsy basket into the bile duct and try to manoeuvre it through the ampulla and into the duodenum. Take care in negotiating the junction between the cystic and common bile ducts in order not to injure the posterior wall of the bile duct.

7. Deploy the basket in the duodenum and gently pull it back through the ampulla and catch stones as the basket is slowly withdrawn along the duct. It is often possible to retrieve several stones with each pass, depending on their size. Repeat the procedure, adding more contrast as necessary until the duct is seen to be clear (Fig. 15.14).

8. For stones lying above the level of the cystic duct insertion, it is necessary to pass the basket proximally, rather than distally, which can be challenging.

9. If the basket cannot be encouraged to enter the common hepatic duct it is often possible to flush the stones into the distal duct by injecting saline. Alternatively, a 3-mm choledochoscope with an instrument channel may also be used, although this is not widely available.

10. Following retrieval of all the stones, completion imaging of the ducts should be obtained either by cholangiography, choledochoscopy or ultrasound and the duct secured in the standard fashion prior to division.

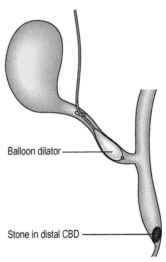

Fig. 15.13 A balloon dilator may be used to enlarge the cystic duct in order to facilitate trans-cystic removal of larger stones. Care should be taken not to rupture the duct wall by injudicious dilatation.

Balloon dilator

Stone in distal CBD

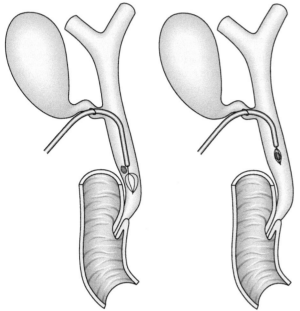

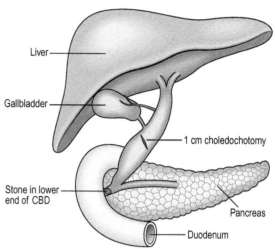

Fig. 15.15 A 1-cm oblique longitudinal choledochotomy should be made in the supraduodenal bile duct to facilitate direct exploration. Care should be taken to minimize mobilization of the duct and subsequent damage to its blood supply and ducts <8–10 mm should not be explored in this manner.

Fig. 15.14 A basket is useful to entrap and remove stones. The basket may be passed through an appropriate choledochoscope, passed through a cholangiogram catheter or simply passed directly down the duct. In all cases, care should be taken to avoid injury to the posterior wall of the bile duct as instruments are inserted.

Direct choledochotomy

1 Do not attempt direct choledochotomy on bile ducts of less than 8–10 mm in diameter. You will cause a postoperative stricture of the duct.

2 Divide the peritoneum overlying the supraduodenal bile duct to expose its anterior surface over a length of around 2 cm.

3 Do not attempt to dissect the duct laterally or posteriorly as you risk injuring its blood supply, resulting in possible postoperative ischaemic stricture formation.

4 Use a laparoscopic scalpel/cutting diathermy to create an oblique or longitudinal dochotomy of around 1 cm in length (Fig. 15.15).

5 Gently insert the tip of the 5-mm laparoscopic sucker to clear bile and small stones.

6 The duct is most easily cleared by the insertion of an ERCP catheter, which should be first passed proximally to the intrahepatic ducts and then distally to the level of the ampulla and the ducts trawled with the balloon inflated in order to eject the stones through the dochotomy.

7 If stones are impacted, it may be necessary to use a lithotripsy basket to ensnare them or even crush them prior to removal.

8 Complete clearance of the ducts can be confirmed by choledochoscopy using a 5-mm instrument, the majority of which, unlike their 3-mm counterparts, contain an instrument channel to ensnare or trawl any remaining stones under direct vision. The choledochoscope should be used with continuous saline irrigation and can be used to push any recalcitrant distal ductal stones onward through the ampulla if they cannot be dislodged proximally.

9 Close the dochotomy carefully with interrupted fine (5/0 or 6/0) monofilament absorbable sutures spaced approximately 3 mm apart, with 2-mm bites on either edge of the divided duct.

10 Some surgeons advocate the use of either a biliary stent or a T-tube to decompress the duct, but these are not strictly necessary. A closed non-suction drain should be placed at the site of the closure. This may drain placed a small amount of bile for a day or two postoperatively, but inevitably dries up quickly provided the closure has been carefully performed. The potential complications of a displaced T-tube or stent may outweigh their benefits in this situation.

Open exploration

1 Use fixed retractors (e.g. Thompson, Bookwalter) to optimize the view of the gallbladder and structures of the porta hepatis.

2 Transcystic exploration may be performed as described above; however, the majority of ducts that are being explored by open surgery are likely to contain 'difficult stones' and success with a trans-cystic approach may therefore be limited.

3 Expose the supraduodenal bile duct as described above. If the duct is difficult to identify then use a 2-ml syringe and a fine needle to aspirate bile from the suspected duct. Then insert fine 5/0 PDS stay sutures on either side of the duct prior to incision using a number 11 scalpel blade.

4 The duct can be explored as above with a combination of balloon catheter, basket and choledochoscope.

5 If stones are impacted distally, it may be possible to dislodge them by bimanual manipulation of the intra-pancreatic portion of the duct, taking care not to squeeze the pancreas too firmly as this may result in pancreatitis.

6 In cases of difficulty, it may be necessary to mobilize the duodenum by dividing the lateral peritoneal attachments (Kocher's manoeuvre) in order to better manipulate the duct.

7 If the stone is stuck fast, make a 3-cm duodenotomy opposite the ampulla and control with stay sutures. Gently insert a catheter from the distal end of the duct in an attempt to dislodge the stone. If this fails and the stone is palpable above the ampulla through the posterior wall of the duodenum, then a direct incision of the duct and sphincteroplasty can be performed (see below). Close the duodenotomy with interrupted absorbable monofilament sutures.

TRANSDUODENAL SPHINCTEROPLASTY

Appraise

1 Endoscopic sphincterotomy has removed many of the indications for transduodenal sphincteroplasty. Although the surgical technique provides complete division of the sphincter muscle to provide a more reliable and longer lasting drainage procedure than the endoscopic alternative.

2 Impacted distal stones, recurrent problems with primary choledocholithiasis and benign ampullary stenosis are the most frequent indications for sphincteroplasty.

Prepare

1 Explain the procedure, including the possible risks of bleeding, infection, biliary or enteric leak, VTE, myocardial events, and chest infection. In the long term, there is a risk of anastomotic stricture or enteric reflux, which could lead to episodes of cholangitis.

2 The patient should have group and save of serum and routine antibiotic prophylaxis at the time of induction of anaesthesia. VTE prophylaxis should be given in line with local policies.

3 The patient should be positioned supine with the upper abdomen overlying a radiolucent section of the operating table.

Action

1 Make a right subcostal incision to enter the peritoneal cavity.

2 Perform a preliminary inspection of the abdominal contents to exclude concomitant disease.

3 Use fixed retractors and gauze packs to expose the lateral border of the duodenum and the porta hepatis, by packing the small bowel and colon downwards.

4 Mobilize the duodenum by performing Kocher's manoeuvre – it may also be necessary to mobilize the hepatic flexure of the colon to facilitate this.

5 Locate the ampulla in the second part of the duodenum by palpation through the lateral duodenal wall.

6 Make a 3-cm longitudinal duodenotomy opposite the ampulla and use small retractors or stay sutures on the margins of the incision to give you an optimal view of the ampulla.

7 Pass a small cannula into the duct and aspirate bile to confirm your position in the duct and to guide you in the direction in which you need to divide the sphincter – generally this will be between the 11 and 1 o'clock position on the ampulla. Place stay sutures in the papilla in the 11 and 1 o'clock positions, tie the sutures and secure with clips.

8 Cut down either onto the cannula or onto a small right angle Lahey forceps placed within the bile duct orifice. Stitch the duodenal wall to the bile duct wall on each side of the divided sphincter and bile duct every 3 mm or so as you advance using fine (5/0 or 6/0) absorbable monofilament sutures.

9 Continue in this manner until all the muscle fibres of the ampulla have been divided along the line of the sphincterotomy. You should have a 'wide-open' view of the pale mucosal lining of the bile duct and a sphincteroplasty between 1 and 1.5 cm in length. Be sure that all bleeding has been controlled and complete the sphincteroplasty by placing a final suture at the apex of the 'V' to stitch the duodenal and biliary mucosa (Fig. 15.16).

10 Be sure that you have identified the major pancreatic papilla – usually around the 6 o'clock position of the sphincterotomy and confirmed by the presence of clear pancreatic juice. Avoid instrumentation of the pancreatic duct, but ensure that it has not been narrowed by any of your sphincterotomy sutures.

11 The bile duct may be explored with a balloon catheter or choledochoscope to ensure that it is clear and then the duodenotomy should be closed with interrupted monofilament non-absorbable sutures. If there is any concern over narrowing the duodenum, then close the duodenotomy transversely as a duodenoplasty rather than longitudinally.

? DIFFICULTY

1. As transduodenal sphincteroplasty is rarely performed outside specialist HPB units, elective procedures and those anticipated to be complex should be referred to a specialist unit.

2. If you have trouble identifying the ampulla, pass a catheter from the common bile duct, which should pass into the duodenum. If a stone is impacted in the ampulla, a catheter from above may help disimpact it when you cut down onto it.

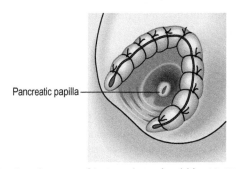

Pancreatic papilla

Fig. 15.16 An adequate sphincteroplasty should be 10–15 mm in length and the duct should be sutured to the duodenal mucosa every 3–5 mm to ensure haemostasis. It is important to identify and protect the pancreatic papilla when fashioning the sphincteroplasty.

ROUX EN Y HEPATICO-JEJUNOSTOMY – BILIARY RECONSTRUCTION

Appraise

1 There are numerous indications for biliary reconstruction, including situations where part of the biliary tree has been excised (such as for cancer operations or choledochal cysts), where the duct has been damaged and cannot be repaired (such as cholecystectomy bile duct injuries) and also where a definitive drainage procedure is required in the case of recurrent bile duct stone formation or benign bile duct stricture.

2 In cases of ductal stone disease where a definitive drainage procedure is required, a formal hepatico-jejunostomy is a far better treatment than hepatico-duodenostomy, which is associated with significant entero-biliary reflux and long-term problems with recurrent cholangitis.

Prepare

1 Explain the procedure, including the possible risks of bleeding, infection, biliary or enteric leak, VTE, myocardial events, and chest infection. In the long term, there is a risk of anastomotic stricture or ascending cholangitis. The former may require biliary balloon dilatations; the latter is treated with antibiotics.

2 If the reconstruction is being performed for a bile duct injury with an associated arterial injury, the risks of stricture are higher and there is also a long-term risk of the development of sepsis/abscess in the affected section of the liver.

Patients with bile duct injury should not undergo reconstruction until full visualization of the biliary tree has been established by cholangiography, vascular injury assessed by IV contrast CT and overt sepsis controlled by antibiotics and drainage of any collections.

3 The patient should have a group and save of serum and intra-operative cholangiography and/or choledochoscopy should be available.

4 Antibiotic prophylaxis should be given at the time of induction of anaesthesia and VTE prophylaxis should be given in line with local policies.

5 The patient should be positioned supine with the upper abdomen overlying a radiolucent section of the operating table.

Action

1 Make a right subcostal or rooftop incision to enter the peritoneal cavity, depending on the patient's build (larger patients may require a rooftop incision).

2 Perform a preliminary inspection of the abdominal contents to exclude concomitant disease.

3 If the gallbladder is still in place, dissect the structures at Calot's triangle and divide the cystic artery.

4 Palpate the lateral edge of the hepatoduodenal ligament to identify an accessory right hepatic artery arising from the superior mesenteric artery. This vessel runs along the lateral border of the main bile duct.

5 Dissect the gallbladder from the liver bed and follow the cystic duct to its junction with the main bile duct.

6 Divide the lateral peritoneum of the hepatoduodenal ligament to expose the bile duct at the level it is to be divided – usually above the level of insertion of the cystic duct and just distal to the biliary confluence.

7 Encircle the bile duct at this level using a right angle Lahey forceps. Pass the instrument behind the bile duct from medial to lateral to minimize risk of injury to the portal vein, which lies behind and medial to the bile duct. Be careful to avoid injury to the accessory artery if present.

8 Pass a nylon tape behind the duct and divide the duct onto the tape with diathermy or knife. Minimize the amount of dissection of the proximal duct in order to protect its blood supply.

9 Suture or diathermize any significant bleeding from the proximal cut end of the duct.

10 The distal duct will be dealt with according to the underlying pathology. For bile duct injuries, it should be dissected down to the upper border of the pancreas, excised and oversewn at that level.

11 Ensure that the proximal ducts are clear by flushing with saline and direct inspection to the level of the second order ducts using a choledochoscope, or by performing a cholangiogram.

12 Release the retraction on the colon and small bowel to identify the Duodenal-Jejunal (D-J) flexure.

13 Use a theatre light angled to transilluminate the jejunal mesentery from above in order to visualize the vascular arcade. Identify an appropriate point to divide the jejunum to provide an optimal blood supply to each end of the bowel, with an adequate length for the Roux loop to reach the bile duct without tension.

14 Find a point where the marginal arcade has good feeding vessels and make a mesenteric window between the feeding vessels on either side of the marginal arcade, before dividing it between clips (Fig. 15.17).

15 Where possible, divide the arcade centrally between the feeding vessels in order to optimize the blood supply to each end of the bowel. You may need to make the division further to the right in order to lengthen the Roux loop if the mesentery is short.

16 Divide the jejunum using a transverse linear cutting stapler and oversew the distal end of the divided bowel (the tip of the Roux loop) with a 3/0 monofilament absorbable suture.

17 The Roux loop is usually best passed through the transverse mesocolon (retrocolic) – assess the lie of the loop in both an antecolic and retrocolic position.

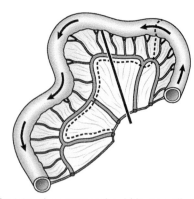

Fig. 15.17 The jejunal mesentary should be transilluminated to identify the best level for division in order to maximize the length of the Roux loop and to preserve the best blood supply to each bowel end.

18 Transilluminate the transverse mesocolon and identify the avascular window to the right of the middle-colic vessels. Open this window with diathermy sufficiently to allow free passage of the Roux loop and its mesentery without any tension.

19 Bring the distal limb of the jejunum through the transverse mesocolon until it sits easily adjacent to the bile duct at the hilum.

20 Start the hepatico-jejunostomy by inserting a series of interrupted double ended 4/0 or 5/0 monofilament sutures along the anterior wall of the bile duct – place the sutures approximately 3–5 mm apart, taking 3-mm bites of the bile duct and mount each suture on a rubber-shod clip, leaving both needles attached and arranging the clips in order of insertion (Blumgart Technique, Fig. 15.18). The first and last suture to be placed should be at each corner of the bile duct.

21 Make an enterotomy in the anti-mesenteric border of the distal end of the Roux loop, so that the loop sits neatly on the bile duct and without tension. The enterotomy should be just smaller than the bile duct and should be divided through the full thickness of the bowel wall.

22 Place further interrupted sutures, inside to out on the posterior wall of the bowel, starting 3–5 mm from the corner of the enterotomy and pass the needle out to inside on the posterior wall of the bile duct in the corresponding position.

23 After each suture is placed, cut off both of the needles and mount each suture on a small clip arranged in order of insertion.

24 At either corner of the enterotomy place the corner bile duct stitches inside to out on the bowel and loop the tails to identify them as the corner stitches (Fig. 15.19).

25 Bring the bowel up to efface the bile duct and tie each of the posterior sutures in order on the inside of the anastomosis – do not tie the corner stitches at this point and trim the loose tails when all the knots have been tied.

26 Now pass each of the anterior wall sutures from inside to out on the bowel, cut off the needles and again mount each suture on a small clip until all the anterior sutures have been placed.

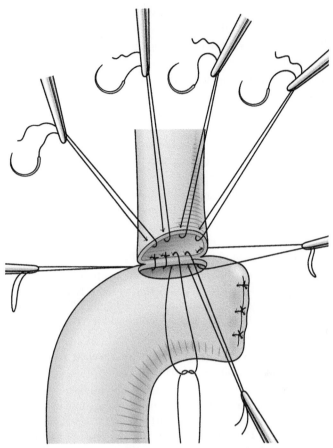

Fig. 15.19 Following insertion of each corner stitch, the posterior wall sutures are placed so that the knots will be tied within the bowel lumen and all of the sutures should be positioned before the knots are tied.

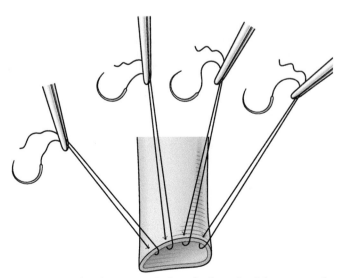

Fig. 15.18 In the Blumgart technique for hepatico-jejunostomy, the anterior bile duct wall sutures are placed first and mounted on rubber-shod artery clips.

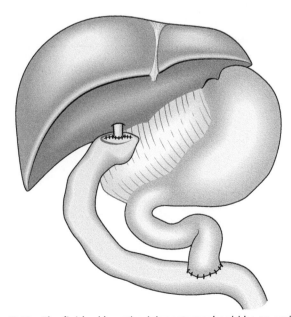

Fig. 15.20 The finished hepatico-jejunostomy should be an end-(of bile duct) to- side (of bowel) anastomosis and is usually passed behind the colon (retrocolic). It is important that the Roux loop lies neatly and without tension.

27 Tie each of the sutures in turn, starting with one of the corner stitches and trim the tails when all knots have been secured.

28 The anastomosis should be sitting squarely without any tension (Fig. 15.20).

29 Intestinal continuity must now be restored by joining the other divided end of the bowel to the distal small bowel. Mark an area on the anti-mesenteric border of the small bowel around 30–40 cm distal to the end of the Roux loop.

30 The entero-enterostomy can be fashioned in a number of ways – we prefer an end-to-side, two layer, continuous sutured anastomosis.

31 Using a 3/0 monofilament absorbable suture: take a bite of the free end of the bowel on the anti-mesenteric border around 10 mm from the staple line and pass the suture through the anti-mesenteric border of the marked small bowel. Tie this suture and place the short end on a small clip.

32 Fashion the outer posterior layer of the anastomosis by suturing the free end of the small bowel, staying about 10 mm from the staple line, to the side wall of the biliary limb. When you reach the mesenteric border, lock the suture and leave the needle attached on a small clip.

33 Use diathermy to excise the staple line and to make a corresponding enterotomy on the adjacent small bowel.

34 Take a fresh suture and start by passing the needle from out to in on the corner of the free end of the bowel and from in to out on the enterotomy, tie this and loop the short end and mount it on a small clip. Continue the inner posterior layer by taking full-thickness bites of the bowel wall on each side; on reaching the end of the posterior layer continue around onto the anterior layer and close this with sero-submucosal bites to exclude and invert the mucosa (Fig. 15.21). Tie the suture to the looped free end when you finish the inner anterior layer and trim the tails.

35 Now simply finish the outer anterior layer by continuing with the free needle from the outer posterior layer and by taking small seromuscular bites to cover the inner layer. Tie the suture to the clipped free end on completion and trim the tails.

36 The Roux loop should be fixed as it passes through the transverse mesocolon to prevent herniation into the supra-colic compartment – do this by suturing the mesenteric and anti-mesenteric border of the bowel wall to the peritoneum of the transverse mesocolon using two interrupted absorbable sutures.

37 Place a non-suction closed tube at the site of the biliary anastomosis and close the abdomen in the standard fashion when all swabs and instruments have been accounted for.

? DIFFICULTY

1. If the bile duct is very small, it may be possible to enlarge the lumen available for the anastomosis by spatulating the anterior wall of the bile duct, using a short longitudinal incision, in order to minimize the risk of postoperative stricture formation.
2. In general terms, ducts smaller than 10 mm are most prone to postoperative complications and bile duct injuries where the first or second order branches of the duct are involved are particularly troublesome.
3. Anastomosis and repair of small calibre ducts should be referred to a specialist HPB unit.

FURTHER READING AND REFERENCES

Ahmed K, Wang TT, Patel VM, et al. The role of single-incision laparoscopic surgery in abdominal and pelvic surgery: a systematic review. Surg Endosc Feb;25(2):378–96.

Al-Ghnaniem R, Benjamin IS, Patel AG. Meta-analysis suggests antibiotic prophylaxis is not warranted in low-risk patients undergoing laparoscopic cholecystectomy. Br J Surg Mar 2003;90(3):365–6.

Attili AF, De Santis A, Capri R, et al. The natural history of gallstones: the GREPCO experience. The GREPCO Group. Hepatology Mar 1995;21 (3):655–60.

Blumgart L. Surgery of the Liver, Biliary Tract and Pancreas. 4th ed. New York: Elsevier; 2006.

Garden OJ. Hepatobiliary and Pancreatic Surgery: A Companion to Specialist Surgical Practice. 4th ed. Edinburgh: Elsevier; 2009.

Gossage JA, Forshaw MJ. Prevalence and outcome of litigation claims in England after laparoscopic cholecystectomy. Int J Clin Pract Dec;64 (13):1832–5.

Gurusamy K, Samraj K, Gluud C, et al. Meta-analysis of randomized controlled trials on the safety and effectiveness of early versus delayed laparoscopic cholecystectomy for acute cholecystitis. Br J Surg Feb;97 (2):141–50.

Gurusamy KS, Samraj K. Primary closure versus T-tube drainage after open common bile duct exploration. Cochrane Database Syst Rev 2007;(1): CD005640.

Gurusamy KS, Samraj K, Fusai G, Davidson BR. Early versus delayed laparoscopic cholecystectomy for biliary colic. Cochrane Database Syst Rev 2008;(4):CD007196.

Gurusamy KS, Samraj K, Mullerat P, Davidson BR. Routine abdominal drainage for uncomplicated laparoscopic cholecystectomy. Cochrane Database Syst Rev 2007;(4):CD006004.

Halldestam I, Enell EL, Kullman E, Borch K. Development of symptoms and complications in individuals with asymptomatic gallstones. Br J Surg Jun 2004;91(6):734–8.

Hugh TB. New strategies to prevent laparoscopic bile duct injury–surgeons can learn from pilots. Surgery Nov 2002;132(5):826–35.

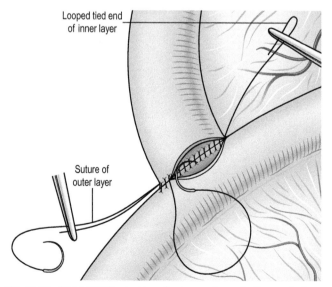

Looped tied end of inner layer

Suture of outer layer

Fig. 15.21 For a continuous two-layer anastomosis, the posterior suture line of the outer layer is positioned first and the suture locked to allow completion of the continuous inner layer (posterior then anterior). The anastomosis is then completed by constructing the outer anterior layer.

Macafee DA, Humes DJ, Bouliotis G, Beckingham IJ, Whynes DK, Lobo DN. Prospective randomized trial using cost-utility analysis of early versus delayed laparoscopic cholecystectomy for acute gallbladder disease. Br J Surg Sep 2009;96(9):1031–40.

Marks J, Tacchino R, Roberts K, et al. Prospective randomized controlled trial of traditional laparoscopic cholecystectomy versus single-incision laparoscopic cholecystectomy: report of preliminary data. Am J Surg 2011;201(3):369–72; discussion 372–3.

Peng WK, Sheikh Z, Nixon SJ, Paterson-Brown S. Role of laparoscopic cholecystectomy in the early management of acute gallbladder disease. Br J Surg May 2005;92(5):586–91.

Perry KA, Myers JA, Deziel DJ. Laparoscopic ultrasound as the primary method for bile duct imaging during cholecystectomy. Surg Endosc Jan 2008;22(1):208–13.

Rai SS, Grubnik VV, Kovalchuk OL, Grubnik OV. Comparison of long-term results of laparoscopic and endoscopic exploration of common bile duct. J Minim Access Surg Mar 2006;2(1):16–22.

Strasberg SM. Laparoscopic biliary surgery. Gastroenterol Clin North Am Mar 1999;28(1):117–32, vii.

Strasberg SM. Avoidance of biliary injury during laparoscopic cholecystectomy. J Hepatobiliary Pancreat Surg 2002;9(5):543–7.

Strasberg SM. Error traps and vasculo-biliary injury in laparoscopic and open cholecystectomy. J Hepatobiliary Pancreat Surg 2008;15(3): 284–292.

Strasberg SM, Eagon CJ, Drebin JA. The "hidden cystic duct" syndrome and the infundibular technique of laparoscopic cholecystectomy–the danger of the false infundibulum. J Am Coll Surg Dec 2000;191(6): 661–667.

Strasberg SM, Helton WS. An analytical review of vasculobiliary injury in laparoscopic and open cholecystectomy. HPB (Oxford) Jan;13(1): 1–14.

Way LW, Stewart L, Gantert W, et al. Causes and prevention of laparoscopic bile duct injuries: analysis of 252 cases from a human factors and cognitive psychology perspective. Ann Surg Apr 2003;237(4): 460–469.

Wilson RG, Macintyre IM, Nixon SJ, et al. Laparoscopic cholecystectomy as a safe and effective treatment for severe acute cholecystitis. BMJ Aug 15 1992;305(6850):394–6.

Pancreas

S.H. Rahman, O. Damrah

CONTENTS

INTRODUCTION

1 Operations on the pancreas are some of the most challenging in abdominal surgery for the following reasons:
- The retroperitoneal position of the pancreas renders it relatively inaccessible: the neck, body and tail lie behind the lesser sac while the head is obscured by the greater omentum and transverse colon. Exposure of the pancreas therefore requires a good deal of mobilization.
- The pancreas is intimately related to major blood vessels, notably the splenic and superior mesenteric veins, which unite to form the portal vein behind its neck. Adherence to the superior mesenteric vessels can make for a difficult dissection in inflammatory or neoplastic disease. The pancreas has a rich arterial supply: the head receives blood from the pancreaticoduodenal arcades and the body and tail from the splenic artery. Its venous drainage to the portal system is by a number of quite large, but thin-walled veins.
- Shared blood supply and close anatomical relationships necessitate the routine removal of adjacent organs as part of a pancreatic resection: thus the spleen is generally included in a distal pancreatectomy. More importantly, the duodenum and lower bile duct are excised during Whipple's procedure, necessitating a complex biliary reconstruction.
- Resection of the head of the pancreas is followed by anastomosis between the pancreatic stump (a solid organ) and a hollow tube (generally the jejunum). If this anastomosis leaks, powerful digestive enzymes are liberated in active form and can cause severe tissue destruction.
- Acute and chronic pancreatitis are amongst the most difficult inflammatory conditions to manage anywhere in the body. Likewise, pancreatic cancer is often advanced at diagnosis and may require an extensive resection.

- Diseases of the head of pancreas commonly present with obstructive jaundice which leads to impaired function of many of the body's systems, notably the kidneys, reticuloendothelial system and coagulation pathways, as well as the liver itself. Thus special precautions are required when undertaking major procedures on such patients.

▶ KEY POINT Expertise

- It follows that you should undertake pancreatic operations only after adequate training in the field and decidedly not if you are inexperienced.

2 Pancreatic imaging has dramatically improved over the last two decades with the routine use of ultrasonography, spiral computed tomography (CT), endoscopic retrograde cholangiopancreatography (ERCP), endoscopic ultrasound, percutaneous transhepatic cholangiography (PTC) and magnetic resonance cholangiopancreatography (MRCP).[1]

Some form of vascular imaging is required prior to pancreatic surgery in order to determine operability and delineate vascular anomalies. Visceral angiography has to a large extent been superseded by CT and MR angiography.

3 Pancreatic endocrine tissue is scattered through the gland in islets described in 1869 by the Berlin physician and anatomist, Paul Langerhans (1847–1888), with a relative preponderance in the body and tail. A major pancreatic resection can impair both endocrine and exocrine function and may cause diabetes and/or steatorrhoea. It is therefore good practice to measure pancreatic function before and after operation, particularly in chronic pancreatitis where there may be pre-existing insufficiency.

4 Pancreatic operations should be covered by appropriate broad-spectrum antibiotics such as a cephalosporin.

EXPLORATION OF THE PANCREAS

Access

1 Examination of the pancreas is usually performed as part of a general abdominal exploration.

2 If examination of the whole pancreas is the major purpose of the operation, select either a bilateral subcostal incision or a curved transverse incision midway between umbilicus and xiphoid and convex upwards.

3 Adequate inspection and palpation of the whole pancreas requires both mobilization of the duodenum and entry into the lesser sac.

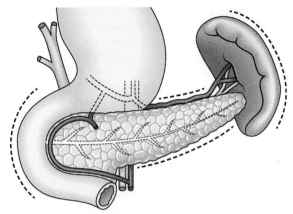

Fig. 16.1 Exposure of the pancreas. The lines of peritoneal incision are shown. The head of the pancreas and uncinate lobe are supplied by the superior and inferior pancreaticoduodenal arteries and the body and tail by the splenic artery.

Assess

1 Mobilize the duodenal loop and pancreatic head by Kocher's manoeuvre (Fig. 16.1). Gently clear the omentum from the anterior aspect of the head of pancreas, which can now be directly inspected and palpated between finger and thumb.

2 Expose the body and tail of the pancreas through the lesser sac, which can be entered through the greater or lesser omentum. Separate the congenital adhesions between the stomach and the pancreas. If necessary, divide the peritoneum along the superior border of the pancreas, so that you can insinuate a finger beneath the gland.

3 The inferior border of the pancreas can also be mobilized by dividing the overlying peritoneum; take care not to injure the superior or inferior mesenteric veins. Trace the middle colic vein downwards to find the superior mesenteric vein.

4 Lying at the splenic hilum, the tail of pancreas is the least accessible part of the gland. It can usually be approached by dividing the greater omentum and retracting the stomach upwards. You may need to divide several short gastric arteries and the attachments of the splenic flexure of the colon from the spleen. If necessary, be willing to divide the peritoneum lateral to the spleen and lift the spleen and tail of pancreas forwards into the wound.

5 Learn to recognize the firm, nodular consistency of normal pancreas by palpating the gland during all upper abdominal operations. You should then be able to differentiate the hard sclerotic gland of chronic pancreatitis or a localized tumour. The pancreatic duct is not palpable unless it is dilated.

6 If you feel a mass in the region of the ampulla, it may assist diagnosis to open the duodenum and directly visualize the pancreatic papilla. Confirm suspected carcinoma at this site by removing a suitable biopsy for immediate frozen-section histology, if endoscopic biopsy has not already provided the diagnosis.

▶ KEY POINTS Access to the pancreas

■ You cannot adequately examine the pancreas without full (Kocher's) mobilization of the duodenum along with exploration of the lesser sac.

■ Mobilize the lateral attachments of the spleen if necessary, to facilitate examination of the pancreatic tail.
■ You may also need to divide the peritoneum along the upper and lower borders of the pancreas.

REFERENCES

1. Fayad LM, Kowalski T, Mitchell DG. MR cholangiography: evaluation of common pancreatic diseases. Radiol Clin North Am 2003; 41:97–114.

PANCREATIC BIOPSY

Appraise

1 No method of biopsying the pancreas is devoid of risk, yet a positive tissue diagnosis is particularly important for the proper management of suspected malignant disease.

2 Cancer in the head of the pancreas usually obstructs the pancreatic duct, leading to chronic pancreatitis in the upstream gland. At operation it can be difficult or even impossible to distinguish the induration of obstructive pancreatopathy from that of malignant infiltration, which may lead to sampling error. Likewise, on pancreatic imaging there is often no sharp distinction between tumour and adjacent pancreatitis.

3 Percutaneous biopsy of the pancreas can be carried out under ultrasound or CT scan guidance by directly inserting a fine needle for cytology, or wider-bore needle for histology, into the mass. In expert hands this is quite a sensitive technique, although more than one pass of the needle may be required to obtain a positive answer. Although percutaneous biopsy of the pancreas is a relatively safe and sensitive technique, as a rule limit it to patients with unresectable tumours or those patients in whom operative treatment is not indicated.[1]

4 At ERCP pure pancreatic juice may be obtained or brushings can be taken from strictures of the bile duct or pancreatic duct. Cytological examination of this material may reveal malignant cells. When pancreatic cancer invades the duodenum, it can be directly biopsied through the endoscope. Endoscopic ultrasound has been increasingly used to guide biopsy of pancreatic lesions, as well as providing valuble information about relationship to major vascular structures.[2]

5 At laparotomy the safest method of confirming the diagnosis of cancer is to sample a site of possible metastasis, usually a liver nodule, peritoneal deposit or lymph node adjacent to the pancreas (see Chapter 17 for the technique of liver biopsy). If there are no obvious metastases, do not hesitate to biopsy the primary pancreatic tumour itself.

6 The usual indication for pancreatic biopsy is to confirm carcinoma in a patient whose tumour is deemed irresectable, since in a resectable case the specimen itself provides ample histological material. Because of the risk of sampling error you must obtain pathological confirmation of carcinoma before closing the abdomen, and this need may govern the choice between fine-needle aspiration biopsy and the use of a Tru-cut needle. In many

hospitals it is easier to obtain urgent frozen-section histology, as from a Tru-cut specimen, than an urgent cytological opinion.

Action

1 Using a fine (18–20G) needle and a 20-ml syringe, aspirate the site of the lesion. Apply strong suction while advancing and withdrawing the needle within the lesion, then release the suction and remove the needle and syringe. Eject the material in the needle track on to a glass slide and make a smear for cytological examination.

2 If the surface of the pancreas is diseased, perform a 'shave' biopsy with a scalpel. Remember the possibility that an inflammatory 'halo' may surround the actual neoplastic tissue.

3 You can obtain a core of tissue for histological examination using a Tru-cut needle. If the lesion is in the head of the pancreas you can approach it transduodenally, avoiding the risk of pancreatic fistulae, or insert the needle directly into the pancreas.

4 If the above techniques are inadequate and a biopsy is essential, incise the gland directly over the lesion and obtain a small piece of tissue. However, it may be better to carry out a formal partial pancreatectomy under these circumstances.

5 The complications of biopsy include acute pancreatitis and pancreatic fistula. If pancreatic juice escapes from the site of incision or the needle puncture, consider pancreatectomy or Roux-en-Y drainage of this area.

REFERENCES

1. Ihse I, Axelson J, Dawiskiba S, et al. Pancreatic biopsy: why? when? how? World J Surg 1999;23:896–900.
2. Varadarajulu S, Eloubeidi MA. The role of endoscopic ultrasonography in the evaluation of pancreatico-biliary cancer. Surg Clin North Am 2010;90(2):251–63.

LAPAROTOMY FOR NECROTIZING PANCREATITIS

Appraise

1 There is absolutely no role for diagnostic laparotomy in patients with acute pancreatitis, given the widespread availability of abdominal CT. Despite this, you may be confronted occasionally by acute pancreatitis during a laparotomy for other suspected pathologies such as small-bowel infarction and leaking abdominal aneurysm.

2 Avoid laparotomy in the first week of acute pancreatitis, as it is too early for a safe, effective debridement and formal resection carries a formidable mortality rate. Laparotomy can often be delayed for several weeks to allow the necrotic tissue to mature, and the vast majority of infective collections can be managed by aggressive radiological drainage. Patients with proven severe gallstone pancreatitis may, however, benefit from early ERCP and stone extraction if ductal calculi are suspected, as this may lower both morbidity and mortality.[1]

3 Laparotomy and debridement for patients with established necrotizing pancreatitis is now reserved primarily for those with infected necrosis.[2] Determine the presence of infection

preoperatively by percutaneous radiological fine-needle aspiration. For necrosis confined predominantly to the left of the neck of pancreas, open necrosectomy has almost completely been superseded by aggressive radiological drainage and video assisted percutaneous necrosectomy in specialist units. Percutaneous radiological drains are inserted under local anaesthetic in the plane between the spleen and splenic flexure of the colon. The tract is subsequently dilated to permit passage of a nephroresectoscope. The necrotic tissue can then be resected using the endoscope and irrigation catheters inserted. Initial publications suggest a reduction in mortality and morbidity with this minimally invasive approach.[3]

Other complications of acute pancreatitis such as pseudocysts, bleeding and abscesses are now often managed radiologically, with surgery reserved for complications not amenable to radiological intervention or in patients with infective necrosis not amenable to percutaneous techniques. Because of the benefits of multidisciplinary care of patients with severe acute pancreatitis, especially access to experienced interventional radiology, such patients should, wherever possible, be cared for in specialist units.

4 If you detect gallstones it is wise to carry out a cholecystectomy after the patient has recovered from pancreatitis but before discharge so as to prevent another acute attack (see Chapter 15). Prior to operation, have the bile duct imaged using either MRCP or ERCP to avoid leaving occult ductal calculi.

Prepare

1 On admission, or following a diagnostic laparotomy, it is helpful to assess the severity of acute pancreatitis using the Ranson or Imrie scoring systems and/or serial measurements of C-reactive protein and white cell count.

2 Hypovolaemia is a consistent feature of acute pancreatitis and may be profound. Make sure that fluid depletion has been fully corrected by intravenous administration of colloid and crystalloid solutions before embarking on the operation. Monitor central venous pressure and urine output during resuscitation in the elderly or those with severe fluid loss.

3 Look for and treat early complications such as hypoxaemia, hypocalcaemia and incipient renal failure. Give prophylactic broad-spectrum antibiotics.

Access

1 If the cause of peritonitis is uncertain, the patient is likely to have a midline incision performed for abdominal exploration. If necessary, extend the incision upwards to permit examination of the biliary apparatus and pancreas.

2 When operating for confirmed pancreatitis, use a transverse incision.

Assess

1 Bloodstained free fluid is usually present in the abdominal cavity in acute pancreatitis. Whitish plaques of fat necrosis are visible on serosal surfaces, especially in the region of the pancreas.

2 Lift up the greater omentum and transverse colon. There is oedema and blackish discoloration of the retroperitoneal tissues.

The pancreas itself is swollen and may be haemorrhagic or even necrotic.

3 Examine the gallbladder and, if possible, the bile duct to determine if these organs are diseased. A more thorough examination is required if the patient has obstructive jaundice.

4 In a case of infected pancreatic necrosis, extensively explore the retroperitoneal tissues to carry out a full assessment.

Action

At laparotomy

1 Once you have made the diagnosis, do nothing unless there is a definite indication. Attempts at debridement of the pancreas at this stage can be disastrous. Formal exploration of the pancreas is usually unnecessary to obtain a diagnosis and may be meddlesome.

2 The management of coincidental gallstones is controversial, so be prepared to seek senior advice. In oedematous (mild) pancreatitis it is correct to carry out cholecystectomy with operative cholangiography and proceed to exploration of the duct and even transduodenal sphincteroplasty, if necessary (see Chapter 15). In haemorrhagic, severe pancreatitis, extensive ductal exploration and duodenotomy are best avoided. If ductal stones are present, remove them gently if possible and leave a T-tube to drain the duct.

3 It is unusual to encounter loculated fluid or pus during the first week of an attack of acute pancreatitis, but drain any such collection to the exterior.

4 Wound dehiscence is common following laparotomy for acute pancreatitis. Take extra care in closing the linea alba or rectus sheath and consider inserting tension sutures.

For infected pancreatic necrosis

1 Enter the lesser sac by dividing the greater omentum. In severe pancreatitis this will expose a large cavity containing pus and necrotic debris. Although the pancreas itself can undergo haemorrhagic infarction in a severe case of pancreatitis, more often the gland is viable and there is peripancreatic necrosis affecting the retroperitoneal fat.

2 Digitally explore the necrotic cavity and remove all dead tissue. The cavity may ramify extensively: be prepared to explore upwards to the diaphragm, downwards behind the left or right colon to the pelvis, backwards to the perirenal areas and forwards into the transverse mesocolon and the root of the small bowel mesentery. Where possible, avoid sharp dissection and use your fingers to separate the solid necrotic material. A blunt-tipped sucker, used gently, provides a good method of atraumatic dissection. Send samples of fluid and necrotic material for bacteriological examination. The main risk is of bleeding, so be gentle but thorough.

3 Check the viability of the small and large intestine. The right colon in particular can become ischaemic following thrombosis of its blood supply. In these circumstances proceed to right hemicolectomy, but do not restore intestinal continuity. Bring out the terminal ileum as an end ileostomy (Chapter 11) and the transverse or descending colon as a mucous fistula, using separate trephine incisions for each stoma. Placement of a gastrostomy

avoids long-term nasogastric intubation and insertion of a jejunostomy tube aids early enteric feeding.[4]

4 Irrigate the retroperitoneal cavity thoroughly with warm saline and secure haemostasis. You must now choose between closing the abdomen with generous drainage and leaving it open as a 'laparostomy'. Each technique has its advocates. The closed technique is easier to manage with regard to nursing care, but up to one-third of patients require one or more repeat laparotomies for further debridement. The open technique allows inspection of the abdominal contents on a daily basis with ready drainage of further collections, but at the expense of a higher incidence of postoperative bleeding and intestinal fistula. For this reason laparostomy should be reserved for the most severe cases and the closed drainage technique used when necrosis is less extensive.

5 In the *closed* technique it is vital to ensure adequate drainage of the retroperitoneal cavity and lesser sac. Place four wide-bore drains, siting two as far posteriorly as possible, one on each side. If the necrotizing process is limited to the lesser sac, it is helpful to 'compartmentalize' the abdomen by suturing the greater omentum to the peritoneum along the lower border of the transverse incision. Postoperatively, the lesser sac can then be irrigated in isolation from the remaining abdominal viscera. Take care closing the abdomen because of the risk of subsequent wound dehiscence. Insert deep tension sutures in severe cases.

6 In the *open* technique make no attempt to suture the abdominal wall. One or two drains may be placed in the depths of the cavity and brought out through stab incisions. Cover the exposed viscera with several packs wrung out in saline. Consider placing a large piece of adherent plastic sheeting over the entire wound to prevent leakage of fluid. Surprisingly, evisceration is seldom a problem.

Aftercare

1 Continue standard supportive measures for acute pancreatitis, with intravenous fluids and nasogastric suction as required. Patients with a severe attack will require total parenteral nutrition. Antibiotic therapy is needed to manage septic complications, the choice of agent being tailored to the organism cultured. Recent evidence suggests that, in cases of severe pancreatitis, early prophylactic antibiotics decrease the incidence of septic complications and there may be a corresponding decrease in mortality rate.[5]

2 All patients with severe acute pancreatitis should be managed in an intensive therapy unit. Ultrasound and CT scans may be used to detect the development of complications, notably pseudocyst, bleeding and infected pancreatic necrosis.

3 Following a closed drainage procedure for necrotizing pancreatitis, institute saline lavage down two of the four drains, using the other two for egress of the fluid. Commence lavage with warm isotonic fluid either at the end of the operation or after overnight recovery, allowing the peritoneum to 'seal'. Infuse between 50 and 200 ml/hour, depending upon the size of the cavity and the degree of contamination. Continue lavage at least until the effluent becomes clean. Monitor the serum albumin level, because prolonged lavage will exacerbate protein depletion. Use clinical judgement and weekly CT scans to assess progress and the necessity or otherwise for repeat laparotomy and debridement.

4 Following laparostomy, inspect the abdominal cavity. Nearly all these patients will require mechanical ventilation in an intensive therapy unit, and the packs can usually be changed in this setting under intravenous sedation without the need to take the patient back to the operating theatre. Remove the packs and examine the abdominal viscera. Gently insinuate your hand into the cavity, drain any pus and tease out any further necrotic tissue. Wash out the cavity and place fresh packs. If the patient's condition improves, consider secondary closure of the abdominal wall at a later date.

> **KEY POINTS** Surgical intervention in acute pancreatitis

- Patients with severe pancreatitis require combined specialist care by surgeons and intensivists.
- In most cases of sterile necrosis, operation is not required but you must be mindful of other complications occurring, such as bowel infarction or gastrointestinal haemorrhage, that need urgent surgical attention.

Complications

1 Infected pancreatic necrosis is a difficult and dangerous condition. The mortality rate is at least 20–30% in most published series. A successful outcome requires good surgical and nursing care which often needs to be continued for several weeks. Supportive measures include intravenous fluids, parenteral nutrition and antibiotics as required.

2 There are many potential complications, and their management can be summarized as follows:
- *Respiratory failure/adult respiratory distress syndrome (ARDS)*. Continue assisted respiration under the supervision of an experienced anaesthetist, and consider tracheostomy after 10–14 days of endotracheal intubation (see Chapter 2).
- *Renal failure*. Haemofiltration or haemodialysis is required unless the infracolic compartment of the abdomen can be used for peritoneal dialysis. Dopamine and dobutamine may be used to improve renal blood flow.
- *Myocardial failure*. Pressor support may be required to maintain an adequate blood pressure and peripheral circulation.
- *Continuing sepsis*. This is the single most important factor underlying multiple organ failure. Persistent high fever and leucocytosis indicate active infection. Remember the possibility of septicaemia from a contaminated central venous line: obtain blood cultures and consider changing the line. Repeat the chest X-ray to look for a focus of infection. Perform ultrasound, CT or isotope scans to image the abdominal cavity, and consider whether percutaneous drainage or repeat laparotomy is needed to deal with further collections.
- *Intestinal failure*. Prolonged ileus is common in patients with abdominal sepsis, especially those on a ventilator. Remember the possibility of colonic or small-bowel ischaemia, which may require repeat laparotomy. Very occasionally prolonged duodenal ileus necessitates a gastroenterostomy. These patients are prone to peptic stress ulceration: institute prophylaxis with topical agents such as sucralfate or intravenously with H2-receptor antagonists or proton-pump inhibitors.

- *Haemorrhage*. Bleeding follows arterial or venous erosion in the wall of the infected cavity and blood may escape into the gut, into the abdominal cavity or via the drains. Resuscitate the patient and, if there is gastrointestinal haemorrhage, consider endoscopy to look for erosive gastritis (see Chapter 10). If there is evidence of intra-abdominal bleeding the patient should have a CT scan with vascular reconstruction. In most instances this reveals the site of bleeding and identifies the feeding vessel. This can then be treated by visceral angiography and transcatheter embolization. If radiology is unsuccessful then a laparotomy may be required, with suture of the bleeding vessel and occasionally formal resection. Such operative procedures carry a high morbidity and mortality.
- *Pancreatic fistula*. Survivors may develop a pancreatic fistula from the abscess cavity along a drain track to the skin. Most of these fistulas heal spontaneously with the passage of time and can simply be managed in the interim by collection into a stoma bag. Manage an intestinal fistula or mixed fistula along standard lines (see Chapter 11).

REFERENCES

1. Fogel EL, Sherman S. Acute biliary pancreatitis: when should the endoscopist intervene. Gastroenterology 2003;125:229–35.
2. Werner J, Uhl W, Hartwig W, et al. Modern phase-specific management of acute pancreatitis. Dig Dis 2003;21:38–45.
3. Carter CR, McKay CJ, Imrie CW. Percutaneous necrosectomy and sinus tract endoscopy in the management of infected pancreatic necrosis: an initial experience. Ann Surg 2000;232:175–80.
4. Al-Omran M, Groof A, Wilke D. Enteral versus parenteral nutrition for acute pancreatitis. Cochrane Database Syst Rev 2003;(1): CD002837.
5. Bassi C, Larvin M, Villatoro E. Antibiotic therapy for prophylaxis against infection of pancreatic necrosis in acute pancreatitis. Cochrane Database Syst Rev 2003;(4): CD002941.

DRAINAGE OF PANCREATIC CYSTS

Appraise

1 True cysts are congenital or neoplastic and are rare. Cysts complicating acute or chronic pancreatitis and pancreatic trauma are 'false' pseudocysts, in that they have no epithelial lining. Both types are best diagnosed by ultrasound and CT scanning of the upper abdomen.

2 Fluid collections around the pancreas are common following acute pancreatitis, but most resolve spontaneously. Drainage is required for an expanding mass, which often causes pain, for vomiting, jaundice or for a mass that fails to resolve or becomes infected. Within 4–5 weeks of the acute attack, the cyst wall is unlikely to be sufficiently mature to take sutures, and external drainage is required. Thereafter, internal drainage becomes feasible, either cystgastrostomy or cystjejunostomy Roux-en-Y. Reserve cystgastrostomy for moderate-sized cysts that are closely applied to the back of the stomach on imaging. Endoscopic and laparoscopic techniques are increasingly employed to avoid open operation for internal cyst drainage.

3 Percutaneous aspiration of pancreatic pseudocysts is becoming increasingly popular. The procedure is carried out under ultrasound or CT control. A pigtail catheter can be inserted for external drainage, or a percutaneous transgastric approach can be used to position a stent in the cystgastrostomy position.[1] Percutaneous

needle drainage is suitable for small cysts discovered in the early weeks after an attack of acute pancreatitis; surgical drainage is more appropriate for large, mature or recurrent cysts and for those that communicate with the pancreatic duct.

4 Sometimes an encysted collection of blood and/or pancreatic fluid may follow blunt abdominal trauma. Traumatic cysts are prone to complications and require early drainage, usually to the exterior.

5 Pseudocysts developing in association with chronic pancreatitis are generally contained within the pancreatic capsule and frequently communicate with the main ductal system. They may develop insidiously with gradual expansion of the pancreas, sometimes at multiple sites, or rapidly after an attack of acute-on-chronic pancreatitis, in which case they contain necrotic material. Endoscopic retrograde pancreatography is a useful investigation as it allows drainage of the dilated pancreatic duct, but may, potentially, introduce infection into the cyst cavity: give prophylactic antibiotic cover. Smaller cysts can be resected together with diseased pancreas or drained into the duct and thence to a Roux loop of jejunum. Treat larger cysts by cystenterostomy unless a preoperative angiogram shows an arterial pseudoaneurysm in the wall, in which case resection may be safer.

6 Never assume that a cystic mass in or adjacent to the pancreas is an inflammatory pseudocyst unless there is clear evidence of acute pancreatitis (for example recent pain and hyperamylasaemia) or a history and imaging consistent with chronic pancreatitis. Cystic neoplasms include serous and mucinous cystadenoma, mucinous cystadenocarcinoma and cystic endocrine tumour. Always obtain a biopsy of the cyst wall at operation, and arrange frozen-section examination if there is any suspicion of neoplasia.[2] Resect neoplastic cysts if possible.

7 Endoscopic internal drainage of a pseudocyst under endoscopic ultrasound guidance is gaining in popularity. With a diathermy wire passed down the operating channel of an endoscope, the endoscopist creates an opening from the cyst into the stomach or duodenum and usually passes several stents to maintain patency.[3] It is even possible to drain a communicating pseudocyst into the duct via a nasopancreatic tube or short pancreatic stent passed per endoscope.

Prepare

1 In patients with a chronic pseudocyst, do not embark on an operation for the cyst without fully investigating the pancreas.

2 Bleeding can be a problem during operations for pseudocyst, so ensure that cross-matched blood is available beforehand.

> **KEY POINTS** Drainage of pseudocysts

- The techniques of percutaneous or endoscopic cystgastrostomy require the posterior wall of the stomach to be adherent to the pseudocyst. This is often not the case in pseudocysts associated with chronic pancreatitis where the lesser sac is patent.
- Furthermore, patients with chronic pancreatitis often have varices around the stomach, adding further hazard to this technique.

Assess

1 After an acute attack of pancreatitis or pancreatic trauma an encysted collection of fluid may be entered on approaching the pancreas. This type of collection is usually best drained to the exterior. The resultant pancreatic fistula does not cause skin excoriation, since the pancreatic enzymes are not activated, and it will nearly always close spontaneously. If a large cyst is palpable within the lesser sac, try to determine whether the posterior wall of the stomach is adherent to the front of the cyst, in which case cystgastrostomy may be appropriate. If not, internal drainage into a Roux loop of jejunum is a satisfactory method of dealing with a mature cyst.

2 During laparotomy for chronic pancreatitis plan your approach according to the operative findings, supplemented by a knowledge of pancreatic ductal anatomy obtained from ERCP or MRCP. A cyst in the head of the pancreas can sometimes be marsupialized into the duodenum. Elsewhere in the gland, cystjejunostomy Roux-en-Y is the best option unless complete resection can be safely achieved.

3 Try and create a good-sized fistula between the cyst and the viscus chosen for internal drainage.

Action

The vast majority of these techniques are peformed laparoscopically, although the exact detail of the laparoscopic approach is beyond the scope of this chapter. Nonetheless, the technique of drainage is the same and shall thus be described.

Cystgastrostomy (Fig. 16.2)

1 This is only indicated for effusions into the lesser sac that have been present for long enough to have developed a fibrous wall. The stoma will probably close once the cavity has collapsed following drainage.

2 After packing off the stomach, make a longitudinal incision through the anterior gastric wall fairly close to the greater curvature and opposite the incisura angularis. Suck out the gastric contents.

3 Now incise the posterior gastric wall for a short distance opposite the anterior gastrotomy. If the cyst is difficult to palpate, a 19

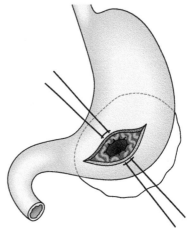

Fig. 16.2 Pancreatic cystgastrostomy. The anterior wall of the stomach is held open by stay sutures. A collection of pancreatic fluid in the lesser sac ('pseudocyst') is drained into the stomach through a posterior gastrostomy.

Gauge needle on a 10-ml syringe is often used to localize the cyst. Deepen the incision and enter the cyst, obtaining samples of the fluid for culture and chemical analysis. Evacuate the contents of the cyst and gently break down any loculi with your finger.

4 Insert a running polyglactin 910 (Vicryl) suture round the margins of the posterior gastrotomy, ensuring a stoma at least 4 cm in diameter. Close the anterior gastrotomy in two layers and close the abdomen with drainage.

Cystduodenostomy

1 Reserve this procedure for a small cyst in the head of pancreas close to the duodenal loop.

2 Make a longitudinal duodenotomy opposite the cyst. Insert a needle into the cyst: aspiration of bile warns you that the bile duct is nearby and you should not proceed.

3 If the aspirate is clear, leave the needle in place and incise the duodenal wall to enter the cyst. Suture the margins of the opening as above. Close the duodenum in two layers, taking care not to narrow its lumen. Close the abdomen with drainage.

Cystjejunostomy (Fig.16.3)

1 This technique is applicable to all types of cyst with walls thick enough for suturing. It is the most likely method to obtain dependent drainage and avoid the potential problem of food debris contaminating the pseudocyst cavity.

2 Mobilize the pancreas. Now incise the anterior wall of the cyst, sample and drain its contents and explore its recesses for any obvious ductal communication.

3 Create a Roux loop of jejunum (Chapter 11) and close the end. Approximate the upper end of the Roux loop to the front of the cyst without tension. Create a generous side-to-side anastomosis between the opening into the cyst and a longitudinal jejunotomy. Use one or two layers of suture according to the thickness of the cyst wall, but use polyglactin 910 (Vicryl) for the inner layer.

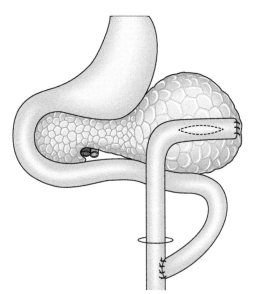

Fig. 16.3 Pancreatic cystjejunostomy. A retrocolic Roux loop of jejunum has been anastomosed to a large cyst within the tail of pancreas.

4 Restore intestinal continuity by jejunojejunostomy at the base of the Roux loop. Drain the abdomen through a stab incision as above.

> ### KEY POINT Drainage versus resection of pseudocysts

- The decision to drain or resect a chronic pseudocyst will depend on several factors: its position in the gland, the general condition of the patient, the patient's endocrine and exocrine function, the presence or absence of varices, the extent of disease in the underlying pancreatic tissue and the degree of suspicion of neoplasia.

Complications

1 Decompression of a pseudocyst into the gut may be followed by haemorrhage if there was a pre-existing pseudo-aneurysm and angiography, whether derived from CT, MRI or visceral angiography, should always be undertaken before drainage of a chronic cyst. If bleeding occurs the patient requires a CT scan, with an emphasis on the arterial phase, to determine the site of origin, proceeding to an angiogram and transcatheter embolization. If this fails, re-operation is required, sometimes with formal resection.

2 Pancreatic fistula is seldom troublesome, because the enzyme content of pancreatic juice is low in patients with chronic pancreatitis. Treat a gastric or intestinal fistula along standard lines.

REFERENCES

1. Vidyarthi G, Steinberg SE. Endoscopic management of pancreatic pseudocysts. Surg Clin North Am 2001;81:405–10.
2. Spinelli KS, Fromwiller TE, Daniel RA, et al. Cystic pancreatic neoplasms: observe or operate. Ann Surg 2004;239:651–9.
3. Beckingham IJ, Krige JE, Bornman PC, et al. Long term outcome of endoscopic drainage of pancreatic pseudocysts. Am J Gastroenterol 1999;94:71–4.

DRAINAGE OF THE PANCREATIC DUCT

Appraise

1 Ductal drainage is preferable to resection for the relief of pain in chronic pancreatitis, since it preserves the remaining functioning tissue. However, only an anastomosis between the pancreatic duct and adjacent viscus that is several millimetres in diameter is likely to remain patent. Therefore do not ordinarily undertake a drainage operation unless the duct is two to three times its normal diameter.

2 The operation of choice is longitudinal pancreaticojejunostomy, which creates a long side-to-side anastomosis between the incised duct and a Roux loop of jejunum. Often this may be combined with a 'coring' out of the head of the pancreas, a so-called 'Frey modification'. An anastomosis between the amputated body of pancreas and a Roux loop is less likely to stay open unless the duct is grossly dilated at the site of transection, in which case it should probably be opened up in the proximal gland. Sometimes it is reasonable to combine conservative distal resection with a limited longitudinal pancreaticojejunostomy.

3 Formerly popular for the treatment of chronic pancreatitis, sphincteroplasty has in fact little to offer. It is reasonable to consider biliary sphincteroplasty (Chapter 15), followed by a similar procedure to widen the orifice of the pancreatic duct, when there is moderate dilatation of the whole duct tapering to a stricture at its orifice, but this is an uncommon situation in chronic pancreatitis. Pancreatic sphincteroplasty may be indicated for patients with recurrent acute pancreatitis or chronic abdominal pain and stenosis in the terminal pancreatic duct. In pancreas divisum, accessory pancreatic sphincteroplasty is sometimes helpful.

4 Drainage of an obstructed distended duct into the back of the stomach (pancreaticogastrostomy) is quite a simple technique that may bring worthwhile relief of pain from irresectable carcinoma of the head of pancreas.

5 Techniques for draining normal-calibre and dilated pancreatic ducts after proximal pancreatectomy (Whipple resection) are considered at the end of this chapter.

Prepare

1 Do not operate on patients with chronic pancreatitis unless you have some experience of this disease and are capable of carrying out pancreatectomy.

2 Ensure that appropriate preoperative imaging and pancreatic function tests have been undertaken.

3 Arrange for cross-matched blood to be available and give prophylactic antibiotics perioperatively.

Access

Operations for chronic pancreatitis require generous access to the upper abdomen. Excellent exposure is afforded by a transverse subcostal incision that divides both recti and is gently curved with an upward convexity.

Assess

1 Expose the pancreas carefully but completely and examine it thoroughly. Is the gland indurated throughout, or is the disease partly localized? Can you feel the pancreatic duct as a soft dilated tube in the body of the gland? Are there any associated cysts? If there is suspicion of carcinoma, obtain a biopsy.

2 Look for evidence of gallstones, which are quite commonly associated with chronic pancreatitis. The bile duct may be slightly dilated, with a thickened, opaque wall. Examine the stomach and duodenum for peptic ulcer disease. Exclude cirrhosis of the liver, portal hypertension and splenomegaly. Perform liver biopsy if the patient is an alcoholic.

> **KEY POINTS** Indications for drainage procedures in chronic pancreatitis
>
> ■ Although drainage procedures are the optimal operations in chronic pancreatitis because they can relieve pain without exacerbating functional insufficiency, they require a 'target' to drain, either a pseudocyst or a dilated duct.
> ■ Otherwise some form of resection is required, tailored to the site of maximal disease.

Action

Pancreatic sphincteroplasty

1 Expose the papilla by a transduodenal approach and carry out biliary sphincteroplasty.

2 Look for the orifice of the major pancreatic duct on the lower lip of the papilla. Magnifying spectacles may be helpful. Pass a soft umbilical catheter (4–6F) and obtain a retrograde pancreatogram if ERCP or MRCP were inadequate. If you cannot locate the orifice, ask the anaesthetist to give an intravenous injection of secretin (1 unit/kg) and look for the flow of pancreatic juice within 30–60 seconds.

3 Divide the common septum between the terminal portions of the bile duct and pancreatic duct for a distance of about 10 mm. Obtain a tiny biopsy if the septum appears scarred. Facilitate the septotomy by placing fine (5/0) sutures on either side of the proposed line of incision, tying them and dividing the septum between them, using straight iris scissors.

4 Suture the mucosa of the pancreatic duct to that of the bile duct using 5/0 polyglactin 910 (Vicryl) sutures.

5 A similar technique should be used for accessory sphincteroplasty, but here it is often necessary to give secretin to identify the tiny ductal orifice.

6 Close the duodenum and leave a drain in the subhepatic space as for biliary sphincteroplasty.

Longitudinal pancreaticojejunostomy (Fig. 16.4)

1 Expose the body, neck and part of the head of pancreas through the lesser sac. It is usually not necessary to mobilize the gland completely.

2 Incise the front of the pancreas between stay sutures at a convenient place in the body of the gland. If the duct is clearly dilated, make the incision in the long axis of the gland. If not, either attempt to localize the duct by aspiration, using a small needle and a 10-ml syringe, or make a small exploratory incision across the axis. Intra-operative ultrasound can be helpful in identifying

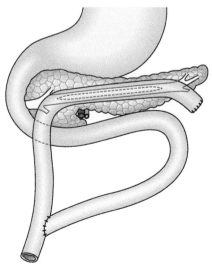

Fig. 16.4 Longitudinal pancreaticojejunostomy Roux-en-Y. The dilated duct is opened widely and a long side-to-side anastomosis is created.

an impalpable duct. If localizing the duct using an aspirating needle, it is possible to cut down along the plane of the needle to open up the duct.

3 On entering a dilated ductal system, aspirate the pale, greyish pancreatic juice. Extend the incision in each direction, using scalpel or pointed scissors, and under-run any major bleeding vessel. Ensure that the gastroduodenal artery is properly controlled where it is divided in the neck of the gland. Open the duct widely from head to tail. Remove all calculi and try to open any cysts into the main duct.

4 Select a Roux loop of jejunum and close its end. Bring the loop through a mesocolic window so that it lies comfortably along the entire pancreas. Insert interrupted Vicryl sutures to approximate the fibrotic 'capsule' of the pancreas and the seromuscular layers of the jejunum. Now make a long jejunotomy to match the incision in the pancreatic duct and place a running all-coats suture between the two, using 3/0 polyglactin 910 (Vicryl). The ductal lining is tough and takes sutures quite well. Finish with an anterior seromuscular layer.

5 Restore intestinal continuity by end-to-side jejunojejunostomy. Close the abdomen with drainage of the pancreas.

Lateral pancreaticojejunostomy (Fig. 16.5)

1 Reserve this procedure for draining a dilated duct in the neck or proximal body of pancreas after distal resection. It may be sensible to open up the duct at the site of transection by incising for a few centimetres through its anterior wall and the overlying pancreas.

2 Fashion a retrocolic Roux loop of jejunum as above and close the end. Make a small subterminal jejunotomy to match the diameter of the duct and insert an all-coats suture, using fine non-absorbable stitches. Tack the peripheral pancreatic substance to the seromuscular layer of jejunum with a second layer of similar sutures.

3 Restore intestinal continuity as usual.

Intubated pancreaticogastrostomy (Fig. 16.6)

1 Examine the body of pancreas for the tell-tale sensation of a dilated duct. Needling the duct or intra-operative ultrasound may be helpful.

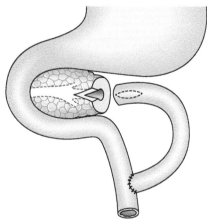

Fig. 16.5   Lateral pancreaticojejunostomy Roux-en-Y. Following distal pancreatectomy a dilated pancreatic duct is opened for a short distance and sutured to the Roux loop.

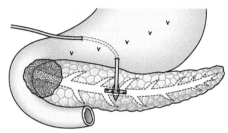

Fig. 16.6   Intubated pancreaticogastrostomy. In an attempt to relieve back pain from an irresectable carcinoma of the head of pancreas, the obstructed pancreatic duct is decompressed into the stomach. The small incisions in the back of the stomach and the front of the pancreas are approximated and the T-tube is brought to the exterior.

2 Make a short vertical incision across the body of pancreas and deepen this until you enter the duct. Insert a T-tube into the duct; suture the gland around the entry of the tube. Make tiny posterior and anterior gastrotomies several centimetres apart. Bring the tube through each wall of the stomach and thence by a stab incision to the exterior. Make sure there are two or three holes in the tube within its intragastric course, and tighten a purse-string suture around the anterior gastrotomy. By traction on the tube, draw the stomach down on to the front of the pancreas, and approximate the two organs with a few tacking sutures.

3 Postoperatively, the T-tube may drain the stomach in preference to the nasogastric tube, but it can usually be clamped with safety after flatus has been passed per rectum.

Complications

1 These are uncommon, but reactive haemorrhage and pancreatic fistula are theoretical risks, as after a cyst drainage procedure (see above).

2 Acute pancreatitis should not follow a sphincteroplasty unless the ductal orifice has been inadvertently occluded.

3 A transient rise in serum amylase following manipulation of the pancreas is of little importance.

LAPAROTOMY AND BYPASS FOR PANCREATIC CANCER

Appraise

1 Ductal adenocarcinoma of the pancreas is both common and difficult to treat. Its cause is largely unknown. Most tumours are irresectable by the time they are diagnosed, and this is particularly so for cancers of the body and tail of pancreas, where early symptoms are scarce and non-specific. When the tumour is within the head of pancreas, the patient may present with obstructive jaundice while the tumour is still relatively small and localized.

2 Some patients with cancer of the head of pancreas require laparotomy to confirm the diagnosis, determine the potential resectability of the tumour and allow a choice to be made between resection and bypass. Despite the scale of the operation required, carry out resection for potentially curable tumours in those of reasonable general health, since this policy offers the only chance of cure. Less aggressive cancers such as neuroendocrine tumour or

cholangiocarcinoma may be difficult or impossible to differentiate from pancreatic cancer on either preoperative or operative assessment, and the same can hold true for chronic pancreatitis.

3 Staging laparoscopy in combination with laparoscopic ultrasound may allow detection of peritoneal deposits, small liver metastases and even portal venous invasion, but the number of patients in whom this will add extra information to that obtained from conventional imaging is controversial. Some authors claim that laparoscopic examination excludes an extra 30% of patients from curative resection. Most series suggest that 14% of patients can be spared an unnecessary laparotomy,[1] and if one considers that laparoscopy may in fact provide the opportunity to institute palliative bypass then this technique of staging becomes attractive.

4 Most patients with cancer of the body or tail of pancreas do not require laparotomy because the tumour either metastasizes or encases the superior mesenteric vessels at an early stage and is therefore seldom resectable.[2] Moreover, jaundice and duodenal obstruction occur late, if at all. Thus optimal management comprises obtaining a tissue diagnosis by means of guided percutaneous needle biopsy, confirming the irresectability of the tumour by CT scan and considering non-operative measures such as radiotherapy and chemotherapy, especially for younger patients and those with troublesome back pain. However, if imaging leaves you in any doubt about the nature or resectability of the tumour, perform laparotomy.

5 Preoperative investigation of a patient with obstructive jaundice starts with liver function tests and ultrasound scan to exclude hepatocellular disease and confirm dilatation of the biliary tree consistent with a 'surgical' cause of obstruction. Ultrasound and CT scan may show gallstone disease, a pancreatic or peri-ampullary mass, nodal or hepatic metastases and major vascular involvement. PTC and ERCP are invaluable for showing the level and the nature of bile duct stricture, but one or other test will generally suffice. PTC gives better visualization of the proximal biliary tree, which is useful for a high stricture, whereas ERCP can provide an additional pancreatogram, which is useful to confirm pancreatic cancer or chronic pancreatitis. If combined with endoscopic ultrasound, this can visualize the adjacent vascular structures and aid in the assessment of operability.[3] Endoscopic-ultrasound-guided fine-needle aspiration can provide a cytological diagnosis without risking tumour seeding outside the pancreas. If preoperative jaundice is not deep and stenting not required, then non-invasive imaging with MR or spiral CT may be sufficient. Delineation of the adjacent venous and arterial anatomy is important both in determining operability and in identification of anatomical anomalies. This can usually be achieved non-invasively using three-dimensional reconstructions of CT,[3] but may require formal visceral angiography. Preoperative percutaneous biopsy is unnecessary in patients who are proceeding to laparotomy.

6 It is debatable whether non-operative stenting or surgical bypass is the better option for irresectable cancer of the pancreatic head. Stenting can be achieved by either the percutaneous transhepatic route or the endoscopic transpapillary route depending on available local expertise. In expert hands the two procedures have similar morbidity and mortality rates equivalent to those of surgical bypass. The recent introduction of expandable metal stents seems likely to reduce the problem of stent clogging, which leads to cholangitis and recurrent jaundice. Metal stents should only be placed if the patient is deemed to be inoperable. The longevity of metal stents is an important consideration because repeated admissions for clearing or replacement of blocked stents can outweigh any advantage gained by avoiding the initial recovery period in hospital that follows a surgical bypass. It is not acceptable simply to stent a patient who might otherwise be suitable for resection without thorough assessment of the case. In general, very elderly or infirm patients and those with advanced carcinoma (metastatic disease) should be managed by non-operative stenting. For younger patients, those with a potentially resectable tumour and those without extensive distal spread or incipient duodenal obstruction, operative bypass is preferable. The ability to perform biliary and gastric bypass by laparoscopic techniques,[4] along with increasing expertise with expandable metal stents in the biliary tract and more recently in the duodenum, means that the surgeon has a wider choice of palliative options and patient selection becomes even more important.

▶ **KEY POINT** Surgery versus stenting

■ If any doubt exists about the diagnosis or the resectability of the tumour then patients should undergo a laparotomy and trial dissection. If unresectability is confirmed, then the option of a double surgical bypass should be considered.

Prepare

1 Patients with prolonged obstruction of the extrahepatic biliary tree tolerate major resectional procedures very poorly. The following specific problems should be anticipated and countered:

■ *Coagulopathy.* If hypoprothrombinaemia is present, give sufficient parenteral vitamin K to restore the prothrombin time of the blood to normal. Routine preoperative administration of vitamin K is a sensible precaution in any jaundiced patient.

■ *Hepatorenal syndrome.* Preoperative rehydration is the simplest and most important precaution. In deeply jaundiced patients, renal failure may be precipitated by intra-operative hypotension, and this should be avoided as far as possible. Catheterize the patient after induction of anaesthesia, ensure adequate hydration and administer intravenous mannitol (40 g) to achieve an osmotic diuresis during the operation.

■ *Sepsis.* Though infected bile is more likely with gallstones than a malignant stricture, 'invasive' cholangiography or operation may provoke infection in any obstructed biliary tree. Both procedures should, therefore, be covered by prophylactic antibiotics.

■ *Malnutrition.* Decreased hepatic synthesis of albumin inevitably follows obstructive jaundice and may not improve until the obstruction has been relieved. Consider parenteral nutrition postoperatively if convalescence is prolonged.

■ *Wound failure.* The healing of wounds is impaired in jaundiced patients. Take particular care with abdominal closure.

2 Preoperative decompression of the obstructed biliary tree is controversial. External transhepatic drainage may improve general health at the risk of various complications (e.g. infection, bile leakage, electrolyte loss). In general, preoperative biliary stents

should be reserved for patients with deep and prolonged jaundice or those with complications such as renal insufficiency and cholangitis. Internal decompression by transhepatic or endoscopic retrograde intubation of the stricture is safer but requires appropriate expertise.

Access

1 Make a transverse bilateral subcostal incision.

Assess

1 If the gallbladder is distended and there is diffuse metastatic spread, indicating that the patient is unlikely to live very long, relieve obstructive jaundice by the simple expedient of cholecysto-jejunostomy (see Chapter 15). If you are in doubt about the patency of the cystic duct, consider obtaining an operative cholecystogram via a Foley catheter inserted into the fundus. If the extent of disease is known preoperatively, patients with carcinomatosis are better served by non-operative stenting, whereas for those with a better prognosis, but irresectable tumours, the common hepatic duct is better for anastomosis since it prevents recurrence of jaundice from encroachment of tumour on the cystic duct.

2 If the tumour is clearly irresectable, but not as advanced, or alternatively, the gallbladder is collapsed or contains calculi, do not use the gallbladder for anastomosis. More lasting biliary diversion is achieved by choledochojejunostomy Roux-en-Y (see Chapter 15), dividing the bile duct above the 'leading edge' of tumour to limit upward spread. Cholecystectomy generally facilitates the operation and is certainly advisable if the gallbladder is obstructed.

3 If the tumour may be resectable and there are no overt metastases, embark upon a trial dissection. If the superior mesenteric and portal veins can be separated from the neck of pancreas, proceed to pancreatoduodenectomy (see next section).

4 *You have decided against resection.* Be sure that you obtain a positive tissue diagnosis by appropriate biopsy with frozen-section confirmation. Consider palliative procedures to relieve jaundice, vomiting and pain. Carry out biliary diversion as described in paragraphs 1 and 2 above. Unless the prognosis is extremely limited, create an antecolic gastroenterostomy (see Chapter 10) to bypass present or future duodenal obstruction (Fig. 16.7). Alternatively, use the same Roux loop for biliary and gastric bypass (Fig. 16.8).

5 Options for pain relief include intubated pancreaticogastrostomy, if the pancreatic duct is clearly dilated, or coeliac plexus block; postoperative radiotherapy may also help. An intraoperative nerve block involves injection of 15–20 ml of 50% alcohol on each side at the level of the diaphragmatic crura. Aspirate the syringe each time to ensure that the needle has not entered the aorta or vena cava. Another option is division of the splanchnic nerves within the chest via thoracoscopic splanchnicectomy. This minimally invasive procedure has been shown to provide pain relief in some patients with pancreatic cancer, although relief is rarely afforded past 6 months.

6 Palliative resection cannot be justified for adenocarcinomas of the pancreas as positive margins are one of the strongest predictors of poor outcome and survival in this patient group is no better than those undergoing bypass alone.

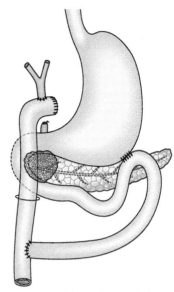

Fig. 16.7 Bypass procedures for an irresectable carcinoma of the head of pancreas. The bile duct is transected well above the tumour, cholecystectomy is performed and biliary drainage is achieved by hepaticojejunostomy Roux-en-Y. An antecolic gastroenterostomy is included.

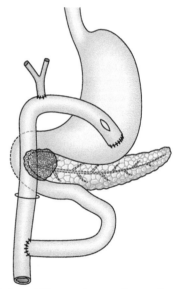

Fig. 16.8 Single-loop biliary and gastric bypass for an irresectable carcinoma of the head of pancreas. This procedure is an alternative to that shown in Figure 16.7.

Aftercare and complications

1 Once the patient recovers from surgery and there is an unequivocal tissue diagnosis, consider the advisability of radiotherapy and/or chemotherapy.

2 There is a low risk of leakage from the biliary anastomosis following palliative bypass. Should the leak persist it should be investigated by fistulography and if necessary PTC, with the option for percutaneous stenting of the anastomosis.

3 Occasionally, patients with advanced carcinoma of the pancreas continue to vomit postoperatively despite one or two patent gastric outlets (i.e. pylorus and stoma). A possible mechanism

for delayed gastric emptying may be autovagotomy caused by extensive lymph-node spread. Exclude a mechanical obstruction by means of barium meal and/or endoscopy and administer prokinetic agents such as metoclopramide, domperidone and erythromycin.

REFERENCES

1. Hennig R, Tempia-Caliera AA, Hartel M, et al. Staging laparoscopy and its indications in pancreatic cancer patients. Dig Surg 2002;19:484–8.
2. Dickinson KJ, Gomez D, Lowe A, et al. Carcinoma of the body of pancreas in evolution: an aggressive disease affecting younger patients? JOP 2007;8(3):312–9.
3. Kalra MK, Maher MM, Mueller PR, et al. State of the art imaging of pancreatic neoplasms. Br J Radiol 2003;76:857–65.
4. Urbach DR, Swanstrom LL, Hansen PD. The effect of laparoscopy on survival in pancreatic cancer. Arch Surg 2002;137:191–9.

DISTAL PANCREATECTOMY

Appraise

1 Distal pancreatectomy is undertaken for chronic inflammation, trauma or tumour in the body and tail of the gland or as part of a radical gastrectomy for carcinoma of the stomach. In chronic pancreatitis indications include scarring and calcification that are predominantly to the left of the midline, ductal stricture in the neck or body of pancreas and a pseudocyst in the body or tail. Visualization of the surrounding vasculature should be performed preoperatively, using CT or angiography, to look for splenic artery pseudo-aneurysm or splenic vein thrombosis. CT scan, ERCP, MRCP and tests of endocrine and exocrine pancreatic function help in assessing the patient and choosing the best surgical option in chronic pancreatitis.

2 In distal hemipancreatectomy the gland is divided in front of the portal vein, but the resection may be extended to include the neck and part of the head of pancreas. Occasionally performed for diffuse pancreatitis, a subtotal pancreatectomy removes upwards of 80% of the gland. Take care to preserve the bile duct and at least one of the pancreaticoduodenal arteries. Anticipate varying degrees of pancreatic insufficiency such as diabetes and steatorrhoea, depending on the functional status of the residual pancreas. In such extensive disease proximal pancreatoduodenectomy or even total pancreatectomy may be better options (see below).

3 *Conventional* distal pancreatectomy includes splenectomy. This procedure is indicated for the limited number of ductal carcinomas that are resectable and for most cases of chronic pancreatitis, especially when associated with severe inflammation, pseudocyst and/or splenic vein thrombosis.

4 *Conservative* distal pancreatectomy involves separating the distal pancreas from the splenic vessels and preserving the spleen. It may be indicated for less severe cases of chronic pancreatitis and for endocrine tumours in the body and tail. It is useful to preserve the immunological function of the spleen and avoid the large dead space that follows splenectomy.

Prepare

1 Distal pancreatectomy can be a difficult and bloody operation. Ensure that cross-matched blood is available.

2 Immunize the patient with the polyvalent anti-pneumococcal vaccine Pneumovax, since these organisms are the most common cause of overwhelming post-splenectomy infection. Current guidelines also include immunization with meningococcal and *Haemophilus influenzae* type b vaccines.[1] Try to give the vaccines 2–4 weeks before operation for maximum effect.

Access

1 Good exposure of the upper abdominal cavity is essential for any type of pancreatectomy: the best access is provided by a transverse subcostal incision.

Assess

1 In operations for chronic pancreatitis the likelihood and extent of resection are indicated by preoperative investigations including endoscopic pancreatography, MRCP, CT and pancreatic function tests. At laparotomy, however, examine the entire gland. Perform operative pancreatography if there is any chance of a dilated ductal system not identified on preoperative imaging, since drainage might be more appropriate than resection in such a case.

2 When operating for upper abdominal trauma, first inspect the liver, spleen and mesentery and deal with any site of bleeding. Pancreatic or duodenal injury should be suspected if there is a retroperitoneal haematoma. Mobilize the duodenum and inspect both surfaces. Enter the lesser sac and examine the pancreas thoroughly. Major contusion or fracture of the pancreatic neck should be treated by distal pancreatectomy.

3 Resection of carcinoma of the body of pancreas is nearly always precluded by direct involvement of the superior mesenteric vessels and/or metastatic spread. Follow the middle colic vein back to find the superior mesenteric vein and establish the relation of this vessel to the tumour. If the main vessels are uninvolved, distal pancreatectomy may be appropriate.

4 Many surgeons remove the left pancreas in a *prograde* fashion, starting with the tail and proceeding towards the midline; this technique is described below. Increasingly, the authors carry out much of the dissection in a *retrograde* fashion, mobilizing and dividing the neck of the pancreas at an early stage and, if possible, securing the splenic vessels before elevating the pancreatic tail and body. The prograde technique is especially useful in chronic pancreatitis, in which extensive retropancreatic fibrosis has obscured the anatomical landmarks of the superior mesenteric and portal veins.

Action

Conventional distal pancreatectomy (Fig. 16.9)

1 Start by freeing the neck of pancreas from the underlying portal vein. Trace the middle colic vein downwards to the root of the transverse mesocolon. To display its junction with the superior mesenteric vein it is necessary to incise the peritoneum along the inferior border of the neck and proximal body of pancreas. In chronic pancreatitis this can be a slow and difficult dissection, and a number of small vessels on the pancreas need to be secured. Once the superior mesenteric vein has been exposed, gently develop the plane between the vein and the pancreas. Pass a finger upwards through this tunnel and expose the tip of your finger by dividing the peritoneum along the superior border of

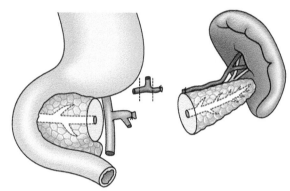

Fig. 16.9 Conventional distal pancreatectomy including splenectomy. Transection just to the right of the portal vein removes about 60% of the gland.

the neck of pancreas. Now that the superior mesenteric and portal veins have been freed, it is safe to proceed to mobilize the tail and body of pancreas towards the midline. Alternatively, continue the dissection to the left to identify, ligate and divide the splenic artery and vein before mobilizing the tail of pancreas (see 'assess' section, paragraph 4). Ligating the splenic artery prior to the vein reduces bleeding and venous congestion within the spleen.

2 In chronic pancreatitis, especially if there is a pseudocyst, the posterior surface of the stomach and the transverse mesocolon and splenic flexure can become adherent to the distal pancreas and need to be dissected free.

3 Mobilize the spleen upwards by dividing its posterior peritoneal attachment, the posterior layer of the lienorenal ligament. The greater omentum will have been partly divided already in entering the lesser sac; now complete the division. Ligate and divide the short gastric vessels. If the spleen is torn during the dissection, ligate its vascular pedicle and complete the splenectomy at this stage.

4 The pancreatic tail lies at the splenic hilum and has already been partly mobilized. Divide the peritoneum along the upper and lower borders of the distal pancreas. Several small vessels need to be ligated or coagulated by diathermy. Continue the dissection towards the midline, lifting the body and tail of pancreas forwards and to the right. Severe chronic inflammation binds the pancreas firmly to its bed, and sharp dissection is needed to free it posteriorly.

5 As the prograde pancreatic dissection approaches the midline, identify the splenic artery as it reaches the posterior surface of the gland near its upper border. Encircle the vessel with a right-angled Lahey forceps and tie it with stout ligatures (2/0 polyglactin 910), doubly ligating on the proximal side. Ideally, the artery should be tied before the vein to prevent congestion of the spleen, but sometimes it is necessary to ligate and divide the splenic vein first if the artery is encased and inaccessible.

6 The splenic vein can be seen running along the posterior surface of the body of pancreas. As it approaches its right-angled junction with the superior mesenteric vein, it is usually joined by the inferior mesenteric vein. Carefully insert a pair of Lahey forceps between the pancreas and the splenic vein. Ligate and divide the splenic vein, if possible preserving the entry of the inferior mesenteric vein. The pancreas can now be lifted gently off the

portal vein. Great care must be taken in the presence of chronic inflammation, since it is easy to tear the veins.

7 Decide where to transect the pancreas: division in front of the portal vein is usual in hemipancreatectomy. Insert 2/0 PDS stay sutures at the upper and lower border of the pancreas at this point and place a soft intestinal clamp across the neck. Divide the pancreas to the left of the clamp and stay sutures and remove the specimen. Be careful not to injure the underlying vein during transection of the gland.

8 Remove the clamp and secure haemostasis. Look for the amputated main pancreatic duct, which normally measures 2–3 mm in diameter at this point. Consider operative pancreatography, and a drainage procedure, if the duct is dilated. Otherwise, under-run the duct with 4/0 PDS and close the pancreatic stump using interrupted 3/0 PDS sutures.

9 Check that the splenic bed and pancreas are dry. Insert one or two tube drains and close the abdomen.

Conservative distal pancreatectomy (Fig. 16.10)

1 The principles of the operation are similar to those for conventional resection, except that an attempt is made to preserve the splenic vessels and spleen. The dissection can be either prograde or retrograde—that is towards, or away from, the midline, or a combination of both. The operation is carried out entirely within the lesser sac without any mobilization of the spleen. This procedure is ideally suited for benign disease and is associated with a significantly lower morbidity rate.[2]

2 Start by freeing the neck and proximal body of pancreas from the underlying great veins as described above. Select the site of pancreatic transection and insert stay sutures on either side approximately 1 cm apart, one pair on the upper border and one pair on the lower border. Place a Kocher's director beneath the pancreas to protect the great veins, then incise through the gland with a scalpel on to the director.

3 Secure haemostasis from each cut surface of the pancreas. Identify the proximal pancreatic duct and under-run it with a 4/0 PDS suture. Oversew the pancreatic stump at this point with interrupted 3/0 PDS sutures.

4 Gently elevate the distal pancreas from the underlying splenic vein. Identify the splenic artery as it passes from the coeliac axis to reach the pancreas to the left of the midline. Proceed slowly to free the pancreas from the splenic vessels, ligating and dividing the several arterial and venous branches that connect them.

5 If the pancreas is very adherent to the splenic vessels, it may help to elevate the tail of the gland and dissect progradely towards

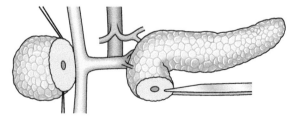

Fig. 16.10 Conservative distal pancreatectomy preserving the spleen. The pancreas is transected at its neck and peeled off the splenic artery and vein from right to left, dividing the numerous vascular branches.

the site of adherence, thereby approaching it from both sides. It is not uncommon to pull a small branch off the splenic artery or vein and then encounter bleeding. Using a sucker to maintain access, close the defect(s) in the vessel with fine sutures (e.g. 4/0 or 5/0 polypropylene). Sometimes the parent vessel has been sufficiently exposed for a soft vascular clamp to be used for temporary control.

6 Complete the dissection, remove the specimen, check for haemostasis and close the abdomen, leaving a tube drain to the pancreatic bed.

Other techniques

1 If there is concern about the extent of distal resection and the potential for endocrine or exocrine failure, then a middle segment pancreatectomy may be performed.[3] Transect the pancreas to the right of the portal vein as described and then, once the gland is mobilized off the splenic vessels, transect it again. Close the proximal stump as for a distal pancreatectomy and anastomose a Roux-en-Y loop of jejunum to the tail (see below).

> ► **KEY POINT** Splenectomy versus splenic preservation in distal pancreatectomy
>
> ■ Although splenic preservation is usually associated with a lower morbidity rate, the risk of major intra-operative blood loss probably outweighs this benefit. If bleeding becomes a problem, then sacrifice the spleen and draw the operation to a close.

> **?** **DIFFICULTY**
>
> 1. Even with a normal pancreas, the conservative technique is seldom easy. Do not attempt it until you have some experience of conventional distal pancreatectomy. If you encounter serious bleeding, it is better to abandon the attempt to preserve the spleen. In fact, it is usually possible to ligate the splenic artery, with or without the vein, yet retain the spleen, provided that the site of ligation is away from the splenic hilum and the short gastric vessels remain intact.
> 2. Bleeding is also the main problem with conventional distal pancreatectomy, especially in severe pancreatitis. If you encounter serious haemorrhage, control it with pressure while taking the usual steps: ensure that access and lighting are optimal and that you have adequate assistance and a functioning sucker. Then remove the pack, identify the source of haemorrhage and control it with sutures. A tear in the splenic vein is usually to blame, and there is a risk that this can extend into the portal vein. It is for this reason that the portal vein is exposed as the first step in the operation, so that any bleeding can be controlled under direct vision.
> 3. If you are uncertain about the security of stump closure, start the patient on octreotide (100 μg three times a day by subcutaneous injection), continued for up to 7 days, to

> decrease pancreatic exocrine secretion. This may reduce the risk of pancreatic fistula and other complications, although it is not supported by all studies.[4]

Aftercare

1 Leave the drain(s) for a minimum of 5 days, especially after splenectomy, then shorten and remove them over a period of 2–3 days.

2 If preoperative pancreatic function was normal, a 50–60% distal resection will seldom precipitate serious endocrine or exocrine insufficiency. In a patient with prediabetes or a more extensive pancreatectomy, the blood glucose should be monitored particularly closely and insulin may be required. In any case, repeat exocrine and endocrine function tests before allowing a patient with chronic pancreatitis to return home.

Complications

1 Even with a drain there is a chance of haematoma in the splenic bed and a subsequent left subphrenic abscess. Suspect the diagnosis if the patient develops fever, leucocytosis and a pleural effusion at the left base. Ultrasound or CT scan will confirm the diagnosis and allow percutaneous drainage of the collection.

2 A few patients develop a pancreatic fistula from the cut end of the pancreas, sometimes after percutaneous drainage of a collection. Provided that there is no ductal obstruction in the head of pancreas – and pancreatic ductal imaging with ERCP, MRCP or ductography should have declared this issue – the fistula will close spontaneously, usually within a month of operation. The somatostatin analogue octreotide may possibly hasten closure of a fistula: if it persists, place a pancreatic stent endoscopically or institute nasopancreatic drainage to encourage closure.

REFERENCES

1. Funk EM, Schlimok G, Ehret W, et al. The current status of vaccination and antibiotic prophylaxis in splenectomy. I: Adults. Chirurgie 1997;68:586–90.
2. Benoist S, Dugue L, Sauvanet A, et al. Is there a role of preservation of the spleen in distal pancreatectomy? J Am Coll Surg 1999;188:255–60.
3. Warshaw AL, Rattner DW, Fernandez-del Castillo C, et al. Middle segment pancreatectomy: a novel technique for conserving pancreatic tissue. Arch Surg 1998;133:327–31.
4. Stojadinovic A, Brooks A, Hoos A, et al. An evidence based approach to the surgical management of resectable pancreatic adenocarcinoma. J Am Coll Surg 2003;196:954–64.

PANCREATICODUDENECTOMY

Appraise

1 Pancreatectomy is undertaken for:
- Carcinoma of the head of pancreas
- Other less aggressive tumours in this region, loosely called periampullary cancers and including distal cholangiocarcinoma, carcinoma of the ampulla, carcinoma of the duodenum and large neuroendocrine tumours of the pancreatic head

■ Severe chronic pancreatitis preferentially involving the head of pancreas and sometimes complicated by bile duct stricture or pseudocyst.

2 All of these conditions can present with obstructive jaundice, which should be managed as previously described. Particularly in pancreatic cancer, attempt to assess resectability before operation using ultrasound, CT scan and/or angiography to determine the size and extent of the tumour, the presence or absence of lymph node and liver metastases and the all-important relationship of the tumour to major vascular structures, notably the portal vein. Vascular imaging is also useful to show anomalies in arterial supply, notably the right hepatic or common hepatic artery arising from the superior mesenteric artery and running up behind the portal vein, which is present in about 25% of patients.

3 Offer pancreaticoduodenectomy for resectable tumours of the pancreatic head, provided that on-table assessment (see below) confirms the absence of distal metastases. There is no absolute upper age limit, but pay particular consideration to patients over the age of 70–75 years because of the extent of the operation required. Palliative procedures for pancreatic cancer have already been described.

4 Neoplastic and inflammatory conditions of the pancreatic head typically present in very different ways. In pancreatic cancer there is a short history of progressive obstructive jaundice with minor or moderate pain, a discrete non-calcified mass on CT scan and an irregular stricture on cholangiography. In chronic pancreatitis there is a long history of abdominal pain associated with weight loss and alcoholism, the jaundice is less severe, remitting or absent and imaging reveals calcification and/or pseudocyst and a smooth tapering stricture in the bile duct. However, the clinical features of the two conditions can overlap sufficiently to be indistinguishable. Resection is the best treatment in either case and obviates the need for biopsy.

5 There is lively debate regarding the best operation for the various conditions described above, but controlled data are scarce. The extent of the operation can be considered under three headings:

■ *The extent of pancreatic resection.* For cancer most surgeons perform hemipancreatectomy rather than total pancreatectomy, but for chronic pancreatitis tailor the resection to the distribution of the disease. This question is considered further under 'Total pancreatectomy'.

■ *The extent of gastroduodenal resection.* The occasional benign tumour of the ampulla and small localized ampullary carcinomas in elderly patients may be suitable for a *transduodenal ampullectomy*, in which the ampulla is circumcised and the terminal portions of bile duct and pancreatic duct are resutured to the duodenal mucosa. The operation of *duodenum-preserving resection*[1] of the head of pancreas has recently been advocated for chronic pancreatitis. The central portion of the head of pancreas is removed, leaving a rim within the duodenal loop, and a Roux loop of jejunum is brought up for anastomosis to the pancreatic duct on either side and sometimes also to the bile duct, if this is strictured or has been entered. With these exceptions, which will not be discussed further because of their limited application, resection of the pancreatic head involves excision of the duodenal loop and terminal bile duct. This *pancreatoduodenectomy* may be accomplished by conventional or conservative techniques, as described below.

■ *The extent of resection of other organs.* The gallbladder is frequently removed in the hope of improving the radical cure of cancer by dividing the bile duct at a higher level. Some surgeons advocate resection of the portal vein en bloc for locally invasive tumour, with end-to-end venous reconstruction. Others are prepared to resect and reconstruct the superior mesenteric artery or even the coeliac axis, while others will carry out a radical lymphadenectomy, removing most of the para-aortic nodes. With the exception of cholecystectomy, all of these procedures increase the duration of the operation and the risk of subsequent complications and death. There is no convincing evidence that these disadvantages are outweighed by improved cure rates.

6 The *conventional* type of pancreatoduodenectomy (Fig. 16.11), described in 1935 by the New York surgeon Allen O. Whipple (1881–1963), includes a distal hemigastrectomy for two largely historical reasons:

■ It removes lymph nodes along the greater and lesser curves of the stomach: these nodes are very seldom involved until the tumour has widely disseminated.

■ Antrectomy reduces the risk of erosive gastritis and postoperative bleeding: pylorus-preserving pancreatoduodenectomy prevents alkaline reflux and modern acid-suppressing drugs give added protection.

Whipple's operation is indicated for carcinoma of the upper portion of the pancreatic head or neck and for chronic pancreatitis complicated by duodenal ulcer disease or duodenal stenosis.

7 The *conservative type* of pancreatoduodenectomy retains the entire stomach and duodenal cap and is termed pylorus-preserving pancreatoduodenectomy (PPPD). This facilitates better postoperative nutrition and weight gain and the duodenal anastomosis is easier to construct, but delayed gastric emptying is sometimes a problem in the early postoperative period, although the delay in return to normal diet would seem to be no different.[2] PPPD is indicated for most patients with chronic pancreatitis and periampullary cancer and for those with pancreatic cancer arising from

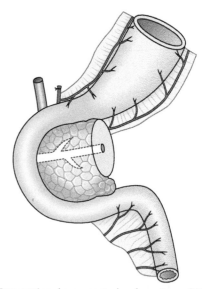

Fig. 16.11 Conventional pancreatoduodenectomy (Whipple's operation). The resection specimen is shown and includes the distal half of the stomach, the duodenal loop and duodenojejunal flexure, the terminal bile duct and the head and uncinate process of the pancreas.

the lower part of the head and uncinate process, providing similar local control and long-term survival.[3]

Prepare

1 Pancreatoduodenectomy is a major undertaking. Detailed pancreatic imaging should be accompanied by thorough assessment of the patient's general health. Ensure that at least 4 units of cross-matched blood are available. Cover the procedure with broad-spectrum antibiotics.

2 The perioperative precautions to be taken in deeply jaundiced patients and the role of preliminary biliary decompression have been discussed earlier.

Assess

As for all major pancreatic operations, the bilateral subcostal approach gives the best access, but a vertical midline or transverse incision can also be employed.

Access

1 In a case of suspected or proven neoplasia, start by making a detailed search for metastatic disease. Look and feel for hepatic metastases, peritoneal seedlings and lymph nodes. Pancreatic cancer spreads first to lymph nodes in the anterior and posterior duodenopancreatic grooves and along the hepatic artery, and then to nodes around the origin of the coeliac axis and superior mesenteric artery. Select one or more suitable metastases for biopsy to confirm the diagnosis. Nodes adjacent to the pancreas can be resected en bloc, but more distant disease means that resection should be abandoned except in highly selected patients, for example those with neuroendocrine cancer.

> **KEY POINTS** Intra-operative staging of pancreatic cancer
>
> ■ Undertake a thorough search for extrapancreatic tumour deposits before attempting resection, including the liver, all peritoneal surfaces, the coeliac nodes and the inferior surface of the transverse mesocolon near the ligament of Treitz.
>
> ■ Sample any suspicious deposits and subject them to frozen-section examination.

2 Ensure that the primary tumour can be mobilized. The usual problem is posterior fixity to the preaortic fascia, which is often heralded by back pain. If the tumour is irresectable by virtue of local invasion or distant metastasis, proceed to bypass surgery. Do not forget to obtain a positive tissue diagnosis before closing the abdomen.

3 In a favourable case, now proceed to establish whether the portal vein is free of the cancer. Preoperative vascular imaging should have clarified this, but there is no substitute for a trial dissection to make sure. Enter the lesser sac by dividing the greater omentum outside the gastroepiploic arcade or elevate the omentum off the transverse colon in the avascular plane. Use the middle colic vein(s) to guide you to the superior mesenteric vein below the neck of pancreas. Carefully divide the peritoneum and fascia

over the vein until the vessel wall is clearly exposed, then use gentle blunt dissection to develop the tunnel upwards behind the neck of pancreas.

4 If the tumour lies close by, or obstructive pancreatitis hampers this dissection, it may be safer to expose the portal vein above the neck of pancreas before proceeding from below. Divide the peritoneum overlying the free edge of the lesser omentum, securing the superficial blood vessels. Identify and expose the common bile duct, encircle it with a right-angled forceps and pass a soft tube around the duct as a sling. Dissect out the gastroduodenal artery, which arises almost invariably from the apex of a right-angled bend (or 'genu') of the main hepatic artery. Sling these vessels also. Now, pulling gently on the slings, separate the structures and dissect deeply between them to expose the front of the portal vein. The gastroduodenal artery can be ligated and divided at this point to provide better exposure to the portal vein.

5 Gently establish the tunnel between the neck of pancreas in front and the portal vein behind, using your two index fingers passed one from above and one from below (Fig. 16.12). As long as you stay directly in front of the vein you will not encounter any pancreatic venous branches. If there is clear-cut invasion of the portal vein, abandon the resection and proceed to a bypass. If not, proceed to pancreatoduodenectomy (see 'Action' below).

6 In a case of chronic pancreatitis carry out a general laparotomy. In particular, examine the liver (and consider biopsy), gallbladder, bile duct, spleen, stomach and duodenum: cirrhosis, gallstones, splenomegaly and peptic ulcer can all be associated with pancreatitis. Mobilize and examine the pancreas from head to tail. It is almost always possible to resect the head of pancreas in chronic pancreatitis, even if a small portion of tissue has to be left to protect the great veins, so a trial dissection as such is unnecessary. The inferior tunnel is often impossible to create safely from below, and it is often easier to create the tunnel from above and divide the neck of the pancreas onto a right-angled clamp passing inferiorly, without first dissecting from below.

7 Sometimes there is a mass in the head of pancreas, but it is impossible to be certain whether it is inflammatory or neoplastic. Remember that induration of the body of pancreas could represent either ductal obstruction by tumour or primary chronic pancreatitis. Resection is the best treatment in either case, so do not waste time with a biopsy. If you have the necessary expertise, proceed to pancreatoduodenectomy. If not, carry out

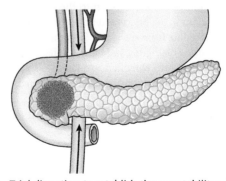

Fig. 16.12 Trial dissection to establish the resectability of a carcinoma of the head of pancreas. One finger is passed along the portal vein from above and another finger along the superior mesenteric vein from below to establish a safe plane behind the neck of pancreas.

a cholecystojejunostomy in the presence of jaundice and then refer the patient elsewhere.

8 Make a choice between conservative or conventional pancreato-duodenectomy. For most patients the standard procedure is now PPPD, and distal gastrectomy should be undertaken only if there is concomitant duodenal disease, if the cancer lies close to the pylorus or if the pancreatitis is so severe that the duodenum cannot easily be separated. There are several different techniques for reconstruction after pancreatoduodenectomy: one is described below.

Action

Conservative pancreatoduodenectomy

1 Once the trial dissection has been completed, you are well under way. In chronic pancreatitis, however, it may require a long and rather hazardous dissection to clear the portal vein. Attempt this procedure only if you have had adequate experience. If you have not already done so, dissect out the structures in the free edge of the lesser omentum. Doubly ligate the gastroduodenal artery, with two ligatures on the proximal side, making sure that you have identified and preserved the main hepatic artery.

2 Begin to separate the first part of the duodenum from the underlying pancreas, securing the numerous vessels that run between the two. Keep close to the duodenal wall, proceeding either towards or away from the pylorus as you prefer. Ligate and divide the right gastroepiploic artery and vein close to their origin on the pancreas. Aim to mobilize the pylorus and the proximal 6 cm or so of duodenum. Apply a light crushing clamp to the duodenum at least 3 cm beyond the pylorus and cut the bowel flush with the clamp, using a non-crushing clamp temporarily to occlude the pylorus. Now suck out the stomach, cover the duodenal stump with a swab wrung out in antiseptic solution and held in place with Babcock's forceps and displace the stomach to the left side of the abdomen. Frozen-section examination of the duodenal resection margin may be necessary and can be carried out at this time. Quickly oversew the distal duodenum so you can remove the crushing clamp.

3 You have now exposed the pancreatic neck and can divide it under direct vision. Complete the mobilization of its upper and lower borders. Insert and tie four stay sutures of 3/0 PDS, one on each side of the proposed line of transection (Fig. 16.13). Place a Kocher's director in front of the portal vein and divide the pancreatic neck on to the director. Apply a soft intestinal clamp to the pancreas on one side or the other if there is marked bleeding from the gland. Stop the bleeding from each cut surface, using diathermy and sutures as necessary. Identify the pancreatic duct, which will often be dilated. In a potential case of cancer take a generous biopsy from the transected neck of pancreas for frozen-section pathology.

4 Proceed to separate the head and uncinate process of the pancreas from the portal and superior mesenteric veins. Tease out, ligate and divide the pancreatic veins, usually one from the superior aspect of the gland and two or three lower down. These are fragile vessels and bleed profusely if damaged. Have fine sutures available such as 4/0 or 5/0 polypropylene (Prolene) to close any holes in the portal vein. Throughout this dissection use your left hand to grasp, steady and retract the head of pancreas. Compress the portal vein using your left hand to control venous bleeding

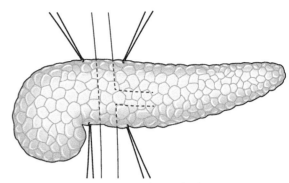

Fig. 16.13 Preparing to transect the neck of pancreas. Stay sutures are placed on the upper and lower borders of the pancreas on either side of the proposed line of transection.

that may occur. This is why it is so important to Kocherize the duodenum prior to creating the portal vein 'tunnel'.

5 Mobilize the bile duct prior to dividing it either low down in chronic pancreatitis or generally at a higher level in carcinoma of the pancreas; in this case perform cholecystectomy. Apply a small vascular clamp or bulldog clip to the bile duct and cut across the duct below this point, taking a culture swab of bile. If a stent is in situ it will have to be removed at this point and can also be sent off for microbiological examination. Frozen-section of the bile duct can be arranged at this point if required.

6 Now free the pancreas from its attachment to the preaortic fascia, ligating and dividing the connective tissue just beyond the gland. Control the specimen during this manoeuvre with your left hand, as before, taking care not to injure the superior mesenteric artery, which can be pulled underneath the vein by traction on the specimen. The divided tissue will contain the inferior pancreaticoduodenal branch(es) of the artery.

> ▶ **KEY POINT** Mobilization of the pancreatic head
>
> ■ During division of the deep attachments of the pancreatic head, it is helpful if the operator's left hand is placed behind the head of pancreas and duodenum in order to elevate the specimen out of the wound, thereby facilitating the dissection and maintaining vascular control in case of venous bleeding. During this procedure care must be taken not to damage the superior mesenteric artery, which can easily be rotated from its normal position and pulled into the field of dissection.

7 Mobilize the ligament of Treitz below the transverse mesocolon. Gently draw the upper jejunum through the congenital retrocolic 'defect' and into the supracolic compartment. Complete the mobilization of the uncinate process. Ligate and divide the mesentery to the duodenojejunal flexure. Complete the resection by dividing the upper jejunum and its mesentery at a convenient point. The end of the jejunal loop is then brought into the supracolic compartment through a window created in the transverse mesocolon, although the congenital retrocolic defect can be used. If the transverse colon mesentery is short you may need to bring the jejunal loop antecolically.

8 You must now embark on the reconstruction, joining the pancreatic neck, bile duct and duodenal stump to the upper jejunum in that order (Fig. 16.14A). First, elevate the body of pancreas posteriorly for about 4 cm, carefully dividing one or two tributaries of the splenic vein. This manoeuvre allows you to create an invaginating anastomosis.

9 *Pancreatic anastomosis.* The technique varies according to the disease process and the calibre of the pancreatic duct:

■ In a patient with cancer (soft gland) and a small pancreatic duct (<3 mm), use a transanastomotic stent and a separate Roux loop to reduce the risk of leakage of activated pancreatic juice from the anastomosis (Fig. 16. 14B). Check that a 4F or 6F infant-feeding tube will pass well down the pancreatic duct (Fig. 16.15). Now introduce the tube, first into the abdomen through a stab incision below the right-hand end of the main wound and then into the upper jejunum through a tiny incision about 30 cm distal to the cut end of bowel; use a long pair of forceps thrust down the bowel to grasp the tube and draw it out. Insert the tube right down the pancreatic duct

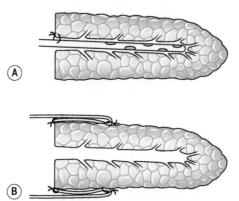

Fig. 16.15 Pancreaticojejunostomy following resection of the pancreatic head: (A) insertion of a transanastomotic stent; (B) two-layer invaginating anastomosis.

and suture it firmly in place with two 3/0 polyglactin 910 sutures that pick up the ductal mucosa. Alternatively, the tube can be secured by transfixing it with a double-ended suture, then passing each needle through the duct and out through the anterior surface of the gland; tie the suture over a small 'buttress' of muscle taken from the abdominal wall.

■ In a patient with cancer and a degree of obstructive pancreatopathy, where both the duct is somewhat enlarged and the gland firmer than normal, a separate Roux loop is unnecessary, as is the transanastomotic stent, because many of the sutures can incorporate the duct and hold it open.

■ In chronic pancreatitis the fibrotic nature of the gland along with the ductal dilatation and the low enzymatic content of the pancreatic juice make serious leakage unlikely, so in this case the anastomosis can be accomplished without the need for a stent.

Use a modified Cattell technique to construct a two-layer duct-to-mucosa anastomosis. The serosa of the jejunal loop is opened carefully so as not to breach the mucosal layer. Starting posteriorly with the outer layer, place a row of interrupted stitches between the pancreatic parenchyma and the jejunal serosa. Take generous bites of pancreas to avoid the sutures cutting out. Once complete, a small enterotomy is made in the jejunal mucosa opposite the pancreatic duct orifice. The pancreatic duct is anastamosed to the mucosa using interrupted 5/0 PDS sutures, being careful not to occlude the duct. Finally, the anterior jejunal serosa layer is anastamosed to the pancreatic parenchyma in a similar fasion to the posterior layer.

If the pancreas is very friable, invaginate the cut end into the end of the jejunal loop (the 'dunking technique'). A single layer of interrupted 3/0 ethibond sutures is used to invaginate the pancreas. Starting posteriorly, place a row of interrupted sutures circumferentially between the outer aspects of the pancreas and jejunum at least 1 cm from the cut edge. When this outer layer of stitches is tied it will draw the jejunum over the pancreas like a sheath. Alternative anastomoses are end-to-side pancreaticojejunostomy (see Fig. 16.16) and end-to-side pancreaticogastrostomy, in which the pancreatic stump is joined to the back of the stomach[5] (Fig. 16.17).

10 *Biliary anastomosis.* Carry out an end-to-side choledochojejunostomy with one layer of interrupted 3/0 polyglactin 910

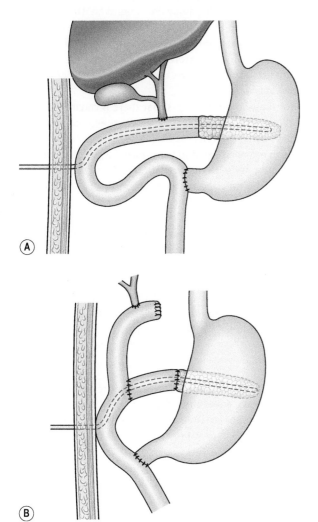

Fig. 16.14 Reconstruction following pylorus-preserving pancreatoduodenectomy (PPPD): (A) the pancreatic anastomosis is protected by a fine-bore tube brought to the exterior and sutured into the duct; (B) if the pancreas is soft and its duct is tiny, it may be safer to perform the pancreaticojejunostomy using a separate Roux loop.

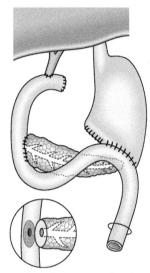

Fig. 16.16 Reconstruction after conventional pancreato-duodenectomy with an end-to-side pancreaticojejunostomy. To create the pancreatic anastomosis (inset), the pancreatic duct is sutured directly to the jejunal mucosa; the anastomosis can be splinted by a fine polythene tube.

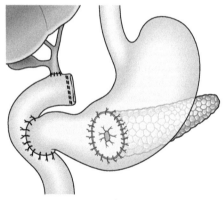

Fig. 16.17 Reconstruction following pylorus-preserving pancreato-duodenectomy (PPPD). Pancreaticogastrostomy has been described as a safe alternative.

sutures. Insert stay sutures in the bile duct, remove the clamp, suck out the bile and secure any bleeding vessels. Now place the posterior row of sutures, tie them and complete the anastomosis anteriorly. In most patients with cancer the anastomosis is easy because the duct is dilated, but in chronic pancreatitis the wall may be thick and the lumen narrow; consider using a fine-bore T-tube inserted through a stab incision in the duct with the lower limb of the 'T' placed across the anastomosis. Bring the long limb of the tube out through a stab incision in the abdominal wall. Another option is to pass a stent as per the pancreatic anastomosis, bringing it out through the same enterotomy. If a pancreatic stent has been used, suture the jejunum to the abdominal wall at the exit point well below the biliary anastomosis.

11 *Duodenal anastomosis.* Check the viability of the duodenal stump and be prepared to sacrifice the terminal 1–2 cm. Try to preserve a minimum of 2 cm of healthy bowel between pylorus and anastomosis. Now carry out a two-layer end-to-side duodenojejunostomy, using 3/0 PDS sutures. The duodenal anastomosis should be 25–30 cm distal to the biliary anastomosis.

Conventional pancreatoduodenectomy

1 The only difference from PPPD is that the distal 30–50% of stomach is resected, together with the pylorus and entire duodenum.

? DIFFICULTY

1. Pancreatoduodenectomy is generally easier in cancer than it is in chronic pancreatitis, when severe inflammatory adherence can make for a particularly difficult dissection. Be prepared to leave a small amount of inflamed pancreatic tissue to protect the portal and superior mesenteric veins if necessary.
2. If bleeding occurs from the portal vein, do not panic. Control the bleeding with packs, try to identify the source and suture it. It is seldom necessary (or easy) to clamp the main portal vein above and below the source of haemorrhage.
3. If, after dividing the neck of pancreas and mobilizing the head, you find invasion of the superior mesenteric vein in the region of the uncinate process, it is occasionally appropriate to resect a short segment of vein en bloc and restore continuity by end-to-end anastomosis. More often it will become apparent that the origin of the superior mesenteric artery is also encased and that the resection is therefore palliative. Mark the residual tumour with metal clips and consider postoperative radiotherapy.
4. If the pathologist reports that there is carcinoma at the transection line in the pancreas, proceed to total pancreatectomy (see below).
5. *The pancreas is soft and the sutures keep cutting out.* Take deeper bites with mattress sutures. Stent the anastomosis and invaginate the bowel thoroughly. If all else fails, perform total pancreatectomy.
6. *There is a low entry to the cystic duct.* Either remove the gallbladder or divide the septum between cystic duct and common hepatic duct to create a common biliary channel for anastomosis.
7. *After PPPD the duodenal stump looks blue.* Resect back towards the pylorus until bleeding is encountered from the end. If the duodenum is clearly non-viable, convert to a conventional Whipple resection.

2 After freeing the portal vein, divide the greater and lesser omentum along the antrum (see Chapter 10). Cut across the stomach between clamps or TA90 staple lines. Now displace the gastric stump to the left to expose the neck of pancreas, and proceed as before.

3 At the end of the operation carry out gastrojejunostomy rather than duodenojejunostomy, as described for Polya gastrectomy in Chapter 10. Use a two-layer anastomosis to create a generous stoma (Fig. 16.18).

Closure

1 Check carefully for haemostasis and consider washing out the upper abdomen. Place two soft tube drains to the region of the pancreatic anastomosis.

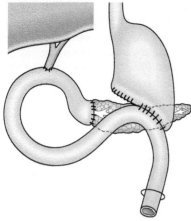

Fig. 16.18   Reconstruction after conventional pancreato-duodenectomy with an end-to-end pancreaticojejunostomy.

2   Consider the need for a feeding jejunostomy, particularly in elderly patients or those with a low preoperative serum albumin level. We use a 14F latex T-tube placed in the infracolic jejunum and sutured to the abdominal wall.

3   Close the abdominal wall in layers, taking particular care to achieve a sound closure in a jaundiced patient in whom impaired healing can be anticipated.

Aftercare

1   Watch the patient closely for the first 48 hours after this major procedure. Check the postoperative haemoglobin levels and correct any anaemia promptly. Monitor the serum amylase level also, together with urea and electrolytes.

2   Keep a close eye on the drain output. Brownish fluid may indicate a developing pancreatic fistula (see below) and a high amylase level in the effluent will confirm this.

3   Pancreatic stents should drain a variable quantity of clear juice but if they slip out into the jejunum the fluid becomes bile stained. Consider performing an X-ray down the tube after 5–7 days. Thereafter, clamp the tube before removing it at 10–12 days.

4   Some surgeons give octreotide routinely for 5–7 days postoperatively (200 μg t.d.s. subcutaneously, or by intravenous infusion), starting immediately before operation. Others reserve the drug for 'high-risk anastomoses', that is those with a soft pancreas and a tiny duct, which are especially prone to leak.

Complications

1   The most serious complication is leakage from the pancreatic anastomosis, which can result in sepsis and serious haemorrhage. The fistula usually declares itself about 5 days postoperatively. If the output is low and the patient's general condition is satisfactory, it is reasonable to consider conservative treatment with antibiotics, octreotide and parenteral nutrition. In the presence of bleeding or sepsis the patient should have a CT scan. If a collection is present it should be drained percutaneously. If bleeding has occurred an arterial reconstruction should be done from the CT and if possible transcatheter embolization performed. If this fails then perform laparotomy. If anastomotic dehiscence is confirmed, the safest measure is to remove the remaining pancreas and to under-run any bleeding from the gastroduodenal artery stump, which lies adjacent to the pancreatic anastomosis.

2   The other anastomoses may also leak, causing biliary or duodenal fistulas, but the consequences are seldom serious unless internal sepsis leads to secondary breakdown of the pancreatico-jejunostomy. Thus conservative measures may suffice to allow spontaneous closure.

3   Reactive haemorrhage, chest infection and wound infection are possible complications of any major upper abdominal procedure.

4   Approximately 10% of patients develop delayed gastric emptying after PPPD and require continued nasogastric intubation. This can be avoided using an antecolic approach to the anastamoses. Institute parenteral nutrition and give prokinetic drugs such as metoclopramide, domperidone and erythromycin. A feeding jejunostomy is particularly helpful in this situation. Carry out a barium study to see if any contrast leaves the stomach and rule out a mechanical obstruction. Gastric tone will eventually recover.

REFERENCES

1. Beger HG, Schlosser W, Siech M, et al. The surgical management of chronic pancreatitis: duodenum-preserving pancreatectomy. Adv Surg 1999;32:87–104.
2. Halloran CM, Ghaneh P, Bosonet L, et al. Complications of pancreatic cancer resection. Dig Surg 2002;19:138–46.
3. Yamaguchi K, Kishinnaka M, Nagai E, et al. Pancreatoduodenectomy for pancreatic head carcinoma without pylorus preservation. Hepatogastroenterology 2001;48:1479–85.
4. Masson B, Sa-Cunha A, Laurent C, et al. Laparoscopic pancreatectomy: report of 22 cases. Ann Chir 2003;128:452–6.
5. Aranha GV. A technique for pancreaticogastrostomy. Am J Surg 1998;175:328–9.

TOTAL PANCREATECTOMY

Appraise

1   Total pancreatectomy has sometimes been recommended for the routine management of resectable cancers on the grounds that it avoids the problems of multifocal ductal carcinoma and potential leakage from the pancreaticojejunostomy. The counterarguments are that it increases the risks of the procedure, conveys no actual survival advantage and renders the patient an obligate diabetic. Reserve the procedure for bulky tumours encroaching on the neck, for cancer in diabetics and for the occasional patient in whom frozen-section examination is positive during partial pancreatectomy. There is no evidence to suggest that total pancreatectomy for cancer provides any survival advantage, and in fact it may be associated with a worse outcome.[1]

2   Total pancreatectomy is occasionally indicated in patients with end-stage chronic pancreatitis and may be combined with pancreatic transplantation, especially if lesser procedures have failed or there is generalized disease with pre-existing endocrine and exocrine failure.[2,3]

3   Completion pancreatectomy may be the wisest move if a fistula develops from a leaking pancreaticojejunostomy anastomosis in a patient requiring re-laparotomy (see previous section).

4 Duodenal resection is virtually always a part of total pancreatectomy.[3] Most of these procedures have been carried out for chronic pancreatitis, and here it is usually possible to preserve the pylorus and sometimes possible to preserve the spleen.

Assess

1 Patients who are candidates for total pancreatectomy should have thorough preoperative investigation to determine the structure and residual function of the gland.

2 At laparotomy the surgeon should assess whether the appearances of the pancreas are consistent with the previous imaging, whether any lesser procedure than total pancreatectomy might be appropriate and whether the stomach or spleen can be retained.

Action

1 The operation is essentially an amalgam of proximal and distal pancreatectomy, as described above. It is generally best to start by freeing the pancreatic neck from the subjacent portal vein, then to proceed with mobilization of the head and conclude by resecting the body and tail. Sometimes you may initially embark on an extended distal resection but decide that the head of pancreas is so diseased that it should also be removed.

2 Following pylorus-preserving total pancreatectomy, the neatest reconstruction is an end-to-end duodenojejunostomy followed by biliary anastomosis a few centimetres downstream (Fig. 16.19).

Aftercare and complications

1 There is no pancreatic anastomosis to leak, but biliary and intestinal fistulas can arise from the other two anastomoses and reactive haemorrhage and subphrenic abscess may occur.

2 The early management of diabetes is not usually difficult provided that glucose and insulin therapy are modulated to avoid hypoglycaemia. Aim to keep the blood sugar on the high side of normal and do not worry about precise control until the patient is eating normally. Involve a diabetologist in the subsequent management and do not allow the patient home until he has

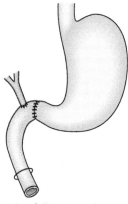

Fig. 16.19 Reconstruction following pylorus-preserving total pancreatectomy. The gallbladder has been included in the resection specimen.

been taught how to measure blood and urine sugar levels and how to self-administer insulin.

3 Exocrine pancreatic supplements will also be required for the rest of the patient's life, the exact dose varying widely from one individual to another. In addition, a low-fat diet and acid-reducing drugs will often be needed to control steatorrhoea and allow proper weight gain.

REFERENCES

1. Ihse I, Anderson H, Andren-Sandberg A. Total pancreatectomy for cancer of the pancreas: is it appropriate? World J Surg 1996;20:288–93.
2. Clayton HA, Davies JE, Pollard CA, et al. Pancreatectomy with islet autotransplantation for the treatment of severe chronic pancreatitis: the first 40 patients at the Leicester general hospital. Transplantation 2003;76:92–8.
3. Fleming WR, Williamson RCN. Role of total pancreatectomy in the treatment of patients with end stage chronic pancreatitis. Br J Surg 1995;82:1409–12.

LAPAROTOMY FOR ISLET CELL TUMOUR

Appraise

1 *Insulinoma* is the commonest islet cell tumour. It is usually solitary and benign. It presents with episodic hypoglycaemia and the diagnosis is confirmed by finding a low blood sugar and inappropriately high serum insulin either spontaneously or after provocation by fasting. Most insulinomas are sufficiently vascular to be localized as a 'blush' on selective pancreatic arteriography.[1] Local excision is sufficient.

2 *Gastrinoma* can arise in the pancreas, the duodenal wall or sometimes further afield. It presents with the Zollinger-Ellison syndrome of intractable peptic ulceration and diarrhoea. The diagnosis is confirmed by finding high basal gastric acid with hypergastrinaemia on radioimmunoassay. The ulcer diathesis should be controlled preoperatively by ranitidine or omeprazole while an attempt is made to localize the tumour by arteriography, endoscopic ultrasonography, contrast-enhanced CT scan and somatostatin receptor scintigraphy. Many gastrinomas are malignant, with lymph node or even liver metastases.[2] The best surgical treatment is to identify and resect all tumour tissue, but subtotal or even total gastrectomy is sometimes required.

3 Glucagonoma, somatostatinoma and other hormone-secreting tumours are rare entities, but a more common condition is the *non-functioning neuroendocrine tumour* of the pancreas. This presents as a relatively slow-growing mass with pain or jaundice or bleeding, and imaging usually shows a sizeable tumour, which is hypervascular and may be calcified or partly cystic. It is often worth resecting these tumours even in the presence of metastases,[3] as sometimes residual disease will respond to chemotherapy.

4 Some patients with islet cell tumour, especially gastrinoma, have coincident tumours of the parathyroid or pituitary gland as a part of *multiple endocrine neoplasia* (MEN I—multiple endocrine neoplasia type I). There is usually a positive family history, and the pancreatic tumours are often multiple.[4]

Assess

1 To find a small islet cell tumour, you must be prepared to mobilize and examine the entire pancreas. Inspect and palpate the anterior and posterior surfaces from head to tail. Even if one tumour has been identified preoperatively and you find it quickly, remember that these lesions can be multiple (especially in MEN I) and continue to examine the rest of the gland. Preoperatively, all attempts should be made at localization, employing CT, MRI, endoscopic ultrasound, isotope scans and provocative arteriography. This latter technique involves injecting calcium into the pancreatic feeding vessels whilst measuring the plasma hormone levels, to determine the part of the pancreas in which the tumour is located.

2 Intra-operative ultrasound scanning can be extremely useful, allowing identification of previously unseen lesions, exclusion of multifocal disease and relationship of tumours to the pancreatic duct, which is important when deciding between resection and enucleation.

3 If you do not find the tumour, repeat the digital examination and the ultrasonography if you have it available. If you are searching for a gastrinoma remember that there may be a tiny tumour in the duodenal wall; mobilize and examine the duodenum thoroughly. There is little role for 'blind' pancreatic resection in the management of insulinoma, unless there has been confident preoperative localization, but you are unable to feel the tumour. It may be better to close the abdomen and reinvestigate the patient using transhepatic portal venous sampling.

4 For large non-functioning tumours, assess the patient at operation as you would for ordinary pancreatic cancer except that the presence of distant metastases should not necessarily preclude resection. You may enucleate liver secondaries or even carry out partial hepatectomy in suitable cases.

Action

1 For insulinoma or gastrinoma in the head or neck of pancreas, *enucleation* is the best option. Incise the pancreas over the tumour and shell the lesion out with a small cuff of normal tissue. Send the lesion for immediate frozen-section pathological examination. Secure haemostasis. If removal of the tumour has left a significant cavity within the gland or if the pancreatic duct is opened it is safer to create a Roux loop of jejunum and suture it to the margins of the defect (Fig. 16.20), otherwise a pancreatic fistula may result. Successful removal of an insulinoma may be followed by rebound hyperglycaemia within 30–45 minutes. A small gastrinoma in the duodenal wall is also suitable for local excision unless metastases limited to pancreaticoduodenal lymph nodes make pancreatoduodenectomy advisable.

2 For an islet cell tumour in the distal body or tail of pancreas, conservative distal pancreatectomy is often the best option.

3 For non-functioning tumours some form of major pancreatic resection is usually indicated.

4 A laparoscopic approach for resection of islet cell tumours has been used and both enucleation and partial resection have been reported.[5] With the addition of laparoscopic ultrasound it may be possible to find moderate-sized tumours but there is no substitute for palpation during open exploration.

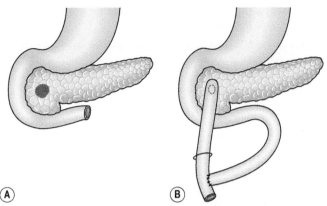

Fig. 16.20 Surgical management of an insulinoma in the pancreatic head: (A) enucleation of the adenoma; (B) a retrocolic Roux loop is brought up and sewn to the margins of the defect.

REFERENCES

1. Geoghegan JG, Jackson JE, Lewis MP, et al. Localization and surgical management of insulinoma. Br J Surg 1994;81:1025–8.
2. Kisker O, Bastian D, Bartsch D, et al. Localization, malignant potential, and surgical management of gastrinomas. World J Surg 1998;22:651–8.
3. Cheslyn-Curtis S, Sitaram V, Williamson RCN. Management of non-functioning neuroendocrine tumours of the pancreas. Br J Surg 1993;80:625–7.
4. Mignon M, Ruszniewski P, Podevin P, et al. Current approach to the management of gastrinoma and insulinoma in adults with multiple endocrine neoplasia type I. World J Surg 1993;17:489–97.
5. Jaroszewski DE, Schlinkert RT, Thompson GB, et al. Laparoscopic localisation and resection of insulinomas. Arch Surg 2004;139:270–4.

MINIMALLY INVASIVE PANCREATIC SURGERY

Appraise

1 Minimally invasive techniques have become increasingly employed for the treatment of pancreatic disease.

2 Laparoscopy has been applied in:
- Enteric drainage of pancreatic pseudocysts and dilated ducts associated with acute and chronic pancreatitis.
- Pancreatic necrosectomy in cases of infected necrosis complicating pancreatitis.
- Enucleation of neuroendocrine tumours; mostly insulinomas.
- Staging of pancreatic malignancy to avoid unnecessary laparotomy in patients with occult metastatic disease not detectable on preoperative imaging; however, it remains controversial whether laparoscopic staging for pancreas cancer should be recommended routinely.[1]
- Laparoscopic gastrojejunostomy and/or choledochojejunostomy in patients with duodenal obstruction and/or jaundice due to unresectable periampullary tumours recognized either on preoperative imaging or during laparoscopic staging.
- Neurolytic coeliac plexus block for chronic pain related to retroperitoneal invasion of tumour mass.

3 Laparoscopic pancreas resection, although it remains technically challenging, is gaining ground as experience mounts in high-volume centres. Various techniques and approaches have been reported, including hand-assisted and robot-assisted techniques,

as well as the use of a minilaparotomy for the reconstructive portion of the operation.

4 Benefits of laparoscopic pancreatic surgery may include decreased wound complications, less postoperative pain, faster return of digestive function, faster return to normal activities and diminished procedure-related inflammatory response and alterations in host immune function.[2]

5 There are no randomized controlled trials to evaluate the outcomes of laparoscopic pancreatic resection for neoplasms in terms of recurrence and survival rates. Since lymphadenectomy is technically achievable, given the excellent visualization, it is, therefore, likely to be a safe and an appropriate operative approach for cancer.[3]

6 A pancreatic duct leak rate comparable to open procedures has been reported after laparoscopic pancreatic resection in patients with pancreatic neoplasms, reflecting the safety and feasibility of this procedure.[4]

> **KEY POINTS** Minimally invasive pancreatic surgery

- Open surgical procedures remain the standard for both benign and malignant diseases.
- Laparoscopic pancreatic surgery requires great expertise and skill and should only be attempted after adequate training in the field. Patient selection is of paramount importance.

Access

1 Usually the patient is placed in lithotomy position.

2 Four or five ports are routinely used and access is obtained via open (Hasson) approach (Fig. 16.21)

3 An angled 30° laparoscope is inserted.

4 A window is created through the gastrocolic ligament using ultrasonic dissection and locking clips. Other forms of energy such as electrocautery can be used.

Action

1 *Drainage of pancreatic pseudocyst:* The cyst is localized by visualization of bulging or by the use of intra-operative ultrasonography. In the case of cystogastrostomy, it can be approached through the lesser sac or an anterior gastrostomy. The anastomosis can be created by endoscopic linear stapler or intra-corporal suturing. The same principles apply for gastric/biliary bypass in cases of unresectable pancreatic malignancy.

2 *Enucleation of neuroendocrine tumours:* The entire pancreas should be explored. Enucleation of the pancreatic mass is achieved by blunt and sharp dissection of the peripancreatic tissue. After completion of the surgical procedure, the pancreatic mass is withdrawn from the abdominal cavity within a plastic retrieval bag.

3 *Staging of pancreatic malignancy:* Careful examination of all peritoneal surfaces including the undersurface of the diaphragm is performed. Intra-operative ultrasonography may be a useful adjunct. Suspicious lesions must be biopsied.

4 *Pancreatectomy:* Laparoscopic distal pancreatectomy is the most commonly performed procedure. En-bloc splenectomy is recommended in cases of malignancy and vascular involvement/thrombosis. Pancreatic mobilization usually proceeds from proximal to distal. The splenic artery and vein must be isolated and clipped or stapled; the pancreatic stump can be managed by use of the endo-GIA stapler or oversewing.

5 *Pancreaticoduodenectomy:* Laparoscopic pancreaticoduodenectomy requires a high level of skill, good patient selection and a great deal of stamina. It is ideal for ampullary tumours, cystic lesions and small cancers in the head of pancreas with no evidence of vascular invasion. The classic Whipple's technique is favoured and a single loop reconstruction is undertaken. The pancreatic stump is invaginated into the jejunal loop using interrupted 3/0 Ethibond. All anastamoses are completed intra-corporeally and the the specimen delivered either through a pfannenstiel incision in females or gridiron incision in males.

REFERENCES

1. Stefanidis D, Grove KD, Schwesinger WH, et al. The current role of staging laparoscopy for adenocarcinoma of the pancreas: a review. Ann Oncol 2006;17:189–99.
2. Kooby D, Gillespie T, Bentrem DJ, et al. Left-sided pancreatectomy: a multicenter comparison of laparoscopic and open approaches. Ann Surg 2008;248(3):438–46.
3. Palanivelu C, Jani K, Senthilnathan P, et al. Laparoscopic pancreaticoduodenectomy: technique and outcomes. J Am Coll Surg 2007;205:222–30.
4. Pierce RA. Outcomes analysis of laparoscopic resection of pancreatic neoplasms. Surg Endosc 2007;21(4):579–86.

FURTHER READING

Bassi C, Falconi M, Molinari E, et al. Duct-to-mucosa versus end-to-side pancreaticojejunostomy reconstruction after pancreaticoduodenectomy: results of a prospective randomized trial. Surgery 2003;134(5):766–71.

Bassi C, Molinari E, Malleo G, et al. Early versus late drain removal after standard pancreatic resections: results of a prospective randomized trial. Ann Surg 2010;252(2):207–14.

Berger AC, Howard TJ, Kennedy EP, et al. Does type of pancreaticojejunostomy after pancreaticoduodenectomy decrease rate of pancreatic fistula? A randomized, prospective, dual-institution trial. J Am Coll Surg 2009;208(5):738–47; discussion 747–9.

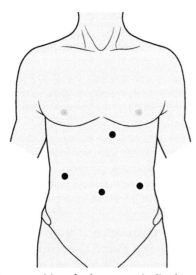

Fig. 16.21 Trocar positions for laparoscopic distal pancreatectomy.

Cahen DL, Gouma DJ, Nio Y, et al. Endoscopic versus surgical drainage of the pancreatic duct in chronic pancreatitis. N Engl J Med 2007;356 (7):676–84.

Conlon KC, Labow D, Leung D, et al. Prospective randomized clinical trial of the value of intraperitoneal drainage after pancreatic resection. Ann Surg 2001;234(4):487–93; discussion 493–4.

Diener MK, Bruckner T, Contin P, et al. ChroPac-trial: duodenum-preserving pancreatic head resection versus pancreatoduodenectomy for chronic pancreatitis. Trials 2010;11:47.

Farnell MB, Pearson RK, Sarr MG, et al. A prospective randomized trial comparing standard pancreatoduodenectomy with pancreatoduodenectomy with extended lymphadenectomy in resectable pancreatic head adenocarcinoma. Surgery 2005;138 (4):618–28; discussion 628–30.

Hwang TL, Chen HM, Chen MF. Surgery for chronic obstructive pancreatitis: comparison of end-to-side pancreaticojejunostomy with pancreatico-duodenectomy. Hepatogastroenterology 2001;48(37):270–2.

Izbicki JR, Bloechle C, Knoefel WT, et al. Duodenum-preserving resection of the head of the pancreas in chronic pancreatitis. A prospective, randomized trial. Ann Surg 1995;221(4):350–8.

Izbicki JR, Bloechle C, Broering DC, et al. Extended drainage versus resection in surgery for chronic pancreatitis: a prospective randomized trial comparing the longitudinal pancreaticojejunostomy combined with local pancreatic head excision with the pylorus-preserving pancreatoduodenectomy. Ann Surg 1998;228(6):771–9.

Köninger J, Seiler CM, Sauerland S, et al. Duodenum-preserving pancreatic head resection – a randomized controlled trial comparing the original Beger procedure with the Berne modification (ISRCTN No. 50638764). Surgery 2008;143(4):490–8.

Koti RS, Gurusamy KS, Fusai G, et al. Meta-analysis of randomized controlled trials on the effectiveness of somatostatin analogues for pancreatic surgery: a Cochrane review. HPB (Oxford) 2010;12(3):155–65.

Lai EC, Lau SH, Lau WY. Measures to prevent pancreatic fistula after pancreatoduodenectomy: a comprehensive review. Arch Surg 2009;144 (11):1074–80.

Lee SE, Ahn YJ, Jang JY, et al. Prospective randomized pilot trial comparing closed suction drainage and gravity drainage of the pancreatic duct in pancreaticojejunostomy. J Hepatobiliary Pancreat Surg 2009;16(6):837–43.

Lin PW, Shan YS, Lin YJ, et al. Pancreaticoduodenectomy for pancreatic head cancer: PPPD versus Whipple procedure. Hepatogastroenterology 2005;52(65):1601–4.

Oláh A, Issekutz A, Belágyi T, et al. Randomized clinical trial of techniques for closure of the pancreatic remnant following distal pancreatectomy. Br J Surg 2009;96(6):602–7.

Pedrazzoli S, DiCarlo V, Dionigi R, et al. Standard versus extended lymphadenectomy associated with pancreatoduodenectomy in the surgical treatment of adenocarcinoma of the head of the pancreas: a multicenter, prospective, randomized study. Lymphadenectomy Study Group. Ann Surg 1998;228(4):508–17.

Poon RT, Fan ST, Lo CM, et al. External drainage of pancreatic duct with a stent to reduce leakage rate of pancreaticojejunostomy after pancreaticoduodenectomy: a prospective randomized trial. Ann Surg 2007;246(3):425–33; discussion 433–5.

Proske JM, Zieren J, Müller JM. Transverse versus midline incision for upper abdominal surgery. Surg Today 2005;35(2):117–21.

Riall TS, Cameron JL, Lillemoe KD, et al. Pancreaticoduodenectomy with or without distal gastrectomy and extended retroperitoneal lymphadenectomy for periampullary adenocarcinoma – part 3: update on 5-year survival. J Gastrointest Surg 2005;9(9):1191–1204; discussion 1204–6.

Suzuki Y, Fujino Y, Tanioka Y, et al. Randomized clinical trial of ultrasonic dissector or conventional division in distal pancreatectomy for non-fibrotic pancreas. Br J Surg 1999;86(5):608–11.

van Santvoort HC, Besselink MG, Bakker OJ, et al. A step-up approach or open necrosectomy for necrotizing pancreatitis. N Engl J Med 2010;362 (16):1491–502.

Wente MN, Shrikhande SV, Müller MW, et al. Pancreaticojejunostomy versus pancreaticogastrostomy: systematic review and meta-analysis. Am J Surg 2007;193(2):171–83.

Winter JM, Cameron JL, Campbell KA, et al. Does pancreatic duct stenting decrease the rate of pancreatic fistula following pancreaticoduodenectomy? Results of a prospective randomized trial. J Gastrointest Surg 2006;10(9):1280–90; discussion 1290.

Zhou W, Lv R, Wang X, et al. Stapler vs suture closure of pancreatic remnant after distal pancreatectomy: a meta-analysis. Am J Surg 2010;200(4):529–36.

Liver and portal venous system

B.R. Davidson, R.S. Koti

CONTENTS

INTRODUCTION

Liver surgery has evolved considerably over the last two decades and can be carried out with a low morbidity and mortality, and often without the need for blood transfusion. Up to 70% of the liver can be resected with a mortality of less than 5%. The surgery is, however, technically complex and should wherever possible be undertaken in specialist centres.

TRAUMA

The liver is the second most common organ injured in abdominal trauma. Blunt liver trauma, for example following road traffic accidents, is more common than penetrating trauma such as stab or gunshot injuries. The mortality is much higher for blunt liver trauma and it increases even more if associated with other visceral injuries. Types of injuries include laceration, contusion, haematoma, vascular injury, bile duct and gallbladder injury. Over the last two decades there has been a paradigm shift in liver trauma management from compulsory operative treatment to non-operative management.[1–4]

Appraise

1 The patient will frequently present in a shocked state: the first priority is to maintain airway, breathing and circulation (ABC), following the principles of advanced trauma life support (ATLS). After ensuring normal cardiorespiratory function, carry out a secondary survey, examining the head, spine, chest and limbs as well as the abdomen. If the external injuries do not explain the degree of shock, assume there is internal bleeding. Stop external haemorrhage by direct pressure, splint any broken limbs, protect a fractured spine, treat a crushed chest by mechanical ventilation and assess any head injury. Now direct your attention to the internal bleeding.

2 Focused assessment sonography in trauma (FAST) is very valuable in diagnosing free intra-peritoneal fluid when performed by trained staff but is not reliable in diagnosing parenchymal injury. An emergency laparotomy is mandatory in the presence of free intra-peritoneal fluid on FAST in a haemodynamically unstable patient. However, if the patient is haemodynamically stable then obtain an urgent contrast enhanced computed tomography (CT) scan to diagnose and grade parenchymal injury. The four quadrant abdominal tap was superseded by diagnostic peritoneal lavage (DPL). However, DPL is often oversensitive and nowadays is performed less frequently due to increased use of FAST and CT. Very few surgeons in the UK now have experience in performing DPL.

3 If you remain in doubt and the patient fails to respond to resuscitation, consider performing an emergency laparotomy.

4 Penetrating injuries and gunshot wounds are treated by laparotomy. Treat conservatively only selected patients with stab injury who are haemodynamically stable and in whom there is no evidence of hollow viscus perforation.

5 Treat conservatively those patients with blunt trauma who are haemodynamically stable, even if there is demonstrable liver injury on CT or ultrasound scan. Monitor the patient with repeated clinical assessment and scans. If the patient becomes haemodynamically unstable or develops signs of peritonitis, proceed to a laparotomy.

6 Interventional radiology is now an important part of liver trauma management. Angiography and hepatic artery embolization is safe and effective in controlling hepatic arterial bleeding. If the patient is haemodynamically stable, consider angiography and embolization if there is extravasation of contrast on CT. This will decrease the number of blood transfusions and may avoid a laparotomy.

> ### ► KEY POINT Emergencies
>
> ■ Blunt trauma in stable patients should be assessed by CT. If the patient fails to respond to resuscitation then perform an emergency laparotomy.

EXPLORATION OF A DAMAGED LIVER

Prepare

1 Have you booked an intensive care unit bed if needed postoperatively?

2 You are about to embark on a major surgical procedure, carrying a high mortality rate. As far as possible, ensure you have an

experienced anaesthetist, competent assistant and experienced scrub nurse. Ensure vascular clamps and sutures are readily available.

3 Maintain good communication with your anaesthetist and scrub team. There is potential for sudden, life-threatening haemorrhage during the procedure. Good team work is essential for achieving a successful outcome.

4 Check the clotting. If coagulopathy is present give fresh-frozen plasma (FFP), platelets and cryoprecipitate as necessary. Watch for the deadly triad of coagulopathy, hypothermia and acidosis. If this is present then surgical control of the bleeding is unlikely to be successful.

5 Pass a bladder catheter. It is essential to monitor urine output and ensure adequate fluid volume replacement during major liver surgery to avoid acute renal failure.

6 Your anaesthetist will place a central venous line, wide-bore peripheral venous lines and, ideally, an arterial catheter to allow constant measurement of arterial pressure. A warming blanket is used to prevent hypothermia.

7 Ensure there are at least six units of blood available, together with FFP and platelets to replace lost clotting products.

Access

1 If you suspect the diagnosis preoperatively, use a transverse incision in the right upper quadrant, extending from a point 2 cm above the umbilicus to a point on the midaxillary line midway between the subcostal margin and iliac crest, with a vertical midline extension to the xiphoid. If necessary extend the incision across the midline transversely in the left upper quadrant. If you need to gain access above the liver, create a second incision in the tenth rib bed from the anterior axillary line to join the original subcostal incision at right angles. This allows you to open the chest, divide the costal margin and so gain control of the inferior vena cava (IVC) above the diaphragm.

2 If you discover the rupture at diagnostic laparotomy through a midline incision, create a transverse lateral extension to the right (as described above) to gain access and assess the need for further extensions.

3 If you discover the rupture through a lower abdominal incision, close it and re-explore the abdomen through an appropriate incision.

4 Use a self-retaining retractor that can be fixed to the operating table and provides forcible upward retraction of the costal margins, such as Thompson's retractor (Thompson Surgical Instruments Inc.). It crucially reduces the need for manual assistance, greatly improves access and usually eliminates the need for thoracic extension of the incision.

Assess

1 There is usually a great deal of blood clot in the peritoneal cavity and probably some fresh bleeding. Remove clot with your hands and a sucker.

2 Look systematically for damage to the liver, spleen, the gut from oesophagus to rectum, pancreas, anterior and posterior abdominal wall and the diaphragm. If necessary, pack the abdominal cavity with sterile packs, removing them serially, inspecting each of the four quadrants in succession.

Action

1 If there is obvious damage to, and haemorrhage from, another intra-abdominal viscus such as the spleen, and that is the primary source of bleeding, surround the damaged area of the liver with large sterile packs and have an assistant apply gentle pressure to control the bleeding. Attend to the lesion in the other organ first, and then turn your attention to the liver.

2 Inspection and palpation of the liver surface will allow you to estimate the extent of the parenchymal injury. Place packs over the superior and inferior surfaces of the liver to compress the laceration or contusion. Remove blood and blood clots to gain adequate exposure of the bleeding area of the liver. The initial packing with compression of the liver parenchyma will control much of the active bleeding. If the patient has coagulopathy, wait with the packs in place until sufficient FFP, platelets or cryoprecipitate have been transfused. Most patients do not require major surgical procedures: attempt only the minimum surgery necessary to control haemorrhage.

3 If initial packing does not control the haemorrhage then perform inflow occlusion (Pringle manoeuvre) by inserting a finger through the opening into the lesser sac behind the hepatic hilar structures and apply a Satinsky or other vascular clamp across them. If you do not have vascular clamps available, carefully apply a non-crushing intestinal clamp. This manoeuvre stops bleeding from branches of the hepatic artery and portal vein.

4 If bleeding persists despite the Pringle manoeuvre, then the bleeding is from the hepatic veins or the inferior vena cava, or the patient may have an aberrant arterial supply such as an accessory left hepatic artery arising from the left gastric artery, or an aberrant right hepatic artery arising from the superior mesenteric artery.

5 Avoid rough handling of sites of injury that are not bleeding at the time of exploration. If the patient is hypotensive there is risk of reactionary haemorrhage when the blood pressure subsequently rises.

> ▶ KEY POINT Remember to stick to essentials
>
> ▪ Your primary aims are, in order: to stop the bleeding, to remove obviously devitalized liver tissue and to stop bile leaks.

6 Explore the liver injury locally and remove any devascularized tissue. If the laceration continues to bleed and extends deeply into the liver parenchyma, gently explore the depth of the wound but avoid creating further damage. This procedure is very important in contusion injuries where major branches of the liver vessels may be ruptured, producing large areas of devascularized tissue. Do not be tempted to explore tears that are not bleeding, since you only encourage further bleeding.

7 Identify bleeding points and ligate them with fine synthetic absorbable material such as polyglactin 910 (Vicryl) or polydioxane sulphate (PDS) or use titanium Ligaclips. Suture-ligate larger vessels with PDS or Vicryl.

8 If there is vascular oozing from a large raw area of liver, cover it with one layer of absorbable haemostatic gauze (Surgicel) and apply a pack. Fibrin sealants such as Tisseel or Tachosil (Baxter) may help in stopping the ooze from a raw surface. Avoid using deep mattress sutures to control such bleeding, since they may produce areas of devascularization, which predisposes to subsequent infection.

9 Although a normal liver can tolerate normothermic ischaemia for up to 1 hour, after clamping the liver hilar vessels it is advisable to release the clamp for 10 minutes every 15 minutes, timed by the clock.

10 Before releasing any vascular clamps after prolonged clamping, warn the anaesthetist so that they may take precautionary measures against the effects of massive acidosis and potassium release, which can cause cardiac arrest.

11 Injuries involving the major hepatic veins close to the suprahepatic inferior vena cava or injuries to the retrohepatic inferior vena cava are very difficult to treat and even in experienced hands they are associated with high mortality. Bleeding from such injuries is not controlled by clamping the liver hilum. Attempt to mobilize the inferior vena cava above and below the liver. Complete mobilization of the right lobe of liver is required to expose the retrohepatic vena cava: identify the caval tear and suture it. Clamping the vena cava above and below the liver in addition to clamping the liver hilum will achieve total vascular isolation of the liver, but do not attempt this unless you are very experienced. Veno-venous bypass can be used to shunt blood from the femoral vein to the internal jugular vein to maintain venous return to the heart when total vascular isolation is attempted. However, expertise in veno-venous bypass is generally available only in specialist transplant units.

12 *Perihepatic packing.* If you cannot achieve control using the described techniques, do not attempt a major resection as an emergency procedure without the assistance of an experienced hepatic surgeon. This is rarely necessary in an emergency and has a high mortality rate. It has been shown in several studies that control is better achieved by packing around the liver with gauze rolls. Do not insert gauze into the depths of a liver laceration. Gently place the packs above, behind and below the liver to compress the bleeding areas (Fig. 17.1).

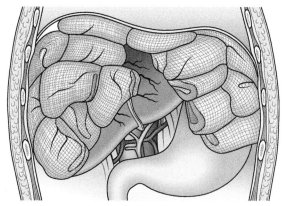

Fig. 17.1 Placement of packs around a ruptured liver. (Adapted from Blumgart LM (ed.). Surgery of the liver and biliary tract. Churchill Livingstone, Edinburgh, p 1230, 1994.)

13 Having gained control with perihepatic packing, close the abdomen. Carry out a contrast-enhanced CT scan and if necessary, a hepatic angiogram. You may then choose to either re-explore in 48–72 hours to remove the packs and re-assess, or transfer the patient to a specialist liver surgery unit.

14 If you encounter torrential bleeding from the liver during the laparotomy, consider autotransfusion using a cell saver system, if available. This will allow you to keep pace with the blood loss whilst attempting to control the haemorrhage.

15 *Is there damage to the extrahepatic biliary tree?* Attempt reconstruction by anastomosing cut ends of the bile duct end-to-end over a T-tube splint inserted through healthy bile duct. Use fine, interrupted absorbable sutures such as 4/0 Vicryl or PDS. If the damage to the duct is excessive, identify the most distal section of duct which is undamaged below the liver and divide it there. Suture-ligate the distal stump of the bile duct. Anastomose the proximal end of the bile duct to the side of a loop of jejunum, preferably a Roux-en-Y loop, using interrupted sutures of fine Vicryl or PDS in a single-layer anastomosis.

16 If the patient is very ill and unstable, there is no urgency in carrying out a biliary anastomosis. Leave a tube drain through the abdominal wall down to the site of biliary leak; the repair can be carried out by an expert at a later date.

Check

1 When you have gained control of the bleeding from the liver, carry out a full, careful and gentle exploration for other intra-peritoneal injuries if you have not done so already. Examine the entire gut from the oesophagus to rectum, paying special attention to the retroperitoneal duodenum, the pancreas and the spleen.

2 When you are certain that haemorrhage is controlled and that other lesions have been appropriately dealt with, inspect the liver once more, unless you needed to pack it to control haemorrhage. If there are devascularized areas, remove them to prevent infection.

> ▶ **KEY POINTS** Decision
>
> ■ If you have had no experience of liver resection then pack rather than resect.
> ■ Either transfer the patient to an experienced colleague or seek advice before re-exploring the liver yourself after a few days, when the patient's condition is stable.
> ■ If you find bile leaking from damaged intrahepatic bile ducts, ligate or suture them.

Closure

1 Before you close, mop the peritoneal cavity dry with surgical swabs, or carry out a gentle lavage with warm normal saline and then suck out all the fluid.

2 Close the abdomen using a standard mass technique.

3 If you have operated on any part of the biliary tract insert a drain, preferably with a closed system. If there is liver parenchymal damage only, then a drain is probably unnecessary in the absence of an obvious biliary leak.

Aftercare

1 Admit the patient to an intensive care unit or high-dependency nursing area.

2 If further operation is required, for example because packs were inserted to control haemorrhage, arrange transfer to a specialist unit if possible. Packs increase the risk of sepsis, therefore give antibiotics whilst packs are in place.

3 Mechanically ventilate the patient electively and maintain the blood gases within normal range until the patient is haemodynamically stable, other injuries have been treated and the core temperature has returned to normal. Correct any remaining electrolyte imbalance. Measure blood sugar hourly and treat any abnormality immediately.

4 Evaluate biochemical liver function daily.

5 Maintain intravascular volume and normal clotting. Transfuse with blood and FFP as required.

6 Maintain urine flow. If it falls below 30 ml/hour, first check that the circulating blood volume is adequate, with normal blood pressure and central venous pressure. If you are in any doubt about this, give a 'fluid challenge' of 250 ml of colloid intravenously. If this fails to stimulate urine flow despite an adequate blood pressure and normal central venous pressure, consider a low-dose dopamine infusion. If this fails to improve urine flow give 40 mg of furosemide (frusemide) intravenously and seek the advice of a renal physician.

7 Give broad-spectrum antibiotics such as a combination of cefuroxime and metronidazole.

8 If gastrointestinal activity does not return within 2–3 days, institute intravenous nutrition.

9 Sudden collapse suggests that the patient has developed further internal bleeding or septicaemia. If this is associated with abdominal swelling, resuscitate with intravenous blood or colloid, and FFP if the clotting screen is abnormal. Order a contrast-enhanced CT scan and return the patient to the operating room if haemorrhage is confirmed.

10 If you suspect septicaemia then order investigations to determine the source. Culture blood, urine and any leaking body fluid; order a chest X-ray and carry out an ultrasound or CT scan of the abdomen to look for an abscess. Give appropriate antibiotics. Drain an intra-peritoneal abscess either by a further operation or by ultrasound-guided needle aspiration. If the patient is very shocked and the diagnosis uncertain, it is safer to re-explore the abdomen than to wait. Intra-abdominal sepsis is very common following liver trauma and devascularized areas of the liver may become necrotic and infected.

> ► KEY POINT It is better to look and see than wait and see

■ If you are in any doubt about further bleeding or sepsis, re-exploration is safer than waiting. If you fail to recognize and treat it, the patient may die.

RE-EXPLORATION

Prepare

1 If arterial injury is suspected due to extravasation of contrast on CT or signs of active haemorrhage in the absence of another source of bleeding, obtain a hepatic arteriogram before re-exploration to allow preoperative embolization and to fully assess any vascular damage: this will allow you to prepare for appropriate surgical management and, if necessary, obtain expert help.

2 Ensure that the patient is stable and correct biochemical and haematological abnormalities. Discuss any clotting impairment with the haematologists and give cryoprecipitate or FFP before surgery.

3 Order six units of blood and some platelets and FFP.

Access

1 Gently and carefully open the previous incision.

2 If the abdomen had been packed at the original laparotomy then soak the packs with saline before you attempt to remove them. Remove them slowly and gently. Send a piece immediately for microbiological culture.

Assess

1 If there is no bleeding from the liver do not mobilize or retract it as this may result in renewed blood loss.

Action

1 Suture-ligate bleeding points with a fine suture or apply haemostats to any obvious bleeding vessels and ligate them.

2 Aspirate any bile collections and attempt to ligate or suture any leaking bile ducts.

3 If major bleeding starts again, attempt to identify the main vessel and suture it. On rare occasions you may carry out lobectomy (see below) if the injury is confined to one lobe.

4 Occasionally, following a severe blunt crushing injury, the damage is so great that no surgical procedure can save the patient's life, even in the most expert of hands.

Closure

1 If you are sure there are no more local problems, perform a warm saline peritoneal lavage, close the abdomen and continue antibiotic therapy, modified as appropriate when culture and sensitivity data are available.

Aftercare

See above.

REFERENCES

1. Piper GL, Peitzman AB. Current management of hepatic trauma. Surgery Clinics of North America 2010;90:775–85.
2. Kozar RA, McNutt MK. Management of adult blunt hepatic trauma. Curr Opin Crit Care 2010 Sep 9 (E-pub ahead of print).
3. Badger SA, Barclay R, Campbell P, et al. Management of liver trauma. World J Surg 2009;33:2522–37.
4. Milla DJ, Brasel K. Current use of CT in the evaluation and management of injured patients. Surgery Clinics of North America 2011;91:233–48.

PRINCIPLES OF ELECTIVE SURGERY

Appraise

> ▶ KEY POINT Caution
>
> ■ Liver surgery is complex and should be carried out in specialist high-volume centres.

1. The commonest indication for liver resection is primary or secondary malignancy. Hepatocellular carcinoma, cholangiocarcinoma, gall bladder carcinoma and colorectal liver metastases are the most frequent indications for liver resection. Benign diseases such as cavernous haemangioma, adenoma, focal nodular hyperplasia and cystic diseases may occasionally require liver resection. Rarely, liver resection may be required for managing liver injuries. Over the last two decades, liver resection has been increasingly used to procure part of the liver from living donors for liver transplantation.

2. The treatment of hepatobiliary cancers should be discussed at a specialist multidisciplinary meeting involving surgeons, hepatologists, oncologists and interventional radiologists.

3. Do not undertake an elective operation on the liver without complete preoperative investigation and a fairly certain working diagnosis. Occasionally, an isolated hepatic lesion may be identified during a scan carried out for another reason. If you discover a lesion in the liver during a laparotomy, carefully consider the risks before trying to excise or biopsy it. Operating on a patient with impaired liver function can be very hazardous and carries a high morbidity and mortality.

4. The preoperative workup should start with a detailed history and physical examination of the patient. Liver resection in the presence of underlying chronic liver disease is associated with increased morbidity and mortality. Look for signs of chronic liver disease on examination.

5. Carry out biochemical liver function tests, blood count and clotting profile. Underlying chronic liver disease should be suspected if there is an elevated bilirubin, low albumin, increased prothrombin time or low platelet count. Check the tumour markers alfa-feto protein (primary liver cancer) and carcinoembryonic antigen (gastrointestinal cancers) if you suspect a malignant lesion. If chronic liver disease is suspected, carry out hepatitis virus and autoimmune antibody screens.

6. Ultrasound (US) is usually the initial imaging modality for patients presenting with abdominal pain or jaundice. US is useful in assessing the size of the liver and bile ducts, confirming gall stones and detection of ascites, and may show a tumour mass in the liver. Computed tomography (CT) and magnetic resonance imaging (MRI) are optimal investigations for characterizing the nature of liver lesions, assessing resectability and tumour staging. CT and MRI may demonstrate features of chronic liver disease or cirrhosis and can accurately quantify the volume of the liver remnant following resection.

7. Angiography demonstrates hepatic vascular anatomy and vascular involvement by tumour, which often dictates whether resection is feasible. CT angiography and MR angiography have high diagnostic accuracy and conventional angiography is rarely used nowadays.

8. When CT and MRI findings are equivocal in the diagnosis or staging of malignancy, PET scan may be of use. However, there is no role for the routine use of PET in the diagnosis or staging of hepatobiliary malignancies.

9. Inadequate volume of the liver remnant can lead to hepatic insufficiency after extended right or left hepatectomies. In such instances, consider preoperative portal vein embolization to increase the volume of the future liver remnant. This is performed in the radiology suite by an interventional radiologist. Through a percutaneous transhepatic route the desired portal vein segments are embolized with embolic agents such as polyvinyl alcohol, foam particles or coils. If radiological expertise is not available surgical ligation of the desired branches of portal vein can be performed, although it complicates subsequent definitive surgery because of hilar scarring.

10. Laparoscopy is an important part of the staging of primary liver and biliary tract malignancies as it can detect peritoneal disease which is often overlooked by both CT and MRI. Tru-cut biopsy of the future remnant liver can be obtained at laparoscopy to exclude underlying parenchymal liver disease.

11. Be cautious about performing percutaneous biopsies of resectable liver tumours. There is now good evidence that malignant cells can seed along the biopsy track. Current CT and MRI technology is highly accurate in diagnosing malignant lesions and histological confirmation is not required prior to resection. Biopsy may be required for histological confirmation of malignancy before commencing palliative treatment in patients with unresectable disease.

12. In patients with liver tumours and a background of chronic liver disease consider wedged hepatic venous pressure (WHVP) measurements. WHVP corrected for inferior vena caval pressure gives an estimate of portal venous pressure: it increases in portal hypertension secondary to chronic liver disease and is an independent predictor of poor outcome after liver resection.

13. Before undertaking any operative procedure on a patient with chronic liver disease, check the blood film, platelet count and clotting profile and correct any abnormality, if possible by giving blood products. Rarely are platelet infusions necessary, but all patients undergoing liver surgery, especially if jaundiced or with severe biochemical dysfunction, benefit from injections of vitamin K_1. If the clotting profile is badly deranged, the patient may need an infusion of FFP and occasionally cryoprecipitate.

BIOPSY OR RESECTION OF A LIVER LESION FOUND AT THE TIME OF LAPAROTOMY

Action

1. Select an area of diseased liver or an edge that presents easily through the incision.

2. Place two mattress stitches of 3/0 Vicryl or PDS on an atraumatic round-bodied needle to form a V, the apex of this pointing towards the hilum of the liver (Fig. 17.2A).

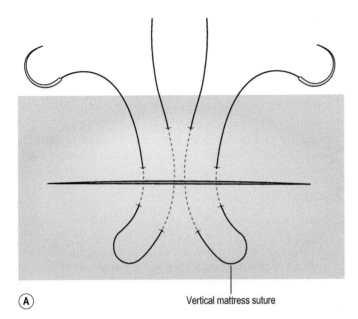

(A) Vertical mattress suture

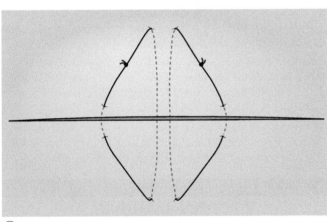

(B)

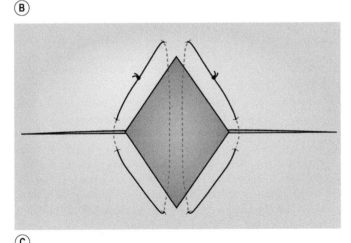

(C)

Fig. 17.2 Technique for wedge liver biopsy: (A) initial placement of two mattress stitches; (B) tie each firmly; (C) remove the wedge of tissue between them.

3 Gently but firmly tie these stitches (Fig. 17.2B) and remove the wedge of tissue between them with a sharp knife (Fig. 17.2C). The cut edges of the liver should be dry. Insert another suture of similar material if haemostasis is not complete or use diathermy coagulation to establish haemostasis.

4 You may also use a Tru-cut needle to take a liver biopsy. If you are not familiar with the needle, rehearse your movements before inserting it into the liver. After removing the needle, check that you have an adequate core of tissue. Gently shake or tease the core of tissue into a pot of formalin, taking care not to crush it. The puncture site occasionally requires a figure-of-eight or Z-stitch with 4/0 Vicryl or PDS to obtain haemostasis.

INFECTIVE LESIONS

BACTERIAL LIVER ABSCESS

Appraise

1 Open surgical drainage of liver abscesses is rarely necessary. The standard treatment is a prolonged course of antibiotics along with aspiration of the pus under ultrasound guidance as the abscess matures or liquefies.

2 Until the exact nature and antibiotic sensitivities of the causative organism are known, administer intravenous broad-spectrum antibiotics such as co-amoxiclav, carbapenem or cephalosporin empirically.

3 Liver abscesses require prolonged treatment which can usually be carried out as an outpatient. Continue antibiotics and US surveillance with admission for US-guided aspiration if clinically septic or the abscess is increasing in size.

4 You may have to aspirate the abscess several times, but if it fails to respond to repeated aspiration and antibiotics or the percutaneous insertion of a drain, then very rarely you may be forced to operate. Localize the abscess first with ultrasound or CT scans. Administer intravenous antibiotics. Cross-match four units of blood and have available FFP. Use intra-operative ultrasound, if available, to identify the site of an intrahepatic lesion.

Access

1 Use a right subcostal incision 3 cm below the costal margin for an anterior abscess.

2 Approach a posterior abscess through the bed of the right posterior 12th rib.

Action

1 Isolate the peritoneal contents from the area of the abscess by packs.

2 Insert a needle into the abscess, aspirate some of the contents to send for immediate examination and culture, including anaerobic culture, to confirm the diagnosis.

3 Incise the abscess and suck out the contents. Gently insert a finger to identify and breakdown all loculi.

4 Wash out the cavity with physiological saline.

5 Insert a tube drain, preferably as a closed system such as a Robinson drain. Pass the distal end of the drain through the abdominal wall at a suitable site, not through the incision.

6 Achieve haemostasis at the edge of the liver incision by using 3/0 Vicryl or PDS mattress sutures on an atraumatic needle or diathermy coagulation.

7 If possible, draw some omentum into the abscess cavity.

8 Close the abdomen.

9 Leave the drain until drainage ceases and the cavity is demonstrably collapsed on ultrasound, CT or a sinogram. Until then continue appropriate antibiotics.

AMOEBIC ABSCESS

Appraise

1 This rarely requires surgical treatment.

2 Positively confirm the diagnosis by identifying amoebae in a fresh aspirate, or a positive serological test (antibodies to Entamoeba histolytica). The presence of amoebae in stools is indicative, but absence of organisms does not exclude the diagnosis.

3 Treatment is with metronidazole, 400–800 mg orally 8-hourly in an adult for 10 days. Resolution of the abscess can be monitored using regular ultrasound screening. If it becomes secondarily infected or is discovered at laparotomy then treat it like any other liver abscess.

HYDATID CYST

Appraise

1 Suspect a hydatid cyst in patients who present with a liver mass and who live or have lived in an endemic area (developing countries, the Mediterranean and Middle East, South America and South Australia). Confirm it by the presence of eosinophilia, positive hydatid serology and classic ultrasound and CT appearances.

2 Past treatment was mainly surgical. There are many reports that percutaneous treatment combined with antihelminthic drug therapy is safe and effective in selected patients with uncomplicated cysts.[1] Consider it only if the cyst does not communicate with the biliary system on ERCP (endoscopic retrograde cholangiopancreatography). Remember that this procedure carries a low but definite risk of anaphylaxis. Administer an initial course of albendazole, followed by Puncture of the cyst under imaging guidance, Aspiration of the cyst contents, Instillation of hypertonic saline into the cyst cavity and then Re-aspiration – the acronym is PAIR. In some centres a sclerosing agent is finally injected into the cyst cavity, followed by a further course of albendazole. Albendazole alone without percutaneous intervention is not considered ideal therapy; use it only if PAIR or surgery is not possible. Surgery, in the form of cystectomy and omentoplasty, is still preferred by many clinicians who feel there is insufficient evidence for the routine use of PAIR. It is certainly the standard treatment for complicated cysts, cysts that communicate with the biliary tree and where percutaneous therapy has failed.

Prepare

1 Give at least a 4-week cycle of albendazole tablets (10 mg/kg/day in divided doses for an adult) before and after surgery to prevent growth of any spilt protoscolices (Greek: protos = first + scolex = a worm). You may administer up to three cycles of 4 weeks each, with a 2-week gap between cycles. Some surgeons additionally cover the perioperative period with another drug, praziquantel.

2 Visualize the biliary tract preoperatively with ERCP if the cyst is close to the liver hilum or if there is any history of attacks of jaundice or cholangitis, suggesting a communication between the cyst and the biliary tree.

3 Have available a scolicidal agent with which to wash out the cyst to kill any remaining scolices. This can be absolute alcohol, 1% cetrimide, or sterile 20% saline, which is the safest. 10% formalin and 0.5% silver nitrate are no longer used as they can cause sclerosing cholangitis.

4 Have available sterile black towels (see below) with which to pack off the surrounding tissues. Some surgeons soak these in scolicidal solution.

5 Warn the anaesthetist to be prepared for sudden anaphylactic shock if there is inadvertent spillage of cyst contents into the peritoneal cavity, although this is rare.

Access

1 Make a transverse incision in the right upper quadrant, extending from a point 2 cm above the umbilicus to a point on the midaxillary line midway between the subcostal margin and iliac crest, with a vertical midline extension to the xiphoid. If possible, arrange for the incision to overlie the cyst.

Action

1 When you reach the cyst, take care in handling it to avoid rupture. It is usually attached to surrounding tissues by fibrinous adhesions which you must gently separate.

2 Isolate the cyst from the rest of the peritoneal contents with packs. Traditionally, these are covered with black towels, which are claimed to make any spilt daughter cysts or scolices more visible.

3 Insert a wide-bore trocar, using a purse-string suture to avoid spillage, into the cyst and carefully aspirate as much as possible of the contained fluid, then fill with hypertonic saline.

> ▶ KEY POINT Avoid spillage
>
> ■ Do not spill any of the cyst fluid, daughter cysts or membranes: they can infect any other part of the abdomen.

4 Aspirate the hypertonic saline through a suction unit without spillage.

5 When the cyst is empty fill it again with a fluid – ideally 20% saline – that will destroy any remaining protoscolices. Leave the fluid in the cyst for at least 10 minutes, then aspirate it and repeat the procedure. The preoperative ERCP should have demonstrated any communications between the cyst and the biliary tree: close them using an absorbable suture such as Vicryl or PDS before irrigating the cavity. Alternatively, place an atraumatic clamp on the extrahepatic bile duct to demonstrate any biliary communication.

6 De-roof the cyst as much as possible – a technique known as saucerization – to allow omentum and other peritoneal contents to fill the cavity easily and so avoid the problems associated with delayed healing and infection of intrahepatic fibrous-walled cavities with a narrow neck. The omentum may be tacked into place with a few absorbable sutures (omentoplasty).

7 The value of inserting a drain into the cyst cavity is controversial. If it is possible to saucerize it then do not drain. If you must leave the cavity with a narrow neck insert a closed drainage system.

8 If you have demonstrated any evidence of communication between the cyst and biliary tree, consider performing an operative cholangiogram to ensure that you have closed it and that the biliary tree is free from any obstructing daughter cysts, which will need to be removed.

9 Ensure that haemostasis is complete. Wash out the peritoneal cavity with large volumes of physiological saline.

Technical points

1 Some surgeons advocate excision of the cyst intact, including the 'pericyst' (Pericystectomy). In some circumstances this is possible, but often cysts are adherent to major vessels and can cause severe bleeding. A formal hepatic resection can also be performed. These operations require experience in liver surgery: attempt them only if you are experienced.

2 If there has been spillage of cyst contents into the peritoneal cavity, washing with sterile water may reduce the likelihood of further infestation because of the toxic osmotic effect of water on the protoscolices.

Postoperative

Watch for hypernatraemia if you have used large volumes of 20% saline.

OTHER CYSTS

Appraise

1 The majority of liver cysts are asymptomatic and are discovered usually on imaging for other pathology. When symptoms develop, they include right upper quadrant abdominal swelling, discomfort or acute pain associated with haemorrhage into the cyst or rupture of the cyst. Symptomatic cysts are usually diagnosed using ultrasound and CT.

2 Massive polycystic disease of the liver is rare, but can cause severe pain. In 50% of patients with polycystic disease there is associated polycystic renal disease. The renal lesions are more commonly associated with organ failure whereas patients with severe polycystic liver disease often have normal liver function. Some patients also have associated pancreatic cysts. These patients should be treated only in major centres since they may ultimately require liver transplantation.

3 Occasionally cysts become infected or develop haemorrhage, producing pain.

4 Liver cyst may also result from a biliary cystadenoma – a benign but premalignant lesion which requires formal resection.

5 Before attempting diagnostic percutaneous aspiration of a cyst, consider if it is hydatid (see section on hydatid cyst) or cystic tumour.

6 Don't operate on liver cysts unless they are symptomatic, a known hydatid cyst or for resection of cystadenoma.

Access

1 Make a transverse incision in the right upper quadrant, extending from a point 2 cm above the umbilicus to a point on the midaxillary line midway between the subcostal margin and iliac crest, with a vertical midline extension to the xiphoid.

Action

1 For a symptomatic large cyst, carefully de-roof it, allowing it to drain freely into the peritoneal cavity. You may gently pack omentum into it. Such a cyst may recur, but can then be treated by percutaneous aspiration or formal resection. If you are experienced in laparoscopic surgery you may elect to de-roof a symptomatic superficial liver cyst by a minimal access approach.

2 Cystadenoma will require formal liver resection (see section on neoplasms below).

REFERENCE

1. Nasseri Moghaddam S, Abrishami A, Malekzadeh R. Percutaneous needle aspiration, injection, and reaspiration with or without benzimidazole coverage for uncomplicated hepatic hydatid cysts. Cochrane Database Syst Rev 2006;(2):CD003623.

NEOPLASMS

Appraise

1 Liver neoplasms can be benign or malignant. Benign liver tumours are usually asymptomatic and incidentally detected on imaging for other pathology. Amongst malignant liver tumours, in the Western world metastases are more common than primary malignancies: the majority of metastases arise from colorectal cancers. Other less common primary sites are pancreas, stomach, lung and breast.

2 Modern CT and MRI have high accuracy in differentiating benign from malignant lesions. AFP, CEA, CA 19-9 levels are valuable but remember these tumour markers have low sensitivity and specificity.

3 Benign liver neoplasms such as haemangioma or focal nodular hyperplasia do not require surgical excision unless they are causing significant symptoms. Hepatic adenomas carry a risk of bleeding and of malignant change and most surgeons advocate resection of adenomas.

4 Malignant liver neoplasm should be considered for surgery since this is the only potentially curative treatment.

5 See the section on principles of elective surgery above for preoperative workup and staging. Remember, preoperative histological confirmation is not necessary if surgical resection is feasible, as biopsy may lead to needle-track tumour dissemination. Remember to obtain histological confirmation of underlying parenchymal liver disease before considering surgery in patients with suspected chronic liver disease.

6 Laparoscopic surgery has evolved significantly. Wedge liver resections of superficial and peripherally located tumours and, left lateral liver resections are commonly performed laparoscopically in most centres. In limited numbers, formal left and right hepatectomies have also been performed in selected centres. Success in laparoscopic major liver resections requires expertise in both liver surgery and laparoscopic surgery.

Prepare

1 Once operability and resectability is confirmed, prepare the patient for liver resection. Crossmatch four to six units of blood. Arrange platelets, fresh frozen plasma and cryoprecipitates to be available intra-operatively or postoperatively.

2 Make certain that clotting is normal. Correct clotting abnormalities preoperatively. Give vitamin K to jaundiced patients.

3 A Thompson type self-retaining retractor is an indispensable tool for liver operations. The retractor is fixed on the side of the operating table and provides forcible, upward retraction of the costal margins, giving safe and adequate access to all surfaces of the liver. Make sure the retractor is available in theatre.

4 Have available vascular clamps and sutures. Intra-operative ultrasound is valuable in planning your surgical strategy. Make sure the appropriate ultrasound probe for liver surface placement is available. Several techniques of parenchymal division are described including clamp crushing (Kelly-clysis), ultrasonic dissector, radiofrequency assisted devices, harmonic scalpel, vascular stapler, etc. Have available the instrument of your choice.

5 Maintain good communication with your anaesthetist. Sudden haemorrhage can occur anytime during the operation. The anaesthetist will insert central venous catheter, arterial cannula and large bore peripheral cannula. Remember, it is the hepatic veins which bleed more than the artery during parenchymal transection. It is now common practice to maintain a low CVP during parenchymal transection to limit bleeding from hepatic vein branches and maintain the patient in the reverse Trendelenburg position to decrease the risk of air embolism from disrupted hepatic veins. The anaesthetist lowers the CVP (<10 mmHg) by fluid restriction and anaesthetic techniques.

6 Pass a urinary catheter to monitor urine output.

7 Discuss and plan postoperative analgesia with your anaesthetist. The upper abdominal muscle cutting incision and costal margin retraction do give rise to considerable postoperative pain. It is common practice now to use epidural analgesia. Make sure the morning dose of subcutaneous heparin is omitted if an epidural catheter is going to be inserted.

WEDGE EXCISION OF SOLITARY LIVER LESION

Access

1 Make a transverse incision in the right upper quadrant, extending from a point 2 cm above the umbilicus to a point on the midaxillary line midway between the subcostal margin and iliac crest.

2 Add a vertical extension in the midline to the xiphoid. If greater exposure is required, a left transverse extension can be added to create a Mercedes-Benz incision.

3 You will rarely need to split the sternum or open the chest through a rib extension.

4 Stitch back the flaps and retract the costal margins with a Thompson self-retaining retractor.

Assess

1 Carry out a general exploration of the abdominal cavity to exclude peritoneal and omental disease, and other intra-abdominal pathology.

2 Explore the liver hilum. Identify the hepatic artery, portal vein and common bile duct and pass a tape around them. This allows a vascular clamp to be applied to control haemorrhage during liver resection – the Pringle manoeuvre.

3 Carefully palpate the entire liver and perform an intra-operative ultrasound examination of the entire liver to identify the number, site and vascular relations of all tumours and exclude additional disease. Open the gastrohepatic omentum and palpate the caudate lobe.

Action

1 Once you make the decision to proceed, mark the lines of parenchymal transection on the liver capsule with diathermy, at least 1 cm away from the macroscopic tumour margin.

2 If you are using hilar clamping (the Pringle manoeuvre, see above), although the normal liver can tolerate up to 60 minutes of warm ischaemia, to reduce hepatocellular damage to a minimum release the clamp for 10 minutes every 15 minutes.

3 Use the device of your choice for parenchymal division. As you divide the parenchyma, vessels and bile ducts will be exposed. Control the exposed vessel with diathermy, clips, ligatures or sutures. Always clip or ligate the exposed bile ducts.

4 Remove the tumour, and clip or ligate any remaining ducts and vessels. Coagulate with diathermy any remaining small bleeding points. Check the raw area for bile leaks and carefully oversew them with fine vicryl or PDS.

5 If the cut surface of the liver is not dry, cover it with absorbable haemostatic gauze (Surgicel) and apply a pack. After 10 minutes, gently remove the pack. The area should be dry. Coagulate any remaining bleeding points.

Check

1 Carefully inspect the cut surface to ensure haemostasis and no bile leaks.

2 Carefully inspect the liver hilum to ensure that no major structures have been damaged.

Closure

1 Once the cut surface of the liver is dry, wash the perihepatic peritoneal cavity with warm saline.

2 You may apply the omentum to the transected surface of the liver. There is no evidence that the traditional practice of inserting a drain offers any advantage.

3 Close the wound using a mass closure suture. Close the skin.

RIGHT OR LEFT HEPATECTOMY

For an extensive discussion of liver resection techniques refer to Blumgart.[1]

Anatomy

1 The liver is divided into two anatomical lobes, each being supplied by its own branch of the hepatic artery, portal vein and hepatic duct. The junction of the two lobes is in the line of the gallbladder bed (Fig. 17.3A). By ligating the hepatic artery and portal vein branches supplying either lobe, it is possible to demarcate the junction between them as a fairly sharp colour change.

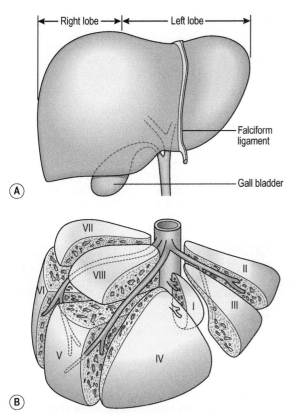

Fig. 17.3 Anatomy of the liver: (A) the main lobes of the liver; (B) diagrammatic representation of the segments of the liver. (Adapted from Launois B, Jamieson GG. Modern operative techniques in liver surgery. Churchill Livingstone, Edinburgh, p 7, 1993.)

2 The liver is further divided into eight segments, described initially by Couinaud[2] in 1957 (Fig. 17.3B). Segment I, adjacent to the IVC, is also known as the caudate lobe, and segment IV, between the falciform ligament and the main lobular division, is known as the quadrate lobe.

3 As a result of the hepatic architecture it is possible to divide the liver through the main plane separating the right and left lobes. It is also possible to remove segments of the liver. Removal of all the liver tissue to the right of the falciform ligament (right lobe plus segment IV) is called an extended right hepatectomy or trisegmentectomy.

4 Removal of segments II and III of the left lobe, that part of the liver to the left of the falciform ligament, is comparatively straightforward and is usually carried out laparoscopically in most units.

Appraise

The size and position of the cancer, the necessity for a clearance margin and the function of the underlying parenchyma will dictate whether a formal hepatic resection (right, left or extended hepatectomy), segmental resection or non-anatomical wedge excision is indicated. The clearance margin is ideally at least 1 cm.

Access

1 Make a transverse incision in the right upper quadrant, extending from a point 2 cm above the umbilicus to a point midway between the subcostal margin and iliac crest on the midaxillary line.

2 Add a vertical extension from the midpoint to the xiphoid. If greater exposure is required, a left transverse extension can be added to create a Mercedes-Benz incision.

3 You will rarely need to split the sternum or open the chest through a rib extension.

4 Stitch back the flaps and retract the costal margins with a Thompson self-retaining retractor.

Action

1 After positioning the self-retaining retractor, perform a full exploration of all abdominal viscera and palpation of the pelvis. Next, divide the falciform ligament on the anterior surface of the liver as far as the suprahepatic IVC using the diathermy. This will allow you to mobilize the liver by dividing right and left triangular ligaments.

2 Divide the peritoneal reflections between the back of the liver lobe and the diaphragm and retract the lobe from the diaphragm and posterior abdominal wall until you see the retrohepatic IVC.

3 The main inflow pedicle to the affected lobe can be controlled extrahepatically prior to parenchymal transection or intrahepatically during parenchymal transection. For extrahepatic control, dissect the hepatic hilum and identify the branches of the hepatic artery, portal vein and bile duct supplying and draining the affected lobe. Identify and dissect the cystic duct and artery and perform a cholecystectomy first as this is the plane of division for a right or left hepatectomy.

4 Divide the artery, duct and portal vein branches supplying the lobe to be removed and oversew or transfix the ends of the vessels with fine prolene and duct with PDS (Fig. 17.4A). Alternatively, you can divide the entire pedicle within the Glissonian sheath with a vascular stapler, which is quicker.

5 Carefully dissect, ligate and divide all hepatic vein branches entering the IVC from the liver. Identify the small veins from segment I (the caudate lobe), entering the IVC. Dissect, transfix or clip and divide them (Fig. 17.4B). Carefully dissect the main hepatic veins (right, middle or left) draining the lobe to be removed; they will be divided later.

6 Return to the anterior surface of the liver. You are now ready to start transecting the liver parenchyma. Inform your anaesthetist that you are about to commence parenchymal transection so that they lower the CVP. You should be able to identify a demarcation line between the devascularized lobe to be removed and the normal vascularized liver which is to remain.

7 Just on the vascularized side of this demarcation line mark your line of parenchymal transection on the liver capsule with diathermy.

8 Use Kelly-clysis or the instrument of your choice, such as the ultrasonic dissector, to divide the liver substance between this incision and the IVC.

9 Ligate or suture with fine prolene or PDS, or clip with titanium clips any vascular or biliary tract structures crossing the line of transection as you encounter them.

10 As your plane of transection goes deeper into the liver parenchyma, you will encounter larger branches of the hepatic veins. Clip and divide these with fine haemostats.

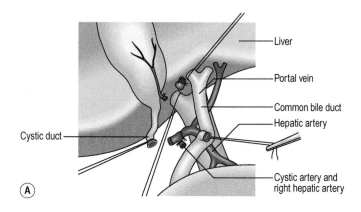

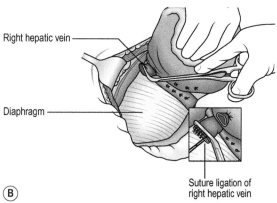

Fig. 17.4   Right hepatectomy: (A) the vessels supplying the lobe to be removed are divided and transfixed; (B) the hepatic veins from the lobe to be removed are divided and oversewn.

11 Finally, clamp the main hepatic veins (right, middle or left) with vascular clamps before dividing them. Use vascular suture to oversew the ends (Fig. 17.4B). You may use an endovascular stapler, if one is available, to divide and staple the hepatic veins.

12 Control any smaller bleeding points by diathermy coagulation.

13 If there is continued bleeding, cover the raw area of the liver with absorbable haemostatic gauze (Surgicel) and apply a pack for 10 minutes.

Check

1 When haemostasis is complete, check the hilar structures to ensure that they are intact.

2 Check that the remnant liver is well perfused with good haemostasis and no bile leaks.

Closure

1 Gently flush the peritoneal cavity with warm saline.

2 Cover the transected area of liver with omentum and close the abdomen. Tube drains may be placed to detect bile leaks postoperatively.

Technical point

1 T-tube drainage of the biliary tract is unnecessary unless you suspect some distal obstruction, or if there has been damage to the common bile duct.

Aftercare

1 The initial postoperative management of these patients is critical, and is best carried out in an intensive care or high-dependency unit for the first 24 hours, or at least until the patient is warm, extubated, self-ventilating and haemodynamically stable.

2 The broad principles of management are as outlined in the aftercare of major liver trauma.

REFERENCES

1. Blumgart LH, editor. Surgery of the Liver, Biliary Tract and Pancreas, vol. 2, 4th ed. Philadelphia, PA: Saunders Elsevier; 2006. p. 1341–451.
2. Couinaud C. Le Foie. Etudes anatomiques et chirurgicales. Paris: Masson; 1957.

SURGICAL MANAGEMENT OF HAEMORRHAGE FROM OESOPHAGEAL VARICES

The most life-threatening complication of chronic liver disease that requires surgical treatment is bleeding from oesophageal varices secondary to portal hypertension. Over the last two decades, the mortality from acute variceal bleeding has decreased because of improvement in general management and expertise in endoscopic and radiological techniques.

Management of a patient with variceal haemorrhage is complex and is ideally undertaken by a specialist team including a medical hepatologist, specialist radiologist and a surgeon.[1,2,3]

Appraise

1 Aim to resuscitate the patient, find the site of the bleeding and stop it. These three processes must be carried out in parallel. The prognosis is directly related to the severity of any underlying liver disease. Minimal hepatocellular damage (Child class A/B) carries a good prognosis; if it is severe (Child class C), the prognosis is poor. As there is no way of predicting which patients will fare badly or well, initially treat them all actively. Generally, patients with Child class A or B disease are likely to respond to standard medical therapy. In patients with Child class C disease the decision to place transjugular intrahepatic portosystemic shunt (TIPSS) needs to be made early in the management.

2 Patients with suspected variceal haemorrhage should be admitted to the intensive care unit.

3 Assess the patient's airway and insert two large-bore peripheral cannulas. Resuscitate by restoring and maintaining circulating volume with intravenous fluids, blood and plasma expanders as necessary. The aim is to maintain haemodynamic stability. Avoid hypervolaemia as this will increase the portal pressure and exacerbate the bleeding. Avoid excess use of saline for fluid resuscitation as this can worsen ascites. Many patients will have coagulopathy which should be corrected fully with FFP, platelets and vitamin K. Recombinant factor VII is expensive and there is no good evidence to support its routine use in the control of variceal haemorrhage.

4 Antibiotic prophylaxis has been shown to reduce the risk of bacterial infections which are associated with recurrence of bleeding. Use norfloxacin, ceftriaxone or ciprofloxacin.

5 Initiate treatment with a splanchnic vasoconstrictor such as vasopressin, or its synthetic analogue Terlipressin, Somatostatin, or

its analogue Octreotide, to reduce splanchnic blood flow, thereby reducing portal flow and pressure. Vasopressin is the most potent vasoconstrictor. Vasopressin can cause myocardial ischaemia, arrhythmias, heart failure, mesenteric ischaemia, limb ischaemia, pulmonary oedema and cerebrovascular accidents, so use it with caution. Be willing to administer simultaneous nitroglycerine sublingually, intravenously or transdermally. Vasopressin is administered as a continuous intravenous infusion at 0.4 units/minute, increasing if necessary to 0.6 units/minute and continuing until bleeding has stopped for 24 hours. Somatostatin, is expensive but is the safest; give it as a 250-µg bolus and a 250–500-µg/hour infusion, continued for 2–5 days if it is beneficial. Generally, terlipressin, somatostatin and its analogue octreotide are considered 'safe' vasoconstrictors. Avoid beta-blockers as they can cause hypotension and blunt the physiological response to shock.

6 Upper gastrointestinal endoscopy is essential to establish an accurate diagnosis since 50% of patients with portal hypertension will have a non-variceal source of bleeding. Endoscopy is the gold standard for diagnosis of variceal bleeding. Patients with severe haemorrhage may need endotracheal intubation for endoscopy.

> ### ▶ KEY POINTS Accurate diagnosis

- Although a previous history and clinical examination may suggest variceal bleed, you must directly visualize the bleeding area before starting treatment.
- Especially alcoholics with known varices bleed from other gastrointestinal lesions.

7 If you confirm variceal bleeding at endoscopy, perform endoscopic variceal banding by placing a constricting rubber band at the base of the varix or perform sclerotherapy by injecting sclerosing agents into or around the varices. Polidocanol, ethanolamine and sodium tetradecyl sulfate are some examples of available sclerosants. Variceal banding is based on the same technique as used for rubber band ligation of haemorrhoids. Although both techniques are equally effective in controlling acute bleeding, banding is preferred to sclerotherapy for acute variceal bleeding because rebleeding occurs less frequently with banding. You need to be experienced in the appropriate techniques.

8 The combination of vasoconstrictor and endoscopic therapy is standard medical therapy for control of acute variceal bleed and is successful in controlling bleeding in up to 90% of patients.

9 In about 10 to 20% of patients standard medical therapy will fail to control variceal bleeding. Consider placement of a transjugular intrahepatic portasystemic shunt (TIPSS) as a salvage procedure. This is performed in the radiology suite by a specialist interventional radiologist. A catheter is passed from the jugular vein into a major hepatic vein, usually the right hepatic vein, preferred because of its size and proximity to the portal vein. A needle is then passed through the catheter and directed from the right hepatic vein, through liver parenchyma into the right branch of the portal vein. The track is then dilated by a forced balloon angioplasty and an expandable, metallic, wall stent

8–12 mm in diameter is placed along the track. This creates a portal-systemic shunt and provides immediate decompression of the portal system. TIPSS is successful in controlling acute variceal bleeding in more than 90% of patients. Problems associated with TIPSS resemble those following surgical shunts, including hepatic encephalopathy (20–40%) and progressive shunt occlusion. TIPSS should be considered as a bridge to subsequent liver transplantation.

10 If TIPSS is not available, decide if the general condition of the patient or the severity of parenchymal liver disease would suggest that surgical intervention is likely to be successful. This can be either a 'veno-occlusive' procedure designed to stop the venous haemorrhage, such as oesophageal transection or oesophagogastric devascularization, or a 'portal decompression' procedure, namely a portal-systemic shunt.

> ### ▶ KEY POINTS Select a procedure within your expertise and available facilities

- Initially prefer a veno-occlusive technique which carries less risk than other procedures. The exact choice of technique depends on your expertise and facilities. It is better to attempt to stop the bleeding initially by a veno-occlusive technique.
- Emergency portal decompression is associated with a 50% mortality rate and a 40% chance of portasystemic encephalopathy in survivors.
- Bleeding from gastric fundal varices is difficult to control by sclerotherapy or banding and, if TIPSS is not possible, operation remains the only effective treatment.

11 Balloon tamponade is now rarely used. It is very effective in temporarily controlling the bleeding in more than 80% of patients but is associated with dangerous complications including oesophageal perforation and aspiration pneumonia and has a 20% mortality rate. Consider balloon tamponade in patients with uncontrollable bleeding in whom a definitive treatment such as TIPSS or shunt surgery is planned within 24 hours. Oesophagogastric tamponade is provided by an oro-gastric triple lumen balloon tube (Sengstaken-Blakemore tube). This has a gastric balloon, an oesophageal balloon and a channel for draining the stomach. In the four-lumen Minnesota version there is also a channel for oesophageal drainage. After passing the tube, inflate the gastric balloon with 250–300 ml of air and apply gentle traction to the tube. This tamponades (French: *tapon* = a plug) the oesophagogastric junction and the fundus. If bleeding continues, as signalled by continuing haematemesis, then connect the oesophageal balloon to a manometer with a 'Y'-connection and fill it with air to a pressure not exceeding 40 mmHg. Deflate the oesophageal balloon for 30 minutes every 4–6 hours and remove the tube after 12 hours. Balloon tamponade is unlikely to be curative: expect half the patients to re-bleed when the tube is removed. It 'buys time' while deciding on more definitive measures.

12 The role of embolization of varices in acute variceal bleeding is controversial. This is performed by an interventional radiologist.

Through a percutaneous transhepatic route, a catheter is inserted into the left gastric vein and the varices are embolized with gelfoam, stainless steel coils, ethanol or tissue adhesives.

OESOPHAGEAL TRANSECTION AND OESOPHAGOGASTRIC DEVASCULARIZATION

Appraise

1. Oesophageal transection and oesophageal devascularization procedures are rarely performed nowadays because of increased use of TIPSS. Also, there is a high incidence of postoperative hepatic encephalopathy following these procedures.

2. Oesophageal transection and re-anastomosis is effective in controlling acute variceal bleeding, but has a lower re-bleeding rate when combined with oesophagogastric devascularization.

3. The portal vessels feeding the varices or the varices themselves can be ligated by a variety of thoracic or abdominal surgical approaches. Oesophageal transection and re-anastomosis is performed using a circular stapling device. If a stapler is not available it is possible to achieve the same effect by transection and sutured re-anastomosis but this is a difficult procedure. The transection is best performed leaving a cuff of 1 cm of stomach attached to the oesophagus, since the gastric wall holds sutures more securely than the oesophageal wall. If you encounter bleeding from gastric fundal varices that stapled disconnection alone will not control, a more extensive devascularization procedure is indicated.

4. Oesophagogastric devascularization may be performed electively to prevent recurrent variceal re-bleeding:
   - When extrahepatic portal hypertension involves thrombosis of the portal, splenic and mesenteric veins so there are no suitable veins into which the portal system can be shunted
   - In schistosomiasis, in which there is mild liver dysfunction with splenomegaly and hypersplenism
   - Where there exists a high probability of encephalopathy with a shunt.

5. Oesophagogastric devascularization may be achieved as described by Hassab. Through a transabdominal route, the distal oesophagus is mobilized, all of its feeding vessels are ligated and disconnected. Splenectomy is carried out, the left gastric (coronary) vein is ligated, and the greater and lesser curves of the entire proximal stomach are devascularized. Sugiura described a more extensive operation which was originally performed as a two-stage procedure. Through a thoracotomy, the lower oesophagus is devascularized and oesophageal transection carried out. After 6 weeks, through an abdominal approach, the stomach is devascularized and splenectomy carried out, followed by vagotomy and pyloroplasty. The procedure has now been modified to a one-stage transabdominal operation. The distal oesophagus is mobilized transhiatally and devascularized, followed by a stapled transection, then gastric devascularization and splenectomy are performed.

6. The technique to be described involves performing a stapled oesophagogastric transection and re-anastomosis in an emergency, together with the outline of a more extensive devascularization should it be necessary.

▶ KEY POINTS Caution

- Because of existing portal hypertension, these procedures are technically demanding. Do not undertake them if you do not have the expertise.
- Before undertaking any procedure for variceal bleeding, consider carefully the possibility that the patient may in due course need a liver transplant.

Prepare

1. This procedure, designed to occlude all veins filling the oesophageal plexus from below, is best carried out using a mechanical circular stapling instrument such as EEA Autosuture or Proximate ILS Ethicon. Have available disposable circular stapling instruments (sizes 25, 28 and 31 or similar) and the accompanying measuring bougies.

2. Have the anaesthetist give prophylactic antibiotics at the start of the operation.

Access

1. Rotate the patient slightly to the right with wedges placed under the left shoulder and left side of pelvis.

2. Use a left subcostal incision 3 cm below the costal margin. An upper midline incision can also be used.

3. Use a Thompson style self-retaining retractor to retract the costal margins.

Assess

1. Aspirate ascitic fluid from the peritoneal cavity and measure the volume carefully. This helps you to calculate subsequent fluid replacement.

2. Carry out a general exploration.

Action

1. Identify the oesophagogastric junction by palpation after the anaesthetist has passed a nasogastric tube.

2. Gently retract the left lobe of the liver from this region using a Deaver retractor. Divide the left triangular ligament.

3. Incise the peritoneum in front of the lower end of the oesophagus, coagulate any bleeding vessels and gently pass a finger behind the oesophagus and immediate peri-oesophageal tissues. Encircle these structures with a tape.

4. Extend the oesophageal mobilization proximally and distally until you can easily pass two fingers around the whole of the lower oesophagus. You do not need to separately identify the vagi unless they prevent adequate mobilization, in which case exclude them from the mobilized tissues.

5. Make a vertical gastrotomy in the anterior stomach wall 10–15 cm from the oesophagogastric junction and insert through this one of the measuring bougies. Start with the 31-mm bougie and introduce it into the lower oesophagus to ensure that the lumen is large enough to accommodate it and thus the 31-mm staple instrument. It usually passes easily but, if not, do not force it; instead try one of the smaller ones.

6 Select a staple gun of the same size.

7 Remove the tape from the lower oesophagus and replace it with a stout thread ligature.

8 Pass a finger through the gastrotomy and into the lumen of the lower oesophagus. Have the anaesthetist slowly withdraw the nasogastric tube until the tip just disappears proximally up the oesophagus.

9 Pass the well-lubricated head of the selected staple gun into the lower oesophagus and separate the anvil from the staple cartridge by adjusting the screw on the handle. Have an assistant steady the instrument and palpate the groove between the separated head and anvil through the wall of the oesophagus.

10 Tie the thread ligature firmly in this groove and cut the ends (Fig. 17.5A): ensure that the ligature is firmly tied.

11 While protecting the lower end of the oesophagus with a hand placed around it, tighten the screw to bring the staple cartridge and anvil together. Check the mobility of the lower oesophagus and fire the staple instrument. Carry out this manoeuvre very gently and carefully to avoid damaging the lower oesophagus, which is usually very delicate, especially following recent endoscopic sclerotherapy.

12 Unscrew the handle of the instrument by two full turns to separate anvil from staple cartridge. Firmly hold the lower oesophagus and, with a gentle twisting motion, remove the instrument via the gastrotomy.

13 Place a large pack into the upper peritoneal cavity in the region of the transection while you inspect the instrument. Separate the anvil and staple cartridge, and remove the anvil and the plastic ring. Within the circular knife blade you will find the resected portion of oesophagus. Remove this and ensure that a complete 'doughnut' of oesophageal wall has been obtained (Fig. 17.5B).

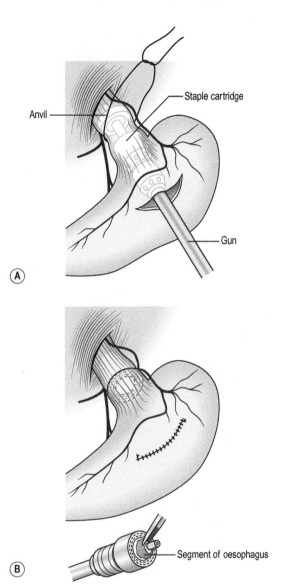

? DIFFICULTY

1. If the doughnut is incomplete, it means that there is a portion of the oesophageal wall that has not been adequately stapled, and patent varices may still be present.

2. When you remove the pack from the upper abdomen, bleeding may not be fully controlled. If so, carefully inspect the anastomosis to identify where the transection is incomplete, or determine the site of bleeding.

3. In both cases insert some additional mattress sutures of Vicryl through the entire thickness of the oesophageal wall to control bleeding from any remaining vessels and seal the anastomosis. If the transection is complete the area will be dry.

Fig. 17.5 Use of EEA staple instrument to carry out oesophagogastric transection: (A) the instrument is passed into the lower oesophagus, the staple cartridge and anvil are separated and a ligature is tied around the entire oesophagus in the groove between the two; (B) after firing the gun the instrument is removed.

14 Pass a finger through the gastrotomy into the lower oesophagus across the line of transection, have the anaesthetist slowly re-pass the nasogastric tube and, with your finger, guide it back into the lumen of the stomach.

15 Close the gastrotomy in one or two layers with absorbable sutures.

16 If there is bleeding from fundal varices, undersew them or carry out gastric devascularization coupled with splenectomy

(Fig. 17.6). Mobilize the spleen as for splenectomy. Ligate and divide the vessels in the splenic pedicle. Identify, dissect, ligate and divide all the short gastric vessels between the greater curvature of the stomach and the spleen. Remove the spleen. Check the rest of the greater curvature of the stomach and dissect, ligate and divide any remaining vessels between it and the diaphragm. On the lesser curve of the stomach identify, ligate and divide any vessels passing to it from the lesser omentum. Continue this dissection down to the region of the antrum. The entire proximal stomach should now be separated from any feeding vessels along its greater and lesser curves. Fortunately, the internal vascularization of the stomach is almost always adequate to prevent any avascular necrosis. Devascularization of the abdominal oesophagus is performed close to the oesophageal wall by ligating and dividing all perforating veins which run transversely. Division of the vagii facilitates the devascularization; because of this, perform a pyloroplasty. If you have preoperatively made the decision to

311

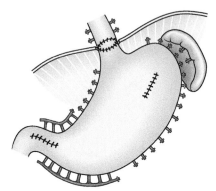

Fig. 17.6   Oesophagogastric devascularization.

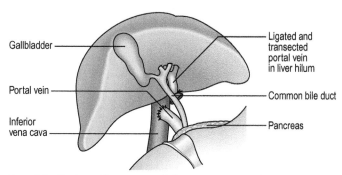

Fig. 17.7   End-to-side portacaval shunt.

perform devascularization, then perform a splenectomy as the first step of the operation; this will greatly improve access to the lower oesophagus and stomach.

Closure

1 Flush the area gently with 2–3 L of warm saline.

2 Close the abdominal incision en masse in the usual way without drainage.

Postoperative

1 Since the stomach has been opened give antibiotics for 48 hours.

2 Arrange initial management in an intensive care unit with the help of medical hepatologists (see section on aftercare following liver trauma and liver resection).

REFERENCES

1. Garcia-Tsao G, Bosch J. Management of varices and variceal hemorrhage in cirrhosis. N Engl J Med 2010;362:823–32.
2. Dooley JS, Lok ASF, Burroughs AK, Heathcote EJ, editors. Sherlock's Diseases of the Liver and Biliary System. 12th ed. London: Wiley-Blackwell; 2011.
3. Garcia-Tsao G, Sanyal AJ, Grace ND, Carey W, Practice Guidelines Committee of the American Association for the Study of Liver Diseases, Practice Parameters Committee of the American College of Gastroenterology. Prevention and management of gastroesophageal varices and variceal hemorrhage in cirrhosis. Hepatology 2007;46:922–38.

PORTAL DECOMPRESSION

This involves creating a surgical shunt to divert blood flow from the portal system to systemic circulation. The aim of the shunt is to achieve profound decompression of the portal system and lower portal pressure, thereby stopping the variceal bleeding.

Appraise

1 Portal decompression can be portacaval, which may be end-to-side or side-to-side (Fig. 17.7), mesocaval, which may be side-to-side or with a synthetic PTFE 'H' graft (Fig. 17.8A), proximal splenorenal (Fig. 17.8B) or distal splenorenal (Fig. 17.8C). The last one, also known as the Warren shunt, is called a 'selective' shunt, as it decompresses only the varix-bearing area of the portal bed. There is no evidence to suggest that any one operation is in the long term any better than any of the others, so choose the

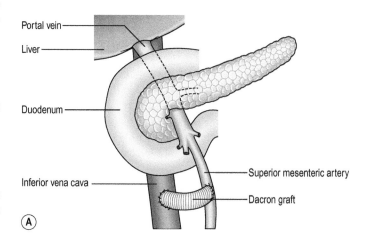

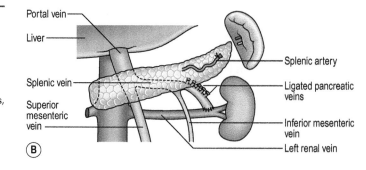

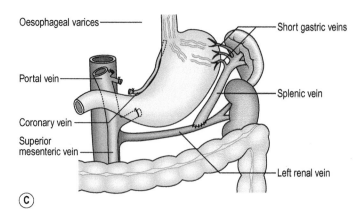

Fig. 17.8   Mesocaval and splenorenal shunts: (A) Drapanas 'H' mesocaval shunt; (B) proximal splenorenal shunt; (C) Warren distal splenorenal shunt.

one with which you have had most experience. In poor-risk patients perioperative mortality is 50%; in good-risk patients, around 5%.

2 The incidence of the major complication, portal-systemic encephalopathy, is similar (20–40% over 1 year) following all of these operations, although it may be less in the early period following the Warren shunt and perhaps following the small-diameter mesocaval shunt.

3 A problem with all shunts is that they are liable to occlude.

4 Do not attempt portal decompression without full preoperative investigations, including consultation with an experienced hepatologist. Investigate liver function, identify the nature of the liver pathology and the vascular anatomy. Patients who tolerate this operation well with minimal encephalopathy are those with good liver function, such as patients with portal vein occlusion, primary biliary cirrhosis or hepatic fibrosis. Do not undertake a shunt operation lightly; there is a risk of encephalopathy and consequent intellectual impairment. Do not undertake it in an emergency situation.

5 Shunt procedures are carried out infrequently now since patients with poor liver function and bleeding oesophageal varices are often candidates for TIPSS in the first instance and liver transplantation in the long term. Therefore the description will be limited to the traditional end-to-side portacaval shunt.

PORTACAVAL SHUNT

Appraise

1 This is the time-honoured operation for achieving portal decompression, although it is now rarely performed. It shunts all the portal blood into the infrahepatic vena cava, reduces the portal hypertension and stops bleeding from oesophageal varices.

2 The problems are:
- There is a high incidence (30–40%) of portal-systemic encephalopathy.
- The operation involves extensive dissection of the liver hilum, which may make subsequent liver transplantation difficult.

3 It is still a very useful operation for treating portal hypertension in patients with good liver function.

Prepare

1 A detailed knowledge of the patient's hepatic and portal vascular anatomy is essential. Modern contrast enhanced CT has replaced portography and provides good images of the splenic, superior mesenteric and portal veins. CT will also show aberrant hepatic arterial anatomy and is reliable in excluding thrombosis in the portal vein.

2 Correct any electrolyte or blood clotting imbalance preoperatively. Order six units of blood, some FFP and platelets, and warn the blood bank that you may need more.

3 Have available vascular instruments and sutures.

Access

1 Place the patient supine on the operating table with slight rotation towards the left.

2 Use a transverse incision in the right upper quadrant, extending from a point 2 cm above the umbilicus to a point midway between the subcostal margin and iliac crest on the midaxillary line, with a midline extension to the xiphoid.

3 Use a Thompson style self-retaining retractor to retract the costal margins.

Assess

1 Aspirate any ascitic fluid.

2 Thoroughly explore the abdomen to exclude any incidental serious intra-abdominal pathology that may make you review the decision to perform a portacaval shunt.

3 If histological assessment of the liver pathology has not been made, take a liver biopsy.

Action

1 Mobilize and retract distally the hepatic flexure of the colon. Mobilize the duodenum using Kocher's manoeuvre by dividing the peritoneal reflection between it and the posterior abdominal wall. Identify and expose the IVC below the liver. There are usually dilated portal-systemic venous anastomotic vessels in this tissue, which may require careful, individual suture ligation. Diathermy coagulation alone is inadequate to secure haemostasis.

2 Incise the edge of the hepatoduodenal ligament between liver and duodenum and identify the portal vein behind the common bile duct.

3 Dissect the portal vein free of attachments from its origin up to its bifurcation. There are frequently one or two branches entering it from the pancreas. Divide and transfix them with a fine monofilament suture. You can gain extra length by gently dissecting the vessel from the pancreas. During this dissection retract the common bile duct anteriorly and to the left, taking care not to damage the blood supply to its wall. Be careful of preserving an aberrant right hepatic artery if it exists, as it lies behind the bile duct and on top of the portal vein.

4 Pass a tape around the portal vein.

5 Dissect the anterior surface of the IVC from the right renal vein to the lower edge of the liver.

6 Clamp the portal vein just above the pancreas with a Satinsky or DeBakey clamp.

7 Clamp and divide the portal vein at the hilum and oversew the hepatic end with 4.0 prolene. Flush the now collapsed segment of portal vein distal to the clamp with a solution of heparin 1:500 000 in physiological saline.

8 Draw the vein to the IVC. Apply a side-biting Satinsky clamp to the anterior surface of the IVC without totally occluding the lumen.

9 Trim the end of the portal vein obliquely so that it will join the anterior wall of the IVC in a gentle curve without kinking.

10 Remove an oval segment of the anterior wall of the IVC the same size as the oblique cut end of the portal vein.

11 Using standard vascular anastomotic techniques, suture the end of the portal vein to the side of the IVC with 4/0 polypropylene or similar vascular suture material. Just before completing the

anastomosis flush the lumen of the portal vein and the occluded segment of the IVC with heparinized saline.

12 Complete the anastomosis. Remove the clamp on the IVC, followed by the clamp on the portal vein.

Check

1 Confirm a good flow through the shunt by feeling for a venous thrill or preferably by observing a measured fall in portal pressure (using a Doppler flow probe or measure portal pressure by manometer) when the clamps are removed. It should be only slightly higher than the IVC pressure.

2 Check that haemostasis is complete.

Closure

1 Close the abdominal wall in a standard manner, without drainage.

2 For a description of other portal-systemic shunts, refer to Blumgart.[1]

Postoperative

Because the liver loses part of its vascular inflow, a degree of hepatic decompensation may develop. To anticipate and manage this:

- Manage the patient initially in the intensive care unit with help from an expert medical hepatologist

- Maintain accurate fluid balance and correct abnormal clotting

- Take steps to prevent or control hepatic encephalopathy. In consultation with the hepatologist prescribe twice-daily phosphate enemas to keep the colon empty, and oral lactulose or lactitol when gastrointestinal activity returns, at a dose producing one or two soft motions a day. Restrict protein intake, starting at 20 g/day and increasing by 10 g every second day. Patients with chronic encephalopathy will probably tolerate no more than 40–60 g/day of protein per day. In some severe cases of portal-systemic encephalopathy the patient needs additional oral non-absorbed antibiotics such as neomycin 1 g four times a day for a week.

REFERENCE

1. Blumgart LH, editor. Surgery of the Liver, Biliary Tract and Pancreas. 4th ed. Philadelphia, PA: Saunders Elsevier; 2007. p. 1635–53.

MANAGEMENT OF ASCITES

- The management of ascites is mainly medical, and consists of a low-sodium diet, fluid restriction, diuretics and concomitant potassium replacement if necessary. Paracentesis with intravenous colloid replacement is the next step if medical management does not succeed. Monitor progress by weighing the patient daily, measuring urine volume and checking for electrolyte imbalances, azotaemia and encephalopathy. If repeated paracentesis is required then the patient should be considered for a TIPSS procedure.

- Another option is a surgical peritoneovenous shunt (LeVeen shunt). This involves placement of a tube extending from the peritoneal cavity to the jugular vein through a subcutaneous track in the anterior chest wall. Interposed in the tube is a one-way valve that opens only to pressure exceeding 2–4 cmH2O and allows drainage of ascitic fluid into the circulation. The Denver version of the shunt has a pumping mechanism within the valve. A peritoneovenous shunt is indicated only in cirrhotic patients with intractable ascites unresponsive to medical therapy. Contraindications include very poor liver function with encephalopathy, infected ascites, coagulopathy and cardiac failure. Complications are common with peritoneovenous shunts, and include shunt blockage, infection, thrombocytopenia and, occasionally, disseminated intravascular coagulation. The operation is rarely performed these days.

18

Spleen

S. Appleton, D. Roy

CONTENTS

Appraisal

1   The spleen is an important organ, with both haematological and immunological functions (Fig. 18.1). Do not lightly remove it. Its haematological functions include the storage, maturation and destruction of red blood cells. Immunologically it produces peptides necessary for the phagocytosis of encapsulated bacteria (*Streptococcus pneumonia*, *Neisseria meningitidis* and *Haemophilus influenza*). It is a site of antibody synthesis and may be a reservoir for monocytes that are mobilized following tissue injury. When possible, conserve at least part of the spleen, as opposed to total splenectomy. This may protect against overwhelming post-splenectomy infection (OPSI).

2   Elective splenectomy is most commonly carried out for idiopathic thrombocytopenic purpura (ITP) and haemolytic anaemias. Splenectomy is also required occasionally for other types of splenomegaly with hypersplenism and rarely for conditions such as cyst, abscess, haemangioma or splenic artery aneurysm. Splenectomy is sometimes carried out as a part of other operations, such as total gastrectomy and distal pancreatectomy. Indications are listed in Table 18.1.

3   The indications, preoperative preparation, surgical principles and aftercare are similar for both open and laparoscopic splenectomy.

4   Laparoscopic splenectomy is the standard approach for elective splenectomy for the majority of patients, with operative duration between 60 and 90 minutes, and a hospital stay between 1 and 2 days. There is controversy about its use when treating patients with very large spleens, in splenic trauma and its adequacy for removal of accessory spleens in ITP.

5   There are no absolute contraindications to laparoscopic splenectomy. Spleen size is a major factor. Massive splenomegaly presents difficulties in access, vision and manoeuvring the spleen. Identification of accessory splenic tissue may be less thorough than in open surgery but the long-term results are same. Obesity, peritoneal adhesions and the presence of inflammation also add to the difficulties.

6   The advantages of laparoscopic splenectomy include less postoperative pain, more rapid recovery and fewer respiratory complications when compared to open splenectomy. Long-term follow-up of patients with ITP and autoimmune haemolytic anaemia, the two most common indications, have shown identical results to the open approach. The rate of conversion to open splenectomy varies from 0% to 19%. Haemorrhage is the most common reason for conversion, followed by difficulty in mobilizing the spleen due to adhesions or spleen size and injury to adjacent organs.

7   Open splenectomy should be reserved for failure of the laparoscopic technique, emergency splenectomy for trauma and when the necessary laparoscopic skills or equipment are not available.

8   Emergency splenectomy is indicated for traumatic rupture of the spleen, mostly following road traffic accidents and other blunt abdominal injuries. Enlarged spleens are at increased risk of rupture, which may occur spontaneously. Classically, patients are shocked, with pain in the left hypochondrium and shoulder-tip and evidence of left lower rib fractures. Urgent laparotomy is required to control bleeding if the patient remains unstable after initial resuscitation.

9   There is an increasing trend to non-operative management of splenic injuries, particularly in children. Lesser splenic injuries can be managed conservatively with vigilant clinical observation and blood transfusion. Appropriate patients are those less than 60 years of age, haemodynamically stable, with a blood transfusion requirement not exceeding 3–4 units and with computed tomography (CT) scan evidence that the spleen has not been fragmented. A grading system for splenic trauma is summarized in Table 18.2.

10   Accidental splenic injury sustained during operations, such as left hemicolectomy, was formerly an indication for splenectomy, but the bleeding can usually be controlled by lesser means. Intra-operative splenic injury occurs in approximately 0.01% of open laparotomies and the incidence increases following reoperative surgery. Up to 10% of splenectomies performed are secondary to iatrogenic injury.

11   Preoperative splenic artery embolization may reduce the risk of intra-operative haemorrhage. This percutaneous radiological technique has been described in conjunction with open splenectomy, primarily in cases of massive splenomegaly. Other advantages of embolization include reduced splenic volume and avoidance of the risk of arteriovenous fistula from stapling across the splenic hilum. Embolization is most frequently performed on the day of surgery to reduce the discomfort associated with splenic ischaemia and infectious complications.

Prepare

1   Vaccinate patients 2 weeks prior to surgery to decrease the risk of post-splenectomy sepsis. Immunize against pneumococcal infections (Pneumovax II 0.5 ml IM/SC, Sanofi Pasteur) and

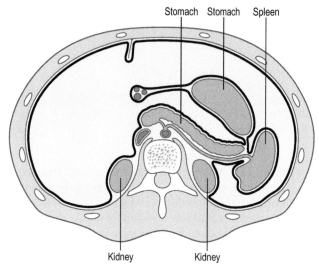

Fig. 18.1 Attachments and relationships of the spleen.

TABLE 18.1 Indications for splenectomy

Red cell causes	Hereditary spherocytosis Sickle cell disease Autoimmune haemolytic anaemia Thalassaemias
White cell causes	Hodgkin's lymphoma Non-Hodgkin's lymphoma Leukaemia
Platelet causes	Idiopathic thrombocytopenic purpura (ITP) TTP
Other causes	Trauma Cysts Abscesses

TABLE 18.2 A grading system of splenic trauma

Grade I: capsular injury not actively bleeding	Non-operative
Grade II: capsular or minor parenchymal injury	Topical haemostatic agent
Grade III: moderate parenchymal injury	Suturing and haemostatic agent
Grade IV: severe parenchymal injury	Partial splenic resection
Grade V: Extensive parenchymal injury	Splenectomy

Haemophilus influenza type b (Hib) and meningococcus group C infections (Menitorix 0.5 ml IM, GlaxoSmithKline).

2 Preoperative percutaneous splenic artery embolization is used in some units to reduce the risk of bleeding or decrease significant splenomegaly.

3 Give antibiotics (first generation cephalosporin) perioperatively. Ensure patients are adequately hydrated before surgery. Pneumatic compression stockings are routinely employed.

4 Correct anaemia, thrombocytopenia and coagulopathies preoperatively. Reserve packed red blood cells for all patients and

platelets for thrombocytopenic patients. Preoperative medical therapy (e.g. IgG therapy or increasing steroids) may elevate platelet count transiently in ITP cases. Give parenteral steroid cover in patients with ITP or other haematological disease on long-term corticosteroids. Involve the haematologist in the pre- and postoperative care of the patient. If the platelet count is low, transfuse platelets intra-operatively after ligation of the splenic artery to prevent rapid sequestration.

5 A nasogastric tube may be needed to decompress a distended stomach, but is not routinely required.

6 Ensure you have explained and documented the advice given to patients on the risks of post-splenectomy sepsis.

LAPAROSCOPIC SPLENECTOMY

Access

1 Position the patient in a left lateral position. This position facilitates retraction of the stomach and omentum away from the spleen and improves access.

2 Create a pneumoperitoneum using a Veress needle technique at the umbilicus or an open technique at the camera port site. Exact port placement depends on the size of the spleen. For a normal-sized spleen place the 11-mm camera port above the umbilicus and to the left of the midline. Place a 5-mm port in the epigastrium and a 12-mm port for stapler and retrieval bag in the left lateral position as shown in Figure 18.2. An additional port for a fan retractor may be necessary.

▶ KEY POINTS Technical considerations

- Before inserting the additional ports, assess whether it is possible to complete the procedure laparoscopically.
- Division of the left triangular ligament of the liver may improve access, but is not routinely necessary.

3 Pass a nasogastric tube to decompress a distended stomach.

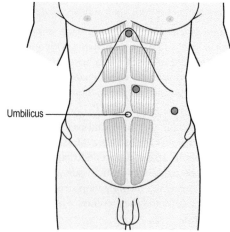

Fig. 18.2 Operating port positions for laparoscopic splenectomy. For larger spleens the lower ports may need to move towards the right iliac fossa.

Assess

1 Perform a systematic exploration looking for splenunculi (small nodules of splenic tissue away from the main body of the spleen), which may be found anywhere in the abdominal cavity, but are commonly located at the hilum of the spleen and adjacent to the tail of the pancreas. When identified, if the splenectomy is performed for conditions in which blood cells are sequestered in the spleen, remove all splenunculi immediately so they are not lost during subsequent dissection.

2 Use scissor diathermy or a harmonic scalpel to divide any omental adhesions to the lower pole of the spleen and the splenocolic ligament.

Action

1 Avoid grasping the spleen directly. Use open Johannes forceps to gently retract the spleen medially. Divide splenic attachments about 1 cm away from the spleen and use these attachments to retract the spleen. Continue the dissection laterally to divide the attachments to the lateral sidewall. Continue the dissection, using the harmonic scalpel or hook diathermy, from the inferior pole of the spleen to the superior pole. As the dissection progresses the spleen becomes more mobile and can be moved medially to expose the back of the splenic hilum.

2 Leave the splenophrenic ligaments at the top of the spleen to stop it falling into the abdominal cavity: these are divided once the spleen has been placed in the retrieval bag, immediately prior to its removal. It is important to clear the back of the splenic hilum carefully at this stage and identify the tail of the pancreas to avoid damaging it at a later stage.

3 Return to the lower pole of the spleen and begin the medial dissection by dividing the serosa over the hilar vessels (Fig. 18.3). As you pass towards the upper pole of the spleen you will encounter the short gastric vessels. Divide these now with the harmonic scalpel. Alternatively, they can be divided together with the hilar vessels using a vascular stapler.

4 A fan retractor may be used by the first assistant from the right upper quadrant position to retract the splenic flexure and, later in the procedure, to retract the stomach away from the spleen.

5 Once a clear view in front and behind the hilum is obtained, place a vascular stapler across the vessels at the hilum of the spleen and divide the splenic artery and vein. Take care to remain close to the spleen as straying medially may damage the tail of the pancreas.

6 A simple approach to the short gastric vessels is to include them in the vascular staple line or reload the stapler and divide them.

7 Once all the vessels are divided, lift the spleen anteriorly to allow division of any remaining posterior attachments using a harmonic scalpel. In cases of massive splenomegaly this manoeuvre may prove difficult, as there is limited room to lift the spleen.

8 At this stage only the superior attachments of the spleen remain. Insert a retrieval bag through the 12-mm port and slip it over the lower pole of the spleen. Divide the superior attachments to allow the spleen to fall into the retrieval bag.

9 Partially withdraw the bag through the 12-mm port and use a finger or sponge holding forceps through the port site to break down the spleen whilst it is still intra-abdominal. Remove the spleen piecemeal from the bag using a combination of sponge holding forceps and a sucker.

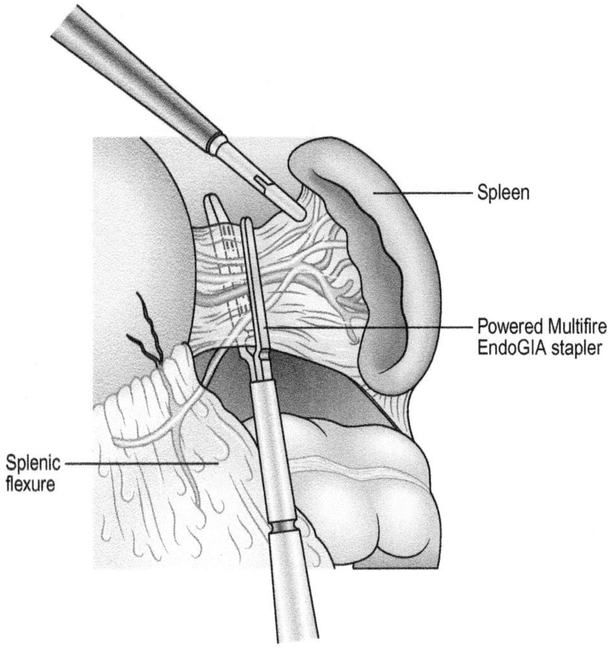

Closure

1 Reinsert the laparoscope and ensure haemostasis using saline lavage. Aspirate the pneumoperitoneum to reduce postoperative shoulder tip pain.

2 Routine drainage is not necessary. Close the fascial wounds in a standard manner.

Fig. 18.3 Transection of hilar vessels.

▶ KEY POINTS Precautions

■ Try to avoid damaging the splenic capsule.
■ While stapling the hilum, take extra care not to injure the fundus of the stomach or the tail of the pancreas. Position the stapler correctly before closing it, because reopening the stapler for repositioning is dangerous and may damage the hilar vessels.
■ Occasionally the stomach is so close to the spleen that a cuff of stomach will be incorporated into the staple line. This should present no problems.

▶ KEY POINTS Accessory spleens?

■ Accessory spleens normally lie deep to the spleen, but may lie in the mesentery. Look for these and remove any if found.
■ At the end of the procedure, search again in the hilar area, greater omentum and ligamentous attachments of the spleen.

1. Do not hesitate to convert the procedure into an open operation if you encounter uncontrollable bleeding, visceral injury, difficulty in handling the spleen, or when dense posterior adhesions are present between the spleen and the diaphragm.

OPEN SPLENECTOMY

ACCESS

1 Make an upper midline or left subcostal incision through the abdominal wall.

2 For large spleens use a full midline laparotomy.

Assess

1 Perform a full exploratory laparotomy, in particular noting the liver and abnormal lymph nodes. Perform biopsies as appropriate.

2 Make a careful search for splenunculi. Remove all splenunculi if the splenectomy is performed for conditions in which blood cells are sequestered in the spleen.

Action

1 Ligate the splenic artery at the beginning of the operation if the spleen is very large or prior to infusing platelets in patients with ITP. Enter the lesser sac by dividing 10 cm of the gastrocolic omentum using diathermy or a harmonic scalpel. Incise the peritoneum at the superior border of the pancreas to identify the tortuous splenic artery. Use a right angle forceps to pass a ligature behind the splenic artery and ligate it in continuity with a large non-absorbable suture.

▶ KEY POINT Reduce the size of a very large spleen

■ Consider injecting 1 ml of 1: 10 000 adrenaline (epinephrine) into the splenic artery immediately before ligating it. This can shrink the size of a massive spleen and facilitate the subsequent dissection.

2 Gently divide omental adhesions to the lower pole of the spleen using diathermy, harmonic scalpel or suture ligation. These adhesions are fragile and bleed easily.

3 Use your left hand to draw the spleen medially and have your assistant retract the abdominal wall laterally.

4 Using scissors, incise the peritoneum that attaches the spleen to the lateral sidewall (Fig. 18.4). Extend this incision up along the lateral border of the spleen towards the diaphragm. Because of its position this cannot always be achieved under direct vision. Extend this incision downwards around the lower pole of the spleen to identify the splenic flexure and separate it from the spleen.

5 Dividing this lateral attachment allows your left hand to gently move the spleen medially and upwards into the abdominal wound. As the spleen is lifted medially take care to identify

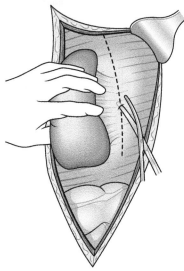

Fig. 18.4 Division of the lateral peritoneum to mobilize the spleen.

and preserve the tail of the pancreas, which must be separated from the splenic hilum.

6 As the spleen becomes more mobile divide the adhesions from the upper pole of the spleen to the diaphragm.

7 Divide the peritoneum over the front of the splenic hilum from the lower pole to the upper pole. The stomach can be very close to the spleen at this point so take care not to damage the greater curve. The short gastric arteries are branches of the splenic artery that run to the fundus of the stomach in this region. Divide them carefully with the harmonic scalpel or by suture ligation (Fig. 18.5).

8 At this stage the spleen should be fairly mobile and attached only by the vessels in the splenic hilum. These can be thinned by careful dissection. Divide the splenic vessels between large clips, such as a Roberts. Several clips may be required to take all the vessels. Be careful not to injure the tail of the pancreas at this point. Divide any remaining peritoneal attachments to remove the spleen.

9 Place a large pack in the splenic bed.

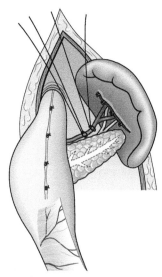

Fig. 18.5 Exposure of the splenic vessels after division of the gastrosplenic ligament and short gastrics.

1. Especially with a massive spleen (larger than 1.5 kg), you may encounter troublesome bleeding from vascular adhesions to the diaphragm or parenchymal tears.
2. Enlarge the incision or ligate the splenic artery above the pancreas to improve control. Alternatively, mobilize the spleen and bring it up to the surface as soon as possible.

Closure

1 Remove the pack, inspect the splenic bed and coagulate any oozing vessels.

2 Examine the ligatures on the main vascular pedicles.

3 Make sure that adjacent viscera are undamaged.

4 Consider a suction drain in the splenic bed if there is any question over haemostasis.

5 Close the abdominal wounds in a standard way.

CONSERVATIVE SPLENECTOMY

Appraise

1 Following splenectomy there is a 1–2% risk of developing overwhelming post-splenectomy infection (OPSI) from encapsulated bacteria, especially pneumococcus, usually within 2 years of operation. Leaving behind viable splenic tissue rather than total splenectomy may reduce this risk by preserving some of the spleen's immunological function.

2 Increasingly, there is a move towards non-operative management of splenic trauma or conservative splenic surgery, particularly in children.

3 Anatomically, there are between three and seven well-defined splenic segments, each with an independent blood supply, which makes a partial splenectomy a practical proposition.

Assess

1 At operation for abdominal trauma, immediately remove a spleen that is either fragmented or avulsed from its vascular pedicle. Under these circumstances consider autotransplantation of splenic tissue by suturing a piece of omentum around a sliver of removed splenic pulp to encourage splenic regeneration (splenosis).

2 If the extent of the damage and bleeding is less severe, gently mobilize the spleen into the wound after dividing its peritoneal attachments. Remove attached clot and examine the organ thoroughly. Decide whether topical haemostatic agents, partial splenectomy or some form of splenic repair is feasible, with or without ligation of the splenic artery or its branches.

3 Capsular tears and other minor injuries can often be controlled by application of a haemostatic agent.

4 Marsupialization (Greek: maryp(p)ion = a pouch; removing the top) of a thin-walled congenital or traumatic cyst avoids splenectomy but there is a risk of recurrence.

Action

1 To avoid the need for splenectomy apply haemostatic applications to superficial lacerations of the capsule or splenic pulp. Full mobilization of the spleen is unnecessary if the damaged area is accessible, but use suction to obtain a clear view. Fibrin glue may be sprayed over the injured site or injected into a splenic laceration. Apply an appropriate disc of haemostatic sponge to the laceration and maintain light pressure until the sponge soaks up the blood and becomes adherent. Gently pack off the area and leave if for 5–10 minutes before checking that you have achieved haemostasis.

2 Deeper or more extensive lacerations may still be suitable for repair. Mobilize the spleen, at least in part. Use synthetic absorbable sutures on a long blunt needle. Take deep bites of splenic tissue on either side of the tear, and tie the sutures snugly. Use omentum or Teflon buttresses to prevent the stitches cutting through (Fig. 18.6A), together with a topical haemostatic agent to control surface bleeding. Alternatively, wrap the organ in an absorbable polyglycolate mesh and suture the edges of the mesh together to envelop the spleen.

3 For partial splenectomy, fully mobilize the organ and carefully dissect in the splenic hilum to identify and ligate the segmental arteries and veins. Incise the capsule of the spleen at the line of ischaemia and use a finger-fracture technique to resect the upper or lower pole (Fig. 18.6B). Secure haemostasis by means of synthetic absorbable sutures or with argon coagulation. Preserve at least 30% of the spleen volume to maintain adequate splenic function.

1. If bleeding continues despite these endeavours, proceed to total splenectomy.
2. Leave a drain to the area of the spleen following conservative operations.

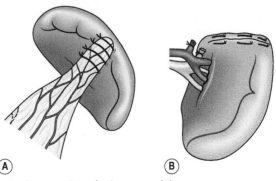

Fig. 18.6 Conservative splenic surgery: (A) greater omentum sutured over a laceration of the splenic pulp; (B) resection of the upper pole of the spleen with ligation of its feeding vessels.

Aftercare

1 Check the haemoglobin, white cell and platelet counts postoperatively. Leucocytosis and thrombocythaemia nearly always ensue, with peaks at 7–14 days. Persistent leucocytosis and pyrexia suggest the possibility of a subphrenic abscess. Consider antiplatelet medication such as aspirin if the platelet count exceeds 1000×10^9 per litre.

2 After an emergency splenectomy, vaccinate the patient once fully recovered. Administer prophylactic antibiotics (cephalosporin based) at induction of anaesthesia. If you have previously overlooked it, start immunization with anti-pneumococcal vaccine. Children should receive prophylactic penicillin for 2 years to prevent post-splenectomy sepsis. Advise adults to take an antibiotic such as amoxicillin at the first sign of any infective illness.

3 Monitor the haemoglobin level and remove the drain, if used, when it ceases to function.

4 Immunological function after splenorrhaphy or partial splenectomy is uncertain, so prophylactic measures should probably be taken against post-splenectomy sepsis.

5 Nasogastric tube and drain is not routinely used after splenectomy. Remove the nasogastric tube if used when gastric aspirates diminish.

Complications

1 Haemorrhage: intra-operative haemorrhage can develop rapidly. Alert the anaesthetist that there is active bleeding. Small splenic tears may be controlled with compression by surrounding tissues and haemostatic diathermy. However, the spleen is an end organ and the quickest way to get control of a difficult situation is to mobilize the spleen and get control of the hilar vessels. In a laparoscopic splenectomy this may require rapid conversion to open surgery. Once the spleen has been mobilized onto the abdominal wall, a soft bowel clamp is applied across the splenic hilum. This will control the situation and allows the anaesthetist time to resuscitate the patient before completing the operation. When the patient is stabilized, the soft bowel clamp can be sequentially removed to ligate the hilar vessels and to make sure that the tail of the pancreas is not damaged.

2 Postoperative haemorrhage is reported to occur in 2–5% of patients after splenectomy. Postoperative bleeding is suspected if the patient becomes unstable or a drain, if used, produces a large amount of fresh blood. If the patient is stable, re-laparoscopy can be undertaken to look for the site of bleeding. The usual sites are the hilar or short gastric vessels. If identified, the bleeding vessel can be clipped or sutured. If the patient is unstable, urgent laparotomy is preferred to control the bleeding site.

3 Overwhelming post-splenectomy infection (OPSI): post-splenectomy sepsis remains the most severe cause of late postoperative morbidity and mortality. Following splenectomy there is a 1–2.5% risk of developing overwhelming septicaemia from encapsulated bacteria, usually within 2 years of operation. The risk is higher in young children (4–10%) and after splenectomy for haematological disease, but fatal cases have also been reported in adults. The mortality rate of post-splenectomy sepsis is higher in children (50%). Though long-term oral antibiotic prophylaxis is controversial, all patients should be thoroughly counselled to seek prompt medical attention, particularly for respiratory illness. Patients should be advised regarding immunization and foreign travel and to carry an information card at all times. All patients should be advised to have yearly influenza immunization.

4 Injury to adjacent organs: the splenic flexure of the colon, the greater curvature of the stomach and the tail of the pancreas are all susceptible to damage during splenectomy. Pancreatic injury following laparoscopic splenectomy resulting in pancreatitis and pancreatic fistula occurs in 1–3% of cases. Laparotomy may be required to inspect the damage. A colonic or stomach injury should be closed using interrupted seromuscular absorbable sutures. Injury to the tail of pancreas may require either primary repair or resection. Undetected pancreatic injury may later present as pancreatic ascites, a subphrenic collection or pancreatic fistula. All such injuries are rare.

5 Thrombocytosis can occur following splenectomy, leading to deep venous thrombosis and pulmonary emboli. Portal vein thrombosis has also been reported. It is a difficult diagnosis to make as symptoms are of vague abdominal pains. We recommend routine subcutaneous heparin prophylaxis and compression stockings in all patients.

6 Respiratory complications such as pneumonia, atelectasis, and pleural effusion are by far the most common morbidity following open splenectomy, occurring in 20–40% of patients. There are fewer respiratory complications after laparoscopic splenectomy with early mobilization and discharge on the second or third postoperative day. Chest infection may result from splinting of the left diaphragm causing atelectasis. Vigorous physiotherapy will help early recovery.

7 Subphrenic collection: this may develop due to minor bleeding or serous oozing from the raw area in the diaphragm and retroperitoneum. If this happens, carefully monitor the platelet count and clotting parameters. A CT (computed tomography) scan is often required to confirm the diagnosis. Subphrenic abscess has been reported in 4% of patients after open splenectomy for all indications in a large series. This complication is less common after laparoscopic splenectomy and in the absence of gastrointestinal trauma. A subphrenic collection can usually be drained percutaneously with antibiotic cover but may occasionally require a laparotomy.

8 Accessory spleens are noted in 15–30% of patients and account for late failure of splenectomy in ITP. The ability to identify accessory spleens using laparoscopic techniques is in question. The initial step during laparoscopic splenectomy is a systematic exploration for accessory splenic tissue. When identified, they are immediately removed because they may be easily lost during the dissection. Preoperative CT is performed by some units to identify these structures.

9 Other sporadic complications include trocar site hernias, wound infection and ileus.

FURTHER READING

Clarke PJ, Morris PJ. Surgery of the spleen. In: Morris PJ, Wood WC, editors. Oxford Textbook of Surgery. Oxford: Oxford University Press; 2001. p. 2755–64.

Cooper MJ, Williamson RCN. Splenectomy: indications, hazards and alternatives. Br J Surg 1983;71:173–80.

Casaccia M, Torelli P, Pasa A, et al. Putative predictive parameters for the outcome of laparoscopic splenectomy: a multicenter analysis performed on the Italian registry of laparoscopic surgery of the spleen. Ann Surg 2010;251(2):287–91.

Department of Health. Department of Health guidance for patients following splenectomy. Available at http://www.dh.gov.uk/assetRoot/04/1135/82/04113582.pdf. Accessed 20/12/2012.

Grahn SW, Alvarez J, Kirkwood K. Trends in laparoscopic splenectomy for massive splenomegaly. Arch Surg 2006;141:755–62.

Habermalz B, Sauerland S, Decker G, et al. Laparoscopic splenectomy: the clinical practice guidelines of the European Association for Endoscopic Surgery (EAES). Surg Endosc 2008;22:821–48.

Kercher KW, Matthews BD, Walsh RM, et al. Laparoscopic splenectomy for massive splenomegaly. Am J Surg 2002;183:192–6.

Kojouri K, Vesely SK, Terell DR, et al. Splenectomy for adult patients with idiopathic thrombocytopaenic purpura. Blood 2004;104:2623–32.

Olmi S, Scaini A, Erba L, et al. Use of fibrin glue (Tissucol) as a haemostatic in laparoscopic conservative treatment of spleen trauma. Surg Endosc 2007;21:2051–4.

Park AE, Birgisson G, Mastrangelo MJ, et al. Laparoscopic splenectomy: outcomes and lessons learned from over 200 cases. Surgery 2000;128:660–7.

Pomp A, Gagner M, Salky B, et al. Laparoscopic splenectomy: a selected retrospective review. Surg Laparosc Endosc Percutan Tech 2005;15:139–43.

Redmond HP, Redmond JM, Rooney BP, et al. Surgical anatomy of the human spleen. Br J Surg 1989;76:198–201.

Schwartz J, Leber MD, Gillis S, et al. Long term follow-up after splenectomy performed for immune thrombocytopenic purpura (ITP). Am J Haematol 2003;72:94–8.

Uranues S, Alimoglu O. Laparoscopic surgery of the spleen. Surg Clin North Am 2005;85:75–90.

Velmahos GC, Zacharias N, Emhoff T, et al. Management of the most severely injured spleen. Arch Surg 2010;145:456–60.

Walsh RM, Brody F, Brown N. Laparoscopic splenectomy for lymphoproliferative disease. Surg Endosc 2004;18:272–5.

Winslow ER, Brunt LM. Perioperative outcomes of laparoscopic versus open splenectomy: a meta-analysis with an emphasis on complications. Surgery 2003;134:647–55.

Breast

M. Keshtgar, D.B. Ghosh

MANAGEMENT OF BREAST SYMPTOMS (Fig. 19.1)

Assessment

1 Management of breast disease involves a multidisciplinary team approach. Interact with and use the expertise of the different members of the team to deliver the best results.

2 Breast pain, lumps, lumpiness, deformity and nipple changes including inversion, bleeding and discharge are the common symptoms that are seen in a breast clinic. Ideally, manage all patients in a triple assessment clinic with facilities for concurrent radiological and cytopathological investigations.

3 Offer all patients with palpable breast lumps and asymmetrical nodularity 'triple assessment'.

4 Triple assessment includes history and clinical examination, breast imaging – mammography, ultrasound or magnetic resonance imaging (MRI), and tissue diagnosis (core biopsy/cytology). Order mammography and/or ultrasound to complement clinical examination for women over the age of 35 years. Order ultrasound examination as the first choice of imaging investigation for women aged below 35 years.

5 Consider MRI scans for patients with lobular carcinoma, young women and those with dense breast tissue, to assess the size and extent of malignant lesions and assessment of the contralateral breast. MRI scans are used as a screening tool in patients who fall in the high risk category for family history of breast cancer in the age groups of 30–40.

6 For discrete breast lumps, ultrasound is useful to differentiate cystic from solid lesions. Obtain a needle biopsy, preferably under image guidance, from all solid lumps. The advantage of core biopsy is that you obtain a definite tissue diagnosis. In malignant lesions it establishes whether the lesion is invasive or non-invasive and determines receptor status. Fine needle aspiration cytology (FNAC) of breast lesions is now used less frequently than formerly. Reserve it for younger patients with clinically benign breast disease and for the assessment of axillary lymph node abnormalities.

7 Breast cysts are common findings, appear suddenly and are of concern to the patient. They are most common before and around the menopause but can occur at any age. Assess and confirm all cysts which appear as a lump with ultrasound. Aspirate and drain the cyst, establishing the diagnosis and 'curing' the condition so you can immediately reassure the patient.

▶ KEY POINTS Caution

■ If the fluid from the cyst is blood stained, or if there is a residual lump, perform core biopsy.
■ Cytology of cyst fluid is worthwhile only if it is blood stained or if there is a residual mass after aspiration.

8 You can leave alone lumps that prove to be benign on core biopsy or cytology. You can offer excision if the woman is above the age of 35, if the lump increases in size or is associated with pain, if the histology is equivocal or if the patient is anxious and requests an excision. As an alternative to observation or excision you can offer a younger patient with a confirmed fibro-adenoma a variety of percutaneous methods such as vacuum-assisted Mammotome excision, laser ablation, microwave or cryo-ablation.

9 Obtain a core biopsy on all lesions that have indeterminate cytology (C3, C4), or inadequate cells (C1). For lesions with core biopsies reported to be equivocal, repeat the core biopsy or undertake formal excision. If a core biopsy/excision biopsy is performed for microcalcification or abnormal calcification a specimen radiograph must be obtained to confirm the presence of calcification and this should also be confirmed on histology, otherwise repeat biopsy must be considered.

10 Frozen section is no longer considered an investigation of choice in breast surgery.

11 Assess patients with a family history of breast cancer and stratify their risks based on published guidelines; in the United Kingdom refer to National Institute for Clinical Excellence (NICE) guidelines for Family History of Breast Cancer. Arrange regular follow-up

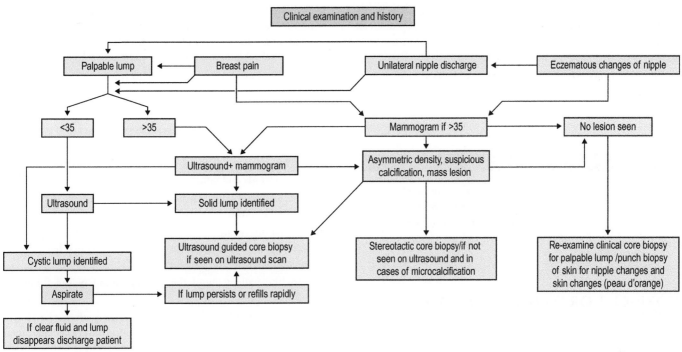

Fig. 19.1 Evaluation and work up of patient presenting with breast symptoms.

including appropriate surveillance investigations based on local guidelines. Organize for all patients who fall in the high-risk category to have risk assessment and genetic counselling.

12 Arrange for patients who fall into a high-risk category for developing familial breast cancer, with BRCA1, BRCA2, CDH1, PTEN, STK11, and TP53 genetic defects to be appropriately counselled for genetic testing. If they prove to be a gene carrier, you can offer a risk-reducing mastectomy with immediate breast reconstruction.

13 A small group of patients present to you with problems related to the breast size and symmetry, including large or small breasts or asymmetry. They are best managed by a trained breast oncoplastic surgeon or in conjunction with a plastic surgeon.

14 You will also be referred male patients with breast symptoms including breast lumps and gynaecomastia (Greek: gynaikos = woman + mastos = breast). Treat male breast cancer like a female breast cancer, except that there is no role for breast conservation surgery.

15 Breast surgery for cancer is based on two important values: careful attention to oncological principles and consideration of the aesthetic and cosmetic outcome.

16 Surgical management of breast cancer has become less radical (Latin: radix = root; by the roots) over the years without compromising the local control or long-term survival.

17 Multimodality treatments of breast cancer, using new generations of drugs, have made a significant impact in improving survival.

BREAST BIOPSY

FINE NEEDLE ASPIRATION CYTOLOGY

1 This procedure is performed in the outpatient clinic and involves insertion of a fine needle (21–23 G) into the lesion and aspiration of cells which are spread on glass slides and stained. This has the advantage of being fast and applicable for all breast lumps and requiring the minimum of special equipment.

2 It has the disadvantage of requiring the special skills of an experienced cytologist and the quality of the aspirate is operator-dependent, demanding experience and skill. Moreover, it is not possible to differentiate between invasive and non-invasive cancer.

3 The cytological aspirate is usually reported as containing no cells (C0), blood and debris or inadequate cells for reporting (C1), benign epithelial cells (C2), atypical cells, probably benign (C3), cells suspicious of carcinoma (C4) or diagnostic of carcinoma (C5).

Action

1 After obtaining verbal consent, attach a 21G (green) or 23G (blue) needle to a 10-ml syringe with or without an extractor gun.

2 Clean the overlying skin then fix the lump between thumb and index finger of the non-dominant hand. If necessary, use ultrasound localization as an aid while performing a FNA.

3 Warn the patient. Insert the needle into the middle of the lump and apply suction to the syringe plunger. Move the needle in several different directions through the lump while maintaining negative pressure. Do not allow the needle point to leave the skin or air enters the needle and the aspirated material is drawn into the syringe.

▶ KEY POINT Pleural damage

■ Avoid penetrating the intercostal space, which may result in bleeding or pneumothorax.

4 Release the pressure and then withdraw the needle. Ask the patient or your assistant to apply pressure to the breast for 2 minutes to avoid haematoma formation.

5 Eject a drop of aspirate onto the end of a dry and clean microscope slide. Gently spread this out with another slide to create a thin smear.

6 Immediately label the slide and ensure that no material falls onto the table, which could then be picked up onto the back of the next set of slides. Spray the slide with, or immerse it in, a fixative. Send the slide for reporting.

7 If you do not succeed in aspirating any cells, repeat the procedure.

CORE-CUT OR 'TRU-CUT' NEEDLE BIOPSY (Fig. 19.2)

Appraise

1 Ideally, remove a core biopsy from every lump. Even if the lump is clinically palpable, where possible employ ultrasound guidance.

2 Core biopsy is a more accurate method of tissue diagnosis, allowing for a definite diagnosis to be based on the results of core biopsy.

3 The receptor status can be performed on core biopsy and decision for hormonal therapy can be made based on that.

4 Drag cytology (touch preparation cytology) obtained from the core samples can be used to give an immediate report similar to cytology.

5 Ductal carcinoma in situ (DCIS) can be diagnosed only on core biopsy.

6 Core biopsy can be performed clinically, under US guidance or under stereotactic control

Action

1 Infiltrate the skin over the lump with 1% lidocaine. Introduce the needle into the skin and superficial tissue to inject the local anaesthetic. Deep infiltration with local anaesthetic can obscure a small lump. Preferably perform this procedure under US guidance.

2 Wait 2 minutes for the anaesthetic to work.

3 Make a small nick in the skin with the tip of a sharp-pointed scalpel (no. 11 blade).

4 Fix the tumour within the breast between finger and thumb, to provide a static target.

5 Prefer to approach the lump from the side to avoid firing the needle backwards and penetrating the chest wall.

6 Insert the core biopsy needle, in its closed position, through the skin incision until you reach the edge of the tumour.

7 A spring-driven automatic biopsy needle can obtain a sample more rapidly than the one obtained by the manual hand driven one and it causes less discomfort for the patient.

8 Warn the patient about the clicking sound before firing the automatic device.

9 If microcalcification is a dominant feature, perform the biopsy under stereotactic mammographic control. X-ray the specimen to ensure you have obtained the correct specimen.

10 Obtain at least three samples in different directions from the lesion and transfer the specimens into small bottles containing formalin and label them appropriately.

11 Dispose sharp objects into appropriate containers.

12 Vacuum-assisted Mammotome biopsy is being used for obtaining cores of tissue from impalpable lesions, or for completely excising small impalpable lesions. Insert a small metallic marker clip if all the microcalcifications have been removed to allow subsequent localization of an abnormal area.

OPEN BIOPSY

Rarely, an open biopsy is required to make a diagnosis. This can be in a form of excision biopsy (lumpectomy) if the lesion is small or incision biopsy if the lesion is large.

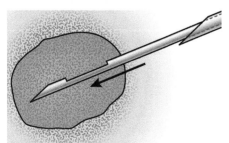
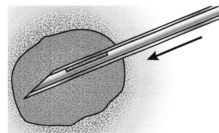
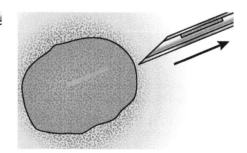

Fig. 19.2 Tru-cut needle.

Reserve the term 'lumpectomy' for a definitive operation to remove a benign lump. Use the term 'wide local excision' for removal of a carcinoma with a zone of normal surrounding breast tissue.

NEEDLE-LOCALIZATION BIOPSY

As a result of national breast-screening programmes there are a large number of screen-detected abnormalities that require surgical excision. As these lesions are not palpable, they require to be localized under mammogram (stereotactic localization) or ultrasound scan. This procedure requires close collaboration with the radiologist.

Prepare

1 Discuss the imaging (mammograms/ultrasound scans) with the radiologist who inserts the localization needle and wire.

2 Discuss the needle-insertion site, direction and depth with the radiologist, and the type of wire used, such as simple hook, Reidy or Nottingham needle. It is helpful if the distance between the needle entry site and the lesion is as short as possible.

3 Ensure that the mammograms are taken in two planes (craniocaudal and medio-lateral oblique) following wire insertion. Check that the images are available in the operating theatre.

4 Frozen section has no role in assessment of biopsy specimen.

Access

Plan a cosmetically satisfactory incision (Fig. 19.3) and estimate the likely surface marking of the lesion from the preoperative mammograms. The incision need not be placed at the point of wire entry. It is useful to measure the length of the wire that is outside. This helps to determine the length of wire inside and helps guide your excision.

Action

1 Raise a skin flap between the chosen site of incision and the needle entry site until you reach the wire in the subcutaneous plane. Grasp the wire with an artery forceps and cut off the excess wire.

2 Follow the wire down towards the site of the lesion by sharp dissection or use the diathermy. Use a scalpel instead of heavy scissors as the latter can bend or inadvertently cut the wire. When using the diathermy for excision, be careful not to activate diathermy whilst it is in contact with the wire, to avoid burning the skin.

3 Once you reach the point of the wire at least 2 cm above the tip (site of the suspected lesion) excise the lesion with an appropriate radial margin (depending on whether the excision is diagnostic or therapeutic). Mark the specimen with metal clips to facilitate orientation and obtain the specimen that was identified by radiography.

▶ KEY POINT Specimen size

■ Do not generally excise diagnostic specimens exceeding 20 g.

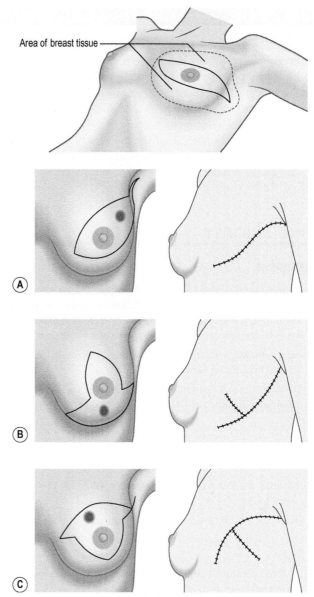

Fig. 19.3   Incisions for removal of a lump from the right breast.

4 Achieve haemostasis, and check the cavity for any residual suspicious tissue.

5 Check the radiograph of the specimen to confirm that it contains the mammographic abnormality. If the lesion is close to a specific margin, excise that specific margin. If the lesion is not visible, you need to re-excise and repeat the specimen radiography until you find it.

6 Close the wound as for excision biopsy.

7 Take extra care to avoid needle-stick injury from the wire. Label the specimen container clearly and warn the pathology staff about the wire and the risk of needle-stick injury.

8 Localization of lesions with radioactive injection (ROLL, radioactive occult lesion localization) is another approach currently used in many centres. Results from a recent study on the use of radioactive seed localization also show significant promise.

PUNCH BIOPSY

Appraise

1 Reserve punch biopsy of the skin for nipple biopsy suspected of Paget's disease, recurrence in the skin following surgery for breast cancer, or in suspected inflammatory cancer (where dermal lymphatics are involved with cancer, giving an appearance of inflammation).

2 Paget's disease starts in the nipple and then moves on to the areola and underlying breast ducts.

3 Always perform a mammogram in Paget's disease to rule out underlying malignancy or DCIS.

Action

1 Clean the area.

2 Infiltrate with 2 ml of 1% lidocaine using a blue needle (size 23 G).

3 Use a 3.5- or 4-mm size punch for performing the biopsy.

4 Use the punch to press on the area where you wish to obtain the biopsy.

5 Hold the obtained tissue with forceps and use scissors or a blade to cut the tissue from the underlying breast.

6 Send the obtained sample to the pathology laboratory in formalin.

7 Compress the area of biopsy for 5 minutes to stop the bleeding.

8 You can apply Steristrips to close the defect left by the punch.

9 Advise the patient to watch for bleeding on discharge.

BREAST ABSCESS

Appraise

1 This develops most commonly during lactation. Empty the affected breast by manual pressure, but encourage the mother to continue breast feeding.

2 Treat early infection with antibiotics alone but do not wait for fluctuation, or widespread destruction of the underlying breast tissue may have developed by then. Start co-amoxiclav early. If an abscess is present clinically or on ultrasound, aspirate it using a wide-bore needle under US guidance and repeat aspiration as necessary.

3 If the skin over the abscess has become thin, drain it under general anaesthesia.

Access

If the abscess cavity is longstanding, you may need to incise and drain it, although this can often be avoided.

Action

1 Site the incision over the point of skin thinning, but if it is near the nipple use a peri-areolar incision.

2 Send pus for culture and antibiotic sensitivities. If necessary, change to the appropriate antibiotic.

3 Introduce a gloved finger into the abscess cavity and rotate it to break down all loculi in a potentially multiloculated cavity.

4 If the cavity allows, introduce a retractor and examine the walls. Stop any bleeding using diathermy.

5 If this is a lactational abscess cavity it is not necessary to obtain biopsy specimens. Otherwise remove a specimen from the cavity to exclude a carcinoma.

6 Ensure that the incision is sufficiently long to allow the wound to heal from the deepest parts upwards, in order to prevent the development of a chronic abscess.

7 Insert a drain if you observe a large residual cavity. Alternatively, loosely pack the cavity.

8 Apply a non-adhesive dressing.

9 Advise the patient to wear a supportive brassiere to diminish the risk of developing a haematoma.

10 Allow bilateral breastfeeding to recommence as soon as it is comfortable.

DUCT ECTASIA AND MAMMARY DUCT FISTULA

Appraise

1 Duct ectasia (Greek: *ex* = out + *tenein* = to stretch; dilatation), is widening of the breast lactiferous ducts and is often related to breast inflammation. It is a benign condition characterized by nipple discharge, swelling, retraction of the nipple or a lump that can be felt.

2 Occasionally, a fistula develops between a duct and the skin at the areolar margin. This discharges pus, and often heals spontaneously before breaking down again. As it is related to smoking, advise abstention.

3 If a mammary duct fistula does not heal, you may need to excise it under antibiotic cover (see below).

Action

1 If there is a fistula, insert a probe through the external opening and hook it up though the nipple. Cut around the areola, extending to no more than a quarter of the nipple and excise the fistulous track to the back of the nipple.

2 Obtain perfect haemostasis.

3 Close the wound with interrupted absorbable sutures.

4 If you are operating to excise the major ducts (Hadfield's operation), you need a longer periareolar incision – but no more than half the circumference of the areola.

5 Ensure that you are beneath the subareolar plexus. Cut the subcutaneous tissue down to the duct system.

6 Use blunt and sharp dissection to reach the plane, circumferentially around the terminal lactiferous ducts, just deep to the areola and nipple. Preferably, use bipolar diathermy. If you are using monopolar diathermy, do so cautiously to avoid nipple necrosis.

7 Divide the ducts close to the nipple and remove them with a conical wedge of tissue including the distal 1–2 cm of the subareolar tissue, as well as the major lactiferous ducts and sinuses.

8 If there is a fistulous tract, ensure that you excise it in its entirety with all the granulation tissue.

9 Send all tissue for histological examination.

10 Insert a small vacuum drain and close the wound with 3/0 subcuticular absorbable sutures or interrupted 4/0 polypropylene.

NIPPLE DISCHARGE AND BLEEDING

Appraise

1 If the nipple discharge is serous (watery), serosanguinous, or frank blood arises from a solitary duct, then manage it as for nipple bleeding (below).

2 Test for blood. This is usually done using Dip-Stix. Nipple discharge can be sent for cytological examination. Intraductal papilloma is the commonest cause of bloody nipple discharge.

3 If one duct is associated with blood-stained discharge and imaging is negative, then a microdochectomy (Greek: small duct cutting out) (Fig. 19.4) may be required.

4 If embarrassing nipple discharge occurs in patients above the age of 45, prefer Hadfield's procedure (excision of major ducts).

5 Multiduct multicolour nipple discharge is often physiological and does not need intervention.

▶ KEY POINT

■ Warn the patient of possible risks including nipple necrosis, loss of nipple sensation and nipple inversion.

NIPPLE BLEEDING

Appraise

1 Determine from which duct the blood is coming.

2 Arrange an ultrasound scan and a mammogram to exclude underlying malignancy.

3 Send the material for cytology; it may yield papillary cells or, very occasionally, carcinoma cells.

4 Consider ductoscopy when this available

5 Surgically explore the breast unless the bleeding occurs during pregnancy, in which case it is frequently bilateral and stops

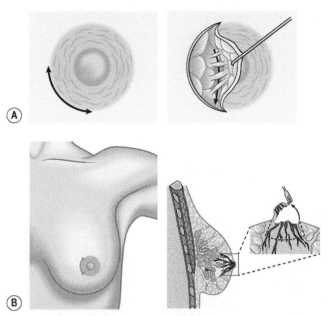

Fig. 19.4 Microdochectomy and Hadfield's procedure of total duct excision.

spontaneously after parturition, or in a patient who is taking anticoagulants.

Prepare

1 Mark the site of the affected duct on a diagram.

2 Discuss the operation and the possible implications with the patient. Warn specifically about alterations in nipple sensation.

3 Mark the site and side of the lesion on the patient with a skin pencil.

Access

1 Perform the procedure either under a local or general anaesthetic.

▶ KEY POINTS Cannulate the duct

■ Cannulate the affected duct with a fine lacrimal probe to assist in dissecting it out.
■ Insert the cannula when the patient is on the operating table.
■ Be careful not to make a button hole in the nipple when dissecting the ducts off the nipple.

2 Infiltrate the area with bupivacaine 0.5% and adrenaline (epinephrine) 1: 200 000 to minimize bleeding and postoperative pain.

3 When you pick up the nipple between finger and thumb, you may feel thickening along one duct, or feel the probe within the duct.

Action

1 Make a circumareolar incision and dissect down to expose the duct.

2 Excise the duct with a small amount of surrounding breast tissue and send it for histology.

3 Secure haemostasis.

Total duct excison (Hadfield's procedure)

1 Make a peri-areolar incision (but no more than three-fifths of the circumference of the areola).

2 Cut the subcutaneous tissue down to the duct system.

3 Use blunt and sharp dissection to reach the plane circumferentially around the terminal lactiferous ducts, just deep to the areola and nipple.

4 Divide the ducts close to the nipple and remove them with a conical wedge of tissue including the distal 1–2 cm of the subareolar tissue, including the major lactiferous ducts and sinuses. Orientate the specimen with marking suture for the pathologist.

5 Take a purse-string suture around the subcutaneous tissue where you have removed a wedge of retroareolar tissue, to prevent sinking of the nipple.

6 You may insert an inverted suture with vicryl from inside the nipple to prevent it from inverting.

7 Close the subcutaneous layer with absorbable sutures and skin with a non-absorbable suture such as prolene or ethilon.

▶ KEY POINT

■ Warn the patient of possible risks including nipple necrosis, loss of nipple sensation and nipple inversion.

FIBROADENOMAS

Appraise

Fibroadenomas are benign lesions, generally found in younger women. There is also increasing detection of fibroadenomas in women above the age of 45.

1 Confirm the presence of fibroadenoma using triple assessment.

2 These lesions are firm, well circumscribed, and mobile.

3 On palpation, a fibroadenoma may resemble a marble rolling under the fingertips.

Action

1 Make an incision depending upon the location of the fibroadenoma. (see Fig. 19.5). Make either a periareolar, submammary or a lateral incision as preferred.

2 If excision biopsy is indicated, prefer a peri-areolar incision. This results in the best cosmetic outcome.

3 Move the fibroadenoma to the site of the nipple–areola complex using your non-dominant hand.

4 With your dominant hand, make a peri-areolar or inframammary incision directly over the fibroadenoma, and excise the lesion through this incision.

5 Excise the fibroadenoma using sharp dissection, staying close to the edge of the lesion.

6 After removing the fibroadenoma pay meticulous attention to haemostasis using electrocautery.

7 Irrigate the wound then approximate the skin edges with a 3/0 or 4/0 Monocryl subcuticular stitch.

? DIFFICULTY

1. Fibroadenomas can be impalpable: ultrasonographic (USG) marking and wire localization may be used in these cases.
2. Fibroadenomas may be difficult to keep steady during excision. It may help to insert a stitch or a 21G needle through it to stabilize it prior to excision.

CARCINOMA AND DUCTAL CARCINOMA IN SITU

Establish the diagnosis preoperatively in all cases, by means of triple assessment. Counsel the patient about treatment options with close involvement of the Breast Clinical Nurse Specialist. Discuss the options of primary breast surgery such as wide local excision or mastectomy, axillary staging with sentinel node biopsy or axillary node dissection. In patients who have a large tumour (larger than 3.5 cm) you may discuss neoadjuvant chemotherapy. Ensure that you document your discussions

When carcinoma has been detected as a result of screening, you will have it confirmed by percutaneous biopsy and, if required, with wire-guided localization.

Appraise

1 The local management of breast carcinoma demands excision of the tumour with clear margins. If the tumour is small in comparison with the total breast volume, achieve this by wide local excision. Up to 20% of breast volume can be removed without significant cosmetic differences being observed by the patient. The long-term survival after wide local excision and radiotherapy equals that of a mastectomy. Some form of axillary surgery is still required to stage the patient and if necessary to treat the axillary disease. The importance of axillary node staging is reinforced by the evidence that adjuvant cytotoxic chemotherapy can reduce the relative risk of death by 20–25% in the node-positive population. A similar benefit is seen in patients who have hormone-responsive tumours, if they are given tamoxifen or the newer generation aromatase inhibitors. Sentinel node biopsy is now the accepted standard of care in staging the axilla (see below).

2 Mastectomy options:

■ Simple or total mastectomy: In this procedure, the entire breast is removed, but the lymph nodes and surrounding muscle are left intact.

■ Modified radical mastectomy: The entire breast, the axillary lymph nodes and the lining over the chest muscles are removed. The muscles remain intact.

■ Radical mastectomy: The breast, lymph nodes, muscles under the breast, and some of the surrounding fatty tissue are removed. This procedure is rarely performed. It is used in cases of extensive tumours where cancer cells have invaded the chest wall.

- Skin-sparing mastectomy (SSM): This is a relatively new surgical technique that may be an option for some patients. During this procedure, you make a much smaller incision, sometimes called a 'keyhole' incision, circling the areola. Even though the opening is small, the same amount of breast tissue is removed. Scarring is negligible and 90% of the skin is preserved. You perform reconstruction at the same time, using expandable implants, tissue from the patient's abdomen or a muscle in the back.
- Subcutaneous mastectomy (skin and nipple-sparing mastectomy): You remove the tumour and breast tissue but leave intact the nipple and the overlying skin. Reconstruction surgery is easier, but take extra care to ensure that no cancer cells are left in the retroareolar tissue.

3 Mastectomy with immediate reconstruction, using either an implant or a myocutaneous flap, is increasingly used by breast surgeons (oncoplastic surgery), sometimes in conjunction with plastic surgery colleagues. This procedure is also valuable in the management of extensive intraduct carcinoma and as a prophylactic procedure in patients with a very strong family history with proven BRCA gene mutation. This is discussed in further detail below.

4 Primary endocrine therapy (tamoxifen or aromatase inhibitors) may be used in frail elderly patients. Primary cytotoxic chemotherapy may be appropriate in otherwise fit patients with locally advanced cancer such as 'inflammatory' carcinoma. In patients with large tumours that are operable by mastectomy, primary (or neoadjuvant) chemotherapy may be used to shrink the tumour and allow breast conservation in up to 50% of cases.

5 Risk-reducing mastectomy is a term used when prophylactic mastectomy is offered to women with a family history of breast cancer that are considered high risk, including the ones with genetic mutations (BRCA1, BRCA2 gene defects).

PAGET'S DISEASE

1 Described by Sir James Paget (1814–1899), this disease frequently presents with a chronic, eczematous rash on the nipple and adjacent areolar skin. Proper recognition of this disorder is required to initiate an appropriate work up (e.g. skin biopsy) for differentiating it from other benign conditions like eczema. When you suspect this disease, perform a biopsy of the nipple area under local anaesthetic to confirm the diagnosis histologically. It may also be possible to do so with imprint cytology of the nipple.

2 When Paget's cells are demonstrated there is usually an underlying intraduct carcinoma, which is invasive in 50% of cases.

3 Mastectomy is usually recommended, but wide excision of the nipple and underlying breast tissue and radiotherapy are possible alternatives in less extensive cases.

BREAST CONSERVATION SURGERY

The aim of breast conservation surgery (BCS) is to provide not only an oncologically safe procedure, but also a good cosmetic outcome with minimal scarring and postoperative deformity. The basic principles lie in planning the right incision and choosing the right procedure for different tumours. Achieve this by using a cylinder

technique in which the tumour, with a clear zone of normal breast tissue, is excised in a cylindrical form from subcutaneous tissue to the pectoralis major muscle, ensuring clear radial and deep margin.

Breast conservation surgery now can be divided into two groups – tumours needing a simple wide local excision and ones requiring an oncoplastic procedure. You make the decision by estimating the tumour to breast ratio and the amount of tissue to be removed. Breast conservation may need to be supplemented with different symmetrization procedures to achieve symmetry with the contralateral breast. These are discussed in the plastic surgery section of this book. This includes mastopexy (Greek: mastos = breast, nipple + pexinai = to fix, fasten), reduction mammoplasty and nipple reconstructions.

Remember that after excision you must ensure the contour of the breast is maintained. Defects created by large excisions or quadrantectomy can be filled either by volume displacement or volume replacement. Glanduloplasty or mobilization of normal breast tissue to fill a defect is volume displacement. Use of fat filling or use of partial flaps (mini-flaps) to cover defects is volume replacement. Detailed discussion of volume replacement procedures is beyond the scope of this chapter; however, basic volume displacement techniques will be described here. Glanduloplasty and glandular remodelling must be considered for all defects that arise from any kind of excision of breast tissue.

WIDE LOCAL EXCISION/ QUADRANTECTOMY

Appraise

This is a therapeutic operation for the excision of a carcinoma, with the removal of clear zone of surrounding breast tissue. As an extra precaution, the cavity walls can be re-resected, thus increasing the chance of achieving clear margins and so reducing the need to return the patient to the operating theatre for a further resection. It does, however, have the potential disadvantage of prejudicing the cosmetic appearance.

Perform simple wide local excision in patients who will lose less than 20% of breast tissue.

Perform quadrantectomy or segmental mastectomy for a larger tumour. The procedure is similar to wide local excision (WLE), but requires the excision of a larger volume of breast tissue. You will need to consider glanduloplasty and various other oncoplastic techniques in this circumstance.

The different incisions for wide local excision are shown in Figure 19.5.

1 The aim is to excise the lesion with an adequate zone of normal breast tissue (at least 1 cm) and producing the least cosmetic defect.

▶ KEY POINT Inadequate surgery

- Excision biopsy consists of removing the suspected lesion with a narrow rim of normal tissue around it. It is insufficient for removal of carcinoma.

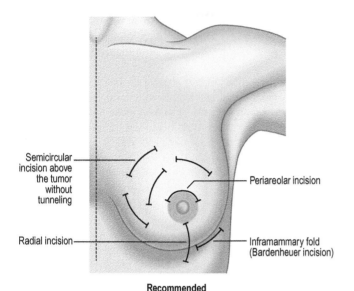

Semicircular
incision above
the tumor
without
tunneling

Periareolar incision

Radial incision

Inframammary fold
(Bardenheuer incision)

Recommended

Fig. 19.5 **The different incisions for wide local excision.**

2 Preliminary excision biopsy is occasionally necessary for a minority of patients with a breast carcinoma in whom the diagnosis cannot be established by preoperative cytology, core-cut needle biopsy and/or mammography. Definitive operation is then required as a second procedure after paraffin-section histological examination.

Prepare

> ### KEY POINT Inadequate surgery

> ■ Recommend all patients undergoing surgery for breast cancer to have deep vein thrombosis prophylaxis including anti-embolic compression TED stockings, together with intermittent pneumatic compression and warming blankets during surgery.

1 Check that the lesion is still present on admission. Occasionally, lesions disappear; this has been seen in certain patients who have been put on neoadjuvant drug therapy. Check also that no new lesion has appeared in either breast.

2 Mark the exact site of the lesion on the breast with the patient lying in the operating position; otherwise you may be unable to find the mass once the patient is anaesthetized.

3 Obtain informed consent for the operation and carefully explain the potential risks.

4 Check that you have the correct patient in the anaesthetic room and are operating on the correct side.

> ### KEY POINT

> ■ If the lesion is not palpable or is a small tumour in a large breast, consider ultrasound marking of lumps near the skin or opt for wire-guided localization.

Access (Fig. 19.5)

1 Incise over the region of the lump. Place the incision to minimize scarring.

2 Peri-areolar incisions heal with least visible scars, but may not always be suitable.

3 Incisions in the medial half of the breast have a tendency to develop keloid scars.

4 Avoid radial incisions except medially.

5 Place the incision within the area of skin that could be included within a mastectomy if it is deemed necessary subsequently. This avoids an unnecessary additional scar to the mastectomy scar.

Action

1 Ensure to excise the lump completely without cutting into it. Use sharp dissection with scissors or knife, or use diathermy whilst dissecting around the tumour.

2 Try not to cut into the specimen. The pathologist needs to report on the margins of excision and so needs to incise the lesion. Palpate the resected specimen to make sure you have removed the palpable abnormality. Excise a zone of normal breast tissue at least 1 cm around the palpable abnormality in all directions.

3 When you are operating on a benign lesion, it is unnecessary to resect cavity margins.

4 Ensure that you obtain good haemostasis. Try using the spray setting, if there is one, on the diathermy machine. Spray diathermy, also called fulguration mode, employs a high voltage. The electrode is held 2–4 mm from the tissue so that the current jumps across the air gap and spreads to create widespread coagulation. It is useful to cauterize small vessels without the need to pick them up in forceps.

Closure

1 In the majority of cases you do not need to introduce a drain. Otherwise insert a small suction drain to reduce the risk of a haematoma.

2 Close the skin using a subcuticular suture of 3/0 absorbable material. Support the closed wound with steri-strips.

> ### KEY POINTS

> ■ As a rule do not approximate the residual breast tissue at the edges of the cavity. However, this may leave an unacceptably large defect.
> ■ If you mobilize the residual breast and approximate the edges with absorbable sutures this restores shape, but it produces a greater loss of volume.
> ■ Avoid radial incisions and curvilinear incisions in the inferior and superolateral quadrant.
> ■ Avoid radial incisions near the areola as they cause severe nipple retraction.

ONCOPLASTIC SURGERY

Oncoplastic surgery is a relatively new field which combines the techniques of plastic surgery with oncologic principles of breast surgery to accomplish satisfactory cosmetic outcomes without compromising oncologic clearance. It is beyond the scope of this chapter to describe in detail every operation that is used in oncoplastic surgery. We shall provide a basic overview with the principles used to decide the type of operation. An advantage of oncoplastic surgery is that breast conservation surgery (BCS) can be performed in certain patients who would otherwise need mastectomy. Wider margins are taken, hence there is less need for re-operations because of involved margins.

Appraise

Two levels of oncoplastic surgery procedures (OPS) have been described: the decision to choose the level of procedure is dependent on the extent of loss of volume relative to the breast, the extent of skin incision and the density of breast tissue – whether it is glandular or fatty in nature. Criteria for choosing the Level I or II procedure are described in Table 19.1.

Level I procedures are performed using the prescribed steps described in Table 19.2 in order to prevent severe deformities that arise due to careless breast operations. The basic principles of a Level I procedure are to choose the correct incision, accomplish dual plane mobilization of breast tissue, complete full-thickness excision of the breast and volume displacement and glanduloplasty. Nipple–areolar complex (NAC) repositioning is performed using de-epithelialization of the peri-areolar skin.

The flow chart (Fig. 19.6) along with the adjoining figures (Fig. 19.7) describes the various operations that can be performed as part of the Level II procedures for OPS. Note that the size of the breasts and the ptosis of the breast determine the choice of the procedure.

AXILLARY SURGERY

■ Axillary nodal status remains the most important prognostic indicator and, combined with the tumour size and grade, it forms the Nottingham Prognostic Index (NPI).

■ All patients with invasive breast cancer must have their axilla assessed preoperatively with an US scan. If nodes are suspicious clinically or on scanning, they must undergo preoperative FNAC or core biopsy to confirm metastatic disease.

■ All node-positive patients on preoperative work up should be offered axillary clearance.

TABLE 19.1 Oncoplastic decision guide

Criteria	Level I	Level II
Maximum excision volume ratio	20%	20–50%
Requirement of skin excision for reshaping	No	Yes
Mammoplasty	No	Yes
Glandular characteristics	Dense	
(reference Krishna Clough)		

TABLE 19.2 Level I OPS: step-by-step surgical approach

Procedure	Result
Skin incision	Allows wide access for excision and reshaping
Skin undermining	Facilitates wide excision and glandular mobilization for reshaping
NAC undermining	Avoids displacement of nipple towards excision defect
Full-thickness excision	Prevents anterior and posterior margin involvement
Glandular reapproximation	Late-occurring deformity is avoided
De-epithelialization and NAC repositioning	Re-centres NAC on new breast mound

■ All patients who are node negative on preoperative work up must be offered sentinel lymph node (SLN) biopsy. SLN is the first node(s) receiving lymph from the primary tumour and accurately reflects the nodal status of the axilla.

■ There are several methods of intra-operative assessment of SLN, using various techniques including the one-stage nucleic acid (OSNA) test, which is an RCR based technology, touch imprint cytology and frozen-section histology.

■ If intra-operative tests are available at your centre, always perform sentinel node biopsy before the breast surgery to save time.

■ If nodes are found to be positive for cancer cells, perform axillary lymph node dissection (ALND) during the same operation.

■ Where results of sentinel node biopsy are available at a later date and positive nodes are detected, patients are recommended to undergo further axillary treatment (completion ALND or axillary radiotherapy).

SENTINEL NODE BIOPSY

The sentinel (Italian: *sentinella* = on guard) node is the first node to which the lymph drainage of the breast goes. With a patient who has a clinically uninvolved axilla, sentinel node biopsy has replaced conventional axillary dissection. The node is identified by injecting a radioisotope (usually technetium-99 m combined with colloidal albumin particles) some hours before operation, combined with a blue dye (Patent Blue V) injected when the patient is on the operating table.

Prepare

1 Discuss with the patient if you intend to proceed to a full axillary clearance if you discover positive nodes, so you have informed consent.

2 Warn the patient about the need for a second operation if the sentinel node is found to be positive subsequent to surgery.

Upper inner	Upper central	Upper outer
Small - Round block S, reduction Medium-Round block S reduction, inferior pedicle/sup pedicle Large -S reduction sup. / inf. pedicle Round block	Small - Round block S reduction Medium-Round block S reduction, inferior pedicle/sup pedicle Large - S reduction . / inf. pedicle Round block	Small - Round block S reduction Medium-Round block S reduction, inferior pedicle/sup pedicle fusiform mammoplasty Large -S reduction sup. / inf. pedicle Round block fusiform mammoplasty

Central and Lower central
Small - Benelli, S Reduction, Vertical mammoplasty Medium-Vertical mammoplasty, Inferior Pedicle Flap and Grisotti Flap Large/Ptotic Breasts-Inferior pedicle flap, Grisotti, Inverted T resection

Lower inner	Lower outer
Small-Superior pedicle mammoplasty/inverted T or vertical scar Medium- Superior pedicle mammoplasty/inverted T or vertical scar Large- Superior pedicle mammoplasty/inverted T or vertical scar	Small-Superior pedicle mammoplasty/inverted T or vertical scar Medium- Superior pedicle mammoplasty/inverted T or vertical scar Large- Superior pedicle mammoplasty/inverted T or vertical scar

Fig. 19.6   Recommended procedures for level II oncoplastic surgery depending on the quadrant of tumour.

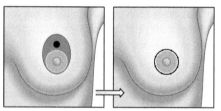

Periareolar mammoplasty
Upper Outer

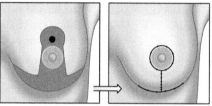

Inferior pedicle mammoplasty
Upper Central

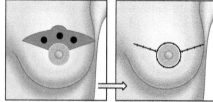

Omega mammoplasty
Central

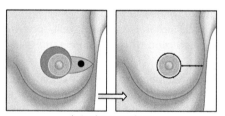

Lateral mammoplasty
Upper Outer

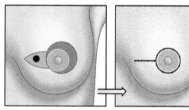

Medial mammoplasty
Upper Inner

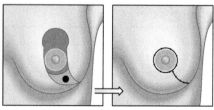

J Plasty
Lower Outer

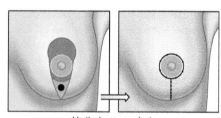

Vertical mammoplasty
Lower Inner

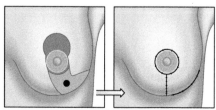

L Plasty
Lower Outer

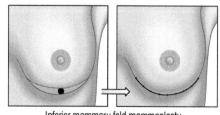

Inferior mammary fold mammoplasty
Lower Central

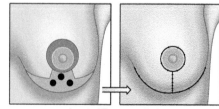

Inverted T mammoplasty
Central

Fig. 19.7   Oncoplastic surgery operations.

3 Mention injection of blue dye carries around 1% risk of allergic reaction and will cause the urine to become green. Warn the patient about the blue staining/tattooing of the skin.

4 Check the lymphoscintigram (if available) for the presence and number of hot nodes in the axilla.

5 If you have intra-operative diagnostic techniques available, perform SLN biopsy before breast surgery.

Access

1 Allow enough time for the blue dye to travel from the injection site to the axilla. This is of the order of 5–10 minutes, therefore inject the dye before scrubbing.

2 Make a short incision over the site of maximum radioactivity as detected by the gamma probe.

3 If no clear signal is obtained, make the incision just below and medial to the edge of the hair-bearing skin.

Action

1 When you open the axilla you usually see blue lymphatic vessels. Follow these to the relevant node. The node can also be localized using the gamma probe, which directs you by the shortest route to the SLN.

2 Gently remove the node without damaging it.

3 When you have excised the SLN, carefully check that there are not other sentinel nodes present.

4 Achieve perfect haemostasis.

5 Close the wound using subcuticular soluble stitches.

Postoperative

1 Following wide local excision and sentinel node biopsy you can usually discharge the patient on the same day.

AXILLARY LYMPH NODE DISSECTION

Appraise

1 Axillary dissection must be performed only as a therapeutic procedure in breast cancer patients with proven axillary disease and has no place as a staging procedure.

2 Level II (up to the medial border of pectoralis minor) or level III (beyond the medial border of pectoralis minor and below the axillary vein) axillary lymph node dissection (ALND) is an operation that is therapeutic, providing local disease control without the need for axillary irradiation.

3 The combination of axillary surgery and irradiation is associated with high risk of lymphoedema.

Prepare

1 Shave the axilla.

2 Warn the patient about the possibility of postoperative numbness or paraesthesia if the intercostobrachial nerve is damaged, and of lymphoedema.

3 Encourage the patient to move the shoulder fully before operation and arrange for her to be taught shoulder exercises to perform after operation.

Access

1 Axillary clearance performed either through an oblique incision just behind, and parallel to, the lateral edge of the pectoralis major muscle provides good access but has the disadvantage of producing an ugly scar and limitation of shoulder abduction. We prefer a transverse incision with its anterior corner at the pectoral edge and the posterior angle just crossing the anterior border of latissimus dorsi, with the arm abducted at 90°. Cosmetically the latter incision produces better result.

2 Use a combination of sharp and blunt dissection at either end of the axillary incision to identify the lateral border of pectoralis major and the anterior border of latissimus dorsi muscles. These landmarks form the anterior and posterior limits of your axillary dissection.

3 Dissect up and down along the lateral border of the pectoralis major muscle and identify the underlying pectoralis minor muscle. Insinuate a finger under the insertion of pectoralis minor to separate it from the underlying structures and have your assistant retract the muscle forwards and medially in order to expose the axillary contents of level II.

4 If you intend to carry out a level III clearance, define both borders of the pectoralis minor muscle. It may be necessary to divide the insertion into the coracoid process but with good assistance it is usually possible to dissect behind the muscle.

5 Flex and abduct the shoulder and flex the elbow so that the forearm lies across the patient's towelled-off face to facilitate exposure of the subpectoral area. Have the arm supported by an assistant or sling it from the crossbar of the anaesthetist's drape support.

> ### ► KEY POINTS Preserve structures
>
> - Carefully follow and preserve the thoracodorsal trunk down into latissimus dorsi muscle and the nerve to serratus anterior (long thoracic nerve of Bell).
> - Also avoid damaging the lateral division of the medial pectoral nerve and the long thoracic nerve.
> - Try and preserve the intercostobrachial nerve if possible.
> - Identify and carefully ligate the angular vein which runs anteriorly into the thoracodorsal trunk.

6 Gently 'stroke' the axillary contents away from the chest wall and off the subscapularis muscle using a gauze swab or 'peanut' swab, to identify the nerve to serratus anterior in the posterior axillary line, and the nerve to latissimus dorsi travelling with the subscapular vessels.

7 Identify the intercostobrachial nerve and dissect it free from the axillary contents (if possible), preserving as many branches as feasible.

8 Now you have defined the limits of the dissection and the nerves, you can complete the removal of the axillary contents.

9 Achieve complete haemostasis.

1. If you are unable to remove the axillary contents without severing the intercostobrachial nerve, do not hesitate to divide it; afterwards inform the patient that she is likely to experience a little numbness on the medial aspect of her upper arm.
2. Axillary vein damage should not happen, but occasionally an over-enthusiastic assistant can tear a vein. Repair this promptly – if necessary ask for help from an experienced vascular surgeon. A short course of postoperative anticoagulation may be required if significant venous injury has occurred.
3. If there is heavy nodal involvement in the axilla excise all the palpable lymph nodes together with any soft tissue disease.
4. Only rarely is tumour found encasing the axillary vein and it is usually fairly easy to dissect off. If you have to leave any tumour behind, mark it with surgical clips to allow planning of any future radiotherapy.

Closure

1. Insert a vacuum drain into the axilla and suture the skin with subcuticular sutures.
2. Personally supervise the dressing of the wound. In particular, squeeze out all blood and air from under the flaps into the vacuum containers in order to avoid the subsequent development of an axillary seroma.
3. Before sending the specimen to the pathology laboratory mark the apex of the specimen with a stitch. This helps the pathologist to orientate around the specimen and subsequently report on it.

SIMPLE MASTECTOMY

Appraise

Indications for performing a mastectomy

1. Patient's choice.
2. Multifocal disease.
3. Recurrence after breast conserving therapy when radiotherapy has already been given.
4. Patients with DCIS more than 4 cm or multifocal DCIS.
5. Women with certain serious connective tissue diseases such as scleroderma, which make them especially sensitive to the side-effects of radiation therapy.
6. Pregnant women who would require radiotherapy (risking harm to the child).
7. A tumour larger than 5 cm that doesn't shrink significantly with neoadjuvant therapy.
8. A cancer that is large relative the breast size.
9. Women who have tested positive for a mutation on the BRCA1 or BRCA2 gene and opt for prophylactic removal of the breasts.
10. Male breast cancer patients.

Appraise

1. Check that the histological diagnosis of breast carcinoma has been confirmed.
2. If the diagnosis rests on positive cytology, ensure that you are satisfied clinically and radiologically about the diagnosis.
3. If axillary ultrasound does not reveal any abnormality, offer sentinel node biopsy and if an abnormal node is detected, after cytological confirmation of involvement with metastatic cancer, proceed with axillary dissection.
4. In case of doubt perform a preliminary biopsy for paraffin sections to be examined.

■ The archaic 'Frozen section? Proceed' operation is no longer acceptable.

Prepare

1. Confirm that the patient has seen the Breast Clinical Nurse Specialist and has had an opportunity to fully discuss her diagnosis and treatment.
2. Breast reconstruction should be available for every patient undergoing mastectomy. Ensure that the patient is aware of this, offered either immediately or as a delayed procedure.
3. Mark the side and site of the carcinoma.
4. Cross-matched blood is seldom necessary, but establish the patient's blood group.
5. With a skin-marking pen, mark the position of the lump. Draw an ellipse for the incision, lying transversely and encompassing approximately 5 cm of skin around the lesion and also the nipple (Fig. 19.5). Mark the patient in standing up position and mark the inframammary crease as well.

Access

1. Position the patient on the operating table in the supine position, with the arm on the operative side extended on an arm board.
2. Prepare the skin and place the towels to allow access to the breast and axilla. Wrap the arm separately to facilitate axillary dissection (see below).
3. If a transverse incision is impracticable, then make an oblique incision, but do not place it high. The current trend is to place the mastectomy incision as low as possible near the inframammary fold, which gives much better cosmetic outcome after delayed reconstruction.
4. Ensure that you will be able to approximate the wound edges at the end of the operation before you make the incisions along your marked lines.

Action

1. Elevate the skin flaps in the plane between subcutaneous fat and mammary fat. This can be facilitated by subcutaneous infiltration with 1:400 000 adrenaline (epinephrine) in saline or 0.25% bupivacaine (Marcaine) and adrenaline (epinephrine).

2 Have your assistant hold up the skin flaps and constantly check the flap thickness. Ensure that the flap is not too thin, resulting in 'button-holing' or ischaemia and not too thick that you leave breast tissue in the flaps.

3 Raise the upper flap to the upper limit of the breast. This is usually 2–3 cm below the clavicle, but varies from patient to patient. A good guide is the second intercostal space.

4 Catch any bleeding points with diathermy forceps and take care not to burn the skin. If skin is inadvertently burned, excise the damaged area (Fig. 19.8). Burnt skin takes many weeks to heal and is painful.

5 Raise the lower flap in a similar manner, to the inframammary fold.

6 Try to preserve the inframammary fold if reconstruction of breast is planned.

7 Place a large tissue forceps, such as Lane's, on the breast which is to be removed, handing it to an assistant to apply traction, thus facilitating the subsequent dissection.

8 Return to the uppermost part of the breast and dissect down until you see the fascia of pectoralis major. Pectoral fascia is taken if the tumour is deeply placed or is attached to the muscle.

9 Proceed in this plane in a downwards direction, identifying and ligating the perforating vessels as they appear (mainly second and third intercostal spaces), before dividing them. This considerably reduces the amount of operative bleeding.

10 If the tumour appears to infiltrate into the pectoralis muscle, then excise a portion of this muscle with the specimen.

11 Continue downwards, elevating the breast alternatively laterally and medially but leaving the axillary tail of the breast in continuity with the axillary contents.

12 Place dry packs under each skin flap.

13 Perform a SLNB or ALND based on the plan for staging the axilla. If you have facilities for intra-operative testing of SLN, perform SLN biopsy before mastectomy.

Closure

1 Insert two vacuum drains, one for the flaps and a second for the axilla.

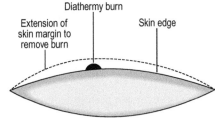

Fig. 19.8 Removal of accidental diathermy burn.

2 Suture the skin edges with subcuticular sutures. If there is a discrepancy between the lengths of the two flaps, close the wound using interrupted sutures placed halfway along the incision then halfway between these lengths and so on, thus avoiding a 'dog-ear' at one end.

3 After completing the closure, activate the vacuum drains and squeeze out all the fluid and air from beneath the skin flaps so that they adhere to the chest wall.

Aftercare

1 Encourage early mobilization to prevent deep vein thrombosis (DVT). Use TED stockings in all patients.

2 All patients must be offered supply and fitting of a breast prosthesis during the postoperative period.

   Artificial breasts are now available that are of a weight and consistency comparable with the removed breast. They change shape with the patient's change of posture and they take on body temperature. It is difficult to identify which is the side of the mastectomy when feeling through a patient's clothes.

3 Make yourself aware of the range and variety of prostheses available. In the UK, under Health Service regulations, any woman is entitled to the type and size of prosthesis of her choice. In addition, these may be replaced as frequently as necessary. If you are unaware of the variety available, delegate the responsibility to the Appliance Officer.

4 Many centres now employ mastectomy counsellors who, as well as providing psychosocial rehabilitation of the patient, are responsible for the physical rehabilitation. This includes the prescription of a soft temporary prosthesis immediately postoperatively, which can be worn for about 6 weeks until the wound is healed and not sensitive and then replaced by the permanent prosthesis worn within the brassiere.

5 Commence active physiotherapy within 24 hours of operation and provide the patient with a list of exercises for abduction of the arm to minimize shoulder stiffness.

SKIN-SPARING MASTECTOMY (Fig. 19.9)

Usually, skin-sparing mastectomy (SSM) is performed with an immediate reconstruction.

Appraise

The common indications for SSM include:

1 Risk-reducing mastectomy in patients with genetic mutations.

2 Patients having mastectomy for DCIS.

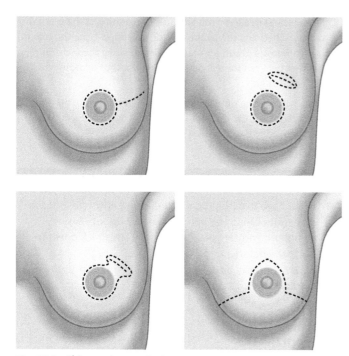

Fig. 19.9 Skin sparing mastectomy.

3 Skin-sparing mastectomy and immediate breast reconstruction (SSM and IBR) is the treatment of choice for early stage breast cancer patients who need or desire a mastectomy.

4 Patients with locally advanced breast cancer or patients with local recurrences after breast conservative surgery (BCS).

Prepare

1 The inframammary fold is delineated preoperatively with a marking pen with the patient in the upright position. The nipple–areolar complex, skin overlying superficial cancers and previous biopsy incisions are marked.

2 Four possible incisions can be used in SSM:
- A type 1 peri-areolar incision with or without lateral extension is useful in non-palpable tumours and smaller breasts.
- Type II SSM is used when a superficial tumour or previous biopsy is in proximity to the areola.
- Type III SSM is used when the superficial tumour or previous incision was remote from the areola. Care must be taken to ensure the viability of the intervening skin.
- A type IV SSM Wise pattern is used in large, ptotic breasts when a reduction is planned on the opposite breast (see Fig. 19.9).

> ▶ KEY POINT
>
> ■ A common problem with the Wise pattern incision is necrosis of the most distal portions of the flap, particularly at the 'T' junction.

Action

1 Place patient in supine position in arms abducted to 90° position.

2 Prepare both breasts and expose the arms to the mid humerus level.

3 Elevate the skin flaps superficial to the enveloping fascia of the breasts. The skin thickness depends upon the body habitus. Keep the cautery in a low blend mode and elevate the skin in a centripetal direction. Use double-pronged skin hooks for skin retraction. If a Wise pattern is used the vertical limbs can be de-epithelialized and used to cover an implant or an expander.

> ▶ KEY POINT
>
> ■ Breast tissue extends closer to the skin in the lower quadrants and the subcutaneous tissue is thicker in the upper, outer quadrant of the breast. In a thin patient, skin flap thickness may be only 2 to 3 mm and transmit light. In the obese patient, the flaps may be 5 to 10 mm in thickness.

4 Superiorly, the breast falls away from the skin as the clavicle is approached. Follow the fascia down to the pectoralis major muscle.

5 Medially, the fascia is not very well defined, stop the dissection at the border of the sternum.

6 Perforating vessels of the internal mammary artery are frequently encountered along the sternal border. Preserve these perforators to improve the blood supply of the skin flap. These vessels can also be used as recipient vessels in free flap breast reconstruction.

7 Inferiorly, follow the superficial layer of the fascia to its junction with the deep layer. The skin is adherent to the anterior abdominal wall at this juncture.

8 Laterally, continue the dissection over the pectoralis muscle toward the humerus, enabling removal of the axillary tail.

9 Use a lighted retractor or an extended electrocautery when the access becomes very deep.

10 Remove the breast by elevating the fascia of the pectoralis major muscle with the specimen. This is best accomplished by dissecting parallel to the muscle fibres.

Closure

1 This will depend upon the type of reconstruction that is performed with a SSM.

> ? DIFFICULTY
>
> 1. SSM is technically more demanding and time consuming than a traditional total mastectomy. Careful handling of the skin flaps is required to prevent ischaemic complications.
> 2. Skin flap viability is assessed clinically if ischaemia of skin is suspected.
> 3. If there is a question of skin perfusion, fluorescein can also be employed.

BREAST RECONSTRUCTION

1 In order to undertake breast reconstruction you need skill in assessing the patient's suitability for the various procedures as well as in the technical performance of a procedure.

2 While most patients with operable breast cancer can now be treated by breast-conserving surgery, careful attention must be paid to patient selection and technique to achieve optimal cosmetic results. All patients undergoing mastectomy should be offered the option of a reconstruction, as either an immediate or a delayed procedure (Table 19.3). Fears about hiding local recurrence or affecting survival are unfounded and have been disproved.

3 The aims of a breast reconstruction are to achieve symmetry, provide a lasting result and satisfy the patient's requirement for a good aesthetic result in terms of shape, form, consistency and size. These demand a skilled, experienced surgeon specializing in breast reconstruction.

4 There are many available techniques including the insertion of a submuscular silicone implant, placement of a tissue expansion device with subsequent implant insertion, implantation of a 'permanent' expander, and autologous tissue transfer using either the latissimus dorsi myocutaneous flap with or without a silicone implant or a myocutaneous flap (DIEP flap or TRAM flap), which has the advantage of not requiring an implant.

5 Consider construction of a new nipple/areola complex and adjustment of the contralateral breast.

6 Loss of more than 20% of the breast volume is associated with a cosmetic defect. Some patients may be suitable for 'fill' procedures such as latissimus dorsi mini-flap without transposition of skin.

BREAST RECONSTRUCTION WITH A 'PERMANENT' TISSUE EXPANDER/ SILICONE IMPLANTS

Appraise

1 Prior chest wall irradiation is a relative contraindication to this procedure.

2 Following mastectomy a breast mound can be recreated using a subpectoral silicone prosthesis. This can be done either at the time of mastectomy or as a delayed procedure at any time later.

3 Note that only a very moderate degree of ptosis can be achieved by an implant and there is a limit to the size of breast mound that can be made. In patients with large and/or ptotic breasts either a myocutaneous flap such as LD with or without implant or DIEP flap may be indicated. Alternatively, the contralateral breast can be reduced or lifted.

> **KEY POINTS** Suitability?
>
> - Involve the breast CNS.
> - Have the patient assessed as to her suitability for breast reconstruction and the choice of method.
> - Show her photographs of your results, let her read any literature on the subject and if possible arrange for her to meet a patient who has had the procedure.
> - This ensures that she has realistic expectations and is likely to be satisfied with the result.

Prepare

1 Discuss the operation and complications with the patient, including any concerns she may have about silicone. You can reassure the patient that the use of silicone implants is safe.

2 Order selection of implants if a bank of implants is not available. To gain enough expertise in reconstruction operations, it is likely you will be working in a unit that has access to all these facilities.

3 Preoperatively, mark the breast borders, including the position of the inframammary fold.

4 Administer antibiotics with induction of anaesthesia.

Action

1 If the procedure is being performed at the same time as mastectomy, following removal of the breast and appropriate

TABLE 19.3 Options for immediate or delayed breast reconstruction

Option	Indications/advantages	Disadvantages
Implant-based reconstruction	■ Good for small breasts with minimal ptosis ■ Single or two operations, low morbidity ■ Cannot be used in irradiated breasts	■ Contracture formation ■ Implant rupture ■ Lifelong risk of infection ■ Implant change may be required
Autologous tissue	■ Most women who undergo a mastectomy are candidates for this type of reconstruction ■ Entails using the patient's own tissues to create a breast mound ■ Avoids the complications of implants ■ Natural feel and texture of tissue	■ Flap failure ■ Longer recovery ■ Donor site complications
Implant plus autologous tissue	■ Can be used in patients with previous radiation ■ Can be used in patients who are too thin or have had previous abdominoplasty	■ All the risks of implants ■ All the risks of autologous tissues

axillary surgery make an incision in the line of the fibres of pectoralis major at about the level of the sixth intercostal space.

2 If the procedure is delayed, open the old mastectomy scar and free skin flaps from underlying fascia and muscle using sharp dissection.

3 Form a pocket between pectoralis major and the underlying ribs and intercostal muscles. Use a combination of blunt and sharp dissection, including diathermy.

▶ KEY POINTS Technical aids

- ■ Make sure you have good lighting. A head-light may be a valuable aid.
- ■ Carefully arrange suitable retraction.
- ■ Maintain good haemostasis.

4 You may need to employ sharp dissection under the fibres of rectus abdominis muscle.

5 Open the implant and soak it in an antiseptic or antibiotic solution. If using an expander, remove all air from the expander. Insert the expander or implant into the submuscular pocket (Fig. 19.10).

6 If using an expander with a port, the tubing is brought out of the submuscular pocket at the lateral side of the chest wall, through pectoralis major muscle. You need to form a subcutaneous pocket using dissecting scissors, well away from the implant.

7 Suture the port in place.

8 Close the pectoralis muscle over the implant. Inflate the implant with saline provided the muscle tension allows this.

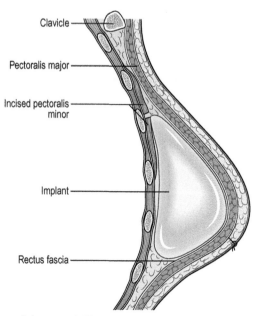

Fig. 19.10 **Subpectoral silicone implant.**

Clavicle

Pectoralis major

Incised pectoralis minor

Implant

Rectus fascia

? DIFFICULTY

1. If the pectoralis muscle is somewhat atrophied in the lower part, it can be completely detached from its lower border and either the muscle can be closed over the prosthesis or it can even be left so that the lower part of the implant is subcutaneous.
2. If you make small holes in the muscle when forming the subpectoral pocket, repair them using absorbable sutures.
3. You may improve the cosmetic result by reconstructing a submammary fold using absorbable sutures from the muscle to the subcutaneous tissue.
4. The use of tissue matrices in implant-based reconstruction has helped achieve an excellent cosmetic outcome.

Closure

1 Insert two vacuum drains, one submuscularly over the implant and the other subcutaneously.

2 Close the wound in two layers uniting subcutaneous tissues deeply and closing the skin with subcuticular sutures.

Aftercare

1 Arrange for the patient to wear a firm brassiere or compression garment for at least 2 weeks.

2 If expanders are used, commence expansion of the prosthesis as an outpatient procedure under sterile conditions. Insert a butterfly needle into the port at the side of the chest wall (or use the magnet to identify the site of the insertion of the needle into the self-sealing prosthesis) and inject 50–100 ml of saline. Repeat this at weekly or longer intervals until you achieve the correct volume to match the opposite breast. Some devices, such as the Becker, require over-expansion for a time.

3 Warn the patient that achieving ptosis can take up to 1 year.

LATISSIMUS DORSI FLAP RECONSTRUCTION

1 The latissimus dorsi is generally a safe flap and is within the expertise of an experienced oncoplastic breast surgeon (see Chapter 33).

2 Develop the ability to think in three dimensions so you can assess which part of the skin, if necessary, needs to be rotated to fill the defect.

3 The flap area can be used without skin to fill large defects.

DEVELOPMENTAL ABNORMALITIES

Appraise

1 Mastitis neonatorum occurs in the first few days of life, is associated with maternal hormones and subsides spontaneously. Rarely, infection supervenes, requiring surgical drainage.

2 Extra or supernumerary breasts and/or nipples are encountered along the milk line from midclavicular region to groin. Do not intervene unless they become involved with a disease process such as may affect normal breast tissue or unless the size is cosmetically unacceptable. Lactation may occur with pregnancy, and carcinoma occasionally arises in a supernumerary breast. Treatment is as for any breast disease.

3 With the onset of puberty, one breast disc may enlarge in a young girl from the age of 8 years onwards. If the disc is excised, no breast will develop on this side of the body; if it is biopsied, the developed breast may be deformed.

> ### ▶ KEY POINTS Preserve children's breasts
>
> - Do not excise unilateral breast enlargements thinking they are neoplasms.
> - Neoplasms are almost unknown before the age of 12 years.
> - See the child again in a few months; usually the other breast disc has begun to enlarge.
> - Reassure the mother and child.

4 In some racial groups (Afro-Caribbean and some Asians), axillary accessory breast tissue can be a problem. This accessory tissue is occasionally removed for cosmesis or if it enlarges extensively during pregnancy. The scars are often unattractive and may become infected, so counsel the patient beforehand.

5 Poland's syndrome is an uncommon congenital chest-wall deformity characterized by unilateral absence of the sternal head of the pectoralis major muscle, deficiency of the breast and nipple, chest-wall deformity and abnormalities of the upper extremity including finger-shortening and syndactyly. Correction is difficult and requires specialist expertise.

6 Breast size is rarely uniform and you may be consulted by patients asking for a procedure to make them even. Should you enlarge the smaller breast or reduce the larger breast? Generally, prefer the latter unless the smaller breast is very undeveloped. Timing is important. The under-developed breast may catch up towards the end of puberty; balance this against the embarrassment that unevenness may cause during this period of a girl's life.

OTHER BREAST PROCEDURES

BREAST AUGMENTATION

This requires insertion of prostheses either in the submammary or subpectoral plane in order to enhance the breast size. This operation is not generally available on the UK Health Service. Take care in counselling these patients. Determine what exactly the patient's expectations are. Unless you are expert, refer these patients to a specialist.

BREAST REDUCTION

This operation is allowed under the National Health Service in patients with symptomatic macromastia and is generally of great benefit to the patient. Increasingly a minimum of about 500 g must be removed on each side before the Health Service is willing to allow the procedure to be undertaken.

From the various techniques that are available you need to make a suitable selection for each patient after discussion of the scars, alteration of nipple sensation, potential loss of the nipple, and prospects of breast feeding. Show pictures of previous patients following this procedure. Warn patients that the breast tissue may grow back.

GYNAECOMASTIA

Appraise

1 This is frequently unilateral and may occur in boys and young men. It usually settles without treatment.

2 If it does not settle, it may be necessary to excise the breast disc on one or both sides. Carry this out through a peri-areolar incision or a round block technique without leaving a noticeable scar, but there is a high incidence of postoperative haematomas. It is best to leave a nubbin of breast tissue attached to the areola for best cosmetic results.

3 Gynaecomastia also occurs in old age, associated with drugs given for hypertension or congestive cardiac failure. Less frequently nowadays it is seen in men treated with high doses of oestrogens for prostatic cancer and in men suffering from alcoholic cirrhosis. Occasionally, subcutaneous mastectomy is indicated if the condition is an embarrassment or is causing pain and tenderness. One of the common causes is cannabis usage.

4 Operations for gynaecomastia are often performed badly and patient dissatisfaction is high. You must warn the patient about the likely outcome and, if you feel that the patient has inappropriate expectations, refer him to a specialist. Newer techniques of endoscopic surgery and liposuction are available.

FURTHER READING

Bostwick J. Plastic and Reconstructive Breast Surgery. St Louis: Quality Medical Publishing; 1997.

Clough KB, Kaufman GJ, Nos C, et al. Improving breast cancer surgery: a classification and quadrant per quadrant atlas for oncoplastic surgery. Ann Surg Oncol 2010;17(5):1375–91.

Curran D, van Dongen JP, Aaronson N, et al. Quality of life of early stage breast cancer patients treated with radical mastectomy or breast conserving procedures. Eur J Cancer 1998;34:307–14.

Dixon M. ABC of Breast Disease. London: BMJ Publishing Group; 1995.

Early Breast Cancer Trialists' Collaborative Group. Effects of radiotherapy and surgery in early breast cancer. N Engl J Med 1995;333:1444–55.

Early Breast Cancer Trialists' Collaborative Group. Ovarian ablation in early breast cancer: an overview of the randomised trials. Lancet 1996;348:1189–96.

Early Breast Cancer Trialists' Collaborative Group. Tamoxifen for early breast cancer: an overview of the randomised trials. Lancet 1998;351:1451–67.

Early Breast Cancer Trialists' Collaborative Group. Polychemotherapy for early breast cancer: an overview of the randomised trials. Lancet 1998;352:930–42.

Fisher B, Redmond C, Poisson R, et al. Eight year results of a randomized trial comparing total mastectomy and lumpectomy with or without radiation in the treatment of breast cancer. N Engl J Med 1989;320:822–8.

Fitoussi A, Berry MG, Couturaud B, Salmon RJ. Oncoplastic and Reconstructive Surgery for Breast Cancer: The Institut Curie Experience. France: Springer; 2008.

Fitzal F, Schrenk P, editors. Oncoplastic Breast Surgery: A Guide to Clinical Practice. New York: Springer; 2010.

Harris JR, Hellman S, Henderson IC, et al. Breast Diseases. Philadelphia: Lippincott; 1987.

Hermon C, Beral V. Breast cancer mortality rates are levelling off or beginning to decline in many western countries: an analysis of time trends, age-cohort and age-period models of breast cancer mortality in 20 countries. Br J Cancer 1996;73:955–60.

Hughes LE, Mansel RE, Webster DJT. Benign Disorders and Diseases of the Breast: Concepts and Clinical Management. London: Bailliere Tindall; 1989.

Jatoi I, Kaufman M, Petit JY. Atlas of Breast Surgery. London: Springer; 2006.

Keshtgar MRS, Ell PJ. Sentinel lymph node detection and imaging. Eur J Nucl Med 1999;26:57–67.

Mariani L, Salvadori B, Marubini E, et al. Ten year results of a randomised trial comparing two conservative treatment strategies for small size breast cancer. Eur J Cancer 1998;34:1156–62.

Silverstein MJ. Ductal carcinoma in situ of the breast. Br Med J 1998;317:734–9.

20

Thyroid

J.C. Watkinson, J.A. Smith

CONTENTS

Appraise

1 Indications for thyroid surgery fall into three categories:
   - Suspected or proven malignancy
   - Benign symptomatic goitre
   - Graves' disease (named after the Irish physician Robert James Graves, who described a case of goitre with exophthalmos in 1835. In Europe the condition is named after Karl von Basedow).

2 All thyroid surgery carries significant potential morbidity. Carefully investigate patients about to undergo surgery and involve the multidisciplinary team to avoid inappropriate or unnecessary surgery. Thyroid surgery is a significant potential source of litigation. As well as counselling your patient, provide clear documentation, especially with regard to potential damage to the recurrent laryngeal nerve and the parathyroid glands.

3 Thyroid surgery is increasingly performed in specialist centres by surgeons with a special interest in thyroid disorders. Closely liaise with endocrinologists and oncologists to achieve satisfactory outcomes. Joint or combined clinics are advocated, particularly for patients with complex disease.

4 It is mandatory to have access to and attend an appropriate multidisciplinary team meeting (MDT) if you regularly undertake malignant thyroid surgery. Familiarize yourself with local arrangements.

5 Be willing to work jointly with other surgical specialists, such as cardiothoracic surgeons, when treating retrosternal extensions.

6 Re-operation in the neck carries significantly increased morbidity. As a result, partial or subtotal thyroidectomy is now less frequently performed in favour of either hemi- or total thyroidectomy. The aim is to leave behind as little thyroid tissue as possible.

7 Audit your results personally, locally and nationally. In the UK results are submitted to the British Association of Endocrine and Thyroid Surgeons (BAETS).[1] The Association publishes audit results and guidelines for managing thyroid disease. Familiarize yourself with the website www.baets.org.uk.

8 Assessment (see Table 20.1).

9 Investigate:
   - *Biochemical evaluation* is mandatory in patients with thyroid disease. Familiarize yourself with and check thyroid function tests (tri-iodothyronine (T3), thyroxine (T4) and thyroid stimulating hormone: TSH), as well as calcium and albumin assays, prior to considering surgery. Undiagnosed or unrecognized thyrotoxicosis can lead to serious consequences during general anaesthesia. Vitamin D levels may be assayed in areas where deficiency is endemic and corrected prior to surgery. Thyroid auto-antibodies may also be requested to screen for the presence of Hashimoto's thyroiditis (first described by Japanese physician Hashimoto Hakaru in Germany in 1912).
   - *Fine needle aspiration cytology* (FNAC) is an efficient and cost-effective method of evaluating thyroid nodules. Diagnostic accuracy is dependent on the experience of the operator,

TABLE 20.1 Assessment in the clinic		
Ask yourself:	History	Examination
Is the patient euthyroid?	Intolerance to heat and cold, weight loss, altered bowel habit, anxiety/depression	Tachycardia, tremor, Graves' eye signs, skin changes
What kind of goitre is this?	Physiologic, toxic	Diffuse, solitary nodule, multinodular
Is a malignant process likely?	Neck pain, hoarseness, family history of thyroid cancer, previous exposure to radiation	Lymph nodal masses, recurrent laryngeal nerve palsy, fixation, Berry's sign (loss of carotid pulsation indicating invasion by tumour)
Does the patient have obstruction?	Dysphagia, shortness of breath, inability to lay flat	Stridor, venous engorgement, Pemberton's sign (Hugh Pemberton, 1946) – facial flushing on raising both arms indicating SVC obstruction
Can the goitre be delivered through the neck?	Longstanding goitre, significant obstructive symptoms	Retrosternal extension

Box 20.1 Performing fine needle aspiration cytology of the thyroid gland

- Gain consent verbally and explain the procedure.
- Position the patient supine with neck extended.
- Prepare the skin with an alcohol wipe and allow to dry.
- Set up the equipment needed (22 or 24 gauge needle, 5 ml syringe, slides or cytology wash).
- Fix the nodule with one hand and pass the needle through the skin into the nodule.
- Aim for between 4 and 6 passes through the nodule before withdrawing back through the skin. Try not to stain the aspirate with blood.
- Smear onto glass slides and allow to either air dry or fix, depending on local protocol.
- Label all specimens.
- Communicate with and gain feedback from the cytopathologist to improve the quality of your technique.
- Audit your own results.

the position and type of nodule and the experience of the cytologist. Increasingly, FNAC is performed under ultrasound guidance which can be particularly beneficial in complex cysts and nodules deep within the gland. Having access to a cytologist and radiologist in the thyroid clinic ('one-stop' clinic), can lead to increased diagnostic accuracy (Box 20.1).

- *Ultrasound scanning* (USS) is the radiological investigation of choice for the thyroid nodule. It can be used in isolation or in conjunction with FNAC. It is increasingly used in the diagnosis and follow-up of thyroid nodules and can give important prognostic information.
- *Computed tomography* (CT) is of particular use in staging of patients with proven malignant disease as well as patients with benign disease with obstructive symptoms. CT can accurately assess tracheal compression, retrosternal extension and aid in the planning of access surgery that may require a thoracotomy.
- *Barium swallow* enables you to assess the extent to which a patient's dysphagia can be attributed to extrinsic compression of the oesophagus by a goitre.
- *Pulmonary function tests* may give information regarding breathlessness related to tracheal compression.
- *Positron emission tomography* (PET) scanning can be useful in the management of suspected recurrent malignant disease. Anatomic detail is improved when used in conjunction with CT (PET-CT).

10 Indications for surgery in nodular thyroid disease:
- Clinical suspicion of malignancy regardless of FNAC
- Repeatedly non-diagnostic cytology (Thy 1)
- Indeterminate or follicular cytology (Thy 3)
- Likely or definitive malignancy (Thy 4/5)
- Patient choice
- Pressure or obstructive symptoms.

11 Your decision to recommend surgery should be based on clinical assessment in conjunction with the FNAC result and findings on imaging studies.

▶ KEY POINTS Risks of surgery

- Fully informed consent is vital. Document the discussion in the notes and in correspondence.
- Use your own department's figures where possible.

Prepare

It is essential to warn the patient about the risks of surgery:

1 *Laryngeal nerve damage.* Recurrent laryngeal nerve damage leads to a weak breathy voice and poor cough, typically described as bovine. Discuss with the patient the risk of temporary (5%) and permanent (0.5–1%) damage to the recurrent laryngeal nerve. Neuraopraxias may take several months to resolve. Referral to a voice therapist may be indicated. For patients with permanent damage, vocal cord medialization procedures may be indicated. Damage to the external branch of the superior laryngeal nerve may lead to subtle changes in voice (typically loss of high-pitched phonation). This is most evident to professional voice users and singers. Always record vocal cord function and occupation preoperatively.

2 *Hypocalcaemia.* Temporary hypocalcaemia occurs in up to 25% of patients following total thyroidectomy. It may be higher in patients with Graves' disease or those with vitamin D deficiency. Permanent hypocalcaemia (requiring replacement with vitamin D and calcium) occurs in 2–5% of cases.

3 *Haematoma.* Haematoma rate is approximately 1%. It is higher in recurrent surgery.

4 *Wound infection.* Occurs in less than 1%.

5 *Poor cosmesis.* Hypertrophic or keloid scar formation can lead to an unsightly scar. Patients with a history of keloid formation should be counselled appropriately. You should consider using steroid injections and meticulous closure to minimize the risk.

MANAGEMENT OF THE SOLITARY THYROID NODULE AND THE DOMINANT NODULE WITHIN A MULTINODULAR GOITRE

1 Nodules within the thyroid gland are common, especially in women. Most are benign colloid nodules and/or cysts. The most common neoplasm of the thyroid gland is the thyroid adenoma. Importantly, follicular adenomas cannot be distinguished from carcinomas on the basis of cytology and as such require further diagnostic evaluation.[3]

▶ KEY POINTS Identification of follicular adenomas

- Follicular adenomas cannot be distinguished from carcinomas on cytology alone.
- They require excision for diagnosis.

2 Thyroid cancer is rare: the incidence is increasing, but in spite of this there is no corresponding increase in mortality. Much of the increase can be explained by subclinical malignant disease

Thy 1	Non-diagnostic
Thy 2	Non-neoplastic
Thy 3	Neoplasm possible (hyperplasia vs. low grade neoplasm)
Thy 4	Suspicious of malignancy
Thy 5	Malignant

detected on routine scanning ('incidentalomas'). Where incidence has increased, 89% of new disease manifests as tumours less than 2 cm in size.[5]

3 The solitary nodule in a euthyroid patient is the most common presentation of thyroid cancer. The malignant risk is independent of nodule size and it ranges between 10 and 20%.[6] The risk of a thyroid nodule being malignant is higher in extremes of age, in males and in those previously exposed to ionizing radiation. Incidental nodules found on PET scanning carry a 30% malignant risk (Box 20.2).[5]

4 Hemithyroidectomy (removal of lobe and isthmus) is the procedure of choice for the solitary thyroid nodule. Cytology is by no means definitive and as such some suspicious lesions will turn out to be benign. There are instances where a total thyroidectomy may be offered but these cases should be discussed at the MDT prior to surgery.

MANAGEMENT OF MALIGNANT THYROID DISEASE

1 Well-differentiated thyroid cancer (papillary and follicular) makes up the majority of cancers of the thyroid gland. By far the commonest is papillary carcinoma, which accounts for approximately 80% of cases.[2] It tends to occur in a younger age group than other thyroid cancers, with mean age at onset 40–45 years. It is often associated with micro and macro metastasis to cervical lymph nodes. The main risk factor for papillary thyroid cancer is ionizing radiation. The prognosis of papillary cancer is good, with 95% survival at 10 years.

2 Follicular carcinoma comprises 10–15% of carcinomas and has a mean age of onset in the 6th decade. It has a good prognosis, although slightly less favourable than papillary.

3 Medullar cancer is a malignancy of parafollicular C cells and makes up 5% of thyroid cancers. It is associated with multiple endocrine neoplasia syndrome (MEN IIa, MEN IIb), which has autosomal dominant inheritance. The RET proto-oncogene is implicated in MEN II and patients with medullary cancer and their relatives should be screened for this genetic mutation. Rule out phaeochromocytoma prior to surgical intervention.

4 Anaplastic (poorly differentiated) thyroid cancer is rare and carries a very poor prognosis. It typically presents with a rapidly expanding mass, often in an older patient. It progresses rapidly to airway compromise and death. Surgery is not indicated and most patients succumb to their disease within 3 months. The differential diagnosis is of thyroid lymphoma, which is eminently treatable: open biopsy may be needed to establish the diagnosis.

5 Treatment of choice for well-differentiated thyroid carcinoma is total thyroidectomy with central compartment nodal clearance. Most patients with papillary or follicular carcinoma then have ablative treatment with radioactive iodine therapy. Once all thyroid tissue is ablated, thyroglobulin can be used as a sensitive marker of recurrence.

MANAGEMENT OF GRAVES' THYROTOXICOSIS

1 Graves' disease demands a multidisciplinary team approach. An endocrinologist, a specialist in nuclear medicine, surgeon and anaesthetist should be involved if surgery is being considered. Treatment options include antithyroid drugs, beta-blocking drugs and radioactive iodine ablation. Surgery is often only recommended when these treatments have failed or were not tolerated by the patient.

2 Surgery may be the preferred option, for example in women planning a family who wish to avoid radioiodine treatment. Preoperatively, discuss the operative risks, including increased rates of hypocalcaemia. You should emphasize that eye signs, such as exophthalmos associated with Graves' disease, may not regress postoperatively. Rarely, in the short term, they may worsen.

3 Total thyroidectomy is the surgical treatment of choice for patients with thyrotoxicosis. Performing subtotal thyroidectomy runs the risk of recurrent disease. Re-operation carries significantly increased risks, therefore consider total thyroidectomy in younger patients where lifetime risk of recurrent disease is higher.

4 Prepare by rendering patients euthyroid with antithyroid drugs such as carbimazole, adjusting the dose for each patient. Alternatively, institute a 'block and replace' regimen. Give large doses of antithyroid drugs and replace using T4, while giving beta-blocking drugs such as propranolol to reduce the risks of thyrotoxic crisis. Alternatively, give beta-blockers to overcome parasympathetic overactivity.

5 Lugol's iodine (containing free iodine, named after the French physician), given orally 1 ml daily for 10 days preoperatively, reduces the vascularity of the gland at operation and in theory should reduce blood loss.

6 Anticipate and avoid life-threatening thyroid crisis by fully controlling thyrotoxicosis, which manifests with hyperpyrexia, tachycardia, agitation and respiratory distress. Manage within an intensive care unit with oxygen, beta-blocking drugs and sodium iodine.

MANAGEMENT OF BENIGN MULTINODULAR THYROID DISEASE

1 Multinodular goitre on its own is not an indication for surgery. Decide to what extent symptoms can be explained by the goitre. Breathlessness or dysphagia may have causes that warrant investigation.

2 Multinodular goitres can have significant extension into the superior mediastinum and in rare cases may be difficult or impossible to deliver through the neck. Rarely, in cases with significant retrosternal component, a sternal split or lateral thoracotomy may be required.

3 Treatment of choice is a hemithyroidectomy or total thyroidectomy, depending on the nature of the goitre and the patient's symptoms.

4 Tracheomalacia (Greek: malakos=soft) may develop after removal of a longstanding goitre, although some doubt its existence. Discuss it with your anaesthetist preoperatively. The patient may require prolonged intubation or tracheostomy.

THYROID OPERATIONS

Prepare

1 Check the patient on the ward and in the anaesthetic room. Check for recent thyroid function test. Brief the team. Consider marking the patient's neck whilst they are awake and in a sitting position to position the incision for best cosmetic results.

Access

Position the patient supine on the table on a head ring with a sandbag between the shoulders. By extending the neck you will significantly improve access. You should take care, however, not to overextend, particularly in elderly patients. A head up tilt on the operating table reduces venous pooling. Apply external pneumatic compression boots to the legs and complete the preoperative phase of the World Health Organization (WHO) surgical checklist:

1 Check the position of the mark on the neck and adjust if needed. The incision gives adequate access to the upper pole vessels. It is typically two finger breadths above the clavicle, but be flexible, depending on the individual characteristics of the patient (Fig. 20.1). Place the incision between the sternomastoid muscles. Adjust the length depending on the size of the goitre.

2 Infiltrate the subcutaneous and subplatysmal layers along the intended incision with 20 to 30 ml of 1:200 000 adrenaline (epinephrine) in normal saline. You should prepare this in advance by mixing 0.5 ml of 1 in 1000 adrenaline (epinephrine) with 100 ml of normal saline. Allow time for it to have an effect prior to cutting.

3 Cut through skin, subcutaneous fat and platysma, taking care not to go deep to platysma where anterior jugular veins may be encountered. Use bipolar diathermy to control bleeding. Lift the platysma muscle of the superior flap upwards, dissecting to identify the subplatysmal plane. Develop the plane by sharp or blunt dissection or using diathermy or harmonic scalpel. By staying in this plane you will avoid damaging the anterior jugular veins and cutaneous nerves which lie superficial to the strap muscles.

4 Raise the upper flap as far as the thyroid cartilage and the lower flap as far down as the sternal notch. When this is completed insert a Joll's or similar self-retaining retractor to the platysma and subdermal tissues at the midpoint of each flap and open it fully to expose the strap muscles. A second Joll's retractor may be used for larger goitres.

5 Identify the pale midline raphe between the strap muscles and incise it allowing access to deeper tissues. Now separate the strap muscles by incising along this line using diathermy or harmonic scalpel, until you see the thyroid gland (Fig. 20.2). At this stage have your assistant retract the strap muscles laterally and lift, while you apply pressure on the thyroid gland, pulling it towards you. Always handle the gland with care, using a gauze swab. Create a tissue plane between the strap muscles and the thyroid gland along its length.

6 Identify a 'cobweb' of fascial layers and divide them by a combination of blunt dissection and diathermy. As the last flimsy layer is divided, the vessels on the surface of the thyroid bulge as the restraining pressure is released from them. Dissection should be completely bloodless. Coagulate small vessels with bipolar diathermy, ligate and divide larger vessels with 3/0 vicryl ties. Divide the sternothyroid muscle (deeper strap) to improve access to the upper pole in larger goitres.

Action

1 Stand on the side opposite to the lesion. Work across the surface of the gland, retracting it medially whilst your assistant retracts the strap muscles laterally and vertically on the strap muscles. Identify the middle thyroid veins if present and ligate them close to the gland, watching for the inferior parathyroid, which may be in close proximity.

2 To allow the gland to be rotated medially and facilitate access to the recurrent laryngeal nerve (RLN) and parathyroid glands, the

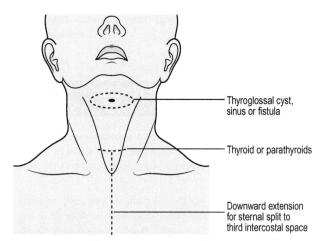

Fig. 20.1 Incisions for operations on the thyroid, parathyroids and thyroglossal lesions.

Thyroglossal cyst, sinus or fistula

Thyroid or parathyroids

Downward extension for sternal split to third intercostal space

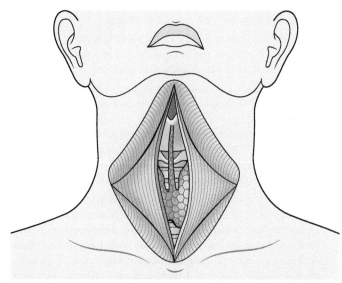

Fig. 20.2 Separation of strap muscles to expose isthmus and larynx.

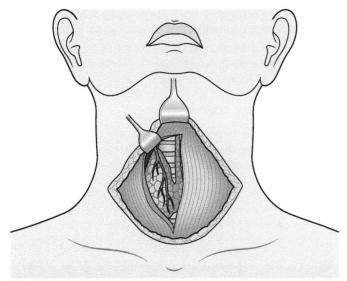

Fig. 20.3 Retraction of strap muscles to expose superior pole and blood supply.

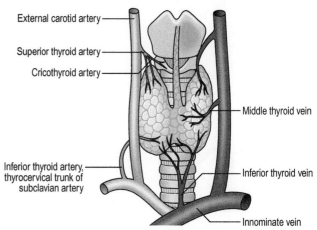

Fig. 20.4 Arterial supply and venous drainage of thyroid.

External carotid artery

Superior thyroid artery

Cricothyroid artery

Middle thyroid vein

Inferior thyroid artery, thyrocervical trunk of subclavian artery

Inferior thyroid vein

Innominate vein

upper and lower poles must be freed and their vessels ligated. This can be achieved in any order. Working towards the upper pole place a small Langenbeck retractor superiorly and a large Langenbeck retractor laterally (Fig. 20.3). Gently push the upper pole of the thyroid laterally and create a tissue plane medially between the cricothyroid muscle and the superior thyroid vessels. Dissect in this plane using a fine haemostat. Coagulate small vessels with bipolar diathermy. By pulling the vessels laterally away from the cricothyroid you minimize the risk of damaging the external laryngeal nerve, as this can be difficult to identify. The external laryngeal nerve runs superiorly in close proximity to the upper pole vessels and usually lies either on, or deep to, the covering fascia of the cricothyroid muscle.

3 Gently dissect free the superior pole vascular pedicle both medially and laterally, using a combination of sharp and gauze pledget dissection. Place a Lahey or similar angled forceps, under direct vision, underneath the superior thyroid vessels. Once the vessels are isolated they can be clipped, divided and tied with 3/0 vicryl, placing two ties on the proximal stump. Clip and tie close to the gland avoiding damage to the external laryngeal nerve. Once the vessels are safely controlled, you can mobilize the gland inferiorly and medially. Look for branching vessels and the superior parathyroid gland, which often lies on the posterolateral portion of the gland. The vascular supply is displayed in Figure 20.4.

4 Move now to the lower pole and divide and ligate lower pole veins close to the gland. Once the upper and lower poles are controlled and dissected, the gland should rotate medially, allowing access to its posterolateral surface. At this stage you can change sides with your assistant and search for the RLN and parathyroid glands.

5 With a gauze swab on the gland, position your assistant to retract the gland medially. The strap muscles can be retracted laterally if needed. Dissect bluntly using a gauze pledget and identify the inferior thyroid artery and parathyroid glands. The RLN lies posteriorly and medially in the tracheo-oesophageal groove. Its position is variable anatomically and arises vertically on the left side, but more lateral to medial on the right. It can be found by

careful dissection using non-toothed forceps and a mosquito artery clip. The RLN usually lies deep to the branches of the inferior thyroid artery, although it can lie in front of, or between, its branches (Fig. 20.5). In 17% of cases the recurrent laryngeal nerve is bifid for 1–2 cm before entering the cricothyroid muscle. The nerve appears white, usually with a small red vessel running on its surface. On the right side only, the nerve may be non-recurrent, coming directly either downwards or laterally across from the main vagal trunk. Once you have identified the nerve, trace it towards the cricothyroid joint, carefully dividing the tissue and small vessels that overlie it.

6 Now with the nerve in full view, look for the tongue-like, pinky-brown, upper parathyroid gland; it is usually adherent to the upper, posterolateral surface of the thyroid (Fig. 20.6). Dissect the parathyroid from the gland using bipolar diathermy preserved on its own blood supply. Once the parathyroids have been preserved, secure the branches of the inferior thyroid artery (Fig. 20.4) on the capsule of the thyroid.

7 The RLN enters the larynx at the cricothyroid joint. At its distal end it is covered by fibres of the lateral thyroid ligament (of Berry). Divide these fibres carefully using a small curved haemostat to create a tunnel parallel to the nerve. Do not apply a sling or retract the nerve. Once the nerve is freed and can be viewed along its entire length, divide the remainder of Berry's ligament by sharp dissection. Dissect across the front of the trachea, separating the gland, using diathermy when necessary. Include the

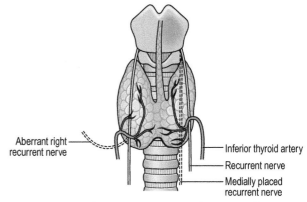

Aberrant right recurrent nerve

Inferior thyroid artery

Recurrent nerve

Medially placed recurrent nerve

Fig. 20.5 Position of recurrent nerves in relation to inferior thyroid artery and some variations.

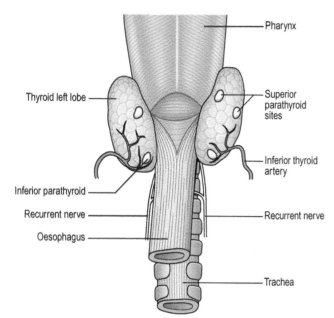

Fig. 20.6 Thyroid and parathyroids seen from behind. Variable positions of parathyroid glands.

isthmus and dissect it out fully. Search for and dissect out a pyramidal lobe if present, up to the level of the hyoid bone.

> ### KEY POINTS Parathyroid glands

- Anatomical position is variable
- Take care when handling the glands as they are sensitive to damage
- Preserve vascular pedicle if possible.

8 The lobe to be removed, and the isthmus are now free. For a total thyroidectomy, repeat the procedure from the opposite side.

9 For a hemithyroidectomy, place artery forceps across the contralateral side of the isthmus, divide the gland and remove the specimen. Oversew the remnant capsule with a running Vicryl suture.

10 Check the anatomy, confirm the viability of the parathyroids. If one parathyroid gland is doubtful, remove it, mince it into small pieces and re-implant it, either in the sternomastoid or a strap muscle, marking its position with a non-absorbable suture. Assiduously seek and seal any bleeding points, checking the position of the nerve at all times. Ask your anaesthetist to perform a Valsalva manoeuvre (described by the 17th Bologna physician Antonio Valsalva) to highlight any occult venous bleeding.

11 Drains are not mandatory following thyroid surgery. They are rarely needed for lobectomies. If required, position a fine tube drain in the same skin crease as the skin incision to improve cosmesis. Secure the drain with a silk suture. Take care not to allow the drain to sit on the nerve as a neuropraxia may occur.

12 Normally remove the drain 12 to 24 hours following surgery.

Closure

1 Approximate the strap muscles with vicryl. Leave a small space inferiorly to allow blood to escape into the subplatysmal space

in the event of bleeding. Close platysma and subcuticular layers with care with an absorbable suture such as 4/0 vicryl.

2 Use staples or subcuticular sutures for the skin closure. Remove staples by the third postoperative day. Remove non-absorbable subcuticular sutures after 1 week.

Postoperative care

1 Closely monitor the patient over the first few hours for respiratory distress that may indicate a haematoma. Haematoma in the thyroid bed can lead to upper airway obstruction as a result of laryngeal oedema. It is a surgical emergency requiring prompt exploration and evacuation in the operating theatre. Faced with a patient in extremis, be prepared to open the wound on the ward to relieve the pressure. Understanding wound closure is vital, as all layers need to be opened to relieve a haematoma in the thyroid bed.

> ### KEY POINTS Postoperative haematoma

- Brief the medical and nursing team regarding recognition of postoperative haematoma
- Identify a problem early, contact the anaesthetist and make arrangement to return the patient to theatre
- Releasing skin clips alone will not decompress the haematoma
- Release all layers of closure – on the ward if necessary.

2 In total thyroidectomy, check calcium on the night of surgery and the following morning. Check the patient for symptoms and signs of hypocalcaemia. Check that you have a protocol for calcium replacement if needed.

RETROSTERNAL MULTINODULAR GOITRE

Appraise

1 Surgery for retrosternal goitre carries a higher risk of damage to the recurrent laryngeal nerve. Explain this when obtaining consent.

2 If you are doubtful about the degree of extension of a goitre obtain cross-sectional imaging to aid decision making.

Action

1 The mediastinum offers little resistance to an expanding goitre and the retrosternal extension can be significant. Most retrosternal extensions are into the anterior and superior mediastinum and can be safely delivered into the neck. Gentle traction along with blunt or finger dissection are often sufficient.

2 Occasionally they extend behind the trachea, enter into the posterior mediastinum and become intimately related to major vascular structures within the chest. Occasionally the blood supply is direct from the aortic arch – so-called thyroidea ima (Latin: ima: =lowest). Bleeding may be difficult to control and require a thoracotomy for access. Anticipate and identify the artery with care before ligating it. Attempt this procedure only if you are experienced.

3 You rarely need to divide the sternum to gain access to the superior mediastinum. If you cannot palpate the goitre in the neck it will be difficult to deliver. A largely intrathoracic goitre shaped like a tear-drop, with a narrow neck and wider, inferior bulk requires a sternal split to release it.

THYROGLOSSAL CYSTS

Appraise

1. These cysts form from incomplete closure of the thyroglossal tract, which extends from the tongue base to the thyroid gland. They are situated between the thyroid and hyoid bone, to which they are intimately related. Although considered midline swellings, they are usually just off the midline to one side and usually present as painless lumps moving on swallowing or protruding the tongue.

2. Excise them both for cosmesis (Greek: cosmeein = to adorn; beautify) and because they occasionally become uncomfortable or infected.

3. Locate the cyst with an ultrasound scan and document the position of the thyroid gland prior to surgery. The mass could be an undescended gland rather than a cyst.

4. Thyroglossal cyst excision (Sistrunk's procedure) was described by the American surgeon Walter Sistrunk in 1920. Any attempt to excise the cyst without removing part of the hyoid bone is likely to result in recurrence.

Access

1. Position the patient as for a thyroidectomy.
2. Make a skin crease incision over the cyst.

Action

1. Dissect out the cyst to define the tract in its upper position.
2. Separate the strap muscles and trace the tract up to the hyoid bone.
3. Strip the muscles off the middle portion of the hyoid bone using monopolar diathermy.
4. Excise the middle portion of the hyoid bone, since thyroglossal tracts have a complex relationship to the back of the body of the hyoid bone.
5. Transect the hyoid bone using small bone-cutting forceps just lateral to the cyst on each side (Fig. 20.7).
6. Follow the tract up into the neck, to the base of the tongue. Excise it as far up as possible. Surgery for recurrent thyroglossal cyst requires wide local excision of skin, subcutaneous tissue, strap muscles and hyoid bone. By performing the procedure in this way you minimize the risk of further recurrence.

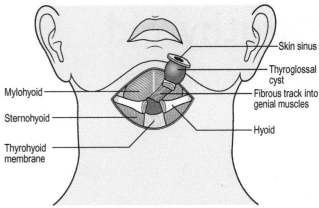

Fig. 20.7   Excision of thyroglossal cyst with sinus, showing excision of hyoid bone.

> ▶ KEY POINTS Removing part of the hyoid
>
> ■ Thyroglossal cysts are always intimately related to the hyoid bone. Remove the central portion to reduce the risk of recurrence.

Closure

1. Re-approximate the strap muscles and the platysma.
2. Insert clips or a subcuticular suture in the skin.

REFERENCES

1. British Association of Endocrine and Thyroid Surgeons BAETS. Available at http://www/baets.org.uk. Accessed Nov 2010.
2. British Thyroid Association. Guidelines on the management of thyroid cancer. Available at http://www.british-thyroid-association.org/Guidelines/. Accessed Nov 2010.
3. Gleeson MJ, editor. Scott-Brown's Otolaryngology, Head and Neck Surgery. 7th ed. London: Hodder Arnold; 2008.
4. Royal College of Pathologists. Guidance on the reporting of thyroid cytology specimens. Available at http://www.rcpath.org/resources/. Accessed Nov 2010.
5. The American Thyroid Association (ATA) Guidelines Taskforce on Thyroid Nodules and Differentiated Thyroid Cancer, Cooper DS, Doherty GM, Haugen BR, et al. Revised American Thyroid Association management guidelines for patients with thyroid nodules and differentiated thyroid cancer. Thyroid 2009;19(11):1167–214.
6. Watkinson JC, Gaze MN, Wilson JA. Stell and Maran's Head and Neck Surgery. 4th ed Oxford: Butterworth Heinemann; 2000.

21

Parathyroid

J.C. Watkinson, D.S. Kim, J. England

CONTENTS

HYPERPARATHYROIDISM AND PARATHYROIDECTOMY

Hyperparathyroidism (HPT) is classified into primary, secondary and tertiary disease. In practice, secondary hyperparathyroidism is nearly always associated with chronic renal failure and its treatment. HPT may be inherited as part of a multiple endocrine neoplasia (MEN) syndrome or less frequently occurs in an isolated form.

A single benign adenoma is the commonest cause of primary hyperparathyroidism (PHPT). The presence of more than one adenoma is rare. In 10–15% of cases hyperplasia of more than one gland is the cause and, very rarely (less than 1%), the cause is a parathyroid carcinoma.

Most parathyroid surgery is carried out for PHPT. The decision when to operate is sometimes difficult since a significant proportion of patients can be treated conservatively by regular monitoring and, in some, symptomatic and biochemical improvement can be achieved with drugs. Furthermore, the majority are apparently asymptomatic patients with the discovery of incidental hypercalcaemia during biochemical analysis. However, the only definitive treatment for hyperparathyroidism remains surgery and with the newer technique of targeted 'minimally invasive parathyroidectomy' (MIP), many argue that surgery should be considered in every case.

Surgery for familial hyperparathyroid syndromes is challenging because of the high incidence of multigland disease. Surgery is seldom required for secondary HPT, but those that persist after correction of the initiating stimulus, i.e. tertiary HPT, require specialized management.

Appraise

1. The multiple symptoms of primary HPT can be summarized by the aphorism 'bones, stones, groans, and psychic moans'. However, 80% of patients are asymptomatic and present incidentally with the finding of hypercalcaemia on routine blood testing for other medical conditions. Very rarely, patients may present with significant bone disease (osteitis fibrosa cystica), most clearly seen on X-rays of the middle phalanges showing subperiosteal bone resorption. This presentation tends to occur more frequently in severe longstanding disease, parathyroid cancer or secondary and tertiary hyperparathyroidism.

2. The biochemical diagnosis of hyperparathyroidism requires the demonstration of persistently raised levels of serum calcium with an associated high serum parathormone (PTH) level, or a level that is inappropriately normal in the presence of high serum calcium levels. Normocalcaemia does not exclude hyperparathyroidism and some patients with renal stones have been shown to have high PTH levels in the presence of a normal serum calcium. Always consider and exclude other causes of hypercalcaemia. In particular, familial hypercalcaemic hypocalciuria (FHH) can be confused with it since it presents a similar biochemical profile. Order urinary calcium estimations to exclude this condition. Hypocalciuria (less than 2 mmol/day) should prompt the diagnosis of familial hypercalcaemic hypocalciuria.

3. You have a responsibility to ensure that, whatever the referral pathway, potential reversible causes of secondary hypercalcaemia (including lithium therapy and vitamin D deficiency) have been excluded, and hereditary conditions identified. The early diagnosis of familial disease is important since the management differs from primary to secondary HPT. The syndromal acronyms are: FHH, ADMH, NSHPT, MEN1, MEN2a, HPT-JT, HPT-IF. (Refer to the landmark article on these acronyms by Marx et al. 2002.)

4. A serum calcium level in excess of 3 mmol/L is an absolute indication for surgery. Consider symptomatic patients for surgery. However, the majority are asymptomatic patients with the discovery of incidental hypercalcaemia during biochemical analysis. A more liberal approach to surgery for asymptomatic patients is developing (see Proceedings of the 3rd International Workshop JCEM 2009).

5. There is increasing evidence that patients aged 70 years or less have a higher mortality with untreated disease and that this can be reversed by successful parathyroid surgery. Cardiac changes have been shown to be reversed after treatment of asymptomatic disease and symptoms of depression and anxiety may be reversed. Loss of bone mineral content has been shown to be partially reversible, an important factor in postmenopausal women.

6. In secondary hyperparathyroidism, elevated calcium levels can make control of dialysis programmes difficult and can produce significant pathological bone change. It is often accompanied by severe pruritus, muscle weakness and sometimes with soft-tissue calcification. The timing and indications for surgery very much rely on the renal physicians.

7. Once the decision to operate has been made, decide the type of operation needed. In primary HPT, this decision depends upon the patient's wishes, your competence in the subspecialty, and the success of preoperative localization.

8 The standard operation is a four-gland neck exploration through a cervical collar incision made in a similar way as for exploring the thyroid (see Chapter 20).

9 In 80% of cases, the causative lesion is a solitary parathyroid adenoma, and successful preoperative localization of such a lesion enables you to offer minimally invasive parathyroidectomy using a targeted approach under general or local anaesthesia.

10 In 15–20% of cases, HPT is caused by parathyroid hyperplasia, which may be genetically predetermined. Here, preoperative imaging is far less successful at localizing the causative pathology, and the four-gland exploration is usually more appropriate. Both the targeted approach and four-gland exploration are performed endoscopically in some centres.

11 Explain in preoperative counselling that the same potential risks exist in parathyroid surgery as can occur after thyroid surgery, including recurrent laryngeal nerve injury. There is also the additional risk of failing to find the gland at the first operation, often because it is ectopic.

▶ KEY POINTS Experienced?

■ Do not attempt parathyroidectomy on an occasional basis.
■ Before embarking on this operation seek special training and experience, especially re-operations.

Prepare

1 An experienced parathyroid surgeon can cure up to 95% of patients without the benefit of preoperative localization, employing the traditional and more extensive four-gland exploration. However, preoperative localization techniques are now commonly used prior to an initial targeted neck exploration. This is in response to the increasing popularity of daycase parathyroidectomy, minimally invasive parathyroidectomy (MIP), and parathyroidectomy under local anaesthesia.

2 Nuclear scintigraphy is seen as the most accurate localization technique. Technetium Tc 99 m sestamibi, either with a subtraction technique using radio-iodine (I^{123}) or used alone in a 'double-phase scan' where the scan is repeated at 2–3 hours, gives the best results. It can localize solitary adenomata in 95% of cases and multigland disease in 80%. The double-phase method relies on the differential washout rate of sestamibi from parathyroid tissue compared to thyroid tissue as a result of the high metabolic rate of the parathyroids, particularly when adenomatous.

3 Ultrasonography is also frequently employed. Results are operator dependent, but in the best hands solitary adenomas can be identified in 93% of cases. Colour Doppler Ultrasound is of limited value when glands are located in the mediastinum.

4 In the detection of ectopic glands, particularly when other tests have failed or following unsuccessful exploration and especially in the identification of suspected mediastinal glands, other forms of imaging may be valuable. Apart from CT or MRI, three-dimensional imaging techniques can be such as single photon emission computed tomography (SPECT). Positron emission tomography (PET) may be carried out either with (^{18}F)-fluoro-2-deoxy-D-glucose or (^{11}C)-methionine.

5 Venous sampling can be employed if less invasive imaging techniques have failed, when planning revision surgery. This involves central venous catheterization and the subsequent collection of blood samples, measuring intact PTH levels, from the draining veins of the thyroid plexus. Intact PTH assays are measured. Although interpretation of results is hampered somewhat by previous surgery(s) it can be very useful in rough localization of the gland(s) by determining the side, whether it is higher or lower in the neck, or likely to be in the superior mediastinum and thus direct the general area of re-exploration.

6 The patient needs to be well hydrated: if the patient has been admitted in a hypercalcaemic crisis then a period of re-hydration is mandatory before attempting surgery.

STANDARD OPERATION: FOUR-GLAND EXPLORATION

Access

1 With the patient in a supine position, and with approximately 30 degrees of reverse Trendelenberg to decrease venous engorgement, extend the neck where possible by appropriate placement of a head ring and sand bag.

2 Make a standard Kocher incision situated midway between the cricoid cartilage and the jugular notch. In most cases it need only be 5 cm long. Continue it through the platysma muscle to the level of the superficial layer of strap muscles. Raise the superior myocutaneous flap to a level at least 2 cm above the cricoid cartilage.

3 Identify the linea alba then separate the strap muscles. Now peel the strap muscles from the ventral surface of one of the thyroid lobes. Begin the search for the parathyroid glands by dislocating the thyroid lobe medially and anteriorly whilst retracting the strap muscles laterally. It is often necessary to divide the middle thyroid vein. Use blunt dissection with pledgets, mosquito forceps and bipolar diathermy division of fine vessels, to maintain absolute haemostasis. In a series of 547 autopsies Gilmour demonstrated that 6% of patients have three and 6% have five glands. In 80% of cases, the position of both the superior and inferior glands on each side is symmetrical – useful to recall when a gland proves difficult to locate.

4 While searching for the superior parathyroid gland the inferior thyroid artery can be readily identified deep to the carotid sheath, usually around the mid-part of the thyroid lobe. Follow it to the thyroid lobe. Now identify the recurrent laryngeal nerve (see Chapter 20). The superior parathyroid glands usually lie behind the upper pole of the thyroid lobe, close to the cricothyroidius muscle. The majority of superior parathyroids are within 1 cm of the cricothyroid joint, above the main branch of the inferior thyroid artery in a plane deep to the recurrent laryngeal nerve. It may be closely adherent to the recurrent laryngeal nerve.

5 The inferior parathyroid glands develop together from the third pouch and descend with the thymus. The majority settle in the neck along this line of descent and separate somewhat from the thymus, which continues into the chest leaving a thyrothymic tract in the neck in which the parathyroid is frequently situated.

6 Mobilize the inferior pole, inspecting particularly in the region of the thyrothymic tract. The gland normally lies on or just below the inferior pole of the thyroid lobe and ventral to the coronal plane of the recurrent nerve. In about 15% of patients it lies distinctly separate from the gland and in the upper pole of the thymus. Its position often allows the excision of an inferior adenoma without recurrent laryngeal nerve identification, provided the dissection proceeds directly on the surface of the gland.

7 The parathyroid glands (often pale brown or tan coloured) are enclosed in an envelope of fat that moves separately from the thyroid. There is usually a small feeding vessel which can be cauterized, ensuring that the gland is not in close proximity to the recurrent laryngeal nerve.

8 During the operation, glands judged macroscopically normal are commonly marked with a Ligaclip. Macroscopically abnormal gland(s) are removed and sent for histology. The procedure can be enhanced by intra-operative frozen section and ioPTH, the latter procedure to confirm cure following a successful dissection, or to point to the need for further exploration.

9 An increasingly difficult problem arises in older people with milder disease forms who are now operated on earlier in their disease process than was previously the case. A solitary adenoma and three 'normal glands' can be difficult to distinguish from hyperplasia affecting mainly one gland with mild hyperplasia of the other three. This requires great judgment, and in case of doubt elect to remove three and a half glands. Similarly, if more than one gland is clearly involved, or if this is hyperplasia either from primary or secondary hyperparathyroidism, then elect to remove three and a half glands, leaving approximately 30–50 mg of functional tissue. We advocate this approach as the best way to minimize the risk of recurrence whilst preserving parathyroid function. Some authorities advocate the removal of all four glands, then place the patient postoperatively on calcium and vitamin D supplements to minimize recurrence and surgical failure.

10 Further intra-operative localization strategies are available:
- Methylthioninium chloride (methylene blue) is a total-body infusion technique. Methylene blue (5 mg/kg body weight) in 5% dextrose is infused an hour prior to surgery: timing of infusion to surgery is crucial. The dye is preferentially taken up by the parathyroids (>90%), particularly when adenomatous or hyperplastic, making their identification easier. Warn the anaesthetist that this may affect oxygen saturation but it is not generally significant. Monitor the patient closely, since the infusion occasionally produces adverse reactions. Anaphylaxis is extremely rare and demands orthodox treatment.
- Gamma probe identification can be carried out on a radioisotope injected preoperatively and selectively concentrated within parathyroid tissue. Technitium 99m sestamibi is the usual choice. Success depends on strict timing between radioisotope injection and time of surgery. It is not in widespread use but has gained some acceptance in MIP.
- Intra-operative PTH (ioPTH) serum assay. In 1987, the development of an immunochemiluminescent assay for human PTH paved the way for intra-operative PTH monitoring (ioPTH) as a reliable indicator of success during parathyroidectomy. An approximate turnaround time of 10 minutes makes ioPTH monitoring a useful tool, particularly in minimal access, localized and daycase resections. In addition,

once an adenoma has been removed, it is unnecessary to biopsy the remaining apparently normal glands to ensure no hypersecreting gland remains, thus avoiding the associated risk of prolonged postoperative hypocalcaemia.

The procedure of ioPTH monitoring varies from centre to centre, depending on the specifics of the immunoassay employed and local experience. An initial baseline blood sample is taken prior to the commencement of surgery (T-0) because it is recognized that manipulation of parathyroid glands intra-operatively can lead to spikes in PTH levels. Further samples are then taken at 5 (T-5) and 10 (T-10) minutes after removal of each gland. Operative success is predicted if either the T-5 or T-10 sample demonstrates a PTH level 50% or greater below the T-0 level. The procedure indicates long-term operative success with about 95% accuracy in single gland disease. However, the results in multigland disease are less reliable, with false-positive reduction in PTH levels occurring in as many as 75% of patients. Although ioPTH has many advantages, the procedure is expensive so that in many institutions, without significant cost decreases, it is unlikely to become routine practice.

> ### ▶ KEY POINTS Description of parathyroid glands
>
> - Parathyroid glands are like little tongues. They are not usually round and globular unless they are significantly enlarged and their consistency is quite different from that of lymph nodes.
> - Lymph nodes very rarely pick up methylthioninium chloride.

? DIFFICULTY

1. After initial bilateral exploration, in the vast majority of cases an adenoma is discovered and no further dissection is necessary even if one or more parathyroids remain hidden. The return from further dissection is likely to be small, with the added risk of de-vascularizing small normal parathyroids. However, when initial exploration is unfruitful further exploration must be undertaken in the most likely ectopic sites.
2. When the upper gland is ectopic it tends to progress inferiorly and posteriorly and may lie in the retro-oesophageal or retro-pharyngeal gutter, having descended posteriomedial to the nerve. This is purely a pulsion effect due to deglutition forcing the enlarging tumour in the direction of least resistance and, in extreme cases, a superior adenoma may be found in the posterior mediastinum.
3. Lower glands, if they become ectopic, go further down to the thymus and are most commonly situated in the anterior mediastinum. A missing inferior gland is thus first sought along the thyrothymic tract and traced into the anterior mediastinum to explore the thymus. However, in ectopia, their position can be far more variable than the superior glands. They may be discovered as high as the carotid bifurcation and associated with failure of thymic

descent, or they may also be found within the carotid sheath (from skull base to aortic level).

4. True intrathyroid parathyroids are very rare and they are usually situated in little clefts in the surface of the gland and careful re-examination of the thyroid lobes may reveal an adherent subcapsular parathyroid. But on some occasions they can be truly within the gland substance itself and in this situation it would be acceptable to perform a hemithyroidectomy. Before proceeding to remove thyroid tissue, unless demonstrated by a clear-cut preoperative localization study, the respective veins should be sampled for ioPTH to give an indication in which side of the neck the adenoma resides, and if none is available, it is then the surgeon's choice.

5. In the event of no adenoma being found after these measures, the exploration should be abondoned with the expectation that the rogue gland is hidden deeper in the mediastinum, requiring additional imaging studies and a targeted revision procedure.

Autotransplantation of parathyroid tissue

To avoid the long-term consequences of hypoparathyroidism, whenever you conclude that there is aparathyroidism following surgery, embark on immediate parathyroid autotransplantation. Some surgeons routinely cryopreserve parathyroid tissue for subsequent autotransplantation if necessary.

Closure

1. Close the wound of the standard cervical incision in the usual way for a thyroid operation.

2. It is not usually necessary to insert drains except in patients subjected to a difficult neck dissection, who may benefit from having a small suction drain for a day or so.

Postoperative

1. The vast majority of patients undergoing parathyroid surgery do not run into problems with hypocalcaemia postoperatively. The small number of patients who do can sometimes be predicted. They are those who have significant bone disease, those who have significant metabolic biochemical disorders and those who start with calcium levels in excess of 3.25 mmol/L.

2. Take baseline calcium and PTH levels at the completion of parathyroid surgery. Take further tests according to patient symptoms. Generally take a further sample the following morning either as an outpatient or inpatient. Where there is the possibility of permanent hypoparathyroidism, check serum calcium and possibly PTH again, approximately twice daily. The trend in serum calcium indicates the likely course of action. The serum calcium levels fall within the first few hours but the time of maximum fall of calcium levels is on the 5th postoperative day, by which time most patients have been discharged. Warn patients of symptoms of tingling in the hands, or of tetany (Greek: teinein = to stretch; muscle twitching, spasm, cramps). Advise them to report back to hospital if they suffer from these symptoms.

3. Asymptomatic hypocalcaemia to a level of about 2 mmol/L does not, as a rule, need any specific treatment and usually spontaneously corrects within 24–48 hours. Calcium levels below 2 mmol/L, or where there are symptoms of hypocalcaemia such as tetany and tingling, are usually treated acutely with a combination of intravenous infusion of 10% calcium gluconate plus oral calcium supplements. In mild cases, oral calcium supplementation alone resolves symptoms and maintains acceptable serum calcium level, although more severe cases require One-Alpha calciferol in addition. Resulting from the advent of short-stay surgery, a downward trend is best managed with supplementation for 1 week or longer with twice-weekly calcium checks. Treatment can be with oral calcium alone (1g tds or 2g bd) if the calcium level hovers around 2 mmol/L and above, otherwise add One-Alpha calciferol; 0.25 μg bd controls most, but some patients require 0.5 μg bd. Patients can safely be discharged on this; then, at follow-up within 1 week or 2 in outpatients, monitor their calcium levels and attempt to withdraw the supplements. Temporary hypoparathyroidism usually lasts only for days or weeks. Consider hypoparathyroidism to be permanent when calcium and/or vitamin D supplementation are still required at 3 months (or at 6 months by some authors).

4. In the case of solitary adenomas it is usual to see patients once more at about 3 months, when they can safely be discharged. Keep under review patients who have hyperplasia, because after some years there is a tendency for the remnant half gland to enlarge and become reactive.

MINIMALLY INVASIVE PARATHYROIDECTOMY

The development of intra-operative PTH assays, the gamma probe and accurate preoperative localization techniques have paved the way for unilateral explorations and single gland-targeted excisions through incisions of 2 cm, aimed at minimizing inpatient stay and patient discomfort. This is particularly so as the predominant pathological cause of primary HPT is the solitary adenoma and hyperplasia is now being recognized as an increasingly rarer entity.

THE LATERAL APPROACH

An incision about 2 cm long is made transversely across the neck just in front of the sternomastoid muscle on the side of the suspected adenoma. It can be placed over the lower or upper pole of the thyroid, whichever seems appropriate. A tissue plane is then created lateral to the strap muscles and between them and the sternomastoid. The omohyoid muscle may require division for optimal exposure. The sternomastoid is retracted laterally, and the medial border of the carotid sheath is then easily dissected to provide an excellent view of the posterolateral aspect of the thyroid gland and the tracheoesophageal groove. During the subsequent parathyroid search, if greater exposure is required, it is a simple matter to divide the overlying sternothyroid muscle, which gives the same exposure as the traditional medial approach.

Having removed the gland you need only to close the platysma and appose the skin incision. The patient can be allowed home later the same day. The small localized lateral cervical incision heals so it is virtually invisible within a few weeks of surgery.

OTHER MINIMAL ACCESS/MINIMALLY INVASIVE TECHNIQUES

These have been developed particularly in Italy and France, using endoscopic equipment to remove a pre-localized adenoma through a minimal incision in the neck (Minimal Access/Video assisted/'Laparoscopic' Parathyroidectomy). The glands can be removed in the same way as for the lateral approach. A successful resection can be effectively confirmed with the use of ioPTH. In some institutions, minimal access video-assisted parathyroidectomy enables a bilateral four-gland exploration through a single medial horizontal 1.5-cm incision.

Other approaches have been described for those patients who feel strongly about not having a scar in their neck. These techniques approach the thyroid and parathyroid glands through incisions made in the axilla or, in some case reports, via a peri-areolar incision, and should not be attempted by the inexperienced surgeon.

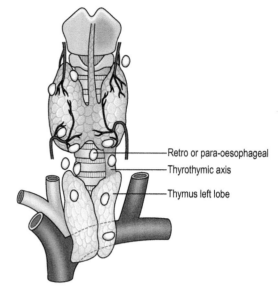

Retro or para-oesophageal
Thyrothymic axis
Thymus left lobe

Fig. 21.1 Various positions for parathyroid glands.

PARATHYROID CARCINOMA

Parathyroid carcinomas are usually associated with extremely high calcium levels and sometimes with a palpable gland in the neck preoperatively. They are commonly diagnosed clinically at operation because they are often seen to invade neighbouring structures, particularly the thyroid gland and, on occasions, the recurrent laryngeal nerve. Indeed, someone presenting with hypercalcaemia and voice changes should always be considered to have a parathyroid carcinoma and counselling should be given preoperatively that there may be risks of permanent changes to the voice.

The usual recommended procedure if parathyroid carcinoma is suspected at operation is to perform a hemithyroidectomy on the same side and also to undertake wide local excision removing all adjacent tissues that are macroscopically affected. This would include any obviously enlarged lymph nodes, but it is not usual at the first operation to recommend radical removal of lymphatic tissue in the neck.

RE-OPERATION

The reasons for surgical failure in order of frequency are: inadequate cervical exploration, failure to diagnose or adequately resect multigland disease, gland ectopia (Fig. 21.1) and the wrong diagnosis. When failure occurs, the first step is to reconfirm the diagnosis. Other possible diagnoses, in particular familial hypercalcaemic hypocalciuria, pseudohyperparathyroidism and sarcoidosis must be excluded. Secondly, the requirement for curative surgery must be re-evaluated and its necessity reconfirmed. Patients without bony or renal complications, or normocalcaemic patients with an elevated PTH, for example, may opt to be observed rather than to undergo further surgery with increased complication rates and decreased cure rates. If re-exploration is judged appropriate, the histological specimens and operative notes from the first exploration should be examined, as these will often help in pointing to the likely location of the missing gland.

In revision surgery, attempts at preoperative localization are mandatory. High resolution ultrasound and technetium sestamibi scanning are the commonest modalities used. If a mediastinal location

is suspected, contrast enhanced CT with technetium sestamibi scanning demonstrate the best sensitivities at 92 and 85%, respectively. MRI and highly selective venous sampling are also sometimes employed, and when other imaging techniques have failed 11C-methionine PET has proved useful, although this modality is not widely available. Ideally ioPTH will be available and if the levels remain high, then intra-operative ultrasound and selective venous sampling are sometimes used. Prior to re-operative surgery, the patient must be made aware of the increased risks to the recurrent laryngeal nerve, of surgical failure and of permanent hypoparathyroidism. Re-operation for persistent or recurrent hypercalcaemia should only be performed by experts, given the higher risks and lower success rate.

FURTHER READING

Bilezikian JP, Khan AA, Potts JT, et al. Guidelines for the management of asymptomatic primary hyperparathyroidism: Summary Statement from the Third International Workshop. J Clin Endocrinol Metab 2009;94:335–339.

British Association of Endocrine and Thyroid Surgeons. Guidelines for the surgical treatment of endocrine disease and training requirements for endocrine surgery. Available at www.baets.org.uk. Accessed Dec 2012.

Marx SJ, Simonds WF, Agarwal SK, et al. Hyperparathyroidism in hereditary syndromes: special expressions and special managements. J Bone Miner Res 2002;17(2):N37–43.

Miccoli P, Berti P, Materazzi G, et al. Results of video-assisted parathyroidectomy: single institution's six-year experience. World J Surg 2004;28:1216–8.

Palazzo FF, Sadler GP. Minimally invasive parathyroidectomy. Br Med J 2004;328:849–50.

Palestro CJ, Tomas MB, Tronco GG. Radionuclide imaging of the parathyroid glands. Semin Nucl Med 2005;35:266–76.

Irvin GL, Molinari AS, Figueroa C. Improved success rate in reoperative parathyroidectomy with intraoperative PTH assay. Ann Surg 1999;229:874–8.

Udelsman R, Pasieka JL, Sturgeon C, et al. Surgery for Asymptomatic Primary Hyperparathyroidism: Proceedings of the Third International Workshop. J Clin Endocrinol Metab 2009;94:366–72.

Adrenalectomy

T.R. Kurzawinski

CONTENTS

INTRODUCTION

Adrenalectomy is not a common operation. It should be performed only in centres performing at least 10–15 cases per year. Care for these patients within a multidisciplinary team comprising an endocrine surgeon, endocrinologist, radiologist and anaesthetist.

Over the last 20 years open adrenalectomy has been largely replaced by a laparoscopic approach. Adrenalectomy is ideally suited to laparoscopic surgery via either a transperitoneal or retroperitoneal approach, which significantly reduces the trauma associated with an open incision and results in less pain, quicker recovery and better cosmetic results. Reserve open adrenalectomy nowadays either for very large or malignant tumours.

> ### KEY POINTS Adrenalectomy is not an operation for 'an occasional adrenalectomist'

- Make sure you have appropriate training in open and laparoscopic techniques and, if you are not experienced, make sure help is available.
- Consult extensively with an endocrinologist and anaesthetist to confirm the correct diagnosis and plan perioperative management. Never, ever, schedule a patient for adrenalectomy without doing so.

ANATOMY

The normal adrenal gland weighs 3–5 g and measures 5x3x1 cm. Both left and right glands lie in the retroperitoneum within the perirenal (Gerota's) fascia, with their posterior surface attached to the diaphragm. They receive arterial blood supply from several small branches of the inferior phrenic artery, aorta and renal artery. The adrenals are not symmetrical: the right is triangular in shape and its short, wide adrenal vein drains medially into the inferior vena cava; the left is more semilunar, with the vein draining downwards into the left renal vein. Each adrenal gland consists of medulla, secreting catecholamines (adrenaline (epinephrine), noradrenaline (norepinephrine) and dopamine), and cortex, secreting cortisol, aldosterone and adrenal sex hormones (Fig. 22.1). Lymphatic capillaries draining the cortex follow arteries while the medulla lymphatics follow veins.

> ### KEY POINTS Identifying the adrenal glands

- **Look for the golden edge**: adrenal has a characteristic golden colour (due to its high lipid content).
- When searching for the adrenal distinguish it from fat (pale yellow) and pancreas (creamy yellow).

Appraise

Before you embark on adrenalectomy, consider:

1. The functional status of the adrenal nodule, as this determines patient preparation before surgery and perioperative management.
2. Look at the size of the adrenal mass and its relation to surrounding organs. This determines your choice of incision and approach. You must review CT or MRI scans yourself and have them available in the operating theatre during surgery.
3. Decide whether you are dealing with malignant or benign pathology.
4. Find out whether this is a sporadic or familial problem.
5. Ensure that surgery is the best treatment and is really necessary.

> ### KEY POINTS Before you operate consider the following

- The function of the adrenal mass determines the patient's management before and after surgery.
- The size of the adrenal mass affects your choice of approach/incision.
- Finding a mutation responsible for familial disease affects the management of not just that patient but his/her whole family.

Indications for adrenalectomy

1. *Phaeochromocytomas* arise from adrenal medulla and secrete adrenaline (epinephrine), noradrenaline (norepinephrine) and dopamine. It is difficult to predict their biological behaviour but 10% of them are malignant and 10% arise from chromaffin cells outside the adrenals (paragangliomas). Most of them are sporadic, but 20–30% are familial and may be bilateral. Patients present with headaches, sweating, hypertension and palpitations. Establish the biochemical diagnosis by measuring catecholamine and metanephrine levels in urine and plasma. CT, MRI and MIBG (meta-iodobenzyl-guanidine) scans are used to assess tumour location and size and to detect possible metastases. Carefully prepare all patients with phaeochromocytomas with α blockade and sometimes β blockade to minimize the risk of hypertensive crisis. During surgery avoid extensive manipulation of the tumour to

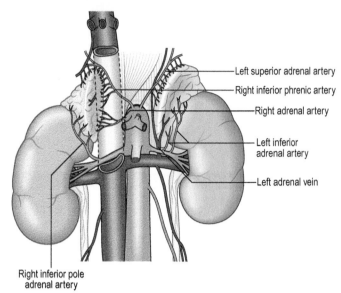

Left superior adrenal artery
Right inferior phrenic artery
Right adrenal artery
Left inferior adrenal artery
Left adrenal vein
Right inferior pole adrenal artery

Fig. 22.1 Anatomy of the left and right adrenal gland.

prevent a sudden rise in blood pressure. You should work with an experienced anaesthetist who is able to control surges of blood pressure during dissection and hypotension after the removal of the tumour.

2 *Primary hyperaldosteronism (Conn's syndrome)* is caused by excess of aldosterone produced by either a solitary adenoma or bilateral hyperplasia of the zona glomerulosa of the adrenal cortex. Patients present with hypertension and low potassium. Biochemical diagnosis is confirmed by an elevated plasma aldosterone concentration and suppressed plasma renin activity. Use CT or MRI scans to identify adrenal nodules, which are usually about 1 cm in size. Adrenal venous sampling is sometimes necessary to differentiate unilateral from bilateral disease. The aim of the treatment is to normalize aldosterone levels and prevent mortality and morbidity caused by hypertension, low potassium, cardiovascular and renal damage. Unilateral adenomas should be treated with adrenalectomy, which corrects hypokalaemia in 98% and improves hypertension in 90% of patients. Patients with bilateral hyperplasia should be treated with mineralocorticoid receptor antagonists (e.g. spironolactone), not surgery.

3 *Hypercorticolism* is caused by excess of cortisol. *Cushing's disease* is caused by pituitary ACTH producing adenomas, which stimulates adrenal production of cortisol. Twenty-five percent of patients are not cured by transphenoidal pituitary surgery and require bilateral adrenalectomy. *Cushing's syndrome* is caused by a cortisol-secreting adenoma or rarely adrenocortical carcinoma and is an indication for unilateral adrenalectomy. Patients present with central obesity, hypertension, diabetes and muscle weakness. They have impaired immunity and poor wound healing. Biochemical diagnosis is made by measuring plasma ACTH and urine cortisol and performing a dexamethasone suppression test. Before surgery hypercorticolism can be controlled with ketaconazole or metyrapone. After bilateral adrenalectomy patients need lifelong treatment with hydrocortisone and mineralocorticoids. The contralateral gland is often suppressed after unilateral adrenalectomy and these patients also need treatment with hydrocortisone for many months.

4 *Adrenocortical carcinoma* is a rare but highly malignant tumour with poor prognosis. 60% of adrenal cancers are hormonally active and can cause Cushing's or virilizing syndromes. Most of these tumours are large at diagnosis and an open approach should be used to resect them. Surgery often needs to be extensive with en bloc removal of adrenal and surrounding organs combined with lymphadenopathy. Tumour spillage must be avoided at all cost to prevent local recurrence.

5 *Adrenal 'incidentaloma'* is a mass discovered by chance during radiological investigations performed for other indications. They are common, with a prevalence of 4–6%. Most of them (70%) are non-secreting adenomas, but about 16% are hyperfunctioning and cause subclinical Cushing's, Conn's or phaeochromocytoma syndromes. Incidentalomas larger than 4–5 cm may represent malignant pathology. Hyperfunctioning and large incidentalomas suspicious of being malignant should be resected.

Prepare

1 With the correct diagnosis established and the perioperative plan discussed with an endocrinologist and implemented, you can now plan your surgical procedure. Depending on pathology you must make a decision:
   - Whether to perform unilateral or bilateral adrenalectomy
   - Which access is best (anterior, lateral, posterior)
   - Whether to perform an open or laparoscopic adrenalectomy.

2 Order perioperative thromboprophylaxis. If MRSA screening is positive use the hospital eradication protocol. Consider giving prophylactic antibiotics – important in Cushing's syndrome.

3 Discuss these decisions fully with the patient while taking a full formal consent.

Access

Lateral approach (Fig. 22.2)

The lateral approach to the adrenal gland is the most popular for both open and laparoscopic techniques. Its main advantage is good access and exposure of the adrenal gland, which allows removal of large and malignant tumours. Potential disadvantages are significant trauma from the incision, including rib excision in the open posterolateral approach, and the need to reposition the patient if you plan bilateral adrenalectomy.

Place the patient in the lateral decubitus position with the affected side uppermost. Stabilize the patient using a 'bean bag', sandbags or supports in front and behind. A strap usually secures the patient's pelvis. Place a pillow between the legs and place the uppermost

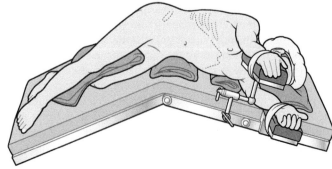

Fig. 22.2 Lateral position for laparoscopic and open adrenalectomy.

arm in a suitable arm rest at the same height as the shoulder. You may 'break' the table (jack-knife position) to maximize the distance between costal margin and iliac crest. Prepare the skin of the chest and abdomen to allow for either extension of the incision or conversion to an open procedure.

Laparoscopic lateral (transperitoneal) approach

1 Tilt the operating table laterally to a position half way between true lateral and fully supine and stand facing the patient's abdomen with your camera operator next to you and scrub nurse opposite.

2 Create a pneumoperitoneum using an open technique (recommended) or Veress needle to achieve a pressure between 10 and 15 mmHg.

3 Insert the first port below the costal margin in the mid-clavicular line and inspect the peritoneal cavity with a 0° or 30° telescope. Insert two or three further ports in the posterior, middle and anterior axillary lines (Fig. 22.3). Use a combination of 5- and 10–12-mm ports, depending on which instruments you are planning to use (e.g. 10 mm for camera, 12 mm for vascular stapler, 5 mm for forceps/diathermy/harmonic scalpel).

4 **Left adrenalectomy** (Fig. 22.3) is usually performed with three ports but a fourth port may be necessary for additional retraction of the spleen and colon:
   ■ Mobilize the splenic flexure by dividing its lateral and superior attachments until you see the upper half of the kidney and lower edge of spleen.
   ■ Mobilize the spleen and tail of pancreas by dividing splenocolic and splenorenal ligaments until, assisted by gentle traction and forces of gravity, they 'flip' medially. Ensure good

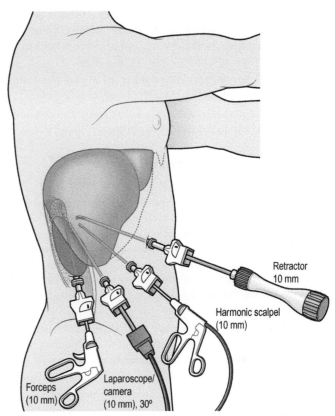

Fig. 22.4 Position of trocars for right laparoscopic adrenalectomy.

access to the adrenal to secure a trouble-free operation and dissect thoroughly and, if necessary, extensively. Be aware of the spleen, colon, pancreas and splenic vein in order to avoid damaging them.
   ■ Identify the adrenal in the perirenal fat and start dissecting it at the upper pole; carry the dissection downwards along both medial and lateral borders. Divide small arterial branches with a harmonic scalpel. Make sure that whole gland is mobilized – the lower limb frequently descends as far as the renal hilum. Do not grasp the adrenal with forceps as it is friable and bleeds easily. Retract by pushing the adrenal or apply forceps to the surrounding fat.
   ■ Identify the left adrenal vein on the inferomedial aspect of the gland as it empties into the renal vein. Divide it between double clips. Be careful not to damage the renal vessels, which may contribute an accessory renal artery to the superior pole.

5 **Right adrenalectomy** (Fig. 22.4) is usually performed through four ports as it is necessary to retract the right lobe of the liver:
   ■ The duodenum and hepatic flexure of the colon do not need to be mobilized routinely as they are retracted by forces of gravity.
   ■ Divide the right triangular ligament and retract the liver medially. Incise the posterior peritoneum along the lateral edge of the inferior vena cava (IVC) and lower edge of the liver and identify the adrenal gland.
   ■ Gently dissect between the IVC and adrenal until you encounter the right adrenal vein. For larger tumours it may be helpful to dissect the lower and lateral aspects of the adrenal first as this helps to retract it and facilitates dissection between the medial edge and IVC.

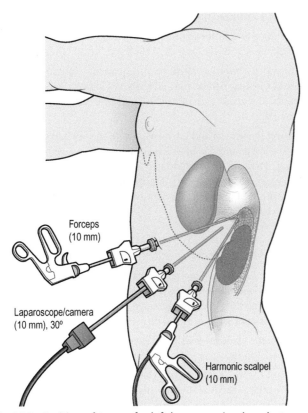

Fig. 22.3 Position of trocars for left laparoscopic adrenalectomy.

■ The right adrenal vein is short and wide. Divide it between double clips or using a vascular stapler. Mobilize the remaining gland from the kidney, liver and posterior muscles by dividing small arteries with a harmonic scalpel.

6 After completely mobilizing the right or left adrenal, place it in a retrieval bag and retrieve it through one of the incisions.

7 Check haemostasis, make sure there is no damage to surrounding organs and close the incisions with stitches.

Open posterolateral approach

1 The technique for left and right adrenalectomy is similar.

2 Make an incision over the eleventh rib from the lateral edge of the paravertabral muscles to the lateral rectus sheath margin. Divide latissimus dorsi and serratus posterior muscles with cutting diathermy and incise the periosteum of the eleventh rib using a diathermy point. Strip the periosteum from the rib throughout its length, freeing the deep attachments to the rib with a gauze swab. Dissect the rib free anteriorly first, elevating it as the dissection proceeds.

3 Cut through the costal cartilage with scissors and remove it. Sweep the pleura superiorly and posteriorly and similarly sweep the peritoneum anteriorly, using gauze swabs.

4 Identify the kidney lying inferiorly. Incise the deep fascia, allowing the retroperitoneal fat to bulge out. Have your assistant retract the kidney inferiorly while you proceed carefully to bluntly dissect the fat above and medial to the kidney.

5 Identify and mobilize right or left adrenal gland as described above, paying attention to haemostasis. Handle the gland gently to avoid disruption and avoid damaging surrounding organs.

6 Close the wound in layers. Take care to close the pleura if it was opened, after asking the anaesthetist to expand the lungs. Drains are not usually necessary. As a rule, order a chest X-ray in the recovery ward to exclude a significant pneumothorax.

> **KEY POINTS** Avoid causing damage to organs surrounding the adrenals

■ Dissect the vena cava and renal veins carefully, especially for larger tumours.
■ Retract gently. Spleen and liver are friable and bleed easily.
■ Colon, duodenum or stomach can sustain thermal damage from diathermy/harmonic scalpel.
■ Do not damage the intercostal neurovascular bundle and underlying pleura.

Posterior (retroperitoneal) approach

Posterior access to the adrenals is an attractive concept, as both glands lie retroperitoneally and this approach can be used for both endoscopic and open surgery. Using the posterior approach, you do not enter the peritoneal cavity and do not need to mobilize or retract intra-peritoneal organs. It is ideal for patients with previous abdominal surgery and adhesions. Bilateral adrenalectomy can also be performed without repositioning the patient. Its main disadvantage is limited working space, which only allows resection of adrenals smaller than 6 cm.

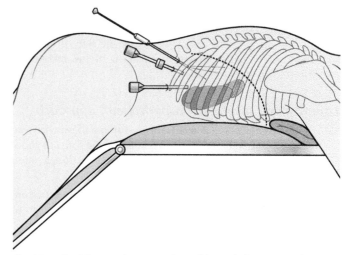

Fig. 22.5 Position on the operating table and placement of trocars post posterior endoscopic adrenalectomy.

Position the patient prone with good support under the shoulders and hips. Place the patient's arms alongside the head, carefully supported. Break the table to tense the lumbar fascia.

Endoscopic posterior (retroperitoneal) approach
(Fig. 22.5)

1 The technique for left and right adrenalectomy is similar.

2 Make an incision between the tips of the eleventh and twelfth ribs and dissect bluntly through the muscles until you can feel the kidney. Insert the first port and create an artificial space using either an inflatable balloon or blunt dissection aided by CO_2 insufflation at a pressure of around 20 mmHg.

3 Introduce two further ports (5 mm) close to the costal margins on either side of the port used for the 0° or 30° camera.

4 Carry the dissection close to the quadrate lumbar muscle to avoid opening peritoneum. Identify the kidney, retract it downwards and dissect perirenal fat until you see the edge of the adrenal.

5 Dissect the ventral and lateral aspects of the adrenal gland by dividing small anterior branches until the adrenal vein is encountered. Division of the adrenal vein between clips or using a vascular stapler greatly increases mobility of the gland. Complete dissection of the adrenal, retrieve it in a bag and close the incisions.

Open posterior (retroperitoneal) approach

1 Make a horizontal incision over the eleventh rib, extended medially and superiorly over the paravertebral muscles. Excise the rib, carefully avoiding damage to the neurovascular bundle at the inferior margin of the rib.

2 Dissect the gland as described above, retrieve it in a bag and close the incision in layers.

3 Try not to damage the pleura, but if you do, reconstitute it at the end of the procedure. Do not insert a chest drain provided you have expressed all the air from the pleural cavity by expanding the lungs at the end of the procedure.

Anterior approach

Use the anterior approach mainly for open adrenalectomy when excising large tumours that cannot be removed laparoscopically because of their size or because they are malignant and invade surrounding organs. This approach provides access to both adrenals, allows extension of the incision into the chest and safe control of major blood vessels if necessary, resection of involved organs and extended lymphadenectomy.

Laparoscopic anterior approach

1 The first laparoscopic adrenalectomies were attempted using this approach but because of technical difficulty retracting structures, identifying the adrenals and controlling bleeding, as well as the duration of the procedure, it has been superseded by the lateral and posterior laparoscopic approaches.

Open anterior approach

1 Use either a transverse (rooftop) or midline abdominal incision.

2 Expose the left adrenal by dividing the lienorenal and lienocolic ligaments and retracting the splenic flexure downwards and spleen and pancreas medially. This provides good access to the adrenal and renal hilum and allows safe dissection of large tumours.

3 Expose the right adrenal by retracting the hepatic flexure of the colon downwards and performing Kocher's manoeuvre to mobilize the duodenum. Divide the triangular ligaments of the right lobe of the liver and retract the liver medially, exposing its 'bare area' and the inferior vena cava. For large and infiltrating tumours encircle the inferior vena cava with tapes placed below and above the liver to provide safe control in case of major haemorrhage or if its resection and graft replacement are indicated.

4 Dissect the adrenal gland carefully and, after removing the tumour, close the abdomen using a mass closure technique. Abdominal drains are rarely required.

Postoperative

1 Postoperative management depends on the functional status of the removed adrenal, the size of the tumour and type of the operation performed (i.e. laparoscopic or open).

2 Patients following laparoscopic adrenalectomy for Conn's syndrome can be nursed on the ward and go home after an overnight stay. Remember to check post operatively potassium and cortisol levels as some patients can suppress cortisol production in contralateral gland. They will require cortisol supplementation. Stop spironolactone and potassium supplementation. Gradually stop other medications for hypertension.

3 Manage most patients after surgery for Cushing's syndrome/disease on the high dependency unit (HDU) overnight because they are often diabetic, obese, require careful fluid and electrolyte management and close cardiovascular monitoring. They also need treatment with hydrocortisone and fludrocortisone.

4 Initial treatment of patients after removal of phaeochromocytoma must take place on the HDU as they require invasive cardiovascular monitoring of blood pressure, careful fluid replacement and may need adrenaline (epinephrine) or noradrenaline (norepinephrine) infusion.

Complications

Conversion of laparoscopic to open adrenalectomy (3–5%) is not a complication and should be the result of dispassionate appraisal of the intra-operative situation. The commonest reasons for conversion are excessive bleeding, difficulty in mobilizing the mass due to its large size, injury to surrounding organs or, especially early on the learning course, the length of operation.

Complications after adrenalectomy (10–15%) may be the result of either suboptimal perioperative management of metabolic and cardiovascular abnormalities caused by functioning adrenal masses or related to the surgical procedure itself.

1 Electrolyte abnormalities and hypertension are common in patients with hormonal syndromes. Correct them perioperatively to prevent cardiovascular incidents and strokes. Anticipate and treat the possibility of postoperative hypotension.

2 Failure to stop medications no longer required after surgery (e.g. phenoxybenzamine after resection of phaeochromocytoma) or prescribe new medications which are essential after adrenalectomy (e.g. hydrocortisone after adrenalectomy for Cushing's syndrome) is a common mistake and can result in re-admission and endanger the patient's life.

3 Bleeding during surgery may be the result of inadequate control of arteries and veins supplying the adrenal, or damage to surrounding structures such as the inferior vena cava, renal veins and arteries, liver or spleen. Carefully dissect and retract and sensibly employ the harmonic scalpel, diathermy, clips or vascular stapler to prevent this complication. Most adrenalectomies can be performed without blood transfusion. Postoperative bleeding is very rare.

4 Perforation of bowel (colon, stomach, or duodenum) may occur during introduction of trocars or adrenal dissection. Repair injuries detected during operation immediately – but the presentation of thermal injury to the bowel may be delayed by 24–48 hours.

5 Pancreatitis or pancreatic leak are rare complications of left adrenalectomy caused by excessive manipulation or damage to the pancreatic parenchyma.

6 Control postoperative pain with appropriate oral or parenteral analgesia; offer patients with large incisions epidural infusion or PCA (patient-controlled analgesia). Long-term pain may result from entrapment of intercostal nerves.

FURTHER READING

Assalia A, Gagner M. Laparoscopic adrenalectomy. BJS 2004;91:1259–74.
Gagner M, Inabnet WB, editors. Adrenal surgery. In: Minimally Invasive Endocrine Surgery. New York: Lippincott Williams&Wilkins; 2002. p. 167–252.

Arteries

D.M. Baker, M. Davis

CONTENTS

INTRODUCTION

Arterial disease and its management is becoming an increasingly specialized field, with training programmes accordingly recognizing this. However, all competent surgeons should be familiar with the basic principles of arterial control, repair and reconstruction.

▶ KEY POINTS Indications for operation

There are three main reasons for operating on an artery:
- Injury
- Aneurysmal dilatation
- Occlusion.

INDICATIONS FOR OPERATION

1 *Injury.* This may result from sharp or blunt trauma secondary to assault or road traffic accident. Iatrogenic injuries are becoming more prevalent as a consequence of percutaneous arterial access for diagnostic procedures and treatments such as coronary interventions. Challenging self-induced injuries are also seen as a result of intravenous drug addiction.

2 *Aneurysm.* This is defined as a pathological, permanent dilatation of an artery. Arterial aneurysms may involve the aorta and/or peripheral arterial system. The three main sites for aneurysms are the abdominal aorta, femoral and popliteal arteries. Most vascular surgeons consider the aorta to be dilated once it is twice its normal diameter; for non-aortic vessels an arterial aneurysm is defined by an increased diameter of 50% or more. Aneurysmal disease secondary to atherosclerosis is responsible for considerable morbidity and mortality in the developed world and the prevalence of abdominal aortic aneurysm is increasing. Vascular disease is rarely localized and it is essential to exclude co-existent pathology in other vessels.

Infected (mycotic) aneurysms are much less common than those caused by degenerative disease. True mycotic aneurysms result from septic emboli of cardiac origin (endocarditis), which may result in multiple aneurysms at different sites. With an ageing population, microbial aneurysmal arteritis is seen more frequently than true mycotic aneurysms; this results from bacterial seeding into diseased arterial intima with subsequent pseudoaneurysm formation, the most common infecting organisms being the Salmonella species, *Escherichia coli*, *Staphylococcus* species and *Klebsiella pneumoniae*. In approximately 25% of cases no organisms are isolated.

3 *Occlusion and stenosis.* Most arterial occlusions result from thrombosis of a diseased vessel and are part of a generalized atherosclerotic process. Surgical intervention is not always necessary and careful assessment and management of risk factors is required before surgery is planned. Less commonly an artery is blocked by an embolus. Sudden occlusion of an otherwise normal major artery may threaten both the limb and the life of the patient and warrants emergency intervention either by embolectomy or dissolution of the occlusion. The management of acute-on-chronic limb ischaemia is quite different: this develops following thrombotic occlusion of a previously diseased vessel and cannot usually be treated effectively with thrombectomy alone.

The sections which follow assume that the patient has already been critically evaluated and the need for operation established.

GENERAL PRINCIPLES

In the United Kingdom (UK), most arterial surgery is now undertaken in specialized vascular centres with access to hybrid operating theatres able to perform combined open and endoluminal techniques. The best results are achieved with a multidisciplinary approach by a team of specialized vascular anaesthetists, vascular surgeons, interventional radiologists and vascular scientists to optimize the care of vascular patients.

In addition, facilities such as cell-saver technology to reduce blood transfusion, point-of-care coagulation testing, intra-operative monitoring and intensive care facilities are paramount to gain good outcomes in vascular patients.

There are instances where arterial surgery needs to be undertaken outwith a vascular centre, where the facilities described above may not be available. It is therefore essential for all surgeons to understand the principles of vascular operations and it is in this context and for the benefit of the generalist that this chapter is written.

EQUIPMENT

Most vascular operations can be performed with the naked eye but it is useful to become familiar with the use of magnifying loupes as they enhance clarity and may result in a technically superior anastomosis, paramount in vascular success. Loupes magnifying to x 2.5 are usually sufficient when performing an anastomosis on vessels of 2–3 mm in diameter such as tibial vessels. For smaller vessels an operating microscope should be considered and is beyond the remit of this chapter.

Instruments

In addition to a general surgical set, including a selection of fixed self-retaining retractors appropriate to the area being operated upon (for example, the Omnitract system), the following instruments are helpful:

1 *Clamps.* A good selection of lightweight vascular clamps is essential. The DeBakey Atraugrip range is suitable for large intra-abdominal and thoracic vessels. For smaller vessels (e.g. femoral, popliteal, subclavian, brachial and carotid arteries), miniature clamps of the Castaneda type designed for paediatric cardiac surgery are ideal. The springs should be gentle and not cause intimal damage. A selection of small 'bulldog' clamps is useful to control bleeding while minimizing arterial damage. Alternatively, control of small distal vessels can be gained with the use of fine nylon loops or smooth, round-ended atraumatic intraluminal catheters.

2 *Dissecting instruments.* Handle arteries gently, and only with non-toothed forceps such as the DeBakey Atraugrip range. Following an initial arteriotomy with an appropriate-sized scalpel blade (a No. 15 for infrainguinal surgery), Pott's scissors angles in two planes are required for lengthening the arterial incisions. For dissection within the vessel, in order to remove adherent thrombus or elevate the plaque in an endarterectomy, Watson-Cheyne and James MacDonald's dissectors are ideal. Long tunnelling instruments are necessary for conveying grafts between unconnected incisions.

3 *Catheters and shunts.* Atraumatic (umbilical) catheters ranging from 3F to 6F in size are useful for intraluminal irrigation and to control small vessels. In addition, a range of the Pruitt type catheters are helpful as they have dual ports to irrigate and occlude vessels. These catheters are particularly useful where heavily calcified vessels may preclude the use of traditional vascular clamps, which may cause iatrogenic injury. A similar size range of Fogarty embolectomy catheters is also required. Catheters with a central lumen allow their introduction over a guidewire under fluoroscopic control, to facilitate intra-operative radiological imaging as well as the instillation of anticoagulant solutions, for example heparinized saline or tissue plasminogen activator (tPA).

It is sometimes necessary to employ an intraluminal shunt as a temporary bypass during reconstruction of a vessel, most commonly in carotid endarterectomy or during arterial and venous reconstruction following trauma. There are two basic types: the Javid and Pruitt-Inihara. A Javid shunt is a tapered plastic tube with a bulbous expansion at each end; these allow large and small ring clamps to be applied to the outside of the vessel once the shunt has been introduced into the artery (see Fig. 23.35).

The second type is a modification of the Pruitt catheter described above, with a balloon at each end to retain it in place and to control bleeding, and a side-arm for withdrawal of blood or air from the lumen.

4 *Endovascular equipment.* For the most part, percutaneous procedures are the remit of the interventionalist and/or the vascular specialist. Procedures may involve both open and endoluminal techniques. It is paramount that procedures involving radiation and contrast medium are undertaken by appropriately trained staff with the requisite certification. For the non-specialist a basic understanding of the guidewires (variety of diameters, thickness, lengths and coatings as well as stiffness, depending on usage, tip shapes and steering capabilities), catheters and sheaths available is all that is required. It is not recommended that surgeons lacking the requisite training and skills undertake these techniques.

5 *Sutures, needle-holders and suture clamps.* Arteries are always sewn with non-absorbable stitches. There are three types:

- Fine monofilament material such as polypropylene (Prolene) has the advantage of being very smooth and slipping easily through the tissues so that a loose suture can be drawn tight. The material possesses a slight 'memory' which can easily be compensated for with familiarity of use. Its main disadvantage is that it has a tendency to fracture with direct handling with metal instruments.
- Braided materials are coated with an outer layer of polyester to render them smooth, for example Ethiflex and Ethibond. Sutures of this type do not slip so easily through the arterial wall but are pleasantly floppy to handle and knot easily.
- PTFE (polytetrafluoroethylene; Gore-Tex) sutures are designed specifically for use with PTFE grafts. PTFE is non-compliant: thus holes in the graft made by the passage of a needle result in more bleeding than occurs with other types of grafts. In PTFE sutures the diameter of the needle is smaller than that of the suture itself, thereby reducing bleeding. This is at the expense of some loss of strength, and the fragility of these needles precludes their use in tough or calcified arteries. The suture material itself is extremely strong and has excellent handling properties.

In general, use the finest suture appropriate for the job; as a rough guide, 3/0 for the aorta, 4/0 for the iliacs, 5/0 for the femoral, 6/0 for the popliteal and 7/0 for the tibial arteries. For very fine work a monofilament stitch is always necessary.

Vascular sutures are usually double-ended sutures and are used accordingly. The end of the suture not being used for the anastomosis is usually attached to a 'rubber shod' clamp-a mosquito or similar clamp with fine tubing cushioning the jaws to prevent damage to the suture. Unprotected clamps should never be applied to monofilament sutures.

To complement the range of sutures a wide selection of needle-holders varying in length should be available; likewise, the tips should reflect the degree of delicacy of the anastomosis being performed.

Solutions

For local irrigation of opened vessels and instillation into vessels distal to a clamp use heparinized saline (5000 units of heparin in 500 ml of 0.9% normal saline).

Grafts and stents

The best arterial substitute is the patient's own blood vessel, usually vein. However, quite often there is no suitable vein available because it is either absent, too small, varicose or damaged by thrombophlebitis. In these circumstances a prosthetic graft has to be chosen:

1 *Dacron.* This is an inert polymer that is spun into a thread and then either woven or knitted; it is available as straight or bifurcated grafts measuring from 5 to 40 mm in diameter. In general, the knitted variety with a velour lining is preferred as its porosity leads to better anchoring of the internal 'neointimal' surface. The original knitted grafts needed to be carefully preclotted with blood taken from the patient prior to the administration of heparin and in an emergency such as a ruptured aneurysm it was necessary to use a woven graft, which leaks less. However, most vascular surgeons now use knitted grafts that have been presealed with bovine collagen, gelatin or albumin. These grafts have very low porosity at the time of insertion and so do not require preclotting. Dacron grafts perform well when used to bypass large arteries with a high flow-rate (e.g. the aorta and iliac arteries) and are the conduit of choice in these situations provided there is no obvious infection present. In general, Dacron grafts are used above the groin and PTFE below the groin. Dacron grafts are available with external ring supports to prevent compression or kinking.

2 *Expanded polytetrafluoroethylene (PTFE)* is more expensive than Dacron, but its performance is superior for reconstruction of small arteries. PTFE grafts are again available with an external polypropylene ring support to prevent compression or kinking of the graft. It is essential to use this type of graft when traversing a joint (for example the knee joint). Further developments in this field include preshaped grafts which are manufactured from PTFE to reproduce an anastomosis of 'ideal' configuration without the need to form a vein cuff at the distal anastomosis. The long-term patency rate is inferior to that of vein grafts.

3 *Biological.* The first arterial substitutes tried were arterial or venous allografts or xenografts but these degraded and were abandoned. Grafts from cryopreserved human umbilical veins have been advocated for bypass procedures in the presence of infection; however they are prone to aneurysmal dilatation and therefore their use is limited.

4 *Compliant grafts.* Prosthetic grafts are stiff and non-compliant and hence their patency is inferior to that of human vessels. Newer grafts developed using nanotechnology have an excellent compliance profile; they are currently in clinical trials and may prove to be a significant new material in the armamentarium of the vascular surgeon.

5 *Stents and stent-grafts.* Metallic stents made from either stainless steel or nitinol may be used as an adjunct to balloon angioplasty in order to maintain patency of a vessel. There are two types: balloon expandable (e.g. Palmaz stent) and self-expanding (e.g. Wallstent). Stent-grafts are used for endovascular aneurysm repair and are made of polyester/PTFE attached to a metal stent (either stainless steel or nitinol, which is a nickel–titanium alloy).

The metal stent provides both radial and longitudinal support, with the aneurysm being excluded from the circulation by the graft material. Endografts are usually self-expanding but balloon expandable devices have been made. All endoluminal stent-grafts rely on being oversized by 10–15% relative to the normal diameter of the artery in which they are placed. One further variable is the proximal fixation method, which usually consists of hooks or barbs which secure the device to the proximal aortic wall to minimize distal migration. Most stent-grafts are either bifurcated aortoiliac or uni-iliac devices and are either one piece or modular in design. If a uni-iliac device is deployed, the contralateral iliac artery has to be occluded, usually with a radiological plug, and a femoro-femoral crossover graft performed to allow perfusion of the contralateral lower limb.

GENERAL CONSIDERATIONS

Antibiotics. Infection is disastrous in vascular surgery and antibiotic cover is essential, particularly if a prosthesis is to be used. The local regimen should be consulted; however, appropriate cover for Staphylococcus should be given intravenously before the first incision is made.

Anticoagulation. Before arteries are clamped systemic anticoagulation should be given, this is calculated at 70 units of heparin per kg (approximately 5000 units of heparin for a standard 70 kg person given intravenously) and is given 2 minutes before arterial clamps are applied. In complex thoracoabdominal open or endovascular procedures the heparin regimen differs and is usually determined and controlled by regular monitoring of the ACCT with appropriate reversal at the end of the procedure.

BASIC TECHNIQUES OF ARTERIAL REPAIR, ANASTOMOSIS AND TRANSLUMINAL ANGIOPLASTY

Arteriotomy

▶ KEY POINTS Longitudinal arteriotomy

Arteries are best opened longitudinally:
- A longitudinal arteriotomy is easier to close and can be extended. However, care needs to be taken to ensure that when the arteriotomy is closed the vessel is not stenosed.
- A transverse arteriotomy is difficult to close because the intima retracts away from the outer layers. This increases the risk of blood tracking in a subintimal plane, which can cause vessel occlusion.

Simple suture

1 Longitudinal arteriotomies in large or medium-sized arteries can usually be closed by simple suture (Fig. 23.1).

2 Use the finest suture material compatible with the thickness and quality of the arterial wall. The aim is to produce an everted suture line that is leak-proof, with apposition of the intima. This is quite different from bowel anastomosis, where the mucosa is

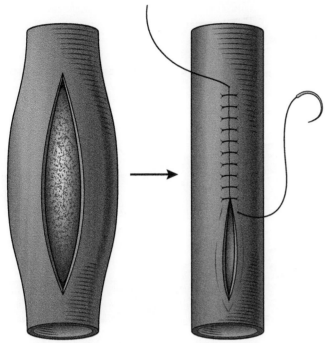

Fig. 23.1 Longitudinal arteriotomy closed by continuous everting arterial suture.

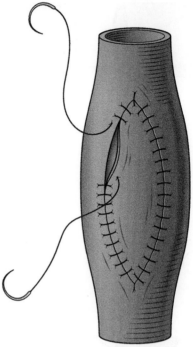

Fig. 23.2 Closure of longitudinal arteriotomy with a patch.

deliberately inverted into the lumen and tension on the sutures is minimal to prevent necrosis of the edges. There is no need to use everting mattress sutures which would narrow the lumen: a simple over-and-over stitch is adequate provided that care is taken to ensure that the intima turns outwards. The needle must pass through all layers of the arterial wall with every stitch. The inner layers must be included to ensure good intimal apposition and to prevent flap dissection, and the outer layers must be included since the main strength of the arterial wall resides in its adventitia. A good surgical assistant who follows your stitches and maintains firm, even tension on the suture at all times is important. Experience is required in order to judge the spacing and size of each bite, and this varies with the size and nature of the artery. Occasionally, for example in aortic aneurysm repair, large irregular stitches may be required but in general evenly spaced regular stitching is best.

Closure with a patch

1 Close vessels of less than 4 mm in diameter with a patch in order to avoid narrowing of the lumen (Fig. 23.2).

2 This technique may also be used to widen the lumen of a vessel that has become stenosed by disease (e.g. the profunda femoris artery). For small vessels use a patch of autologous vein. Do not use the proximal end of the long saphenous vein for this purpose. Use either a segment taken from the ankle, a tributary or a piece of vein from another site (e.g. an arm vein). For larger vessels prosthetic material (either Dacron or PTFE) or bovine or equine patches may be used. When cutting the patch to shape, always ensure that the ends are rounded rather than tapered to a sharp point: this prevents narrowing of the lumen caused by clustering of sutures at the pointed end. After shaping the patch use a single double-ended stitch commencing close to one end and working around each side. Do not finish the stitching at

the apex as knots here are at risk of causing significant narrowing: carry one of the sutures around to the other side to complete the closure and tie the knot a short distance to one side. This technique permits direct vision of the internal suture line and allows final trimming of the patch to be delayed until closure is nearly complete in order to ensure a perfect match for size.

End-to-end anastomosis

1 For small delicate arteries this is accomplished most safely by applying the principles of the triangulation technique originally described by Carrel.[1] Join the vessels with a suture placed in the centre of the back or deepest aspect of the anastomosis (Fig. 23.3). Be sure to tie the knot on the outside. Place two more sutures so as to divide the circumference of the vessels equally into three. Any disparity in calibre can be compensated for at this stage. If the vessel is small it is better to insert interrupted sutures to prevent narrowing. Use the three original stay sutures to apply gentle traction and to rotate the vessel and facilitate exposure of each segment of the anastomosis in turn. Complete the back two segments first, leaving the easiest segment at the front to be finished last.

2 For larger vessels it is permissible to use continuous sutures. Cut the ends of the vessels to be joined obliquely then make a short incision longitudinally to create a spatulated shape and reduce the risk of narrowing at the anastomosis.

3 A different technique of end-to-end anastomosis, the inlay technique, is routinely used in open operations for aneurysms (see below).

End-to-side anastomosis

1 This is the standard form of anastomosis for bypass operations. It should be oblique and its length should be 2–2.5 times the diameter of the lumen of the graft. To avoid narrowing the lumen, it is important that the end of the graft is fashioned into a spatulated

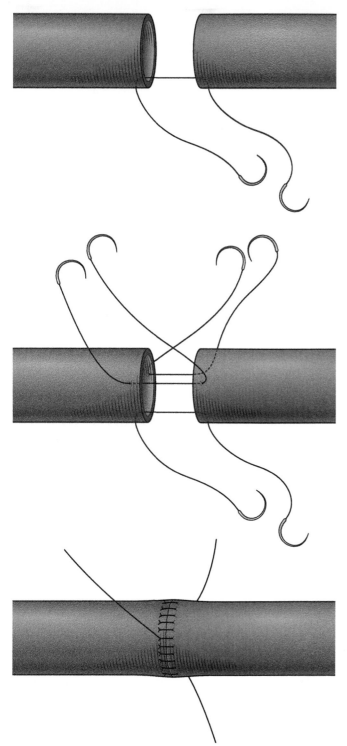

Fig. 23.3 **End-to-end anastomosis by the triangulation technique.**

shape, which on completion of the anastomosis has a smooth curved 'cobra-head' appearance rather than an angulated 'V' appearance. The end of the anastomosis in the angle with the native vessel is referred to as the 'heel' and the other end as the 'toe'. Place a double-ended stitch at the heel and another at the toe and run sutures along each margin, ending with a knot at the halfway point on each side. Alternatively, start with a double-ended suture at the heel and leave the toe free. Run the suture up each side to beyond the midpoint and then place the suture

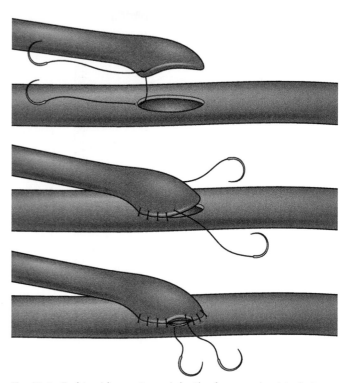

Fig. 23.4 **End-to-side anastomosis by the four-quadrant technique.**

in a 'rubber-shod' clamp to prevent damage. Take a new double-ended suture and start at the toe end and suture around the apex towards the midpoint on either side and then tie to the previously retained threads. This is sometimes known as the 'four-quadrant technique' (Fig. 23.4), and has the advantage of keeping the inside of the suture line in view as much as possible.

The 'toe' and 'heel' are the most crucial points of an end-to-side anastomosis. To ensure that the toe is completed as smoothly as possible, offset the starting point of the 'toe', suturing a few millimetres to one side or the other of the apex. In order to further reduce the risk of causing a stricture at this point, some surgeons prefer to place a few interrupted sutures around the toe. It is essential that this end of the anastomosis is performed under direct vision and to ensure that each stitch is placed carefully without causing narrowing.

2 A stricture of the heel may be avoided by stenting the vessel with an intraluminal catheter of appropriate size until this portion of the anastomosis is complete. An alternative method is the 'parachute' technique (Fig. 23.5). This is particularly useful where access is difficult and good visualization of the anastomosis is impaired, but it is applicable to most situations. With the graft and the recipient artery separated, place a series of running sutures between them at what will become the heel of the anastomosis. These sutures are then pulled tight as the vessels are approximated.

▶ KEY POINTS 'Parachute' technique

■ It is essential to use a monofilament suture with this method.
■ Limit the number of loops to a maximum of eight before approximating the anastomosis.

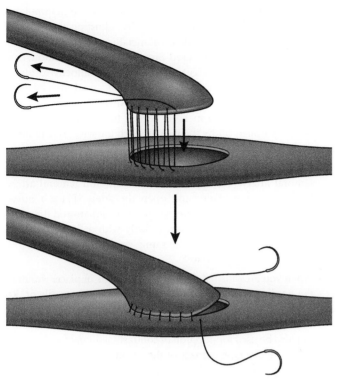

Fig. 23.5 End-to-side anastomosis by the parachute technique.

Transluminal angioplasty (Fig. 23.6)

1 Angioplasty is performed by appropriately trained vascular interventionalists. Most patients with symptoms secondary to peripheral arterial occlusion are now treated with endoluminal techniques rather than open surgery. Prior to offering patients transluminal angioplasty, optimize the patient's risk factors with best medical therapy, cessation of smoking and a supervised exercise programme.[2]

It is paramount to consider these patients in the context of a multidisciplinary meeting. Most surgeons and radiologists will not offer angioplasty to patients with calf claudication as the risks may outweigh the benefits. Angioplasty and, if required, placement of a stent may be warranted in patients with buttock claudication with iliac stenosis, as the risks of emboli and consequent limb loss are lower. Patients with critical ischaemia and tissue loss should be considered for an endoluminal approach.

Patients with diabetes mellitus may present with challenging long occlusions extending from superficial femoral to crural vessels in tandem with significant co-morbidites. In these patients an endoluminal approach may be offered in isolation or in conjunction with surgical revascularization: subintimal angioplasty may be preferred to a transluminal approach; however, this should not be undertaken without due consideration and by an experienced endovascular specialist. Specialist equipment such as the 'Outback' catheter and 'Ree kross' balloon can achieve endoluminal revascularization of long occlusions and may result in a successful outcome in patients with critical limb ischaemia or tissue loss who may not be candidates for traditional surgery.

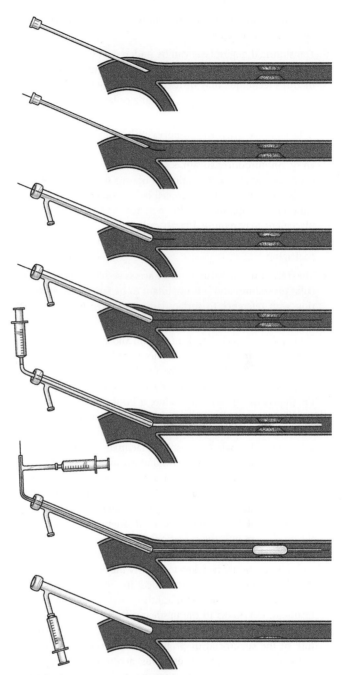

Fig. 23.6 Percutaneous angioplasty.

2 Essential requirements are fluoroscopy with 'subtraction' and 'road-mapping' functions and skilled radiographic assistance. Use a radiolucent operating table.

3 Ensure all operating theatre staff are properly protected against radiation.

4 In the case of elective procedures ensure that patients are prescribed antiplatelet therapy at least 48 hours prior to the procedure. Minimize contrast-induced renal damage by ensuring adequate rehydration with intravenous fluids pre and post procedure.

5 Consider giving mild sedation and oxygen; ensure regular non-invasive monitoring of blood pressure, heart rate and

oxygen saturation. Well-chosen music in the operating room may help patients to relax.

6   Transluminal angioplasty can be undertaken percutaneously or using an open technique to expose the relevant artery. Be aware that this technique may be used concurrently with open arterial reconstruction (for example, iliac angioplasty and femorodistal bypass).

7   If the chosen entry vessel cannot easily be palpated consider using ultrasound to locate the vessel, allowing accurate single puncture entry. An introducer sheath is always used and permits repeated endovascular access with minimal trauma to the vessel. The size of sheath required is determined by the procedure to follow – balloon angioplasty usually requires a 4–7F sheath; stent placement may require a larger catheter. All manufacturers recommend the appropriate sheaths on their instructions and packaging.

8   The common femoral artery is the access vessel for most endovascular procedures and it is important to be familiar with its position with reference to surface landmarks (see Exposure of the common femoral artery, below).

9   For percutaneous access, clean the skin and apply drapes as for an open procedure. Inject a small amount of local anaesthetic at the chosen puncture site and make a nick in the skin with a no. 11 scalpel blade. While palpating the common femoral artery with the fingers of one hand introduce a Potts-Cournand or similar needle. These needles have a central trocar that allows blood to 'flashback' into a chamber on the hub when the lumen of the vessel is entered. Angle the needle to facilitate access of the guide wire in the direction required and to avoid puncture of the back wall or creation of a false lumen and dissection. For infrainguinal procedures, puncture the artery just distal to the inguinal ligament, allowing room to manoeuvre the tip of the needle within the lumen of the common femoral artery whilst negotiating the guide wire into the superficial femoral artery. Note that the inguinal ligament lies approximately 2 cm proximal to the groin crease. Care should be taken to identify the landmarks accurately in all patients: do not be misled in obese patients whose groin crease will be significantly lower than the inguinal ligament. For access to the upstream iliac arteries the puncture site may be a little lower, but take care to avoid unintended puncture of the superficial or profunda femoris arteries. When no pulse is palpable or percutaneous access is difficult use an ultrasound-guided arterial puncture technique. Alternatively, 'cut-down' onto the common femoral artery under local infiltration anaesthesia.

10 When 'flashback' occurs you should observe strong pulsatile flow from the needle. Unless there is severe inflow obstruction, the absence of pulsatile flow from the needle indicates that the tip is not properly positioned within the lumen. Do not attempt to advance a guide wire, but re-position the needle to gain access to the arterial lumen.

11 When satisfied with the position of the needle, advance a short J guide-wire down the trocar (normally a suitable wire is packaged as a part of the introducer set) and check with fluoroscopy. A guide-wire that is within the lumen passes without resistance: if resistance is encountered do not apply force as this is likely to result in dissection of the subintimal plane. Stop, withdraw the guide-wire and readjust the position of the needle. For downstream procedures the guide-wire must be manipulated into the superficial femoral artery by adjusting the angle of the needle. This requires that stiff metallic rather than soft plastic or Silastic needles are used. Simple fluoroscopy without contrast is usually sufficient to guide this manoeuvre, but if persistent difficulty is encountered obtain a road-map by injection of contrast through the needle. Never pass a hydrophilic guide-wire through a metallic needle: the hydrophilic coating will be stripped off by the needle when the wire is withdrawn, with potentially dire consequences.

12 If angioplasty is to be performed through the exposed common femoral artery (see Exposure of the common femoral artery, below), do not clamp and open the artery. Place a purse-string suture of 5/0 polypropylene (Prolene) around the artery before puncturing the vessel directly with a Potts-Cournand needle. Then proceed in the same way as for a percutaneous procedure.

13 When you are satisfied that the guide-wire is in place, withdraw the needle and insert the introducer sheath with its dilator. Remove the dilator. Flush the sheath with heparinized saline through the side channel, which is fitted with a tap. This channel can also be used for injection of contrast medium in order to obtain an angiographic image of the lesion.

14 Withdraw the short guide-wire and replace it with the wire chosen to navigate the lesion to be treated. The size of guide-wire required is indicated on the packaging of the balloon catheter – most often 0.035 inches in diameter for peripheral arterial procedures. Introduce it through the sheath floppy end first, using the small plastic introducer cone that comes with the wire to penetrate the valve. If difficulty is encountered in crossing the lesion use a hydrophilic guide-wire. Always wipe the guide-wire with a swab soaked in heparinized saline after removing a catheter as dried blood on the surface obstructs the smooth passage of a subsequent catheter.

15 If navigation of the guide-wire has been difficult, pass an appropriately sized catheter across the lesion and obtain an angiogram to ensure that the natural lumen has been entered beyond the lesion before passing a balloon catheter. If a subintimal space has been entered consider abandoning the procedure.

16 For most applications select a balloon catheter of 4 cm in length. For accurate sizing of the balloon obtain an angiogram using a measuring catheter with 1 cm markings. Match the size of the balloon to the diameter of the unstenosed artery. However, this degree of precision is not normally necessary: for lesions in the superficial femoral artery balloons with a diameter of 6 mm, and for iliac lesions 8 mm, are usually appropriate. Be cautious when selecting catheters for female patients with small arteries.

17 Use a hand-operated syringe driver to inflate the balloon to a pressure of 5–10 atmospheres with a 50/50 mixture of contrast medium and saline. Observe the shape of the balloon as it inflates; 'popping' of the 'waist' caused by the stenosis indicates that the plaque has given way and, usually, a satisfactory outcome. It is not necessary to maintain inflation of the balloon for more than a few seconds but a second inflation helps smooth the irregularities of the flow surface that result from splitting and fissuring of the plaque.

18 Obtain a completion angiogram to assess the final result. Remember that some irregularity of the flow surface at the site of angioplasty is usual. This tends to remodel naturally within a few weeks. Also, dilatation may continue to occur at the angioplasty site for a short time. If a significant stenosis remains, or if a large intimal flap has developed following iliac artery angioplasty, consider the use of an intraluminal stent. Stents do not perform well in arteries below the groin and should only be used in exceptional circumstances.

19 Following withdrawal of the introducer sheath apply digital pressure to the puncture site for a minimum of 10 minutes, and longer if needed, before applying a dressing and moving the patient. Give clear instructions to the nursing staff regarding duration of bed rest prior to mobilization to minimize haematoma and pseudoaneurysm formation. If the artery has been exposed, tie the purse-string suture to secure haemostasis or apply clamps and proceed with the open procedure.

20 Unless contraindicated, prescribe subcutaneous heparin or low-molecular-weight heparin postoperatively. Monitor peripheral perfusion and the groin for signs of haematoma or formation of a false aneurysm. Ensure post procedure antiplatelet therapy is continued indefinitely.

REFERENCES

1. Carrel A. La technique operatoire des anastomoses vasculaires et de la transplantation des visceres. Lyon Med 1902;99:114–52.
2. Basil trial. www.basiltrial.com.

EXPOSURE OF THE MAJOR PERIPHERAL ARTERIES

Common femoral artery

1 The common femoral artery needs to be exposed more frequently than any other vessel in the body and it is important to know how to do this swiftly and correctly (Fig. 23.7).

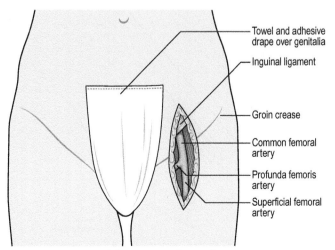

Fig. 23.7 **Exposure of the common femoral artery.**

▶ **KEY POINTS** Anatomy

■ The surface marking of the artery is at the midinguinal point (i.e. halfway between the anterior superior iliac spine and the pubic symphysis). Remember these landmarks as the artery is not always palpable.
■ The common femoral artery is related anatomically to the inguinal ligament; do not be influenced by the position of the groin crease, which can be 2–3 cm distal to the common femoral artery (more in an obese patient).

2 The position of the groin crease does not correspond to that of the inguinal ligament, but lies distal to it by 2–3 cm.

3 The midpoint of the incision should roughly correspond to the groin crease. Inexperienced surgeons tend to make the incision too low. When limited exposure of the common femoral artery is required (e.g. access for an endovascular intervention), it is permissible to use a transverse incision, which heals better and less painfully than a vertical incision crossing the groin crease. Position a transverse incision two fingers breadth above the groin crease.

4 Deepen the incision through the subcutaneous fat, taking care not to cut across any lymph nodes. Expose the femoral sheath and incise it longitudinally to expose the artery. The femoral vein lies medially and must be protected, but the femoral nerve on the lateral side lies in a deeper plane and is not usually at risk. However, do not be over zealous with positioning of a self-retainer, as the nerve can easily be stretched and a neuropraxia ensues.

5 Dissect a length of the common femoral artery and without undue force pass a Lahey clamp around the back of the artery in order to draw through a plastic sling. Gently lift the artery with the sling and identify its branches and its bifurcation into the superficial and profunda femoral arteries. Isolate these similarly with slings. Take care to avoid damage to the profunda vein, a tributary of which always passes anterior to the main stem of the profunda artery. For a more extensive exposure of the profunda femoris artery divide this vein between ties.

6 If exposure of the greater saphenous vein is required at the same operation make a 'lazy-S' incision, commencing vertically over the artery at the inguinal ligament and then deviating medially over the vein in the upper thigh.

7 Transection of the many lymphatics in the femoral triangle may cause a troublesome lymphocele or lymphatic fistula after the operation. There is no sure way of avoiding this, but approach the artery from its lateral rather than its medial side and gently reflect any lymph nodes and visible lymph vessels off the femoral sheath with minimal damage. If there are any obvious lymph leaks at the time of surgery suture the lymphatic channels closed with 6/0 Prolene.

Popliteal artery

1 The popliteal artery can be exposed above and below the knee by medial approaches. Prior to embarking on this surgery decide which part of the artery needs to be accessed and consider how the patient should be positioned on the operating table. The most inaccessible part lies directly behind the joint line and if

its exposure at this level is required a posterior approach is essential (see paragraph 4 below).

2   To expose the supragenicular part of the artery the patient is placed supine with adequate support to flex the lower thigh and knee; a longitudinal incision is then made over the medial aspect of the lower thigh (Fig. 23.8). If you intend to perform a bypass with a saphenous vein graft, mark the vein before surgery; otherwise the incision should correspond with the anterior border of the sartorius muscle – the tendency is to place this incision too anteriorly. Deepen the incision to expose the sartorius muscle, which is retracted posteriorly to reveal the neurovascular bundle enveloped by the popliteal fat pad. The artery lies on the bone and the nerve lies some distance away with the vein in between. The popliteal artery is always surrounded by a plexus of veins, which must be carefully separated and divided in order to avoid troublesome bleeding.

3   In order to expose the infrageniculate popliteal artery, make an incision on the medial aspect of the calf along the border of the gastrocnemius muscle (Fig. 23.9). To optimize exposure to this area the tendons of sartorius, semitendinosus and gracilis can be divided. If the greater saphenous vein is to be harvested identify the vein first along an appropriate length before

continuing the dissection between the medial head of gastrocnemius and the tibia to reveal the neurovascular bundle. The vein is exposed first and this has to be lifted carefully away to give access to the artery. By dividing the soleus muscle along its attachment to the medial border of the tibia it is possible to expose the origin of the anterior tibial artery and the whole extent of the tibioperoneal trunk through this incision. If necessary, completely divide the medial head of gastrocnemius; this results in little functional disability.

4   If exposure of the whole length of the popliteal artery is required it is better to use a posterior approach. With the patient placed prone, make a 'lazy-S' incision (medial proximally to lateral distally) through the popliteal fossa. Deepen the incision through the popliteal fascia and fat pad and define the diamond between the hamstring muscles above and the two heads of gastrocnemius below; then follow the lesser saphenous vein into the neurovascular bundle. In a posterior approach the popliteal artery will be superficial, with the vein and nerve lying deeper.

Tibial arteries

1   The proximal end of the anterior tibial artery is relatively inaccessible, but the remainder of this vessel and its terminal dorsalis pedis branch can be readily exposed through lateral or anterior incisions made directly over the vessels. Retract the tibialis anterior and extensor digitorum longus muscles anteriorly to reveal the artery lying on the interosseous membrane (Fig. 23.10). If exposure of the proximal anterior tibial artery is required this can be achieved very effectively by excision of the upper part of the fibula with disarticulation of the proximal tibiofibular joint. The common peroneal nerve, which winds around the neck of the fibula, must be protected carefully. This approach destroys the lateral ligament of the knee and, while this is well tolerated in elderly, relatively immobile patients, it is best avoided in younger and fitter individuals.

2   The peroneal artery can also be exposed through a lateral incision following removal of a segment of fibula. The peroneal artery lies directly deep to the fibula: it is accompanied only by vein and has

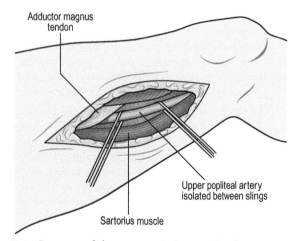

Fig. 23.8   **Exposure of the suprageniculate popliteal artery.**

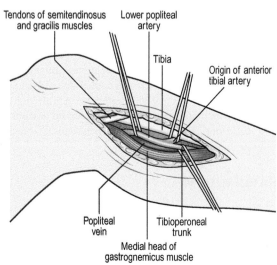

Fig. 23.9   **Exposure of the infrageniculate popliteal artery.**

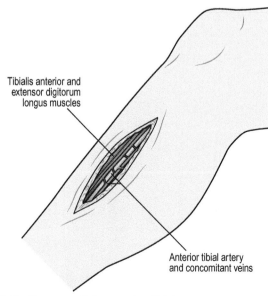

Fig. 23.10   **Exposure of the anterior tibial artery.**

no neurovascular bundle. Take care to divide and tie the veins which interdigitate around the artery. Do not be tempted to use diathermy to gain haemostasis. In most cases, however, it is preferable to expose this vessel by a medial approach (see below).

3 To expose the posterior tibial artery, make a longitudinal incision on the medial aspect of the calf centred over the junction between gastrocnemius muscle and its Achilles tendon. Incise the deep fascia and develop the plane between the gastrocnemius and soleus muscles to reveal the posterior tibial vessels and nerve lying on the surface of soleus beneath a layer of fascia (Fig. 23.11). Alternatively, the posterior tibial artery and its terminal lateral plantar branch may be exposed by an incision made directly over it, as it lies behind the medial malleolus where it is covered only by deep fascia, and then following it into the foot.

4 To expose the peroneal artery by a medial approach, split the lateral fibres of soleus and flexor hallucis longus muscles. This reveals the artery surrounded by its concomitant veins in the depths of the wound.

Subclavian artery

1 Make a transverse incision 1 cm above the medial third of the clavicle; divide the platysma muscle in the same plane (Fig. 23.12). This exposes the clavicular head of the sternocleidomastoid muscle, which is divided, and also a fat pad containing the scalene lymph nodes. Dissect and retract this fat pad superiorly off the surface of the scalenus anterior muscle. Identify the phrenic nerve, which passes obliquely from lateral to medial across the front of this muscle to lie along the medial border of its tendon and usually separated from it by a few millimetres. Pass the blade of a MacDonald's dissector behind the tendon of scalenus anterior muscle, in such a way as to protect the phrenic nerve, and divide the tendon by cutting down on to the dissector with a pointed scalpel blade. Retraction of the muscle superiorly exposes the subclavian artery with its vertebral, internal mammary and thyrocervical branches. The first thoracic nerve root and the lower trunk of the brachial plexus cross the first rib above and posterolateral to the artery. The subclavian vein is deep to the clavicle and is not normally seen through this approach. On the left side the thoracic duct enters the confluence of the internal jugular and subclavian veins. If it is damaged, ligate it to prevent the development of a troublesome postoperative chylous fistula.

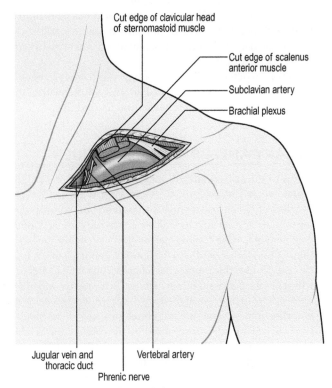

Fig. 23.12 Exposure of the subclavian artery.

Labels: Cut edge of clavicular head of sternomastoid muscle; Cut edge of scalenus anterior muscle; Subclavian artery; Brachial plexus; Jugular vein and thoracic duct; Phrenic nerve; Vertebral artery

2 Extensive exposure of the subclavian artery can be obtained by excision of the inner two-thirds of the clavicle, although this is rarely necessary. The two most common operations on the subclavian artery are carotid-subclavian anastomosis or bypass for a proximal occlusion (subclavian steal syndrome) and repair of a subclavian aneurysm (this is usually a misnomer since most so-called subclavian aneurysms involve the first part of the axillary artery). The former is usually completed without difficulty through the approach described above, and the latter is most conveniently accomplished with separate incisions above and below the clavicle to expose the subclavian and axillary arteries (see below).

3 Operations that involve direct exposure of the origin of the subclavian artery have been largely superseded by extrathoracic bypass procedures (carotid-subclavian and subclavian-subclavian bypass). On the rare occasions when direct exposure is considered essential this is best achieved by splitting the manubrium and upper sternum.

Make a right-angled incision with a horizontal component above the medial third of the clavicle and a vertical component in the midline over the manubrium and upper sternum. Complete the supraclavicular exposure of the artery as described above. Deepen the vertical incision through the subcutaneous tissue and periosteum. The periosteum is extremely vascular and diathermy is required to seal the small arteries. Commencing at the suprasternal notch, open a retrosternal plane by finger dissection, and then, with a sternal chisel and hammer or a properly protected reciprocating saw, divide the manubrium and sternum in the midline and spread the edges with a self-retaining retractor. Dissection of the thymus and anterior mediastinal fat is necessary to expose the arch of the aorta and the origins of the supra-aortic vessels. The innominate vein is stretched across the upper part of the incision and must be protected. It is not usually necessary to

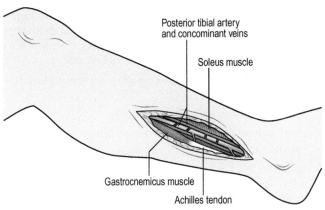

Fig. 23.11 Exposure of the posterior tibial artery.

Labels: Posterior tibial artery and concominant veins; Soleus muscle; Gastrocnemicus muscle; Achilles tendon

divide the sternal tendon of the sternocleidomastoid muscle. Close with peristernal wire or strong nylon sutures, taking care to avoid damage to the internal mammary and intercostal arteries when inserting them.

The origin of the left subclavian artery, which arises far back on the aortic arch, can also be exposed through a posterolateral thoracotomy through the bed of the second or third ribs.

AXILLARY AND BRACHIAL ARTERIES

1 Access to the axillary artery is most often required for axillofemoral bypass and occasionally for subclavian aneurysm repair (see above). For an axillofemoral bypass procedure consider placing the arm in abduction to facilitate estimating the length of the graft required. Make a horizontal incision 1 cm below the lateral third of the clavicle, and split the fibres of pectoralis major muscle (Fig. 23.13). This exposes the infraclavicular fat pad, beneath which lies the pectoralis minor muscle. Divide the tendon of this muscle close to its origin at the tip of the acromion process. Some branches of the acromiothoracic vessels may need to be divided. Find the axillary artery surrounded by the cords of the brachial plexus, which must be carefully protected. The axillary artery can be a friable vessel and care should be taken when slings and clamps are applied. Care should also be taken when performing an anastomosis that the back wall of the artery is not inadvertently incorporated in to the suture line.

2 The proximal brachial artery is found in the groove between biceps and brachialis muscles on the inner aspect of the upper arm (Fig. 23.14). At this point it is still enclosed by cords of the brachial plexus joining to form the median nerve, which crosses it obliquely from the lateral to the medial side. These structures must be carefully separated from it.

3 It is more frequently necessary to expose the bifurcation of the brachial artery in order, for example, to perform a brachial

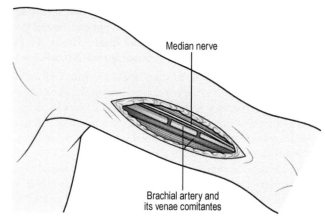

Fig. 23.14 Exposure of the proximal brachial artery.

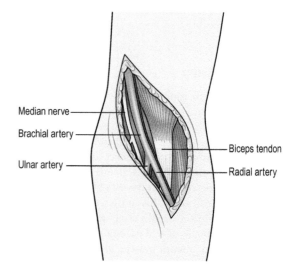

Fig. 23.15 Exposure of the distal brachial artery.

embolectomy. To do so, make a 'lazy-S' incision (medially proximally and laterally distally) in the antecubital fossa, followed by division of the biceps aponeurosis (Fig. 23.15). Distal extension of this incision permits the radial, ulnar and anterior interosseous arteries to be followed into the forearm.

TYPES OF OPERATION

Details of the techniques used to repair or bypass damaged or diseased arteries will be included within the relevant descriptions of specific arterial operations (see below). However, it is useful at this point to summarize the range of procedures available:

1 Direct repair, interposition grafting and patch grafting for arterial trauma

2 Surgical embolectomy or thrombectomy

3 Thrombolytic therapy, percutaneous suction and mechanical embolectomy

4 Endarterectomy, which, with the exception of carotid endarterectomy, has now been largely supplanted by bypass surgery as the treatment of choice for occlusive disease

5 Bypass grafting

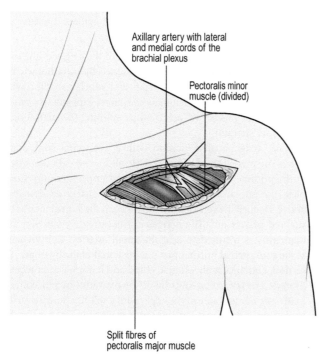

Fig. 23.13 Exposure of the axillary artery.

6 Percutaneous and intra-operative (adjunctive) dilatation angioplasty and endovascular stenting for occlusive arterial disease. The basic technique involves the use of a guide-wire and a balloon dilatation catheter.[1] Devices exist to assist recanalization of resistant occlusions, including lasers, rotational guide-wires, high-frequency electrocoagulation ablators and various types of atherectomy catheters. None of these has yet found a major role in the routine management of vascular disease, and lasers in particular, despite increasing technological sophistication, have so far proved disappointing. The use of balloon catheters (some with drug elution) has, however, made a major impact in recent years and in vascular centres the majority of patients with occlusive disease are treated by these methods

7 Inlay grafting for aneurysms

8 Endovascular stent-graft repair of aortic and peripheral aneurysms.

QUALITY CONTROL

Success in arterial surgery demands technical perfection and this must always be assured as far as is practically possible by appropriate assessment before the patient leaves the operating room. Omission of this step results in a high incidence of early postoperative occlusion and is therefore unacceptable. It is important to appreciate that the presence of a palpable pulse in a graft gives no indication whatsoever that it is technically satisfactory. There may be no mean forward flow through the graft and yet it will be pulsatile to palpation. Acceptable methods available for assessing vascular reconstructions at operation include the following:

1 *Completion angiography.* This continues to be the 'gold-standard' method. State of the art fluoroscopy is ideal but for infrainguinal reconstructions 'on-table' angiography is performed very easily using the simple X-ray equipment available in all standard operating theatres. Angiography allows graft and anastomotic assessment.

Place an X-ray plate wrapped within a sterile Mayo tray cover directly beneath the limb, and take an exposure while injecting 15–20 ml of contrast medium into the proximal end of the graft. Apply a clamp proximal to the injection site during exposure to obviate the necessity for accurate timing of the exposure. Observe proper radiation protection measures during this procedure and further reduce the radiation dose to yourself by interposing a long length of connecting catheter (for example an arterial line) between the syringe and the injection site.

For more proximal reconstructions, special X-ray equipment is required but other methods of quality control may be effective.

2 *Intra-operative Doppler flowmetry.* Intra-operative Doppler probes give an indication of flow and some can also give a waveform tracing which is helpful in ascertaining stenoses. It is also possible to use a simple hand-held Doppler probe placed in a finger of a sterile surgical glove with gel to assess flow.

3 *Angioscopy.* Fibreoptic endoscopes of little more than 1 mm in diameter are now available. Inserted at one end, such instruments will allow direct inspection of the interior of a graft and anastomosis. However, such instruments traumatize the flow surface and are expensive and for these reasons have been largely abandoned.

4 A satisfactory arterial reconstruction for occlusive disease restores either normal or improved blood flow to the distal circulation, and confirmation that this has occurred is a minimal requirement. The return of palpable pulses to vessels downstream of the

reconstruction, for example in the pedal arteries, is a valuable sign and there are a number of simple and inexpensive devices available to supplement clinical assessment, including strain gauge and photoplethysmographs (digital pulse monitors), toe temperature probes, flat and hand-held Dopplers and pulse oximeters.

REFERENCE

1. Gruntzig A, Kumpe DA. Technique of percutaneous transluminal angioplasty with the Gruntzig balloon catheter. Am J Radiol 1979;132:547–52.

ARTERIAL OPERATIONS

▶ KEY POINTS Factors for success

There are three basic prerequisites for success in arterial surgery. Although the relevance of each varies according to specific circumstances it is a valuable discipline to include an appraisal of all three factors when planning any arterial reconstruction:

■ An unimpeded inflow tract – the run-in.
■ An adequate outflow tract – the run-off.
■ An efficient recanalization or bypass – the conduit.

REPAIR OF ARTERIAL INJURY

Appraise

Arterial trauma may occur as an isolated event but more often it occurs in association with other injuries, for example fracture of long bones. Under these circumstances there is a danger that the symptoms of ischaemia may be masked and therefore go unrecognized until irreversible tissue damage has occurred. Always assess the distal circulation in cases of fractured long bones or disarticulation injuries, especially those that involve the elbow or knee.

1 Arterial injury is manifest by:
■ Bleeding, either externally or with the formation of a large haematoma
■ Acute ischaemia with pallor, coldness, loss of sensation, muscle tenderness and weakness, absent pulses and absent or damped Doppler signals with reduced systolic arterial pressure in distal vessels.

2 Suspicion of arterial injury is an indication for urgent angiography (CT angiography or digital subtraction angiography), except for haemorrhage, in which case proceed directly to surgical exploration unless you are in a centre which can offer radiological options such as embolization.

3 Angiographic discontinuity of a major limb vessel always requires urgent surgical exploration. Occlusion of a single tibial or forearm vessel is usually tolerated without ischaemic damage and does not as a rule require reconstruction.

4 Beware the concept of 'arterial spasm'. It is true that the smooth muscle of arteries contracts protectively in response to injury so that an important vessel may appear quite small both angiographically and on direct inspection. However, luminal

discontinuity is always due to a mechanical fault and demands surgical repair. Never attempt to treat such lesions with vasodilator drugs.

5 In the case of multiple injuries, co-operate closely with colleagues of other specialities in planning surgical treatment. Repair of damaged major arteries always takes precedence over orthopaedic fixation of fractures. However, there is a danger that vascular anastomoses may disrupted during subsequent manipulation of fractures. In these circumstances it may be advisable to restore vascular continuity initially by inserting a temporary intraluminal plastic shunt, and completing the repair once the fractures have been stabilized, when the length of the arterial defect can be accurately measured. Always check for venous disruption as well as arterial damage.

6 *Run-in*. This is not usually a problem in arterial trauma.

7 *Run-off*. There is a risk that blood clot may form and occlude vessels distal to the site of injury. The procedure must include measures to deal with this problem (see below), otherwise the run-off vessels are usually normal.

8 *Conduit*. In the case of limb injuries this is either the original artery repaired directly or an interposition graft of autologous vein. Since only short segments are required, problems are rarely encountered in finding a vein of suitable quality and calibre. If there has been extensive injury to both artery and major veins consider harvesting a segment of vein from the opposite leg or upper limb.

9 For closed injuries to major arteries (e.g. iliac, subclavian) with tearing or rupture of the vessel consider endovascular repair with a covered stent in hospitals with facilities for this type of procedure (see Endovascular repair of aortic and peripheral aneurysms, below).

Prepare

1 Once the presence of major arterial injury has been established, undertake surgical exploration without delay.

2 Have blood and blood products available and correct hypovolaemia. Inform the blood bank of major haemorrhage so that appropriate products can be made available.

Access

1 In the case of limb injury, prepare and drape the limb so as to permit direct inspection of skin perfusion and palpation of pulses distal to the site of injury.

2 Consider also the possibility that a segment of healthy undamaged vein of suitable size may need to be harvested for construction of a graft.

3 First, gain proximal control of the artery and then gain distal control. This requires a skin incision that extends well beyond the confines of the injury. Make this incision along the axis of the injured vessel and directly over it.

4 Do not enter the haematoma until the vessel has been dissected and controlled by passing rubber slings around it proximally and distally.

Assess

1 On entering the haematoma there may be brisk fresh bleeding, in which case apply clamps at the proximal and distal control points already prepared.

2 If there is complete disruption of the artery find the ends and apply soft clamps. It is unlikely that they will be actively bleeding at the time of exploration.

3 The traumatized vessel will be damaged some distance proximally and distally from the principal site of injury, therefore trim each end back a few millimetres at a time until normal undamaged intima is seen.

4 Assess the length of the defect. Attempt direct end-to-end anastomosis only if there will be no tension. In most cases it is more prudent to insert an interposition graft of autologous vein, even if this is only a centimetre in length.

5 If the artery is in continuity there may be bruising of the adventitia at the site of injury and absence of downstream pulsation. These are sure signs of internal disruption. The intima and inner layers of the media split transversely and the edges roll back to form a flap, which obstructs flow, causing secondary thrombosis. It is never sufficient, therefore, to simply inspect the outer surface of such a vessel and it is totally unacceptable to treat such lesions by topical application of vasodilator substances. Excise the damaged segment completely, cutting back each end of the artery as before to find healthy intima.

6 Active arterial bleeding usually signifies incomplete disruption or a lateral wall defect that inhibits protective retraction and constriction of the vessel.

Action

1 Before commencing repair of the artery check for adequate inflow and backflow. If either is inadequate pass a Fogarty catheter distally and proximally to withdraw any propagated clot and then instil heparinized saline.

2 If there are associated orthopaedic injuries consider inserting a temporary intraluminal shunt (see above).

3 The adventitia tends to prolapse over the end of a normal artery that has been cut across. Trim this back to prevent it intruding inside the anastomosis.

4 If direct end-to-end anastomosis is possible, accomplish it by the triangulation technique (see Basic techniques) and in most cases employ interrupted sutures in preference to continuous.

5 If the defect is too great to permit direct repair, harvest a segment of vein of appropriate size. Remember to reverse the vein to avoid obstruction to blood flow by competent valves. Complete the proximal anastomosis first, in end-to-end fashion, using the triangulation technique with interrupted sutures for small or inaccessible vessels or the oblique overlap technique for larger vessels. Apply a clamp to the distal end of the graft and allow arterial pressure to distend it in order to determine the optimum length to avoid both excessive tension and kinking. Finally, complete the distal anastomosis.

6 A small puncture or lateral wall defect, as may result from iatrogenic injury following arterial access for investigation or treatment, may be repaired by direct suture or by closing the arteriotomy with a patch.

1. Technical difficulty may be encountered in effecting satisfactory end-to-end anastomoses, usually because of awkward access. Under these circumstances the ends of the artery may be ligated and the area of trauma bypassed with end-to-side anastomoses at remote, more accessible, sites.
2. Magnification is advisable for small vessel anastomoses.
3. If there is any doubt about the effectiveness of the repair, obtain an on-table angiogram.
4. Recurrent thrombosis despite a technically satisfactory repair warrants immediate systemic heparinization.
5. It may be difficult to decide whether or not to repair associated damage to veins. As a rule, repair major axial veins such as the femoral vein and, in the case of near-amputation of a limb, restore continuity to two veins for each artery repaired. Construct venous anastomoses obliquely and with interrupted sutures.

Closure

1 Where possible, effect primary closure of the incision with suction drainage.

2 In the case of blast injuries and other causes of extensive skin and soft-tissue damage, observe the general principles of wound management. Where primary closure is either not possible or inadvisable, always cover the arterial repair with healthy viable tissue, which in practice usually means a muscle flap.

Aftercare

1 Except in cases where continued bleeding is a serious problem, maintain anticoagulation with heparin for several days.

2 Arrange regular half-hourly observation of the distal circulation during the immediate postoperative period and be prepared to re-explore immediately in the event of recurrent occlusion.

Complications

1 Early thrombosis or bleeding at the site of the repair demands immediate re-exploration and re-assessment.

2 A false aneurysm may result from a contained anastomotic leak and this also requires early re-exploration and repair.

3 The risk of associated deep venous thrombosis is high, so take appropriate preventative measures.

4 Repair of arterial injuries in young, healthy people is usually very successful and long-term disability associated with ischaemia is rare.

SURGICAL EMBOLECTOMY

Appraise

1 Embolic occlusion of a major artery results in acute ischaemia, which, if not relieved quickly, may progress to irreversible tissue damage and limb loss.

2 The differential diagnosis is from acute thrombosis occurring within an already diseased artery. Differentiation between these two conditions may be impossible on clinical grounds alone, especially since embolization is nowadays more commonly associated with ischaemic heart disease than valvular stenosis, and most patients therefore have generalized arteriosclerosis.

3 On examination, if there is an immediate threat to the viability of the limb with loss of power and movement and a neurosensory deficit then immediate surgical exploration is required irrespective of the cause.

4 Revascularization of a limb that is already totally non-viable invariably has fatal consequences due to reperfusion injury and is absolutely contraindicated. Urgent amputation may be life-saving.

5 Under other circumstances urgent angiography is indicated to establish the diagnosis and to permit proper appraisal of the various options for treatment.

6 Surgical embolectomy is indicated for embolic occlusion of:
 ■ The common femoral artery and vessels proximal to the groin (e.g. saddle embolus)
 ■ The brachial and axillary arteries.

7 For patients in whom there is no immediate threat to the viability of the limb, more distal emboli, such as those in the popliteal artery, are more appropriately treated by thrombolytic therapy.

8 Surgical embolectomy can be performed under local anaesthesia but general anaesthesia is preferable in the absence of serious anaesthetic risk.

9 Run-in, run-off and conduit usually are not relevant to surgical embolectomy in the absence of associated arterial disease.

Prepare

1 The urgency of the situation dictates that preoperative preparation must be limited. Treatment may be required for heart failure or dysrhythmia.

2 Commence systemic anticoagulation with therapeutic doses of heparin.

Access

1 For lower limb emboli, expose the common femoral artery (see Exposure of the major peripheral arteries, above).

2 For upper limb emboli, expose the brachial artery in the antecubital fossa (see above).

Action

1 Make a short longitudinal arteriotomy. In the case of the femoral artery make this directly over the origin of the profunda artery.

2 Select an embolectomy catheter of a size appropriate to the vessel: 3F for axillary and brachial arteries, 4F for the superficial and profunda femoral arteries and 5F for the aortic bifurcation.

3 A number of different makes of embolectomy catheter are available. Choose one with a central irrigating lumen that permits injection of heparinized saline or X-ray contrast medium into the vessels beyond the balloon.

4 Pass the uninflated catheter proximally through the vessel beyond the clot. Inflate the balloon and withdraw the catheter slowly while adjusting the pressure within the balloon to accommodate changes in the diameter of the vessel. Avoid severe friction between the balloon and the arterial wall since this can cause intimal damage to the vessel.

5 Instruct an assistant to control bleeding from the vessel during this process by applying gentle traction to the rubber sling previously placed around it.

6 Repeat the procedure until no more thrombus is retrieved and adequate forward arterial flow is obtained from the vessel. Avoid unnecessary passages of the catheter.

7 Instil heparinized saline into the artery and gently apply a clamp.

8 Repeat the same procedure distally.

9 Fill the vessels with heparinized saline and close the arteriotomy. Directly suture the common femoral artery; consider using a small vein patch for the brachial artery.

? DIFFICULTY

1. *The catheter will not pass proximally or forceful forward bleeding is not obtained.* This can be due to pre-existing arterial disease or to the catheter having been introduced in a subintimal plane. Avoid direct aorto-iliac reconstruction under these circumstances if at all possible and perform either a femoro-femoral crossover or an axillofemoral bypass.

2. *The catheter will not pass distally.* Obtain an on-table angiogram. This may show embolus impacted at the popliteal bifurcation and in the tibial arteries, or evidence of atherosclerotic occlusion. Instil a small amount of a thrombolytic agent (streptokinase, urokinase or tPA) locally through a small catheter advanced to the site of occlusion.[1] Then pass a small Fogarty catheter 15 minutes later; more embolus may be retrieved. Alternatively, expose the infrageniculate popliteal artery to enable Fogarty catheters to be introduced directly into the tibial vessels. This requires the administration of a general anaesthetic. If there is a longstanding atherosclerotic occlusion of the superficial femoral artery, restoration of blood flow to the profunda system alone is likely to be sufficient to save the limb. However, if distal perfusion remains poor, then proceed to femoropopliteal bypass. Where facilities for intra-operative fluoroscopy exist, as an alternative to exposure of the popliteal artery for retrieval of emboli from the tibial arteries, pass the embolectomy catheter over a guide-wire negotiated into each vessel in turn. Assess the result by angiography.

Closure

1 Close the wound in layers with interrupted skin sutures or clips after instituting suction drainage.

2 Be willing to perform calf fasciotomies.

Aftercare

1 Arrange long-term anticoagulation therapy to prevent recurrent embolization for younger patients, but in the very elderly weigh the risks of this strategy against the benefits.

2 Evaluate and treat the underlying cardiac disease.

PERCUTANEOUS THROMBOLYTIC THERAPY AND THROMBECTOMY

Appraise

See Surgical embolectomy.

Prepare

1 Prior to the administration of thrombolytic therapy it is mandatory to ascertain that patients have no contraindication to it. Haemorrhagic pathologies, bleeding tendency, recent surgery and intracardiac thrombus are a few of the contraindications.

2 Streptokinase is antigenic and may induce severe anaphylactic shock if administered more than once. Therefore ascertain that the patient has never received streptokinase previously. Urokinase and tissue plasminogen activator (tPA) may be given repeatedly without risk of this specific complication but are more expensive.

3 Administer systemic anticoagulation with heparin.

4 Provision needs to be made for these patients to be cared for in a specialized unit with close monitoring for the duration of thrombolytic therapy.

Action

1 Puncture the common femoral artery with a Potts-Cournand needle and pass a short guide-wire into the superficial femoral artery.

2 Remove the needle and insert an introducer sheath over the wire.

3 Under X-ray control advance a long guide-wire through the vessel beyond the embolus.

4 Pass a small-bore catheter over the guide-wire so that the tip enters the clot.

5 Withdraw the guide-wire and infuse the thrombolytic agent according to the manufacturer's instructions. Because the agent is infused locally into the thrombus relatively small amounts are required. The high incidence of serious bleeding complications associated with systemic administration is thereby reduced.

6 After 30–60 minutes ascertain by X-ray the progress of clot lysis and advance the catheter again over a guide-wire into the embolus. Lysis may occur over a period of hours or may need to continue for 24–48 hours, with repeated angiography to assess progress and repositioning of the wires. This requires close nursing supervision of the patient, with fastidious care of the intra-arterial lines and infusions.

7 More rapid and efficient lysis of thrombus can be achieved by the 'pulse-spray' technique. This involves pulsed high-pressure injection of the thrombolytic agent through a catheter with multiple side holes.

8 At the end of lysis, withdraw the catheter and apply pressure to the puncture site in the groin for a minimum period of 10 minutes to ensure haemostasis.

9 Thrombosed infrainguinal bypass grafts are best treated by mechanical thrombectomy in preference to thrombolysis. This avoids haemorrhagic complications and is associated with a reduced risk of embolization of fragmented thrombus into the peripheral vascular bed. The most effective device employs the Bernouilli effect to break up and aspirate the thrombus.

A larger sheath is required and excessively prolonged application may induce haemolysis. In most cases adjuvant percutaneous angioplasty will be necessary to deal with causative stenotic lesions due to anastomotic intimal hyperplasia or progressive atheroma. Mechanical thrombectomy is not available in all hospitals.

? DIFFICULTY

1. The embolus may fragment and impact in more distal vessels. Further administration of the thrombolytic agent may be effective but it must be infused directly into the clot.
2. Alternatively, small fragments may be removed by suction applied to a larger catheter (suction embolectomy). Provided that the viability of the limb has been secured, small residual fragments of this type may be of no consequence and they may lyse spontaneously.

Complications

1. In order to minimize haemorrhagic complications, monitor coagulation tests repeatedly and adjust the dose of thrombolytic agent accordingly.

2. There is a risk of blood clot forming around the catheter itself, therefore maintain heparin anticoagulation throughout the procedure. It is imperative that any arterial lines in situ have continuous infusions to prevent clot formation.

3. Groin haematomas will usually resolve spontaneously but expanding haematomas and false aneurysms require surgical repair.

4. Thrombolysis can cause spontaneous haemorrhage at other sites (for example brain, retroperitoneum), so careful monitoring of the patient is required.

REFERENCE

1. Parent FN, Bernhard VM, Portos TS, et al. Fibrinolytic treatment of residual thrombus after catheter embolectomy for severe lower limb ischaemia. J Vasc Surg 1989;9:153–60.

AORTOBIFEMORAL BYPASS

All aortic operations have features in common. These will be described in detail here and will not be repeated in subsequent sections.

Appraise

1. The indications for aortobifemoral bypass have decreased considerably since the advent of effective percutaneous angioplasty.

2. It is an appropriate procedure for total aortic occlusion, severe aortic bifurcation disease or diffuse widespread aortoiliac disease in patients with critical limb ischaemia or severely disabling claudication.

3. Localized iliac disease, stenoses or short occlusions can be treated by balloon angioplasty dilatation.

4. Manage extensive unilateral iliac disease by either a unilateral extraperitoneal bypass or a femoro-femoral crossover graft (see below).

5. *Inflow.* Ensure a graft takes its blood supply from an area of the aorta with adequate inflow and assess and consider the position of the proximal clamp, especially in the presence of calcified plaque which may be at risk of rupture.

6. *Outflow.* Very commonly patients with severe symptoms have multilevel disease with involvement also of the femoropopliteal arteries. The profunda femoris artery is nearly always patent but may be stenosed at its origin. There is evidence that the long-term patency of aortofemoral grafts is affected adversely when only one of the run-off vessels is patent.[1,2] Consider concomitant femorodistal bypass, particularly in patients with critical ischaemia. In all other patients it is probably better to confine the operation to the proximal bypass initially and then appraise the merits of a second distal bypass at a later date. However, always correct any profunda origin stenosis at the time of aortofemoral bypass.

7. *Conduit.* Use a bifurcated polyester Dacron graft – either 14 mm × 7mm, 16 mm × 8 mm or 18 mm × 9 mm, depending on the diameter of the native vessels.

Prepare

1. The major risk associated with aortic surgery is that of cardiac complications. It is, therefore, appropriate for patients to undergo cardiac risk assessment before surgery. This might include evaluation of myocardial perfusion, measurement of left-ventricular ejection fraction and coronary angiography. Poor function might result in:
   - Surgery not proceeding
   - A lesser procedure being offered (e.g. an extra-anatomic bypass)
   - Intensive care facilities being arranged for postoperative care
   - Coronary artery disease being treated first.

2. For patients with known myocardial impairment it is essential to optimize left ventricular preload and afterload during the procedure; consider the need for trans-oesophageal monitoring.

3. On induction of anaesthesia and prior to skin incision administer intravenous broad-spectrum antibiotic.

4. The patient is fully anaesthetized with total muscular relaxation and placed supine on the operating table.

5. Insert arterial, central venous and peripheral venous lines in all patients and consider trans-oesophageal monitoring.

6. Insert a 14F urinary catheter.

7. Prepare the entire area from the level of the nipples to mid-thigh. Cover the genitalia with a small towel and apply an adhesive drape allowing access to the whole of the abdomen and both inguinal regions.

Access

1. Expose the common femoral arteries first.

2. The abdominal aorta may be exposed through a vertical midline incision, a transverse supra-umbilical incision or an oblique muscle-cutting incision in the flank with an extraperitoneal approach. There are advantages and disadvantages associated with each of these. When only one intra-abdominal arterial anastomosis is anticipated, as, for example, in an aortobifemoral bypass, a transverse incision made directly over

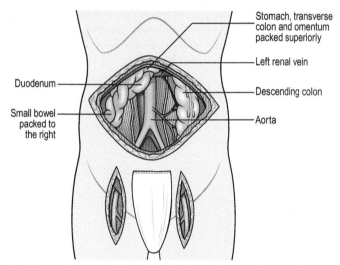

Duodenum

Small bowel packed to the right

Stomach, transverse colon and omentum packed superiorly

Left renal vein

Descending colon

Aorta

Fig. 23.16   Exposure of the abdominal aorta for aortofemoral bypass.

the site of the anastomosis gives adequate exposure and heals well with less postoperative pain than a vertical incision (Fig. 23.16).

Make the incision 2 cm above the umbilicus and extend 2–3 cm beyond the rectus sheath on each side. Divide the rectus muscles with diathermy in the same line as the skin incision. Locate and divide the superior epigastric arteries on both sides. Open the posterior rectus sheath and the peritoneum together; vessels in the edge of the falciform ligament should be ligated.

3   Perform a laparotomy and check all abdominal contents to exclude the presence of major pathology (e.g. malignancy) which may influence the decision to proceed.

4   Note the presence of other pathologies such as gallstones or peptic ulcer but do not attempt surgical treatment of these at the time of aortic reconstruction.

5   Displace the omentum and transverse colon superiorly, and the small bowel with its mesentery to the right. A self-retaining retractor system such as Omnitract allows the bowel to be retained within the abdomen, protected by large moistened abdominal packs behind retractor blades.

6   The aorta lies beneath the posterior parietal peritoneum with the duodenum anterior to it. Incise the peritoneum around the left margin of the duodenum and displace it superiorly and to the right to expose the aorta. This is usually crossed in the upper part of the dissection by the left renal vein, but beware, as occasionally the renal vein may travel behind the aorta.

7   Continue dividing the peritoneum inferiorly to the right of the inferior mesenteric artery to expose the aortic bifurcation and both common iliac arteries (Fig. 23.16). Consider the amount of dissection that needs to be performed in order to minimize damage to the nervi erigentes in this region.

Assess

1   Palpate the aorta and the iliac arteries to determine the extent of the disease. If there is a very localized block, consider endarterectomy or a local aortoiliac bypass. More commonly the disease is not localized and an aortobifemoral bypass is required. At this juncture select an appropriate area for the proximal anastomosis,

avoiding as far as possible large calcified plaques. The segment between the renal vein and the inferior mesenteric artery is usually the most favourable.

2   If there is a total occlusion of the aorta, it is most appropriate to transect it and construct an end-to-end anastomosis with the graft. If the aorta is not totally occluded then many surgeons prefer to construct an end-to-side (onlay) anastomosis in order to preserve perfusion through the natural vessels into the internal iliac arteries. If the external iliac arteries are occluded then an end-to-side anastomosis is preferred as there may be no retrograde flow from the distal anastomoses into the iliac system, and ischaemia of the pelvic organs and buttocks may otherwise ensue.

3   Assess the inferior mesenteric artery. If it is a large vessel with a widely patent aortic ostium then preserve it carefully.

Action

1   In order to perform the proximal anastomosis choose an aortic clamp to either occlude the aorta completely, by applying a straight aortic clamp vertically down the sides of the aorta to the spine or by partially occluding the aorta and creating a window anteriorly through which an arteriotomy is performed. In occlusive disease there may be numerous collaterals, so take care not to damage these. If the occlusive disease is close to the take off of the renal arteries then consider gaining suprarenal control by exposing and gaining control of the aorta below the diaphragm. This is achieved by dissecting adjacent to the lesser curve of the stomach, taking care to avoid damage to the oesophagus.

2   Select a bifurcated Dacron graft of appropriate size to match the internal diameter of the aorta (see General principles) or, if performing an onlay technique, choose a graft which will allow adequate flow distally.

3   Give heparin 5000 IU intravenously and allow 3 minutes for it to circulate before applying the arterial clamps.

4   When performing thrombectomy of the infrarenal aortic stump take care to dissect a plane between the thrombus and aortic wall using a MacDonald's or similar dissector. Dissection in the subintimal plane carries a risk of obstruction of the renal arteries by an intimal flap and must be avoided at all costs.

5   The body of bifurcated grafts is always much longer than is required. Trim away the excess, leaving only 1–2 cm, otherwise the 'legs' of the graft will come off at a sharp angle and may kink.

Construct an end-to-end anastomosis with 3/0 polypropylene sutures (Fig. 23.17).

6   If an end-to-side anastomosis is considered appropriate (Fig. 23.18) and the aortic wall is soft it may be possible to apply a partially occluding clamp of Satinsky type. If the aorta is calcified it may be easier to apply two clamps, one above and the other below the anastomosis, but back-bleeding will occur from lumbar arteries, in this case on opening the aorta; control these vessels first with sutures. A bifurcated graft of 16 mm × 18 mm size is usually most appropriate. Cut the graft obliquely, removing the excess from the body. Construct an end-to-side anastomosis with 3/0 polypropylene sutures.

7   On completion of the aortic anastomosis apply clamps to each limb of the graft and release the aortic clamp to test its integrity. Additional interrupted sutures may be required at this stage. Once the integrity of the suture line has been secured instil

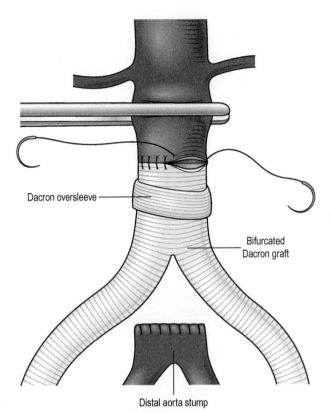

Dacron oversleeve

Bifurcated
Dacron graft

Distal aorta stump

Fig. 23.17   Aortic anastomosis: end-to-end technique.

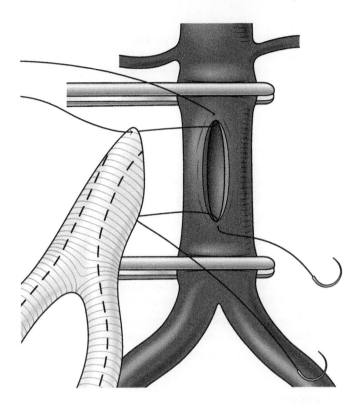

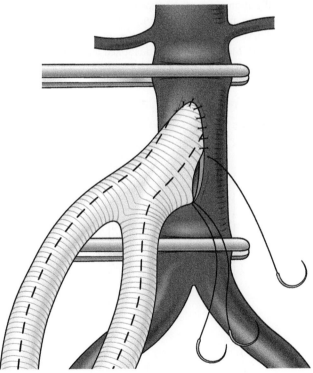

Fig. 23.18   End-to-side 'onlay' anastomosis.

heparinized saline into the graft and reapply an arterial clamp distal to the suture line.

8   Make retroperitoneal tunnels through which to pass the limbs of the graft to the groin incisions. Do this by inserting a finger from the groin to the lateral side of the femoral artery in order to avoid damage to the vein. Insert a finger of your other hand beneath the peritoneum at the aortic bifurcation, ensuring that it passes beneath the ureters, and tunnel both fingers gently until they meet. Then pass a tunnelling instrument from the groin through this channel, attach the limb of the graft and gently deliver each limb to the femoral region.

9   Apply clamps to the common, superficial and profunda femoral arteries and make a longitudinal arteriotomy. If there is a profunda origin stenosis extend the arteriotomy towards the profunda artery to allow an endarterectomy to be performed and to allow the hood of the graft to be sutured across this region to optimize flow to the profunda femoris.

10   Apply gentle traction to the limb of the graft, sufficient to just draw out the crimping, then trim it obliquely to the required length and construct an end-to-side anastomosis with 5/0 polypropylene sutures. The distal anastomoses may be constructed simultaneously by two surgeons, but the graft should be vented through one of the anastomoses prior to completion in order to eliminate any clot that may have formed during clamping.

11   Tell the anaesthetist 2–3 minutes before you are ready to release the clamps, in order to ensure the patient is adequately filled and to reduce the effect of ischaemia reperfusion injury.

12   Close the posterior parietal peritoneum over the graft. If there is difficulty, cover the graft with omentum to avoid adhesion and erosion of the bowel with the attendant risk of late graft infection.

?   DIFFICULTY

1.   Calcification in the wall of the aorta may prevent effective application of a clamp, or it may fracture and penetrate the wall, causing a tear, or it may not allow passage of a needle. It is important to avoid large calcified plaques and

occasionally it may be necessary to apply a clamp at the level of the diaphragm above the visceral arteries. It is often possible to place sutures around calcified plaques. Exercise caution in removing such plaques because this may result in an extremely thin and friable aortic wall. Carefully repair rupture of the wall by a fractured plaque with adventitial sutures, if necessary buttressed by pledgets.

2. Beware of trying to close suture-line tears of the aorta with more stitches since this often makes matters worse. Reapply the clamps and carefully place an adventitial mattress suture buttressed with a pledget across the tear (Fig. 23.19).

Closure

1 Close the abdominal wound in layers, using a non-absorbable nylon stitch for the anterior rectus sheath.

2 Cover the groin anastomosis with two layers of 2/0 synthetic absorbable sutures and subcuticular absorbable sutures for the skin.

3 Drains are not normally required.

Aftercare

1 Carefully monitor cardiac, respiratory and renal function and observe the peripheral circulation. Preoperatively, a decision should have been taken as to whether intensive care monitoring is required. Most patients can be looked after satisfactorily in a high-dependency area on a general ward.

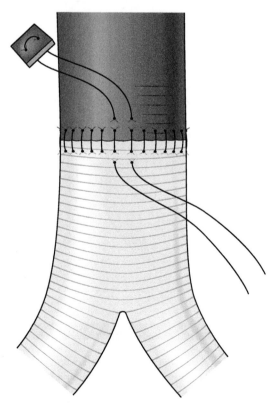

Fig. 23.19 Dacron buttress to control suture line or needle-hole bleeding.

2 Most patients develop a postoperative ileus and may require parenteral fluid support for 4–5 days.

3 The incidence of postoperative chest infection is particularly high in this group of patients; therefore ensure that they receive regular physiotherapy.

4 Maintain deep venous thrombosis prophylaxis.

5 Following discharge from hospital, patients require follow-up visits in the outpatient clinic at about 6 weeks, 6 months and 1 year. The late occlusion rate for these grafts is low and follow-up beyond 1 year is usually not required.

Complications

Remember five potential complications in particular:

1 *Haemorrhage.* A suspicion of intra-abdominal bleeding postoperatively demands immediate re-operation. 'Haematological' bleeding due to the effect of the heparin or other coagulopathy should be corrected accordingly, usually with infusions of fresh frozen plasma and platelets.

2 *Graft occlusion.* This results either from embolization of material trapped above the aortic clamp that was not flushed out or from a technical fault at one of the suture lines. This also requires immediate re-exploration. Try passing a Fogarty catheter from the groin first and ensure adequate inflow. Recurrent occlusion may indicate an outflow problem and requires either refashioning of the distal anastomosis or even a distal bypass procedure.

3 *Renal failure.* Application of a juxtarenal clamp nearly always results in some temporary impairment of renal function secondary to embolization. There is no evidence that the routine administration of renal dopamine, mannitol or other diuretic is of any benefit. Renal tubular necrosis may occur postoperatively if there has been excessive blood loss with associated hypotension. It usually recovers but haemodialysis or haemofiltration may be required. Total anuria immediately after operation may indicate occlusion of both renal arteries. Immediate imaging (Duplex ultrasound and CT aortography) is required and if there is absence of renal perfusion then urgent re-exploration with a view to renal artery reconstruction is required; however, the prognosis is often poor.

4 *Myocardial infarction.* This is the most common cause of postoperative mortality and close monitoring is advised.

5 *Infection.* This occurs in 2–3% of aortic grafts and can often be disastrous, resulting in loss of either life or limb. It may become manifest any time from days to years after operation. The symptoms are fever, backache and perhaps a purulent discharge from the wound. If nothing is done, a fatal haemorrhage occurs sooner or later. Computed tomography (CT) and microbiological culture of perigraft fluid are useful diagnostic tests. Occasionally infection is confined to one groin, in which case conservative management with antibiotics may be adequate. If the wounds in the groin dehisce surgery may be required to debride necrotic and infected tissue as well as systemic antibiotics; a sartorial flap may be raised to achieve adequate coverage of the arterial anastomosis. If the whole graft is infected it must be removed and replaced with an extra-anatomical axillofemoral bypass tunnelled and anastomosed away from the previous site of infection: a challenging procedure for the surgeon

and possibly a devastating situation for the patient. Occasionally, graft infection is associated with erosion of the gastrointestinal tract (usually the duodenum) by the graft and this may result in formation of an aortoenteric fistula. Assume that gastrointestinal bleeding in a patient who has previously had an aortic graft is due to an aortoenteric fistula until proven otherwise. There is no reliable diagnostic test and the diagnosis is therefore made by a process of elimination. Urgent surgical treatment is essential but what form this should take is a matter of some controversy. If the graft is grossly infected it should certainly be removed completely. However, there are many reports of aortoenteric fistulae with local contamination alone being treated successfully by simple closure of the fistula reinforced by an omental patch. Increasingly an endovascular approach is being used, either as a temporizing measure or permanently, to treat aortoenteric fistulae.

REFERENCES

1. Harris PL, Cave-Bigley DJ, MacSweeney L. Aortofemoral bypass and the role of concomitant femorodistal reconstruction. Br J Surg 1985; 22:317–20.
2. Harris PL, Jones D, How T. A prospective randomised clinical trial to compare in-situ and reversed vein grafts for femoropopliteal by-pass. Br J Surg 1987;74:252–5.

UNILATERAL AORTOFEMORAL/ ILIOFEMORAL BYPASS

Appraise

The indication for this operation is unilateral iliac artery occlusive disease (see Aortobifemoral bypass).

Prepare

See Aortobifemoral bypass.

Access

1 Expose the common femoral artery.
2 Make a gently curved incision in the flank extending from the costal margin superiorly to the lateral edge of the rectus sheath 2–3 cm above the inguinal ligament inferiorly (Fig. 23.20).
3 Divide the external oblique muscle and aponeurosis in the line of its fibres.
4 Cut the internal oblique and transversus muscles in the line of the incision using diathermy. Take care not to open the peritoneum. Repair any inadvertent holes immediately.
5 With finger dissection open up the retroperitoneal space and displace the peritoneal sac and its contents medially. The ureter usually displaces with the peritoneum. Identify it and protect it.
6 Identify the aortic bifurcation and the common and external iliac arteries. Use a fixed self-retaining retractor system to aid exposure.

Assess

Technically, it is easier to make the proximal anastomosis to the common iliac artery than to the aorta. Assess whether or not this is feasible by palpation of the vessels.

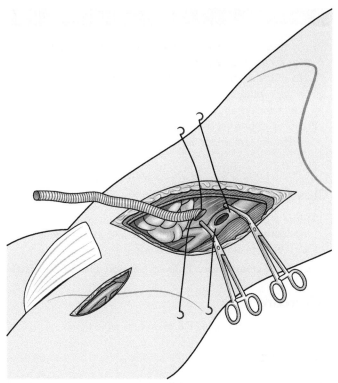

Fig. 23.20 Extraperitoneal iliofemoral bypass.

Action

1 Select a straight Dacron graft of appropriate size. One of 8 mm in diameter is usually most appropriate, but occasionally grafts that are slightly larger or smaller may be required.
2 Administer heparin and allow 3 minutes for it to circulate.
3 For an anastomosis to the common iliac artery apply a clamp to the origin of this vessel and another one at a suitable point distally.
4 For an aortic anastomosis it may be possible to apply a partially occluding clamp of the Satinsky type. If the aorta is calcified, this is unsafe so apply occluding clamps to the aorta and both common iliac arteries; alternatively, consider using the occlusion balloons on an embolectomy catheter.
5 Make a longitudinal arteriotomy approximately 1.5 cm in length.
6 Take the previously prepared Dacron graft and trim the end obliquely to match the length of the arteriotomy.
7 Construct an end-to-side anastomosis with a continuous 4/0 polypropylene suture.
8 Apply a clamp to the graft just beyond the anastomosis and release the arterial clamp to test the suture line. Reinforce it if required (see Aortobifemoral bypass).
9 By finger dissection make a channel through to the groin incision, keeping to the lateral side of the artery to avoid damage to the vein. Draw the graft through this channel using either a tunnelling instrument or a straight aortic clamp.
10 Trim the graft to length and construct an end-to-side anastomosis to the common femoral artery with 5/0 polypropylene sutures (see Aortobifemoral bypass).

1. In obese patients access may be difficult, especially for an aortic anastomosis. Tilt the table away from you to shift the abdominal contents out of the way, make a generous incision and use a fixed self-retaining retractor system.
2. Aortic or arterial calcification can be a cause of major difficulty (see under aortobifemoral bypass).

Closure

1 Close each muscle layer separately, with interrupted sutures for the transverses and internal oblique and a continuous suture for the external oblique aponeurosis.

2 Close the groin incision in layers (see Aortobifemoral bypass).

Aftercare

See Aortobifemoral bypass, but recovery is more rapid.

Complications

1 In addition to those described for aortobifemoral bypass, beware of acute arterial occlusion in the opposite limb.

2 Application of clamps at or close to the aortic bifurcation is associated with a high risk of embolic occlusion or thrombosis in the other common iliac artery. This must be checked for and corrected before anaesthesia is reversed.

3 Try passing a Fogarty catheter from the groin first. If this is not successful then consider performing a femoro-femoral crossover graft. Occasionally, a radiological approach with iliac angioplasty and stent insertion is possible.

MINIMALLY INVASIVE AND TOTALLY LAPAROSCOPIC AORTIC RECONSTRUCTION

Appraise

1 Minimally invasive techniques for reconstruction of the abdominal aorta and iliac arteries are being developed with the aim of minimizing surgical trauma, recovery time and postoperative complication rates.

2 Totally laparoscopic procedures are undertaken by a retroperitoneal approach, with or without gas insufflation. Special instrumentation including aortic clamps has been designed for the purpose. The technical aspects of the operation are based upon the principles of other established laparoscopic procedures.

3 Minimally invasive operations performed through short (8 cm) incisions using retractors designed specifically for the purpose represent a compromise between the conventional open and laparoscopic approaches. 'Hand-assisted' laparoscopic reconstruction is a further variation on this theme.

4 Obese patients and those with calcified aortas are not suitable for these procedures. Otherwise, the factors to be considered preoperatively are the same as those for aortofemoral bypass (see above).

5 Facilities for immediate 'conversion' to conventional open surgery in case of haemorrhage or other critical intra-operative complications are essential.

6 These procedures are currently performed in a few vascular centres by surgeons with specialist skills in these fields. Laparoscopic vascular surgery requires a high level of laparoscopic skill and should only be undertaken by trained and competent enthusiasts.

FEMORO-FEMORAL BYPASS AND ILIOFEMORAL CROSSOVER BYPASS

Appraise

1 These are alternative procedures to iliofemoral bypass for unilateral iliac artery disease and the results are comparable in terms of graft patency. Femoro-femoral bypass is virtually a subcutaneous procedure and if necessary it can be carried out under local anaesthetic in very unfit patients (Fig. 23.21).

Iliofemoral crossover bypass has the important advantage of leaving the groin and femoral artery on the donor side undisturbed for possible future procedures. The angle between the graft and the donor artery is also in line with the direction of blood flow and this may have haemodynamic advantages. It is a more invasive operation than femoro-femoral bypass and requires a regional or general anaesthetic.

2 *Inflow.* Adequacy of inflow is a crucial factor for the success or failure of these operations as well as their effect on the perfusion of the donor limb. Reliance on subjective assessment of angiograms is unsafe and some objective test is therefore helpful. Intra-arterial cannulae are connected to pressure transducers in order to record pressure waves from radial and femoral arteries. If there is a pressure gradient under resting low-flow conditions, this represents inadequate inflow. If the diagnosis is in dispute, a bolus of papaverine 20 mg is then injected into the femoral artery by means of a three-way tap connected to the pressure line. This causes regional vasodilation and accelerates the blood flow into the limb. A radial to femoral pressure gradient in excess of 20 mmHg developing

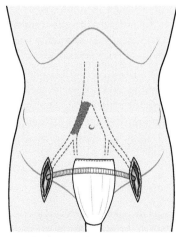

Fig. 23.21 Left-to-right femoro-femoral crossover graft.

under high flow conditions is evidence of significant inflow stenosis.

There are three options possible following a positive pressure test:

- Abandon the operation completely
- Treat the inflow stenosis by balloon angioplasty dilatation either before or during the operation (see below) and then proceed with the femoro-femoral bypass
- Convert to an axillofemoral bypass.

3 *Run-off.* See Aortobifemoral bypass.

4 *Conduit.* It is necessary to use a prosthetic graft for this purpose, and 8-mm diameter externally supported Dacron or expanded PTFE grafts are most suitable.

Action

1 For femoro-femoral bypass expose both common femoral arteries.

2 For crossover iliofemoral bypass expose the common femoral artery in the recipient limb. On the donor side expose the external iliac artery by making a transverse incision 3–5 cm above the inguinal ligament and entering the retroperitoneum as previously described.

3 Select an 8-mm graft.

4 By finger dissection create a tunnel between the two incisions. For femoro-femoral bypass make a subcutaneous tunnel just above the superior pubic rami using blunt dissection to avoid damage to the bladder. In the case of a crossover iliofemoral bypass make an extraperitoneal tunnel passing deep to the rectus muscles. Draw the graft into the tunnel using either a tunnelling instrument or a large aortic clamp.

5 Give intravenous heparin and allow 3 minutes for it to circulate.

6 Apply clamps to the femoral or iliac arteries and make longitudinal arteriotomies.

7 Trim the ends of the graft obliquely to match the length of the arteriotomies.

8 Fashion end-to-side anastomoses on both sides with 5/0 Prolene or Gore-Tex sutures as appropriate (see General principles). Flush the graft and arteries before completing the anastomoses.

Closure

Close both wounds carefully in layers, ensuring haemostasis and thus avoiding the need for drains.

Complications

1 In addition to the risks of haemorrhage, occlusion and infection (see Aortobifemoral bypass) the main concern is the possibility of ischaemia in the donor limb.

2 Provided that the procedure described here has been followed correctly, inflow obstruction should have been eliminated, but there remains the risk of thrombosis or embolization in the distal vessels.

3 Acute ischaemia requires immediate re-exploration. Less severe ischaemia warrants angiography with a view to further elective surgery.

AXILLOFEMORAL BYPASS

Appraise

1 Indications for axillofemoral bypass are:
- Critical lower limb ischaemia in a patient with severe bilateral aortoiliac occlusive disease who is medically not fit for an aortobifemoral bypass (see Aortobifemoral bypass)
- Infection of a previously inserted aortobifemoral bypass
- Long-term patency rates for axillofemoral grafts are approximately 50% those of aortobifemoral grafts. Axillobifemoral grafts have better patency rates than axillounifemoral grafts.

2 *Run-in.* Although occlusive disease is unusual in the upper limb arteries it is slightly more common on the left than the right side. Therefore, other considerations being equal, use the right axillary artery as the donor vessel. If critical ischaemia is confined to one leg and brachial artery pressures are equal, then use the axillary artery on the same side for the donor vessel.

3 *Run-off.* See Aortobifemoral bypass.

4 *Conduit.* Preformed axillobifemoral grafts with either right or left side-arms are available. When using a preformed graft, trim it in such a way as to ensure that its length from the junction of the side-arm to the distal anastomosis is as short as possible. The reason for this is that the velocity of flow in the graft is potentially halved beyond this point, with a greater risk of thrombosis in this segment. When constructing the bypass from separate axillofemoral and femoro-femoral components, use a 10-mm diameter graft for the former and an 8-mm graft for the crossover. Construct the crossover bypass first (see above, Femoro-femoral bypass) and anastomose the distal end of the axillofemoral component to it in end-to-side fashion. When infection of a pre-existing aortobifemoral graft is the indication for operation consider impregnating the graft with antibiotic. This is prepared by soaking the graft in a solution of rifampicin before implantation. An effectively treated graft turns uniformly brown in colour. A Dacron graft impregnated with silver, which is intended to resist infection, is also available commercially.

Prepare

1 General anaesthesia is required, with the patient supine on the operating table. The procedure can be performed under local anaesthetic with sedation being used for graft tunnelling.

2 It is necessary to prepare the skin and arrange the drapes in such a way as to make available the whole of the trunk and both legs to mid-thigh level. Place the donor arm in abduction so that there is no tension on the anastomosis to the axillary artery in this position. Use adhesive drapes to hold the towels in place.

3 Ensure that the anaesthetist places radial or brachial arterial lines on the side that is not going to be clamped.

4 Give prophylactic antibiotics as for aortobifemoral bypass.

Action

1 Expose the axillary artery and both common femoral arteries (Fig. 23.22; see Exposure of the major peripheral arteries).

2 Select 10-mm and 8-mm Dacron grafts of appropriate length or a preformed axillofemoral graft.

379

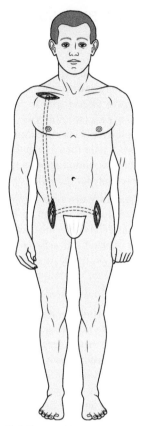

Fig. 23.22 Right axillobifemoral bypass.

3 If possible, it is better to avoid making additional incisions over the course of the graft. Use a long tunnelling instrument inserted from the upper (axillary) incision. Pass it deep to the pectoralis major muscle and then subcutaneously in the anterior axillary line, finally curving forwards above the anterior superior iliac spine to the ipsilateral groin incision. Attach the end of the main stem of the graft to the tunneller and then draw it through to the upper incision. When using a preformed graft continue to pull it through until the junction with the side-arm lies at the upper end to the groin incision.

4 Pass the side-arm or femoro-femoral component through a subcutaneous suprapubic tunnel (see Femoro-femoral bypass).

5 Administer heparin and allow 3 minutes for it to circulate.

6 Apply clamps to the axillary and femoral arteries and make longitudinal arteriotomies approximately 1.5 cm in length.

7 When gauging the length of the graft, having the arm abducted ensures that there will be no tension on the anastomoses in this position.

8 Considerable time is saved if the anastomoses are constructed simultaneously. Trim the ends of the graft obliquely to match the length of the arteriotomies and complete the anastomoses in end-to-side fashion with 5/0 polypropylene suture.

9 Test each anastomosis, flush the graft and fill it with heparinized saline before finally releasing the clamps. Open the circulation into one leg at a time in order to reduce the risk of reperfusion injury.

Closure

1 Carefully close all three wounds in layers.

2 Drains are not usually necessary.

Complications

1 Occasionally, seromas develops around these grafts and unless they become infected this should be allowed to settle spontaneously and not aspirated.

2 The risk of occlusion by thrombosis is greater than for other proximal bypass procedures. If this occurs, re-establish patency by thrombectomy, ensure there are no technical errors and commence long-term anticoagulation. An important cause of occlusion is angulation due to tension on the axillary artery and this should be corrected during secondary intervention.

ILIAC ARTERY ANGIOPLASTY AND STENTING

Appraise

1 Localized stenoses and short occlusions in the common iliac artery respond well to angioplasty. The addition of an intraluminal stent is indicated when:
- The stenosis is resistant to angioplasty or recurs immediately due to elastic recoil
- Treatment is being undertaken for a recurrent lesion.

2 This procedure may be undertaken as a sole therapeutic intervention and it has largely replaced open surgery for the management of localized iliac artery disease. Increasingly, angioplasty is being used in tandem with surgery to secure an adequate inflow in anticipation of an infrainguinal arterial reconstruction, in which case it may be undertaken percutaneously or intra-operatively through the exposed common femoral artery.

Prepare

1 When undertaken percutaneously, prepare the skin and drape the patient as for open iliofemoral bypass (see above).

2 When undertaken intra-operatively, prepare the patient as for a femorodistal bypass (see below).

Access

Either

1 Puncture the common femoral artery percutaneously. If there is no pulse palpable in the common femoral artery employ ultrasound guidance (see Basic Techniques, Transluminal angioplasty).

Or

1 Expose the common femoral artery (see Exposure of the major peripheral arteries). Insert a 5/0 polypropylene purse-string suture into the front of the artery to aid post-procedure haemostasis.

Assess

1 Puncture the common femoral artery through the purse string and insert a sheath in a proximal direction (see Basic techniques, Transluminal angioplasty).

2 Use a 0.035 inch J-wire to cross the lesion under fluoroscopic control.

3 Pass a 'pigtail' angiography catheter over the wire and, using a pump injector, obtain a digitally subtracted angiogram to visualize the lesion.

4 For further assessment of the lesion record 'pull-through' pressure measurements. Having crossed the lesion with a straight 4F angiography catheter over the guide-wire, connect it to a pressure transducer to record intraluminal pressure. Withdraw the catheter slowly through the stenosis and record the pressure gradient across it. Any pressure gradient under low-flow conditions is significant. For more accurate assessment repeat the process following injection of a vasodilator (e.g. papaverine 30 mg) intra-arterially into the limb (see above, Femoro-femoral bypass, Assess).

Action

1 Select a balloon catheter of appropriate size using the preoperative angiogram as a guide (see Basic techniques). A balloon with an inflated diameter of 8 mm and length of 4 cm is often appropriate; it is essential not to over-dilate the artery.

2 Obtain another angiogram to create a 'road-map'. This allows a 'live' image of the balloon catheter to be superimposed over a stored image of the lesion to assist accurate positioning of the balloon.

3 Position the balloon over the guide-wire across the lesion and inflate it to the pressure as recommended by the manufacturer.

4 Use dilute contrast medium to dilate the balloon.

5 Observe the balloon by fluoroscopy as it expands. 'Popping of the waist' signals a good outcome.

6 Replace the balloon catheter with an angiography catheter and obtain a check angiogram to assess the result. If 'pull-through' pressure measurements were made prior to angioplasty repeat these now to ensure that the pressure gradient has been abolished.

7 Remove the introducer sheath and proceed with the femorodistal bypass procedure.

? DIFFICULTY

1. *Unable to cross the lesion with the guide-wire.* Try again with a low friction, hydrophilic wire. Alternatively, through an access sheath in the contralateral common femoral artery direct a low-friction hydrophilic guide-wire over the aortic bifurcation with suitably shaped guiding catheters and attempt to cross the lesion in an antegrade direction. If these methods fail or the wires pass subintimally abandon the procedure. Opt for open iliofemoral or femoro-femoral bypass to overcome the inflow obstruction.

2. *The lesion is resistant to dilatation or there is a persistent stenosis due to intimal flap formation.* Use an intraluminal stent. For short, hard lesions use a balloon-expandable Palmaz stent. For longer lesions consider using a self-expanding Wallstent.

3. *Lesions at the origin of the common iliac artery do not dilate adequately because displacement of the balloon is accommodated by compression of the opposite iliac*

artery. There is also a risk that the patency of the contralateral common iliac artery may be compromised. Insert balloon catheters into both common iliac arteries and inflate them simultaneously. This is known as the 'kissing balloons' technique.

Complications

Rupture of the iliac artery needs either the prompt deployment of a covered stent or surgical repair. (See also Basic techniques and Balloon angioplasty dilatation for femoropopliteal occlusive arterial disease.)

FEMOROPOPLITEAL AND INFRAPOPLITEAL SAPHENOUS VEIN BYPASS

Appraise

1 Chronic occlusion of the superficial femoral artery alone seldom if ever results in critical limb ischaemia.

2 Most stenoses or short occlusions in the superficial femoral artery can, if deemed appropriate, be treated successfully by percutaneous balloon angioplasty dilatation.

3 The patency rates of long femorodistal bypass grafts are not sufficiently good to warrant their application for non-critical disease.

4 The indications for elective femorodistal bypass surgery are critical limb ischaemia associated with extensive superficial femoral, popliteal and tibial artery occlusive disease, or extremely disabling intermittent claudication. Vascular trauma constitutes a frequent indication for emergency femorodistal bypass.

5 *Inflow.* An unimpeded inflow is an essential prerequisite for a successful outcome. Objective assessment is essential (see Femoro-femoral bypass) and an additional procedure to enhance inflow (e.g. iliac artery angioplasty) may be required.

6 *Run-off.* Poor run-off is a major cause of femorodistal graft failure. It is essential to carefully select the site of the distal anastomosis in order to optimize outflow capacity. When the popliteal artery is visualized angiographically this vessel should normally be used. However, even with digital enhancement, preoperative angiographic assessment of tibial vessels may be unreliable, especially in the presence of critical ischaemia; the absence of images of these vessels on such films must not be accepted as evidence that they are definitely occluded. Objective tests such as pulse-generated run-off assessment[1] have been largely abandoned. Preoperative Duplex ultrasound will help the planning of these procedures and identify patent distal vessels. Surgical exploration of the distal vessels and on-table angiography is the only reliable method for confirming non-operability. (See also Femoropopliteal and infrapopliteal prosthetic bypass.)

7 *Conduit.* There are two established methods for using the saphenous vein for femorodistal bypass grafting. These are the reversed and the in-situ techniques. A third method, the non-reversed transposed-vein technique, combines features of both of the original methods. Clinical evidence for the superiority of one of these

methods over the others is lacking. Indeed, randomized studies to date indicate that reversed and in-situ grafts perform equally well in both femoropopliteal and infrapopliteal situations.[2] Reversed vein grafts are associated with fewer complications. The quality of the vein itself, and particularly its diameter, does have an important effect on outcome. This can be assessed preoperatively by Duplex scanning. If the saphenous vein is inadequate (less than 3 mm in diameter or varicose), alternative sources of autologous vein should be sought (consider the short saphenous or arm veins) or a decision may be made to use a prosthetic graft. It is worthwhile deferring the definitive decision regarding a prosthetic graft until the vein has been exposed surgically. An ideal vein has few divisions, is free from postphlebitic thickening of the wall and has a fairly uniform diameter of not less than 4 mm. Unfortunately, not many conform to the ideal and clinical judgement has to be exercised in determining acceptability.

8 Note that longer grafts fare less well than shorter grafts and it is permissible in the absence of significant disease in the superficial femoral or popliteal arteries to use a distal donor site as a means of shortening a graft. Most grafts, however, should originate from the common femoral artery.

Prepare

1 Mark the course of the long saphenous vein with indelible ink before operation. If it is not visible on simple clinical examination use a Doppler ultrasound flow probe to follow its course or alternatively arrange for the vein to be 'mapped' by vascular scientists.

2 The leg is shaved, together with the pubic area and lower abdomen.

3 Under general or regional anaesthesia, the patient lies supine on the operating table. The knee of the affected leg is flexed to about 45° with the hip flexed and slightly externally rotated. Swab the whole area from the umbilicus to the ankle. Enclose the foot in a sterile transparent plastic bag. Place towels under the leg and over the abdomen. Retain the position of the towels over the genitalia and upper thigh with an adhesive drape.

Access/assess

1 Expose the common femoral artery and the proposed site for the distal anastomosis. If there is concern regarding the patency of the distal receiving vessel, consider performing an on-table angiogram. Ideally, this should communicate directly with the primary pedal arch.

2 Expose a sufficient length of the saphenous vein from the groin to the anticipated distal anastomosis by making an incision directly over it. If possible, leave intact skin bridges along the length of the vein harvest to reduce postoperative morbidity and skin breakdown. Assess its suitability for use as a graft (see above, Appraise).

Action

Reversed saphenous vein graft

1 This is the standard procedure first performed successfully by Jean Kunlin in Paris in 1942.[3]

2 Completely mobilize and remove the long saphenous vein. Ligate the tributaries with fine material a millimetre or so away from their junction with the main trunk to avoid any possibility of narrowing the graft. Transfix the saphenofemoral junction with a stitch.

3 Insert an umbilical catheter into the distal end of the vein, which will become the proximal end of the graft, and with a clamp at the other end gently distend it with heparinized blood (5000 IU of heparin in 50 ml of blood; Fig. 23.23). Secure any untied tributaries with fine ligatures and any small tears with 6/0 polypropylene mattress or figure-of-eight sutures inserted transversely.

4 Take great care to handle the vein gently at all times. Do not pick it up with metal instruments, do not apply clamps to it (except at the very end during distension – this will be trimmed away prior to construction of the anastomosis), do not overdistend it, do not allow the vein to desiccate. A traumatized segment of vein may become the site of fibrous stricture formation following implantation and threaten the long-term patency of the graft (see below). Indicate the orientation of the vein by marking it with indelible ink.

5 Using a long tunneller, place the reversed vein in a route alongside the natural artery through the subsartorial canal and popliteal fossa but outside the abductor magnus tendon. Make sure it passes between the medial and lateral heads of the gastrocnemius muscle to enter the popliteal fossa. In the calf, place it in the plane between the gastrocnemius and soleus muscles. Note that it is technically easier to enter this plane with the tunneller inserted from the distal incision and advanced proximally than it is the opposite way round. If the distal anastomosis is to be made to the anterior tibial artery, cross the interosseous membrane just below the popliteal fossa, taking care to avoid damage to the plexus of veins in this area.

6 Be meticulous and ensure that the vein does not become twisted when laying it in its tunnel. Check that this has not occurred by gently distending it with heparinized blood after insertion.

7 Give intravenous heparin and allow 3 minutes for it to circulate.

8 The anastomoses may be completed simultaneously if two surgeons are available. Otherwise apply clamps to the femoral arteries, make an arteriotomy 1–2 cm in length, trim the graft and construct an end-to-side anastomosis with 5/0 polypropylene sutures. Allow the graft to run and check the anastomosis for haemostasis then apply a gentle clamp just proximal to the distal anastomosis, having confirmed correct vein orientation for the distal anastomosis. To assess flow within the graft open the vein graft and allow free flow of blood into a kidney dish for 5 seconds, measure this volume and calculate flow per minute: a flow rate of greater than 180 ml/minute is satisfactory.

9 Distally, treat the vessels gently and select the least traumatic clamps for haemostasis to allow the anastomosis to be sutured. Consider using slings as these may cause less damage. (see General principles).

10 Make an arteriotomy in the recipient vessel about 1 cm in length. Trim the vein graft obliquely to match the length of the arteriotomy and complete the anastomosis in end-to-side fashion with either 6/0 polypropylene for the popliteal artery or 7/0 polypropylene for the infrapopliteal arteries. Prior to distal clamp removal and restoration of blood flow remove the clamp from the vein graft and expel air and old blood then complete the anastomosis.

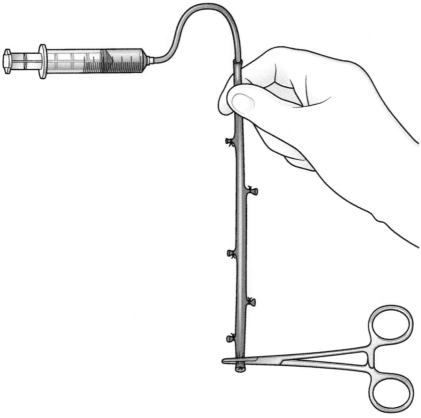

Fig. 23.23 Distending the reversed vein graft with heparinized blood.

11 Remove all clamps. Observe the appearance of the graft, the recipient artery and the perfusion of the foot within the transparent plastic bag.

12 Consider performing completion imaging before closure of the wounds.

? DIFFICULTY

1. *The vein is inadequate.* Short narrow segments can be resected and replaced with interposition grafts of autologous vein from other sites. If the whole vein is inadequate or missing (having been removed previously), consider using arm veins. This is often possible for femoropopliteal bypass, but impractical for longer grafts. It is preferable to use autologous vein rather than prosthetic graft in terms of patency. Use a prosthetic graft only if there are no adequate autologous veins available. (Fig. 23.24).

2. *The graft is twisted.* If this occurs despite all precautions, divide the graft at a convenient and readily accessible point, undo the twist and reanastomose the ends by the triangulation technique with 6/0 polypropylene sutures.

3. *Completion angiogram shows a technical error at the distal anastomosis.* Take down and reconstruct the anastomosis.

4. *Completion angiogram shows embolic occlusion of the run-off vessels.* Pass a small Fogarty catheter through a short incision in the graft made directly over the distal anastomosis.

In-situ saphenous vein graft

1 In this operation most of the vein is left undisturbed in its natural bed and the valves are destroyed by the passage of a valvulotome (Fig. 23.25).[3,4]

The potential advantages over the reversed operation are:

- It retains its viability and those properties of the vein that depend upon its viability – most importantly an antithrombotic flow surface and a compliant muscular wall
- The natural taper of the vein matches more closely that of the recipient artery, thereby facilitating the anastomoses and possibly conferring some haemodynamic benefits
- It is claimed (but not proven) that smaller veins can be made to function more successfully by this technique than by the reversed method[3]
- Because the graft lies subcutaneously it is easily assessed by simple clinical examination.

    On current evidence these advantages would seem to be more theoretical than practical but many surgeons prefer the in-situ operation, particularly for infrapopliteal bypass.

2 Expose the vein throughout the required length (using skin bridges if possible) and tie in continuity all visible tributaries, ensuring that the vein itself is not narrowed by placing the ligatures a millimetre or so away from the main trunk. Consider preserving the most proximal large tributary in the thigh to allow access of a cannula for on-table angiography later.

3 Carefully dissect the saphenofemoral junction and ligate and divide all tributaries at this level. Perform a flush ligation of the saphenofemoral junction to maximize the length of vein available. Mobilize the proximal 5–6 cm of the saphenous vein.

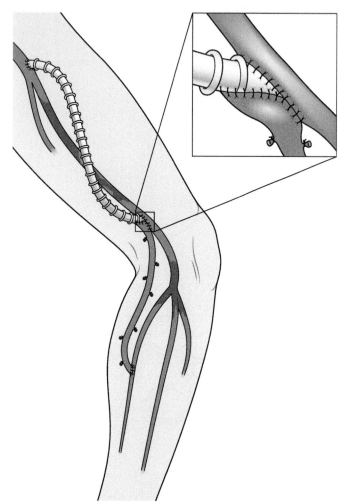

Fig. 23.24   Composite PTFE/autologous vein graft.

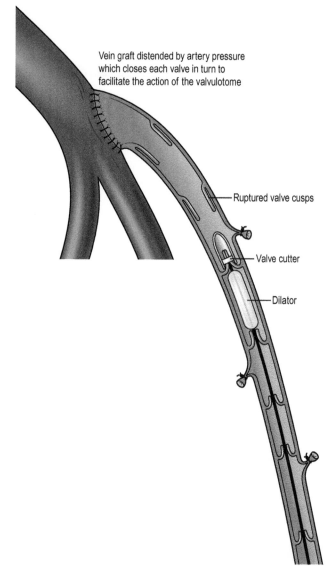

Vein graft distended by artery pressure which closes each valve in turn to facilitate the action of the valvulotome

Ruptured valve cusps

Valve cutter

Dilator

Fig. 23.25   In-situ vein graft. Mode of action of Hall's valvulotome.

4   Give heparin and allow 3 minutes for it to circulate before application of arterial clamps.

5   With the leg straight, find the point on the femoral artery to which the proximal end of the saphenous vein can be anastomosed without tension. Apply clamps and make a short arteriotomy at this site.

6   Open the proximal end of the saphenous vein, find the first valve and excise its cusps under direct vision with fine scissors.

7   Construct the proximal anastomosis end-to-side with 6/0 polypropylene sutures and release the clamps, allowing the arterial pressure to distend the graft to the level of the first competent valve.

8   Mobilize the distal end of vein and divide it, allowing sufficient length for trimming prior to construction of the anastomosis.

9   Select a valvulotome of appropriate size. The valvulotome must not impact within the vein and it must not under any circumstances be used as a dilator. Most commonly, the smallest (2.5 mm diameter) instrument will suffice. Pass the valvulotome proximally through the graft to the upstream anastomosis and then withdraw it slowly (Fig. 23.25). Gently tug it as it catches on each valve to break the valve cusps and repeat this process after rotating the valvulotome through 90° to ensure that each of the cusps is ruptured. As the valve is made incompetent, arterial pressure closes the next in line, which once again facilitates the action of the valvulotome. Vigorous pulsatile bleeding on final

withdrawal of the instrument indicates that all of the valves have been rendered incompetent. If this does not occur, pass the valvulotome again but try to avoid repeated unnecessary passages of the instrument. The absence of pulsatile bleeding despite destruction of the valves is due to persistence of a large perforating vein. Sometimes the presence of a localized palpable thrill will locate it, but if not it can be identified with an on-table angiogram.

10   Apply a soft clamp to the graft. Trim the distal end and complete the distal anastomosis in an end-to-side manner using 6/0 polypropylene for the popliteal artery or 7/0 polypropylene for the infrapopliteal arteries.

11   If the distal anastomosis is to be made to the anterior tibial artery, it is necessary to mobilize a sufficient length of the vein to allow it to be routed through the interosseous membrane to the lateral side of the calf.

12   For anastomosis to the infrageniculate popliteal artery the end of the vein should simply be turned into the popliteal fossa and a short anastomosis constructed to make a T-junction. An attempt to make this anastomosis oblique is likely to result in kinking and obstruction of the graft.

13 Consider performing a completion angiogram to confirm graft patency and run off and if necessary to locate and ligate residual tributaries.

1. *Short vein.* The anatomical relationship between the saphenofemoral junction and the common femoral bifurcation may be such that even after mobilization the saphenous vein will not reach the common femoral artery without tension. Construct the proximal anastomosis to the superficial femoral or profunda arteries. A limited endarterectomy may be required to ensure a satisfactory inflow.

2. *On-table angiography shows an intact valve cusp.* Use a tributary to re-introduce the valvulotome, or partially take down the distal anastomosis and re-pass the valvulotome. If both of these are technically difficult, a small incision may be made in the graft itself but great care must be taken not to cause any narrowing upon closure.

3. A tributary protected by a valve at its junction with the main vein will not be visualized on intra-operative angiography. If this valve should later become incompetent under arterial pressure a fistula will develop. Involvement of a superficial tributary causes the development of a painful patch of inflammation in the affected skin, which may progress to skin necrosis. The appearance of these changes postoperatively, with an associated overlying bruit, is an indication to return the patient to theatre for ligation of the offending tributary. This can be performed under local anaesthesia.

4. See also difficulties associated with reversed saphenous vein bypasses.

Non-reversed transposed saphenous vein graft

1 This method combines features of both the reversed and in-situ techniques.

2 The vein is excised completely and re-sited as appropriate in order to bypass an arterial occlusion. However, it is not inverted.

3 The valves are destroyed by passage of a valvulotome as previously described.

Closure

1 Close the incisions with absorbable sutures in the subcutaneous tissues and a subcuticular absorbable suture. Use two layers of subcutaneous sutures to cover the femoral anastomosis and place a suction drain in the proximal and distal wounds.

Aftercare

1 Note the state of perfusion of the foot and mark the position of palpable or Doppler-audible pulses.

2 Evidence of deteriorating perfusion and loss of pulses warrants immediate re-exploration and re-assessment of the graft.

3 Keep the knee slightly flexed for 24 hours. Allow mobilization on the first day. Swelling of the leg is almost invariable after a successful reconstruction. Reassure the patient that this will resolve but may take several weeks to do so. In the meantime encourage leg elevation when resting.

4 A postoperative vein graft surveillance programme using Duplex ultrasound is worthwhile, as 20–30% of grafts develop intimal hyperplastic strictures within the first 6–9 months after implantation and these strictures are associated with a three-fold risk of occlusion during the first 12 months. Prophylactic treatment of such strictures, either by open surgery or balloon angioplasty dilatation, improves secondary patency rates by 10–15% at 12 months.[4] Arrange surveillance scans at regular intervals for the first year. Strictures that require treatment are:

■ Those that occur at the first screening interval

■ Those causing a stenosis equivalent to a two-thirds reduction on the cross-sectional area of the graft or reduce the flow in the graft to below 40 cm/s

■ Those that show evidence of progression.

Treat short strictures in the body of the graft or at the distal anastomosis by balloon angioplasty dilatation. For maximum effect, higher than normal inflation pressures may be required (up to 20 atmospheres). Treat strictures over 1 cm in length and those at the proximal anastomosis by patch angioplasty, interposition grafting or jump grafting.

5 Except where specifically contraindicated, all patients should receive regular daily low-dose aspirin or clopidogrel as an antithrombotic agent and all patients should be prescribed a statin.

REFERENCES

1. Beard JD, Scott DJ, Evans JM, et al. Pulse generated run-off, a new method of determining calf vessel patency. Br J Surg 1988;75:361–3.

2. Harris PL, Jones D, How T. A prospective randomised clinical trial to compare in-situ and reversed vein grafts for femoro-popliteal by-pass. Br J Surg 1987;74:252–5.

3. Hall KV. The great saphenous vein used in-situ as an arterial shunt after extirpation of the vein valves. Surgery 1962;51:492–5.

4. Leather RP, Powers SR, Karmody AM. A re-appraisal of the in-situ saphenous vein arterial bypass. Its use in limb salvage. Surgery 1979;86:453–61.

FEMOROPOPLITEAL AND INFRAPOPLITEAL BYPASS WITH PROSTHETIC GRAFT

Appraise

1 The best prosthetic grafts perform almost as well as saphenous vein grafts when anastomosed to the popliteal artery above the knee. However, below the knee they are not nearly as effective as vein grafts and, if the distal anastomosis is to a single tibial or peroneal artery, patency rates at 2 years of approximately half those of veins are to be expected. Furthermore, when prosthetic grafts occlude they often result in loss of the distal run-off, with a high risk of limb loss.

2 Use of prosthetic grafts below the knee is justifiable only if there is no autologous vein available and must be strictly limited to those patients in whom the alternative to reconstruction is amputation.

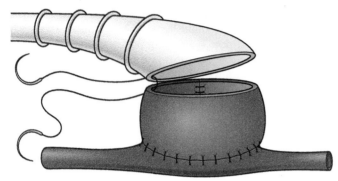

Fig. 23.26   The Miller cuff.

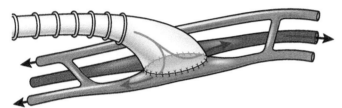

Fig. 23.27   An adjuvant arteriovenous fistula at the distal anastomosis.

3 *Inflow.* See Saphenous vein bypass.

4 *Outflow.* One reason why prosthetic grafts perform less well than autologous vein grafts is that they require a higher velocity of blood flow through them to prevent blood clot forming on the flow surface (a higher thrombotic threshold velocity). A restricted outflow tract is therefore less well tolerated. Attempts have been made to overcome the problem by creating an adjuvant arteriovenous fistula (Fig. 23.27) at or close to the distal anastomosis, thereby augmenting the run-off, but clinical trials indicate that this manoeuvre does not have sufficient value to justify its routine use.[1]

A second problem with prosthetic grafts is that platelets react with the alien flow surface. This causes them to adhere, particularly at the distal anastomosis, restricting the outflow further either by initiating thrombosis formation or by the later development of subintimal hyperplasia. The unnatural end-to-side configuration of the anastomosis itself probably also contributes by causing excessive flow disturbance. In order to try to overcome this problem the distal anastomosis has been modified by means of vein patches or cuffs.[2,3] These adjuvant techniques are of proven benefit in terms of short- and long-term graft patency.

5 *Conduit.* Use an externally supported PTFE graft.

Prepare

1 Commence antiplatelet therapy at least 48 hours before operation.

2 Give prophylactic antibiotic cover by administration of a broad-spectrum agent at the time of induction of anaesthesia.

3 For positioning of the patient and preparation of the limb see Femoropopliteal saphenous vein bypass.

Action

1 Expose the common femoral artery and distal recipient vessel as previously described.

2 Select a graft of either 6 mm or 5 mm internal diameter and, using a long tunnelling instrument, pass it between the two incisions (see Reversed saphenous vein graft).

3 Give intravenous heparin and allow 3 minutes for it to circulate before the application of arterial clamps.

4 Construct end-to-side anastomoses to the common femoral and popliteal or tibial arteries using 5/0 and 6/0 sutures, respectively. If a PTFE graft has been chosen, consider using PTFE sutures.

5 If it has been decided to incorporate an interposition vein cuff at the distal anastomosis use the following technique:

Miller cuff (Fig. 23.26).[2] Obtain a 3-cm length of autologous vein: the distal end of the saphenous vein from the ankle is suitable. Open the vein longitudinally to make a flat strip. Make an arteriotomy 1 cm in length, and suture the strip of vein to the edges of the arteriotomy using 7/0 polypropylene sutures for a tibial artery or 6/0 polypropylene for the popliteal artery. Commence the stitch in the middle of one side and suture the vein to the whole circumference of the arteriotomy. Then trim the excess of the vein strip away and complete the cuff by suturing the free edges together. Finally trim the graft to match the size of the vein cuff and construct an oblique end-to-end anastomosis with a continuous 6/0 polypropylene suture.

6 If a precuffed PTFE graft is used it is essential not to trim or adjust the shaped end of the graft in any way. Match the length of the arteriotomy to that of the 'cuff' and not vice versa. When using a precuffed graft it is helpful to perform the distal anastomosis before the proximal anastomosis and to draw the graft from the distal to the proximal wound during the tunnelling procedure.

? DIFFICULTY

Note that all anastomoses to tibial arteries must be technically immaculate. Use umbilical catheters of suitable size as stents and fine suture material. Magnification is essential (see General principles).

Closure

1 Close the wounds in layers with drainage as for saphenous vein bypass.

Aftercare

1 Detailed observation of peripheral perfusion and distal pulses, as for saphenous vein grafts.

2 Maintain aspirin antiplatelet therapy throughout and continue indefinitely.

Complications

1 *Early thrombotic occlusion.* In the event of early thrombosis of the graft, return the patient to theatre immediately for thrombectomy and careful reappraisal.

▶ KEY POINT   Decision-making

■ Avoid repeated over-zealous re-exploration of grafts that are doomed to failure; early amputation is better for the patient.

2 Late occlusion of a prosthetic graft warrants a new angiogram. It is often due to subintimal hyperplasia at or close to the distal anastomosis.

The options are:
- Thrombolysis of the graft and dilatation of the outflow tract by balloon angioplasty
- Operative thrombectomy with patch angioplasty or a jump graft at the distal anastomosis
- A combination of thrombolysis and surgical treatment.

Although PTFE grafts can usually be re-opened it is sometimes preferable to replace the whole graft, particularly when it has been occluded for more than 3 weeks. The patency of grafts re-explored for occlusion is reduced and graft replacement has to be considered in the context of up-to-date imaging to assess patent distal vessels.

3 In common with other prosthetic grafts there is a risk of infection (see Aortobifemoral bypass).

PERCUTANEOUS BALLOON ANGIOPLASTY DILATATION FOR FEMOROPOPLITEAL OCCLUSIVE ARTERIAL DISEASE

Appraise

1 Percutaneous techniques are increasingly being used as the first-line treatment for femoral occlusions. Good results are being achieved following treatment of long femoral lesions using a deliberate subintimal technique.[4] The use of novel long balloons for long lesions and wires to improve re-entry into the lumen are increasingly replacing traditional open surgery. It should be emphasized that these approaches should be performed by those with special skills and training.

2 Localized calcified lesions of the common femoral artery, the distal external iliac artery or proximal superficial femoral artery are usually best treated surgically with an endarterectomy or jump graft.

Prepare, action and aftercare

See Basic techniques.

Complications

1 Arterial rupture and acute thrombosis, if not managed with a covered stent or aspiration of clot, will require urgent surgical intervention.

2 Expanding groin haematoma, if not stabilized with pressure, may require surgical intervention.

3 Be aware of the possibility of retroperitoneal haemorrhage if the patient shows signs of hypovolaemia without obvious blood loss. This is most likely to occur if arterial puncture was made proximal to the inguinal ligament. Urgent resuscitation followed by surgical repair under general anaesthesia is required.

4 Occasionally, a false aneurysm develops at the puncture site. In the first place, attempt treatment by manual compression using Duplex ultrasound scanning to localize the communication with the arterial lumen. It may be necessary to apply pressure for 30 minutes or more but this technique is usually successful even when applied some weeks after the procedure.

In certain circumstances, direct injection of thrombin can be used under ultrasound guidance to occlude the false aneurysm. Alternatively, undertake open repair under local or general anaesthesia.

5 Stents in the superficial femoral artery tend to cause excessive myointimal hyperplasia and are rarely successful in the long term, therefore their use should be limited.

REFERENCES

1. Hamsho A, Nott D, Harris PL. Prospective randomised trial of distal arteriovenous fistula as an adjunct to femoro-infrapopliteal PTFE bypass. Eur J Vasc Endovasc Surg 1999;17:197–201.
2. Miller JH, Foreman RK, Ferguson L, et al. Interposition vein cuff for anastomosis of prosthesis to small artery. Aust N Z J Surg 1984;54:283–6.
3. Taylor RS, MacFarland RJ, Cox MI. An investigation into the causes of failure of PTFE grafts. Eur J Vasc Surg 1987;1:335–45.
4. Bolia A, Fishwick G. Recanalisation of iliac artery occlusion by subintimal dissection using the ipsilateral and the contralateral approach. Clin Radiol 1997;5:684–7.

REPAIR OF ABDOMINAL AORTIC ANEURYSM – OPEN SURGERY

Appraise

1 The infrarenal abdominal aorta is the commonest site for aneurysms. These are dangerous lesions, death being the likely outcome in the event of rupture. The rate of growth and the risk of rupture increase exponentially with the diameter of the aneurysm. Therefore, unless the patient is gravely ill from other causes, any aneurysm wider than 5.5 cm should be considered for intervention. The UK Small Aneurysm Trial showed that for smaller aneurysms conservative management with regular surveillance by ultrasound is preferable to operation.[1]

2 With improvements in anaesthetic management and progressive modification of surgical technique, the mortality rate associated with elective aneurysm surgery is less than 5% in the best centres. In the UK Small Aneurysm Trial the in-hospital mortality rate was 5.8%. Endovascular aneurysm repair (EVAR) is accepted internationally as a safe treatment for abdominal aortic aneurysms (AAA) greater than 5.5 cm in diameter, as a result of almost 15 years of experience of the technique. The EVAR and DREAM Trials confirmed a significant reduction in aneurysm-related mortality of 60%, which is maintained at 4 years after implantation. NICE Guidelines issued in 2006 stated 'the current evidence on the efficacy and short-term safety of stent-graft placement in AAA appears adequate to support the use of this procedure provided that the normal arrangements are in place for consent, audit and clinical governance'. In the EVAR 1 Trial endovascular aneurysm repair resulted in a 30-day mortality rate of 1.7 % compared with 4.7% following open surgery.

The important open surgical principles are:
- Minimal dissection
- Inlay technique of anastomosis
- Use of straight rather than bifurcated grafts whenever possible.

3 Emergency operation is indicated for a patient with an aneurysm who develops severe abdominal or back pain with or without circulatory collapse, unless he is already moribund. The mortality

associated with emergency aneurysm surgery is between 30% and 60%. The overall risk of death from a ruptured aneurysm is, however, higher as approximately 50% of patients die before reaching hospital.

Prepare

1 Confirm the diagnosis by ultrasound scanning. Computed tomography (CT) with intravenous contrast is essential in order to make precise anatomical measurements if endovascular repair is being considered (see below, Endovascular repair of abdominal aortic aneurysm).

2 Detailed assessment of cardiac risk is essential before elective operation (see Aortobifemoral bypass).

3 Preoperative assessment of respiratory and renal function is also required.

4 For elective cases the patient is fully anaesthetized with total muscular relaxation. Arterial, central venous and transoesophageal monitoring are sited and a urinary catheter is positioned in the bladder. The use of a cell saver to minimize blood transfusions is helpful. The patient is placed on the operating table with a warming blanket to minimize heat loss. The entire area from the nipples to mid-thigh is prepared. A small towel is placed over the genitalia and an adhesive drape is applied so as to allow access to the whole of the abdomen and both inguinal regions.

5 For emergency cases, all essential vascular access lines and the urinary catheter are inserted and the abdomen prepared and draped prior to the induction of anaesthesia. The administration of a muscle relaxant may release tamponade of a retroperitoneal haematoma, with re-bleeding and catastrophic circulatory collapse. Therefore the anaesthetist must not commence anaesthesia until you indicate that you are ready to proceed. While preoperative preparations are being made, maintain the blood pressure at a low level: a systolic pressure of 60 to 80 mmHg is ideal. 'Permissive' hypotension reduces the risk of sudden catastrophic haemorrhage. Good venous access lines are essential at an early stage but, except in dire emergency, do not infuse fluid to augment the blood pressure until an aortic clamp has been applied.

6 Give a broad-spectrum intravenous antibiotic with induction of anaesthesia as prophylaxis against graft infection.

Access

1 Make a midline incision extending from the xiphisternum to the pubis, skirting the umbilicus.

2 Check the abdominal contents to exclude the presence of some other condition, such as malignant disease, which might alter the decision to operate on the aneurysm. Note the presence of gallstones or peptic ulcer for future reference only.

3 Displace the omentum and large bowel superiorly and the small bowel with its mesentery to the right. Cover with large moist abdominal packs and retain in place with the blades of a fixed self-retaining retractor system (Omnitract; Fig. 23.28).

4 The duodenum lies across the upper part of the aneurysm and must be displaced. To do this, make an incision in the parietal peritoneum to the left of the duodenum, which is then mobilized

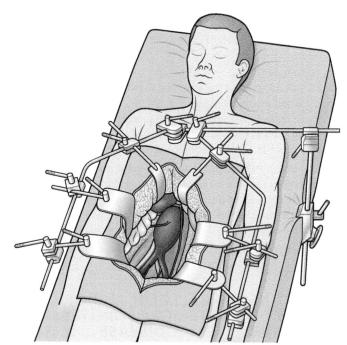

Fig. 23.28 Exposure of the abdominal aorta for resection of an aneurysm.

upwards and to the right. This completed, place deep narrow retractor blades on each side of the aorta, to expose the neck of the aneurysm and the renal vein crossing it.

5 Continue the incision of the peritoneum longitudinally over the surface of the aneurysm, passing to the right of the inferior mesenteric artery and across the bifurcation.

6 Position additional packs and retractor blades to expose the whole aneurysm and both common iliac arteries (see Fig. 23.28). Identify and protect the ureters on each side as they cross the iliac vessels.

7 In the case of an emergency operation for rupture, try to avoid 'crash-clamping' of the aorta without first mobilizing the duodenum and identifying the renal vein. If there is no free bleeding, proceed calmly with the first steps as described above. The presence of a haematoma distorts the anatomy and it is essential to dissect a plane close to the wall of the aorta. Once the neck of the aneurysm has been identified, carefully make a space on each side to accommodate the jaws of a straight clamp and apply this immediately from the front (Fig. 23.29). Then proceed with the remainder of the dissection. If there is free bleeding, obtain control initially by manual pressure against the vertebral column while an assistant packs away and retracts the abdominal contents. In extreme difficulties either apply a clamp at the level of the diaphragm after opening the lesser omentum and splitting the muscular fibres of the crus or use a balloon-occlusion catheter inserted through an incision in the aneurysm itself.

Assess

1 Confirm the position of the neck of the aneurysm relative to the renal arteries: 95% of aneurysms are infrarenal. The minority of aneurysms that involve the visceral arteries, and particularly those extending into the chest, require much more complex and dangerous surgery. Most of these can be diagnosed preoperatively and should be referred to a specialized unit for further assessment and treatment.

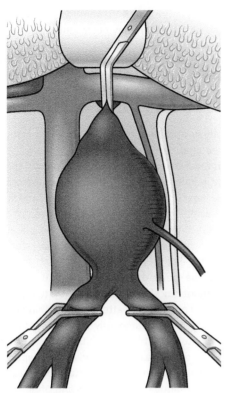

Fig. 23.29   Application of clamps.

2 The left renal vein, which crosses above the neck of most aneurysms, does not usually need to be divided: it can be mobilized to give additional proximal access. If necessary, it can be divided: this should be done well over to the right in order to preserve outflow from the kidney via the adrenal and gonadal veins. Even so, it has been demonstrated that renal function can be affected adversely.

3 Assess the aortic bifurcation and the iliac arteries. A minor degree of ectasia of the iliac arteries can be accepted and it should be possible to use a straight graft in 60–70% of patients. A bifurcated graft is required if the common iliac ostia have been separated by the aneurysm or if one or both of the iliac arteries are grossly aneurysmal. Occasionally, very severe calcification at the aortic bifurcation makes suturing at this site impossible.

4 Assess the inferior mesenteric artery. Usually it is totally occluded. However, if it is widely patent it is advisable to observe the effect of temporary clamping of this vessel on the bowel circulation before it is finally sacrificed. Ligate it close to the aorta or suture the ostium from within the sac in order to preserve its connections with the superior mesenteric artery via its ascending colic branch.

5 Decide whether to use a straight or bifurcated graft and of what size.

Action

1 Make no attempt to encircle either the aorta or the iliac arteries. To do so risks trauma to veins with serious venous bleeding.

2 Carefully dissect a narrow space on each side of the aorta and of both common iliac arteries to permit access for the jaws of straight or slightly angled clamps applied from the front.

3 In elective cases only, give heparin intravenously and allow 3 minutes for it to circulate before closing the clamps. Stabilize the aortic clamp by a ring of nylon tape around the handles of the clamp and tethered to the arm of the retractor or by the use of an assistant's hand. Apply only sufficient pressure to occlude blood flow and no more (see Fig. 23.29).

4 Open the aneurysm longitudinally and proximally towards the neck of the aneurysm. 'T' the aortic side walls gently to aid with the reformation of the aortic wall. Scoop out the laminated thrombus, degenerate atheromatous material and liquid blood it contains. These contents sometimes bear an alarming resemblance to pus. Most aneurysms are in fact sterile, but about 10% yield a growth of organisms on culture.

> ### ▶ KEY POINT Infection
>
> ■ Infection? Always send a specimen to the laboratory for microbiological analysis.

5 Control back-bleeding from patent lumbar and median sacral arteries with figure-of-eight sutures of 3/0 polypropylene (Prolene) applied from inside the sac. Insertion of a Travers retractor to hold open the sac is often useful in order to display the ostia of the lumbar arteries and subsequently to facilitate the anastomoses (Fig. 23.30).

6 If a bifurcated graft is to be used, remember to trim it to leave only 3–4 cm of the main trunk above the bifurcation (see Aortobifemoral bypass.).

7 Using 3/0 polypropylene sutures, construct an end-to-end anastomosis to the proximal aorta. This is done from within the sac by

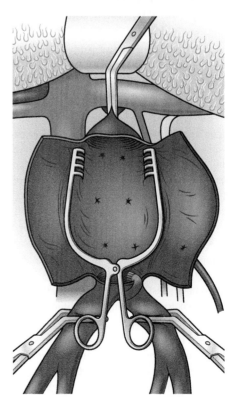

Fig. 23.30   Use of a Travers retractor to display the interior of the aneurysm sac.

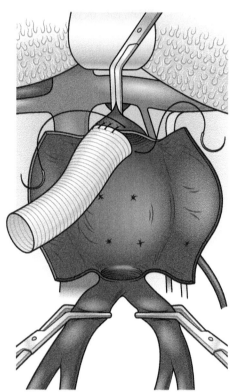

Fig. 23.31   The inlay technique of anastomosis.

the inlay technique (Fig. 23.31). Start suturing to one side of the midline at the back of the graft (see Basic techniques) to create a new back wall; it is usually easier to tie the graft down rather than use a parachute technique. Stitch from graft to aorta and take large bites to include all layers of the aortic wall each time. Finish in the midline anteriorly.

8 Apply a soft clamp to the graft and gently release the aortic clamp to test the anastomosis. Place additional sutures or pledgeted sutures as required.

9 If a straight tube is to be used, construct a similar anastomosis at the aortic bifurcation.

10 If a bifurcated graft is necessary, it may be possible to construct an end-to-end anastomosis by the inlay technique to the iliac bifurcation on both sides. Alternatively, transect the iliac arteries and construct a standard end-to-end anastomosis or pass the limbs of the graft through tunnels to the groin for end-to-end anastomosis to the common femoral arteries (see Aortobifemoral bypass). Try to ensure that one of the internal iliac arteries is perfused orthogradely if at all possible.

11 Before completion of the distal anastomosis flush the graft to eliminate any blood clots and also to ensure that the recipient vessels bleed back satisfactorily. If this is not the case pass embolectomy catheters to retrieve any distal blood clots.

12 Give the anaesthetist several minutes warning before releasing the clamps and reperfuse one leg at a time in order to minimize reperfusion injury. In the case of a bifurcation graft the anastomosis on one side may be completed and this limb perfused before the second anastomosis is constructed. A slight fall in blood pressure on release of a clamp is reassuring evidence that the limb is in fact being adequately perfused.

13 Prior to closing ensure that all anastomoses are blood-tight and that there is no bleeding from any other source. Fold the redundant aneurysm sac over the graft and fix it with a number of synthetic absorbable sutures. Make sure that the graft is covered completely to minimize the risk of aortoenteric fistula in the future.

? DIFFICULTY

1. Difficulty in obtaining control of bleeding from a ruptured aneurysm. See Access.
2. The left renal vein is torn during application of the clamp. If possible, repair the vein with 4/0 or 5/0 non-absorbable sutures. The vein may, if necessary, be ligated and divided (see Access). Bleeding from the region of the gonadal or adrenal vein is best controlled by packing in the first place, and sometimes this will be sufficient. If not, apply stitches later.
3. A tear of the iliac veins can produce torrential venous bleeding, the source of which is difficult to identify. If this defect cannot quickly be repaired with sutures, apply local packing and pressure and attend to something else for a while. It may stop spontaneously or be more easily controlled later. Use sutures buttressed with Dacron pledgets.
4. The neck of the aorta is ectatic and its wall papery thin. It is usually possible to crimp a large aorta into a smaller graft by the inlay technique of anastomosis and often this is preferable to extending the operation into the suprarenal aorta. If the aorta will not hold stitches, which cut out or tear, it is necessary to transect the aorta and construct an end-to-end anastomosis with a circumferential Dacron buttress and Dacron oversleeve (see Aortobifemoral bypass).
5. Suturing is impeded by calcification in the wall of the vessels. See Aortobifemoral bypass.
6. The bowel appears ischaemic on completion of the operation. Re-implant the inferior mesenteric artery.
7. Venous bleeding occurs from inside the aneurysm on opening the sac. This signifies an aortocaval fistula. Close the defect from inside the sac with large sutures. If torrential venous bleeding is encountered, secure control first with intraluminal balloon catheters inserted proximally and distally into the cava through the defect.
8. There is gross perianeurysmal fibrosis (inflammatory aneurysm). This places at risk structures that are adherent to it—especially the duodenum, the left renal vein and the ureters. Continue the dissection with care. It is often possible to find a safe plane within the wall of the aneurysm, which may be up to 1 cm thick (the 'onion-skin' technique). However, if it seems dangerous to proceed it may be more prudent to withdraw, close the abdomen and refer the patient to a specialist unit for further assessment. There is no strong evidence that steroids are of benefit in this situation.

Closure

1 Close the posterior parietal peritoneum over the sac, making sure that the duodenum and small bowel cannot gain access to the graft or suture lines, with a risk of late graft infection or aortoenteric fistula.

2 Perform a mass closure of the abdomen with a permanent suture rather than an absorbable suture as there is a higher incidence of incisional hernia in patients with aneurysms, thought to be related to a connective tissue abnormality. Drains are not normally indicated.

Aftercare

1 Following an emergency operation it is a good policy to maintain positive-pressure ventilation for 12–24 hours after operation. This ensures adequate oxygenation of the blood during a period of potential cardiovascular instability and is also considerably more convenient and kinder to the patient if he has to be returned to theatre for any reason.

2 Maintain cardiac monitoring for as long as is indicated until stability is achieved.

3 Frequently, patients develop a postoperative ileus and require nasogastric suction and intravenous infusions.

4 Deep venous thrombosis prophylaxis is necessary until full mobility is re-established.

5 After an uncomplicated recovery the patient is usually ready for discharge from hospital 6–8 days after operation, depending on their co-morbidities.

Complications

There are six important potential complications to remember:

1 *Haemorrhage.* Early re-exploration is mandatory upon the suspicion of continuing internal bleeding. It may be arising from the anastomosis or from other sources such as a torn mesenteric vessel. 'Haematological' bleeding due to heparin or other coagulopathy can be recognized by appropriate tests and must be corrected with appropriate blood products.

2 *Occlusion.* This results either from embolization of material trapped above the aortic clamp that was not flushed out, from thrombosis in the distal vessels during clamping or from a technical fault at one of the suture lines. Try passing a Fogarty catheter proximally and distally from the groin first, but be prepared to re-explore the graft if this is unsuccessful.

3 *Renal tubular necrosis.* This is common following rupture of an aneurysm and is due to prolonged hypotension. It may be part of a multiple organ failure syndrome, in which case the prognosis is very poor. Isolated renal tubular necrosis often recovers, although a period of support by haemodialysis or haemofiltration may be required. Total anuria immediately after the operation suggests the possibility of occlusion of both renal arteries. Arrange urgent Duplex ultrasound to assess renal perfusion and consider whether re-exploration is indicated, with a view to renal artery reconstruction. Such decisions can only be made on an individual patient basis.

4 *Adult respiratory distress syndrome (ARDS).* This is unfortunately not uncommon following emergency operations for ruptured aneurysm, particularly if there has been massive blood loss. It usually becomes apparent within 24 hours but can develop more insidiously over a few days. Mechanical ventilatory support with a high concentration of inspired oxygen and positive end-expiratory pressure is often required to maintain adequate blood gases. The prognosis is generally poor, especially if secondary infection follows.

5 *Myocardial infarction.* See Aortobifemoral bypass.

6 *Graft infection.* See Aortobifemoral bypass.

REFERENCE

1. The UK Small Aneurysm Trial participants. Mortality results of randomised controlled trial for early elective surgery or ultrasound surveillance for small abdominal aortic aneurysms. Lancet 1998;352:1649–55.

REPAIR OF THORACIC AND THORACOABDOMINAL ANEURYSMS

Appraise

1 While repair of a localized aneurysm of the descending thoracic aorta is a relatively straightforward operation, extensive thoracoabdominal aneurysms (type 2) represent a formidable challenge to the vascular surgeon. Both of these procedures require vascular and cardiothoracic surgical facilities and expertise and should therefore be confined to a few highly specialized units. It is inappropriate to describe them in detail here, but knowledge of the principles involved is important.

2 The application of a clamp to the thoracic aorta dramatically increases the afterload on the heart and is likely to precipitate acute left ventricular failure. At the same time the abdominal viscera and the spinal cord are deprived of a blood supply, with a high risk of multiple organ failure and paraplegia.

3 Left heart bypass using an external pump obviates both of these problems.

4 Perfusion of the spinal cord during clamping of the thoracic aorta is a function of intra-arterial pressure, which is reduced, and cerebrospinal fluid (CSF) pressure, which increases. The insertion of a spinal drain as part of the anaesthetic preparation is helpful and allows monitoring and maintenance of the cerebrospinal fluid pressure at a low level (10 cmH$_2$O). This helps to maintain perfusion of the spinal cord and reduces the incidence of paraplegia.

5 Surgical repair of extensive thoracoabdominal aneurysms without left heart bypass and CSF tapping carries risks of death and paraplegia, both in the order of 20%. Application of the above measures reduces these risks by half.

Prepare

1 CT angiography is required to build up a precise picture of the extent of the aneurysm preoperatively.

2 A rigorous preoperative assessment including assessment of the cardiac, pulmonary and renal systems is also mandatory.

3 Following the administration of general anaesthesia, a double lumen endotracheal tube is inserted by the anaesthetist and arterial and venous lines are inserted. Transoesophageal monitoring is also usually established. The urinary bladder is catheterized.

4 A spinal drain is inserted and connected to a reservoir, the height of which can be adjusted to maintain CSF pressure at the desired level.

5 The patient must be positioned on the table to permit both left thoracotomy and exposure of the abdominal aorta. Support the chest in a left lateral position but rotate the pelvis forward so that the trunk is twisted slightly. Correct positioning of the patient is vital to allow access to the chest and to the abdomen.

6 Prepare and drape the whole of the chest, abdomen and both groins.

Access

1 For thoracic aneurysms make an incision over the fifth intercostal space. For thoracoabdominal aneurysms make an incision over the sixth or seventh space and extend it across the costal margin to the midline of the abdomen and then inferiorly to the pubis. Divide the diaphragm around its margin to permit the wound to be opened widely with a rib retractor and to preserve its function. Do not split the diaphragm into the aortic hiatus. Reflect the spleen, pancreas and left colon to the right to expose the abdominal aorta. The kidney and suprarenal gland may also be reflected or left in situ. Alternatively, the incision in the abdomen can be extended to allow access to the retroperitoneum, thereby removing the need for visceral medial rotation. Using this incision does, however, limit access to the right common iliac artery.

2 Expose the left common femoral or external iliac artery to permit arterial line access for the extracorporeal pump.

Assess

1 Confirm the extent of the aneurysm and decide upon the site of the anastomoses and clamps.

2 Expose the left pulmonary vein at the hilum of the lung in preparation for insertion of a venous cannula for the extracorporeal circulation.

Action

1 When all dissection has been completed administer heparin to achieve full anticoagulation.

2 Establish left heart bypass (left atrium to left common femoral artery).

3 Apply clamps. In the case of extensive aneurysms isolate the proximal site of anastomosis with clamps in the first place in order to maintain uninterrupted perfusion of the viscera for as long as possible.

4 Open the aneurysm, extract the thrombus and assess the intercostal arteries.

5 The artery of Adamkewicz that supplies the spinal cord usually arises from one of the intercostal arteries between D8 and D12 level. Widely patent intercostal arteries at this level should be preserved and reimplanted into the graft within a patch of aorta. Smaller intercostal arteries at other levels may be oversewn.

6 Select a graft (usually 28 or 30 mm or may be larger) and complete the proximal anastomosis with 3/0 polypropylene by an end-to-end inlay technique (Fig. 23.32).

7 Apply a clamp to the graft and check the anastomosis for leaks. Have a low threshold to buttress the entire anastomosis with either buttressed sutures or a ring of Teflon which is sutured concurrently with the native thoracic aorta and graft.

8 Pass the distal end of the graft through the aortic hiatus in the diaphragm.

9 After applying distal clamps, open the remainder of the aneurysm and verify the position of the visceral arteries. Implant these and

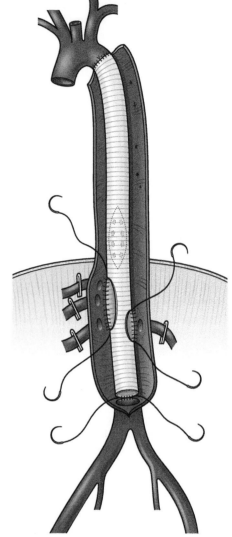

Fig. 23.32   Inlay technique for repair of thoracoabdominal aortic aneurysm.

the intercostals, if patent, using aortic patches. Usually it is possible to include the coeliac axis, superior mesenteric and right renal arteries in one patch (Carrel patch), leaving the left renal artery to be implanted separately. Perfusion of the viscera can be maintained with additional cannulae from the cardiac pump, thereby reducing warm ischaemia time.

As an alternative to constructing an aortic patch bearing the abdominal visceral arteries, use a graft incorporating branches of each of the visceral arteries (Coselli graft). This obviates the risk of subsequent aneurysmal dilatation of the patch.

10 Finally, complete the distal aortic or iliac anastomoses and release the clamps.

11 When satisfactory haemostasis has been achieved discontinue left heart bypass, remove the cannulae, repair the access vessels and reverse full heparinization.

12 Close the aneurysm sac over the graft.

13 Close the wound in layers, taking care to repair the diaphragm. Two chest drains are inserted superiorly and inferiorly to drain blood and to allow lung expansion.

Aftercare

1 Maintain ventilation for 12 hours or until indices indicate that independent ventilation will be possible.

2 Ensure coagulopathy is treated aggressively.

3 Maintain spinal fluid drainage for 48–72 hours.

4 Remove chest drains when drainage has ceased.

Complications

1 Haemorrhage, anuria, adult respiratory distress syndrome, myocardial infarction. See Repair of abdominal aortic aneurysm.

2 Paraplegia. Ensure that CSF pressure is optimized. Infarction of the spinal cord is irreversible, therefore rehabilitation with moral and physical support is the essential and only appropriate response to established paraplegia.

ENDOVASCULAR REPAIR OF ABDOMINAL AORTIC ANEURYSM

Appraise

1 The first reported operation to repair an abdominal aortic aneurysm by endovascular deployment of a stent-graft combination within the aneurysm sac was undertaken by Parodi in 1990.[1] Since then the technology of endovascular stent-grafts has evolved rapidly and there are now a large number to choose from.

2 Endovascular aneurysm repair has the attributes of a minimally invasive operation. The procedure itself carries a very low risk and the recovery time is much shorter than that associated with conventional open operation.

3 For 'fixation' the endograft relies upon a stent, with or without hooks or barbs attached, and for 'seal' to exclude the aneurysm sac from the circulation it relies upon firm contact between the fabric of the graft and the vessel wall at each end. These functions demand the existence of a 'neck' of at least 15 mm in length between the lower renal artery and the start of the aneurysm and adequate distal 'landing zones'.

4 It is essential to match the size of the endograft to that of the vessels within which it is to be implanted. Over-sizing of the diameter of the stent-graft relative to that of the arteries, in the order of 10–20%, is necessary to ensure adequate fixation and seal. Devices with a proximal neck diameter of up to 36 mm are available.

5 The length of the device is critical also. It is permissible to cross the renal arteries with an uncovered stent but in order to achieve an effective seal it is necessary to position the top of the covered part of the stent immediately below the renal arteries without overlapping their ostia. Distally it is permissible to cross one but not both internal iliac arteries.

6 Access for the device is via the common femoral artery and it is essential that the iliac arteries can permit the passage of the introducer systems. Iliac arteries should measure 7 mm or greater and should not be too tortuous or heavily calcified. If the iliac arteries preclude the passage of the introducer systems then either a conduit can be performed on to the distal common iliac artery (10-mm Dacron graft) or a 'trial by angioplasty' can be performed to dilate the vessel.

7 Bifurcated endografts are now the norm and may be one-piece or modular designs, which are assembled in situ during the operative procedure.

8 Aneurysms of the descending thoracic aorta can also be repaired successfully by straight endografts introduced from the groin or via the abdominal aorta or an infrarenal aortic graft. The risk of operative complications, including paraplegia and death, appears to be much lower than that associated with open repair.

9 All endovascular procedures require a significant degree of accurate planning with CT imaging and investment in a full range of consumables and devices. Fenestrated and branched endoluminal devices, which permit endovascular repair of aneurysms in the visceral or thoracoabdominal region, are only undertaken by specialist vascular units and are not the remit of this chapter.

Prepare

1 The clinical indications for endovascular repair are similar to those for open repair (see above). However, some patients who are unfit for the open operation may be able to tolerate the less-invasive endovascular procedure.

2 For accurate measurements of the aneurysm and adjacent arteries and assessment of the access route, obtain CT scans in a dynamic format which can be viewed on a work station. Angiograms performed with an intraluminal measuring catheter in situ (calibrated angiograms) may provide useful additional information, but modern dynamic CT angiography obviates the need for this invasive test in all but a few patients. Be sure that the minimal anatomical criteria, as defined by the device manufacturer, are satisfied.

3 Preoperative assessments of cardiac, respiratory and renal function are required as for open aneurysm repair (see above).

4 General anaesthesia is to be preferred. If regional anaesthesia is used, facilities for general anaesthesia must be immediately available in case conversion to open repair becomes necessary.

5 Place the patient supine upon a radiolucent operating table and prepare as for open aneurysm repair, including the administration of a broad-spectrum antibiotic on induction of anaesthesia (see above).

6 Consideration as to the positioning of the imaging equipment is also required.

Access

1 For endovascular repair with a bifurcated endograft, access to both common femoral arteries is required. Although percutaneous access is possible with some types of device, the benefit is marginal and it is recommended that the common femoral arteries are exposed on both sides. Because the exposure required is limited, use short transverse incisions placed one finger's breadth above the groin crease and directly over the femoral pulse, rather than a classical vertical incision. It is not essential to dissect the profunda femoris artery. Apply Silastic loops or nylon tapes to the common femoral artery.

2 The choice of side of access for the body and ipsilateral limb of the device is dependent upon the anatomical configuration and distribution of disease in the iliac arteries and the direction of any angulation of the neck of the aneurysm.

3 Having exposed the common femoral arteries, give heparin 5000 IU intravenously.

4 Through the contralateral common femoral artery position a pigtail angiography catheter within the aorta just above the expected level of the renal arteries (see above, Basic techniques, for steps required). Obtain an angiogram to determine precisely the position of the renal arteries relative to bone structures or a radio-opaque measuring scale placed under the patient.

5 Via the ipsilateral side pass an angiography catheter over a standard 0.035 inch guide-wire into the suprarenal aorta. Through this catheter exchange the standard guide-wire for a long, super-stiff guide-wire (for example, a Lunderquist) and position it in the ascending aorta. Remove the catheter and introduce the stent-graft over the wire.

6 Manoeuvre the X-ray equipment to ensure that the origin of the renal arteries is in the centre of the image as viewed on the screen, taking into account the angulation of the aneurysm. This step is essential to avoid error when positioning the stent-graft.

7 Via the angiography catheter on the contralateral side obtain an angiogram and mark the position of the lowest renal artery.

8 Carefully adjust the position of the endograft within its introducer sheath so that the upper margin of the fabric of the graft is aligned with the lower border of the lowest renal artery.

9 Under fluoroscopic control deploy the body of the graft according to the procedure specified by the manufacturer. Usually, fine adjustment of the position of the device is possible after deployment of the upper one or two rows of the stent and another angiogram may be obtained at this stage. However, remember to withdraw the angiography catheter into the sac of the aneurysm before deploying the device fully.

10 It is now necessary to pass a guide-wire into the short leg (contralateral limb) on the body of the graft from the opposite groin. Radio-opaque markers are located at strategic points on the device for guidance. Withdraw the angiography catheter from the sheath in the common femoral artery and replace it with a catheter with a shaped end (e.g. cobra) or multipurpose-angled, to assist manipulation of the wire into the limb under fluoroscopic control.

11 Successful cannulation of the contralateral limb can be confirmed by checking that the guide-wire has been advanced into the lumen of the device by passing a pigtail catheter over the wire and observing that it can be rotated within the device without catching or deforming.

12 Exchange the standard 0.035 inch guide-wire for a super-stiff wire advanced well above the renal arteries.

13 Advance the second limb within its introducer system over the super-stiff wire and position it within the short limb on the body of the device under fluoroscopic control using, as a guide, the radio-opaque markers sutured on the stent-grafts provided for this purpose. When you are satisfied with the position deploy the second limb in accordance with the manufacturer's instructions. Modern modular stent-grafts are provided with a choice of limbs of different lengths and diameters.

14 Depending on the manufacturer's recommendations, consider using an intraluminal balloon to gently mould the stent-graft and its components.

15 The basic procedure is now completed (Fig. 23.33) but it is essential to obtain a completion angiogram to ascertain that the position of the device is satisfactory and especially to identify 'endoleaks'. When satisfied with the angiographic appearances remove all sheaths, catheters and guide-wires, close the femoral arteriotomies with 5/0 polypropylene sutures and restore blood flow to both limbs.

18 Close the groin incisions and check to ensure that the peripheral circulation is satisfactory.

? DIFFICULTY

1. Tortuous or calcified iliac arteries may obstruct access of the introducer sheath carrying the device. It is often possible to straighten the iliac arteries by applying gentle traction upon the external iliac artery from the groin. Dilate any focal stenoses with a balloon catheter. Consider deployment of a Wallstent. Large flexible sheaths with long tapered 'nosecones' are available (Cook) and these can often be negotiated through access vessels that will not permit passage of the device. The introducer system for the device may then be advanced through the sheath. If the external iliac arteries are too small to permit passage of an introducer sheath of sufficient size, take one of the following three actions: (a) expose one common iliac artery through an oblique incision in the iliac fossa and an extraperitoneal approach and suture to it a Dacron tube graft (8 or 10 mm) to function as a 'conduit' through which the larger component (main body) of the device is introduced into the aorta; (b) 'convert' to open repair of the aneurysm; (c) abandon the procedure altogether.

2. It may be impossible to manipulate a guide-wire into the short leg from the second groin. Pass a wire over the bifurcation of the graft from the first groin using a specially shaped, Sos-Omni, catheter and catch the end within the iliac artery using a 'goose-neck' snare to withdraw it through the sheath in the second groin. Advance catheters over the wire from both groins to push the loop well up before carefully withdrawing it to position the end within the aorta. Alternatively, use a brachial approach to advance a wire through the device to the second groin. Again, use a goose-neck snare to capture the wire and withdraw it through the sheath in the groin.

3. *Completion angiography demonstrates an 'endoleak'.* This is defined as 'persistence of blood flow outside the lumen of the endoluminal graft but within the aneurysm sac or adjacent vascular segment'. The presence of an endoleak indicates that the sac is still pressurized and therefore that a risk of rupture persists. Flow in the aneurysm sac visualized on completion angiography may originate from: (a) one or more of the anastomoses (type 1 endoleak); (b) retrograde perfusion from patent lumbar or inferior mesenteric arteries (type 2 endoleak); (c) incomplete seal between the modular parts (type 3 endoleak); or (d) graft porosity (type 4 endoleak). Of these, types 1 and 3

Continued

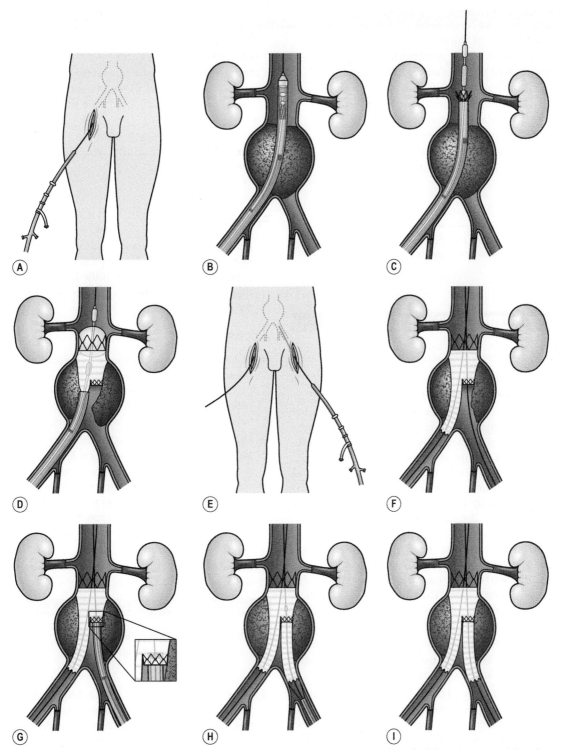

Fig. 23.33 Endovascular repair of abdominal aortic aneurysm with a modular endograft. (A) Guide wire and sheath is introduced via a common femoral artery; (B) Main body is introduced via a common femoral artery and advanced to the level of the renal arteries; (C) The first tow covered stents are deployed and position vis a vis the renal arteries are checked; (D) If the position of the device is satisfactory deployment proceeds until the contralateral limb is open; (E) Access is gained via the contralateral common femoral artery; (F) The contralateral iliac limb is delivered via the femoral artery and the body of the stent graft is cannulated; (G) The contralateral iliac limb is delivered via the artery and advanced to ensure adequate overlap within the main body of the stent graft; (H) The contralateral iliac limb is fully deployed to land in the common iliac artery; (I) A moulding balloon is used to ensure graft expansion and adequate sealing sites.

? DIFFICULTY—cont'd

are the most important and should be corrected either by balloon dilatation of the 'anastomosis' or, if this fails, by insertion of a Palmaz stent or an 'extender cuff'. The patient must not be allowed to leave the operating table with a large proximal type 1 endoleak because these are the most dangerous of all. Anecdotal evidenceindicates that an unresolved proximal type 1 endoleak is associated with a higher risk of rupture than anuntreated aneurysm. Most type 2 endoleaks

resolve spontaneously due to thrombosis of the vessel. Furthermore, clinical studies have demonstrated that they are rarely the cause of adverse postoperative events. Therefore no further intervention is required if a type 2 endoleak is diagnosed from the postoperative angiogram.

4. If, for any reason the endograft cannot be deployed or it is found to be grossly malpositioned, convert the procedure to an open repair.

REFERENCE

1. Parodi JC, Palmaz JC, Barone HD. Transfemoral intraluminal graft implantation for abdominal aortic aneurysms. Ann Vasc Surg 1991;5:491–9.

REPAIR OF POPLITEAL ANEURYSM

Appraise

1   After the abdominal aorta, the popliteal artery is the second most common place for aneurysms to occur. Sixty per cent are bilateral.

2   Popliteal aneurysms are dangerous because of their tendency to thrombosis with peripheral embolization. Initially, mural thrombus develops within the aneurysm and, possibly because of repeated flexion of the knee joint, fragments break away and embolize into the distal vessels. Because the emboli are small this process can occur insidiously so that the peripheral vascular bed gradually silts up until the aneurysm itself suddenly thromboses completely. Reconstructive surgery is often impossible because of the absence of patent vessels distally to receive a graft, and acute ischaemia from thrombosis of a popliteal aneurysm frequently results in loss of the limb. It has been suggested that thrombolytic therapy prior to operation may give better results than surgery alone. There is also a risk of haemorrhage from rupture of popliteal aneurysms but this is much less common.

3   Most popliteal aneurysms should be operated upon electively even if asymptomatic, especially when they contain intraluminal thrombus, which can be identified by ultrasound scanning.

4   Endovascular repair of popliteal aneurysms with a covered endoluminal stent or endograft is an option that can be considered in patients with co-morbidites which preclude open surgery. Good long-term results are being achieved with nitinol stents, which have flexibility and endurance.

5   Proximal and distal ligation of the aneurysm in combination with a bypass graft, by a medial approach, is the traditional approach preferred by many surgeons. The technique is the same as for femoropopliteal bypass graft, with ligation of the aneurysm proximally and distally. The conduit of choice is the long saphenous vein, which is usually of good calibre. Some studies have shown that up to one-third of aneurysms treated by this method continue to expand due to pressurization of the sac by geniculate collateral arteries.[1] Therefore, a direct posterior approach with insertion of an inlay graft is discussed below.

Prepare

1   Position the patient prone on the operating table. The short saphenous vein can be harvested for use as a bypass with the patient in this position, but if the long saphenous vein in the thigh is to be used, first harvest the vein and prepare it with the patient supine.

Access

1   Make a vertical 'lazy-S' incision over the popliteal fossa. Incise the popliteal fascia and fat pad in the same line to expose the 'diamond' defined by the hamstring muscles above and the two bellies of the gastrocnemius muscle below (see Exposure of the major peripheral arteries, Popliteal artery, above).

2   The popliteal artery lies medial and deep to the popliteal vein. Most aneurysms originate 1 or 2 cm distal to the adductor opening and terminate proximal to the anterior tibial branch. Divide any veins draining the gastrocnemius muscle, which may be found crossing the distal popliteal artery to gain access to the popliteal vein. Take care to protect the sural, lateral popliteal and common peroneal nerves, all of which are particularly vulnerable.

3   Pass silastic loops around the popliteal artery proximal and distal to the aneurysm.

▶ KEY POINT Control

■ Note the basic principle of obtaining control of the artery above and below the lesion.

4   The short saphenous vein arises behind the lateral malleolus at the ankle and takes a posterolateral course to enter the popliteal vein at a variable point above the level of the knee joint. In its distal half it is subcutaneous but penetrates the deep fascia to become subfascial proximally. Identify it in the distal popliteal fossa and trace it distally by incising the skin and deep fascia overlying it. Take great care to avoid injury to the sural nerve that runs alongside it. Harvest an adequate length and prepare it for use as a reversed vein graft (see Basic principles).

Action

1   Give intravenous heparin to the patient.

2   Apply clamps proximal and distal to the aneurysm.

3 Incise the aneurysm longitudinally along its whole extent. Oversew vessels that are back-bleeding into the sac, using 4/0 polypropylene figure-of-eight sutures placed across their orifices.

4 Inlay a reversed autologous vein graft with end-to-end anastomoses by the parachute method, using 4/0 or 5/0 polypropylene sutures. The distal limit of the aneurysm may be obscured by the nerves crossing it, making an inlay anastomosis difficult and therefore unsafe. In this case transect the popliteal artery distal to the aneurysm and construct a direct end-to-end anastomosis.

5 Close the wound in layers with a suction drain to the popliteal fossa.

? DIFFICULTY

1. Peripheral embolization from the aneurysm may have occluded the distal vessels.
2. Make an anastomosis to the distal popliteal artery or the tibioperoneal trunk if at all possible. Otherwise, surgical exploration of the tibial arteries and an on-table angiogram may be required to identify the optimal site to receive the bypass.

CAROTID ENDARTERECTOMY

1 Controversy surrounding this operation was dispelled by the publication of two randomized clinical trials in the early 1980s – one from Europe[2] and the other from America.[3] Both trials showed a significant benefit from surgery for patients with transient cerebral ischaemic attacks and a stenosis at the origin of the internal carotid artery of greater than 70%. Those with a mild stenosis of less than 30% fared better with medical therapy than with surgery, while no clear-cut conclusions could be drawn regarding those with a moderate stenosis of between 30% and 70%. A change in practice in the UK, with aggressive investigation and treatment for transient ischaemic events and cerebral infarction with Hyper Acute Stroke Units, has changed the treatment pathways such that it is now recommended that carotid endarterectomy should be performed within 14 days of the acute event; in some centres surgery within 48 hours is being achieved, the emphasis being on the need to prevent further embolic events from the carotid pathology.

2 The main indication for carotid endarterectomy is, therefore, transient cerebral ischaemic attacks and proven cerebral infarcts with an internal carotid artery stenosis greater than 70%.

3 Patients who have suffered a complete stroke and show no improvement in their neurological symptoms are not thought to gain any benefit from this surgery.

4 Surgical intervention for 'strokes in evolution' has potential to prevent or limit the effects of completed stroke in some patients, but there is also a risk of aggravating the condition and this indication is therefore controversial.

5 There is little convincing evidence that patients with symptoms of vertebrobasilar insufficiency benefit from carotid endarterectomy.

6 Total occlusion of the internal carotid artery is a contraindication to surgery.

7 Do not forget that carotid endarterectomy is a prophylactic operation. It will not improve symptoms due to a previous stroke but, in patients with symptomatic lesions of greater than 70%, it will reduce the risk of the patient suffering another ipsilateral stroke from approximately 20% within 3 years to 2% over the same period.

8 Because it is a prophylactic procedure, the complication rate associated with the operation must be extremely low. The justification for carotid endarterectomy is based on the assumption of a combined operative mortality and stroke rate of less than 5%. It is, therefore, essential that those undertaking this operation should maintain an accurate audit of their results and be prepared to refer their patients elsewhere if they cannot achieve this level of performance.

9 Endovascular approaches to the treatment of carotid artery disease have been disappointing, with unacceptably high stroke rates despite the use of cerebral protection devices. At the time of writing carotid endarterectomy remains the 'gold standard'.

Prepare

1 Duplex scanning accurately diagnoses the presence of internal carotid artery stenosis. Conventional carotid angiography carries a risk of stroke of approximately 1% and is normally to be avoided. If detailed imaging of the carotid artery and intracranial vessels is required, CT or magnetic resonance angiography is used.

2 CT scanning of the brain confirms whether or not the patient has suffered infarction (not haemorrhage) prior to surgery being considered.

3 Dual antiplatelet therapy (aspirin and dipyridamole) is usually commenced as soon as a cerebral infarct has been diagnosed and should be continued after the operation.

4 Under either general or regional anaesthesia the patient is placed supine on an operating table and the head of the table is raised slightly in order to reduce pressure in the neck veins (reverse Trendellenberg position). The patient's head, supported on a head ring, is turned slightly to the opposite side with the neck extended. The preparation and towelling include the pinna, which is bent forwards and supported in this position by an adhesive drape. This is to allow access for the sternomastoid muscle to be raised from the mastoid process should exposure of the artery be required at a high level.

5 Local anaesthesia in the form of a regional cervical plexus block has the advantage that the patient is able to cooperate in order to identify impaired cerebral perfusion and the need for a cerebral protection shunt (see below). However, general anaesthesia is preferred by many surgeons and patients. A randomized trial of general or local anaesthetic (GALA Trial) did not demonstrate any significant difference in terms of clinical outcome for either method.

Access

1 Make an oblique skin incision along the anterior border of the sternomastoid muscle extending from the mastoid process to the sternoclavicular joint (Fig. 23.34). Divide all subcutaneous tissue and the platysma muscle in the same line. Cutaneous nerves crossing the line of the incision must be sacrificed and this will leave an area of permanent numbness beneath the line of the jaw. The great auricular nerve should, however, be preserved.

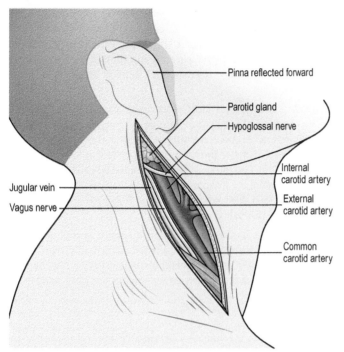

Jugular vein

Vagus nerve

Pinna reflected forward

Parotid gland

Hypoglossal nerve

Internal carotid artery

External carotid artery

Common carotid artery

Fig. 23.34 Exposure of the carotid arteries.

2 Mobilize the anterior border of the sternomastoid muscle and retract it posteriorly.

3 Identify the facial vein and divide it between ligatures. This allows the internal jugular vein to be displaced posteriorly. There may be additional venous tributaries that need to be divided. In the upper part of the incision mobilize the jugular lymph nodes and retract them posteriorly. Take care to avoid damage to the hypoglossal nerve, which sometimes loops surprisingly low into the neck and may be quite superficial. Find the ansa hypoglossi (also known as the ansa cervicalis) nerve on the surface of the carotid sheath and trace it upwards to locate the hypoglossal nerve. The ansa hypoglossi, which supplies the strap muscles, may be cut without any discernible functional disability. Incision into the lower pole of the parotid gland results in troublesome bleeding; therefore, dissect a plane posterior to this structure. The digastric muscle lies beneath it but does not impede access to the artery.

4 Open the carotid sheath initially towards the lower end of the incision to expose the common carotid artery. The vagus nerve lies posteriorly and deep to the artery and is not usually at risk, but its position should be noted so that it can be safeguarded. Pass a nylon tape or rubber sling carefully around the common carotid artery. Expose the carotid bifurcation and trace the internal carotid artery, which lies posterior to the external artery superiorly. It is important to remember that the artery may contain loose thrombotic or atheromatous material which could be dislodged by rough handling, with dire consequences. Therefore, use gentle sharp dissection and do not occlude or otherwise manipulate the vessel until you are ready to apply clamps. Dissecting the tissues off the vessel rather than vice versa is good surgical technique in this situation. Identify and protect the hypoglossal nerve, which must sometimes be lifted off the artery and gently retracted with a soft rubber sling. A small artery and vein loop backwards over the hypoglossal nerve and these should be divided to allow the

nerve to be displaced forwards. Clear as much of the artery as possible distal to the bifurcation and very carefully pass a narrow sling around it.

5 Dissect the origin of the external carotid artery and its superior thyroid branch. Pass a single rubber sling around both of these vessels. A single sling used in this way ensures that the ascending pharyngeal artery, which arises from the posterior aspect of the internal carotid artery close to its origin, is also controlled. If slings are placed around the superior thyroid and internal carotid arteries separately, troublesome back-bleeding may be encountered from this vessel following arteriotomy and during dissection of the atheromatous plaque.

6 You are now ready to clamp the arteries, but before proceeding make sure that you know what you are going to do about protecting the brain from ischaemic damage during clamping and that all the necessary instruments are readily to hand.

Cerebral protection

1 The majority of patients will tolerate prolonged clamping of the internal carotid artery without suffering ischaemic damage to the brain, but it is essential to employ a policy that will protect the minority who are at risk.

2 The use of temporary plastic shunts (see General principles) has entirely replaced controlled hypothermia as the method of choice. They are simpler and safer.

3 Shunts may be used routinely or selectively. If used selectively, some test must be employed to identify those in whom they are needed. These include:

- *Internal carotid artery stump pressure measurement.* After the administration of heparin, clamps are applied to the external and common carotid arteries and the pressure in the internal carotid artery is measured with a needle probe connected to a transducer. The pressure measured in this way provides an assessment of the adequacy of the collateral circulation through the circle of Willis. Different criteria have been applied, but a mean pressure in excess of 60 mmHg with a good pulsatile pressure wave pattern is often said to indicate adequate perfusion of the relevant hemisphere. If these criteria are met, then the operation proceeds without a shunt. If not, a shunt is inserted first.

- *Transcranial Doppler.* A substantial reduction in the velocity of blood flow in the middle cerebral artery and loss of 'pulsatility' indicates the need for a shunt. Transcranial Doppler is also very effective for the detection of particulate emboli and can therefore guide the surgeon during his dissection and manipulation of the arteries. Post-endarterectomy on-table Duplex scanning is an excellent tool for quality control and can also guide the surgeon as to whether the procedure is adequate or if there is residual stenosis requiring further attention while the patient is on table. Emboli detected postoperatively are a predictor of stroke and are an indication for anticoagulation with low-molecular-weight dextran.

- *Operate under local anaesthesia.* This is now the preferred method in many centres, local anaesthesia being administered in the form of a regional cervical plexus block. The patient holds a compressible 'squeaky toy' in his contralateral hand and is asked to squeeze it at intervals. If he is unable to do so or if his ability to speak is lost, a shunt is inserted to restore adequate perfusion of the ipsilateral cerebral hemisphere.

4 In certain circumstances a shunt is required and this is described below. There are small risks associated with shunts related to intimal damage to the artery and air emboli. However, these risks become negligible with familiarity of use.

Action

1 Select the arterial clamps and make sure they are immediately available, together with the Javid shunt and associated large and small ring clamps. Apply a Spencer Wells haemostat to the centre of the shunt.

2 Give heparin intravenously in a dose of 1000 IU for each 10 kg body weight and allow 3 minutes for it to circulate.

3 Apply clamps to the internal carotid, the common carotid and external carotid arteries in that order.

4 Make a longitudinal arteriotomy commencing on the common carotid and extending into the internal carotid beyond the distal limit of the atherosclerotic plaque.

5 Insert the Javid shunt into the common carotid artery and retain it with the larger ring clamp (Fig. 23.35). Temporarily release the Spencer Wells clamp and allow a little bleeding from the end of the shunt to ensure that it is completely filled and that all air has been ejected. Make a loop with the shunt and insert the other end into the distal internal carotid artery, ensuring that it enters freely without catching and that no air becomes trapped in the process. Apply the ring clamp and, after checking again to ensure there is no air trapped within the shunt, release the Spencer Wells clamp. There are at least 3 or 4 minutes of safe clamping time and without hurrying it usually takes less time than this to initiate flow through the shunt.

6 While an assistant holds open the loop of the shunt, commence the endarterectomy. Using a MacDonald's or Watson-Cheyne blunt dissector, find the plane in the common carotid artery. Develop this around the whole circumference and then cut the 'core' across neatly. Continue the endarterectomy distally and define the ostium of the external carotid artery. It may be best to terminate the endarterectomy here by cutting across it but the atheroma may extend for only a few millimetres into this vessel, in which case it often lifts out cleanly.

The most important part of the endarterectomy is its termination in the internal carotid artery. In most cases the atheroma 'feathers' away and the plaque lifts out without leaving any edge. If the atheroma does continue distally in this vessel and the plaque must be cut across, place a number of Kunlin sutures across the edge in order to prevent any chance of internal flap dissection (Fig. 23.36). This should rarely be necessary.

7 Once the core has been removed pay meticulous attention to the endarterectomized surface of the artery, recovering all loose flakes and strands, and flush it with heparinized saline (see General principles).

8 Close the arteriotomy with a patch. Simple closure without a patch may be acceptable if the diameter of the internal carotid artery is exceptionally large; which is sometimes the case in male patients. However, there is good scientific evidence to support the routine use of patches and there should, therefore, be few exceptions to this practice. Vein patches are associated with a risk of spontaneous rupture in this situation, with catastrophic consequences; therefore, patches of prosthetic materials are preferred. These are now manufactured specifically for this purpose. Roll the loop of the shunt towards the proximal end of the arteriotomy and commence the closure in the internal carotid. Use 6/0 polypropylene sutures. Finally, clamp the shunt and remove it. Re-apply clamps to the carotid vessels and complete the closure of the arteriotomy. Flush all vessels before tightening the last stitches.

9 *Declamping.* Remove the clamp from the internal carotid artery, allow blood to fill back into the bifurcation, displacing air through the suture line, and then re-apply the clamp to the internal carotid more proximal than previously placed, at the level of the bifurcation, to maximize flow into the external carotid artery and minimize emboli to the internal carotid artery. Remove the

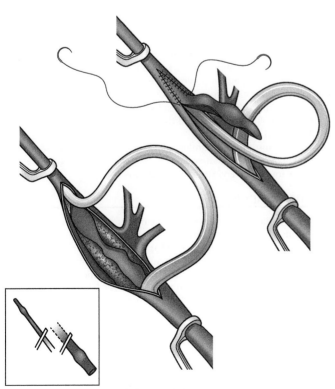

Fig. 23.35 Application of the Javid shunt.

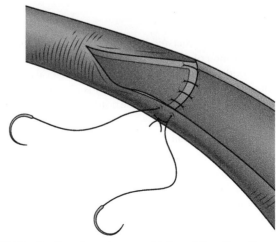

Fig. 23.36 Kunlin sutures to prevent internal flap dissection.

clamp from the external carotid and then from the common carotid. After three or four heart beats, finally remove the clamp again from the internal carotid artery. The purpose of this declamping procedure is to ensure that any retained air bubbles or small fragments of thrombus pass harmlessly into the external carotid and not into the brain.

? DIFFICULTY

1. The carotid bifurcation is situated high in the neck and it may be difficult to mobilize a sufficient length of the internal carotid artery for satisfactory control.
2. You can expose more of the vessel by extending the incision behind the ear onto the mastoid process. Raise the sternoleidomastoid muscle from its attachment and divide the digastric muscle. If necessary, excise the tip of the styloid process, but avoid damaging the facial nerve.
3. Usually it is sufficient to tunnel beneath the digastric muscle. You may also improve access by using a Pruit-Inahara shunt, which is retained with an intraluminal balloon rather than an external clamp.

Closure

1. Use a continuous 2/0 absorbable suture for the platysma muscle and a subcuticular suture for skin closure. Consider whether a small suction drain is needed (it may not be).
2. Reverse the heparin only if bleeding is excessive. Consider whether blood products are required if the patient is on dual antiplatelet therapy and has significant oozing.

Aftercare

1. Observe the pulse rate and blood pressure at quarter-hourly intervals for the first hour, half-hourly for 2 hours and then hourly.
2. Observe and chart neurological signs quarter-hourly for the first 3 hours.
3. If a drain was inserted, consider removal within 24 hours.
4. Discharge home when stable, usually on the second postoperative day.
5. Continue aspirin antiplatelet therapy indefinitely.

Complications

1. *Postoperative bradycardia and hypotension.* This may be associated with stimulation of the nerve to the carotid body. There is, however, no evidence that injecting the nerve with a local anaesthetic agent, as advocated by some surgeons, is of value. Administer atropine at intervals to increase the heart rate and cautiously give more fluid intravenously.
2. *Postoperative hypertension.* This must be controlled, if excessive, by the administration of appropriate drugs.
3. *Stroke.* If the patient develops a sudden severe neurological defect within the first few hours after operation this may be due to thrombotic occlusion of the artery. Scan the artery with Duplex ultrasound. If there is no flow in the artery or the results are

equivocal, return the patient to theatre immediately and re-explore the vessel. A less-severe neurological defect should simply be observed since it is likely to be transient and due to other causes.

4. *Neck haematoma.* A large tense haematoma is a potential cause of airways obstruction due to a combination of compression and laryngeal oedema and is dangerous. All wound haematomas of any size should be drained by re-opening the wound under local anaesthesia. Do not wait for a stridor or other evidence of airway obstruction before taking action.

5. *Cranial nerve lesions.* Temporary dysfunction of the hypoglossal or cervical branch of the facial nerve caused by retraction is common. Trauma to the hypoglossal nerve causes deviation of the protruded tongue to the ipsilateral side. Recovery within a few days is usual but, if permanent, most patients adapt well. Injury to the vagus nerve is manifest by hoarseness. In severe and permanent cases Teflon injections into the vocal cord by an ENT surgeon may help. The glossopharyngeal nerve is rarely damaged since it lies above and deep to the carotid bifurcation. However, injury to it is potentially troublesome since the patient may have difficulty in swallowing.

6. *Late occlusion of the internal carotid artery.* Surveillance by Duplex scanning shows that approximately 12% of carotid arteries become occluded within 5 years of endarterectomy. This is due to subintimal fibrous hyperplasia; it occurs slowly and is almost invariably asymptomatic. It must nevertheless be regarded as an undesirable outcome. Antiplatelet agents may help and there is evidence that the incidence is reduced by the routine application of patch closure rather than direct suturing of the arteriotomy. The indication for late surgical re-intervention is restenosis without total occlusion, accompanied by recurrent transient cerebral ischaemia symptoms. Such a lesion is likely to be due to recurrent atheroma rather than subintimal fibrous hyperplasia.

REFERENCES

1. Kirkpatrick UJ, McWilliams RG, Martin J, et al. Late complications after ligation and bypass for popliteal aneurysm. Br J Surg 2004;91:174–8.
2. European Carotid Surgery Trial Collaboration Group. MRC European Carotid Surgery Trial: interim results for symptomatic patients with severe (70–90%) or with mild (0–29%) carotid stenosis. Lancet 1991;357:1235–43.
3. National Institute of Neurological Disorders and Stroke. Clinical alert: benefit of carotid endarterectomy for patients with high grade stenosis of the internal artery. Stroke 1991;22:816–7.

FURTHER READING

EVAR Trial Participants. Endovascular aneurysm repair versus open repair in patients with abdominal aortic aneurysm (EVAR Trial 1): randomised controlled trial. Lancet 2005;365(20):2179–86.
EVAR Trial Participants. Endovascular aneurysm repair and outcome in patients unfit for open repair of abdominal aortic aneurysm (EVAR Trial 2): randomised controlled trial. Lancet 2005;365(20):2187–92.
The United Kingdom EVAR Trial Investigators. Endovascular repair of aortic aneurysm in patients physically ineligible for open repair. N Engl J Med 2010;362(20):1863–72.
The United Kingdom EVAR Trial Investigators. Endovascular repair of aortic aneurysm in patients physically ineligible for open repair. N Engl J Med 2010;362:1872–80.

Veins and lymphatics

M. Davis, D.M. Baker

CONTENTS

MANAGING LEG SUPERFICIAL VENOUS DISEASE (VARICOSE VEIN SURGERY)

Appraise

■ *Definition*

'Varicose veins' of the leg are classified according to their size:

1 Trunk (true) varicose veins are large tortuous dilated protruding superficial veins. They result from superficial venous incompetence due to valvular damage.

2 Reticular veins are small (2–3 mm), protrude and do not blanch on pressure.

3 Thread or spider veins are small (<1mm) intradermal subcutaneous veins, which blanch on pressure. Both reticular and thread veins result from alterations in the subcutaneous collagen, probably with local venous incompetence.

Trunk varicose veins can be both unsightly and produce symptoms; reticular and thread veins are unsightly but otherwise asymptomatic.

■ *Treatment indications*

The indications for treatment are to manage either venous complications or varicose vein symptoms. In general, the former are medically indicated, but the latter are to improve quality of life and therefore dependent on the patient's wishes.

Venous complications where varicose vein surgery may help include:

1 bleeding from varicose veins, which may occur as a result of trauma from sports, such as rugby, or at the delicate ankle skin secondary to venous hypertension

2 superficial thrombophlebitis which can be secondary to minor trauma to varicose veins as well as other causes such as malignancy. When the thrombus extends to near the saphenofemoral or popliteal junction urgent intervention is indicated to prevent progression. If not, intervention should be considered once the acute phlebitis has settled.

3 Ankle venous hypertensive skin changes. These include frank ulceration as well as lipodermatosclerotic skin thickening with haemosiderin pigmentation; the term does not apply to the age-related development of thread veins at the ankle. Treating any superficial venous incompetence will reduce the risk of ulcer recurrence, although it does not improve the rate of ulcer healing.

Varicose veins symptoms where surgery may help include:

1 Aching: Varicose veins produce a deep dull heavy aching fullness in the legs, which comes on when standing and is eased by elevating the leg or wearing support stockings. Any other leg discomfort is probably not due to venous disease, and venous treatment will not improve the discomfort.

2 Throbbing: The varicose veins can throb, and some patients refer to a sensation similar to water trickling down the leg.

3 Itching: The enlarged veins can itch, especially in warm conditions. This is worsened when eczematous skin changes develop.

4 Night cramps: These can be associated with varicose veins, although there are several other causes and intervention is not usually considered if this is the sole symptom.

5 Cosmesis: In Western society, especially amongst women, it is common to expose the legs.

6 Ankle oedema: This can also be associated with varicose veins, although there are many other causes and treatment solely for this symptom should generally be avoided.

■ *History and examination*

Despite the presence of trunk varicose veins, a careful history and examination are important to confirm that:

1 The symptoms match the signs and therefore the indications for treatment (as outlined above).

2 The veins are primary and not secondary and associated with a vascular malformation or more complex aetiology. Hints that the varicose veins may not be simple and primary include a history of leg fracture; repeated DVTs; venous or leg complications from abdominal surgery and pregnancy; abnormally placed varicose veins (such as laterally along the leg, vulval, or abdominal wall varices); erythematous leg birth marks, leg or foot size discrepancy.

■ *Investigations*

1 *Hand held Doppler*

Use of the hand held Doppler in the clinic adds little.

2 *Duplex colour ultrasound*

This is the mainstay of leg venous disease investigations. In both the deep and superficial leg venous systems it is used to determine:

- Venous flow: An occluded vein suggests the presence of thrombosis.
- Valve competency: Two-directional Doppler flow on calf compression and release indicates incompetence.
- Vein wall compliance: A patent vein that is difficult to compress on direct pressure suggests wall scarring, as occurs following phlebitis or a DVT.
- In complex cases the Duplex ultrasound scan will help define the venous anatomy and distinguish between low and high flow arteriovenous malformations.

Duplex ultrasound machines are becoming cheaper and more portable, and a Duplex scan should be considered before any leg venous surgical intervention.

3 *Magnetic resonance venography (MRV)*

MRV is reserved for complex venous disease, in particular when determining the distribution of a leg venous malformation or investigating suspected pelvic varices.

4 *Venography*

Reserved for treating (not investigating) complex malformations and pelvic varices.

- *Treatment options*

All varicose vein symptoms (apart from cosmesis) and complications of venous disease can be managed with compression hosiery, either graduated compression stockings or bandaging, usually to below the knee. However, continuous long-term compliance is necessary and this can be a considerable nuisance to the patient.

Do not carry out varicose vein surgery if the long saphenous vein forms an important collateral channel for obstructed deep veins. Arterial insufficiency is also a relative contraindication to varicose vein surgery.

20–30% of varicose vein operations are for persistent or recurrent varicosities following saphenous surgery.

There are three surgical steps to superficial venous disease intervention:

1 Dislocation of the superficial venous system from the deep venous system
2 Removal of the incompetent saphenous vein
3 Avulsion of the varicosities.

Specific surgical management of incompetent perforator branches connecting the superficial saphenous system to the deep veins of the leg is no longer undertaken, as perforator incompetence is usually reversed by the saphenous vein operation.

There are three ways of undertaking steps one and two:

1 Physically removing the saphenous vein (surgical ligation and stripping)
2 Thermally ablating the saphenous vein, the heat coming from an endovenous laser or radiofrequency source
3 Use of a sclerosant chemical to occlude the saphenous vein, which may be endovenous catheter-directed.

Medium-term results for varicose vein recurrence are comparable between the techniques. All techniques can be undertaken under local or general anaesthetic and are limited by the number of associated avulsions that are to be undertaken. Pain during the procedure is reportedly lower for radiofrequency ablation and the procedure quicker for sclerotherapy, but all allow return to work within a few days. Sclerotherapy probably has a higher incidence of haemosiderin skin pigmentation. It is wise to be familiar with all techniques and adopt the one best suited to the patient and your financial budget.

Preparation

1 Carefully re-examine patients admitted for varicose vein surgery. Confirm or exclude incompetence in the long and short saphenous veins and in the calf perforating veins.
2 Skin mark with an arrow the origin of the saphenous vein incompetence in the groin or popliteal fossa.
3 With the patient standing, mark all prominent varicosities with indelible pen as 'tram-lines' on either side of the vein to avoid 'tattooing' through the incision.
4 Preoperative marking with Duplex scanning is useful for locating the termination of the short saphenous vein and the sites of incompetent perforating veins.
5 Consent the patient for the planned procedure, warning of the risks of recurrent varicose veins, bleeding, wound infection, scarring and numbness from cutaneous nerve neuropraxia. With recurrent varicose veins warn of the risk of worsening ankle oedema.
6 Ensure that the equipment, including the ultrasound machine, is available and working.

HIGH SAPHENOUS VEIN LIGATION (TRENDELENBURG'S OPERATION) AND STRIPPING OF LONG SAPHENOUS VEIN

Appraise

1 Perform the operation, which was described by Friedrich Trendelenburg of Leipzig (1844–1924) in 1890, on patients with varicose veins who have long saphenous reflux at the groin.
2 Avoid the operation if the long saphenous vein is a collateral channel for obstructed deep veins.

Prepare

1 Have the skin of the groin and leg shaved before the operation.
2 Place the patient supine in the Trendelenburg position with approximately 30° of head-down tilt, both legs abducted by 20° from the midline and the ankles lying on a padded board. This allows easy access and reduces intra-operative haemorrhage (Fig. 24.1).
3 Prepare all exposed surfaces of the limb from the foot to the groin and up to the level of the umbilicus with aqueous 0.5% chlorhexidine acetate solution, while an assistant elevates the leg by lifting the patient's foot.

Access

1 Make an oblique incision just below and parallel to the inguinal ligament in the groin crease, over the saphenofemoral junction, which is lateral to the femoral pulse and medial to the adductor tendon/pubic tubercle (Fig. 24.2).

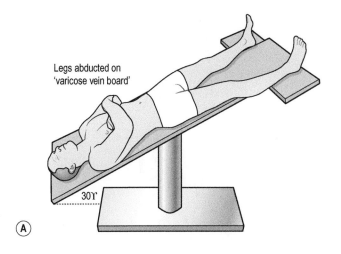

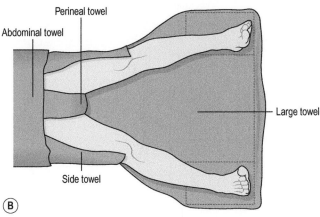

Fig. 24.1 The Trendelenburg position. (A) Head-down tilt. (B) Leg abduction.

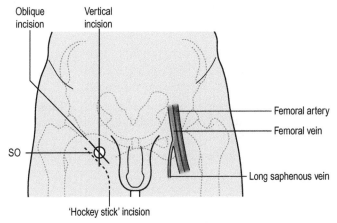

Fig. 24.2 Placing of incisions for access to veins in the groin. Three incisions are shown: vertical, straight oblique, and oblique 'hockey stick' curved. SO, saphenous opening.

2 Deepen the incision through the subcutaneous fat, which is spread by digital retraction, divide Scarpa's fascia and hold it apart by the insertion of a self-retaining retractor such as West's. Modify the length of incision depending on the build of the patient.

Action

1 Dissect the long saphenous vein out of the surrounding fat. Pass a controlling large tie around the vein and trace it upwards and

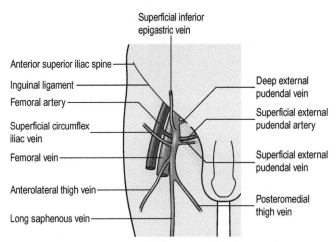

Fig. 24.3 The termination and tributaries of the long saphenous vein in the groin.

towards the saphenofemoral junction. The perivenous plane is simple to open and is bloodless when entered.

2 Dissect out all tributaries that join the long saphenous vein near its termination, ligating them with 3/0 absorbable suture before dividing them. The superficial inferior epigastric vein, the superficial circumflex iliac vein, and the superficial and deep external pudendal veins all join the saphenous trunk near its termination. In addition, the posteromedial and anterolateral thigh veins terminate close to the saphenofemoral junction (Fig. 24.3). One or more of these veins may join together before emptying into the saphenous trunk.

? DIFFICULTY

1. The long saphenous vein normally emerges as a dark-blue tube in the centre of the dissection as the subcutaneous fat is freed from its surface. If it is difficult to find, trace a smaller tributary back to the main trunk.
2. If bleeding occurs, it can appear significant as the hole is relatively small. Avoid repeated cautery with the diathermy or blindly applying artery clips. Pack the wound with a small swab and gain further control by applying direct external pressure to the femoral vein above and below the saphenofemoral junction. Reassess the situation: is it time to summon experienced vascular help? Set up the suction and warn the anaesthetist – it may only be a small tributary or it could be the femoral vein! Slowly move the swab, revealing different areas of the wound, until the bleeding point is found. Judiciously clip or superficially under-run the bleeding point.

---

3 After these tributaries have been divided, approach the saphenofemoral junction. The long saphenous vein dips down through the cribriform fascia over the foramen ovale to join the femoral vein. The femoral vein tends to be a lighter colour. Carefully separate the subcutaneous fat from the vein by blunt dissection to follow its path. Display the femoral vein for approximately 1 cm above the saphenofemoral junction, and clear any small

tributaries entering from either side. Dissecting the femoral vein downwards risks damaging the superficial external pudendal artery, which may pass either anterior or posterior to the saphenous vein. If damaged, ligate and divide it with impunity.

> ### ► KEY POINTS Anatomy of the saphenofemoral junction

- A variable number of tributaries join the long saphenous vein as it approaches the femoral vein.
- Occasionally the anterolateral and posteromedial thigh veins terminate independently into the femoral vein, giving the appearance of a double saphenous vein.
- The long saphenous vein may occasionally be truly bifid with one channel joining the femoral vein below the saphenous opening.
- Do not ligate or divide any large vessel until you have displayed the full anatomy of the long saphenous, its tributaries and its junction with the femoral vein.
- It is easy to mistake the femoral artery for the long saphenous vein, with disastrous consequences if it is inadvertently stripped.

4 Ligate the long saphenous vein in continuity with 2/0 absorbable suture, flush with the saphenofemoral junction, and divide it. For greater safety doubly ligate or transfix the saphenous stump. Alternatively, oversew the termination with a 3/0 polypropylene continuous suture.

5 Place a strong ligature around the divided distal end of the long saphenous trunk and hold it up to occlude retrograde blood flow, then make a small transverse venotomy below the ligature and introduce a disposable plastic stripper with a blunt tip into the saphenous vein. Gently manipulate the tip of the stripper downwards until it is a hand's breadth below the knee, where it may remain in the saphenous vein or pass into a tributary (Fig. 24.4). If it will not pass, withdraw the stripper and re-insert it with a rotational action. Tie the ligature at the top end to prevent blood from leaking out of the divided long saphenous trunk.

6 Make a short oblique incision in one of the skin crease tension lines, 1 cm in length, over the palpable tip of the stripper. Ensure that the incision is large enough to allow the head of the stripper to pass. Palpate the vein containing the stripper and dissect it off the saphenous nerve.

7 Make a small side-hole in the vein through which the tip of the stripper can be delivered. Tie the proximal end of the stripper to the long saphenous vein with a strong, long length of suture.

8 Strip the long saphenous vein from the groin to the knee with steady downward traction (invert strip). Ease the stripper and the bunched up vein through the lower incision. Clamp the attached long saphenous vein and any tributaries, divide and ligate it with 2/0 polyglactin.

9 Prevent excessive bleeding from the stripper track by gently rolling a swab along the course of the vein before applying bandages. Some surgeons apply a sterile tourniquet to the leg to prevent excessive haemorrhage.

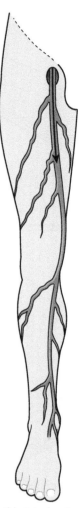

Fig. 24.4 Passage of a flexible intraluminal stripper in the long saphenous vein. Note the tributary below the knee into which the stripper may pass, leaving the main vein.

Closure

1 Inject 10 ml of 0.5% marcaine into the wound.

2 Appose the subcutaneous tissues and fascia with 2/0 absorbable sutures. Close the skin with 3/0 subcuticular sutures and apply Steri-Strip tapes.

3 Apply compression bandages to the whole leg to avoid haematoma formation.

Postoperative

1 Keep the leg elevated 15° above the horizontal in bed.

2 Encourage early mobilization after applying additional compression bandages over the bandages put on in the theatre. This reduces haematoma formation and provides better support when the patient stands. Thromboembolism prophylaxis stockings do not provide sufficient compression.

3 Advise the patient to walk rather than stand still or sit with the feet down.

4 Discharge fit patients on the day of surgery with advice on compression stockings, exercise and adequate hydration postoperatively.

1. The passage of the stripper may be impeded by competent valves, varicosity or false passages into small tortuous tributaries. Attempts to forcibly pass the stripper often end in perforation of the vein wall. If you encounter resistance, withdraw the stripper and re-pass it, twisting the free end to rotate the tip and facilitate negotiating irregularities in the vein.

2. If there is a hold-up around the knee, try flexing and extending the knee to aid the passage of the stripper, at the same time applying gentle external compression over the tip of the stripper to prevent it from passing into superficial tributaries.

3. If these measures fail, leave the stripper in situ. Pass a second stripper into the long saphenous vein from below the knee, then gradually withdraw the first stripper ahead of the advancing stripper passed from below.

4. If neither stripper will bypass the obstruction, cut down over the tips of both strippers. You may be able to re-direct one stripper through the cut-down incision and pass it down the vein, but if this fails strip out the two halves of the vein leaving a short residual portion between the two incisions. Alternatively, forcibly avulse this segment of residual vein.

SAPHENOPOPLITEAL LIGATION AND STRIPPING

Appraise

1. This is indicated if there is gross dilatation and reflux in the short saphenous trunk or its tributaries.

2. The location of the saphenopopliteal junction is very variable and, in a third of cases, the short saphenous vein enters the popliteal vein above or below the middle of the popliteal fossa.

3. Preoperative Duplex scanning and marking of the saphenopopliteal junction provide accurate information about the termination of the short saphenous vein and its proximal tributaries.

■ When you identify the saphenopopliteal junction, mark it on the skin.

4. Carry out short saphenous vein ligation first if you intend to strip the long saphenous vein under the same anaesthetic.

Prepare

1. Place the patient prone, with pillows under the chest, midriff and pelvis. This demands careful supervision from the anaesthetist to ensure that ventilation is maintained and the patient is safely placed on the operating table with adequate pressure area support.

2. If under general anaesthetic, place the operating table in 30° of head-down tilt and slightly abduct the legs to ease access.

Access

1. Make a 3-cm transverse incision at the site of preoperative marking in the popliteal fossa. Dissect down to the fascia and look for the blue of the vein deep to this. Divide the fascia transversely over the vein.

Action

1. Find the short saphenous vein in the popliteal fossa and dissect it from the surrounding fat and accompanying sural nerve, which is usually laterally placed.

2. Follow the short saphenous vein cranially as it dips down to the popliteal vein. Dissecting onto the popliteal vein can be difficult and risks damaging neighbouring structures. It is therefore wise to ligate the saphenous vein with an absorbable 2/0 suture as it dips down, and not at the popliteal vein junction. Ligate the saphenous vein more caudally and divide between the ligatures. Doubly ligate the stump of the short saphenous vein with 2/0 absorbable sutures.

3. In 2.5–10% of patients there is a tributary joining the short saphenous vein from above, known as the vein of Giacomini; carefully divide it between ligatures.

4. Stripping the short saphenous vein is not always undertaken:
   ■ If it is, place a strong ligature around the divided end of the short saphenous trunk and hold it up to occlude retrograde blood flow, make a small transverse venotomy and introduce a disposable plastic stripper into the saphenous vein.
   ■ Gently manipulate the tip of the stripper downwards until it is a hand's breadth above the lateral maleolus. Make a 1-cm vertical incision in a skin crease tension lines over the palpable stripper tip. Dissect the sural nerve off the vein containing the stripper. Deliver the stripper through the vein.
   ■ Tie the proximal end of the stripper to the short saphenous vein with a strong, long length of suture and strip the saphenous vein with steady downward traction.
   ■ Ease the stripper and the bunched up vein through the lower incision.
   ■ Clamp the attached saphenous vein and any tributaries, divide and ligate it with 2/0 polyglactin.

Closure

1. Irrigate the wound with 0.5% marcain local anaesthetic.

2. Use a continuous 2/0 absorbable suture to close the fascia and prevent herniation.

3. Close the skin with a 3/0 subcuticular suture and Steri-Strips.

Complications

1. These are similar to those of long saphenous vein surgery but with an additional risk of damage to the popliteal artery, vein and nerve during popliteal dissection. This is particularly likely if there has been previous knee surgery, such as a total knee replacement, as the anatomy may be distorted.

2 The sural nerve is easily damaged unless you gently dissect it free from the vein at the ankle. For this reason, some surgeons never strip the short saphenous vein. There is no controlled trial to settle this controversy and the subject remains a matter of opinion.

ENDOVENOUS THERMAL ABLATION OF THE LONG SAPHENOUS VEIN

Appraise

1 Endoluminal radiofrequency ablation (VNUS closure system) and endovascular laser treatment have been introduced as minimally invasive alternatives to ligation and stripping of the saphenofemoral or saphenopopliteal veins.

2 Both techniques aim to thermally damage the vessel intima, causing fibrosis and ultimately obliteration of the long saphenous vein trunk.

3 Under ultrasound guidance a catheter is percutaneously passed up the long saphenous vein from just below the knee to within 2 cm of the saphenofemoral junction. To dissipate heat produced by the laser or radio waves, local anaesthetic and saline solution is infiltrated around the long saphenous vein. The heated catheter is slowly withdrawn, closing the vein behind it.

4 The procedure needs to be undertaken under aseptic conditions, but is often performed in a treatment room rather than main operating theatre, especially if under local anaesthetic.

Prepare

1 Be happy with the layout of the theatre, in particular the positioning of the ultrasound machine and radiofrequency/laser equipment. Often it is easiest to sit on the side opposite the leg being treated, facing the machinery, which is on the same side as the affected leg. It is helpful to have the scrub nurse and trays on the same side as you at the foot end, ready to help feed guide-wires.

2 Check all equipment is available, working and compliant. Ensure the staff understand the procedure.

3 With the patient supine in a negative Trendelenburg position with approximately 30° of head-up tilt, prepare all exposed surfaces of the limb from the foot to the groin and up to the level of the umbilicus with aqueous 0.5% chlorhexidine acetate solution, while an assistant elevates the leg by lifting the patient's foot.

Action

1 The long saphenous vein is cannulated at the level of the knee. The ultrasound probe (Linear 38 mm Transducer) is placed in a sterile sleeve with sterile ultrasound jelly on the leg (use lots of it). At a depth of less than 4 cm the long saphenous vein is identified as a black hole in transverse section. The patency and size of the vein along its length from the saphenofemoral junction to below the knee is confirmed.

2 A one-part hollow needle is then inserted into the vein under ultrasound guidance. Initially attempt to cannulate the vein distally towards the foot, because if this fails and the vein goes into spasm, a more proximal part of the vein can still be used. Before attempting a second pass, flush the needle with normal saline.

You will know you are in the vein because blood flows freely from the needle.

3 Pass the guide-wire through the needle up into the saphenous vein. Occasionally, veins are small and a hydrophilic guide-wire is needed.

4 Confirm the guide-wire is in the vein by seeing the white dot in the black hole of the vein on ultrasound.

5 Pass the sheath over the guide-wire into the vein. Occasionally, a small nick in the skin is necessary to get the sheath through. Once the sheath introducer is removed, check there is good back-bleeding and flush the sheath.

6 Next insert the radiofrequency/laser catheter up the vein to within 2 cm of the saphenofemoral junction. This is ensured by measuring the distance on the patient and the catheter (in some cases the catheter has a light on its tip which can be seen through the skin) and by ultrasound identification of junction and catheter tip.

7 To dissipate the heat produced by the radiofrequency/laser catheter tip, local anaesthetic and saline solution is infiltrated around the long saphenous vein. Place the patient in Trendelenburg position with approximately 20° of head-down tilt. Under ultrasound guidance, starting at the knee and working towards the groin, inject saline around the vein. Adequate tumescence is achieved when on ultrasound the vein with the contained catheter is sitting free of surrounding tissues in a sea of saline. Some systems have a temperature probe at the tip, which falls to room temperature as tip tumescence is achieved. In total about 500 ml of saline is used.

8 The machine is then armed and the heat delivered at the catheter tip. Appropriate eye protection is worn by staff and patient before activating the laser. The catheter is slowly withdrawn, closing the vein behind it. Whether this is a continuous withdrawal or pulsed depends on the system used. Digital pressure is applied along the length of the vein treated to ensure good contact with the catheter, which is confirmed with ultrasound.

9 Following the procedure it is the surgeon's preference as to whether multiple avulsions are also undertaken. The lower limb is dressed with compression bandaging or hosiery.

? DIFFICULTY

1. If it is difficult to cannulate the long saphenous vein, increase the degree of head up to maximize venous pooling and attempt to cannulate in a fresh area of vein using a fresh, flushed, finer cannulating needle. Once in the vein, if there is any back-bleeding use a hydrophilic fine wire to cannulate the vein.

ENDOVENOUS THERMAL ABLATION OF THE SHORT SAPHENOUS VEIN

Appraise

The technique is similar to that for the long saphenous vein. Under ultrasound guidance a catheter is percutaneously passed up the short saphenous vein from a hand's breath above the ankle to within 2 cm of the saphenopopliteal junction. To dissipate heat produced by the radiofrequency/laser, local anaesthetic and saline solution is infiltrated around the short saphenous vein. The heated catheter is slowly withdrawn, closing the vein behind it.

ULTRASOUND-GUIDED FOAM SCLEROTHERAPY

Appraise

1. The foam causes an inflammatory reaction in the vein wall, destroying the vein lumen and blocking the vein.

2. When consenting the patient, ensure they are aware of the risks of superficial thrombophlebitis (sometimes treated subsequently by stab incisions over the vein and removing the clot), brown pigmentation, deep vein thrombosis, skin ulceration, allergic reaction to sclerosant and visual disturbances. Stroke has been reported in only two cases, due to high volume injection and a patent foramen ovale.

3. It is usually best to use foam sclerotherapy for patients with moderate-sized incompetent saphenous veins. It is therefore best suited to residual incompetent saphenous vein branches.

4. The procedure is undertaken in a clinic treatment room and not in theatre.

5. Rigorous compliance with compression for several days is vital for success.

Action

1. With the patient supine in negative Trendelenburg position, under aseptic conditions, the incompetent long saphenous vein is identified using ultrasound and cannulated in the calf as described above.

2. The sclerosant is foamed by passing 5 ml of sclerosant (Fibrovein 1%) back and forth between two 20-ml syringes, each containing 10 ml of carbon dioxide plus oxygen, via a three-way tap.

3. The leg is elevated and all blood removed from the collapsed long saphenous vein by milking the vessel from knee to groin.

4. The sclerosant is then injected slowly via the cannula into the saphenous vein. Its course along the vein is monitored by ultrasound. During this the patient is asked to bend their ankles up and down to increase the blood flow in the deep veins.

5. When the foam has filled the entire saphenous vein, the top end of the vein is compressed with the ultrasound probe to keep the foam in the superficial veins.

6. Once enough foam has been injected, the needle(s) are removed and pieces of sponge applied to the leg along the course of the long saphenous vein, followed by a bandage to compress the treated veins (such as Panalast or Colband). A full thigh-length elastic compression stocking is then put on top of this, with a waist attachment to ensure it stays in place.

7. The sponge, bandage and stocking are kept on continuously for 5 days. After this the sponges and bandage are removed and the stocking worn for a further 7 days.

AVULSION OF SUPERFICIAL VARICOSITIES

Appraise

1. Excise large branch veins that are not in close proximity to the saphenous or perforator systems to prevent unsightly local recurrences and provide a satisfactory cosmetic result.

2. Carefully mark out the superficial varicose veins preoperatively in the standing patient, as varicosities are not visible when the patient is anaesthetized and the legs are elevated.

Action

1. Make minute stab incisions over the course of tributaries in the direction of skin tension lines. Draw out a loop of vein by gentle blunt dissection, using specially designed hooks or mosquito artery forceps.

2. Divide the loop between mosquito forceps and tease out the vein in either direction by exerting steady traction and gentle blunt dissection under the skin with fine mosquito forceps.

3. Employ a gentle circular motion on the forceps to help separate the tethering fibrous tissue from the vein.

4. Release traction when the vein starts to stretch, and at this point ligate both ends. Alternatively, continue the traction until the vein breaks, controlling bleeding by local pressure until traumatic venospasm develops.

5. Place incisions 5 cm apart along the course of each tributary. This technique can be used to remove a long segment of varicose vein through 3–5 small incisions.

? DIFFICULTY

1. Reduce local blood loss by performing the avulsions after the limb has been exsanguinated with a tourniquet.

Closure

1. Use Steri-Strip tape to close the avulsion incision.

SURGICAL MANAGEMENT OF RECURRENT VARICOSE VEINS

Appraise

1. *Recurrent varicose veins* are veins that have become varicose after the original treatment. In contrast, *residual varicose veins* refer to those that were not treated at the original procedure (Fig. 24.5).

2. The causes of recurrent veins include:
   - Disease progression, with the development of new venous incompetence between the deep and superficial venous system
   - Inadequate primary procedure, if the tributaries are left unligated, especially in the presence of a dual saphenous system that was not recognized or removed
   - Development of new bridging channels (neovascularization): collaterals may develop following simple ligation, reconnecting the deep veins to the saphenous vein.

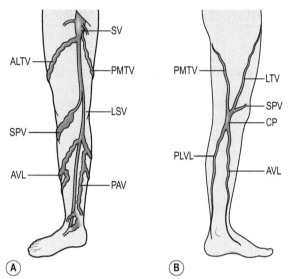

Fig. 24.5 (A) The major superficial tributaries of the long saphenous vein which become varicose. Note that the long saphenous vein itself rarely becomes varicose. (B) The superficial veins on the lateral aspect of the leg. These usually drain into the long saphenous system and are a common site for postoperative recurrences. ALTV, anterolateral thigh vein; AVL, anterior vein of leg (accessory saphenous vein); CP, crossing point; LSV, long saphenous vein; PAV, posterior arch vein; PLVL, posterolateral vein of the leg; PMTV, posteromedial thigh vein; SPV, superior patella vein; SV, saphenous vein.

3 The indications to treat recurrent varicose veins are similar to those for primary varicose veins, but the risk of complications is higher.

4 Diligently examine the varicosities, looking carefully for the scars of a previous operation.

5 Duplex ultrasound is essential to detect reflux in the saphenous veins and in large calf perforators.

6 The same techniques are available for removing incompetent veins as are employed for primary veins (described above). However, open surgical re-exploration, although technically more complete, can be difficult and lead to complications. Recurrent varicose veins are often thin-walled, multiple and easily damaged. Haemorrhage from torn veins can be severe. Persistent lymph leak can occur and damage to local structures such as nerves and vessels is a risk. *For this reason, if possible, an endovenous ablation or sclerotherapy occlusion is the treatment of choice.*

OPEN SURGERY FOR GROIN RECURRENCES

Access

1 Operate for recurrent varicose veins under general anaesthesia.

2 Position the patient as for the primary procedure.

Action

1 Make an adequate incision to ensure good operative access. Incise in the groin crease centred on the saphenofemoral junction, 5 cm in length, extending laterally over the femoral pulse.

2 To reduce the risk of bleeding employ an approach through previously undissected tissue planes, which enables anatomical landmarks and vascular control to be established before tackling the recurrent varices. Expose the anterior surface of the femoral artery to facilitate access to the femoral vein.

3 Approach the saphenofemoral junction from the lateral side through relatively normal tissues. Open the femoral sheath to expose the anterior surface of the femoral artery.

4 Carefully dissect medially and expose the anterior surface of the femoral vein. Dissect it clean and locate the saphenofemoral junction.

5 Clear the saphenous stump on all sites close to the femoral vein until you can pass a Lahey forceps around it. Ligate it with 2/0 absorbable suture before dividing it. For added safety, transfix the stump.

6 Ligate all tributaries individually with 2/0 absorbable suture and divide them.

7 Strip the long saphenous vein if it is still present and avulse all superficial varicose veins in the usual manner.

Closure

1 Close the subcutaneous tissue with interrupted 2/0 absorbable sutures.

2 Close the skin with 3/0 subcuticular sutures and Steri-Strip tape.

Complications

1 Second operations are always more difficult than the primary procedure. If you do not fully display the anatomy it is easy to damage the major vessels.

2 Take care not to damage the femoral nerve during the lateral approach.

3 Lymphocele or lymph fistula may develop postoperatively, but usually resolves spontaneously.

SAPHENOPOPLITEAL RECURRENCES

Appraise

1 Arrange for the saphenopopliteal junction and short saphenous vein to be marked preoperatively using Duplex ultrasound.

Access

1 Make a vertical or S-shaped incision across the centre of the popliteal fossa.

2 Enter the popliteal fossa through a posterior approach and identify the popliteal artery and vein before ligating the varices.

Action

1 Deepen the incision through the subcutaneous tissues.

2 Identify the popliteal artery and vein well above the previous scar tissue and trace them down until you are able to identify the stump of the short saphenous vein.

- Avoid damaging the nerve, which lies superficial to the popliteal vessels.

3 Divide and ligate all the tributaries entering the popliteal vein, and especially the stump of the short saphenous vein.

4 Strip out any residual short saphenous vein or perform multiple avulsions.

Closure

1 Close the subcutaneous tissue with interrupted 2/0 absorbable sutures.

2 Close the skin with 3/0 subcuticular sutures and Steri-Strip tape.

Technical point

- Tourniquets reduce blood loss during varicose vein surgery and so shorten the duration of the operation. There is also a lesser incidence of postoperative haematoma. They may, however, cause nerve damage.

OPERATIONS FOR DEEP VEIN THROMBOSIS

Appraise

1 **There are very few indications for open deep vein surgery.** Anticoagulant treatment is commonly used for the treatment of deep vein thrombosis (DVT).

2 There are two forms of deep vein intervention:
- Venous thrombectomy is usually performed to remove a fresh (less than 5 days old), loose and non-adherent thrombus.
- Insertion of filters to 'lock in' thrombus and prevent pulmonary embolism.

3 Operations are not indicated when the thrombus is more than 5 days old, fixed or totally occlusive. Surgery is also inappropriate when the thrombus is confined to the calf. These patients are best treated with anticoagulants.

4 Treat the uncommon complication of venous pregangrene (phlegmasia caerulen dolens) and gangrene by catheter-directed thrombolysis or venous thrombectomy.

5 Procedures to lock in the thrombus are indicated if anticoagulation is an unacceptable risk, e.g. prior to major abdominal surgery, or ineffective, especially when repeated pulmonary emboli occur despite adequate anticoagulant treatment.

6 Procedures to lock in the thrombus are thought to lower the mortality from pulmonary embolism in patients with loose propagated thrombus extending into the femoral or abdominal veins, although this has never been tested in a prospective randomized trial.

ILIOFEMORAL VENOUS THROMBECTOMY

Prepare

1 Be warned this can be a significant operation for surgeon and patient.

2 Commence treatment dose intravenous heparin before going to theatre.

3 Have a radiographically-placed IVC filter in situ (see below).

4 Patients are usually unwell and general anaesthetic is preferred, using endotracheal intubation and positive-pressure ventilation to stop any loose thrombi being propagated to the lungs, thus preventing intra-operative embolism.

5 Position the patient supine with the legs abducted on a radiolucent operating table.

6 Insert an indwelling urinary catheter to prevent phlebography from being obscured by the accumulation of dye in the bladder.

Access

1 Make a vertical incision over the femoral vein, extending from the midinguinal point to the centre of the thigh for 15–20 cm.

2 Divide the subcutaneous fat down to the deep fascia. The long saphenous vein lies medially, and can be traced up to the saphenofemoral junction.

3 Incise the deep fascia over the femoral vein in a vertical direction and gently dissect the femoral vein from the femoral artery on its lateral border. Use sharp dissection and avoid handling the vein if it contains loose thrombus.

4 Gently pass Silastic slings around the femoral vein above and below the profunda femoris vein, which is also snared.

Assess

1 Confirm the presence of thrombus within the femoral vein by gentle finger palpation.

Action

If thrombus is present in the iliac vein

1 Tip the operating feet down (30°) to ensure caudal blood flow in the vein and minimize the risk of pulmonary embolism.

2 Administer 5000 units of heparin and make a short transverse venotomy. When the loose thrombus has been flushed out of the venotomy by retrograde flow, pass a large Fogarty venous thrombectomy catheter (size 6–8 F) into the inferior vena cava. Inflate the balloon with contrast medium and withdraw it under fluoroscopic control while reducing the balloon diameter until it lies against the orifice of the common iliac vein. Beware of inadvertent insertion into a lumbar vein. Tighten the Silastic tubing around the catheter to prevent troublesome back-bleeding.

3 Pass a second large Fogarty catheter past the iliac thrombus, inflate the balloon and withdraw it to extract the thrombus. Repeat this until no further thrombus is obtained (Fig. 24.6).

4 When all the thrombus appears to have been removed, deflate the caval balloon slightly and withdraw it to remove any loose thrombus that it has trapped.

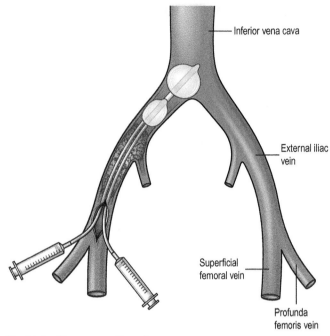

Fig. 24.6 Iliac venous thrombectomy.

5 Infuse heparinized saline into the iliac vein and ensure that all the thrombus has been removed. Confirm this using completion phlebography.

6 Residual thrombus may be compressed against the vein wall by deploying a stent.

7 Remove any distal thrombus by the technique described above and close the venotomy with a continuous 6/0 polypropylene suture.

8 Close the wound in layers. Continue systemic anticoagulation postoperatively.

If thrombus is present in the femoral vein

1 Give 5000 units of heparin.

2 Apply bulldog clamps on the proximal femoral and superficial femoral veins. Pass a suitable Fogarty venous thrombectomy catheter (4–5F) through a transverse venotomy as far distally as competent valves allow. The catheter rarely passes far down the leg.

3 Pull up the Silastic sling to prevent back-bleeding while the catheter is passed and withdrawn.

4 Inflate the catheter balloon and withdraw it slowly, pulling out the loose thrombus.

5 Thrombus must also be removed by manual compression applied along the line of the veins of the calf and thigh muscle or by applying a sterile Esmarch bandage around the limb. Distal thrombus can theoretically be removed using a Fogarty venous thrombectomy catheter passed through a tibial vein.

6 When no more thrombus can be obtained, close the venotomy with a 6/0 polypropylene suture and the wound in layers.

Postoperative care

1 Keep the patient on subcutaneous, low-molecular-weight heparin and allow mobilization while wearing a compression stocking on the day after surgery.

2 Start an oral anticoagulant until therapeutic range is achieved. The required duration of oral anticoagulation is variable and will be determined by the pathology identified.

3 Advise the patient to wear graduated compression stockings to prevent the development of post-thrombotic syndrome.

INSERTION OF VENA CAVAL FILTERS

Appraise

1 There is no indication for open caval clipping. However, it is helpful to remember in times of uncontrollable caval bleeding secondary to trauma that the IVC can be ligated with only a 30% incidence of lower limb oedema.

2 The insertion of a vena caval filter should only be considered when there is a contraindication to anticoagulation (for example imminent surgery, intolerance of or side-effects to warfarin or pulmonary embolus despite adequate anticoagulation).

3 Vena cava filters (Fig. 24.7) are inserted percutaneously into the inferior vena cava, via the groin or internal jugular vein over a guide-wire under local anaesthesia, rather than by open surgical insertion.

4 Some filters are temporary and consideration should be given to when they should be removed.

Access

1 As when inserting a central line, with the patient in a head down position and under ultrasound guidance, percutaneously cannulate the right internal jugular vein using a hollow needle through

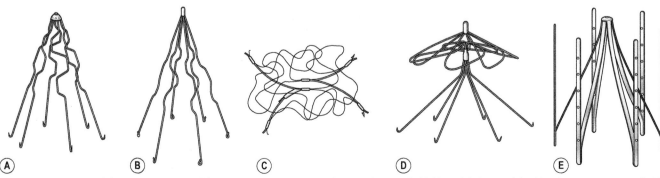

Fig. 24.7 Diagram of the permanent caval filter modules: (A) the stainless steel Greenfield filter; (B) the modified hook titanium Greenfield filter; (C) the birds' nest filter; (D) the Simon nitinol filter; (E) the Venea Tech filter.

a small incision placed over the sternomastoid muscle, 2 cm above the clavicle. Pass a guide wire through the needle into the vein and with fluoroscopy confirm its position into the superior vena cava, atrium and inferior vena cava.

2. Pass a dilating sheath over the guide wire if necessary.

3. Insert the catheter containing the filter over the wire through the sheath, and screen it into the inferior vena cava using an image intensifier.

4. Prevent blood loss by placing a finger over the sheath, but keep the patient head down to prevent air entry.

5. When the catheter lies in the vena cava below the renal veins, deploy the filter, which attaches to the side-wall of the cava by a series of tiny barbs around its periphery. These barbs are designed to prevent the filter from migrating, which is the major complication of the procedure. Incorrect siting of the filter may also be a problem. The mode of filter deployment depends on the filter used: many are re-deployable if positioning is not perfect.

Postoperative

1. Maintain intravenous heparinization for a minimum of 48 hours after the procedure unless there is a strong contraindication.

2. All patients who have had a severe deep vein thrombosis need to wear graduated compression elastic stockings to prevent the development of post-thrombotic syndrome and venous ulceration in the future.

> ▶ KEY POINT Indications?
>
> ■ Consider catheter directed thrombolysis and insertion of caval filters in patients with severe leg swelling or a pulmonary embolus.

OPERATIONS FOR VENOUS ULCER AND POST-THROMBOTIC SYNDROME

Appraise

A plethora of operations have been described to treat saphenous and communicating vein reflux to prevent recurrent venous ulceration in post-thrombotic limbs: all have been unsuccessful.

Saphenous transposition (Palma operation)
(Fig. 24.8)

1. This is valuable for symptomatic venous claudication but use it only:
   - ■ When the femoral venous pressure rises on exercise
   - ■ In the absence of naturally developed suprapubic collateral channels, which are often massive.

2. Dissect the contralateral saphenous vein down and mobilize it until it can be taken through a suprapubic tunnel to anastomose it to the common femoral or profunda femoris vein of the opposite limb, thus providing a collateral channel for a single blocked iliac segment.

3. Patency of the bypass may be improved with an arteriovenous fistula.

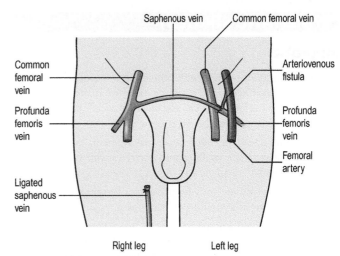

Fig. 24.8 Saphenous transposition.

Valve repair, replacement, autograft insertion and plastic venocuffs

Attempts to repair, replace, strengthen and autograft valves have all been unsuccessful and should not be considered.

SPLIT SKIN GRAFT FOR VENOUS ULCERATION

Appraise

1. A useful adjunct to venous ulcer management and should be considered in clean wounds that are slow to heal despite optimum wound care and compression bandaging.

Prepare

1. The ulcer base should be optimized by bed rest and intensive antiseptic cleaning.

2. The procedure is performed under local anaesthesia. Ensure that the ulcer is clear of infection by microscopy and culture before attempting grafting. Prepare the ulcer by excising the basal tissues with a Humby or Braithwaite knife, using tangential excision, until healthy tissue is reached.

3. Meshed split skin grafts (2:1 ratio) should be applied to the dry base using staples. 'Postage stamp' or pinch grafts can be used as an alternative.

4. Reapply compression dressings in theatre. Failure to do so will result in graft loss. If the leg is very oedematous despite pre-grafting compression, a negative-vacuum pump dressing can be applied over the graft, under the compression bandage.

Postoperative

1. Review the wound **personally** at 48 to 72 hours. Remove the dressings carefully. Aggressively treat any exudates and slough. Re-dress and maintain compression.

LYMPHATIC SURGERY

Appraise

1 The majority of patients with primary and secondary lymphoedema respond readily to active conservative treatment. Regular leg elevation, elastic support and massage are all that are needed to maintain an acceptable level of swelling.

2 If, despite adequate conservative management, the patient develops severe limb swelling that interferes with mobility, consider operative treatment.

3 Such surgery should only be performed by lymphoedema specialists as part of a multidisciplinary team.

4 Perform bilateral isotope or contrast lymphography in patients considered for lymphatic surgery. This displays anatomical information about the site and cause of the lymphatic impairment and may help to select the appropriate surgical procedure. Most patients with primary lymphoedema have slowly progressive distal lymphatic hypoplasia. A smaller number suffer progressive fibrosis of the proximal lymph nodes, leading to obstruction. The distal lymphatics also slowly disappear in these patients. A few have obstruction of the thoracic duct, and a few have megalymphatics with valvular incompetence.

5 Surgery for lymphoedema can be divided into two broad approaches:
   ■ *Reduction operations.* The lymphoedematous subcutaneous tissue and skin are excised; these procedures can be used to treat all forms of lymphoedema.
   ■ *Bypass operations.* These procedures have not found widespread acceptance in clinical practice. They bypass sites of localized lymphatic obstruction, and are suitable for patients with a proximal occlusion and normal distal lymphatics. The mesenteric bridge operation may be applicable for patients with obstruction of the femoral or pelvic lymph nodes. Lymphovenous anastomosis has also been proposed as a means of bypassing lymphatic obstruction. These will not be considered further.

6 Fully inform the patients about the surgery that is proposed for them. They should have a realistic appreciation of the expected functional and cosmetic results (Fig. 24.9). Patients must understand that lymphatic surgery is palliative, and further surgery may be necessary at a later date.

REDUCTION OPERATIONS

Prepare

1 Minimize swelling prior to surgery with a period of bed rest and limb elevation and by compression bandaging.

2 Eradicate sepsis prior to surgery. Swab possible sites of infection on admission and send for microscopy and culture. Antibiotics are prescribed selectively. Clean the limb twice daily in an antiseptic bath, paying special attention to the skin creases. Tinea pedis commonly develops between swollen lymphoedematous toes. Take a skin scraping if the diagnosis is suspected and prescribe a suitable antifungal treatment such as terbinafine.

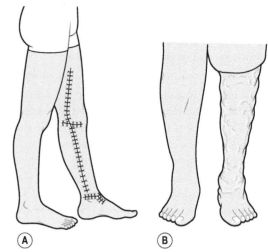

Fig. 24.9 Cosmetic results of reduction operations: (A) Homans' operation; (B) Charles' operation.

3 Perform reduction operations under general anaesthesia with the patient in a supine position.

4 Position the limb to facilitate operative access. For procedures on the medial side of the leg, elevate the limb to about 30–45° and widely abduct it. This is best achieved by inserting a Kirschner wire through the calcaneum and connecting a metal stirrup to the wire on each side of the foot before elevating the leg with a pulley system. Lower the foot of the operating table and flex the contralateral knee. Stand on the medial side of the leg, between the limb and the operating table.

5 To reduce blood loss, place a tourniquet around the upper thigh and inflate it to 350 mmHg after the limb has been exsanguinated with an Esmarch bandage. Note the time of tourniquet application.

CHARLES' OPERATION

Action

1 Described by the English surgeon R.H. Charles in 1912, it aims to excise the lymphoedematous skin and subcutaneous tissue between the knee and the ankle, including the dorsum of the foot. This is the procedure of choice when the skin is greatly thickened and abnormal. Preserve skin cover over the knee and the ankle in order to retain the mobility of these joints (Fig. 24.10).

2 Cover the exposed deep fascia of the leg with split skin grafts taken from the trunk or from the contralateral limb.

3 Take darts of redundant skin and subcutaneous tissue from the medial and lateral sides of the leg at the knee and ankle to prevent a marked 'step' effect and an ugly appearance similar to pantaloons.

4 Staple the skin grafts to the deep fascia and cover them with non-adherent dressings and thick cotton wool held in place with crepe bandages.

5 Plan to maintain elevation of the limb for 1 week, before removing the bandages and inspecting the limb.

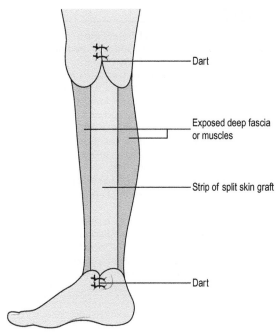

Fig. 24.10 Charles' leg reduction operation.

Complications

1 Delayed healing may be a problem if the split skin graft fails to take.

> ▶ KEY POINT Spare skin
>
> ■ Take spare skin grafts at the initial operation; these can be applied to unhealed areas in the ward at a later stage.

2 Hypertrophic and keloid scars sometimes develop in the grafted skin. Hypertrophic scarring is often associated with chronic infection: treat it by regular cleansing and antibiotics. Prominent tissue can be shaved off with a skin-graft knife. Keloid scars may need to be excised and re-grafted.

3 The Charles' operation is very effective at reducing the excessive bulk of lymphoedematous tissues around the leg and improving mobility. The final appearance is, however, often bizarre, with swollen feet and thighs joined by a narrow calf.

HOMANS' OPERATION

Appraise

1 John Homans (1877–1954) was Professor of Surgery at Harvard, Boston. Lymphoedematous swelling of moderate severity in limbs with relatively normal skin is best treated by the operation he described.

2 The operation is usually first performed on the medial side of the limb, but the tissues on the lateral side can also be reduced. If you intend to operate on both sides, stage the procedures over 3 months, otherwise skin viability is compromised if the excision extends beyond half the circumference of the limb.

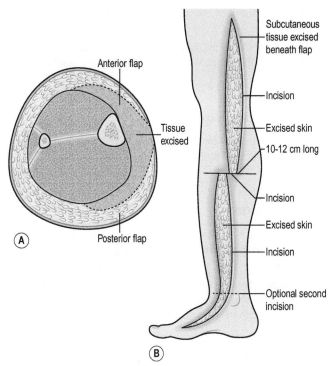

Fig. 24.11 Homans' medial leg reduction operation. (A) The skin flaps. (B) Longitudinal and transverse incisions.

3 Aim to excise lymphoedematous subcutaneous tissues and redundant skin from one side of the limb. When the limb is viewed in cross-section the excised tissues appeared wedge-shaped (Fig. 24.11A).

4 Raise the skin flaps first, then excise the underlying fat. Overlap the skin flaps to decide how much redundant skin needs to be excised.

Action

1 Make a longitudinal incision from a hand's breadth below the knee to a similar distance above the ankle, beginning just behind the posterior border of the tibia, ending anterior to the medial malleolus. Transverse incisions may also be necessary at each of the longitudinal incisions (Fig. 24.11B).

2 Raise skin flaps in an anterior and posterior direction, increasing in thickness towards the base of the flap. Extend the flaps for 10–12 cm around the leg or as far as the midline in each direction.

3 Excise all the underlying subcutaneous tissue not included in the skin flaps down to the deep fascia. Excise any superficial veins and cutaneous nerves with this block of tissue.

4 Overlap the flaps and mark the redundant skin to be excised, allowing for primary closure of the incision. Having excised the skin, if necessary, trim the skin flaps in a longitudinal direction. Excise darts at the ankle and knee to avoid dog-ears. The darts should meet the transverse incision at a different point from the longitudinal incision to reduce the chance of wound breakdown. The upper dart may be extended a considerable distance up the limb towards the groin to allow a simple wedge excision of the skin and subcutaneous tissues of the thigh, as shown in Figure 24.11.

5 Close the skin with interrupted sutures or staples over suction drains.

6 Apply a non-adherent dressing to the suture lines and dress the whole limb from the base of the toes with cotton wool and crepe bandages.

Postoperative care

Nurse the patient with the foot of the bed elevated 10°. Take down the dressing and remove the drains after 1 week, then mobilize the patient.

Complications

1 Although the early results appear good, many patients develop recurrent limb swelling, eventually approaching preoperative dimensions.

2 Repeated reduction surgery may be necessary. Combined with good elastic stocking support, this often produces an acceptable limb, although its size is rarely normal.

3 Skin necrosis, infection and haematoma formation are all recognized problems.

> ► KEY POINTS Skin-flap necrosis
>
> ■ Avoid haematoma formation by meticulous haemostasis.
> ■ Do not risk skin-flap necrosis; avoid cutting the flaps too thin or extending the undermining too far.

FURTHER READING

Adam DJ, Bello M, Hartshorne T, et al. Role of superficial venous surgery in patients with combined superficial and segmental deep venous reflex. Eur J Vasc Endovasc Surg 2003;25:469–72.

Amarigi SV, Lees TA. Elastic compression stockings for prevention of deep vein thrombosis. Cochrane Database Syst Rev 2000:(3). CD001484.

Barwell JR, Davies CE, Deacon J, et al. Comparison of surgery and compression with compression alone in chronic venous ulceration (ESCHAR study): randomised controlled trial. Lancet 2004;363:1854–9.

Browse N. Diseases of the Veins. 2nd ed. London: Arnold; 1999.

Burnand K. The New Aird's Companion in Surgical Studies. 2nd ed. Edinburgh: Churchill Livingstone; 1998.

Campisi C, Boccardo F, Zilli A, et al. Long-term results after lymphatic-venous anastomoses for the treatment of obstructive lymphedema. Microsurgery 2001;21:135–9.

Corrales NE, Irvine A, McGuiness CL, et al. Incidence and pattern of long saphenous vein duplication and its possible implications for recurrence after varicose vein surgery. Br J Surg 2002;89:323–6.

Dwerryhouse S, Davies B, Harradine K, et al. Stripping the long saphenous vein reduces the rate of reoperation for recurrent varicose veins: five-year results of a randomized trial. J Vasc Surg 1999;29:589–92.

Elias M, Frasier KL. Minimally invasive vein surgery: its role in the treatment of venous stasis ulceration. Am J Surg 2004;188:26–30.

Kalra M, Gloviczki P. Surgical treatment of venous ulcers: role of subfascial endoscopic perforator vein ligation. Surg Clin North Am 2003;83:671–705.

Serror P. Sural nerve lesions: a report of 20 cases. Am J Phys Med Rehabil 2002;81:876–80.

Zamboni P, Cisno C, Marchetti F, et al. Minimally invasive surgical management of primary venous ulcers vs. compression treatment: a randomized clinical trial. Eur J Vasc Endovasc Surg 2003;25:313–8.

Zierau UT, Kullmer A, Kunkel HP. Stripping the Giacomini vein: pathophysiologic necessity or phlebosurgical games? Vasa 1996;25:142–7.

25

Sympathectomy and the management of hyperhidrosis

D.M. Baker

ASSESSMENT OF HYPERHIDROSIS

Appraise

1 Hyperhidrosis is uncontrolled profuse sweating. It is classified as either local, affecting only specific areas, or general, affecting most parts of the body. It affects up to 2% of the population, and there is probably a genetic predisposition. The axillae are affected in 60% of cases, the palms (often with the feet) in 30%, the head and neck in 10% and the rest of the body, especially under the breasts in females and groins in 5%. Even in localized cases of hyperhidrosis more than one localized area is often affected.

2 It is a social problem. Confirm the diagnosis is of *hyperhidrosis* (hyper = over + hidros = sweat) and not a complaint of malodour or other dermatological problems such as hydradenitis suppurativa (chronic infection of the apocrine sweat glands). In general those with hyperhidrosis do not have body malodour and the sweat is clear and profuse. Examine each potentially affected area to confirm this.

3 *Identify an underlying cause.* Primary causes tend to result in generalized rather than localized hyperhidrosis. Endocrine causes include thyroid dysfunction and progesterone/oestrogen imbalance, as occurs with polycystic ovary syndrome or the menopause. Take blood samples on the first consultation. Head injury or the use of certain medications can also produce hyperhidrosis.

4 *Determine the severity of the hyperhidrosis* by determining specific occasions when hyperhidrosis is a problem. Sweating may occur at a lower than usual ambient temperature and may be precipitated during social confrontation. It is not always necessary to use a social anxiety psychological scoring systems to demonstrate this, but determining the use of avoidance techniques indicates the degree of severity. Axillary sweaters often prefer wearing black or dark tops, doubled so sweat stains do not show. They insert tissues or commercially purchased pads and avoid loose singlets. Palm sweaters may carry a hand-held article to avoid shaking hands on greeting and hold hands only outside in the cold. True plantar sweaters wear loose, regularly replaced shoes, because sweat rots the fabric. Forehead sweaters tend to avoid spicy foods.

For research purposes the degree of sweating within a heated ambience can be assessed by the weight increase of applied blotting paper.

5 Arrange a sensitively conducted psychological assessment, clarifying its potential benefits. Emphasize that hyperhidrosis is a life-long problem capable only of alleviation by intervention, not cure.

> ▶ KEY POINTS
>
> ■ Hyperhidrosis, although debilitating, is a social problem.
> ■ Make decisions regarding intervention with a fully informed and involved patient.

MANAGEMENT OF HYPERHIDROSIS

1 Aim to treat both the physical and psychological effects. Tailor the range of proffered management to the site, severity, awareness of involved area and perceived severity of disability. Involve the fully informed patient in planning management, fully aware of the implications, actively concurring. Re-discuss the planned treatments and potential side-effects before you embark on a new treatment.

2 Patients with localized hyperhidrosis will usually have tried over-the-counter antiperspirants, often aluminium salt-based. The low pH of these can produce skin irritation, but if they are effective further treatment is not necessary. For primary generalized hyperhidrosis consider oral medications, in particular anticholinergic drugs, such as propantheline or glycopyrrolate (Robinul). After warning of potential anticholinergic side-effects, such as headaches, nausea, urinary hesitancy, blurred vision and palpitations, start with a morning low dose and build up. It is usually best taken in the morning as clients find it is effective for only 4 to 6 hours. Do not normally prescribe it for localized hyperhidrosis except as an adjunctive.

3 Iontophoresis is a 'home based' machine method of reducing localized hyperhidrosis. The treatment involves immersing the affected feet or hands area in baths of shallow tap water or placing a wet pad in the axilla. The machine discharges an electronic current through the water which is channelled to the affected area by placing two electrodes in contact with the patient to form a circuit. Iontophoresis can also be used to deliver a chemical through the skin by adding glycopyrolate to the solution. Published results are good, but compliance is often poor, as the bulky machine has to be used regularly. This is time consuming and in practice results are variable.

SUBDERMAL INJECTION OF ATTENUATED BOTULINUS TOXIN (BOTOX)

Appraise

1 subdermal injection of Botox, by its localized anticholinergic action, is very successful at reducing hyperhidrosis. The effect lasts for 6 months as the acetylcholine vesicles regenerate.

2 It is used predominantly to manage axillary hyperhidrosis; its use in palmar or plantar hyperhidrosis often requires a local nerve block as the subdermal injections are uncomfortable. Ensure that you are fully trained in how to deliver ulnar and median blocks: repeated general anaesthesia instead is not appropriate. There is a small risk of infection which could result in palmar fasciitis, and the injections can lead to localized fingertip numbness. Botox injection to the forehead and hairline has some effect on reducing the sensation of facial sweating.

Action

1 Define the area of hyperhidrosis by painting the affected region with iodine and, when dry, sprinkling starch powder over it. The affected area will be a blackened colour. Mark the outer margins of the area and then mark out a 1-cm square grid within it (Fig. 25.1).

2 Ensure that the Botox solution is drawn up beforehand; 4 ml of 2% lidocaine is added to 100 units of Botox and drawn up into four 1-ml syringes with fine needles (as used by insulin-dependent diabetics). Deliver a 0.1 ml dose to the centre of each grid. Work smoothly and quickly over a couple of minutes.

3 The patient is free to leave 30 minutes later after ensuring there are no systemic side-effects, which are rare.

> ▶ KEY POINTS Performing palmar nerve blocks (Fig. 25.2)
>
> ■ Document a thorough neurovascular examination.
> ■ Place a small roll under the wrist to extend it slightly.
> A. Median nerve block

■ Insert a 23–25 G needle perpendicular to the skin, 2–3 cm proximal to the distal wrist crease between the palmaris longus (PL) and flexor carpi radialis (FCR) tendons, angled slightly to place the needle tip beneath PL.

■ The PL and FCR tendons can be identified by the patient pinching the thumb and little finger together. If PL tendon is absent, inject 5 mm to the ulnar side of FCR tendon.

■ Pass the needle 1–2 cm through the fibrous flexor retinaculum. Aspirate to prevent intravascular injection. Inject 3–5 ml of 1% lidocaine. If there is resistance to injection or paraesthesia on needle insertion, the needle should be repositioned more medial to avoid intraneuronal injection. To include the palmar branches, a small weal of anaesthetic is placed subcutaneously as the needle is withdrawn and massaged over the wrist.

B. Palmar branch of ulnar nerve block

■ Identify the flexor carpi ulnaris (FCU) tendon.

■ Insert a 23–25 G needle 2–3 cm proximal to the distal wrist crease at the ulnar aspect of the FCU tendon, directing the needle radially under the tendon for 1–1.5 cm.

■ Aspirate to prevent intravascular injection. Inject 3–5 ml of 1% lidocaine. If paraesthesia is not elicited, then direct the needle toward the ulna bone, deep to FCU tendon, and inject the anaesthetic as the needle is withdrawn.

■ Wait at least 10 minutes before starting the botox injections

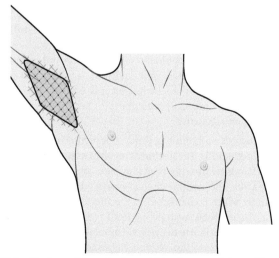

Fig. 25.1 Mark a grid on the hyperhidrosis area of the axilla so that the Botox is evenly distributed over the affected area.

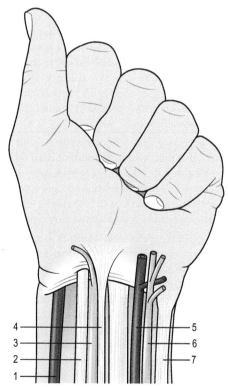

Fig. 25.2 Anatomy of the wrist. 1. Radial artery, 2. Flexor carpi radialis, 3. Median nerve, 4. Palmaris longus, 5. Ulnar artery, 6. Ulnar nerve, 7. Flexor carpi ulnaris.

LOCALIZED AXILLARY SWEAT GLAND ABLATION

There are two surgical approaches in common usage.

HURLEY-SHELLEY OPERATION

Appraise

Traditionally this technique involved removing the axillary skin and undertaking primary closure. It is only considered if there are other dermatological problems, as the wounds are often large and slow to heal, occasionally reducing the range of shoulder movement due to excessive scar tissue.

LOCALIZED RETRODERMAL AXILLARY CURETTAGE

Appraise

This technique is a day-case/clinic procedure that greatly reduces the degree of axillary sweating in 65% of sufferers.

Preparation

Under either general or local anaesthetic, the sterile draped patient lies supine with their hand up over their forehead so that the axilla is exposed.

Action

1 Make a small skin crease incision less than 0.5 cm in the mid axilla.

2 Through the incision inject about 200 ml of normal saline with 15 ml of 1% lidocaine and adrenaline subdermally, using a long needle and syringe. This tumescence lifts the skin off the underlying adipose tissue of the axilla.

3 A curette (3 mm) is then passed through the incision just deep to the skin out to the margin of the hairline. With the roughened edge faced upwards and the curette tenting the skin, it is withdrawn towards the incision, abrading the underside of the skin and destroying the subdermal structures. The procedure is repeated in a sweeping fashion clockwise around the incision so that all the hyperhidrosis area is treated. Take time to ensure that all areas are treated and take care not to make the skin too shallow and button-hole it, or pass the curette too deep and damage deeper structures.

4 A steri-strip over the wound is sufficient. Place a gauze swab in the axilla and secure it firmly with wide adhesive tape.

Aftercare

Send the patient home with instructions to remove the compression dressing in 24 hours and review them in clinic in 1 week.

Complications

1 Bruising does occur, but excessive bleeding should not.

2 Small fibrotic bands may be felt in the axilla and look like stretch marks. They usually resolve in 1 month, especially if the area is massaged.

3 Pigmented discoloration of the axillary skin may occur.

4 Localized reduced axillary sensation may persist.

5 Skin loss is rare, and tends to occur at the site where the skin was button-holed during the procedure.

THORACOSCOPIC SYMPATHECTOMY

Appraise

1 The only clear indications for thoracic sympathectomy are localized palm and axillary hyperhidrosis and facial blushing.

2 Other possible indications are rarer and not clearly defined:
- Consider thoracoscopic sympathectomy for digital artery vasospastic disorders producing pre-gangrenous skin changes, but only as an adjunctive measure. Severe Raynaud's-like symptoms (Maurice Raynaud, Parisian physician 1834–1881) result from significant connective tissue diseases such as scleroderma. Treatment is usually by intravenous vasodilators. Digital artery thrombosis secondary to a cervical rib requires rib excision.
- Sympathectomy may also benefit patients with post-traumatic pain or causalgia (Greek: kausis = burning + algos = pain) and acrocyanosis (Greek: akron = point, tip + kyanos = blue; blue extremities).
- Angina-like pain from terminal coronary artery branch stenosis in the absence of significant main coronary artery disease is a rare indication for thoracoscopic sympathectomy. Undertake it with caution as it can be technically challenging.

3 Although there is a sympathetic innervation to the arteries of the skin and muscle of the limbs, and following sympathetic blockade skin blood flow increases, there is a modest rise only in muscle flow. There is therefore no role for sympathectomy in managing peripheral arterial disease.

▶ KEYPOINT Anatomy

- Acquire intimate familiarity with the sympathetic anatomy.

4 The sympathetic nervous system is a two neurone system. The cell body of the pre-ganglionic neurone is in the spine cord. Its fibres pass through the ventral roots of the spinal nerves, travel in the sympathetic chain and synapse in the ganglia. The sympathetic ganglia lie in a chain running over the heads of the ribs. Postganglionic fibres from the cell bodies in the ganglia pass to the corresponding spinal nerves to enter the limb in one or other of the major nerve trunks. The sympathetic fibres to the arm synapse in ganglia T2–3 (T2 for the hand and T2 + 3 for the axilla). The upper (T1) ganglion fuses with the inferior cervical ganglion to form the stellate ganglion. Damage to the sympathetic stellate ganglion produces a Horner's syndrome (Johann Horner, Zurich ophthalmologist 1831–1886, described ptosis – drooping of the eyelid, myosis – contracted pupil, enophthalmos – eyeball recession, and anhydrosis – dry eye).

5 Several approaches to the upper thoracic sympathetic chain have been described including transaxillary and anterior (supraclavicular), but the thoracoscopic method is the only one regularly undertaken.

Prepare

1 Personally obtain fully informed consent, repeating the counselling to plan the procedure and its alternatives. Warn about compensatory sweating, Horner's syndrome, postoperative pain, the possibility of a chest drain and of conversion to an open procedure and 10% failure rate.

2 Order a preoperative chest X-ray for all patients to exclude any pulmonary disease, which may make the establishment of a pneumothorax difficult.

3 Undertake surgery one side at a time to guard against the small risk of bilateral pneumothorax. Occasionally, unilateral surgery has a bilateral effect. Also, if compensatory sweating follows unilateral operation, the patient can decline surgery on the other side.

Access

1 Perform the procedure under a general anaesthetic. A standard endotracheal tube is almost always sufficient, rather than using a double-lumen tube.

2 Position the patient in a supine position with a small sandbag under the operation side. Bring this side to the edge of the table. Place the arm over the patient's face, held in place with wool and crepe bandaging onto a right angle bar. This resembles someone lying on a beach guarding his eyes from the sun (Fig. 25.3).

3 Through the mid-axillary line at the base of the axillary hairline, make a small 1-cm incision between ribs 3 and 4.

4 Establish an artificial pneumothorax using a Veress needle inserted through the wound after fully informing the anaesthetist.

5 Slowly insufflate 1 L of carbon dioxide into the pleural space.

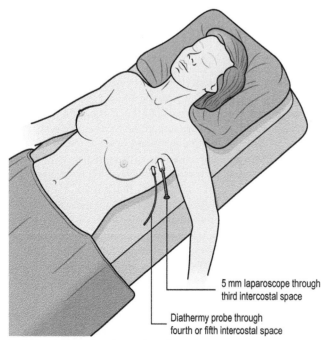

Fig. 25.3 Positioning the patient for a thoracoscopic sympathectomy.

5 mm laparoscope through third intercostal space

Diathermy probe through fourth or fifth intercostal space

► KEY POINTS

- Never undertake bilateral thoacoscopic procedures: the patient may develop a pneumothorax on the first side while the second lung is deflated, with potentially fatal consequences.
- Do not introduce the gas rapidly or you may produce a profound bradycardia as the mediastinum shifts away from the needle.

6 Through the same 1-cm incision introduce a 10-mm 'laparoscopic' port between the ribs. Use an optical port that allows the penetration to be watched under direct vision. Introduce the thoracoscope, usually 0 degrees deflection with a central channel through which to pass instruments. If further access is necessary, insert a 5-mm port below and to one side of the telescope port.

Assess

1 Confirm your orientation (Fig. 25.4). Place the scope looking in the top lateral corner, which is a safe area. Make sure the ribs run horizontally. Follow the ribs medially until you see the sympathetic ganglia and chain lying on the necks of the ribs. The highest rib you see on either side is the second, although in the tall, thin patient the first rib may be visible.

2 Ensure the lung is collapsed. If not, slightly raise the insufflation pressure. Wait a few moments while the lung collapses with the patient in a head up position. This position also decompresses any little veins which may run over or near to the rib heads.

3 Carefully divide the occasionally encountered pleural adhesions, exerting minimal traction.

4 Identify the first rib. Ask the anaesthetist to palpate the rib in the supraclavicular fossa. If you see it covered by the palpating finger, avoid operating on the chain at that level so as to avoid creating a Horner's syndrome.

Action

1 With a blunt (non-diathermy) probe, identify the third rib by tapping it. Identify the ganglia by pushing against them gently with the probe to confirm their soft consistency and glistening surface. If adhesions obscure the view over the third rib, you can easily

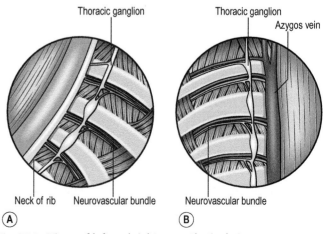

Thoracic ganglion

Thoracic ganglion

Azygos vein

Neck of rib   Neurovascular bundle

Neurovascular bundle

Ⓐ   Ⓑ

Fig. 25.4 Views of left and right sympathetic chain.

identify the chain by visualizing the fourth or fifth rib and following the chain superiorly.

> ▶ KEY POINT Anatomy

■ In the right chest the azygos vein may lie close to the sympathetic ganglia and it can be of a considerable diameter (see Fig. 25.3).

2 Identify the lowest and most effective diathermy setting by creating a preliminary burn over the rib away from the nerve and to get 'under' the pleura. Lift the pleura up and carefully dissect the third thoracic ganglion free over the rib, using sharp dissection. Having cleanly dissected the nerve over the third rib, divide it under direct vision. Alternatively, use the diathermy hook to lift the chain away from the rib before dividing it with diathermy. Now position the inferior cut end of the chain below the rib to avoid later regeneration of the sympathetic chain.

> ▶ KEY POINT Horner's syndrome

■ Horner's syndrome should not occur with a thoracoscopic method as the first rib with the T1 ganglion is not visualized.

3 Clipping of the sympathetic chain is possible and is reputed to achieve the same result in both hyperhidrosis and facial flushing. A theoretical advantage is that the clips can be removed later if complicating side-effects are intolerable.

4 If any of the small veins around the chain start to bleed, apply direct pressure with the non-diathermy probe to the pleura over the vessel away from the cut edge. Wait. The bleeding will stop. Now wash the pleural cavity with saline.

5 Place 40 ml of 0.25% marcaine into the pleural cavity.

6 Withdraw the port and thoracoscope to the chest wall. Turn off the insufflation and open the gas inlets, while watching the lung inflating with the assistance of the anaesthetist. Confirm that the fluid in the pleural cavity is a clear small amount of local anaesthetic and not blood stained. Remove the scope as the fully inflated lung confirms no significant pneumothorax.

7 Close the small wounds with a stitch or plastic adhesive strip.

8 Do not routinely insert chest drains.

Aftercare

1 Examine a chest X-ray in the recovery area to identify any residual pneumothorax. A small pneumothorax is acceptable and is usually re-absorbed within 24 hours. Chest drains are not needed routinely.

2 Return the patient to the ward and discharge several hours later.

3 Forbid flying or diving for 1 month.

Complications

1 Immediate complications include damage to intrathoracic structures requiring thoracotomy. Pneumothorax, which may be under tension, requires the insertion of a chest drain. Pain is variable, occasionally severe, but usually only discomfort on deep breathing.

2 Delayed complications include failure to resolve symptoms and compensatory sweating. These may develop many years after surgery. Compensatory hyperhidrosis, usually on the chest and back, occurs in 50% of patients. It varies from trivial to devastating. There are no clear markers of who will suffer, but it is more likely in generalized hyperhidrosis patients

The 'Harlequin' effect, when half the face blushes and sweats and the other half does not, can be distressing, Usually, if it occurs after bilateral operations, it is not significant.

More rarely, especially if the chain was divided at a high level, the patient complains of nasal congestion and eye lid drooping of a Horner's syndrome. Thoracoscopic sympathectomy has virtually abolished this complication. The highest rib that can be directly viewed intrapleurally via the thoracoscope is the second rib. If you need to go to a high-placed ganglion, as for facial sweating, avoid using diathermy and employ sharp dissection alone to isolate the ganglion over the neck of the highest, most easily viewed rib. This is safe, and Horner's syndrome should not occur.

> ? DIFFICULTY

1. If the patient becomes bradycardic or hypotensive because of mediastinal shift, or the oxygen tension falls precipitately, stop the surgical procedure, offer to reduce the pneumothorax and allow the anaesthetist to re-inflate the lung. It is best to abandon the procedure if the anaesthetist is apprehensive about the patient's condition.

2. Transient Horner's syndrome may occur if you employ a too high-powered diathermy current, or if you cause damage above the level of the second rib.

3. Haemorrhage may occur as a result of intercostal vessel trauma or damage to the azygos vein during diathermy. Have available a suction device that can pass through the insertion tube and long enough to reach across the hemithorax.

4. Adhesions within the chest may cause you to abandon the procedure. However, most adhesions are amenable to division with a combination of sharp dissection and diathermy.

5. Judicious tipping of the patient in the head-up position may allow you to complete the procedure even though the patient is unable to tolerate one-lung anaesthesia.

LUMBAR SYMPATHECTOMY

Appraise

1 This may be carried out as an open operation or non-operatively by injecting phenol into the lumbar chain. A laparoscopic approach has been described but it is difficult to obtain good results. Phenol injection has largely superseded open surgery.

2 The number of lumbar ganglia varies, but there are usually four on each side. The second and third ganglia are removed at operation.

3 Avoid this technique in males because of the risk of causing impotence. Some authors claim that to preserve normal ejaculation the first lumbar ganglion on at least one side must be left intact.

4 The clinical indications for lumbar sympathectomy are vague:

- *Hyperhidrosis* of the feet is cured by lumbar sympathectomy. The procedure is rarely undertaken, but it demands a surgical sympathectomy.

- *Peripheral vascular disease* in patients with non-reconstructable occlusive atherosclerotic disease and thromboangiitis obliterans (Buerger's disease – Leo, New York physician 1879–1943). Rest pain or toe dry gangrene may benefit from a chemical sympathectomy. Rest pain is relieved in 60% for up to 3 years, and further benefit may be obtained by repeated phenol injections. There is no improvement in the subsequent amputation rate.

- *Raynaud's syndrome.* Lumbar sympathectomy may be a last resort in Raynaud's phenomenon due to scleroderma or haematological disorders such as polycythaemia, cold agglutination, cryoglobulinaemia and sickle-cell disease, where ulceration of the toes has occurred and medical measures have failed.

- *Causalgia.* Also called reflex sympathetic dystrophy, this burning pain associated with hypersensitivity and vasomotor disturbance is usually a consequence of trauma to a somatic nerve.

- *Cold injury.* Freezing of the foot at temperatures below -1 °C (frostbite) is associated with arterial spasm and capillary sludging. The resultant tissue loss may be diminished by early sympathetic blockade or sympathectomy. Sympathectomy is not beneficial for feet exposed to the cold at temperatures above freezing (trench foot).

- Other indications for lumbar sympathectomy are acrocyanosis and erythromyalgia.

SURGICAL LUMBAR SYMPATHECTOMY

Access

1 Place the patient supine with a sandbag beneath the side of the operation to give a 20° tilt.

2 Make an 8–10-cm transverse incision at the level of the umbilicus, starting just medial to the linea semilunaris.

3 Incise the lateral border of the rectus sheath. Split the external oblique muscle and incise the internal oblique with cutting diathermy. Carefully separate the transversalis fascia and muscle without entering the peritoneum. Remember that the peritoneum is tougher laterally.

Action

1 Sweep the peritoneum away from the muscle using finger and swab dissection, continuing this mobilization posteriorly and medially until you expose the aorta on the left or the inferior vena cava on the right.

2 Repair any holes created in the peritoneum before proceeding further. Place a Deaver retractor over the peritoneum laterally and have it pulled firmly to open the retroperitoneal space in front of quadratus lumborum and psoas muscles, while avoiding entering the wrong plane behind these muscles.

3 Lift the ureter forwards with the peritoneum out of harm's way. Other structures to avoid which may be confused with the sympathetic chain are the genitofemoral nerve, which runs on the anterior aspect of psoas, the psoas minor tendon and para-aortic lymphatics – identifiable because they are more friable than the sympathetic chain (Fig. 25.5).

4 The sympathetic chain on the left is the easiest to approach as it lies on loose areolar tissue alongside the aorta and can be palpated as a ganglionated cord against the vertebral bodies, where it runs just anterior to the origin of psoas. It passes anterior to the lumbar vessels and posterior to the iliac vessels.

5 On the right side it lies behind the inferior vena cava, which is retracted gently with the tip of the Deaver retractor. Avoid tensing and tearing the lumbar veins, which occasionally pass in front of the sympathetic trunk on this side and can be a source of troublesome bleeding if not recognized and controlled with haemostatic clips.

6 Lift the chain forwards with a nerve hook, diathermize and divide the rami communicantes, then excise the segment containing the second and third ganglia, after applying haemostatic clips, from the lower border of L2 to the lower border of L4.

Closure

1 Check haemostasis and, if necessary, place a drain in the retroperitoneal space.

2 Repair the muscles in layers with absorbable sutures.

3 Close the skin.

Aftercare

1 Postoperative ileus is brief unless a retroperitoneal haematoma forms, when it may be prolonged. The haematoma may need draining, but usually peristalsis is restored after 48 hours of a conservative regime.

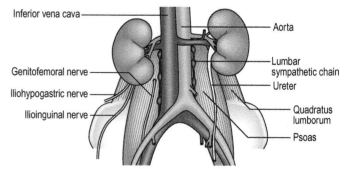

Fig. 25.5 The lumbar sympathetic chain runs down the sides of the bodies of the lumbar vertebrae immediately posterolateral to the inferior vena cava or aorta. The genitofemoral nerve and ureter are important structures that must be avoided.

2 Some patients experience post-sympathectomy neuralgia, a burning pain extending into the thigh. The explanation is unknown, but it resolves after a few weeks.

3 Men in whom both first lumbar ganglia are inadvertently removed will have dry orgasms as a result of damage to the ejaculatory mechanism.

4 Some patients suffer from symptoms of orthostatic hypotension following lumbar sympathectomy.

CHEMICAL LUMBAR SYMPATHECTOMY

Action

1 Position the patient sitting with the legs dependent.

2 Insert a 21 G spinal needle at the level of the upper border of L3, a hand's breadth away from the midline. Under X-ray or CT image guidance, direct it towards the lumbar vertebral body and reposition as necessary until it just slides off the anterior surface of the vertebra (Fig. 25.6). Aspirate it to ensure that it is not in a blood vessel.

3 Inject radiographic contrast fluid and check the needle position with an image intensifier.

4 If the position is correct, inject 7.5 ml of 7.5% phenol in 50% glycine and nurse the patient sitting for 6 hours to allow the heavy phenol solution to track downwards to bathe the sympathetic trunk, rather than laterally to damage the somatic nerves.

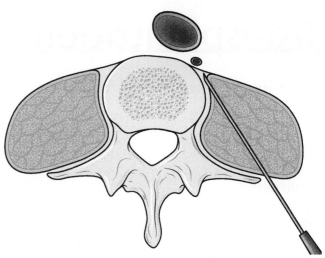

Fig. 25.6   In this posterior approach to chemical lumbar sympathectomy the retroperitoneal space can be located by a sudden loss of resistance to air injection as the needle is advanced through the psoas fascia.

Aftercare

1 Self-limiting post-sympathetic neuralgia may occur, as after surgical sympathectomy.

2 Some patients experience pain down the medial side of the thigh if the phenol tracks laterally around the somatic nerves of the lumbar plexus.

26

Transplantation

K. Rolles

INTRODUCTION

1   Solid whole-organ transplantation has been one of the main events in the evolution of 20th and 21st-century medicine. A kidney transplant offers a quality of life unattainable by long-term dialysis, and the lack of long-term artificial support for end-stage disease of the liver, heart and lungs makes it likely that there will be a demand for organ transplantation into the foreseeable future.

2   Immunosuppressive agents that reduce or abolish graft rejection are vital to the success of organ transplantation. Ciclosporin, acting by calcineurin inhibition within T-cell lymphocytes, blocks progression of the cell cycle from G_0 to G_1 and the production of interleukin 2. In the early 1980s, when used alone or with steroids it improved the 2-year graft survival following kidney transplantation from 50% to 75–80%. Newer drugs include tacrolimus, rapamycin and mycophenolate mofetil. Other interesting molecules differing in their mode of action are leflunomide, brequinar, mizoribine, deoxyspergualin.

   In addition, a number of biological agents such as antibodies to various antigens present on human lymphocytes are available, although so far they have not proved to be any more efficacious than pharmacological agents. Ciclosporin and tacrolimus given long term are associated with nephrotoxicity and neoplasia, especially of the skin and lymphoid tissue, so it is desirable that the dose is progressively reduced. There is evidence that in some cases graft acceptance, without the continued use of immunosuppression, can develop in the long term, but these cases are, unfortunately, not yet predictable.

3   The donor pool comprises:
   Brain-stem dead, heart-beating 'cadavers' – over 80% of solid-organ donors, usually providing multiple organs.
   Non-heart-beating cadavers, providing suitable organs for kidney and increasingly for liver transplantation, occasionally lung transplants but not for hearts.
   Living related donors, such as identical twins, siblings, parents, children, first-order cousins, providing excellent donor organs for kidney transplants; and, with appropriate techniques, segments of livers, pancreas and lung can be grafted.
   Living unrelated donors: spouses, partners, friends, altruists and paid donors (the latter illegal in the UK).

4   The success of organ transplantation has resulted in a shortage of solid organs for transplantation. There are almost 8000 patients waiting in the UK and 70 000 in the USA. The shortfall results in part from cultural, religious, financial, legal and political conditions and varies in different countries. In addition, permission to remove organs after death is usually determined by prior consent of the donor or of the surviving relatives. In some countries, although not in the UK, potential donors are required to 'opt out' – that is, state while alive that they refuse to have organs removed – otherwise it is assumed that they permit it. In the UK 'opt out' legislation is currently being debated. Other discussions taking place include the practicalities and ethics of xenotransplantation (Greek: *xenos* = strange, foreign) – the use of animal organs – and cloning (using nuclear replacement technology) as a means of providing auto-transplantable tissues.

5   Brain-stem death must be established before organs are removed from a mechanically ventilated patient with irreversible cerebral destruction. If the plasma electrolytes or blood gases are abnormal, or if there is suspicion of drug intoxication, organ donation is not pursued. The diagnosis must be made by qualified medical practitioners independent of the transplant team, carrying out the examination individually on two separate occasions. The following signs must be absent:
   - Pupillary reflexes
   - Corneal reflex
   - Caloric response
   - Gag reflexes
   - Spontaneous breathing when disconnected from the ventilator under hypercarbic conditions monitored by blood gases.

6   Tissue transplantation has been successfully practised for many years, including the cornea, which as a 'privileged site' evokes no rejection and requires no immunosuppression. Bone and skin are also transplanted, but essentially serve to provide a non-cellular matrix into which recipient cells can grow as the donor cells are destroyed. Immunosuppressive agents are again unnecessary.

THE MULTIPLE ORGAN DONOR

Appraise

It is possible to remove both kidneys, the liver, the pancreas, the small bowel, the heart and both lungs for transplantation from a single donor using techniques that will not interfere with the immediate function of the transplant organs in their respective recipients.

Donor screening and exclusions

1. Exclude potential donors if there is any possibility of transmitting to potential recipients the following:
   - AIDS/HIV
   - Hepatitis B
   - Hepatitis C
   - Malaria
   - Tuberculosis
   - Rabies
   - Creutzfeldt-Jakob disease (CJD)
   - Glioblastoma multiforme
   - Other extracerebral malignancy.

   Screen all prospective donors for antibodies to HIV-1 and HIV-2, hepatitis C and hepatitis B surface antigen and core antibody. Do not use positive donors.

2. Scrutinize the social history of the donor as far as possible. Exclude prospective donors with a clear history of intravenous drug abuse, prostitution or homosexuality.

Prepare

1. The ventilated heart-beating brain-dead donor may be physiologically unstable, requiring inotropes to maintain systemic vascular resistance and other pharmacological agents such as pitressin or desmopressin (des-amino-des-aspartate-arginine vasopressin, DDAVP) to control diabetes insipidus. Carefully maintain fluid balance, so be willing to institute invasive monitoring such as Swan-Ganz catheterization and direct arterial pressure measurements. Pulse oximetry and cardiac monitoring are essential. Have available body-warming equipment to compensate for hypothermia.

2. Have an anaesthetist in attendance. A general anaesthetic is unnecessary, but give a neuromuscular blocking agents such as curare before making the first incision, to prevent muscular spasms and spinal reflexes, which may be induced by the surgical procedure.

3. Blood loss during the surgical procedure may profoundly destabilize the donor's cardiovascular status and you must therefore take great care to minimize blood loss at all times. Have available 4–6 units of cross-matched bank blood for use during the surgical procedure.

4. The donor surgical team must be self-sufficient and provide surgical instruments, cannulae, sterile bags for the excised organs, ice, cooling fluids, preservation fluids and cardioplegic solution.

> **KEY POINT** Avoid blood loss
>
> - Strictly maintain complete haemostasis.

Access

1. Make a midline incision from the jugular notch to the symphysis pubis.

2. Split the sternum longitudinally with a Gigli saw. Leave the pericardium and pleural cavities intact if possible.

3. Retract the sternal edges with a self-retaining retractor after securing haemostasis by liberal application of bone wax.

Assess

1. Perform a detailed inspection of all abdominal contents to exclude unsuspected pathology, the incidence of which increases in proportion to age. Absolute contraindications to proceeding with organ retrieval are peritoneal contamination due to ruptured bowel and the presence of disseminated intra-peritoneal cancer. Cirrhosis of the donor liver precludes transplantation of that organ.

2. Focal abnormalities found in one or more sites in the abdomen or chest need not prohibit organ retrieval, but remove biopsy specimens of all suspicious lesions for histological examination. You must not re-implant retrieved organs before excluding malignancy histologically.

Action

1. Commence careful dissection of the structures in the free edge of the lesser omentum leading to the porta hepatis. Ligate and divide the common bile duct just above the duodenum. Dissect and control the portal vein with a rubber sling. Carefully search for abnormalities of the hepatic arterial supply. Seventeen per cent of donors have an accessory or aberrant right hepatic artery passing to the porta hepatis posterior to the portal vein and common bile duct. Twenty-three per cent have an accessory left hepatic artery arising from the left gastric artery. Identify these variations early and preserve the vessels.[1]

2. Mobilize the duodenum by Kocher's manoeuvre. Isolate the inferior vena cava above the renal veins and below the liver, and control it with a nylon tape.

3. Divide the peritoneal attachments of the liver, starting with the left triangular ligament and proceeding to the falciform ligament, thus exposing the anterior surface of the suprahepatic vena cava (Fig. 26.1).

4. Divide the right triangular ligament and continue by dividing the upper and lower layers of the coronary ligament while progressively dislocating the liver upwards and to the left, thus separating the liver from the bare area of the diaphragm. Ligate and divide the right adrenal vein, which has now been exposed, and continue dissecting to free the retrohepatic vena cava from the posterior abdominal wall. Achieve complete mobilization of the vena cava by dividing the peritoneum of the right side of the lesser sac. Divide the remnant of the lesser omentum, leaving the liver attached by its blood vessels only.

5. Begin mobilization of the right kidney by dissecting the peritoneum from its anterior surface and controlling the right renal vein and vena cava below the renal vein with rubber slings.

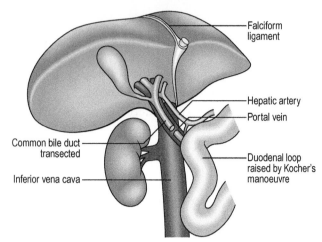

Fig. 26.1 Removal of donor liver. The liver has been dislocated upwards; the common bile duct has been transected low down.

6 Gently lift the kidney from the renal fossa and sweep away surrounding fatty tissue to expose the renal artery or arteries and vein, and control them with further rubber slings.

7 Dissect the ureter with plenty of surrounding connecting tissue down as far as the pelvic rim and then divide it (Fig. 26.2).

8 Repeat the procedure for the left kidney. In addition, ligate and divide the left adrenal and gonadal veins. Also identify, ligate and divide the large lumbar vein opening into the posterior aspect of the left renal vein.

9 Expose and control the lower aorta just above the bifurcation, for subsequent cannulation and flush-cooling of the liver and kidneys.

10 Dissect and control the superior mesenteric vein below the transverse mesocolon for later cannulation of the portal vein and flush-cooling of the liver.

11 Mobilize the pancreas at this stage if it is required. Completely divide the gastrocolic and gastrosplenic omentum. Retract the stomach to expose the pancreas. Divide the lienorenal ligament and, using the spleen as a 'handle', carefully mobilize the tail and

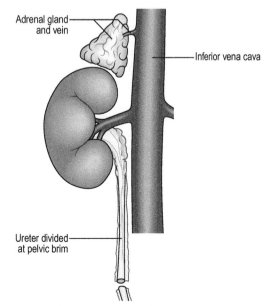

Fig. 26.2 Dissection of the donor kidney on the right.

the body of the pancreas, working towards the midline. Dissect and control with a rubber sling the origin of the splenic artery at the coeliac axis.

12 The cardiac surgical team should now prepare the required thoracic organs for removal. When all the dissections have been completed give 30 000 IU of heparin intravenously. Place a cannula (size 16–20 F) in the portal vein via the superior mesenteric vein and place another in the infrarenal abdominal aorta. Place a third cannula in the infrarenal vena cava.

13 Stop mechanical ventilation. Stop circulation with cardioplegic solution infused through the aortic root. Start flush-cooling of abdominal organs via the portal and aortic cannulas using 3–6 L of University of Wisconsin solution (Viaspan) at 4 °C. Simultaneously exsanguinate the donor via the inferior vena caval cannula to ensure venous decompression and thus effective flush-cooling of the abdominal organs.

14 Following removal of the thoracic organs by the cardiac surgical team wait until the abdominal organs are visibly pale and palpably cold before removing them by dividing the remaining vascular connections. Follow the coeliac axis and the renal arteries back to the aorta. In each case excise a rim of aorta – a 'Carrel patch'.

15 Remove all cannulas. Suck out all free fluid and make a careful watertight wound closure using continuous 0 or no. 1 nylon.

ORGAN PRESERVATION

1 Cool the organs in situ by infusing large volumes of isotonic cold crystalloid solution such as Viaspan, thus reducing the temperature of the perfused organs to 8–15 °C.

2 Excise the organs when they are visibly pale and palpably cold. Flush them through once more with approximately 1 L of a preservation solution (University of Wisconsin solution for the liver and Marshall's hypertonic citrate solution for the kidneys) which will equilibrate throughout the extracellular space of the organ during the preservation period.

3 Double-wrap the organs in sterile bags and place them in boxes of ice where they will remain until re-implantation. Cooling continues to approximately 0 °C in ice over the next few hours.

4 Currently used preservation solutions are hypertonic, contain non-diffusible large anions and usually have a high potassium content corresponding with that of intracellular fluid. These solutions are more effective than physiological saline for cold preservation of organs because they prevent cell swelling and intracellular electrolyte loss during the hypothermic inactivation of the sodium pump.

5 Immediate life-supporting function can be expected from a kidney that has been preserved in one of these solutions for up to 24 hours. Between 24 and 72 hours viability will be preserved but, because of acute tubular necrosis, delayed function is likely.

6 Immediate life-supporting function is an absolute prerequisite for the transplanted liver or heart, thus reducing the safe preservation time dramatically. For the liver, University of Wisconsin solution is clearly the best preservation solution, allowing preservation time for up to 20 hours. For the heart, 4–6 hours is currently the safe limit.

7 Record on the forms provided the donor's demographic details, blood group, anatomical abnormalities and time of circulatory

arrest. Record the type and volume of preservation solution used. Arrange for samples of donor spleen and lymph node to accompany each organ, together with the copy of the data form, to its final destination.

TISSUE TYPING

1 Despite 30 years of clinical organ transplantation, the role of human leucocyte antigen (HLA) matching remains controversial and enigmatic. At least four different gene loci on chromosome 6 code for the human major histocompatibility complex (MHC) and are known as HLA A, B, C and D. Currently, antigens that are cell-surface gene products, usually glycoproteins, of the A B and D loci are routinely determined and matched for donor and recipients in renal transplantation.

2 For renal transplantation from closely related donors such as a parent or sibling, graft survival appears to be directly related to the degree of HLA matching, whereas in the unrelated cadaver donor situation, kidneys fully matched at the A, B and D loci (six antigens) enjoy outstandingly good survival, but any lesser degree of matching significantly prejudices survival.

3 In liver transplantation and heart transplantation no convincing relationship has yet been demonstrated between HLA matching and graft survival. Donors and recipients are usually paired on the basis of ABO blood group compatibility only.

KIDNEY TRANSPLANTATION

Appraise

1 Donor kidneys for transplantation may be obtained from:
- *Living related donors* – usually confined to those with close genetic links such as mothers and fathers, sisters and brothers and, occasionally, first-order cousins. The results of living related kidney transplantation have always been superior to those of cadaver kidney transplantation. In the UK, the Human Organ Transplant Act 1989 stipulates that for any proposed living related organ donation genetic relationship between the donor and the recipient must be established by DNA fingerprinting before the transplant can legally proceed.
- *Living unrelated donors* – a small but increasing number of transplants have been performed between related, but not genetically linked, individuals such as husbands and wives and vice versa. Close friends may also donate. Before a living unrelated donation can legally take place in the UK, a dispensation from the Human Tissue Authority must be obtained, and is a statutory requirement.
- *Unrelated brain-stem-dead heart-beating cadaver donors* – organs are removed immediately following arrest of the circulation. Eighty per cent of all kidney transplants occurring in the UK are based on this type of donor.
- *Unrelated non-heart-beating cadaver donors* – kidneys may be used from a donor following a cardiac standstill as long as the kidneys can be safely removed and cooled within 60 minutes of circulatory arrest. This type of donation is often associated with delayed initial function of the transplant kidney due to acute tubular necrosis.

2 Kidney transplantation currently offers the best chance of long-term survival combined with near-normal quality of life for those suffering from end-stage chronic renal disease.

3 The cost of a well-functioning kidney graft, or any other organ graft, is lifelong treatment with non-specific immunosuppressive agents. Ultimately, the main threat to long-term survival of the kidney graft recipient is likely to be the complications of long-term immunosuppressive therapy in the form of infections and an increased incidence of neoplasia. In addition, hypertension and accelerated cardiovascular disease are commonly seen. After 5 years, recipient death with a functioning graft is the commonest cause of graft loss.

4 End-stage renal disease of all types comprises the indications for renal transplantation. Chronic glomerulonephritis accounts for 60% of all cases of chronic renal failure. Diabetic nephropathy, refluxing pyelonephritis, polycystic disease and previously failed kidney grafts are the other main indications for transplantation.

LIVING RELATED KIDNEY DONATION

Appraise

Remember, the donor has volunteered to undergo a major surgical operation, with all its potential attendant morbidity, which is not of any personal benefit. The altruistic donation of one kidney leaves the kidney donor in a higher risk group for the future with respect to the development of renal failure.

Donor kidneys may be retrieved by the open approach, usually through a muscle-cutting loin incision or, increasingly more frequently, laparoscopically.

THE OPEN APPROACH

Prepare

1 Perform HLA tissue typing and ABO blood grouping. Ensure compatibility with the recipient. Screen for hepatitis B and C and HIV. Demonstrate proof of genetic relationship between donor and recipient by DNA fingerprinting (restriction fragment length polymorphism).

2 Perform diethylenetriamine pentaacetic acid (DTPA) scan to ensure that each of the potential donor's kidneys contributes roughly 50% to total renal function. Gross functional asymmetry between the two kidneys will prohibit donation.

3 Perform an aortogram with selective views of both renal arteries, or magnetic resonance angiography. A kidney with a single renal artery is desirable. Multiple renal arteries supplying both kidneys prohibit kidney donation.

4 Ensure that kidney preservation solutions, ice, organ bags, and cannulae are available for the operative procedure.

Access

1 Place the anaesthetized donor on the operating table in the lateral position.

2 Make a 20-cm muscle-cutting loin incision over the 12th rib. Gain access to the retroperitoneal space through the bed of the 12th rib. Take care to avoid the pleura, which is attached to the medial half of the upper border of the 12th rib. Sweep the peritoneum forward, keeping it intact.

Action

1. Carefully dissect the kidney free of its perirenal fat and the adrenal gland and gently draw it up into the wound to facilitate dissection of the renal pedicles.

2. Dissect both renal vein and renal artery and control each with a soft rubber sling. On the left side divide and ligate the gonadal vein and the adrenal vein. Look for a large lumbar vein entering the posterior aspect of the renal vein. Ligate and divide it. Mobilize the renal vein fully to its confluence with the inferior vena cava.

3. Dissect the renal artery to the aorta. On the right side this requires elevation and retraction of the inferior vena cava and necessitates ligation and division of one or more lumbar veins.

4. Dissect the ureter to the pelvic brim. Ligate it distally at this point and divide it.

5. When attached by its blood vessels only, confirm that the kidney is undergoing diuresis. Give 30 g of mannitol intravenously. Apply vascular clamps to the renal vessels and rapidly excise the kidney. Take it to a side trolley and rapidly flush-cool via the renal artery using a kidney preservation solution at 4 °C. Continue perfusion of the kidney until the effluent from the renal vein is clear and the kidney is palpably cold.

6. Double-wrap the kidney in sterile polythene bags and place it in a bag of ice until the time for reimplantation.

7. Carefully ligate the cut donor renal vessels and close the loin incision in layers, inserting a silicone tube drain.

THE LAPAROSCOPIC APPROACH

This may be performed extraperitoneally through the loin or, more usually, transperitoneally through an anterior approach. Four or five ports are used and the excised kidney is delivered through a 6-cm Pfannenstiel incision. The procedure may be conducted entirely laparoscopically or 'hand-assisted' by inserting a hand through the suprapubic incision.

TRANSPLANTATION OF THE DONOR KIDNEY

Appraise

1. Eighty per cent of renal transplants performed in the UK use unrelated 'cadaver' donor kidneys. Less than 20% of kidney transplants are donated by a close living relative.

2. 'Cadaver' kidneys are exchanged between transplant centres on the basis of clinical need and tissue matching.

3. Organ exchange and transport are arranged by a central distribution agency, the UK Blood and Transplant Authority.

4. Organs are transported in boxes of crushed ice by special courier.

Prepare

1. Before commencing the recipient operation carefully check the information sheet accompanying the donor kidney, paying particular attention to ABO blood group compatibility and any anatomical abnormality recorded.

2. Ensure that an immunological cross-match is negative between recipient serum and donor lymphocytes from the spleen and lymph node samples accompanying the kidney. A positive cross-match absolutely prohibits transplantation as it demonstrates preformed antibodies in the recipient's serum that are capable of killing donor lymphocytes. If the transplant were to proceed in the face of a positive cross-match, the kidney would be hyper-acutely rejected.

3. Remove the kidney from its box of ice and check its anatomical details. Some dissection of excess donor tissues may be necessary. Perform this on a sterile trolley. Ensure that you have an adequate source of light and an assistant. When the dissection is completed, replace the kidney in sterile bags and pack it away once again in the box of ice.

KIDNEY TRANSPLANT OPERATION

Appraise

1. The donor kidney is re-implanted into the right or left iliac fossa and vascularized from the iliac vessels. This is an example of heterotopic (Greek: *heteros* = other + *topos* = a place) transplantation, as the kidney is not re-implanted into its normal anatomical—orthotopic (Greek: *orthos* = straight, right)—position.

2. The reasons why this heterotopic position is most appropriate are:
   - It provides easy access to the iliac vessels
   - The blood supply of the donor ureter is entirely derived from the renal vessels and it should therefore be kept short
   - The implanted kidney is usually easily palpable and amenable to percutaneous procedures such as biopsy, with relatively low risk.

Prepare

1. Ensure the prospective recipient is normokalaemic (*kalium*, modified Latin from Arabic *quail* = potash, potassium).

2. Have a central venous pressure line inserted and cautiously rehydrate the recipient. Most chronically dialysed patients are under-hydrated and hyperkalaemic.

Access

1. Place the patient on the operating table in the supine position.

2. Pass a urinary catheter and attach it to a 1-L bag of saline via an infusion line.

3. Make a 'hockey-stick' incision starting 1 cm above the symphysis pubis and curving laterally to the pararectal line. Proceed vertically up the pararectal line to just above the level of the umbilicus. Incise the abdominal wall along the pararectal line and make an extraperitoneal approach to the external iliac vessels. Ligate and divide the inferior epigastric vessels. Control the spermatic cord with a nylon tape.

4. Insert a self-retaining ring retractor, such as Denis Browne's, and adjust it to provide full access to the operative field.

Action

1. Mobilize both the external iliac artery and vein and control them with nylon tapes. Carefully ligate and seal the perivascular lymphatic vessels with diathermy.

2. Remove the prepared donor kidney from ice.

3. Perform an end-to-side anastomosis between the renal vein and the external iliac vein using continuous 5/0 polypropylene or PDS (polydioxane sulphate).

4. Perform an end-to-side anastomosis between the donor renal artery and the external iliac artery using similar suture materials.

5. Remove the clamps from the iliac vessels, thus perfusing the graft and secure haemostasis.

6. Fill the bladder with physiological saline from the previously attached infusion line to distend it and help identify the bladder in the pelvis.

7. Spatulate the end of the ureter, pass below the spermatic cord and perform an anastomosis to the dome of the bladder using continuous 4/0 synthetic absorbable suture such as PDS. Fashion a submucosal tunnel by incising the bladder muscle down to the mucosa over a 2-cm distance in line with the ureter. Lay the distal ureter in the groove created and close the bladder muscle loosely over the top of the ureter using interrupted absorbable sutures. Test the anastomosis by refilling the bladder with saline (Fig. 26.3).

8. Take a renal biopsy before closing the wound in layers over a large silicone tube drain.

Postoperative

1. Leave the urethral catheter in situ for a minimum of 5 days.

2. Ensure meticulous fluid replacement to maintain a urine output of more than 100 ml/hour.

3. Perform daily full blood count, blood urea, electrolyte and creatinine estimations.

4. Record the patient's weight and fluid balance accurately.

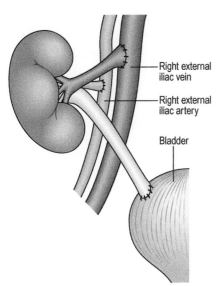

Fig. 26.3 Renal transplantation. The renal vessels have been united end-to-side to the external iliac vessels. The ureter is joined to the dome of the bladder.

Complications

1. *Delayed function* of cadaver grafts occurs in up to 40%, due to acute tubular necrosis. Acute tubular necrosis results from ischaemic injury to the kidney graft, which may occur in the donor before removal, during the preservation period, if it is excessively long, or during the implantation period, if this is excessively long. Acute tubular necrosis is confirmed on DTPA scan and renal biopsy and usually resolves within 6 weeks.

2. *Vascular thrombosis* may occur rarely (approximately 5%), leading to infarction and loss of the graft, which must then be removed. A transplant nephrectomy requires removal of all donor tissue, reconstitution of iliac vessels by vein patch if necessary and oversewing of the bladder.

3. *Urinary leakage* may occur as a result of terminal ischaemic necrosis of the donor ureter. Operative intervention is almost always necessary. Reimplant the ureter into the dome of the bladder or perform uretero-ureterostomy to the recipient's own ureter.

4. *Acute cellular rejection* is seen in up to 80% of cases within 1 week of transplantation. Clinically there is oliguria, pyrexia and a rising creatinine and blood urea. You should obtain histological confirmation by percutaneous biopsy. Give antirejection therapy, usually high-dose steroids, to suppress the immune response. In a small minority of cases rejection is uncontrollable and results in infarction of the graft leading to the need to remove it.

Results

1. For living related donor kidneys, graft survival is over 95% at 1 year and 85% at 5 years.

2. Cadaver kidney graft survival is 90% at 1 year and 70–75% at 5 years.

LIVER TRANSPLANTATION

Appraise

1. More than 200 000 liver transplants have been performed in over 250 liver transplant centres worldwide since Starzl reported the first liver graft in 1963. The introduction of ciclosporin in 1979 was associated with a significant improvement in both short-term and long-term survival following liver grafting. The longest surviving recipient of a liver graft is now more than 43 years post-transplant.

2. Auxiliary heterotopic transplantation of the liver for non-malignant cases of liver disease has had its proponents from time to time. The problems of creating sufficient space for an extra liver, or part of a liver, kinking of the vascular anastomoses and the development of malignancy in the recipient's own liver have precluded its widespread adoption. Auxiliary partial orthotopic liver transplantation, described by Gubernatis,[2] is an interesting technical variant where a donor right or left lobar graft is implanted orthotopically following resection of the same lobe of the recipient's own acutely failing liver. The expectation here is that full recovery of the recipient's native liver will occur so that the grafted lobe may subsequently be removed or abandoned and immunosuppression withdrawn. This expectation is not always achieved.

3 Orthotopic liver transplantation as originally described and practised required the removal of the recipient's own liver together with the retrohepatic inferior vena cava between the renal veins and the diaphragm. For very small recipients, usually children, transplantation of part of a larger liver, obtained either by splitting a cadaver graft or by left hemihepatectomy of a living related donor, requires the recipient's own retrohepatic vena cava to be left in situ. For children, the partial liver graft usually consists of segments 2 and 3 and possibly 4 of the donor organ. For adults, a partial graft consisting of segments of 5, 6, 7 and 8, whether obtained from a 'split' cadaver graft or from a living related donor, usually provides sufficient functional liver cell mass. A graft weight to recipient body weight ratio of 0.8–1% is essential to immediately sustain life. Alternatively, using volumetry based on three-dimensional computed tomography (CT) or magnetic resonance imaging (MRI), the living donor graft should be 40% of the recipient's calculated standard liver volume. Leaving the recipient's own vena cava in situ also allows the option of a single cavocaval side-to-side anastomosis (the so-called piggy-back technique). Several large series of living related donor liver transplants have recently been reported demonstrating excellent outcomes for both adult and paediatric recipients but also showing significant early morbidity for both donor and recipient. Biliary tract complications currently occur in up to 36% of recipients and 20% of donors. Donor mortality appears to be just under 1% at present, an unacceptably high figure in the view of many surgeons. I shall describe the original orthotopic liver transplant procedure.

4 In 70% of cases transplantation is for end-stage chronic liver disease due to cirrhosis arising from a variety of different causes such as primary biliary cirrhosis, primary sclerosing cholangitis, post-hepatitic cirrhosis, autoimmune chronic active hepatitis and alcohol-related liver disease. In approximately 12% it is for primary hepatic malignancy and in another 10% for acute liver failure resulting from fulminant hepatitis, acute (drug) poisoning or idiosyncratic drug reactions. Metabolic diseases account for 6% of cases, including:

■ Where the liver is itself a target organ of the metabolic abnormality such as Wilson's disease, α_1-antitrypsin deficiency and tyrosinosis

■ Where a hepatic enzyme defect leads to damage and failure of other organs such as primary hyperoxaluria, familial hypercholesterolaemia and some forms of familial amyloidosis. Here, liver transplantation is used as a highly effective form of gene therapy.

Prepare

1 Carry out a full biochemical, haematological, bacteriological and virological screen including hepatitis viruses A-G. Replicating HBV must be suppressed by antiviral treatment with lamuvidine or adefovir to prevent post-transplant recurrence in the graft, which may cause its rapid destruction. Similarly, HCV may be treated to suppress or eliminate it preoperatively with interferon and ribavirin, if time and liver function permit.

2 Magnetic resonance angiography and cholangiography are required to assess the vasculature and biliary tract of the recipient liver. An occluded portal vein may be a relative contraindication to transplantation, although transplantation may still be possible if the splenic vein or the superior mesenteric vein is patent and accessible.

3 Perform lung function tests and carefully evaluate cardiac function. Measure pulmonary artery pressure and perform cardiac output studies followed by a detailed anaesthetic assessment.

4 Assess the neuropsychiatric state, including CT scans of the brain.

5 Control ascites, oesophageal varices and encephalopathy by maximizing medical treatment.

6 Immediately before operation have 20 units of blood, fresh-frozen plasma and platelets cross-matched. Give prophylactic broad-spectrum antibiotics at the induction of anaesthesia.

7 Inspect the donor liver graft before starting the recipient operation.

Access

1 Make a bilateral subcostal incision, if necessary with upward extension to the xiphoid. Pin back the abdominal wall flaps so created to the lower chest wall.

2 Insert a Thompson retractor system to elevate the lower costal margin.

Assess

▶ KEY POINTS Unsuspected co-existent disease?

■ Examine the intra-peritoneal contents carefully.
■ Do not proceed if you discover extrahepatic tumour.
■ Remove a biopsy section of suspect tissue for frozen-section histology.

Resect

1 Dissect the structures in the free edge of the lesser omentum leading to the porta hepatis.

2 Ligate and divide the common bile duct as close as possible to the porta hepatis.

3 Dissect and control the common hepatic artery and portal vein with rubber slings.

4 Dissect the infrahepatic vena cava above the renal veins and control it with a nylon tape.

5 Divide the peritoneal attachments of the liver, starting with the left triangular ligament and proceeding to the falciform ligament, thus exposing the anterior surface of the suprahepatic vena cava.

6 Progressively dislocate the liver from the hepatic fossa while dissecting the liver from the bare area of the diaphragm.

7 Completely mobilize the retrohepatic vena cava from the posterior abdominal wall, ligating and dividing the right adrenal vein.

8 Apply vascular clamps to the vascular connections of the liver and excise it, maximizing the length of vessels for the subsequent reimplantation of the new graft (Fig. 26.4).

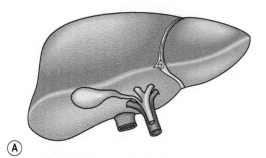

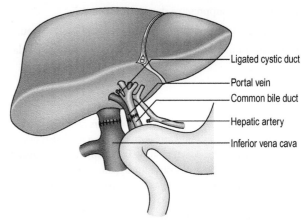

Fig. 26.5 Diagrammatic appearance of donor liver in situ after completing the anastomosis; the first anastomosis, of the superior cut end of the recipient vena cava to the upper end of the donor intrahepatic cava, is not visible. The gallbladder of the donor liver has been removed.

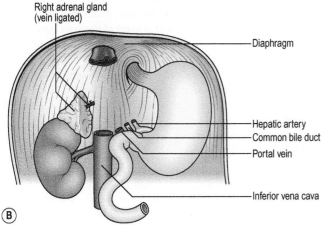

Fig. 26.4 Diagram of recipient liver resection: (A) the removed liver with divided common bile duct, portal vein, hepatic artery and inferior vena cava; (B) the bed for the donor liver. The duodenal loop is mobilized by Kocher's manoeuvre.

> ▶ KEY POINTS Cirrhotic liver fracture?

- Liver fracture during mobilization of the liver results in rapid blood loss.
- Clamp the portal vein, hepatic artery and infrahepatic vena cava to reduce blood loss.
- You can now divide the clamped structures and complete the retrohepatic dissection in a bloodless field.

9 In recipients with borderline renal or cardiac function institute veno-venous bypass during the anhepatic period, inserting percutaneously placed cannulas in the left femoral vein and left internal jugular vein. Flows of up to 3 L/minute are observed, which support cardiac output and effective renal perfusion during the anhepatic period.

Replace

1 Remove the new liver from ice.

2 Begin the reimplantation with the suprahepatic vena caval anastomosis using a continuous 2/0 polypropylene (Prolene), polydioxanone (PDS) or polyester (Merseline) suture. Follow this with the infrahepatic vena caval anastomosis, using a continuous 3/0 polypropylene suture. Before completing the infrahepatic anastomosis insert a 16 F flexible cannula into the retrohepatic vena cava for subsequent flushing of the liver.

3 Anastomose the donor and recipient portal veins end-to-end using 5/0 polypropylene. Before completing this anastomosis flush out the graft via the portal vein with 500 ml of 5% human albumin solution at room temperature. This removes air and

preservation fluid from the liver, which escapes through the retrohepatic caval vent.

4 Complete the anastomoses of the portal vein and infrahepatic vena cava and remove clamps from the infrahepatic vena cava, suprahepatic vena cava and portal vein in that order, thus perfusing the new graft with portal-venous blood (Fig. 26.5).

5 Reconstruct the hepatic arterial supply as an end-to-end anastomosis between the donor and recipient common hepatic arteries using interrupted 6/0 polypropylene.

6 Reconstruct the biliary tract as an end-to-end, duct-to-duct anastomosis using interrupted 5/0 PDS. Splinting is not necessary. Use a 50-cm Roux loop of upper jejunum if there is no recipient common bile duct, as in biliary atresia or primary sclerosing cholangitis.

7 Perform a donor cholecystectomy and a liver biopsy.

8 Check thoroughly for haemostasis, inspecting all anastomoses and placing extra sutures when necessary, and then close the abdomen in layers, inserting two large silicone tube drains.

Postoperative

1 Transfer the patient to the intensive care unit.

2 Continue ventilation until the patient's cardiovascular condition is stable.

3 Carefully monitor temperature, blood pressure, pulse, central venous pressure (CVP), ECG, pulmonary artery wedge pressure, cardiac output and systemic vascular resistance.

4 Monitor haemoglobin, haematocrit (maintaining at 30%), potassium, calcium and magnesium, blood gases, blood lactate and pH.

> ▶ KEY POINT Graft function?

- Increasing blood lactate levels and acidosis are indicative of poor early graft function.

5 Measure and replace fluid losses, including urine output, abdominal drainage and nasogastric losses.

6 Begin immunosuppressive therapy immediately.

7 Cover with broad-spectrum antibiotics for at least 48 hours.

8 Check liver function tests and coagulation profiles twice daily.

Complications

1 Bleeding may occur within the first 24 hours resulting from vasodilatation as the patient warms up. Bleeding may also occur as a result of poor synthesis of clotting factors by the new graft. Correct any coagulation abnormalities with fresh-frozen plasma, platelets and cryoprecipitate as necessary. If bleeding continues, intra-abdominal haematoma may accumulate sufficiently to cause tamponade, resulting in hypotension and anuria. Re-explore the abdomen to evacuate haematoma and improve haemostasis as much as possible. The retrohepatic area, particularly in the region of the right adrenal, is a common site for postoperative bleeding.

2 A right pleural effusion develops in nearly all patients during the first postoperative week. Treat it expectantly unless it rapidly increases in size or causes compression or collapse of the underlying lung. In this case aspirate it or insert an underwater-seal drain.

3 Vascular occlusion is a rare (5–10%) but serious complication, particularly in the first few postoperative weeks. Hepatic arterial thrombosis may lead to extensive patchy infarction of the graft or acute liver failure, requiring urgent re-transplantation. Portal vein thrombosis may be clinically silent. Hepatic arterial thrombectomy or thrombolysis is rarely of benefit, but portal vein thrombectomy is frequently effective.

4 Diagnose acute rejection on biopsy in up to 80% of grafts within the first postoperative week. Treat it by increasing immunosuppression, for example giving 1 g of methylprednisolone (Solu-Medrone) intravenously once daily for 3 days. Repeat the biopsy to assess the response.

5 Send samples of urine, saliva, faeces, blood and appropriate skin swabs every 48 hours for bacteriological and virological surveillance.

> ### ▶ KEY POINT Infection?
>
> ■ Infection under high-dose immunosuppressive cover is serious and could be fatal.

6 Perform a HIDA (hepatobiliary imidodiacetic acid) scan 10–14 days postoperatively to assess the integrity of the biliary tract. Proceed to ERCP (endoscopic retrograde cholangiopancreatography) or transhepatic percutaneous cholangiography if the HIDA scan is equivocal. If there is a small leak at the anastomosis it may heal following careful stenting or nasobiliary drainage inserted endoscopically. Large biliary leaks are usually associated with a substantial infrahepatic bile collection and may signify donor duct necrosis. Reconstructive surgery using a Roux loop is usually the best approach. For an obstruction of the anastomosis, once again temporary stenting may suffice if it is possible to pass a stent across the obstruction; otherwise proceed to reconstructive surgery, performing a choledochojejunostomy using a 50-cm Roux loop.

Results

1 An 85% 1-year patient survival and 65% 5-year patient survival are currently being achieved by most major liver transplant centres. A recurrence rate of about 65% at 5 years for those transplanted for malignant disease of the liver underscores the poor long-term prognosis of transplantation for malignancy, but still compares well with resectional surgery for primary liver cancer.

2 Chronic rejection of the graft occurs in up to 10% of liver transplant recipients, appearing histologically as progressive dropout of liver parenchymal cells and loss of portal tract bile ducts. These changes are due to a progressive obliterative arteriopathy, where the lumina of the major arteries of the graft become progressively obstructed by the accumulation of foamy macrophages of recipient origin. Re-transplantation is the only solution. The falling incidence of chronic rejection seen in recent years has been attributed to more effective immunosuppressive drugs and a more proactive approach to liver graft dysfunction through biopsy.

REFERENCES

1. Michels NA. The hepatic, cystic and retroduodenal arteries and their relations to the biliary ducts. Ann Surg 1951;133:503–23.
2. Gubernatis G, Pichlmayr R, Kemnitz J, et al. Auxiliary partial orthotopic liver transplantation (APOLT) for fulminant hepatic failure: first successful case report. World J Surg 1991;15:660–6.

PANCREAS TRANSPLANTATION

Appraise

The development of microangiopathy, nephropathy and neuropathy appears not to be inevitable among diabetic patients, but may occur in individuals despite ostensibly good blood sugar control by exogenous insulin. Against this backdrop the rationale for pancreatic transplantation has been as an approach to the treatment of diabetes mellitus whereby prevention, arrest or reversal of the long-term complications of diabetes may be achieved.

Transplantation of pancreatic tissue has been performed both clinically and experimentally by two different approaches:

1 Transplantation of the whole or part of the pancreas as a solid vascularized organ graft, which includes both endocrine and exocrine components of the gland.

2 Transplantation of the insulin-producing tissue only – the islets of Langerhans.

VASCULARIZED GRAFTS

Appraise

1 No single technique has been universally adopted in the 40 years since Kelly performed the first vascularized graft in 1966.[1] The question of whether it is better to graft the whole pancreas or a segment comprising the body and the tail of the organ is still unresolved, but the balance of opinion now favours the whole-organ graft. Those who advocate the whole-organ preparation claim that it is beneficial to engraft as much of the donor endocrine mass as possible, thus minimizing islet exhaustion due to too small a graft, as in the segmental technique. Those advocating

the simpler segmental graft claim that it is a lower-morbidity, lower-mortality procedure for the recipient. Other controversial areas include:

- Thrombosis of the graft
- Drainage of exocrine secretion
- The diagnosis and treatment of rejection.

2 Despite these technical difficulties the results of pancreas transplantation have improved substantially over the last decade. In recent years, the most favoured technique is that of transplanting the whole pancreas of the donor into the left or right iliac fossa of the recipient, draining the pancreatic exocrine secretion directly into the bladder, as described by Sollinger et al.[2] These authors also found that a fall in the urinary amylase output from the graft was an early marker of impending graft rejection, indicating the need for antirejection therapy. More recently, because of sometimes insurmountable bladder problems with frequency, dysuria and cystitis, many surgeons have reverted to pancreatic duct drainage into a Roux-en-Y loop of jejunum.

Achievements

1 A well-functioning pancreas graft exerts good control of blood glucose excursions without dietary restrictions and 24-hour blood glucose profiles are normal or near normal.

2 Glucose-tolerance curves show an abnormal pattern of insulin release leading to a slower return of blood glucose to basal levels.

3 Glucose-tolerance curves are similar whether the pancreatic graft venous effluent is drained into the systemic circulation or into the portal circulation, but plasma insulin levels are at least twice as high in those with a systemic venous drainage. Glycosylated haemoglobin values (HbA_{1C}) are maintained within the normal range.

4 Evidence for pancreas transplantation altering the natural history of the secondary complications of diabetes is slowly emerging. Diabetic nephropathy in transplanted kidneys appears to be prevented by a well-functioning pancreas graft. There are also some reports of improved peripheral nerve conduction time following pancreas transplantation. In general, retinopathy is not objectively improved but many patients with diabetic eye problems have found an improvement in acuity.

Techniques

1 The artery and vein of the pancreas graft are anastomosed end-to-side to the common iliac artery and vein of the recipient.

2 For the whole-organ graft some 'bench' surgery is required at a separate sterile work table.

3 An interposition graft comprising the donor common iliac artery bifurcation is anastomosed to the splenic artery and the superior mesenteric artery of the graft so that only a single anastomosis to the recipient artery is required. In addition, a 6-cm length of donor duodenum is retained and anastomosed to either the dome of the bladder or a loop of jejunum to provide exocrine drainage. The graft is placed intra-peritoneally. In contrast, the segmental graft requires no bench procedure and is usually placed extraperitoneally. Exocrine drainage is into a Roux loop or obturated by duct injection with Neoprene.

Results

1 More than 20 000 pancreas grafts have now been reported worldwide; 94% of these have been associated with a kidney graft. In 80%, the pancreas is transplanted simultaneously with a kidney from the same donor. In 14%, a successful pancreas transplant is followed some months later by a kidney transplant, usually from a third-party donor. Only 6% of pancreas transplants are performed alone.

2 1-year patient survival is currently 95%, with a graft survival of over 80%. The use of the new immunosuppressants, such as tacrolimus and mycophenolate mofetil, appears to have significantly improved outcome in recent years.

ISLET CELL TRANSPLANTATION

Avoidance of major surgery, graft thrombosis and pancreatic exocrine secretion management difficulties readily makes islet transplantation an attractive option. Islet grafting can be accomplished by percutaneous placement, and purified islets are in theory more amenable to immunological modulation prior to transplant. In practice, however, islet cell transplantation has its own major difficulties. Specifically these include:

1 Efficient separation of islet tissue from the whole pancreas

2 Preservation of the islet tissue

3 The most appropriate site for islet implantation

4 Rejection of the islet graft.

Nevertheless, as a result of much experimental work performed over the last two decades, the techniques of islet separation and preservation are much improved. It is estimated that, to render an insulin-dependent diabetic normoglycaemic by means of an islet graft, approximately 10 000 islets per kilogram of the recipient's body weight are necessary. The efficiency of current separation techniques is such that more than one donor is usually necessary for each islet cell transplant. Intraportal or intrasplenic injection appear to be the favoured sites of placement for islet grafts at present, but excellent islet survival has been reported in rodents following placement beneath the renal capsule. Islet rejection remains a problem. In addition to T- and B-cell-mediated immunological mechanisms, it is likely that scavenging mechanisms, such as phagocytosis by macrophages, assume an important role in islet graft destruction.

Several hundred attempts at human islet cell grafting have been reported over the years, with insulin independence achieved for a few days only. However, a clinical programme of islet transplants using intraportal injection and achieving excellent insulin independence rates at up to 5 years has been reported recently by workers at Edmonton, Alberta. Highly efficient islet separation techniques, immediate transplantation of the prepared islets into the portal vein by transhepatic or transjugular injection, and the use of the powerful immunosuppressive drugs tacrolimus and sirolimus have been the main factors underpinning this remarkable success.

REFERENCES

1. Kelly WD, Lillehei RC, Merkel FK, et al. Allotransplantation of pancreas and duodenum along with the kidney in diabetic nephropathy. Surgery 1967;61:827–33.

2. Sollinger HW, Kalayoglu M, Hoffman RM, et al. Results of segmental and pancreaticosplenic transplantation with pancreaticocystostomy. Transplant Proc 1985;17:360–2.

SMALL-BOWEL TRANSPLANTATION

Appraise

1 Transplantation of the small bowel may be indicated for small numbers of adults and children who have suffered massive small-bowel loss and are unable to sustain body weight by either enteric feeding or total parental nutrition. In most countries the demand for small-bowel transplantation to date has been low. In small children, transplantation of the liver together with the small bowel has produced better results than transplantation of the small bowel alone.

2 Lillehei was the first to report the technical feasibility of small-bowel transplantation in the dog.[1] Several attempts at human small-bowel transplantation followed, with extremely poor results. The introduction of ciclosporin A in 1978 revived interest in clinical small-bowel transplantation and this has been reinforced by the development of new agents such as tacrolimus and mycophenolate mofetil. Many major transplant centres now have modest series of small-bowel grafts, but graft survival longer than 3 years remains a rare event.

   Major clinical problems are:
   - Immunological rejection of the graft
   - Septicaemia due to bacteriological translocation across the graft during rejection episodes
   - Fluid and electrolyte losses from the graft
   - Graft-versus-host disease, which may be fatal
   - Technical problems, including vascular thrombosis and torsion of the graft pedicle.

3 Small-bowel grafts can be obtained from cadaveric donors or from living related donors. The potential of careful and close HLA matching in grafts taken from living related donors may prove critical for the long-term survival of the small-bowel graft.

4 Access to the recipient's major abdominal blood vessels may be very difficult as candidates for small-bowel transplantation have invariably undergone numerous previous surgical procedures.

5 Implantation of the graft is straightforward, with the superior mesenteric artery of the graft anastomosed end-to-side to the recipient abdominal aorta and the vein anastomosed to the inferior vena cava, or the portal vein if available.

REFERENCE

1. Lillehei RC, Goott B, Miller FA. The physiological response of the small bowel of the dog to ischaemia including prolonged in vitro preservation of the bowel with successful replacement survival. Ann Surg 1958;150:43–54.

HEART TRANSPLANTATION

Appraise

1 Eight years after the first successful series of orthotopic heart transplants in dogs, carried out by Lower and Shumway,[1] Barnard,[2] using the same technique, performed the first human heart transplant in 1967. The wave of worldwide enthusiasm for human heart grafting that followed Barnard's contribution was almost totally dissipated by 1970, when it had become clear that the development of a successful surgical technique had preceded the development of suitable immunological means and immunosuppressive agents to monitor and prevent graft rejection.

2 Heart transplantation continued in a very few centres over the following decade. The introduction in 1980 of ciclosporin A, a potent new non-steroidal immunosuppressant, sparked a second wave of worldwide enthusiasm, which has been sustained and has established heart transplantation as an extremely effective therapy for various types of end-stage heart disease. More than 50 000 transplants have now been performed.

Indications

1 Ischaemic heart disease and its complications, due to coronary artery insufficiency

2 Cardiomyopathy of various types

3 Some cases of congenital heart disease.

Contraindications

1 Pulmonary hypertension

2 Other systemic disease or infection

3 Age greater than 55 years.

Donor and recipient matching criteria

1 ABO compatibility.

2 Negative direct lymphocytotoxic cross-match; that is, donor cells not killed by recipient serum.

3 Body weight of donor and recipient within 10% of each other.

4 Cold preservation time of donor heart not exceeding 4 hours.

Technique

1 Perform a median sternotomy.

2 Establish full cardiopulmonary bypass, placing cannulae in the superior and inferior vena cava transatrially and a return cannula in the ascending aorta.

3 Apply aortic and pulmonary artery clamps and excise the recipient's heart across a transatrial plane just dorsal to the atrial appendages. Leave the posterior atrial wall with the orifices of the systemic and pulmonary veins intact. Divide the aorta and pulmonary trunk just distal to their respective valves.

4 Insert a cannula (12–14 F) in the left ventricle, through the apex of the myocardium, to act as a vent.

5 Implant the new heart, which consists of more of the donor atria in order to preserve the sinoatrial node.

6 Perform left and right atrial anastomoses, followed by aortic and pulmonary artery anastomoses, using continuous polypropylene sutures.

7 On completion of the anastomoses, release the aortic clamp and allow the heart to fill via the coronary circulation, displacing air through the left ventricular vent.

8 When all air is displaced, clamp and remove the vent, release all other clamps and snuggers and reduce bypass flow rate. If the

heart does not restart spontaneously, apply a direct current (DC) shock if necessary.

9   Place temporary pacing wires in the donor right atrial wall and stop bypass. Remove cannulae.

10   Repair the pericardium and close the chest with pericardial drainage.

Rejection

Perform transjugular endomyocardial biopsies regularly – initially every 3–5 days to detect and treat rejection as early as possible.

Results

One-year survival is 85–90% in most large centres; 5-year survival is currently 75%.

REFERENCES

1. Lower RR, Shumway NE. Studies on orthotopic transplantation of the canine heart. Surg Forum 1960;11:9–18.
2. Barnard CN. The operation. S Afr Med J 1967;41:1271–4.

HEART–LUNG TRANSPLANTATION

The first reported human heart–lung transplant was performed by Cooley in 1968.[1] The recipient survived only 4 hours after surgery. Further attempts were reported by Lillehei in 1969 and Barnard in 1971, with similar short-term survival.

Reitz, working at Stanford, California, performed the first heart–lung transplant under ciclosporin immunosuppression in 1981.[2] This patient survived 5 years. Heart–lung transplantation is now a well-established therapy for certain cardiopulmonary disorders.

Indications

1   Primary pulmonary hypertension

2   Pulmonary hypertension secondary to Eisenmenger's syndrome

3   Cystic fibrosis

4   Emphysema.

Whether heart–lung transplantation will be succeeded by single or double lung transplants for cystic fibrosis and emphysema remains to be seen. The potentially serious disadvantage of heart-lung grafting for end-stage lung disease is that a healthy, well-functioning recipient heart is excised (and used for another heart recipient) to be replaced by an allograft that is susceptible to the many complications of allotransplantation, including the risk of both acute and chronic graft rejection.

Donor and recipient matching

1   This is similar to that for heart transplantation. Size matching of the donor lungs to the recipient thoracic cage is very important, as over-inflation occurs if the lungs are relatively too small and inadequate ventilation occurs if the lungs are too large.

2   Donor organs are much more difficult to obtain than hearts alone. Many potential donors are precluded on account of pulmonary infection due to mechanical ventilation. Thus, in view of size matching and scarcity of suitable uninfected donors, a potential heart–lung recipient may need to wait a long time before transplantation.

Technique

1   Make a median sternotomy.

2   Establish full cardiopulmonary bypass as described for heart transplantation.

3   Excise both lungs and heart of the recipient, separately if necessary.

4   Take care not to damage the phrenic nerves or the vagal trunks.

5   Leave the posterior wall of the right atrium intact and in continuity with the superior and inferior vena cavae.

6   Carefully insert the donor heart–lung block.

7   Anastomose right atrium, trachea and aorta in that order, using polypropylene sutures and venting the right and left ventricles as described for the heart graft.

8   On filling the heart by releasing the aortic clamp, the cardiac cycle usually starts spontaneously.

9   Remove vents and withdraw bypass.

10   Close the chest with appropriate pericardial and pleural drainage.

Results

Currently, 1-year patient survival is 78%, with a 5-year survival of 50%. These results are the same for patients undergoing transplantation for cystic fibrosis and for the other indications.

REFERENCES

1. Cooley DA, Bloodwell RD, Hallman GL, et al. Organ transplantation for advanced cardiopulmonary disease. Ann Thorac Surg 1969;8:30–46.
2. Reitz BA, Burton NA, Jamieson SW, et al. Heart and lung transplantation. Autotransplantation and allotransplantation in primates with extended survival. J Thorac Cardiovasc Surg 1980;80:360–71.

FURTHER READING

Advisory Group on the Ethics of Xenotransplantation . Animal tissues into humans: recommendations and report. London: Department of Health; 1996.

Bismuth H, Houssin D. Reduced size orthotopic liver transplantation in children. Surgery 1984;95:367–70.

Campbell KWS, McWeir J, Ritchie WA, et al. Sheep cloned by nuclear transfer from a cultured cell line. Nature 1996;280:54–66.

Couinaud C. Controlled hepatectomies and exposure of the intrahepatic bile ducts. Paris: Couinaud; 1981.

Lancet. Diagnosis of brain death (editorial). Lancet 1976;ii:1069–70.

Medawar PB. The behaviour and fate of skin autografts and skin homografts in rabbits. J Anat 1944;78:176–99.

National Institutes of Health Consensus Development Conference. Statement: liver transplantation 1983. Hepatology 1984;4 (Suppl. 1):1075–105.

Starzl TE. Experience in Hepatic Transplantation. Philadelphia: Saunders; 1969.

Strong RW, Lynch SV, Ong TH, et al. Successful liver transplantation from a living donor to her son. N Engl J Med 1990;322:1505–07.

Warnock GL, Kneteman NM, Ryan EA, et al. Long term follow-up after transplantation of insulin producing pancreatic islets into patients with type I (insulin dependent) diabetes mellitus. Diabetologia 1992;35:89–95.

27

Thorax

E. Lim, A. Sadri

CONTENTS

ACCESS

POSTEROLATERAL THORACOTOMY (Fig. 27.2)

Appraise

1 This approach is most commonly used for pulmonary resection.

2 It allows access to the anterior, middle and posterior mediastinal structures, including the oesophagus.

Access

1 Operate with the patient under general anaesthetic. Ensure that a double lumen endobronchial tube is in place.

▶ KEY POINT

■ If there is a possibility of pneumonectomy, check that the double lumen tube is sited in the contralateral bronchus.

2 Position the patient in the lateral decubitus position (Fig. 27.1), arm at 90 degrees in the 'praying' position, back flush with edge of operating table. Support the patient with sandbags or a vacuum suction bean bag, strapped to the table for additional security if necessary. Apply padding to bony prominences, for example place a pillow between the knees.

3 Break the table to increase the distance between the rib spaces.

4 If necessary shave the skin, then prepare the chest, extending down to the operating table on both sides, up to the neck and down to the umbilicus. Apply the drapes.

5 Identify the tip of the scapula. Initially, start the incision approximately 2 cm below the tip of the scapula, and approximately 5 cm anterior to it, extending along the intercostal space to between the scapula and the spine. If necessary, extend the incision during the operation. Deepen the incision down to the dermis, followed by diathermy through the superficial fat down to the

latissimus dorsi fascia. Two Langenbeck retractors are used to expose the muscle and diathermy slowly through it layer by layer. Grasp with forceps and cauterize any visible blood vessels. Once through the latissimus, place a finger on the interspaces above and below the rib, and apply diathermy directly down to the rib. Pick up the anterior fascia with the cold tip of the diathermy, slide two fingers into the space and apply diathermy onto the finger. Repeat for the posterior aspect.

6 Check with the anaesthetist to ensure lung isolation – ventilation is undertaken by the single contralateral lung).

7 Count the ribs and correctly identify the interspace to incise it. The standard position is the 5th interspace (between the 5th and 6th ribs), corresponding to the line of the oblique fissure. Diathermy in a posterior to anterior direction through the intercostal muscles, to ensure that you stay on the superior border of the lower rib.

8 Visualize the pleura and puncture it with the cold tip of the diathermy. Insert your finger into the pleural space to ensure that the lung is not adherent and to protect the lung from the diathermy, and apply diathermy onto the finger.

9 Resect a small section (1 cm) of lower rib using a costotome at the most posterior aspect if you need to increase access. Insert a swab at the posterior osteotomy site to achieve haemostasis.

10 Introduce a suitable retractor, such as Finocheitto's or two Tudor-Edwards retractors, with a medium and small blade on each.

11 Using the long tip diathermy extend the incision anteriorly and posteriorly with diathermy through the intercostal muscle.

Before closure

1 After achieving haemostasis, check for air leaks which may require attention.

2 Pour warm saline - or water in the presence of malignant disease – into the thoracic cavity and ask the anaesthetist to gently re-inflate the lung. Air leaks are revealed by bubbling.

3 After securing air leaks, insert one or two (28–32F) chest drains, through separate stab incisions anterior to the mid-axillary line.

4 Secure the drains with a purse-string suture so that the nurses can tie the purse string when the drains are removed.

Closure

1 Close the rib interspace incision with a pericostal suture such as 1 PDS. Take care not to catch the lung, intercostal vessels or drains in the sutures. Ensure that the lung inflates fully and in the correct orientation before you tie the pericostal sutures.

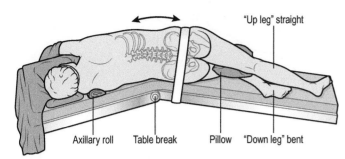

Fig. 27.1 The lateral decubitus position.

2 Close the muscle layer with a continuous suture such as 0 PDS.

3 Close the subcutaneous fat with a continuous suture such as 2/0 Vicryl.

4 Close the skin with a subcuticular stitch, using 3/0 Vicryl or metal clips. Cover it with an occlusive dressing.

> ▶ **KEY POINTS** Important structures

- Acquire intimate critical anatomical knowledge of the layers of the thoracic wall to gain access.
- The main neurovascular bundle lies in the costal groove on the lower border of each rib. However, an accessory neurovascular bundle may also exist near the superior border of each rib.
- Achieve lung collapse on the correct side of the operation to avoid damaging it during thoracotomy.

ANTERIOR THORACOTOMY (Fig. 27.3)

Appraise

This is a commonly used incision for minimal access lobectomy, and a standard incision for lobectomy in some practices.

Prepare

1 Ensure that a double lumen endotracheal intubation is in place.

2 Position the patient similarly to a posterolateral thoracotomy except that the patient lies in a slightly more supine position.

Action

1 Make the incision in the 4th/5th interspace from the mid-axillary line anteriorly, following the line of the intercostal space.

2 As a rule the incision is below the pectoralis major muscle, but it may need to be divided, accessing the chest in the same manner as a posterolateral thoracotomy.

Closure

See Posterolateral thoracotomy.

AXILLARY THORACOTOMY (Fig. 27.4)

Appraise

1 This is the incision of choice for access to the sympathetic chain in the upper thorax, and is used by some surgeons to undertake pleurectomy.

2 It is not suitable for resecting bulky tumours, sleeve resections or radical pneumonectomy.

> ▶ **KEY POINTS** Interspaces

- Access upper lobe lesions through the 4th interspace.
- Access lower lobe lesions through the 5th interspace.

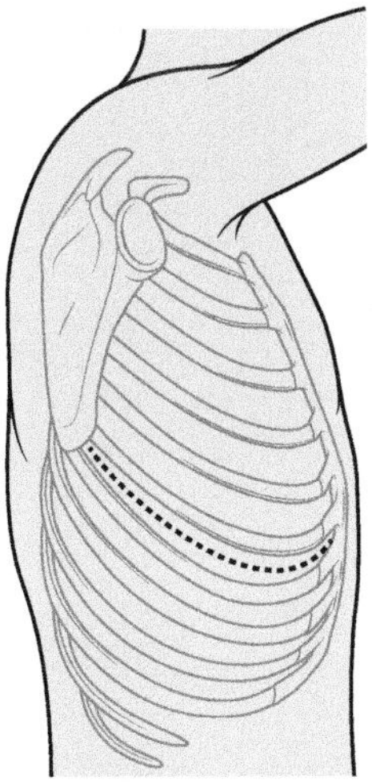

Fig. 27.2 Right lateral thoracotomy incision.

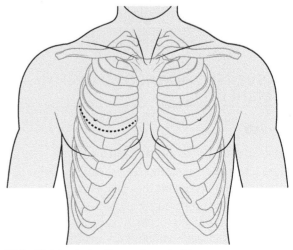

Fig. 27.3 Right anterior thoracotomy incision.

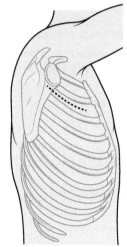

Fig. 27.4   Right axillary thoracotomy incision.

Prepare

Position the patient in a lateral decubitus position with the arm abducted at 90 degrees and supported on an armrest.

Action

1 Make the skin incision in the desired interspace, continued down to the anterior border of the latissimus dorsi.

2 Retract the latissimus dorsi posteriorly and split the serratus anterior muscle in the direction of its fibres.

3 Access the rib interspace in the same manner as a posterolateral thoracotomy.

Closure

See Posterolateral thoracotomy.

▶ KEY POINT Dangers

■ Do not split the serratus anterior too far posteriorly as this may damage the long thoracic nerve and result in a winged scapula.

TRANSVERSE THORACOTOMY (CLAMSHELL) (Fig. 27.5)

Appraise

1 This is an alternative to median sternotomy.

2 Utilize it when you require simultaneous bilateral thoracic access; for example, for penetrating chest injuries.

3 Through it, you can achieve digital control of penetrating wounds, cross-clamping of the thoracic descending aorta or pulmonary hilum, and internal cardiac massage.

4 It is relatively quick and simple to perform.

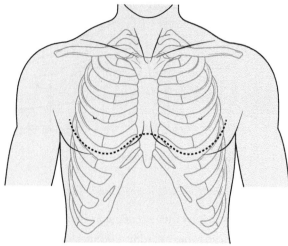

Fig. 27.5   Transverse clamshell incision.

Prepare

In the presence of trauma the patient may be intubated with a single lumen endotracheal tube in a supine position.

Action

1 Make the incision over the 4th or 5th interspace extending to each posterior axillary line.

2 Beware of the internal thoracic vessels, each of which lies approximately 1 cm lateral to the sternal edge. Identify and ligate them.

3 Transect the sternum transversely with an oscillating or Gigli saw.

4 A midline incision in the pericardium allows access to the heart.

ANTERIOR MEDIASTINOTOMY (Fig. 27.6)

Appraise

This commonly provides access for biopsy of lymph nodes and anterior mediastinal masses. The incision also allows access to the subaortic region on the left (a common site for metastasis of left upper lobe lesions), the anterosuperior aspect of the hilum, the lung and pleura.

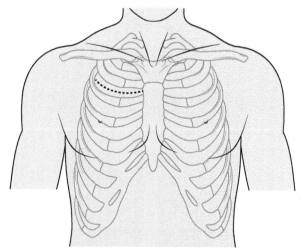

Fig. 27.6   Right anterior mediastinotomy incision.

Prepare

1 Perform the procedure under general anaesthesia with the patient supine and with double lumen endotracheal intubation.

Action

1 Make a 5–6-cm transverse incision just lateral to the sternum at the 2nd or 3rd intercostal space.

2 Split the pectoralis major transversely and identify the intercostal space. A section of costal cartilage can be resected to allow better access but this is rarely necessary. Identify and attempt to preserve the internal thoracic vessels.

3 Dissect off the mediastinal pleural reflection from the sternum and retract it laterally. Use finger dissection to identify the aorta and pulmonary artery. Identify lymph nodes and assess masses for fixation to surrounding structures. Biopsy tissue under direct vision using a mediastinocope or a thoracoscope.

4 If required, open the pleura and obtain a lung biopsy: drain the chest if lung biopsy is performed.

> ▶ KEY POINTS Structures at risk of injury

> ■ You have entered an area containing many structures at potential risk.
> ■ Be aware of the internal thoracic artery and vein, superior pulmonary vein, main pulmonary artery, aorta, vagus nerve and phrenic nerve.

VIDEO-ASSISTED THORACOSCOPIC SURGERY

Appraise

1 Diagnostic applications of video-assisted thoracoscopic surgery (VATS) include cancer staging, lung and pleural biopsy.

2 Therapeutic uses include drainage of fluid such as an effusion, empyema, blood, pleurodesis (Greek: desis = a binding together), pleurectomy, lung resection and sympathectomy.

Prepare

1 Position the patient as for posterolateral thoracotomy, with the operating table counter-flexed to increase the space between the ribs and to ensure that the hip does not restrict downward angulation of the camera.

2 Thoracoscopes range from 5–10 mm in diameter with varying degrees of lens angulation (0, 30 and 45 degrees). The standard scope is a 10-mm, 0 degree scope.

3 Your position depends on the site of the pathology. Place the monitor so that you, the site of pathology, and the monitor are aligned to allow you to look straight ahead when operating.

4 Vision is facilitated by white balancing of the camera and application of an anti-fog solution (e.g. FRED® – fog reduction elimination device).

Action

1 Correlate the initial port insertion with preoperative imaging. If you are undertaking VATS for a pleural effusion, you can use a needle and syringe to aspirate for fluid to ensure a safe position for entry.

2 Insert the camera port first. For indications such as pleurodesis the site of insertion is the junction between the middle and lower thirds of the chest. For indications such as management of pleural effusion place the incision a hand's breadth above the costal margin (corresponding to the dome of the diaphragm).

3 Insert all other ports under direct vision (Fig. 27.7).

4 The length of VATS port incisions is similar to the diameter of the port (e.g. 11.5 mm). A Roberts' forceps can be used as a retractor. Use diathermy all the way to the pleura. Ensure that the lung is isolated (see posterolateral thoracotomy above) before entry to the pleural cavity. Perform a finger sweep to confirm safe entry into the chest.

5 Instrument ports are inserted under direct vision using the scope. They are positioned to triangulate the lesion to facilitate easier dissection.

6 Rotation or tilting of the operating table can improve visualization by allowing the lung to drop away from the area to be examined.

CHEST DRAINS

1 Intercostal chest tube drainage with an underwater seal is a simple, effective and occasionally life-saving method to eliminate air or fluid in the pleural cavity.

2 Knowing when and how to insert a chest drain and its subsequent management is an important skill for all surgeons.

PERCUTANEOUS/SELDINGER CHEST DRAIN

Appraise

1 This versatile percutaneous technique involves passing the drain over a guide-wire and was devised by the Swedish radiologist

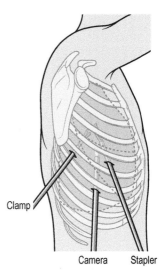

Fig. 27.7 Port and camera position for video-assisted thoracic surgery.

Sven-Ivar Seldinger in 1953. It is relatively atraumatic compared to the open technique and is easy to learn.

2 Seldinger chest drains may be used to manage pneumothoraces (small air leak) or pleural effusions.

3 The disadvantage of Seldinger drains is that insertion is blind. You cannot use a finger sweep to ensure that there are no adhesions and so avoid lung injury. The size of drains available is smaller when compared to open chest drains. There is also the possibility of losing the guide-wire in the pleural cavity.

Prepare

1 In elective situations, have adequate imaging available (chest X-ray, ultrasound or CT) to confirm the site of drain insertion.

2 Ultrasound is particularly useful to identify a safe site for the entry point of a Seldinger drain for effusions, as it can identify the position of the diaphragm and the presence of any loculations. It is important to carry out the procedure with the patient in the same position as when the scan was performed.

3 Position the patient lying supine at 45 degrees with the arm resting on the side of the patient (Fig. 27.8), or sitting leaning forwards.

Action

1 Ensure all equipment is present before starting. Seldinger chest drains come in pre-packaged sterile sets.

2 If possible, have a nurse or assistant helping you.

3 Before starting, confirm the site for drain insertion. Review the chest X-ray and percuss the chest to establish the fluid level.

4 Create a wheal of local anaesthetic over the point of entry. Continue deeper into the pleural space (confirmed by a flash back of fluid or bubbles) and withdraw slightly to anaesthetize the pleura.

5 Introduce the trocar attached to a syringe into the intercostal space and advance it slowly while aspirating on the syringe.

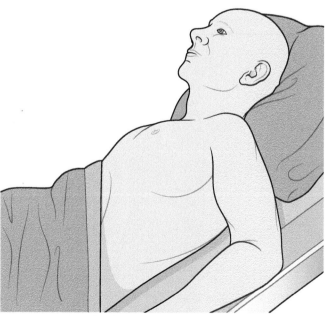

Fig. 27.8 Position for chest drain insertion.

A 'give' may be felt as the parietal pleura is punctured or fluid may be aspirated. As soon as fluid is aspirated stop advancing the needle. Remove the syringe and introduce the guide-wire.

6 Remove the needle over the guide-wire. Never let go of the guide-wire. Next, introduce the dilator over the guide-wire. If the entry point is too tight, widen it with a scalpel.

7 Remove the dilator and pass the chest drain over the guide-wire. Then remove the guide-wire, connect the drain to an underwater seal and suture the drain in place with a horizontal mattress stitch.

OPEN/SURGICAL CHEST DRAIN

Appraise

Open/surgical chest drains can be used in any situation requiring drainage of the chest cavity.

Prepare

1 Ensure that the patient has had a full explanation of the procedure and that all necessary equipment is present before embarking on the operation. If the patient is unwell arrange for adequate monitoring to be organized.

2 Position the patient lying supine at 45 degrees with the arm resting on the side of the patient.

3 Before preparing and draping the operation area, mark the position of the drain. The quadrangle of safety is bounded posteriorly by the posterior axillary line, anteriorly by the lateral border of pectoralis major muscle and overlies the 3rd to 5th intercostal spaces. Usually the 4th intercostal space is chosen just anterior to the mid-axillary line.

Action

1 It is best to perform a 3-level intercostal (field) block prior to starting the procedure. Advance the needle to identify the rib immediately above the chosen intercostal space and 'walk it' down the rib until you feel soft tissue. Angle the needle 45 degrees upwards and infiltrate 2–3 ml of local anaesthetic. Using the same method, inject a further 2 ml in the targeted intercostal space to block the intercostal nerve anteriorly and also in the intercostal nerve of the space above and below the targeted intercostal space (Fig. 27.9).

2 Infiltrate 1–2 ml of local anaesthetic to create a wheal over the marked intercostal space. Make an incision to easily admit one finger.

3 Allow sufficient time for the anaesthetic to take effect.

4 Bluntly dissect through the subcutaneous tissue until you reach the deep fascia and intercostal space.

5 Use a Roberts' clamp to gently spread the intercostal muscles superiorly from the lower margin of the intercostal space. This ensures that the neurovascular bundle is not damaged. Once the parietal pleural is reached a 'pop' or feeling of 'giving way' is sensed. A finger sweep is gently performed to dilate the tract and to detect any adherent lung tissue.

6 Once satisfied that there is no adherent lung tissue, introduce a 28–32F drain into the pleural space without a trocar. Direct it

8 Ensure that you see fogging in the drain, bubbling or swinging of the fluid level to indicate that the drain lies in the pleural space.

MANAGEMENT OF CHEST DRAINS

1 Confirm correct tube placement within the pleural cavity by noting the three signs of fogging of the tube, respiratory swing and bubbling.

2 Obtain a chest X-ray after drain insertion to ensure correct position, lung expansion and to screen for complications such as a new effusion from bleeding. Position the drain bottle below the level of the chest, otherwise fluid will siphon into the chest.

3 Inspect chest drains daily for patency, function, air leakage, and volume and character of the drainage.

4 Assess patency by inspecting for bubbling or swinging of the fluid within the tube with respiration.

5 Air leakage is indicated by the presence of bubbling within the underwater seal. Assess air leakage with the patient disconnected from wall suction and coughing.

6 Note the amount of the fluid collected in the last 24 hours along with its character.

7 Remove drains when there is no air leak for 24 hours, the lung is fully expanded on a chest film and there is an acceptable drainage volume. Obtain a chest X-ray after removal to ensure lung expansion and no accumulation of fluid.

8 If an air leak persists, you may discharge the patient with a chest in situ that is attached to a bag with a portable flutter-valve system (Portex® ambulatory chest drain bags, Smiths Medical USA).

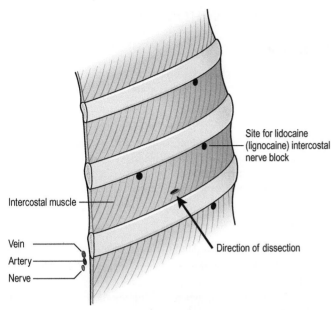

Site for lidocaine (lignocaine) intercostal nerve block

Intercostal muscle

Vein

Artery

Nerve

Direction of dissection

Fig. 27.9 Chest wall anatomy and sites for an intercostal field block.

apically or basally. Advance it until you feel a change of resistance as the drain abuts the pleural apex of diaphragm. Patients may experience pain in the neck or shoulder as the tip of the drain hits the apex. In such cases, withdraw the drain until symptoms disappear.

7 Connect the drain to the underwater seal. Secure the drain with a horizontal mattress, using a double throw to secure the initial tie. Next, tie a knot around the tubing to secure the drain. The horizontal mattress acts as a purse string to secure the wound after drain removal (Fig. 27.10).

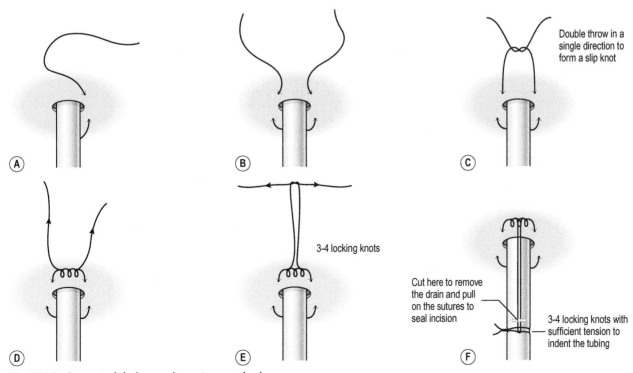

(A)

(B)

(C) Double throw in a single direction to form a slip knot

(D)

(E) 3-4 locking knots

(F) Cut here to remove the drain and pull on the sutures to seal incision

3-4 locking knots with sufficient tension to indent the tubing

Fig. 27.10 Suggested drain securing suture method.

Complications

1 Perforation of the lung can occur with forceful insertion of the chest tube. Warning signs are bleeding and brisk air leak.

2 Lacerations to the intercostal vessels can present and bleed profusely. If this occurs, you may be required to institute fluid resuscitation and possible surgical exploration in theatre.

3 Entry in the abdominal cavity is a possibility. If you detect this, do not remove the drain. Immediately consult a general surgeon.

> **KEY POINTS** Cautions with chest drain

- Never clamp a bubbling chest drain. This indicates a continuing airleak and may result in tension pneumothorax.
- Control drainage of large pleural effusions (e.g. 1 L/hour) to reduce the risk of re-expansion pulmonary oedema.

BRONCHOSCOPY

Bronchoscopy is the application of fibreoptic scopes to visualize the airways. It can be both diagnostic and therapeutic (Fig. 27.11).

Appraise

1 Bronchoscopy (Greek: bronchos = windpipe) is a valuable tool for seeking the cause of an unresolving cough, the onset of stridor or wheeze, haemoptysis, the cytology of sputum and inspecting known or suspected airway obstruction. It allows broncho-alveolar lavage, the staging of oesophageal and air tumours and assists in elucidating abnormal findings on chest radiology.

2 Therapeutically, it permits airway clearance of sputum, the removal of foreign bodies and disobliteration of tumour using diathermy or laser.

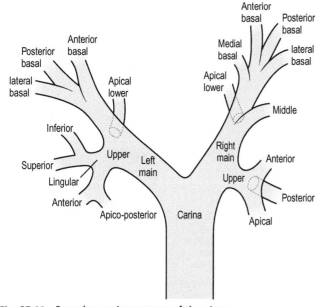

Fig. 27.11 Bronchoscopic anatomy of the airway.

FLEXIBLE BRONCHOSCOPY

Appraise

1 Examine the bronchial tree and vocal cords prior to surgery. It can be performed as a day-case procedure.

2 Identify endobronchial lesions and obtain biopsies and brushings of abnormal respiratory epithelium.

3 Bronchial washings produce samples for cytology in suspected malignancy. Transbronchial lymph node aspiration and lung parenchymal biopsies can be performed for staging lung cancer and diagnosis of lung disease, respectively.

Prepare

1 Gain informed consent. Stop oral intake for 4 hours prior to the procedure in case a general anaesthesia or deep sedation is required.

2 The patient can sit, but where possible should be placed in a supine position. Give supplemental oxygen and monitor oxygen saturation.

Action

1 Spray topical xylocaine into the nasal passage. Wait for it to act before introducing the fibreoptic telescope into the nose. Spray further xylocaine from the side arm of the scope as it is advanced, to anaesthetize the hypopharynx, larynx and vocal cords.

2 Progressing from the trachea, visualize the entire tracheobronchial tree.

Complications

These occur in only 1.7% of cases and mortality is 0.1%. They include respiratory arrest, pneumonia, airway obstruction, cardiac arrhythmias, bleeding, vasovagal attack and aphonia. Transbronchial biopsy carries an additional (10%) risk of pneumothorax.

RIGID BRONCHOSCOPY

Appraise

1 This allows a wide range of therapeutic procedures to be carried out. It provides a valuable method of removing foreign bodies, treating haemoptysis, dilating strictures and for disobliterating endobronchial tumours.

2 Perform it using general anaesthetic. Teeth, mouth and airways are at risk of trauma. There is poor visualization of smaller airways and of obtaining biopsies from the upper lobe.

3 Order a chest X-ray after the procedure to screen for complications. Monitor the patient in a high dependency unit.

Prepare

1 Gain informed consent. Fast the patient overnight in preparation for a general anaesthetic.

2 Position the patient supine with the head and neck extended.

Action

1 Ensure the patient is pre-oxygenated and the eyes taped.

2 Place two fingers of the non-dominant hand on the hard palate with the thumb positioned above to protect the upper incisors. Introduce the rigid scope under direct vision through the mouth with the bevel facing forwards. Correctly positioned, the incisors should be 'biting' into your fingers and thumbs without any contact with the bronchoscope.

3 Once past the base of the tongue, gentle apply forward pressure to identify the epiglottis and elevate this with the instrument. The vocal folds are not visible until the epiglottis is adequately elevated. Rotate the bevel 90 degrees and advance the tip of the bronchoscope between the vocal folds.

4 Provide intermittent jet ventilation through the bronchoscope to maintain gas exchange. Use a straight telescope to inspect the main and lower lobe airways. To visualize the right and left upper lobe bronchi, position the bronchoscope immediately proximal to the upper lobe orifice and use a 90 degree telescope.

5 Identify and assess endobronchial masses or invasive disease of the lower trachea. Note the site and length of stenoses. Record paralysis of the vocal cords.

6 At the end of the procedure, ask the anaesthetist to take control of the airway before you withdraw the bronchoscope.

CERVICAL MEDIASTINOSCOPY

Appraise

1 This is a common diagnostic procedure for mediastinal lymph node biopsy. The nodes accessible to mediastinoscopy are the paratracheal, subcarinal and occasionally the tracheobronchial nodes.

2 Be cautious, particularly in the presence of a large goitre, an aneurysm of the brachiocephalic artery, a previous neck incision, superior vena cava obstruction and anterior mediastinal pathology due to inaccessibility.

Prepare

1 General anaesthesia is required. Position the patient supine with a head ring, neck extended and a sandbag between the shoulders. This brings the trachea from the mediastinum into the neck.

2 Prepare the chest from chin to the umbilicus in case emergency sternotomy is required.

Action

1 Make a 2–3-cm transverse midline incision, one finger's breadth above the sternal notch. Open up the vertical plane between the strap muscles. Incise the pretracheal fascia in the midline and visualize the tracheal ring. If the isthmus of the thyroid obstructs the view it can be retracted or ligated.

2 Introduce a finger deep to the pretracheal fascia and along the anterior surface of the trachea and continued to the full length of the finger. Note the trachea is directed inferiorly and posteriorly.

3 Insert the mediastinoscope on the anterior surface of the trachea. The anatomic orientation is defined by the relationship to the trachea. Carry out blunt dissection using a specific mediastinoscopy rigid suction and diathermy device.

4 Define the edges of lymph nodes and any masses by blunt dissection, to differentiate them from vascular structures. Biopsy specimens by grasping and gently twisting them with the grasping forceps. Avoid excessive pulling. The mass may be adherent to and tear a major vessel.

5 Achieve haemostasis with diathermy and packing with a swab. Approximate the strap muscles with absorbable sutures and close the skin with a subcuticular suture.

6 Nurse the patient in a high dependency unit. Obtain a chest X-ray to screen for complications, which occur in 2% of patients. They include haemorrhage, tracheal, oesophageal or thoracic duct injury. Recurrent laryngeal nerve may ensure or pneumothorax.

LUNG RESECTION

SUBLOBAR/WEDGE RESECTION

Appraise

1 Sublobar resection is a non-anatomic resection used for lung (parenchymal) biopsy, biopsy of discrete lesions within the lung and excision of metastates.

Access

1 Thoracotomy or VATS.

2 The choice of access depends on the indication for surgery. For lung parenchymal biopsy or removal of a limited number of superficial nodules employ VATS. When nodules are small, deep seated or multiple, thoracotomy allows lesions to be identified by palpation.

Action

1 After entry into the chest, make a thorough inspection to ensure that you have identified all areas of disease. If the patient has multiple lesions, address each separately.

2 Perform VATS resection using an endoscopic stapler. This simultaneously seals and cuts the lung. Several stapling devices are available for wedge resections. By inserting converging staple lines on either side of the lesion, you can resect the lesions and lung as a triangular wedge of tissue, with a clear margin.

3 Undertake open resection using precision diathermy, resecting the mass as a hemisphere of lung with clear margins. Oversew and close the defect with 3/0 Prolene using a horizontal mattress suture, followed by an over-and-over layer.

4 After haemostasis, check for air leak by pouring warm saline/water into the pleural cavity and reconnect the lung to the ventilator circuit. Suture the leaking lung surface, identified by the presence of bubbling.

LOBECTOMY

Appraise

1. The principles of lobectomy are mobilization of the lobe, fissure dissection, and management of the vessels and bronchus.

2. There are minor variations, depending on the lobe for resection.

3. Obtain lung function tests prior to any lung resection to establish whether the patient has enough respiratory reserve to withstand the loss of lung tissue postoperatively.

Access

1. Lobectomy may be performed via a posterolateral thoracotomy or VATS.

Action

1. After entering the pleural cavity, mobilize the lobe by dividing any adhesions between the lung and chest wall: use diathermy if they are vascular or a sponge on a stick if avascular.

2. Assess if there is chest wall involvement. If so, you may need to carry out an en bloc resection including the chest wall.

3. We prefer to undertake a systematic nodal dissection. This is initially facilitated by incising the mediastinal pleura in the right paratracheal fossa, between the phrenic and vagus nerves, to access stations 2 and 4. Alternatively, incise over the left para-aortic mediastinal pleura, to access stations 5 and 6. We continue systematic nodal dissection and hilar mobilization by defining the subcarinal space – station 7 – and the para-oesophageal nodes – station 8 – then free the inferior pulmonary ligament – station 9.

4. Define, by sharp and blunt dissection, the pulmonary vein corresponding to the lobe of interest. Encircle it with a 3-mm cotton tape.

5. Now examine the fissure and locate the pulmonary artery within the fissure. On the right, the upper lobe artery usually corresponds to the posterior edge of the junction between upper and middle lobe, and the lower lobe artery usually corresponds to 1 cm anterior to the posterior junction between middle and lower lobes.

6. Once you have identified the pulmonary artery in the fissure (mild lung inflation may assist in defining the planes when the fissure is poorly developed), clearly define the anterior and posterior limits along with any branches and their destination. On the right, the posterior fissure is completed by blunt dissection from the pulmonary artery to the bifurcation of the upper lobe and bronchus intermedius. On the left, the posterior fissure is completed by dissection along the pulmonary artery. Pass a cotton tape between pulmonary artery and posterior fissure and elevate the lung. Staple it with a linear stapler. The anterior aspect of the oblique fissure is completed by dissection between the pulmonary artery and the two pulmonary veins, whilst the anterior aspect of the horizontal fissure is completed by dissection between the pulmonary artery and the bifurcation between upper and middle lobe vein.

7. If the tumour has crossed a fissure, a bilobectomy or pneumonectomy may be required.

8. The pulmonary arteries are dissected from their fibrous sheath. When an adequate length of the vessel has been exposed, pass a right-angled clamp (Lahey or O'Shaughnessy clamp, depending on size of the vessel) to encircle the vessel and to draw round it a ligature (2/0 or 3/0 Neurolon). Tie the arterial branches with two ligatures, one proximal and one distal to the point of division. Alternatively, use a vascular stapler to staple the arterial branches.

9. Clamp the pulmonary vein with two right-angled clamps (Ronald Edwards), divide it and transfix it using a 2/0 Ethibond suture, over-sewn. Alternatively, apply a vascular stapler to staple the vein.

10. Clamp the bronchus and divide it using a right-angled clamp (Ronald Edwards), and undertake bronchial closure using a 3/0 Prolene horizontal mattress sutures (to-and-fro), followed by an over-and-over layer of 3/0 Prolene. Alternatively, use a thick bronchial stapler.

11. After removing the lobe, test the integrity of the bronchial closure by filling the chest with saline and reconnecting the lung to the ventilator circuit. Over-sew sources of bubbles with sutures.

12. Before closing, insert drains through stab incisions anterior to the mid-axillary line.

13. Common branching patterns of the right pulmonary artery are truncus anterior (posterior ascending, apical and anterior), posterior ascending, middle lobe, superior segmental and common basal artery.

Right upper lobectomy

1. Begin with a systematic nodal dissection, mobilizing the lung and defining the fissures.

2. Incise the mediastinal pleura around the right hilum. Begin inferiorly to the azygos vein. Inferior to the azygocaval junction is the upper border of the right pulmonary artery. Using pledgets, dissect out the superior arterial trunk and define the apical and anterior segmental branches (a recurrent posterior branch may be present).

3. Define the azygous vein and make an incision between the vagus and phrenic nerves, over the surface of the trachea, to expose the paratracheal lymph nodes. If possible, resect them as a tissue block.

4. Rotate the lung medially and continue to incise the pleural reflection posteriorly (inferior to the azygos vein), over the right main bronchus.

5. Define the right main bronchus, upper lobe bronchus and bronchus intermedius. Usually there is an interlobar lymph node in the bifurcation between the upper lobe and bronchus intermedius. Note that the pulmonary artery is immediately anterior to this, and that the node usually lies on the posterior surface of the pulmonary artery!

6. Define the inferior border of the bronchus intermedius, which is the subcarinal fossa and remove the lymph nodes in the fossa.

7. Continue to incise the pleural reflection along the oesophagus and remove any station 8 lymph nodes.

8. Ask an assistant to use a swab on a Rampley's forcep to retract the diaphragm, and divide the inferior pulmonary ligament, all the way to the inferior vein. Remove any lymph nodes from station 9.

9 The superior pulmonary vein lies anterior to the artery. Mobilize the vein using sharp dissection, through the fascia. Use pledgets to define the vein and to separate it from the middle vein. Define the posterior aspect using pledgets, and gently pass a blunt O'Shaughnessy clamp behind the vein with a tape to isolate the superior vein, leaving the middle lobe vein in situ.

10 Identify the pulmonary artery within the fissure. For an upper lobectomy we prefer to identify the artery at the confluence of the oblique and horizontal fissure. Once the artery is identified, define it using pledgets and also clearly define the branches to each lobe.

11 Use a finger and thumb to identify the tissue plane between the bifurcation of the airway and the surface of the artery. Pass a tape across this and apply a linear stapler to complete the posterior fissure (Fig. 27.12).

12 From the anterior surface of the pulmonary artery, carefully identify the middle lobe arterial branches and also a plane superior to the middle lobe arteries to the bifurcation between the upper and middle lobe vein. Pass a tape across this and apply a linear stapler to complete the horizontal fissure.

13 Now assess the vascular and bronchial structures to ensure that a lung resection can be undertaken with clear margins. Once a commitment to perform an upper lobectomy is made, we prefer to begin with ligation of the pulmonary arterial branches before the vein, to avoid venous engorgement.

14 Define the arterial branches to the upper lobe and doubly ligate (two proximal, one distal), using a 2/0 or a 3/0 ligature, depending on the size of the branch.

15 Divide the vein and bronchus as described above.

16 Finally, ligate the middle lobe to the lower lobe to prevent torsion.

Middle lobectomy

1 Middle lobectomy is commonly performed in association with either upper or lower lobectomy for tumours that cross fissures.

2 Proceed as described for the upper lobectomy to incise the pleural reflections.

3 Identify and tape the middle lobe vein.

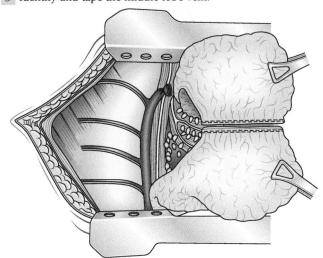

Fig. 27.12   Right upper lobectomy.

4 Complete the fissure as described for the upper lobectomy. In addition, complete the anterior aspect of the oblique fissure.

5 Ligate the arterial branches (usually 1 or 2) to the middle lobe.

6 The middle lobe bronchus is usually only clearly visible after the middle lobe artery has been divided.

Right lower lobectomy

1 Proceed as described for the upper lobectomy to incise the pleural reflections and to perform a systematic nodal dissection.

2 When developing the inferior pulmonary ligament, define and tape the inferior vein.

3 When developing the fissure, note that the pulmonary artery usually lies 2 cm anterior to the confluence between the horizontal and oblique fissures.

4 Develop the posterior aspect of the oblique fissure as described for an upper lobectomy and the anterior aspect is completed.

5 Define and ligate the common basilar artery and the superior segmental artery.

6 Divide the vein and bronchus as described for a lobectomy.

Left upper lobectomy

1 Retract the upper lobe inferiorly and incise the pleural reflection on the surface of the pulmonary artery. Identify the vagus and the recurrent laryngeal nerve. Resect any lymph node in the paraortic (station 6) and aorto-pulmonary window (station 5).

2 Continue to incise the fascia posteriorly and define the posterior aspect of the pulmonary artery. Inferior to the artery lies the left main bronchus.

3 Incise the pleural reflection between the aortic arch and the bronchus to define the subcarinal fossa and resect any lymph nodes (station 7).

4 Continue to incise the fascia along the oesophagus and resect any lymph nodes (station 8).

5 Incise the inferior pulmonary ligament.

6 Define the superior pulmonary vein by sharp dissection through the fascia and pledgets. Pass a blunt O'Shaughnessy behind the vein, with a tape used to isolate the vein.

7 Develop the fissure by identifying the pulmonary artery within the fissure and clearly identify the branches to the upper and lower lobes. Completely separate the posterior and anterior fissure using a linear stapler. This may be made easier by developing the posterior aspect of the pulmonary artery (Fig. 27.13).

8 Now assess the vascular and bronchial structures to ensure that a lung resection can be undertaken with clear margins.

9 Define and doubly ligate the arterial branches to the upper lobe (two proximal, one distal), using a 2/0 or a 3/0 ligature depending on the size of the branch.

10 Divide the vein and bronchus as described for a right upper lobectomy.

Left lower lobectomy

1 Begin as described for a left upper lobectomy to the point of completing the fissure.

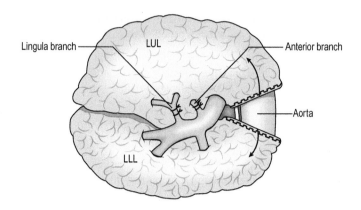

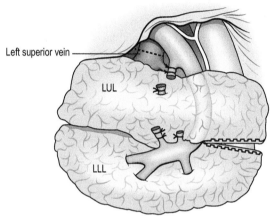

Fig. 27.13 Left upper lobectomy.

2 Define and ligate the common basilar artery and the superior segmental artery.

3 Divide the vein and bronchus as described for a lobectomy.

SEGMENTECTOMY

Appraise

1 This is an anatomic excision of a named bronchopulmonary segment with its pulmonary arterial branch and venous drainage.

2 It is an option for an anatomic resection in patients with poor pulmonary reserve.

Prepare

1 A standard posterolateral approach is used, with the patient under general anaesthetic with single lung ventilation. You require a detailed knowledge of the bronchial and vascular anatomy to perform this operation.

Action

1 The hilar structures are identified and the oblique fissure dissected to reveal the vasculature.

2 Isolate the corresponding segmental bronchus and artery. Ligate vessels feeding the segment for excision only, otherwise pulmonary infarction may occur.

3 Before dividing the bronchus, deflate and inflate the segment to help delineate the intersegmental planes.

4 If you are performing segmentectomy for infection, make sure to ligate the bronchus first, to avoid contamination.

5 After ligation of the artery and bronchus, exert traction on the bronchus, and remove the segment in a retrograde manner. The pulmonary veins run in the intersegmental plane and provide a guide for dissection. Ligate these veins as you free the segment.

6 Examine the remaining raw surfaces for air leaks. If the segmentectomy has been performed accurately, air leaks are minimal.

PNEUMONECTOMY

Appraise

1 This is indicated for bulky, centrally located tumours and for severely degenerative lung secondary to ongoing chronic infection.

Prepare

1 Expose using a posterolateral thoracotomy through the 5th intercostal space.

2 Make a thorough inspection of local metastatic spread of the disease into adjacent structures. If spread has occurred, pneumonectomy is futile.

3 Make a final intra-operative assessment to determine whether a lobectomy or sleeve lobectomy can be safely performed, thus preserving lung tissue. If not, then proceed to pneumonectomy.

Action

Left pneumonectomy

1 Make a circumferential incision around the mediastinal pleura to expose the hilum. Preserve the phrenic nerve if not involved with disease.

2 Use pledget dissection to identify the main pulmonary artery, and place a tape around the artery to gain control.

3 Proceed with dissection as described for a left upper lobectomy, to the point of identifying the main bronchus. Pass a tape around the main bronchus.

4 Prepare both pulmonary veins and pass a tape around each vein.

5 Now assess the vascular and bronchial structures to ensure that a lung resection can be undertaken with clear margins.

6 Clamp the main pulmonary vein with two right-angled clamps (Ronald Edwards), divided and transfixed using a 2/0 Ethibond suture and over-sewn. Alternatively, use a vascular stapler to staple the artery.

7 Clamp both pulmonary veins with two right-angled clamps (Ronald Edwards), divided and transfixed using a 2/0 Ethibond suture and over-sewn. Alternatively, use a vascular stapler to staple the veins.

8 Divide the artery and apply a 2/0 Ethibond suture ligature.

9 Dissect the bronchus, making sure to avoid removing the adventitia. This would impair healing and may lead to increased risk of fistula formation. Free the bronchus up to the level of the carnia and divide it just distally.

10 Clamp and divide the bronchus using a right-angled clamp (Ronald Edwards), and close the bronchus using 3/0 Prolene horizontal mattress to-and-fro sutures. Follow this by an over-and-over layer of 3/0 Prolene. Alternatively, use a thick bronchial stapler.

11 Achieve haemostasis, insert a chest drain that is clamped on extubation and released for 1 minute every hour. This is to assess for bleeding and to prevent mediastinal shift.

Right pneumonectomy

1 Make a circumferential incision around the mediastinal pleura to expose the hilum. Reflect the azygos vein superiorly from the right main bronchus.

2 Manage the artery, veins and bronchus similarly to a left pneumonectomy.

Postoperatively

1 Order regular chest X-rays to ensure that the pneumonectomy space gradually fills. Any drop in the air fluid level may indicate a bronchopleural fistula.

2 Air-fluid levels in the post-pneumonectomy space may suggest infection and require thoracocentesis (Greek: kentesis = a pricking; drainage).

PLEURODESIS AND PLEURECTOMY

1 Pleurodesis (Greek: desis = a binding) is fusion of the parietal and visceral pleura, thus obliterating the space between the lung and chest wall. Pleurodesis is commonly employed in cases of recurrent effusions secondary to malignancy and for pneumothorax. It is mainly indicated for treating a prolonged air leak, or failure of lung re-expansion, for recurrent pneumothorax. For fluid management, success from pleurodesis is not complete pleural fusion but the prevention of re-accumulation of enough pleural fluid to cause symptoms.

2 Pleurectomy is the surgical excision of the parietal pleural to promote adhesion of the lung to the chest wall.

CHEMICAL PLEURODESIS

Appraise

1 A cost-effective method of managing a symptomatic malignant pleural effusion is by instilling a sclerosing agent into the pleural cavity after drainage of fluid and re-expansion of the collapsed lung.

2 Talc slurry or powder is the most effective and commonly used sclerosing agent, achieving pleurodesis in 95% of cases.

3 Talc pleurodesis can cause a fever for up to 72 hours, be very painful and cause a rise in serum C-reactive protein. Talc pleurodesis is associated with a 1% risk of respiratory failure.

Prepare

1 Prior to talc instillation insert a basally directed chest drain, so that all the effusion is drained in a controlled manner and the lung fully expanded. This is so that the lung is in contact with the chest wall and has the maximum chance of adhering.

Action

1 After inserting an intercostal tube and draining all pleural fluid, obtain a chest radiograph to check the position of the chest drain and to ensure full expansion of the lung.

2 Be willing to administer analgesics and supplemental oxygen prior to talc instillation.

3 Mix 2–3 g of talc with 30 ml of normal saline. If not contraindicated, add up to 30 ml of 1% lidocaine to the slurry for analgesia.

4 Instil the talc slurry through the chest tube and clamp it for 1 hour.

5 Connect the chest drain to the wall suction to ensure approximation of the lung to the chest wall.

6 Remove the drain when the daily output is <2 ml/kg/day.

SURGICAL PLEURODESIS

Action

Talc insufflation

1 Access the pleural cavity by VATS. If talc insufflation is to be performed for malignant pleural effusion, first completely aspirate the effusion. If it is being performed for pneumothorax, carry out an examination for any bullae that may require excision.

2 Insert the talc insufflator into the chest and under video guidance distribute talc powder evenly to all areas of the thoracic cavity.

3 Insert two chest drains and place them on suction during the postoperative period.

PLEURAL ABRASION

1 Access the pleural cavity by VATS or mini-thoracotomy.

2 Perform the pleural abrasion with a diathermy scratch pad attached to a sponge holding forceps introduced into the chest through an incision in the 5th or 6th intercostal space on the anterior axillary line.

3 Rub the parietal pleural until it oozes. The pleural abrasion limits are the thoracic mammary artery anteriorly and the sympathetic chain posteriorly.

4 Inspect the lung for bleeding and check for air leaks. Insert two chest drains and place them on suction during the postoperative period.

PLEURECTOMY

Appraise

1 This can be performed by VATS or posterolateral thoracotomy and requires one-lung ventilation. It is indicated in patients with pneumothorax or malignant pleural effusion refractory to nonsurgical management.

Action

1 Access the chest using a limited thoracotomy through the 5th or 6th intercostal space.

2 Strip the pleura, commencing in the plane between the parietal pleura and the extrathoracic fascia, at the margins of the intercostal incision, before inserting the rib spreader.

3 Strip the parietal pleura circumferentially towards the mediastinum, taking care to avoid injury to the sympathetic chain, recurrent laryngeal nerve and the stellate ganglion.

4 The limits of the pleurectomy are the 3rd rib superiorly, the internal mammary artery anteriorly, the diaphragm inferiorly and the sympathetic chain posteriorly.

DECORTICATION

Appraise

1 This is performed when there is inadequate evacuation of haemothorax, empyema, or pleural effusions with incomplete expansion of the underlying lung. The result is the formation of thick fibrous tissue on the lung surface (fibrothorax).

2 Fibrothorax is managed by decortication, the peeling or stripping of a constricting membrane from the pleural surfaces. This allows the lung to fully expand and improves gas exchange.

3 Rule out mesothelioma and malignancy before proceeding to decortication.

Prepare

1 Carry out bronchoscopy prior to decortication to rule out bronchial obstruction which may inhibit expansion of the lung.

Action

1 For decortication of the upper part of the lung, access through the 3rd/4th intercostal space provides best access. The 6th/7th intercostal space is used for decortication of the lower lobe. Evacuate the pleural cavity of debris.

2 Begin with incision of the fibrous peel and locate the plane between the fibrous peel and grey glistening visceral pleura using a spatula. Multiple layers may have to be incised before the visceral pleura is reached. Use a finger and swab to peel off the fibrous sheet.

3 If the wrong plane is dissected, excessive air leaks and bleeding will result as the visceral pleura is stripped. Re-expansion of the lung can be used to facilitate dissection.

4 Insert two intercostal drains and place them on suction postoperatively.

Head and neck

M.P. Stearns

GENERAL PRINCIPLES

■ Details of anatomy tend to be more important in the head and neck than in other regions. Numerous structures are crowded into a small volume and many of them, such as the facial nerve, perform important functions. Some are vital to life itself, such as the recurrent laryngeal nerve and the internal carotid artery. Refresh your memory of the local and neighbouring anatomy before performing a new or unfamiliar operation. Before embarking on any major procedure consider seeking advice from, or collaborating with, a plastic, thoracic, dental or neuro-surgeon or otolaryngologist.

■ The airway may be threatened by the accumulation of blood, by laryngospasm, etc., so insist on endotracheal intubation for all but the simplest procedures.

■ Gastrointestinal complications such as peritonitis, paralytic ileus and disturbances of water and electrolyte balance are rare, as is thrombo-embolism.

■ Postoperative chest complications occur following direct interference with respiratory passages or after long operations but are less common than following abdominal or thoracic surgery.

■ Even massive resections of tissues are therefore well tolerated. Infection is uncommon and healing is usually by first intention.

When skin grafting is necessary to repair a defect, the grafts take well. Good healing is evidence of the good blood supply enjoyed by the territory, the corollary being that the principal operative hazard, after damage to important anatomical structures, is primary haemorrhage.

MINIMIZE BLOOD LOSS

1 Discuss likely blood loss with the anaesthetist, who may decide to use hypotensive anaesthesia, lowering the arterial blood pressure by such agents as ganglion blockers. If you do operate under hypotension, remember the increased risk of reactionary haemorrhage shortly after the wound has been closed, so delay closure until you are certain that the blood pressure has been restored to normal.

2 Venous bleeding is more difficult to control than arterial. Venous pressure, and therefore venous bleeding, can be minimized by paying careful attention to posture. Position the patient so that the area being operated on is at a higher level than the heart. Carefully protect local veins from direct pressure resulting from clumsy positioning of the head, neck or shoulders, and the presence of supports or towels, etc. If it is necessary to divide a large vein draining the operative area, postpone this step in the operation to the latest possible moment. The anaesthetist helps to reduce venous pressure by maintaining the clearest possible airway and by keeping arterial carbon dioxide tension normal or below normal.

3 Control blood vessels before dividing them; in this way you obviate excessive blood loss from, for example, a haemostat slipping off the cut vessel. For sizeable vessels, pass two ligatures with an aneurysm needle and tie them around the vessel before dividing the vessel between them.

▶ KEY POINT Anatomy

■ Acquire a detailed knowledge of the anatomy in order to anticipate encountering vessels so that you can control them before cutting them.

4 Many surgeons infiltrate the skin and subcutaneous tissues with a solution of 1:200 000 adrenaline (epinephrine) in normal saline, thereby producing vasospasm and reducing bleeding.

5 Diathermy is a valuable aid to haemostasis, but use it carefully. It stops bleeding by coagulating the tissues at more than 1000°C, potentially causing extensive destruction. Cutting diathermy produces high-intensity energy over a small sphere from the active electrode; coagulating current produces a lower intensity over a larger sphere. It is traditional to use the cutting current to incise

tissues and the coagulating for producing haemostasis, on the principle that the larger zone of action of the coagulating current compensates for any small inaccuracy in identifying the bleeding point. Use the cutting current for haemostasis, having first made sure that each bleeding point has been accurately identified; this discipline reduces unnecessary tissue destruction to a minimum.

6 After the operation, use suction drainage to obliterate the dead space under the skin flaps, thereby reducing the risk of secondary haemorrhage and haematomas. Note that in the neck a haematoma is a potentially lethal complication, because of its possible effect upon the patency of the airway.

> ### ▶ KEY POINTS Threats to the airway
>
> ■ After any extensive procedures, especially those involving resection of the lower jaw, ask yourself whether such factors as an unstable tongue or laryngeal oedema might be a particular threat to the maintenance of the airway in the postoperative period.
> ■ Be prepared to perform a temporary tracheostomy in such circumstances.

REPLACE BLOOD LOSS

1 Before operation, ensure that every patient has been asked about any history of a bleeding tendency, that a haemoglobin estimation has been performed and that blood has been taken for grouping and serum saved in case cross-matching becomes necessary.

2 With regard to which cases require blood to be cross-matched before the operation, it is difficult to lay down rules. Much depends upon your experience and that of the anaesthetist. Blood transfusion is rarely necessary for conservative parotidectomy under good hypotensive anaesthesia, but, if you are an inexperienced operator, working with normotensive anaesthesia, have 2 units of blood cross-matched and have 4 units cross-matched before an extensive resection involving bone and/or block dissection of the cervical lymph nodes.

3 Normally, the anaesthetist controls blood replacement during the operation. The principles are accurate measurement of the blood loss by weighing swabs and measuring the volume of the contents of the sucker bottle, with prompt and complete replacement, preferably monitored by the measurement of central venous pressure or of urine output.

PAROTIDECTOMY

Appraise

1 Assess a parotid lump before operation by careful clinical examination. Pain and facial nerve palsy are diagnostic of malignancy unless tuberculosis is suspected. Fine-needle aspiration cytology is accurate in about 85% of cases,[2] but the role of needle biopsy is debatable. Small discrete masses usually require surgical rather than conservative management.[3] Most parotid neoplasms are benign.[4]

2 The facial nerve and its five main branches run through the substance of the parotid gland and are at risk in parotidectomy.

3 Plan to expose the facial nerve and its branches at an early stage of any parotidectomy and over a sufficiently wide area to ensure that the required resection is achieved without cutting the nerve (conservative parotidectomy). However, if the object of your operation is to remove a lump in the parotid with a wide margin of normal tissue, you will sometimes find that this condition is impossible to fulfil; an adequate margin cannot be achieved unless you sacrifice the whole nerve (radical parotidectomy) or one or more of its branches (semi-conservative parotidectomy).[5]

4 If the decision is not clear-cut whether to sacrifice the main nerve, lean towards radicalism in elderly males, conservatism in young females. Biopsy the lump, and ask for an immediate histological opinion on frozen sections, provided:
   ■ You take extreme precautions against spreading the tumour in taking the biopsy: parotid tumours are notorious for their tendency to implant
   ■ Your pathologist is an expert in the histopathology of parotid lesions.[6]

5 Repair any gap you produce in the facial nerve system by immediate primary suture, if possible, or by bridging the defect with a free cable graft, taken as a routine from the great auricular nerve at the beginning of the operation. Ignore any damage to the fifth (cervical) branch.

6 Operations for recurrent parotitis not due to parotid calculus (i.e. the group of conditions known as Sjogren's or sicca syndrome) may require total conservative parotidectomy.

Prepare

1 If you confirm a malignant tumour, discuss the implications with the patient, especially if there is a prospect of sacrificing part or all of the facial nerve.

2 Check that male patients are clean-shaven on the side of the tumour.

3 Have the patient lying near your side of the operating table. Tilt the top half of the operating table upwards until the external jugular vein collapses. Extend the patient's head on the neck, turn it away from you and place it on a head-ring to stabilize it, with a sandbag, or similar, under the shoulder

4 To protect the patient, and protect yourself from charges of negligence, monitor the facial nerve. Insert needle electrodes into the ipsilateral frontalis and mentalis muscles to record electromyographic signals from them, producing audible and visual signals when the facial nerves supplying them are stimulated. The nerve monitor can also be used as an aid to identify a doubtful nerve or to confirm that the nerve is intact by demonstrating a signal on stimulating the nerve.

5 Ensure that the patient's eyes are protected from possible damage by lotions used in the skin preparation. Clean the skin over the area shown in Figure 28.1.

6 Place the towels to leave exposed only the area shown in Figure 28.1. Push some ½″ ribbon gauze (which is added to the swab count) into the external auditory meatus with a pair of artery forceps and then discard them.

7 Ask the anaesthetist to maintain the patient in hypotension if possible.

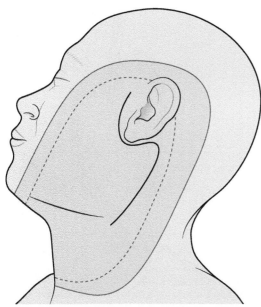

Fig. 28.1 The standard S-shaped cervicofacial incision for parotidectomy. Clean the skin of the area enclosed in the continuous line and towel up so as to leave exposed the area enclosed by the dotted line.

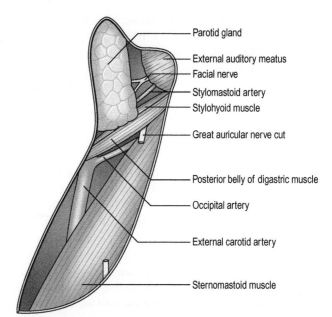

- Parotid gland
- External auditory meatus
- Facial nerve
- Stylomastoid artery
- Stylohyoid muscle
- Great auricular nerve cut
- Posterior belly of digastric muscle
- Occipital artery
- External carotid artery
- Sternomastoid muscle

Fig. 28.2 The S-shaped incision has been deepened in the upper third (in front of the ear) to the bony external auditory meatus, and in its lower third to the stylohyoid muscle. This leaves a bridge of tissues in front of the mastoid that must be whittled away to expose first the stylomastoid artery, then the facial nerve.

Access

1 Follow the standard S-shaped cervicomastoid-facial incision (Fig. 28.1). The lower, cervical part lies in the upper skin crease of the neck, extending forwards to the external jugular vein. The upper, facial, part lies in the skin crease at the anterior margin of the auricle, extending upwards to the zygoma. Between these two parts, the mastoid part of the incision curves gently backwards over the mastoid process. If you intend to remove a lump in this area, exaggerate the posterior curve to encompass the lump. Make the incision in three parts from below upwards, stopping all bleeding before proceeding to the next part. In this way you avoid bleeding from the upper part of the wound obscuring your field lower down.

2 Start by making the cervical part of the incision. Incise skin, fat and platysma.

3 Identify the external jugular vein near the anterior end of the wound, and two branches of the great auricular nerve vertically below the anterior margin of the auricle (Fig. 28.2). Preserve the vein but sacrifice the thinner, usually more anterior, branch of the nerve. Dissect free but do not yet excise, about 4 cm of the thicker branch of the nerve.[7] The nerve runs upwards towards the ear and breaks up into two or three branches; if possible, include a centimetre of each branch with the segment of stem excised.

4 Facilitate the dissection by placing a row of artery forceps on the subcutaneous fat of the upper margin of the wound. Have your first assistant, standing opposite you, to lift the forceps. Identify the anterior border of the sternomastoid muscle. Follow the border upwards and posteriorly towards the mastoid process, as far as the incision permits. Deepen the dissection to expose in turn the posterior belly of the digastric and the stylohyoid muscles, proceeding at this stage only as far as is convenient.

5 Perform the mastoid part of the incision and deepen it on to the sternomastoid muscle. Continue to expose the anterior border of

the muscle right up to the mastoid process. Place more artery forceps on the upper subcutaneous border of the wound and have your assistant pull the superficial part of the lower pole of the parotid gland forwards from the anterior border of the sternomastoid. Friable, yellow parotid tissue forms the visible aspect of the anterior margin of the incision.

6 Continue to expose the posterior belly of the digastric and the stylohyoid muscles upwards towards the mastoid process as far as is convenient at this stage.

7 Create the facial part of the incision and deepen it along the anterior surface of the cartilaginous external auditory meatus by pushing in an artery forceps and opening the blades in an antero-posterior plane. Deepen this plane until you can feel the junction between the cartilaginous and bony external auditory meatus (Fig. 28.2).

8 You now have a large S-shaped incision in which two deep cavities, one in the neck and one in front of the ear, are separated by a bridge of tissue where the dissection has not been deepened to the same extent, in front of the mastoid process. Whittle away these tissues piecemeal; push a closed, curved artery forceps from the upper cavity downwards at 45° towards the lower cavity so that the tips emerge. Separate the tips of the artery forceps and cut the tissue between them. Concentrate on defining the region where the anterior border of the sternomastoid and the two deeper muscles reach the anterior surface of the mastoid process. The dissection approaches the region of the facial nerve, so take increasing care. Remove smaller bites of tissue. Have the diathermy apparatus turned to the lowest mark.

9 The signal that you are close to the facial nerve is to identify the stylomastoid artery running downwards and forwards in the same general direction as the facial nerve. Control it with ligatures or with diathermy coagulation and divide it. Continue the dissection and about 3 mm deeper you will find the facial

nerve trunk. It is 3–6 mm in diameter, white but with fine red vessels visible on its surface, and it bifurcates 1–2.5 cm below the base of the skull.

10 Further steps depend upon the exact operation you wish to perform.

SUPERFICIAL PAROTIDECTOMY

Appraise

1 You cannot determine clinically that a lump in the parotid gland is confined to the superficial part, so cannot determine beforehand to perform a superficial parotidectomy.

2 The definite indication for superficial parotidectomy is therefore recurrent parotitis from a stone in the parotid duct at a site inaccessible from the mouth.[8]

3 You must remove as much parotid tissue and as long a length of parotid duct as you can reasonably achieve, otherwise there is a risk of recurrent flare-up of the residual infected tissues.

Access

1 Employ the cervicomastoid-facial S-shaped incision.

2 Expose the main trunk of the facial nerve and its primary bifurcation.

Action

1 Choose either the upper or the lower main division of the nerve to start the dissection, whichever seems the most convenient. Aim to reflect forwards the parotid tissue superficial to the facial nerve and its five branches until you reach the anterior margin of the gland.

2 Place the closed blades of fine, gently curved mosquito forceps, concavity superficial, along the exposed division of the nerve and in contact with the nerve.

3 Push the forceps points along the surface of the nerve for about 5–10 mm into the region where the nerve is still unexposed (Fig. 28.3).

4 Parotid tissue is tough, requiring a surprising amount of force to split it. Separate the points of the artery forceps and elevate the whole instrument to tauten the overlying tissue bridge. Divide the bridge with scissors, exposing a further few millimetres of the nerve.

5 Repeat the manoeuvre, following the more posterior nerve at any bifurcation. You eventually reach beyond the margins of the parotid gland – at the zygoma if you have followed the upper division, beyond the external jugular vein if you have followed the lower division.

6 Repeat the process with the other main division of the facial nerve and its most posterior branch. You have now exposed the facial nerve trunk and its temporal and cervical branches.

7 The zygomatic branch arises from the upper division, the mandibular from the lower division, and there are at least two buccal branches, one from each division, and sometimes a third, usually from the lower division. Working from the periphery towards the centre of the gland, follow the other main nerve branches forwards to the anterior margin of the parotid gland, that is along a

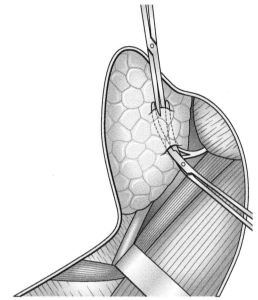

Fig. 28.3 The trunk of the facial nerve and its primary bifurcation have been exposed. When the scissors divide the bridge of tissue covering the blades of the forceps, a further segment of the upper division of the nerve will become visible.

vertical line halfway between the anterior and posterior borders of the masseter muscle.

8 Reflect the skin from the anterior flap until you reach the superior and anterior margins of the gland. With a little more dissection along the nerve branches you will free the gland except for the parotid duct.

▶ KEY POINTS Caution

■ Do not reflect the anterior skin flap at an earlier stage than this.
■ A deeply placed tumour may, by the pressure of its expansion, cause atrophy of the superficial glandular tissue, so that the facial nerve lies close to the skin.
■ In these circumstances the nerve is in danger of being cut if skin flap reflection is attempted too early.
■ This caution does not apply when operating on an inflamed gland.

9 Dissect the parotid duct forwards to the anterior border of the masseter muscle, where it turns medially to perforate the cheek and reach the mouth. Free from it the closely applied buccal nerve branches, then tie the duct at the anterior border of the masseter with an absorbable suture and cut the duct. The excision is complete.

▶ KEY POINTS Pay attention to the nerves

■ If there is a bleeding point so close to the facial nerve that you are afraid that an attempt at stopping the bleeding with artery forceps or diathermy may injure the nerve, ask your assistant to press on the point with a swab and turn your attention to dissecting another part of the facial nerve system. When you return to the original spot the bleeding will probably have stopped.

- The fifth, cervical, branch is not cosmetically important as it supplies only a part of the platysma. However, do not be tempted to sacrifice it at an early stage of the operation: the fourth, mandibular, branch often arises very far forwards from the fifth branch. Make quite certain, therefore, that you have identified and preserved the fourth branch before you consider sacrificing the fifth. The fourth branch takes a very long route, dipping behind the angle of the jaw into the submandibular region of the neck before turning upwards and medially to reach the lower lip. Damage to this branch produces the ugly deformity of loss of the vermillion show of the lower lip.
- You will encounter several cross-communications between the five branches of the nerves. Preserve these if you find it easy to do so, but otherwise do not hesitate to cut them.
- Two of the buccal branches are intimately related to the parotid duct. Carefully separate and preserve them before you dissect the duct.

Checklist

1. Has the anaesthetist raised the blood pressure to normal for the patient or at least greater than 100 mmHg? If not, you risk a high incidence of reactionary haemorrhage. Restore the table to the horizontal position to ensure that any tendency to bleeding becomes immediately manifest. You can ask the anaesthetist to perform a Valsalva manoeuvre to check for any bleeding points.

2. Have you removed the ribbon gauze from the external auditory meatus?

Closure

1. Close the skin with interrupted Vicryl sutures and a continuous 4/0 monofilament nylon blanket suture.

2. Always insert a suction drain via a stab incision 5 cm below the cervical end of the incision.

PAROTIDECTOMY FOR A LUMP IN THE PAROTID REGION

Appraise

1. Most lumps in the parotid region are parotid tumours, and most of the tumours are benign adenomas.[9] Also, most lumps are clinically unremarkable, that is they present no features that enable you to distinguish between non-neoplastic, neoplastic benign and neoplastic malignant lumps.[10] The well-recognized ability of adenoma cells to implant if shed into the wound renders a preliminary open biopsy inadvisable. However, fine-needle aspiration cytology does not seem carry an associated risk of implantation.

2. Controversy besets the decision as to whether to remove the lump with a wide margin of normal tissue after exposing and protecting the facial nerve, or whether to enucleate the lump in the hope of preserving the nerve. The available evidence suggests that enucleation does not reduce the incidence of permanent damage to the facial nerve and that the incidence of recurrence after enucleation and radiotherapy is unacceptably high.[1] Standard management in the UK, the universal management in the USA, is for excision of an unremarkable lump with the widest possible margin of normal tissue, with exposure and preservation of the facial nerve unless the tumour is invading it, or a branch of it. In this case the lump is malignant, so sacrifice the nerve element.

Access

1. Employ the cervicomastoid-facial S-shaped incision.

2. Expose the main trunk of the facial nerve and, if possible, its primary bifurcation. Dissect forwards along the nerve or along its upper and lower divisions. It is soon evident whether the lump is in the part superficial to the facial nerve, or deep to the nerve, and whether the nerve trunk or main divisions run into the lesion rather than being pushed aside by it.

Assess

1. Perform superficial, conservative, parotidectomy, as previously described, if the lump is superficial to the facial nerve.

2. Perform total conservative parotidectomy if the lump is deep to the facial nerve.

Action

1. Dissect under the trunk, divisions and branches of the facial nerve. With a nerve hook and some nylon ribbon, gently lift the nerves off the underlying deep part of the parotid gland until there is clear space between the nerves and the whole of the deep part of the gland.

2. Identify the external carotid artery and companion vein if there is one, at the upper border of the stylohyoid muscle. Ligate and divide the artery and companion vein.

> **KEY POINTS** Anatomy

- Ensure the artery is the external, not the internal, carotid artery.
- Identify the occipital branch that arises from the external carotid artery at this level running backwards and upwards along the lower border of the stylohyoid muscle.
- Confirm that the artery enters the lower pole of the deep part of the parotid gland.

3. Mobilize the deep part of the parotid and its contained lump by working from the anterior and posterior parts of the gland towards the centre and from its lower pole upwards. Aim to mobilize the deep part so as to remove it above or below the facial nerve system, or between the two main divisions in the region of the bifurcation, whichever is most convenient (Fig. 28.4).

4. Facilitate mobilization of a lower pole containing a large tumour by dividing the stylomandibular ligament, of which the anterior

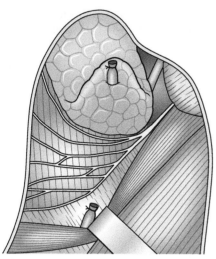

Fig. 28.4 Mobilization of the deep lobe of the parotid gland. The external carotid artery (and companion veins, not shown) has been divided at the lower pole of the gland, and the latter has been turned upwards to be delivered (in this case) above the main trunk of the facial nerve.

insertion is into the angle of the jaw. If necessary, fracture the styloid process to gain more room.

5 Continue to mobilize the deep parotid off the masseter muscle and mandible anteriorly, and the bony external auditory meatus posteriorly. As you approach the upper part of the gland, identify the termination of the external carotid artery at the upper pole where it bifurcates into the superficial temporal artery and the maxillary artery. Tie to divide these arteries and their accompanying veins. The deep parotid is now free and you can remove it.

RADICAL PAROTIDECTOMY

Perform this operation with sacrifice of the facial nerve if this, or its main divisions, are surrounded by tumour.

ACTION

1 Reflect the skin forwards to the anterior margin of the gland.

2 Find the external carotid artery at the lower pole of the gland and divide this and its companion vein between ligatures.

3 Divide the trunk of the facial nerve and mobilize the posterior aspect of the whole gland off the cartilaginous and bony external auditory meatus.

4 Divide the facial nerve branches at the anterior border of the gland and mobilize the whole gland backwards off the masseter muscle and the posterior border of the mandible.

5 Mobilize the whole gland from below upwards. Doubly ligate and divide the superficial temporal and maxillary arteries at the upper pole of the gland and remove the freed whole gland with its contained facial nerve system.

6 A semi-conservative parotidectomy may be performed, sacrificing one or more branches of the facial nerve but preserving at least one of the upper four branches, to preserve an adequate margin round the lump. Repair the cut branches end-to-end if the cut ends will meet; otherwise bridge the gap or gaps using the segment of greater auricular nerve you obtained earlier, with the finest available suture material (usually 8/0 or 10/0).

1. The intention is to remove the lump with an adequate margin of normal tissue and this demands constant concentration.
2. Frequently feel the parotid and intended specimen to ensure that you are not too close to the lump.
3. To assist in preserving the margin, modify the incision as necessary to avoid cutting directly through skin onto the swelling. In case of doubt, be willing to include a layer of extraparotid tissues such as sternomastoid or other muscles, a slice of cartilage or a sliver of bone from the external auditory meatus.
4. If you are unable to control the maxillary veins before dividing them they retract under cover of the zygoma and bleeding may be troublesome. Insert deep sutures to obliterate this plexus of veins.

REFERENCES

1. Hobsley M. A Colour Atlas of Parotidectomy. London: Wolfe Medical Publications; 1983.
2. Al-Khafaji BM, Nestok BR, Katz RL. Fine-needle aspiration of 154 parotid masses with histologic correlation: a 10 year experience at the University of Texas MD Anderson Cancer Center. Cancer 1998;84:153–9.
3. McGurk M, Hussain K. The role of fine needle aspiration cytology in the management of the discrete parotid lump. Ann R Coll Surg Engl 1997;79:198–202.
4. Hibbert J, editor. Laryngology and head and neck surgery. In: Scott Brown's Otolaryngology, vol. 5. Oxford: Oxford University Press; 1997. 5/20, page 6.
5. Stevens KL, Hobsley M. The treatment of pleomorphic adenomas by formal parotidectomy. Br J Surg 1982;69:1–3.
6. Hobsley M, Thackray AC. Salivary glands. In: Hadfield JG, Hobsley M, Morson BC, editors. Pathology in Surgical Practice. London: Edward Arnold; 1985, p. 22–34.
7. Christensen NR, Jacobsen SD. Parotidectomy: preserving the posterior branch of the greater auricular nerve. J Laryngol Otol 1997; 111:556–9.
8. Suleiman SI, Thomson JPS, Hobsley M. Recurrent unilateral swelling of the parotid gland. Gut 1979;20:1102–8.
9. Hobsley M. Salivary tumours. Br J Hosp Med 1973;10:553–62.
10. Hobsley M. Sir Gordon Gordon-Taylor: two themes illustrated by the surgery of the parotid gland. Ann R Coll Surg Engl 1981;63:264–9.

EXPLORATION OF THE LOWER POLE OF THE PAROTID

Appraise

1 The exploration may be used to determine if a lump in the neck is or is not in the lower pole of the parotid gland. The lower pole of the gland extends well down into the neck behind the angle of the jaw and is separated anteriorly from the submandibular salivary gland only by a thickened sheet of fascia, the stylomandibular ligament.

2 The procedure can be employed to obtain a large piece of tissue from the gland for histological examination.

Access

1. Make the incision in the upper skin crease of the neck, starting just in front of the external jugular vein, extending backwards to a point vertically below the lowermost tip of the mastoid process.

2. Identify the external jugular vein and expose the two divisions of the greater auricular nerve. Sacrifice the thinner division of the nerve. Mobilize the thicker division, but preserve it for the moment; you may sacrifice the thicker division later.

3. Define the anterior border of the sternomastoid muscle. Place a row of artery forceps on the subcutaneous fat of the upper margin of the wound and have your assistant raise this edge off the muscle.

Assess

If you are exploring for a lump that may be in the lower pole, you can now determine whether the lump moves upwards with the parotid in the upper leaf of the incision, or whether it lies on a deeper plane between the sternomastoid and the posterior belly of the digastric or deeper muscles.

? DIFFICULTY

If you are still unable to decide on the location of the lump, extend the incision upwards, with a curve convex posteriorly, across the mastoid process to reach the point where the anterior margin of the lobule of the auricle reaches the face (see Fig. 28.2). Continue raising the flap of skin and superficial parotid forwards off the anterior border of the sternomastoid muscle. The greater exposure enables you to decide the position of the lump.

Action

1. If the lump is in the parotid, continue the operation as a parotidectomy for a lump. Even if the lump seems very superficial, do not be tempted to excise it locally. To safeguard the facial nerve and ensure complete removal of the lump, you must carry out a formal parotidectomy after exposing the trunk of the facial nerve.

2. If the lump is not in the parotid, remove the lump, leaving the parotid untouched.

3. If you aim to take a generous biopsy of the parotid, undertake step 1 in Access above. Deepen this cervical part of the dissection to expose the posterior belly of the digastric and the stylohyoid muscle. Define these muscles up to the region of the mastoid process.

4. You will find that a large portion of the lower pole of the parotid gland is now elevated with the anterior skin flap. You can remove a large biopsy of this mobilized portion without risk to the facial nerve.

Closure

1. Ensure that haemostasis is complete.

2. Close the skin only.

3. Always insert a suction drain through a separate stab incision 5 cm below the midpoint of the cervical part of the incision.

OPERATIONS ON THE PAROTID DUCT ORIFICE IN THE MOUTH

Appraise

1. Stomatoplasty (Greek: *stoma* = mouth + *plassein* = to form or reform) is used to enlarge the parotid duct orifice,[1] either to enable a calculus in the parotid duct to be passed more easily or to prevent a stricture forming at the orifice after the duct has been explored, for example to remove a stone from the duct.

2. Two branches of the facial nerve are closely applied to the parotid duct in the cheek and may even wind around the duct. Therefore, do not pass ligatures round the duct to prevent a stone from escaping or to assist retraction; contrast this with the procedure for removal of stone from the submandibular duct.

Access

1. Ask the anaesthetist to use a per-nasal endotracheal tube, thereby leaving the mouth free for your manipulations. Also ask him to pack the pharynx around his tube, as a precaution against blood from the mouth being aspirated into the lungs.

2. Fix the patient's mouth open with a dental prop or Ferguson's forceps inserted between the teeth or gums of the jaws on the side opposite to your operation. Place a strong silk suture into the tip of the tongue and have your assistant use it to retract the tongue towards the opposite side.

3. Identify the papilla on which the parotid duct opens on the inside of the cheek, immediately opposite the second upper molar tooth. Take an atraumatic 2/0 absorbable synthetic stitch on a half-circle (30 mm) cutting needle and put a stitch into the mucosa and underlying muscle of the cheek, about 5 mm above the papilla. Do not tie this stitch; cut it so that each end is 15 cm long, and grip the ends of the stitch with a pair of artery forceps (Fig. 28.5).

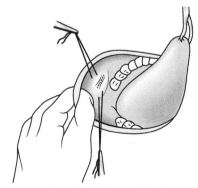

Fig. 28.5 The approach to the right parotid duct orifice. The dental prop in the left side of the mouth is not shown. The tongue is retracted to the opposite side with the towel clip. The operator pulls the angle of the mouth towards himself and at the same time pushes the cheek inwards to make the papillary region prominent inside the mouth; the assistant helps in achieving the latter effect by pulling on the two stay sutures. The dotted line indicates the incision to be made through the mucosa of the cheek and the mucosa of the wall of the duct.

4 Insert a similar stitch about 5 mm below the papilla. Have your assistant pull on the two stitches, thereby elevating the region of the papilla towards you.

Access

1 Feel the region of the papilla with two fingers of one hand, exerting counter-pressure with the fingers of the other hand applied to the external aspect of the cheek. Can you feel a stone?

2 Identify the parotid duct orifice using a lacrimal duct dilator, which is a fine probe with a slight bend at each end in the shape of an elongated letter 'S'. To facilitate this manoeuvre, use one hand to guide the dilator and, with the other, pull the angle of the mouth forwards towards you with your thumb working against the metacarpo-phalangeal joint of your index finger, and push the cheek inwards with the fingertips.

3 At this stage, you are ready to remove a stone from the parotid duct, or to proceed immediately to stomatoplasty, as indicated by your findings.

REMOVAL OF STONE FROM THE PAROTID DUCT: INTRAORAL APPROACH

Action

1 If you can feel the stone at the orifice, keep the papillary region pushed inwards into the mouth by the manoeuvre just described and cut down on the stone with a short-bladed, long-handled scalpel. Start the incision at the orifice of the duct and carry it horizontally backwards for 1 cm.

2 When you have deepened the incision sufficiently, the stone becomes visible. Grasp it with fine-toothed dissecting forceps, and lift it out of the duct. You will find that your incision has divided two layers of mucosa, the lining of the inside of the cheek and the inner lining of the wall of the parotid duct.

3 If you cannot feel a stone in the duct, pass the lacrimal duct dilator into the orifice and along the duct for 2 cm. Get your assistant to hold the dilator steady, keep the papillary region of the cheek pushed inwards into the mouth with your other hand and cut down on the dilator, carrying the incision from the orifice of the duct horizontally backwards for 1 cm.

4 Explore the duct as far back as possible by passing the lacrimal duct dilator. You may be able to feel a stone grating on the tip of the probe. If you do, try milking the stone forward by digital pressure on the parotid gland and duct from outside. This manoeuvre is not often successful, but is worth trying.

5 Whether or not you found and removed the stone, complete the operation by fashioning a large parotid duct orifice.

PAROTID DUCT STOMATOPLASTY

Action

Enlarge the orifice of the parotid duct. To do this, pass a lacrimal duct dilator into the duct for 1–2 cm, get your assistant to hold it steady, keep the papillary region of the cheek pushed inwards into the mouth with your other hand and cut down on the dilator. Take the incision from the orifice of the duct horizontally backwards for 1 cm. Remove the dilator.

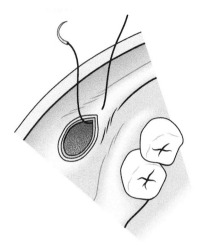

Fig. 28.6 Sewing together the two layers of the mucosa, of the cheek and of the duct. The stitch shown is the first of six or eight that will be inserted at intervals all around the periphery of the now enlarged stoma of the parotid duct.

Closure

You will find that your incision has divided two layers of mucosa, the lining of the inside of the cheek and the inner lining of the wall of the parotid duct. Unite these two layers with a series of interrupted, 3/0 absorbable synthetic sutures around the margins of the incision (Fig. 28.6).

Checklist

1 Make sure all bleeding has stopped.

2 Remove the stay sutures above and below the duct orifice and the suture from the tongue, and check that bleeding does not continue from the puncture wounds.

3 Ask the anaesthetist to remove the pharyngeal pack. If the pack has been effective, there will be no blood on the deeper part of the pack.

4 Remove the dental prop or Ferguson's forceps.

REFERENCE

1. Suleiman SI, Thomson JPS, Hobsley M. Recurrent unilateral swelling of the parotid gland. Gut 1979;20:1102–8.

REMOVAL OF STONE FROM THE SUBMANDIBULAR DUCT

Appraise

1 Do not attempt this operation unless the stone is easily palpable well forward in the floor of the mouth and its presence has been confirmed by radiological investigation.

2 If the stone is more posterior and can only just be felt in the floor of the mouth, or if the submandibular salivary gland is clearly chronically infected, then remove the whole gland together with the stone and as much duct as possible (see the description of excision of submandibular salivary gland for sialolithiasis, below). If there is any possibility of this situation arising, obtain the patient's informed consent.

3 A stone easily accessible in the anterior part of the duct may slip back into the gland during manipulations in the region of the

duct. To prevent this happening, gain control of the duct behind the stone with a ligature under-running the duct at an early stage of the operation.

Access

1 Ask the anaesthetist to pass a nasal endotracheal tube and to pack off the pharynx.

2 Keep the patient's mouth open with a dental prop or Ferguson's forceps inserted between the teeth or gums of the molar region of the contralateral side of the mouth.

3 Grasp the tip of the tongue with a black silk suture and have your assistant retract the tongue towards the contralateral side.

Assess

1 Inspect and feel the submandibular duct in the floor of the mouth. Make sure that the stone is present and where you expect it to be, well forward in the duct.

2 If you cannot feel the stone, do not explore the submandibular duct. Either the stone has passed spontaneously or it has fallen back along the duct into the gland. In the latter circumstance, you should be able to feel it by bimanual palpation via the neck and the floor of the mouth simultaneously. If you can feel the stone in the gland, try to milk it forwards into the duct. If you fail to milk it forwards, the only method of removing the stone safely is to remove the whole salivary gland with it by the cervical route.

> ► KEY POINTS Check before proceeding
>
> ■ Is this larger operation justified by the duration and severity of the patient's symptoms?
> ■ Did you obtain the patient's signed consent for the larger operation?
> ■ If the answer to both these questions is 'yes', proceed to submandibular sialoadenectomy for sialotothiasis.

3 If the stone is probably, and maybe visibly, situated well forward in the submandibular duct, proceed as below.

Action (Fig. 28.7)

1 Insert an atraumatic 0 monofilament nylon stitch on a 30-mm half-circle cutting needle under-running the submandibular duct, immediately proximal to the stone. Do not tie it. Cut it so that each end is 15 cm long, grasp the two ends in the jaws of a pair of artery forceps, to be drawn upwards and proximally along the duct by your assistant. This kinks and obliterates the lumen, preventing the stone from slipping backwards into the gland.

2 Insert a similar stitch, with a deep bite, vertically into the floor of the mouth in the midline between the terminations of the ridges marking the right and left submandibular ducts for your assistant to pull towards you and to the contralateral side.

3 Identify the orifice of the ipsilateral submandibular duct by passing a fine lacrimal duct dilator through the orifice. With the dilator in place, attempt to leave the terminal 0.5 cm of the duct intact.

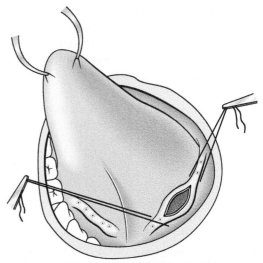

Fig. 28.7 Cutting down on the stone through the mucosa of the floor of the mouth and the muscle and mucosa of the wall of the duct. The duct is steadied, and counter-pressure exerted against the scalpel blade by the two stay sutures, while traction on the proximal one prevents the stone slipping proximally into the gland.

4 With a small-bladed, long-handled scalpel, cut boldly down on to the stone along the length of the duct.

5 Lift out the stone with fine-toothed dissecting forceps.

6 Leave open the linear incision in the anterior wall of the duct.

7 If the stone is impacted at the orifice of the duct, try milking it backwards along the duct, so preserving the integrity of the duct orifice. If you are forced to slit open the orifice, complete the operation by performing a stomatoplasty, sewing the duct lining to the mucosa of the floor of the mouth to leave an enlarged (0.5 cm) orifice, exactly as in the operation of parotid duct stomatoplasty.

Checklist

1 Make sure all bleeding has stopped.

2 Remove the two stay sutures, and the towel clip from the tongue, and check that bleeding does not continue from the puncture wounds.

3 Ask the anaesthetist to remove the pharyngeal pack. If this has been effective, there will be no blood on the deeper part of the pack.

4 Remove the dental prop or Ferguson's forceps.

SUBMANDIBULAR SIALOADENECTOMY

SUBMANDIBULAR SIALOADENECTOMY FOR CALCULOUS DISEASE

Appraise

1 The mandibular (fourth) branch of the facial nerve dips down into the neck behind the angle of the jaw and then curves upwards and medially to cross superficial to the posterior part of the submandibular salivary gland on its way to the angle of the

mouth. This branch is therefore at risk during submandibular sialoadenectomy.

2 The facial artery and vein lie in a groove on the deep aspect of the posterior pole of the superficial lobe of the gland. The vessels are so intimately bound to the gland that you should not attempt to dissect them away from it.

3 The gland has a superficial and a deep lobe; the separation is not complete, the two portions being continuous around the posterior edge of the mylohyoid muscle.

Access

1 Ask the anaesthetist to provide hypotension if possible.

2 Lay the patient close to your side of the table, positioned with head-up tilt from the waist, sufficiently steep to cause collapse of the external jugular vein. Turn the patient's head away from you, with the head extended on the neck, stabilized on a head ring and a sandbag under the shoulder.

3 After cleaning the skin and applying towels, make an incision through skin and platysma in the upper skin crease of the neck, about 5 cm below the lower border of the mandible, extending from a point 2 cm lateral to the anterior midline of the neck to a point vertically below the angle of the jaw.

Action

1 Identify by palpation the inferior border of the submandibular salivary gland.

2 Deepen the cervical incision in the direction of the inferior border of the gland until you expose the border.

3 Keeping as closely as possible to the surface of the gland, dissect all around the superficial lobe until it is free except for the area where it becomes continuous with the deep lobe. During the course of this dissection, you meet the facial artery and vein both at the lower and upper borders of the posterior pole of the superficial lobe (Fig. 28.8).

4 Preferably ligate and divide the artery and vein separately, at both the upper and the lower borders, leaving a segment of each vessel remaining attached to the gland. If you keep very close to the superficial surface of the gland, you stand little chance of injuring the mandibular branch of the facial nerve, which is retracted upwards by your assistant within the superficial flap of tissues. You may be able to see the thread-like marginal mandibular

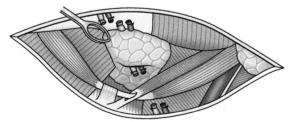

Fig. 28.8 Excision of submandibular gland for calculous disease. The superficial lobe of the submandibular salivary gland has been mobilized by dividing the facial vessels above and below the gland (they are adherent to the deep aspect), and the beginning of the deep lobe can be seen. The deep lobe extends forwards deep to the mylohyoid muscle, and the duct starts at the anterior end of the lobe. Deep to the deep lobe lies the lingual nerve.

nerve as it lies on the deep surface of platysma. The nerve can be stimulated with a disposable nerve stimulator: the lower lip will twitch or an action potential will be recorded if a nerve monitor is being used.

5 Apply a pair of tissue forceps to the gland as it dips deep to the posterior border of the mylohyoid muscle. Have your assistant pull the gland laterally and retract the posterior border of the mylohyoid medially while you free the deep part of the gland from the deep surface of the mylohyoid by blunt dissection. At this stage you may be able to feel the stone stuck in the duct at the point where the duct leaves the anterior pole of the deep lobe.

▶ KEY POINTS Caution

- Do not dissect further forwards at this stage, even if it seems technically easy.
- If you do you may damage the lingual nerve where it crosses the lateral-superficial-aspect of the duct.

6 Now have your assistant retract the deep portion of the gland medially, that is round the edge of the mylohyoid muscle. Dissect by blunt dissection along the deep surface of the deep lobe, separating it from the hyoglossus muscle on which it lies. Keep very closely to the gland, because it also lies in contact with the lingual nerve. You can recognize the nerve as a rather broad (7.5 mm) thin band of white tissue, running forwards and medially on the hyoglossus and a little above the level of the submandibular duct.

7 At the anterior pole of the gland you may again feel the calculus, since this is the most common site, and see the commencement of the duct. Now dissect forwards along the duct, taking special care not to damage the lingual nerve as it crosses the superficial aspect of the duct from above downwards, and then winds right round the lower border of the duct to cross its medial aspect from below upwards.

8 Free the duct as far forwards as possible, nearly to its termination in the mouth. Tie the duct distally with an absorbable synthetic ligature, and cut it across. Remove the duct and gland with the contained stone.

Closure

1 Check that haemostasis is perfect when the anaesthetist has raised the blood pressure sufficiently.

2 Close the wound in two layers, with 4/0 absorbable synthetic for the platysma, 6/0 nylon for the skin.

3 Insert a suction drain through a separate stab incision 5 cm below the middle of the wound.

SUBMANDIBULAR SIALOADENECTOMY FOR TUMOUR

Appraise

1 If a submandibular salivary gland swelling is not due to a calculus, assume it to be due to a tumour. Fine-needle aspiration cytology may aid the diagnosis.

2 With clear-cut evidence that the tumour is malignant, a radical submandibular sialoadenectomy with resection of a segment of the mandible (a 'commando' operation) may be performed, outlined at the end of the chapter.

3 If there is no evidence of malignancy, assume that the tumour is a mixed salivary tumour and aim to remove the submandibular salivary gland with a wide margin of normal tissue, so as to ensure completeness of the excision and to guard against any implantation recurrence.

4 Warn the patient of possible weakness of the angle of the mouth and the lower lip, loss of general sensation and taste from the ipsilateral half of the anterior two-thirds of the tongue and subsequent development of wasting and paralysis of the ipsilateral half of the tongue.

Access

1 Make a skin crease incision through skin and platysma in the upper skin crease of the neck, extending from 2 cm lateral to the anterior midline of the neck to a point vertically below the angle of the jaw. Do not hesitate to extend this incision in either direction to facilitate removing a large tumour.

2 Deepen the incision towards the lower border of the submandibular salivary gland, but stop a few millimetres short of actually exposing the gland.

Assess

By palpation, bimanually if necessary, determine the exact site and extent of the tumour in the gland. In particular, decide whether the tumour reaches the superficial aspect of the superficial lobe, because if it does you may need to modify the plane of your dissection.

Action

1 Dissect free the superficial aspect of the superficial lobe. If the tumour does not reach this aspect, it is acceptable to dissect close to the gland, preserving the mandibular branch of the facial nerve in the overlying platysmal flap as described in the similar operation for sialolithiasis. If the tumour does reach this superficial aspect, perform the mobilization in a plane more remote from the gland. Try to identify the mandibular branch of the facial nerve and preserve it, provided that this does not jeopardize your margin around the tumour. Divide the facial vessels between ligatures, well above and below the posterior pole of the gland.

2 Continue the mobilization of the superficial and deep lobes as described in the corresponding operation for sialolithiasis, but wherever the tumour reaches the surface of the salivary gland make certain of your margin by excising the neighbouring normal tissue. This policy usually only entails the sacrifice of fibres from such muscles as the anterior belly of the digastric anteriorly, the intermediate tendon of the digastric and the stylohyoid muscle inferiorly, the stylomandibular ligament posteriorly and the mylohyoid, stylohyoid, hyoglossus and posterior belly of the digastric medially.

> ### ▶ KEY POINTS Fate of the nerves

> ■ The lingual nerve is an intimate relation of the deep portion of the submandibular gland.
> ■ If possible preserve all or part of the nerve, but occasionally it must be sacrificed to ensure complete tumour excision.
> ■ If the hypoglossal nerve is intimately related to the inferior border of the gland it may also need to be sacrificed.

3 Dissect the submandibular duct forwards as far as possible, tie and divide it, and lift out the block of tissue.

Closure

1 Check that the anaesthetist has restored the blood pressure to an acceptable level while you ensure that haemostasis is perfect.

2 Close the wound with two layers of skin sutures.

3 Insert a suction drain via a separate stab incision 5 cm below the middle of the wound.

EXCISION BIOPSY OF A BASAL CELL CARCINOMA OF THE FACE

Appraise

1 A basal cell carcinoma (rodent ulcer) may be treated by operation or by radiotherapy. If you choose to resect it you must excise it with a wide margin of normal tissue, both around the lesion and deep to it. A 'wide margin' means preferably 1 cm, but in regions where skin is precious, for example near the eye, 0.5 cm is acceptable.

2 If the ulcer is small, in a region where there is plenty of redundant skin, excision and primary closure may be possible. Otherwise you may need to apply a skin graft, preferably a full-thickness graft, as the cosmetic result following split skin grafting on the face is unacceptable. There are two suitable free full-thickness donor sites. Facial surgeons can rotate flaps to cover large defects, but do not attempt these unless you are experienced with the techniques.

Assess

1 Carefully assess by inspection and palpation the extent of the lesion and the required area of excision. It is not yet possible to determine required depth of excision.

2 Plan the excision taking into account the relaxed skin tension lines.[1] After the excision, you may then be able to close the defect by primary suture with the scar lying in the skin crease.

> ### ▶ KEY POINTS Lesions near eyes and nose

> ■ Take care when excising tumours near the eyes and nostrils.
> ■ Excisions in these areas often result in cosmetic and functional defects.
> ■ If possible refer such tumour resections to specialists.

Action

1. Mark out the oval of skin that you intend to excise.

2. Cut vertically through the skin along the oval line, until superficial fat is clearly visible everywhere in the wound.

3. Deepen the incision at one end of the oval. Raise the skin at one end with toothed forceps, using a clean scalpel or scissors including some subcutaneous tissue near the lesion.

4. At this stage you will find it easier to decide by palpation how deeply the lesion extends. Make sure that your plane of cutting is sufficiently deep to give a wide margin of normal tissue below, as well as all round, the tumour.

5. Complete the excision by starting again at the opposite end, meeting the other excision deep to the lesion.

6. Inspect the wound for bleeding and stop it with diathermy.

7. Take a single sheet of petroleum jelly (Vaseline) gauze, lay it on the wound and cut out a piece the shape and size of the wound as a pattern for cutting a full-thickness (Wolfe) graft of skin.

8. Lay the pattern on the chosen donor site. The loose skin immediately below the clavicle and the groove between the side of the head and the medial aspect of the posterior part of the pinna make suitable donor sites. Cut out a full-thickness area of skin corresponding in size and shape to the pattern, with minimal subcutaneous fat. Cut off any remaining fat using a sharp scalpel. Sew up the defect in the donor area.

9. After ensuring there is no residual bleeding following ulcer excision, lay in the graft. Stitch in the graft using interrupted non-absorbable sutures, tying the knots so that they lie on the surrounding intact skin rather than on the skin graft. You should produce sufficient tension in the graft to discourage haematoma without an excess that would produce a strangulation effect on the graft with consequent necrosis.

10. Tie-over sutures over a pad of acriflavine wool or similar can be used as a pressure dressing over full thickness grafts. These will reduce the risk of haematoma formation under the graft.

Checklist

1. Dress the donor site.

2. Check that the specimen, properly labelled and accompanied by the appropriate request forms, is sent to the histopathologist. It is helpful to place a stitch at one end of the specimen so that the pathologist can orientate it and provide information on any areas of inadequate tumour clearance.

REFERENCE

1. Borges F. Elective Incisions and Scar Revision. Boston: Little Brown; 1973.

LOCAL EXCISION OR BIOPSY OF AN INTRAORAL LESION

Appraise

1. Small lesions in the surface of the oral mucosa, whether on cheek, tongue, palate, floor of mouth or inner surface of the lips, are best dealt with by excision biopsy, removing a sufficiently wide margin of normal tissue to ensure that excision is complete.

2. Make sure, however, by careful palpation beforehand, how deeply the lesion penetrates beneath the mucosa. Remember that you must achieve an adequate margin of normal tissue on the deep aspect of the lesion as well as around it.

3. The oral tissues are very vascular, so take special precautions to minimize haemorrhage and so prevent aspiration of blood into the lungs.

Access

1. Ask the anaesthetist to pass a laryngeal mask or an endotracheal cuffed tube and to inflate the cuff. A further precaution against aspiration of blood is to have the pharynx packed with 2.5-cm ribbon gauze.

2. Fix the patient's mouth open with a dental prop or Ferguson's forceps inserted between the teeth or gums of the molar region on the side opposite to the lesion.

3. Position the patient with a head-up tilt of about 15°, sufficient to cause the external jugular vein to collapse. Use a head-ring to stabilize the position of the head.

Assess

1. Palpate the lesion carefully again to assess its depth. Tissues often feel different when the patient is anaesthetized, making you change your decision about the depth of penetration of the lesion.

2. If you are still sure that you can remove the lesion with a wide margin of normal tissue on all aspects, and without producing deformity or serious loss of function, proceed to excision biopsy, or if you are doubtful, biopsy the lesion (vide infra).

EXCISION BIOPSY

Action

1. Form a mental picture of the exact position and shape of your incision.

2. The area around that to be excised or biopsied can be injected with dental local anaesthetic using 1:80 000 adrenaline (epinephrine) in 2% lidocaine. This will help reduce bleeding.

3. Use a 3/0 absorbable suture on a half-circle 30-mm or 50-mm cutting needle, according to the depth of bite required, insert a stitch through the tissues near each end of your proposed incision. The stitches must traverse the tissues far enough from the incision that they will not be cut when you make the incision. Match the depth of stitch to the required depth of excision. Leave the two ends of each untied but held in four artery forceps.

4. Excise the lesion with at least a 5-mm margin in all directions. Make the wound roughly oval or in the shape of an ellipse, the direction of the long axis of the oval being dictated by the need to minimize damage to neighbouring structures. Do this as speedily as possible, as you cannot control bleeding until the excision is complete.

5. Pull each stitch end across the wound towards the opposite end of the other stitch, forming a cross. This controls the worst of the bleeding if your assistant maintains traction on the stitch ends.

6 Inspect the excised specimen with the naked eye. Does the excision appear complete? Excise more if necessary.

7 If excision appears complete, tie the stitches in the form of the cross, as your assistant has been holding them.

8 Complete haemostasis using diathermy and further sutures if necessary while maintaining a clear field with the sucker.

BIOPSY

Appraise

Decide where you will take your biopsy. Plan to excise the rim of the lesion in continuity with a generous portion of the neighbouring normal tissue. In general, the excised piece is oval with its long axis at right angles to the margin of the lesion.

Action

1 Insert one or two deep sutures of 3/0 absorbable material through normal tissues on either side of your proposed excision, and leave the ends untied. Do not insert sutures into the lesion itself, since this may spread neoplastic cells.

2 Excise the specimen, taking care not to cut your sutures.

3 Tie the suture or sutures. Usually this stops all bleeding, but if it fails to do so, use diathermy or insert more sutures.

Checklist

1 Was there any blood on the deeper parts of the pharyngeal pack? If there was, monitor the possibility of chest complications later.

2 Are you sure that the specimen has been correctly bottled and labelled, that the request form for the pathology department has been accurately filled out and that you are satisfied with the arrangements for conveying the specimen to the laboratory?

3 Should you send part of the specimen for bacteriological examination, if the lesion could due to infection including tuberculosis? Remember that any such sample must be sent in a sterile container without formalin.

PARTIAL GLOSSECTOMY

Appraise

1 Excise small lesions of the anterior two-thirds of the tongue with a carbon dioxide laser.

2 Excise larger lesions with a wide margin: since tumour planes in the tongue are indiscrete, a 0.8-mm margin is required.

> ► KEY POINTS Preserve tongue functions
>
> ■ The tongue's important functions include speaking, mastication and deglutition.
> ■ Preserve mobility as far as possible.
> ■ Preserve length, especially of the tip, in preference to width or thickness.

3 We shall describe a wedge excision of the tip of the tongue.

Access

1 Prepare the patient as for a local excision biopsy of an intraoral lesion.

Assess

1 Palpate the lesion and its surroundings carefully. Do not forget the neck and postnasal space.

2 Decide the width and length of wedge that you need to remove to ensure a wide margin of normal tissue around the lesion.

Action

1 Use a dental prop to keep the mouth open. If you are right-handed, stand on the patient's right. If you are left-handed, reverse all references to side in these instructions.

2 Lay your left index finger along the dorsum of the tongue, your thumb along the ventral aspect, to the right of the right-hand margin of your proposed excision. Squeeze the tongue (Fig. 28.9A).

3 Have your assistant, standing on the patient's left, squeeze the tongue between the index finger and thumb, to the left of the left-hand margin of your proposed excision.

4 Excise the wedge carrying the lesion, using a hand-held carbon dioxide laser or cutting diathermy, if available. If you use a knife, the digital pressure of your assistant and yourself minimizes bleeding.

5 Insert a series of interrupted absorbable 3/0 sutures to approximate the muscles in the deeper parts of the defect (Fig. 28.9B). Temporarily relax the fingers, first on one side and then on the

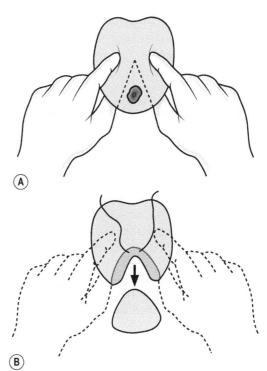

Fig. 28.9 Digital pressure method for controlling bleeding: (A) the index finger and thumb on each side are applied just outside the margins of the proposed excision (indicated by the lines); (B) the start of the repair – the deepest suture has been inserted.

other, to assess the efficacy of these sutures in stopping bleeding from the deeper parts of the wound. Insert further sutures to close the mucosa along the dorsal and ventral surface of the tongue, and to stop bleeding from the superficial layers.

WEDGE EXCISION OF THE LIP

Appraise

1. Early tumours of the lip can be removed with a wide margin by this operation.

2. Particularly in elderly people, up to one-third of the length of the lip can be removed in this way with an acceptable functional and cosmetic result.

3. In a young patient, or if the length of lip to be excised exceeds one-third, various plastic operations are available (see Chapter 33); these are more difficult than they appear, so attempt them only if you are expert.

Assess

1. Inspect and palpate the lesion and its surroundings with care.

2. Decide on the width and length of wedge necessary to remove the lesion with a clear margin of 0.5–1.0 cm of normal tissue.

Action

1. Cut out the wedge, taking the full thickness of the lip, using bipolar diathermy to control the bleeding, if it is available. Alternatively control bleeding with finger pressure. Use mosquito artery forceps and absorbable ties to control bleeding from the labial artery.

2. Close the defect with three layers of interrupted sutures: 3/0 absorbable sutures for the muscle and for the mucosa, and very fine monofilament non-absorbable sutures for the skin and the vermilion border.

> ### ▶ KEY POINT Appearance of the lip
>
> - Pay especial attention to the accuracy with which you join the two edges of the vermilion border and the mucocutaneous junctions. To assist with this it is helpful to 'tattoo' the vermilion border, near the proposed excision, with methylene blue dye, using a green hypodermic needle. This will aid approximation of the vermilion borders without leaving a 'step defect'.

EXCISION OF SUPRAHYOID (SUBMENTAL) CYST

Appraise

1. A *cystic*, subcutaneous swelling in the midline of the neck above the level of the hyoid bone may be a thyroglossal cyst or a simple lesion such as a dermoid cyst. If the lump moves on swallowing and on protrusion of the tongue, it is likely to be a thyroglossal cyst; if it does not, it is likely to be a dermoid cyst. Of course lymph nodes do occur in this area, and a solid suprahyoid swelling is in all probability a lymph node.

2. The distinction between the two types of cystic lesion can be difficult. Ultrasound scanning of lesions in this area is important in the diagnosis of the lesion and most importantly to confirm that a thyroid gland does exist (in the normal situation). When operating on a lump you have diagnosed as a dermoid cyst, always look for evidence of a track upwards towards the tongue or downwards towards the hyoid. If you find such evidence, you must alter your diagnosis to thyroglossal cyst and change your operation accordingly.

Access

1. The patient lies supine, with the upper half of the table angled sufficiently upwards to cause the external jugular veins to collapse. Extend the head on the neck but flex the cervical spine on the thoracic spine. Achieve this by placing a sandbag under the shoulders and use a head ring. This position facilitates access to the front of the neck, without putting the strap muscles and the superficial tissues on stretch.

2. Clean and disinfect the skin from the level of the mouth to the clavicles, and laterally from the anterior midline of the neck to the posterior border of each sternomastoid muscle.

3. Towel up to expose the lesion and a surrounding margin of 5 cm in all directions. Stick the disposable drapes to the skin of the neck around the exposed area.

4. Make a transverse, skin crease, incision centred over the lump and extending 2–3 cm past its borders on either side. Deepen this through the skin and superficial fascia, and achieve haemostasis using diathermy.

5. With a clean No.15 knife-blade, deepen the incision through the platysma and then through the fascial layers until you reach the surface of the lesion.

6. Raise flaps of skin and the other superficial tissues upwards and downwards using a combination of sharp and blunt dissection, to expose the whole of the superficial aspect of the lump.

Action

1. Using fine, curved artery forceps, open up the plane between the surface of the lump and the surrounding fascia. Continue what should prove a relatively bloodless dissection in all directions until you expose the deep aspect of the lesion.

2. In the region of the deep aspect, be particularly careful not to miss any fibrous extension of the wall of the cyst, either penetrating the median raphe between the underlying right and left mylohyoid muscles on its way to the tongue, or passing downwards towards the hyoid bone.

3. Assuming that you find no such extensions, complete the dissection of the deep aspect to free the lump.

Closure

1. Check haemostasis. Have the table flattened so that bleeding points manifest themselves and can be sealed rather than bleed after the skin is closed.

2. Insert a suction drain 2.5 cm below the incision near either the right or the left extremity of the wound and arrange the tube to lie along the length of the wound. Make sure that there are

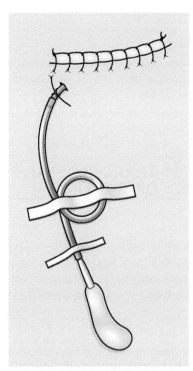

Fig. 28.10 Some details of the closure. Blanket stitch gives firm, side-to-side apposition along every millimetre of the incision, ensuring that the incision is airtight. The suction/drain tubing is stitched to the skin using a clove hitch to ensure that the tube cannot slip in or out. Two strips of Elastoplast strapping or paper tape are used to fix the tubing. The first fixes a loop so that pulling on the end of the apparatus does not pull the tube out of the wound. The drainage tube is connected to a vacuum system such as Redivac.

several side-holes in the part of the tube that is left lying within the wound. Stitch the tube to the skin to maintain the optimal position. Tie the ends of the suture around the tube, firmly anchoring it. Ask the anaesthetist to remove the sandbag.

3 Close the skin with a continuous blanket or a subcuticular suture which may be monofilament nylon or an absorbable material (Fig. 28.10). Skin apposition must be perfect along the whole length of the wound not only to promote healing, but also to create an airtight wound so that the suction drainage can work efficiently, and to achieve the best cosmetic result possible.

4 Connect the drainage tubing to the suction bottle (Fig. 28.10). Check that after the air has been evacuated from the wound the system is airtight.

EXCISION OF THYROGLOSSAL CYST, SINUS AND FISTULA

Appraise

1 The isthmus and part of the lateral lobes of the thyroid gland originate at the foramen caecum (Latin: *caecus* = blind), at the junction of the posterior third and anterior two-thirds of the tongue, and during fetal life migrate downwards to reach their definitive position anterior to the upper end of the trachea. The course of this migration is midline, first through the tongue itself and between the muscles of the submental region, then closely applied to the hyoid bone, or even through it; at this stage the tract loops upwards and

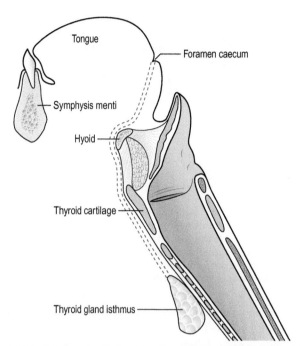

Fig. 28.11 Midline sagittal section through the mouth and neck to show the path taken by the thyroid between the foramen caecum at the base of the tongue and the definitive position of the gland. Note the intimate relationship between the track and the posterior aspect of the body of the hyoid, and the angle at which the suprahyoid portion of the track inclines.

backwards for a short distance before again turning downwards to the isthmus of the thyroid gland (Fig. 28.11).

2 Any part, or all of this thyroglossal tract may persist. Persistence of the whole tract produces a fistula between the mouth and the neck, but this is rare. The sinus, which is more common, is an opening in the skin near the level of the thyroid isthmus connecting with a track that proceeds upwards for a variable distance towards the foramen caecum. The most common lesion is the cyst, which may lie at any point in the track but most often in the region of the hyoid bone, and which may have associated with it a variable stretch of persistent track both upwards and downwards.

▶ KEY POINT Complete excision

■ Whatever the exact position of the lesion, ensure that all persistent portions of the track are excised, otherwise recurrence is inevitable.

3 The intimate relationship between the track and the body of the hyoid necessitates excision of a segment of the bone from the midline to make sure that this portion of the track has been excised.

4 Operations are described separately for (a) a thyroglossal sinus and (b) a thyroglossal cyst lying just below the body of the hyoid.

EXCISION OF THYROGLOSSAL SINUS

Access

1 Make a symmetrical elliptical collar incision at the level of the opening of the sinus, circumcising the sinus with an oval of skin and also excising any skin scarred by infections of the track.

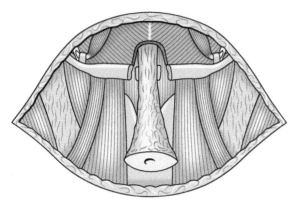

Fig. 28.12 Flaps of skin with platysma have been raised, leaving the opening of the sinus surrounded with an ellipse of skin. The track has been cored out to the body of the hyoid, the central portion of the bone has been detached in continuity with the track, and a cylinder of muscle is cored out in the midline from the submental muscles in a direction backwards and upwards at 45° (see Fig. 28.11).

2 Raise flaps of skin and platysma together; the lower flap need be raised for only 2–3 cm, but the upper flap must be raised in the midline to a level at least halfway between the hyoid and the symphysis menti (Fig. 28.12).

Action

1 Dissect the oval of skin and superficial fascia and the fibrous tissue around the upward track from the sinus opening, raising a tube of tissues containing the track. At this and every subsequent stage, be careful to keep a margin of tissue between your instruments and the track itself. The tract can be injected with methylene blue dye to assist in identifying its path.

2 The opening of the sinus may be situated above the thyroid isthmus, in which case you may be able to feel a fibrous cord, representing the lowest part of the track, running downwards from your dissected tube. Dissect this cord and follow its lower end downwards to the thyroid isthmus to include it in your specimen.

3 Continue coring out the upper part of the track upwards until you reach the level of the hyoid bone. Pass a blunt dissector, such as Macdonald's, deep to the body of the hyoid and gently separate the bone from the attached muscles and the underlying thyrohyoid membrane for a distance of about 1 cm, centred on the midline. Use bone-cutting forceps to excise this segment of bone, leaving it in continuity with the track.

4 Above the hyoid, the track plunges through the median raphe of the mylohyoid muscles in a direction sloping at 45° backwards and upwards. It traverses the deeper submental muscles to reach the foramen caecum. Have your assistant put an index finger in the mouth and push the base of the tongue downwards towards you. Core out a cylinder of muscle in the direction described to complete the dissection of the track.

5 The uppermost part of the track is practically never patent, and indeed may not be palpable even as a fibrous cord, but it is wise to extend this procedure for 2 cm deep to the mylohyoid. If necessary, be prepared to continue until you are separated from the mouth and your assistant's finger by only the mucous membrane covering the tongue. Cut across the core of muscle and remove the whole dissected track. The upper part of the dissection can be ligated with an absorbable suture.

Closure

1 Achieve haemostasis.

2 Suture the defect in the submental muscles in one or more layers. Repair any midline defect in the strap muscles produced by coring out the track.

3 Insert a suction drain via a separate stab incision in the lower flap.

4 Close the skin.

EXCISION OF THYROGLOSSAL CYST (SISTRUNK'S OPERATION)

Access

1 Make a symmetrical collar incision, centred over the cyst.

2 Raise the skin flaps (including platysma muscle), downwards to the lower margin of the cyst and upwards to a point in the midline, halfway between the body of the hyoid and the symphysis menti.

Action

1 Dissect all around the superficial aspects of the cyst. As you approach the deep aspect, separate the sternohyoid muscles in the midline to facilitate the view of the deep aspect.

2 Search for any downward extension of the track as a fibrous cord in the midline. If you find one, follow it as far downwards as you can feel it, or to the isthmus of the thyroid gland, and excise it separately.

3 Mobilize the cyst upwards on its deep surface. You will find that it is intimately adherent to the body of the hyoid bone in the midline.

4 Resect 1 cm of the body of the hyoid as described above, in continuity with the cyst.

5 Complete the excision by the coring-out procedure of the muscles of the submental region as described above.

Closure

This is the same as after the excision of a thyroglossal sinus.

OPERATIONS FOR BRANCHIAL CYST, SINUS AND FISTULA

Appraise

1 Portions of the first or second branchial (Greek: *branchion* = a gill) clefts may remain patent, usually the second cleft. The complete lesion is a fistula with one opening in the pharynx near the posterior pillar of the fauces and the other in the skin at the junction of the middle and lower thirds of the anterior border of the sternomastoid muscle. The complete fistula is not as common as a branchial sinus, where the lower opening and the main track are present but the track does not communicate at its upper end with the pharynx.

2 A branchial cyst is a cystic spherical swelling deep to the junction of the upper and middle thirds of the sternomastoid muscle and becoming superficial at the anterior border of the muscle. There has been considerable debate about the nature of these swellings which may not in fact be congenital in origin but represent cystic degeneration of a lymph node. A large branchial cyst can

encroach on what is clinically the parotid region. In such a case, be careful to proceed in a manner that enables you to carry out a formal parotidectomy if necessary (see Exploration of the lower pole of the parotid). The description given in this section assumes that the clinical diagnosis of branchial cyst is straightforward and that there is no possibility that the swelling is a parotid tumour.

3 Finally, the first arch remnant may give rise to a cyst in the parotid region, or the cyst may communicate as a sinus posteriorly with the cartilaginous external auditory meatus or anteriorly with an opening in the skin of the submandibular region, or there may be a complete fistula between the submandibular region and the external auditory meatus. The simple cyst cannot be distinguished clinically from other lumps in the parotid region, and you will remove it by a conservative parotidectomy, with full exposure and identification of the facial nerve. If the cyst communicates with the external auditory meatus, you may find during the parotidectomy that a cartilaginous extension from the external auditory meatus runs into the cyst. You can cut across this funnel of cartilage and leave the resulting defect open, then proceed with the parotidectomy; after the facial nerve is well exposed you can close the cartilaginous defect by sewing soft tissues together over it without danger to the facial nerve.

4 The operations described in detail in this section are those for a typical (second cleft) branchial sinus or fistula and branchial cyst.

EXCISION OF BRANCHIAL SINUS OR FISTULA

Appraise

The extent of the sinus may be demonstrated radiographically by injection of radio-opaque dye into the mouth of the sinus.

Access

1 Put the patient in a supine position, with the upper half of the operating table tilted upwards sufficiently to cause the external jugular vein to collapse. Turn the patient's head to the opposite side.

2 Clean and disinfect the skin from the level of the mouth to the clavicle, and from the anterior midline of the neck to as far posteriorly as can be reached.

3 Towel up to leave exposed an area from the jaw above to 5 cm below the opening of the sinus below and from the anterior midline of the neck to the anterior border of the trapezius posteriorly.

4 Inject methylene blue dye into the sinus using a syringe attached to a lacrimal cannula. This will stain the sinus tract, facilitating its identification during the dissection.

5 Make an elliptical incision (Fig. 28.13) in the skin around the opening of the sinus; the long axis of the incision should be horizontal, in the skin crease, and about 1–2 cm long, while the short axis should give sufficient clearance above and below the margins of the opening.

6 With a clean knife-blade, deepen the incision through the subcutaneous tissue and the platysma. Exert traction on the skin ellipse with tissue forceps or a stitch, and you should be able to feel the track from the lower aspect of the wound as a fibrous cord running upwards along the anterior border of the sternomastoid, deep to the deep investing cervical fascia.

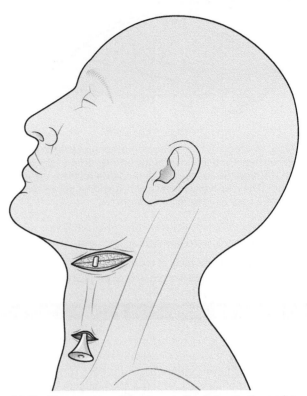

Fig. 28.13 The opening of the sinus or fistula low in the neck is circumcised with an elliptical incision and the track is cored out upwards by incising the deep fascia. At the level of the hyoid, a second incision is made and the mobilized track is drawn upwards through the second incision.

7 Dissect upwards on all aspects of the track, coring it out from the fascial planes of the neck. To facilitate this dissection, raise the upper skin flap in the plane deep to the platysma and incise the deep fascia upwards along the anterior border of the sternomastoid, superficial to the track.

8 If the track can be palpated to ascend higher in the neck than you can comfortably expose through your incision, make a further horizontal skin crease incision with the skin knife at the level of the hyoid bone, extending from 2 cm short of the anterior midline of the neck to the anterior border of the sternomastoid – a step incision. Use the clean knife to deepen this incision through subcutaneous tissue and platysma, and then elevate the lower flap in the plane deep to the platysma until you can pass a pair of long curved artery forceps downwards through the upper incision to grasp the skin ellipse at the lower end of the track. Pull the skin ellipse upwards under the skin-bridge between the two incisions so that it presents at the upper incision. You now have comfortable access to complete the dissection.

Action

1 Continue the dissection of the track upwards. Remember that the most efficient way of finding the direction of the track is to feel the fibrous cord with your fingers.

2 The usual course of the track is between the external and internal carotid arteries and then deep to the posterior belly of the digastric muscle. Divide the digastric at its intermediate tendon anteriorly and 2 cm behind the track posteriorly, having identified and preserved the hypoglossal nerve. When you have excised

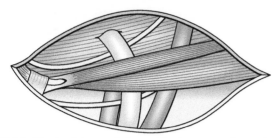

Fig. 28.14 The track is now followed further upwards, passing between external and internal carotid arteries deep to the posterior belly of the digastric, to merge with the fascia covering the middle constrictor. The glossopharyngeal and hypoglossal nerves run between the track and the middle constrictor.

the segment of muscle between these points, it is easy to follow the track upwards to its termination.

3   Deep to the posterior belly of the digastric, the track lies superficial to the middle constrictor muscle of the pharynx (Fig. 28.14).

▶ KEY POINTS Anatomy

■ Avoid damaging the hypoglossal nerve, running forwards between the track and the middle constrictor at the level of the lower border of the digastric.
■ Look out for, and preserve, the glossopharyngeal nerve, which runs a similar course about 1 cm higher up.

4   Immediately above the glossopharyngeal nerve, the track swings forwards and its fibrous sheath blends with the aponeurosis covering the middle constrictor. At this point there may be a connection between the interior of the track and the lumen of the pharynx, but it is not important to discover whether such a connection exists. Simply apply two pairs of artery forceps to the track where it blends with the muscle, cut between the forceps, and tie off the pharyngeal end.

? DIFFICULTY

The really difficult technical problem is the sinus in the submandibular region with a track extending into the parotid region, with or without a palpable cyst in the parotid region. If you operate only occasionally in the parotid region do not lightly attempt to operate on this condition. For this reason the procedure will be described in principle only:

1. Commence as for a superficial parotidectomy and take it to the stage where the cervical and mandibular branches of the facial nerve have been exposed well forwards along their course, at least to the anterior border of the parotid gland itself.
2. Circumcise the submandibular sinus and dissect the track backwards into the parotid region.
3. If, as is usual, the track is superficial to the facial nerve, complete the operation by performing the superficial parotidectomy. Occasionally, however, as you dissect the track backwards you see it run into the deep part of the parotid, and you must perform a deep or total conservative parotidectomy.

Closure

1   Insert a drain through skin and platysma via a point just below the lower incision, and lay the part of the tube within the wound up through the bed of the track to the middle constrictor.

2   Repair the vertical incision in the deep fascia with fine silk or absorbable synthetic ligature. Check haemostasis carefully, especially in the tunnel between the upper and lower incisions.

3   Close the skin incisions, fix the tube to the skin and attach the tube to suction as described for the excision of suprahyoid, submental cyst.

EXCISION OF BRANCHIAL CYST

Access

1   Make a horizontal, skin crease, incision at the level of the lesion, which is at the junction of the upper and middle thirds of the sternomastoid, extending from 1 cm anterior to the anterior margin of the lesion to halfway between the anterior and posterior borders of the sternomastoid.

2   Deepen the incision through subcutaneous tissue and platysma, and reflect the flaps upwards and downwards in the plane deep to the platysma, to the upper and lower margins of the lump.

3   Incise the deep, investing cervical fascia over the lump in a direction parallel to the anterior border of the sternomastoid.

4   Use a self-retaining retractor to separate the upper and lower flaps of skin and platysma. Have your assistant retract the anterior border of the sternomastoid posteriorly. You now have excellent access to the swelling.

ACTION

1   Using careful blunt dissection wipe away the intervening areolar tissue to display the wall of the cyst. Continue the dissection around the superficial aspect of the cyst and then proceed around the deep aspect of its lower pole.

2   Immediately deep to the cyst lies the beginning of the external and internal carotid arteries. Be careful not to damage these or the vagus nerve lying behind the internal carotid artery.

3   The cyst wall is often very thin; try not to damage it, as it is easier to be certain that you have removed the whole cyst if it remains intact throughout the operation. If you leave fragments of the wall behind, the lesion may recur.

4   Continue the dissection upwards behind the cyst, mobilizing it from the middle constrictor muscle. Note and preserve the hypoglossal nerve, running forwards between the cyst and the middle constrictor at the level of the lower border of the posterior belly of the digastric, and 1 cm higher up the glossopharyngeal nerve, running in the same direction and in the same plane (Fig. 28.14 shows the relevant anatomy of this area).

5   Sometimes the cyst does not extend much above the level of the posterior belly of the digastric, but often it does extend considerably upwards, deep to the posterior belly. In such a case retract the muscle to gain access to the superior end of the cyst. Very occasionally it may be necessary to excise a segment of

the posterior belly, from the middle tendon in front to the posterior margin of the cyst behind, so that the dissection can proceed safely upwards on both superficial and deep aspects of the cyst.

6. Rarely, at the deep aspect of the cyst above the level of the glossopharyngeal nerve, you find a fibrous track arising from the cyst and blending with the fascia covering the middle constrictor, rather like the top end of a branchial fistula. Divide this track between two pairs of curved artery forceps and tie the end attached to the muscle. Usually, you will find no evidence of this track and the simple blunt dissection around the cyst is sufficient to free it. Remove the cyst.

Closure

1. Check for bleeding. Use diathermy to stop bleeding points, with special care not to damage the nerves you have demonstrated during the dissection. Insert a drainage tube via a skin puncture 2 cm below the incision.

2. Repair the deep fascia along the anterior border of the sternomastoid with absorbable sutures, such as Vicryl.

3. Close the skin and apply suction to the drain.

EXCISION BIOPSY OF CERVICAL LYMPH NODE

Appraise

1. Usually this operation should not be performed under local anaesthesia if general anaesthesia is available, provided that you are sure of the nature of the node and its relation to underlying structures. For example, a tumour arising from the brachial plexus may present as a cervical lymph node. In this case, having an awake patient during the dissection may be helpful. Cervical lymph nodes may feel superficial yet lie deeply in the neck, and the dissection to remove them may be much more difficult than you expect.

2. Depending on the position of the lymph node, neighbouring structures may be at risk during the operation. An example commonly encountered is the accessory nerve, either in the anterior triangle of the neck at the junction of upper and middle thirds of the anterior border of the sternomastoid muscle, or in the posterior triangle at the junction of the middle and lower thirds of the sternomastoid.

3. Handle lymph glands very gently during dissection. Rough handling is likely to distort the internal structure of the node and make histological interpretation difficult.

4. The operation described here is for a lymph node lying under cover of the anterior border of the sternomastoid muscle near the junction of its upper and middle thirds. The principles illustrated can be applied to an operation on a lymph node anywhere else in the neck.

Access

1. Position the patient supine, with the upper half of the operating table tilted upwards sufficiently to cause the external jugular vein to collapse. Turn the patient's head to the opposite side.

2. Clean the skin from the level of the mouth to the clavicle and from the anterior midline of the neck to as far posteriorly as can be reached.

3. Towel up to leave exposed a circular area of radius about 5 cm around the palpable lymph node.

4. Make an incision across the palpable lump and extended for 1 cm beyond its margins in both directions, in the direction of the lines of skin tension, in this case roughly horizontally, with a slight convex curve downwards. Deepen this incision through skin and platysma.

5. Achieve haemostasis with diathermy coagulation.

Assess

1. Feel the lump carefully again. Is it covered only with fascia or is any other structure between your fingers and the swelling?

2. If the intervening tissues are fascia only, deepen your incision through these tissues with a clean scalpel until you can see the surface of the lymph node itself.

3. If there is some structure other than fascia in the way, you must move it out of the way, excise it or cut through it so as to reach the surface of the lymph node. Exactly what you do depends upon the nature of the structure. The commonest in this particular site is the anterior border of the sternomastoid muscle. Usually it is easy to spread apart the edges of the wound in the skin and platysma with retractors, to divide the fascia where it joins the anterior border of the muscle over a distance of about 3 cm and retract the anterior border of the muscle laterally. The fascia overlying the lymph node can now be incised.

Action

1. Dissect the lymph node free from its surroundings. A good way to do this is to lay a small, curved artery forceps along the surface of the node, with the curve of the forceps corresponding with the curvature of the surface. Insert the tips of the blades of the forceps between the gland and the free edge of investing fascia where you have cut it in order to reach the swelling. Gently push the forceps further along this plane and then separate the blades, thereby stripping the fascia off the lymph node. Cut the fascia with scissors between the separated blades of the forceps, so as to increase the exposure.

2. Repeat this process of combined blunt and sharp dissection all over the superficial aspect of the lymph node. Minimize bleeding by sealing the vessels using diathermy before you cut them. A dry field facilitates the dissection.

3. During this superficial clearance, there is no need to handle the lymph node at all. As you approach the deep aspect, it becomes necessary to push the gland in one direction so that you can free it in that area of its bed from which you are displacing it. This manipulation is likely to damage the gland; be very gentle, and use a finger rather than a metal instrument.

4. Somewhere in this deep aspect you will nearly always find a fairly large feeding artery to the gland. In this region also it is easy to damage neighbouring important structures such as the accessory nerve, because the exposure is limited by the overhanging gland. The safe rule is to cut only tissues that you can see perfectly.

5 When you have completed the dissection deep to the lymph node, it lies free. Remove the node, cut it into two equal parts, put one into a container that will later be filled with formol saline and sent for histological examination. Put the other into a sterile empty container so that it can be sent for culture, including for tuberculosis. Ensure that both specimens are properly labelled.

Closure

1 Ensure complete haemostasis. Ask the anaesthetist to flatten the operating table; this change of posture raises venous pressure and sometimes starts bleeding, and it is better that this should happen while you have the wound still open than after you have sewn up.

2 Sew up any deep muscle that you have had to divide and platysma, using 2/0 absorbable sutures.

3 If the wound seems perfectly dry it may not be necessary to use a surgical drain, but if in doubt do use a small vacuum drain.

4 Close the skin wound using a subcuticular absorbable suture or a blanket stitch using monofilament nylon.

Postoperative

1 Is there any sign of a haematoma forming?

2 Are the two portions of the specimen being properly dealt with?

SCALENE NODE BIOPSY

Appraise

1 The pad of fat lying superficial to the lower end of the scalenus (Greek: *skalenos* = uneven; usually a triangle with unequal sides) anterior muscle contains a number of small lymph nodes that are often involved, even if they are not palpably enlarged, by diseases of the lungs or mediastinum.

2 If the nodes on the left side are palpable, or if the intrathoracic disease being investigated involves only the upper lobe of the left lung, perform the biopsy on the left side. In all other circumstances perform the biopsy on the right side, since the glands on the right side are much more likely to be involved.

Access

1 Position the patient and drape as for cervical lymph node biopsy.

2 Make a 5-cm horizontal skin-crease incision 2.5 cm above the clavicle, extending from the anterior border of the trapezius muscle to the posterior, lateral, border of the clavicular head of the sternocleidomastoid muscle. Deepen the incision through the platysma muscle.

3 Divide between ligatures the external jugular vein and its tributaries. The main vein runs vertically just deep to the platysma, about the middle of the incision.

4 Divide the clavicular head of sternomastoid by gently passing a blunt dissector, such as a Watson-Cheyne, deep to the muscle and cutting down upon the dissector. Make the cuts in successive small portions, so that you can prevent troublesome bleeding from veins within the muscle. Remember also that your dissector is close to the internal jugular vein, and accordingly take care over this manoeuvre.

Action

1 Retract the margins of the wound with a self-retaining retractor. The fat pad lying superficial to the scalenus anterior muscle is now visible, but it may be overlain by the transverse cervical vessels just above the clavicle. Push these vessels downwards, grasp the fat pad with plain dissecting forceps immediately above the vessels and cut horizontally into the fat pad until the fascia covering the scalenus anterior becomes visible. Lift the fat pad upwards and with scissors or knife elevate the fat pad off the fascia from below upwards (Fig. 28.15).

2 Important structures form the bed of the fat pad and you must take care not to damage them. Lying on the anterior surface of the scalenus anterior muscle, but deep to the fascia, is the phrenic nerve, running more or less vertically downwards but with a trend from lateral to medial. Medial to the scalenus anterior is the internal jugular vein, lateral to the muscle lies the brachial plexus.

3 As the elevation continues, retract the omohyoid muscle upwards; the muscle crosses the upper part of the field obliquely, running in a superomedial direction.

4 When you have freed the fat pad as far as you can conveniently push the omohyoid, cut through the upper end of the pad to remove it completely.

5 Check haemostasis. Note whether lymph is accumulating in the wound. This complication is, of course, more likely on the left side. It is important to find the damaged lymphatic duct or thoracic duct and tie it off.

Closure

1 Repair the clavicular head of sternomastoid with fine sutures.

2 Drain the wound by a suction drain via a separate stab incision.

3 Sew up the skin.

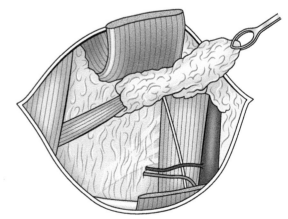

Fig. 28.15 Scalene node biopsy. Flaps of skin with platysma have been raised, the clavicular head of sternomastoid divided. The fat pad covering the scalenus anterior is excised between the transverse cervical vessels below and the omohyoid muscle above. Damage to the brachial plexus, phrenic nerve and internal jugular vein must be avoided.

OPERATIONS ON TUBERCULOUS CERVICAL LYMPH NODES

Appraise

1. You may encounter tuberculous cervical lymph nodes in three main surgical situations:
   - An undiagnosed lump
   - A mass that is biopsied to establish the diagnosis but does not disappear with chemotherapy
   - A cold abscess.

2. The removal of an enlarged, undiagnosed lymph node in the neck has been described. Remember to send half of the specimen for culture, including culture for acid-fast organisms, as well as the other half for histology. If the histology demonstrates tuberculosis, consult a physician regarding chemotherapy or, if one is not available, start triple therapy, combining three common drugs such as streptomycin, isoniazid and rifampicin, while awaiting the reports on culture of the organisms and sensitivity tests upon them.

3. Biopsy a larger mass of lymph nodes. When a histological report of tuberculosis has been received, start chemotherapy. Usually under its influence the mass shrinks and disappears. If not, suspect that the organisms are not sensitive to the combination of drug that you are using.
   Operate if:
   - The mass of infected glands becomes larger
   - The centre of the mass becomes fluctuant, indicating a cold abscess
   - The skin becomes involved and threatens to break down.

4. Aspirate a cold abscess, inserting a hypodermic needle through uninvolved skin at some distance from the lesion so as to produce a long oblique track to minimize the risk of sinus formation. Send the material for culture and sensitivity tests. However, if all or most of the lesion is solid, embark on open operation as described later.

5. Sometimes, though not often now in countries with a high standard of primary health care, you may see a lesion that has already progressed to the stage of a cold abscess, or skin involvement with inflammatory changes and scar formation or even sinuses.

> ▶ KEY POINTS Confirm the diagnosis before treating
>
> - No matter how typical the clinical picture, confirm the diagnosis of tuberculosis by biopsy.
> - It is unthinkable to subject a patient to several months of chemotherapy without a definite diagnosis.

6. In these circumstances, since the material obtained by aspiration of a cold abscess often fails to confirm the diagnosis, carry out open operation.

Principles of open operation

1. Make a horizontal skin-crease incision over the swelling, of a generous length to provide adequate exposure.

2. Modify the incision where necessary to excise all affected skin.

3. Reflect flaps of skin and platysma upwards and downwards to the limits of the involved lymph nodes.

4. Divide the investing fascia of the neck in the region of any fluctuant area or areas, entering the abscesses and evacuating their contents.

5. If the main purpose of the operation is to confirm the clinical diagnosis, scrape the walls of the abscess cavity with a curette to obtain generous portions of the granulation tissue for culture and histology.

6. If the main purpose of the operation is to excise infected glands that have proved resistant to chemotherapy, dissect out as many of the involved lymph nodes as is technically possible. This is a difficult operation, because the lymph nodes tend to be adherent to neighbouring structures that are functionally important and must be preserved.

7. It is not possible to detail more than the principles, nor detail all the difficulties and dangers that you may encounter. These depend on the exact site of the involved lymph nodes. For example, the lymph nodes of the anterior triangle may be adherent to the jugular vein, the common carotid artery and its two branches, and the vagus nerve. The jugulodigastric group may be adherent to the hypoglossal, accessory and glossopharyngeal nerves. Involved lymph nodes in the posterior triangle may lie around the lower part of the accessory nerve.

8. When you have completed the excision, ensure that you have achieved meticulous haemostasis and then close the skin, if possible without drainage. If much skin has been excised, some rearrangement of the skin flaps may be necessary to achieve primary closure.

RADICAL NECK DISSECTION OF CERVICAL LYMPH NODES

Appraise

1. Many carcinomas of the head and neck metastasize to the cervical lymph nodes. Whatever the best mode of treatment for the primary tumour, whether surgery or radiotherapy, control of affected cervical lymph nodes is best obtained by excising them.

2. Your intention is to remove a block of connective tissue containing the nodes from the anterior and posterior triangles, extending from the clavicle below to the base of skull above.

> ▶ KEY POINTS Operation is futile unless:
>
> - The primary growth is cured or curable.
> - There are no metastases at more distant sites.

Access

1. If you are removing the primary growth at the same time, extend the standard approach for parotidectomy, glossectomy, mandibulectomy or laryngectomy appropriately, to create flaps that lay open the neck on the side of the growth.

2. If you are performing the block dissection as a separate procedure following apparent cure of the primary tumour, create a modified Y-shaped incision with equal limbs (Fig. 28.16).

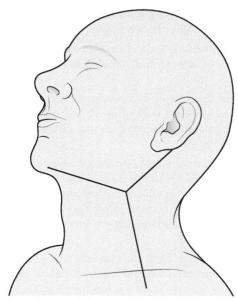

Fig. 28.16 Block dissection of the neck. The incision.

3 Reflect the flaps to expose the entire neck from clavicle to mandible and mastoid and from midline backwards to trapezius. There are many different incisions available, all of which give good exposure and closure. The MacFee approach of two parallel transverse incisions gives limited exposure and should only be used in specialist or experienced hands.

Action

1 Divide the clavicular and sternal heads of the sternomastoid just above their insertions. Gently dissect the lower end of the internal jugular vein, separating it from the common carotid artery and, deep to that, the vagus nerve. Be careful on the left side not to damage the thoracic duct. Ligate and divide the vein, placing two stout non-absorbable ligatures on the lower stump and use a transfixion stitch on the lower end to prevent accidental loss of the suture and subsequent air embolism.

2 Divide the inferior belly of omohyoid and extend the dissection laterally just above the clavicle to the anterior border of trapezius.

> ▶ KEY POINT Caution
>
> ■ Beware an unusually high subclavian vein.

3 Deepen the dissection to the prevertebral fascia covering the scalenus muscles and brachial plexus. Find the plane by blunt dissection.

4 In front of the trachea divide the thyroid isthmus and inferior thyroid veins, so that the hemithyroid gland and strap muscles, first divided above the clavicle and sternum, can be stripped upwards. Ligate and divide the inferior thyroid vessels, preserving the recurrent laryngeal nerve unless a laryngectomy has already been carried out. Head and neck surgeons do not perform hemithyroidectomy unless the primary tumour lies close by, such as laryngeal carcinoma, or the tumour arises in the thyroid.

5 Now dissect the block upwards, taking the hemithyroid gland, sternomastoid, internal jugular vein and all connective and lymphoid tissues from the anterior and posterior triangles. Clean the tissues

off the trapezius border and leave the brachial plexus, prevertebral fascia, scaleni, vagus and phrenic nerves, thoracic duct, carotid vessels, trachea and oesophagus intact. Try and preserve the accessory nerve as it enters the trapezius and dissect it superiorly through the sternocleidomastoid muscle. At the top of the wound divide the sternomastoid again and carefully cut the deeper fascial planes until, drawing the specimen forwards, you can find and dissect again the upper end of the internal jugular vein. Ligate and divide it as near as can be carried out at the skull base.

6 Cut the deep fascia close to the lower border of the mandible and clear the contents of the submental and submandibular triangles. Divide Wharton's duct so that the submandibular gland can be removed as part of the block excision. If necessary, be prepared to take the lower pole of the parotid gland, remembering you will probably sacrifice the cervical branch of the facial nerve. Leave intact the lingual and hypoglossal nerves.

7 You need to ligate sundry large veins such as the common and posterior facial, and, as you work downwards, the remaining vascular attachments near the external carotid artery that must be doubly ligated and divided are the facial and sternomastoid arteries. Divide the upper attachments of the sternohyoid and sternothyroid muscles, and the accessory nerve at its entry into the sternomastoid. Divide a few residual shreds of carotid sheath and the specimen is free (Fig. 28.17). Occasionally, you must sacrifice the external carotid artery in the same block.

Technical

1 If it is not necessary to remove the thyroid gland, preserve the sternothyroid and sternohyoid muscles.

2 In selected cases of 'floor of mouth' cancer, clearance may be limited to the upper half of the neck.

3 If there are bilateral metastases, preserve the internal jugular vein on one side, if possible. Separate the two block dissections by a period of not less than 6 weeks.

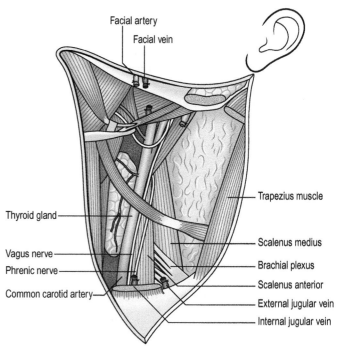

Fig. 28.17 Neck dissection completed.

4 Modified radical neck dissection preserves the sternomastoid muscle, accessory nerve and internal jugular vein. It is now the usual mode of treatment for metastatic neck disease.

Closure

1 Ensure complete haemostasis.
2 Ensure the adhesion of the skin flaps by meticulous skin closure and use continuous vacuum drainage to encourage primary healing.

RADICAL PAROTIDECTOMY WITH BLOCK DISSECTION

1 Patients with proven malignant disease of the parotid gland require a formal block dissection in continuity with the parotidectomy. The posterior end of the upper skin flap is modified by prolonging it as the mastoid-facial part of the standard parotidectomy incision (Fig. 28.18A).

2 Frequently, the disease spreads posteriorly to involve the external ear, and anteriorly to involve the mandible in the region of the angle. Remove the pinna and the posterior part of the mandible, including the ramus and the body as far forwards as the second molar tooth, in continuity with the rest of the excised tissue. The modification of the skin incisions is shown in Figure 28.18B.

3 Widely sacrifice any area of skin infiltrated by the tumour. Reflect the upper flap well forwards to expose the masseter muscle and clear the mandible of the buccinator muscle, forwards to the second molar socket.

4 If the patient is edentulous, now clear the medial aspect of the body without opening the oral mucosa. If the molars are present, cut the mucosa in their vicinity to free them from the mouth. Divide the body through the socket of the second molar tooth.

5 Now free the inner aspect of the ramus from the temporalis muscle, which is attached to the coronoid process, and the pterygoid muscles – the lateral attached to the mandibular condyle, the medial to the mandibular angle. Divide the masseter from the zygoma at the upper border of the coronoid and condylar processes to free the bone and attached lower portion of the masseter, and then continue the dissection posteriorly to remove the whole parotid. If indicated, also resect the zygomatic arch. Closure of the skin flaps can be difficult after this operation, if you need to sacrifice much infiltrated skin. A better option is to accept inevitable skin loss and replace skin and subcutaneous soft tissues with a free vascularized or pedicled myocutaneous flap.[1]

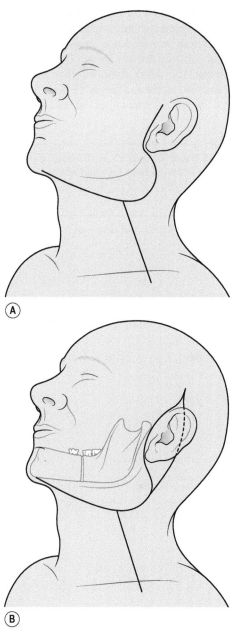

Fig. 28.18 (A) Modified Y-incision for block dissection to include radical parotidectomy. The posterior limb becomes prolonged as the upper two-thirds of a formal parotidectomy incision (see Fig. 28.1). This incision is also suitable for the 'commando' operation, provided that the anterior limb is extended fully to the symphysis menti. (B) Modified Y-incision for block dissection with excision of the pinna and radical parotidectomy. The portion of the mandible to be removed if the tumour extends close to that bone is indicated.

RADICAL SUBMANDIBULAR SIALOADENECTOMY WITH RESECTION OF SEGMENT OF MANDIBLE AND BLOCK

DISSECTION

1 An operation involving resection of a segment of the body of the mandible in continuity with a block dissection of the cervical lymph.

2 Proven malignant disease of the submandibular gland requires resection of the neighbouring segment of mandibular body to achieve a wide clearance. Another indication is carcinoma of the floor of the mouth or of the tongue adjacent to the mandible.

3 The incision is of the type shown in Figure 28.18A, without the posterior parotid extension and with the anterior end of the upper incision prolonged to reach the symphysis menti. Obtain good exposure with wide elevation of the upper flap to the upper border of the body of the mandible.

4 After the excision, repair the mucosa and muscles of the floor of the mouth and submandibular region. The defect in the body of the mandible can be immediately repaired with a titanium prosthesis, provided that the area has not been irradiated. Alternatively, accept the defect. Provided that the region of the symphysis menti is intact, a gap in the body does not produce a severe deformity or instability of the lower jaw.

REFERENCE

1. Gallegos NC, Watkin G, Cook HP, et al. Further evaluation of radical surgery following radiotherapy for advanced parotid carcinoma. Br J Surg 1991;78:97–100.

FURTHER READING

Fleming WB. Infections in branchial cysts. Aust N Z J Surg 1988;58:481–3.

Freidberg J. Pharyngeal cleft sinuses and cysts and other benign neck lesions. Pediatr Clin North Am 1989;36:1451–69.

Jesse RH, Ballantyne AJ, Larson D. Radical or modified radical neck dissection: a therapeutic dilemma. Am J Surg 1978;136:516–9.

Jones AS, Cook JA, Phillips DE. Squamous cell carcinoma presenting as an enlarged cervical lymph node: the occult primary. Cancer 1993;72:1756–61.

Micheau C, Klijanienko J, Luboinski B, et al. So called branchiogenic carcinoma is actually cystic metastases in the neck from tonsillar primary. Laryngoscope 1990;100:878–83.

Radkowski D, Arnold J, Healy GB. Thyroglossal duct remnants: preoperative evaluation and management. Arch Otolaryngol Head Neck Surg 1991;117:1378–81.

Razack M. Influence of initial neck node biopsy on the incidence of recurrence in the neck and survival in patients who subsequently undergo curative resectional surgery. Journal of Surgery and Oncology 1977;9:347–52.

Orthopaedics and trauma: amputations

N. Goddard, R. Brueton

INTRODUCTION

Approximately 5500 amputations are performed each year in England. The number steadily increases as the population ages; 75% of the patients are over 60 years of age, and 65% are men.

> ### KEY POINTS Aims of amputation
>
> - The prime intention is to excise all pathology.
> - The second aim is to restore maximal limb function.

Appraise

1. The main indications for amputation are:
   - Vascular disease—arterial or venous
   - Diabetes (diabetes and vascular disease together account for about 85% of amputations)
   - Trauma (10%)
   - Tumours (3%)
   - Infection (now only responsible for 1.5% of amputations)
   - Neurological causes such as nerve injury and its secondary effects
   - Congenital problems.
2. Major upper limb amputations are rarely required (only 3% of the total).

GENERAL PRINCIPLES

Appraise

1. If you are in any doubt about the necessity for amputation, obtain a second opinion from a senior colleague.

> ### ▶ KEY POINTS Anticipate
>
> - Before elective operations contact the regional limb-fitting centre, when possible, for advice on the best level and type of procedure.
> - Remember, you will obtain the best results by drawing in the informed involvement of a trained team, including nurses, physiotherapists, occupational therapists, prosthetists and social workers.

2. Operate using general anaesthesia whenever possible.
3. The level of amputation and type of prosthesis are influenced by:
   - Viability of soft tissues
   - Underlying pathology
   - Functional requirements
   - Comfort
   - Cosmetic appearance.
4. Energy conservation is an important consideration when planning lower-limb amputation and the chosen level is crucial. Energy expenditure following bilateral below-knee amputation is still less than that of a unilateral above-knee amputation. Plan to preserve every possible dynamic structure, including the knee joint and the epiphysis in children.
5. Appraise the blood supply of the limb clinically by looking for skin colour changes, shiny atrophic appearance and lack of hair growth. Feel for skin temperature changes. Be willing to order transcutaneous Doppler recordings and measurement of the ankle-brachial index, thermography, radioactive xenon clearance and transcutaneous PO_2 measurements.
6. Assess the bone by taking plain radiographs in two planes, tomograms or a radioisotope bone scan. In the presence of bone or soft-tissue malignancy, ensure that the diagnosis has been confirmed with a biopsy. Computed tomography (CT) and magnetic resonance imaging (MRI) are essential in fully staging the lesion and assessing the necessity for amputation. Limb-sparing surgery has recently become more feasible, provided the correct indications are followed under guidance from expert tumour surgeons.

Prepare

1. As the surgeon performing the operation it is your personal responsibility to obtain consent and explain possible complications. Fully inform the patient of the proposed operation.

Obtain consent to amputate, if necessary, more proximally than you intend.

2 Give prophylactic antibiotics: penicillin (or erythromycin) plus one other broad-spectrum antibiotic. Swab and culture any wounds preoperatively.

3 Clean the limb and seal off the infected or necrotic areas.

4 Arrange for the disposal of the limb after amputation to the pathology department or straight to the incinerator.

5 Clearly mark the limb with indelible marker.

Action

General techniques

1 Use a tourniquet except in peripheral vascular disease. Exsanguinate the limb by elevation for 2–4 minutes rather than using an Esmarch bandage.

2 Prepare the skin and apply the drapes.

> **KEY POINTS** Skin flaps

- Mark the proposed skin flaps preoperatively.
- They should be approximately as long as the base is wide at the level of bone section.
- Leave them too long rather than too short.
- If amputation follows traumatic injury, preserve all viable skin to create an adequate stump.
- In the presence of vascular disease do not undermine the edges of the flaps.
- Handle the flaps gently.

3 Wherever possible, include underlying muscles in the flap (myoplastic flap) since this greatly improves the skin blood supply and covers and protects the stump. Muscles provide power, stabilization and proprioception to the stump. In emergency cases remove all dead muscle (this avoids gas gangrene) and leave viable muscle (red, bleeding and contracting). In elective cases cut the muscle with a raked incision angled towards the level of bone section.

4 Double-ligate major vessels with strong silk or linen thread. Ligate other vessels with absorbable material such as polyglycolic acid (Dexon).

5 Gently pull down nerves, divide them cleanly and allow them to retract into soft tissue envelopes. Ligate major nerves with a fine suture prior to and just above the site of division. This stops bleeding from accompanying vessels and decreases neuroma formation.

6 Prepare to cut the bone at the appropriate level. Remember that the stump must be long enough to gain secure attachment to the prosthesis and to act as a useful lever but short enough to accommodate the prosthesis and its hinge or joint mechanism. Divide the periosteum and cut the bone with a Gigli or power saw. During bone section, cover the soft tissues with a moist pack and irrigate afterwards to remove bone dust and particles from the soft tissues. Round-off sharp bone edges with a rasp.

7 Check that the flaps will approximate easily.

8 Release the tourniquet and secure haemostasis.

9 Insert a suction drain.

10 Suture the flaps together without tension, starting with the muscle. Handle the skin carefully and close it with staples if available, or interrupted nylon sutures.

11 In the presence of infection or if you have any doubt about the viability of the flaps, approximate the muscles loosely over gauze soaked in saline or proflavine to prevent them from contracting. Do not close the skin. Plan delayed primary closure at 5–7 days.

Aftercare

1 Apply a well-padded compressible but not crushing dressing, using either cotton wool or latex foam. Hold this in place with crepe bandage taking care to avoid fixed flexion or other deformity of neighbouring joints.

2 Except in cases with infection or doubtful flap viability, apply a *light* shell, maximum four layers, of plaster of Paris over the dressing. This makes the patient more comfortable and able to be more mobile in bed. In specialist centres a prosthetist can apply a rigid dressing to which a temporary pylon can be attached, allowing early ambulation.

3 Leave the dressing undisturbed if possible for 10 days.

> **KEY POINTS** Inspect the wound if there is

- Increasing pain.
- Seepage of blood or pus through the dressing.
- Rising temperature and pulse.

4 Order regular physiotherapy to prevent joint contractures.

5 Encourage mobilization and use of the stump as soon as the patient is comfortable.

6 When the wound has healed and sutures have been removed, apply regular stump bandaging to maintain the shape of the stump.

7 As soon as possible refer the patient to the local limb-fitting centre if you had not already done so before operation.

Special situations

Amputations in children

Children's amputations present their own special problems:

- Growing bones at the site of amputation will overgrow by apposition, not related to growth at the proximal growth plate. You may need to revise the bone to prevent skin problems.

- If possible, always preserve epiphyseal growth plates.

- Perform a disarticulation more distally rather than an amputation through a long bone at a more proximal level if at all possible. The disarticulation prevents terminal overgrowth of the bone.

- Children suffer less than adults from the complications of amputation such as phantom pain, neuroma, etc. They adapt amazingly well to prostheses if fitted correctly at an early age.

- Amputations of accessory digits in children:
    Certain cultures discriminate against children with accessory toes of fingers while other cultures applaud them. Sensitivity is needed and the wishes of the child and parents must be respected.

Accessory digits, and if necessary the associated metacarpals or metacarpals, should be amputated according to the principles described below.

- Amputations of lower limbs with congenital tibial and fibular dysplasia in children:
  - Congenital tibial and fibular dysplasia is frequently bilateral and presents with shortened lower limbs and a child who is crawling on the ground.
  - The whole tibia may be missing, in which case the child is weight bearing through the distal femur.
  - The distal tibia may be absent, in which case the child is weight bearing on the end of the proximal tibia.
  - In either event, there will be a pad of hard skin over the end of the functioning weight bearing bone with a flail distal segment that includes the foot with or without remnants of fibula or tibia.
  - Discuss the possibility of making a prosthesis immediately and during subsequent growth.
  - Discuss amputation with the parents.
  - Use the principles of lower limb amputation discussed below.
  - Bring the already present pad of hard skin over the end of the distal bone as an anterior flap to provide a good weight-bearing surface.
  - A major psychological advantage is that the child can now have eye to eye contact with his peers at the same level.

Decision making for amputations in major trauma

1 Objective criteria help predict amputation following lower extremity trauma. The Mangled Extremity Score (MESS) is one such system. It uses four significant criteria of skeletal/soft-tissue injury, limb ischaemia, shock and patient age.

2 Such systems help you to discriminate between salvageable limbs and those better managed by primary amputation.

Complications

Haematoma

> KEY POINTS Prevention of haematoma

- Avoid by meticulous haemostasis at the time of amputation.
- Double-ligate major vessels.
- Prevent infection, which may cause secondary haemorrhage.
- Never close the stump before releasing the tourniquet.

1 Haematoma in the stump predisposes to infection and greatly delays prosthetic fitting.

2 Drain collections of blood by aspiration or a small incision. Perform this in the operating theatre under sterile conditions, not on the ward. Local anaesthesia is usually sufficient.

3 If there is clearly uncontrolled haemorrhage, apply firm compression and elevate the limb while you make arrangements to explore the stump under a general anaesthetic.

Infection

1 Amputation stumps are more at risk of infection than most other surgical wounds. The stump tissues are often poorly vascularized, there are often infected lesions in the distal extremity, and patients are often frail and elderly, with poor resistance to infection.

2 Give prophylactic antibiotics to all lower-limb amputees. Choose antibiotics that are active against Clostridia, *Escherichia coli* and staphylococci.

3 Handle all soft tissues with care and avoid leaving dead muscle and long sections of denuded cortical bone in the stump.

4 Treat wound infections promptly with antibiotics. Incise and drain any collection of pus.

5 If a chronic sinus fails to dry up with a course of antibiotics lasting up to 6 weeks, explore the stump under general anaesthesia. You will usually find a focus of infection such as a small bony sequestrum or a lump of infected suture material.

Flap necrosis

1 Prevent this complication by carefully assessing skin viability prior to amputation and by handling all skin edges and flaps with the utmost care. Use a myoplastic flap wherever possible as this always has a better blood supply.

2 Treat small areas of wound necrosis conservatively. The wound often granulates beneath the patch of blackened, sloughing skin, which eventually separates spontaneously.

3 Major flap necrosis requires either a wedge resection, down to and including bone, or re-amputation to a higher level.

Joint contractures

> KEY POINTS Susceptibility to joint contractures

- The hip and knee joint are particularly prone to contractures.
- The elderly and immobile and those with serious head injuries, prolonged coma or chronic pain are most at risk.

1 Treat or prevent mild contractures by early active and passive exercises, place the joints in a corrective posture, fit a prosthesis that retains the position, and encourage mobilization. For example, regularly lying the patient prone discourages hip contractures.

2 Severe contractures may require serial plasters or surgical release; otherwise, applying a prosthesis is likely to be impossible and useless.

Neuroma

1 All cut ends of nerves form neuromata but they are painful only if trapped in scar tissue or exposed to repeated trauma. Ensure that transected nerves lie deep within the normal tissues of the limb, proximal to the end of the stump.

2 Treat painful neuromata by resecting the neuroma together with a length of the affected nerve, well away from the area of scar tissue.

Phantom limb sensation

1 Always warn the patient before amputation about the likelihood of still feeling that the missing part of the limb is present. Do not introduce the concept of phantom pain, however.

2 After amputation, reassure the patient that this feeling will gradually fade away. Meanwhile warn against attempting to use a limb that is not present.

Phantom pain

1 This complication is most common with proximal rather than distal amputations, in patients who had severe pain before amputation and in those who have been in contact with other patients with phantom pain.

2 The cause is unknown and the pain is untreatable even by nerve section or cordotomy. Be continually optimistic and supportive, and remember that this distressing symptom occasionally leads to suicide. Involve the whole team in giving the patient support and encouragement.

Failure to use a prosthesis

1 Patients most likely to adapt to a prosthesis are those who have the physical ability, mental capability and the determination to do so. The most adaptable are those who were able to stand and walk, with or without aids, shortly before operation.

2 In both the upper and lower limbs, the higher the amputation the less likely it is that a prosthesis will be used. If the energy expenditure in a wheelchair is less than on a prosthesis, it requires a determined patient to get out of the wheelchair.

> ### ▶ KEY POINTS Facilitating the use of a prosthesis
>
> ■ The earlier a prosthesis is applied, the more likely it is to be used.
> ■ In specialist centres, rigid casts are applied to the stump to which a prosthesis can be attached. Patients are mobilized within 48 hours of operation.
> ■ Advantages of early application are reduced postoperative oedema, considerably reduced pain, profound psychological benefits, fewer complications of immobility such as joint contracture and osteoporosis, shorter hospital stay, earlier maturation of the stump and earlier return to full social activities.

HINDQUARTER AMPUTATION

Appraise

1 This radical operation is usually performed for malignant disease of bone or soft tissue of the pelvis or upper thigh. It is beyond the scope of anyone except a skilled and especially experienced expert.

2 It is included to demonstrate the principles if you are an assistant. The detailed steps were described by Gordon-Taylor and Monro.[1]

3 The incision is shown in Figure 29.1. The external iliac, deep epigastric and internal iliac branch vessels are divided, as are the femoral, obturator and sciatic nerves. The pelvis is sectioned at the symphysis pubis and upwards from the greater sciatic notch to the iliac rim. The anterior portion of the pelvis is freed and removed with the hindquarter, and the wound is closed.

REFERENCE

1. Gordon-Taylor G, Monro R. The technique and management of hindquarter amputation. Br J Surg 1952;39:536–41.

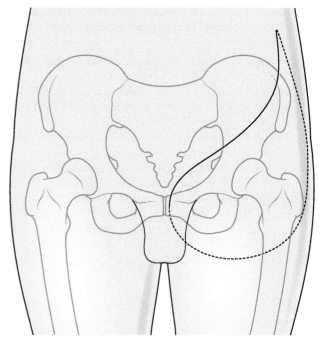

Fig. 29.1 Incision for hindquarter amputation.

ABOVE-KNEE AMPUTATION

Appraise

Decide on the level of the amputation, bearing in mind the following considerations:

■ The longer the femoral stump the better the control of the prosthesis.

■ Do not transect the femur lower than 15 cm above the knee joint; this allows room for the hinge mechanism of the prosthesis. If the stump is longer, the artificial knee joint is lower than on the normal leg. This is most marked when the patient sits.

■ Always perform a myodesis (Greek: *desis* = a binding together), anchoring a muscle group to the femur. This prevents the femur from migrating through the stump, resulting in skin necrosis; it also makes it difficult for the patient to control the prosthesis during walking.

■ If there is fixed flexion deformity at the hip, fashion a shorter stump in order to fit into a prosthesis.

■ If the patient is unlikely to walk after amputation, leave a short stump if the hip is stiff.

If possible, do not amputate through the femur in children, since this removes the lower, growing end of the bone.

Action

1 Place the patient supine with a sandbag beneath the buttock.

2 Use a tourniquet if there is room for it without interfering with the operative area.

> ### ▶ KEY POINT Your position
>
> ■ Operate from the opposite side of the table from the affected leg. This gives you better access to, and elevation of, the stump during the operation.

3 Mark out equal anterior and posterior flaps, their bases sited at the proposed level of bone section.

4 Deepen the incision to the deep fascia, allowing the skin to retract slightly. From this level divide the anterior muscles with a raking cut aimed at the level of bone section.

5 Identify the femoral vessels beneath the sartorius muscle and doubly ligate them. Pull down the femoral nerve, ligate it with a fine suture and then cut it cleanly, allowing it to retract.

6 Divide the periosteum around the whole femur at the level of proposed section. Cut through the bone with a Gigli or amputation saw, protecting the soft tissues as previously described.

7 Now retract the distal femoral fragment and locate the profunda femoris vessels in the tissues behind the femur. Ligate them, then identify the sciatic nerve. Pull it down gently, ligate it and then divide it cleanly, allowing it to retract.

8 Complete the division of the posterior muscles using a raking cut to match the anterior flap.

9 Remove the limb.

10 Secure haemostasis.

Closure

1 Round off the end of the bone with a rasp.

2 Now turn your attention to the flaps, which should be roughly equal in size and thickness. They are composed of muscle and skin and are called myoplastic flaps. Perform a myodesis after drilling a small hole in the posterior cortex of the femoral stump. Draw and fix the quadriceps muscle over the end of the bone with absorbable sutures. Suture the remaining muscles to the quadriceps, attempting to retain roughly equal tension in all the muscle groups.

3 Insert a suction drain.

4 Close the skin with interrupted nylon sutures plus adhesive such as Steri-Strip tapes.

5 Apply a well-padded compression dressing and hold it in place by taking two or three turns of crepe bandage round the waist. Be careful, however, to avoid pulling the stump into a position of flexion with the dressing.

Aftercare

1 Remove the drain at 48 hours.

2 Encourage maximum mobility as soon as the patient is comfortable. Ensure regular physiotherapy is given, including prone lying to prevent a flexion contracture at the hip.

3 Inspect the wound at 10 days and remove the sutures when healed.

4 Apply a firm stump bandage daily thereafter to mould the stump into a roughly conical shape.

5 Arrange for the fitting of a temporary pylon by the third or fourth week and plan for definitive limb-fitting between the sixth and twelfth week.

BELOW-KNEE AMPUTATION

Appraise

1 Carefully assess the viability of the soft tissues of the lower leg when considering amputation at this level, looking for evidence of peripheral vascular disease, diabetic gangrene or trauma.

> **KEY POINTS** Flap lengths?

- Use a long posterior flap, or a skew flap, in peripheral vascular disease, diabetes and trauma.
- Equal flaps are suitable for amputating tumours or for severe acute infection.

2 Do not consider this amputation in the non-ambulant patient but otherwise always try to preserve the knee.

3 The optimal level for tibial section is a third of its length. Do not make it longer than this or the resulting flaps will not contain sufficient muscle to maintain its viability. The minimum length is 6 cm. If there is a fixed flexion deformity of the knee then the required tibial lengths are as indicated in Table 29.1.

Access

1 Seal off any infected, gangrenous areas by enclosing them in a polyethylene bag.

2 Employ general or epidural anaesthesia.

3 Apply a tourniquet to the thigh unless the amputation is for peripheral vascular disease.

4 Place the patient supine on the operating table with a padded, inverted bowl underneath the proximal tibia.

5 Mark the skin flaps (Fig. 29.2).

Action

1 Start the anterior incision at the base of proposed bone section, cutting transversely round each side of the leg to a point two-thirds of the way down each side. Then take the incisions distally on each side, passing slightly anteriorly to a point well below the length that is likely to be required.

2 Join the two incisions posteriorly.

3 Deepen the longitudinal incisions down to deep fascia. Anteriorly incise straight down to bone and then on to the interosseous membrane. Ligate the anterior tibial vessels at this point.

4 Elevate the periosteum of the tibia for 1 cm proximal to the level of section. Divide the tibia using a Gigli or amputation saw. Bevel the anterior half of the tibial stump with the saw and a rasp. Divide the fibula 1 cm proximally and bevel the bone laterally.

5 Use a bone hook to distract the distal part of the tibia. Divide the deep posterior muscles of the calf at the same level as the tibia. At

TABLE 29.1 Required tibial length for below-knee amputation in cases of fixed flexion deformity of the knee

Fixed flexion deformity	Tibial length
35°	6–10 cm
15°	10–15 cm
5°	>20 cm

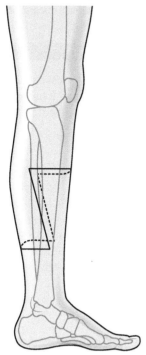

Fig. 29.2 Incision for below-knee amputation.

this stage identify and ligate the posterior tibial and peroneal vessels. Cleanly divide the posterior tibial nerve, allowing it to retract.

6 Use a raking cut through the soleus and gastrocnemius muscles down to the end of the posterior flap. Remove the limb.

Closure

1 Complete the smoothing and bevelling of the tibia and fibula using bone nibblers and a rasp.

2 Bevel the gastrocnemius and soleus medially and laterally, and trim the excess skin to fashion a rounded, slightly bulbous stump.

3 Release the tourniquet and secure haemostasis.

4 Insert a suction drain brought out medially through the wound.

5 Bring the posterior flap forwards over the bone and suture it anteriorly to the deep fascia of the anterolateral group of muscles, using a strong absorbable suture.

6 Close the skin, preferably with closely placed staples, or with interrupted nylon sutures and adhesive strips such as Steri-Strip tapes. Do not leave any 'dog-ears' laterally.

7 Apply a dressing of gauze and sterile plaster wool, then apply gentle compression of the stump with a crepe bandage. Apply a further layer of plaster wool and then a light plaster cast to mid-thigh level. Mould the plaster over the femoral condyles to prevent it from slipping down. Do not use plaster if there is any infection.

Aftercare

1 Elevate the leg.

2 Remove the drain at 48 hours by gently pulling it out of the top of the plaster cast.

3 Mobilize the patient early but retain the plaster cast undisturbed for at least 10 days.

4 Remove the sutures at 14 days.

5 Apply a daily stump bandage.

6 Arrange for daily hip and knee physiotherapy.

7 As soon as the wound has fully healed arrange for the fitting of a temporary pylon, either patellar-tendon-bearing or ischial-bearing, depending on the quality of the stump. Now arrange for definitive limb-fitting.

SYME'S AMPUTATION

Appraise

1 This was described by James Syme (1799–1870), Professor of Surgery in Edinburgh, in 1842, as an alternative to below-knee amputation. Transmetatarsal and tarsometatarsal amputation is occasionally required for severe trauma. For elective amputation, Syme's amputation is functionally superior.

> ▶ KEY POINTS Benefits of Syme's amputation
>
> ■ Properly performed, Syme's is the best amputation of the lower limb.
> ■ The stump is end-bearing with good proprioception and the modern cosmetic prostheses are very light and comfortable.

2 Ensure that there is adequate circulation in the foot. The posterior tibial pulse must be palpable. The skin of the heel must be of good quality.

3 Carry out a Syme's or through ankle amputation, if possible, in preference to a below-knee amputation where there has been an associated amputation of the ipsilateral arm. It is possible to weight bear directly on the Syme's stump, for instance in the night, obviating the need to attach the BK prosthesis, which is difficult to achieve with one arm.

Action

1 Place the patient supine with the foot extending beyond the end of the table.

2 Apply a tourniquet to the thigh.

3 With the foot and ankle in a neutral position, mark the skin flaps (Fig. 29.3). The plantar flap runs from the tip of the lateral malleolus across the sole (curving slightly forward) to a point just below the medial malleolus. The dorsal flap joins the ends of the plantar incision at an angle of 45° from the line of the tibia.

4 Deepen the incision in the plantar flap down to the bone. On the dorsum, divide the extensor retinaculum and pull down the extensor tendons, dividing them as high as possible.

5 Open the ankle joint, plantar-flex the foot and divide the medial and lateral collateral ligaments from within. Take care to avoid the posterior tibial nerve and artery on the medial side.

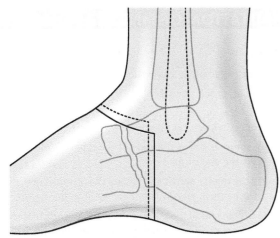

Fig. 29.3   Incision for Syme's amputation.

6   Dislocate the talus downwards and open the posterior capsule of the ankle, exposing the posterosuperior surface of the os calcis and the anterior surface of the tendo achilles.

7   With a periosteal elevator, reflect periosteum and soft tissue from the medial and lateral sides of the os calcis down to the inferior surface of the bone. Continue this dissection so as to free the inferior surface.

8   Detach the long plantar ligament from the tuberosity of the os calcis and continue until you reach the plantar incision. The proximal end of the bone is now free except for the insertion of the tendo achilles. Carefully divide this from above downwards, keeping close to the bone. Avoid buttonholing the skin flap behind the tendon.

9   Now remove the foot.

Closure

1   Turn the heel flap backwards and upwards and free the malleoli and distal centimetre of tibia. Remove the malleoli and a thin slice of tibia with a saw.

> ### ▶ KEY POINT Ensure a flat platform
>
> ■ Make sure your tibial cut is at right-angles to the line of the bone and that you leave the subarticular bone intact.

2   Round off the bone edges.

3   Release the tourniquet and secure haemostasis.

4   Insert a suction drain.

5   Suture the heel flap to the margin of the dorsal incision in two layers with subcutaneous synthetic absorbable material such as polyglycolic acid (Dexon) and interrupted nylon to skin. Begin skin closure in the middle and continue to each end.

6   Ensure that the heel flap remains centred over the cut end of the tibia. The flap may be secured with adhesive such as Steri-Strip tapes.

7   If the heel flap is very unstable, transfix it percutaneously with a Kirschner wire or Steinmann pin passed up into the tibia.
Ensure that the Kirschner wire is bent to 90 degrees outside the stump to prevent its proximal migration into the skin of the flap, so becoming buried.

8   Apply a well-padded pressure dressing and retain this either with adhesive strapping to the upper calf or a lightweight above-knee plaster cast.

Aftercare

1   Elevate the leg.

2   Remove the drain at 48 hours but do not disturb the dressing.

3   If you have not transfixed the heel flap, inspect the wound at 5 days to check the position of the flap. Otherwise, inspect the wound at 14 days, when the sutures and the percutaneous pin may be removed.

4   Carefully apply a stump bandage thereafter and arrange the fitting of a prosthesis as soon as the swelling has subsided, usually at 2–4 weeks.

RAY AMPUTATIONS OF THE FOREFOOT

Appraise

1   Indications for ray amputation are:
   ■ Gigantism. This may affect the 2nd or 3rd rays and the corresponding toes. The feet are too large to fit shoes and cosmetically inappropriate. In this case, a wedge of the forefoot containing the abnormal digits needs to be excised
   ■ Congenital extra rays, with or without the corresponding digits, producing a wide foot
   ■ Diabetic or neuropathic foot. Often associated with a plantar ulcer under the metatarsophalangeal joint (MTPJ), with osteomyelitis of the adjacent metatarsal (MT) and proximal phalanx.

Action

1   Use a tourniquet.

2   In the case of gigantism:
   ■ Mark out a dorsal and ventral wedge to include the affected rays
   ■ Excise the wedge of the forefoot, disarticulating the MT at the tarsometatarsal joint (TMTJ) or dividing the MT at its base
   ■ Close the wedge, approximating the remaining adjacent MTs with strong Vicryl
   ■ Close the skin and elevate until wound healing.

3   Congenital additional rays. If the ray is buried between normal MTs expose it through a dorsal longitudinal incision and excise it. Approximate the adjacent MTs.

4   Diabetic ulcers:
   ■ Approach through the sole and remove all infected tissue
   ■ This includes the chronic infected fibrous cavity and the dead bone of the MT and/or proximal phalanx
   ■ Leave the wound open. Apply a vacuum pump if available or dress until the wound has closed by secondary intention.

AMPUTATION OF THE TOES

Appraise

1. Avoid amputating single toes if possible. Neighbouring toes tend to develop secondary deformity and take more weight.

2. Remove all the toes (nicknamed the 'Pobble' operation, from a poem by the English humourist Edward Lear, 1812–1888) if there are multiple painful, fixed deformities or if several toes are gangrenous.

3. Ray resection of toes may be required for gangrene or diabetes.

4. If you need to amputate the great toe, try to preserve the attachments of the short flexor and extensor tendons on the proximal phalanx.

Action

1. Use a tourniquet after exsanguination.

2. Mark out a racquet incision for amputation of individual toes. For amputation of all the toes use a transverse incision, passing across the root of the toes on the plantar aspect, that is overlying the proximal phalanx, and across the MTPJ on the dorsum. The eventual scar should lie dorsally.

3. Take the flaps straight down to bone and dissect off the proximal phalanx.

4. Preserve the base of the proximal phalanx if possible, dividing the bone just distal to the insertion of the capsule. This creates a small wound cavity, which heals quickly, and the amputation does not damage the transverse MT ligaments. Alternatively, perform a careful disarticulation.

5. Secure haemostasis.

6. Close the skin with interrupted nylon sutures.

7. Apply a bulky compression dressing, passing a few turns of crepe bandage round the ankle to hold the dressing in position.

Aftercare

1. Elevate the leg.

2. Remove the sutures at 10 days and mobilize the patient.

3. Where individual toes have been amputated, ask the chiropodist to supply a toe spacer.

4. Where all the toes have been amputated, order a special insole that incorporates a combined MT and cavus support, together with a cork toe-block faced with sponge rubber.

THE UPPER LIMB

1. Many of the indications for amputation in the hand have changed in recent times as a result of improvements in surgical method, prosthetics and plastic surgery. These techniques require special expertise.

2. Some of the operations are suitable for semi-elective use, provided you adhere to the principles of soft-tissue and wound management.

3. Here we shall consider only some of the common and simpler procedures.

AMPUTATION OF FINGERS

Action

1. Use an exsanguinating tourniquet.

2. Place the arm on a side table.

3. Mark the incision, which should be placed so that the scar will lie on the dorsal aspect and the stump will be covered by volar skin.

4. Do not suture together the ends of the extensor and flexor tendons over the end of the bone.

5. Identify the digital nerves and isolate them from the vessels before dividing them cleanly, 1 cm proximal to the stump.

6. Round off the end of the bone and remove the articular cartilage and prominent condyles when performing a disarticulation.

7. Reduce the bulk of the fibrofatty subcutaneous tissue to allow the skin edges to be brought together without difficulty.

8. Release the tourniquet and secure haemostasis before closure.

9. Avoid tight skin closure, otherwise painful and ischaemic torsion may develop as a result of postoperative swelling. Some soft tissue retraction occurs during the first 2 months but do not, on this account, leave excessive slackness of the stump; this causes an unsightly, unsupported soft-tissue mass.

10. Apply a compression dressing of gauze and narrow crepe bandage.

AMPUTATION THROUGH THE DISTAL PHALANX

If less than one-quarter of the length of the nail remains, the patient may be troubled later by an irregular hooked nail remnant. Therefore, ablate the nail bed and excise the lateral angles as completely as possible.

DISARTICULATION THROUGH THE DISTAL INTERPHALANGEAL JOINT

1. Incise the skin in the midlateral line on either side of the neck of the middle phalanx. Join these two incisions across the dorsum at the level of the joint and across the volar pulp 1 cm distal to the flexor crease (Fig. 29.4).

2. Dissect back the fibrofatty tissue to reveal the digital vessels and nerves, the extensor expansion and the flexor tendon in its sheath.

3. Divide the extensor and flexor tendons at the level of the neck of the middle phalanx and allow them to retract.

4. Ligate the digital vessels and divide the nerves proximally.

5. Divide the capsule and collateral ligaments to complete the amputation.

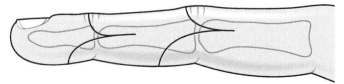

Fig. 29.4 Incision for disarticulation through interphalangeal joints.

6   Shape the head of the middle phalanx using bone nibblers and close the wound as described above.

AMPUTATION THROUGH THE MIDDLE PHALANX

Proceed as above but retain the attachment of the flexor digitorum superficialis to bone.

DISARTICULATION THROUGH THE PROXIMAL INTERPHALANGEAL JOINT

Proceed as above but fashion a volar flap 1.5–2 cm long.

AMPUTATION THROUGH THE PROXIMAL PHALANX

We do not advise amputation of a single digit at this level. Disarticulation at the metacarpophalangeal joint is preferable except in special circumstances, such as multiple amputations.

DISARTICULATION THROUGH THE METACARPOPHALANGEAL JOINT

Assess

1   As a rule, employ this operation only for the middle and ring fingers. It is particularly suitable for the hand of a man doing manual labour, since a powerful grip can be retained.

2   The two disadvantages are the obvious deformity and a gap between the fingers through which small objects in the hand may fall.

3   Disarticulation of the index or little fingers at this level leaves the metarcarpal head projecting and unprotected. Oblique amputation through the metacarpal shaft is preferable.

Action

1   Mark the skin incisions, which should lie over the proximal part of the proximal phalanx on each side, leaving sufficient skin to permit full abduction of the other fingers without tension in the cleft.

2   Join the incisions anteriorly just distal to the flexor crease and posteriorly over the metacarpal head with an extension along the line of the metacarpal (Fig. 29.5).

3   Complete the amputation as described above.

AMPUTATION THROUGH THE SHAFT OF THE METACARPAL

Action

1   Use the same skin incision as for a disarticulation in the middle and ring fingers.

2   For the index and little finger use an incision along the midlateral aspect of the radial, or ulnar, border of the hand from the junction of the proximal and middle thirds of the metacarpal to the metacarpophalangeal joint (Fig. 29.5). Fashion a larger palmar

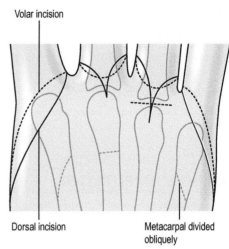

Volar incision

Dorsal incision

Metacarpal divided obliquely

Fig. 29.5   Incision for disarticulation through a metacarpophalangeal joint and for amputation through a metacarpal.

flap and a smaller dorsal flap and joint the incisions in the cleft at the level of the web.

3   Amputate the middle and ring fingers by dividing the metacarpal cleanly through the neck, taking care not to splinter the bone.

4   Amputate the index and little fingers by exposing the middle third of the metacarpal, stripping the muscular attachments and dividing the bone obliquely with a power saw. Smooth the edges of the bone and allow the muscles to fall back over the stump. Divide the digital nerves to the radial border of the index or the ulnar border of the little finger in the proximal part of the wound.

MAJOR UPPER-LIMB AMPUTATIONS

Appraise

These are fortunately rarely required, usually for trauma, occasionally for malignancy, severe infection and congenital abnormalities or deformities. Except in an emergency, obtain a second opinion.

> ▶ KEY POINTS Forearm amputations in children
>
> ■ Following forearm amputation in children, the bone will not grow in proportion to the rest of the body.
> ■ Following above-elbow amputation, the humerus continues to grow and indeed may require revision with time.

Prepare

1   Whenever possible operate using general anaesthesia and an exsanguinating tourniquet.

2   Place the patient supine with the arm on a side table.

3   Rest the arm on an inverted bowl just proximal to the site of the amputation.

Aftercare

1 Remove the drain at 48 hours.

2 Start physiotherapy to the remaining joints in the limb at 48 hours.

3 Remove the sutures at 10 days.

4 Refer to the local limb-fitting centre as soon as the wound has healed.

BELOW-ELBOW AMPUTATION

1 Mark out equal dorsal and volar skin flaps with their bases at the junction of the middle and lower third of the ulna, approximately 17 cm distal to the olecranon process.

2 Ensure that the arm is supinated on the table without any torsional strain below the elbow. If you do not avoid this, the cut flaps will be drawn into an oblique position by the elasticity of the skin.

3 Reflect the flaps deep to the deep fascia. Cut the muscles and tendons with a slightly raked incision aimed at the level of the bone section.

4 Incise the periosteum circumferentially at the level of section and divide the bones with a Gigli or a power saw.

5 Identify and ligate the main vessels. Gently pull down the nerves and divide them cleanly as high as possible.

6 Release the tourniquet and secure haemostasis.

7 Insert a suction drain.

8 Close the deep fascia over the bone ends using interrupted synthetic absorbable material such as Dexon. Close the skin with interrupted fine nylon sutures plus Steri-Strip tapes.

ABOVE-ELBOW AMPUTATION

1 Mark out equal anterior and posterior flaps with their bases 20 cm from the tip of the acromion process of the scapula.

2 Retain as much length of the upper humerus as is possible in the presence of an ipsilateral amputation of the lower limb. This will facilitate the use of a crutch in the axilla.

3 Reflect the flaps deep to the deep fascia.

4 Divide the muscles with a raking incision down to bone.

5 Divide the bone with a Gigli or power saw.

6 Ligate the main vessels. Pull down the nerves and shorten them by about 2.5 cm so that they retract into the depths of the wound.

7 Release the tourniquet if present and secure haemostasis.

8 Insert a suction drain.

9 Close the deep fascia over the bone using synthetic absorbable material such as Dexon. Close the skin and apply a compression dressing.

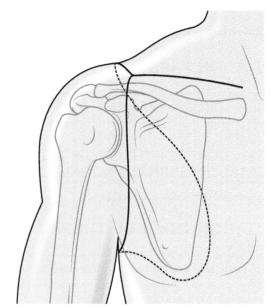

Fig. 29.6 Incision for forequarter amputation.

FOREQUARTER AMPUTATION

Appraise

1 This is beyond the scope of all but the highly skilled, especially experienced surgeons. It is included merely to demonstrate the extent of the excision, usually for extensive tumour, if you are an assistant. There are two methods available: the posterior approach described by Littlewood (Fig. 29.6) and the anterior approach of Berger (1887), which is preferred.

2 The clavicle is divided, the vessels including the subclavian artery and axillary vein are divided, as are the trunks of the brachial plexus. The attaching muscles are divided, including pectoralis major and minor, trapezius, latissimus dorsi, levator scapula rhomboids and serratus anterior.

3 The forequarter, including the scapula, is removed and the wound closed.

FURTHER READING

Angel JC, Weaver PC. Amputations. In: Bentley G, Greer III RB, editors. Rob and Smith's Operative Surgery. 4th ed. Orthopaedics Part 1. London: Butterworths; 1979.

Anonymous. Symposium on Amputations. Ann R Coll Surg Engl 1991;73:133–76.

Gerhardt JJ, King PS, Zettl JH. Amputations. Immediate and Early Prosthetic Management. Bern: Hans Huber; 1982.

Helfet DL, Howey T, Sanders R, et al. Preliminary results of the Mangled Extremity Severity Score. Clinical Orthopaedics 1990;256:80–6.

Thompson RG. Complications of lower extremity amputation. Orthop Clin North Am 1972;3:323.

Tooms RE. Amputations. In: Crenshaw AH, editor. Campbell's Operative Orthopedics. St Louis: Mosby; 1987. p. 597–646.

Orthopaedics and trauma: general principles

N. Goddard, R. Brueton

CONTENTS

PREOPERATIVE PREPARATION

Appraise

1. Most elective orthopaedic operations are carried out on otherwise healthy patients, but always assess the patient's fitness for operation beforehand. When operating for trauma, ensure that the patient is adequately resuscitated.

2. Postpone elective operations until any concomitant illness such as a chest or urinary infection or hypertension has been corrected. This is especially so if one is contemplating implanting a prosthetic device (e.g. a total joint replacement).

3. Correct blood loss and dehydration before emergency operations.

4. *Antibiotics*. It is recommended practice usually to administer an antibiotic intravenously at the time of induction of anaesthesia, followed up by two further doses at 8-hourly intervals, making three doses in all. The choice of antibiotic depends upon the nature of the operation, the likely infecting organism and the patient's potential sensitivity. It is usual to use a broad-spectrum antibiotic (e.g. cefradine 500 mg t.d.s.) or an agent that has a potent anti-staphylococcal activity.

▶ KEY POINTS Avoid bone infection at all costs

- Infection of bone and non-living implants is a potentially catastrophic complication.
- Give prophylactic antibiotics for all but the most minor operations on bone, when an implant is used, and if there is an open wound.

5. *Anticoagulation*. The routine use of prophylactic anticoagulants for major orthopaedic operations, particularly on the hip joint, is controversial. The current consensus from the British Orthopaedic Association[1] is that, while chemical agents (e.g. heparin and warfarin) may reduce the incidence of deep venous thrombosis, death from other causes may be increased and there is no reduction in the rate of fatal pulmonary embolism. Anticoagulant therapy itself may also lead to excessive intra- or postoperative bleeding complications and ultimately jeopardize a total joint replacement. However, where there is a previous history of thromboembolic disease it is advisable to give heparin 5000 IU subcutaneously twice daily. If the patient is already fully anticoagulated, aim to reduce the international normalized ratio (INR) to <2 over the perioperative period, maintaining the patient on intravenous heparin infusion and reverting to oral anticoagulation when the patient is mobile – hopefully within 24–48 hours.

6. *Anaesthesia*. General anaesthetic is appropriate for most orthopaedic procedures, especially for prolonged operations when a tourniquet is used. Under some circumstances (e.g. a patient with rheumatoid arthritis), it may be preferable to operate under a regional block (spinal, epidural, axillary). Some procedures (e.g. carpal tunnel decompression) may be performed using a local anaesthetic wound infiltration. In addition, local anaesthetic is a useful adjunct in postoperative pain relief. In our opinion Bier's block, while theoretically safe, provides an unsatisfactory operative field for anything but the simplest of procedures.

TOURNIQUETS

Appraise

- Most orthopaedic operations on the limbs, especially the hand, are facilitated if performed in a bloodless field using a pneumatic tourniquet. It has been said that attempting to operate on a hand without a tourniquet is akin to trying to repair a watch at the bottom of an inkwell!

■ Use a tourniquet with caution if the patient suffers from peripheral vascular disease or if the blood supply to damaged tissues is poor. Peripheral vascular disease, however, is not an absolute contraindication to the use of a tourniquet.

▶ **KEY POINTS** Dangers of exsanguination

■ Do not exsanguinate the limb in the presence of distal infection, suspected calf vein thrombosis or foreign bodies, so as to avoid propagating the infection, dislodging any blood clot or shifting the foreign body.
■ Take care when exsanguinating an injured limb or a limb that is fractured.

Action

1 Apply a pneumatic tourniquet of appropriate size over a few turns of orthopaedic wool around the proximal part of the upper arm or thigh.
2 Exsanguinate the limb either by elevation (Bier's method) or with a soft rubber exsanguinator (Rhys-Davies). If the latter is not available, use an Esmarch bandage, but take particular care if the skin is friable, as in a patient with rheumatoid disease. A stockinette applied over the skin prior to exsanguination reduces the likelihood of shear stresses and potential skin damage.
3 Secure the cuff and inflate until the pressure just exceeds the systolic blood pressure for tourniquets on the upper limb, and to twice the systolic blood pressure for tourniquets on the lower limb. In practice, 200 mmHg is appropriate for the upper limb and 350 mmHg for the leg. Higher pressures are unnecessary and may cause soft-tissue damage by direct compression, especially in thin patients. Never allow the pressure to exceed 250 mmHg in the arm or 450 mmHg in the leg.
4 If the tourniquet is accidentally deflated or slips during the operation, allowing partial or complete return of the circulation, deflate the cuff completely, re-position and re-fasten it and elevate the limb before re-inflating the cuff.

▶ **KEY POINTS** Precautions with tourniquets

■ Record the time of inflation of the tourniquet and the duration of its application, which must be kept to a minimum by careful planning of the operation.
■ Exsanguination after preparing the skin can save 5 minutes or more of ischaemic time.
■ 60–90 minutes is usually regarded as a safe period for an arm.
■ Up to 3 hours is acceptable, but not desirable, for the leg.
■ If necessary, temporarily release and then re-inflate the tourniquet, but be prepared for a poorer operative field.

5 We prefer to release the tourniquet and achieve satisfactory haemostasis before closing the wound. Some surgeons, however, prefer to close and dress the wound prior to tourniquet release. Under these circumstances a drain is usually necessary and any plaster must be split.

Aftercare

1 On completion of the operation always ensure that the circulation has returned to the limb. Locate and mark the position of the peripheral pulses to facilitate subsequent postoperative observations.
2 Reduce the likelihood of swelling by applying bulky cotton wool and crepe bandage dressing for at least 24 hours after the operation. Encourage and supervise active exercises. A good orthopaedic maxim is 'Don't just lie there – do something!'

SKIN PREPARATION

Elective surgery

1 There should be no break or superficial infection in the skin of a limb or the area of the trunk that is to be operated on. If necessary, postpone the operation until any wound has healed or infection has been eradicated.
2 Instruct the patient to bathe or shower within 12 hours of the operation using an antiseptic soap. Preoperative shaving is a matter of personal preference, but should be performed as late as possible and by an expert. Poor preoperative shaving may result in multiple skin nicks, which in turn become colonized with bacteria, increasing the risk of postoperative infection.
3 Mark the limb or digit to be operated on with an indelible marker. Give instructions to re-mark it if the mark is accidentally erased before the operation.
4 Prepare the skin with either iodine or chlorhexidine in spirit or aqueous solution. Iodine solutions are more effective skin antiseptics but are also the most irritant. Avoid pooling of alcohol-based solutions beneath a tourniquet or diathermy pad, with an attendant risk of explosion.

Emergency surgery

1 Prepare the skin in the anaesthetic room after induction of anaesthesia.
2 Cover open wounds with a sterile dressing held in place by an assistant.
3 Clean the surrounding skin with a soft nail brush and warm cetrimide (Savlon) solution, removing ingrained dirt and debris.
4 Remove the dressing and clean the wound itself in similar fashion to remove all dirt and debris, controlling bleeding by local digital pressure.
5 Irrigate the wound with copious volumes of physiological saline. A pulsed lavage system may be extremely helpful in this regard.
6 Complete the cleansing and irrigation of the wound in the theatre as part of the definitive surgical treatment.

REFERENCE

1. British Orthopaedic Association. Total Hip Replacement: a Guide to Best Practice. London: BOA; 1999.

OPEN WOUNDS

1 Resuscitate the patient, if necessary, according to ATLS (advanced trauma life support) principles and guidelines before dealing with an open wound.

2 Take a culture swab from the wound and send it for culture and sensitivities. This may be useful in the management of later infection.

> ### ▶ KEY POINTS Initial management
>
> ■ Clean open wounds in the accident and emergency department and cover them with an iodine-soaked dressing.
> ■ Leave this dressing undisturbed and do not repeatedly uncover the wound to inspect it until the patient is in theatre.
> ■ This will significantly reduce the rate of wound infection.

3 If possible take a Polaroid or digital photograph of the wound prior to the dressing being applied, to give you (or the treating surgeons) an idea of the extent and configuration of the underlying wound and to avoid disturbing the dressings unnecessarily.

4 Stop the bleeding by applying local pressure. Elevate the limb if necessary. Do not attempt blind clamping of any bleeding vessels, to avoid damaging adjacent structures.

Appraise

1 Determine how the wound was sustained and whether it is recent and clean or long-standing and dirty, and if it is superficial or deep. The longer the period since the injury and the deeper and dirtier the wound, the greater the need for antibiotics and tetanus prophylaxis.

2 Consider what structures may have been damaged and test for the integrity of arteries, nerves, tendons and bones.

3 Make an initial assessment of skin loss or damage and look for exit wounds following penetrating injuries.

4 An X-ray will show the extent of bone damage and the presence of radio-opaque foreign bodies (remember that not all foreign bodies are radio-opaque).

5 Always request X-rays of the skull, lateral cervical spine, chest and anteroposterior views of the pelvis in multiply injured patients, but do not let this delay treatment.

6 Depending on the extent of the wound, carry out further assessment and treatment without anaesthesia or with regional or general anaesthetic. Avoid local infiltration anaesthesia.

Prepare

1 Give a broad-spectrum antibiotic, unless the wound is clean, superficial and recent in origin.

2 If the wound is dirty, deep and more than 6 hours old, give 1 g of benzylpenicillin, and 0.5 ml of tetanus toxoid intramuscularly if the patient has been actively immunized in the past 10 years.

3 If the patient has not been actively immunized, give 1 vial (250 units) of human tetanus immunoglobulin in addition to the toxoid. Ensure that further toxoid is given 6 weeks and 6 months later.

4 Clean the wound and prepare the skin, as described above.

5 Apply a proximal tourniquet when appropriate.

Assess

1 Gently explore the wound, examining the skin, subcutaneous tissues and deeper structures. Follow the track of a penetrating wound with a finger or a probe to determine its direction and to judge the possibility of damage to vessels, nerves, tendons, bone and muscle. If you suspect muscle damage, slit open the investing fascia and take swabs for an anaerobic bacterial culture. Decide into which category the wound falls, since this determines the subsequent management.

2 Simple clean wounds have no tissue loss, although all wounds are contaminated with microorganisms, which may already be dividing. In clean wounds seen within 8 hours of injury, the bacteria will not yet have invaded the tissues.

3 Simple contaminated wounds have no tissue loss. However, they may be heavily contaminated and if you see them more than 8 hours after the injury, they can be assumed to be infected. Late wounds show signs of bacterial invasion, with pus and slough covering the raw surfaces, and redness and swelling of the surrounding skin. Although there is no loss of tissue from the injury, the infection will result in later soft-tissue destruction.

4 Complicated contaminated wounds result when tissue destruction (e.g. loss of skin, muscle or damage to blood vessels, nerves or bone) has occurred, or foreign bodies are present in the wound. Recently acquired low-velocity missile wounds fall into this category since there is insufficient kinetic energy to carry particles of clothing and dirt into the wound.

5 Complicated dirty wounds are seen after heavy contamination in the presence of tissue destruction or implantation of foreign material, especially if the wound is not seen until more than 12 hours have elapsed.

6 High-velocity missile wounds deserve to be placed in a category of their own. For instance, when a bullet from a high-powered rifle strikes the body it is likely to lose its high kinetic energy to the soft tissues as it passes through, resulting in extensive cavitation. Although the entry and exit wounds may be small, structures within the wound are often severely damaged. Muscle is particularly susceptible to the passage of high-velocity missiles and becomes devitalized. It takes on a 'mushy' appearance and consistency and fails to contract when pinched or to bleed when cut. If the bullet breaks into fragments or hits bone, breaking it into fragments, the spreading particles of bullet and bone also behave as high-energy particles. The whole effect is of an internal explosion. In addition, the high-velocity missile carries foreign material (bacteria and clothing) deeply into the tissues, causing heavy contamination.

The risk of tetanus and gas gangrene is increased when the wound is sustained over heavily cultivated ground in which the organisms abound. Devitalized ischaemic muscle makes an excellent culture medium. As haematoma and oedema formation develop within the investing fascia, tissue tension rises, further embarrassing the circulation and causing progressive tissue death. Although handgun bullets, shotgun pellets, shrapnel from shells and fragments from mine, grenade and bomb explosions have a relatively low velocity, they behave as high-velocity missiles when projected into the tissues from nearby. When a shotgun is fired close to the body, the wad and the pellets are carried in as a single missile.

7 Open fractures can be classified in a variety of ways. Probably the most widely accepted is the Gustilo classification, which is particularly useful in discussing soft-tissue reconstruction:

- Type I: an open fracture with a cutaneous wound <1 cm.
- Type II: an open fracture with extensive soft-tissue damage.
- Type IIIA: high-energy trauma irrespective of the size of the wound. There is adequate soft-tissue coverage of the fractured bone, despite extensive soft-tissue lacerations or flaps.
- Type IIIB: there is an extensive soft-tissue injury with loss of tissue, accompanied by periosteal stripping and bone exposure. These wounds are usually associated with massive contamination.
- Type IIIC are open fractures associated with vascular and/or neurological injury requiring repair.

Action

1 Stop all bleeding. Pick up small vessels with fine artery forceps and cauterize or ligate them with fine absorbable sutures. Control damage of major arteries and veins with pressure, tapes or non-crushing clamps, so as to permit later repair.

2 Irrigate clean simple wounds with copious volumes of sterile saline solution without drainage. Do not attempt to repair cleanly divided muscle with stitches but simply suture the investing fascia. Close the skin accurately.

> ### ▶ KEY POINTS Infected wounds
>
> - Never close an apparently simple infected wound immediately.
> - Take a swab for culture.
> - Remove any retained foreign material, radically excise and debride any dead or devitalized tissue and drain any potential pockets of infection.
> - Systemic antibiotic or local instillations may be started but will not make up for poor technique.
> - Pack the wound with gauze soaked in sterile isotonic saline solution and cover with an occlusive dressing. Plan to renew the packing daily until the wound is clean and produces no further discharge.
> - Provided there is no redness or oedema of the surrounding skin, close the wound by delayed primary suture, usually after 3–7 days.

3 Complicated contaminated wounds can be partially repaired after excising the devitalized tissue. Once bone stability has been achieved, damaged segments of major arteries and veins should be repaired by an experienced surgeon, using grafts where appropriate. Loosely appose the ends of divided nerves with one or two stitches in the perineurium, so that they can be readily identified and repaired later when the wound is healed and all signs of inflammation have disappeared. Similarly, identify and appose the ends of divided tendons in preparation for definitive repair at a later date. Do not remove small fragments of bone that retain a periosteal attachment or large fragments whether they are attached or unattached. Excise devitalized muscle, especially the major muscle masses of the thigh and buttock. Remove

foreign material when possible. Some penetrating low-velocity missiles are better left if they lie deeply, provided damage to important structures has been excluded. Remove superficial shotgun pellets. Low-velocity missile tracks do not normally require to be laid open or excised, but do not close the wound. Excise damaged skin when the deep flap can be easily closed, if necessary by making a relaxing incision or applying a skin graft. Do not lightly excise specialized skin from the hands; instead leave doubtful skin and excise it later, if necessary, on expert advice.

4 Stabilize any associated fracture. It may be possible merely to immobilize the limb in a plaster cast, cutting a window into it so that the wound can be dressed. An open fracture, however, is not an absolute contraindication to surgical stabilization using the appropriate device (plates and screws, intramedullary nails), but such should be undertaken only by an experienced trauma or orthopaedic surgeon. In an emergency situation it is preferable to use temporary skeletal traction and external fixator.

5 Complicated dirty wounds require similar treatment of damaged tissues such as nerves and tendons, but do not attempt to repair damaged structures other than major blood vessels. Pack the wound and change the dressing daily until there is no sign of infection, then close the skin by suture or by skin grafting.

6 Lay open high-velocity missile wounds extensively. Foreign matter, including missile fragments, dirt and clothing, is carried deeply into the wound, so contamination is inevitable. Explore and excise the track, since the tissue along the track is devitalized, lay open the investing fascia over disrupted muscle to evacuate the muscle haematoma and excise the pulped muscle, leaving healthy contractile muscle that bleeds when cut. This leaves a cavity in the track of the missile.

7 Mark divided nerves and tendons for definitive treatment later. Excise the skin edges and pack the wound with saline-soaked gauze. Treat any associated fracture as described above. Change the packs daily until infection is controlled and all dead tissue has been excised. Only then can skin closure be completed and the repair of damaged structures be planned.

EXTERNAL FIXATION

There are many types of external fixator, ranging from the simple unilateral frame (Denham, Orthofix), multilateral frames (Hoffman) through to the more complicated circular frames (Ilizarov) and hybrid devices. The essential feature of the external fixator is that it provides a stable reduction of any fracture by using percutaneously introduced wires or pins into the bone, which are then attached to an external frame.

The Ilizarov and similar circular frames are beyond the scope of this chapter, but in an emergency you should be familiar with the principles involved, and the techniques of applying a simple unilateral frame. Such a frame is constructed from one or more rigid bars which are aligned parallel to the limb and to which the threaded pins that are drilled into the fragments of bone are attached. In the more sophisticated devices (Orthofix, AO, Monotube, Hoffman) this is done by clamping the pins to universal joints, which allow the position of the fragments to be adjusted before the clamps are finally tightened. In the simplest form, here described, the pins are held to the bar with acrylic cement (Denham type; Fig. 30.1).

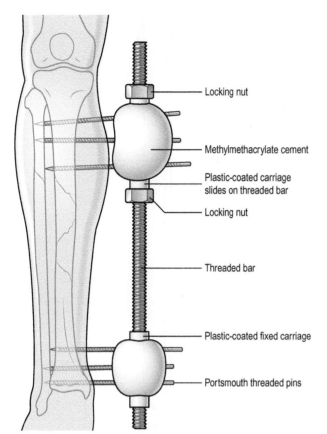

Fig. 30.1 The Denham external fixator.

Prepare

1 Treat the wound as outlined above.
2 Reduce the fracture, either open under direct vision, or closed using an image intensifier.
3 Maintain the reduction using bone clamps, traction or temporary wires.

Action

1 Make a stab wound through healthy skin proximal to the fracture site, bearing in mind the possible need for subsequent skin flaps.
2 Drill a hole through both cortices of the bone, approximately at right-angles to the bone, with a sharp 3.6-mm drill. Take care in drilling the bone that the drill bit does not overheat, which may in turn cause local bone necrosis leading to the formation of ring sequestra with subsequent loosening and infection of the pins. Measure the depth of the distal cortex from the skin surface.
3 Insert a threaded Schantz pin into the drill hole so that both cortices are penetrated.
4 If possible, insert two more pins approximately 3–4 cm apart into the proximal fragment and three pins into the distal fragment in similar fashion. Biomechanically, the stability of the fixator is enhanced if there are three pins in each of the major fragments, with the nearest pin being close to the fracture line.
5 Loosen the locking nuts that hold the carriages on to the rigid bar and hold the bar parallel to the limb and 4–5 cm away from the skin.

6 Place one carriage opposite the protruding ends of each set of three pins and adjust the locking nuts to hold the carriages in position.
7 Fix the pins to the carriages with two mixes of acrylic cement for each carriage, moulding the cement around the pins and the carriage, maintaining the position until it is set.
8 Remove any temporary reduction device and carry out the final adjustment on the locking nuts to compress the bone ends together.
9 Dress the wound.

Aftercare

1 Keep the pin tracks clean and free of scabs and incrustations by daily cleaning with sterile saline or a mild antiseptic solution. A rigorous regime will minimize the risk of pin-tract infection and premature pin loosening.
2 An external fixator is essentially only a temporary measure before definitive treatment can be carried out. It is seldom used as the sole method of fracture management and should, therefore, be removed at a time when the wound is healthy, at which time it may be possible to definitively stabilize the fracture.
3 Fixator removal is simple. Cut the pins with a hacksaw or bolt cutters and then unscrew them. The acrylic cement can be removed from the carriages, which may be used again.

OPEN (COMPOUND) FRACTURES

Appraise

1 Assess the patient according to ATLS principles and resuscitate as necessary.
2 Manage the wound as outlined above.
3 X-ray the bone to determine the pattern of the fracture and to decide on the appropriate method of reduction and fixation.

Prepare

1 Anaesthetize the patient.
2 Prepare the skin.
3 Clean the wound.

Action

1 Explore and reassess the wound.
2 Expose and assess the fracture. Remove only small and completely unattached fragments of bone. Retain any bone that has a remaining periosteal attachment, as this bone is potentially still viable.
3 Free the bone ends from any adjacent fascia and muscle through which they may have buttonholed.
4 Wash away any blood clot and other debris.
5 Strip the periosteum for 1–2 mm only from the bone ends to allow accurate reduction without the interposition of soft tissues.
6 Using a combination of traction, bone clamps, levers and hooks, reduce the major fragments into an anatomical position. If necessary, extend the original wound to improve access.

485

7 If the fracture is stable, immobilize in a plaster cast after definitive treatment of the wound. Leave a window in the cast to permit wound inspection and changes of dressings.

8 Apply an external fixator when the wound is contaminated or there is extensive skin loss.

> ▶ KEY POINTS Fixation?

> ■ If the fracture is unstable and there is a simple, clean wound, then it may be appropriate to internally fix the fracture.
> ■ If there are multiple injuries or if the wound is contaminated an external fixator may be more appropriate.
> ■ Do not forget the possibility of immediate amputation if the limb is severely mutilated with associated neurovascular injuries (Gustilo grade IIIB or C).

SKELETAL TRACTION

Appraise

1 Temporary skeletal traction can be applied using skin traction, and, indeed, this is the method of choice when using a Thomas splint for immobilization of a femoral fracture as a first aid measure. For prolonged treatment insert a traction pin through the tibia or calcaneus. Other sites such as the olecranon or metacarpals are occasionally used.

2 Skeletal traction is a simple and safe method of immobilizing a limb after injury or operation. It may be seen as a temporary measure, as definitive treatment, or as a supplement to treatment. With the more widespread use of increasingly sophisticated internal fixation devices, skeletal traction is less frequently employed as a definitive method of treating long-bone fractures. Skeletal traction requires careful supervision and adjustments to remain effective.

3 There are two types of pin in common usage (Fig. 30.2). Each has a triangular or square butt, which inserts into a chuck, and a trocar point. The Steinmann pin is uniform throughout but the Denham pin has a short length of screw thread wider than the main shaft near its centre, which screws into one cortex of the bone and minimizes sideways slip during traction.

Prepare

1 Clean the skin and drape the limb, leaving about 10 cm exposed on either side of the site of entry.

2 Anaesthetize the skin, subcutaneous tissue and periosteum on both sides of the bone at site of entry and exit of the pin with 1% lidocaine.

3 Make sure that the pin selected fits the sockets in the stirrup.

Action

1 To insert the pin through the upper tibia, make a 5-mm stab incision in the skin on the lateral side of the bone 2.5 cm posterior to the summit of the tibial tuberosity; this avoids damage to the common peroneal nerve when a medial approach is used. If the

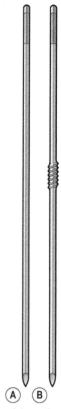

Fig. 30.2 (A) Steinmann pin; (B) Denham pin.

tibial plateau is fractured, make the nick and insert the pin 2.5–5 cm distally.

2 To insert the pin through the calcaneus, make a 5-mm stab incision in the skin on the lateral side of the heel 2.5 cm distal to the tip of the lateral malleolus.

3 Introduce the point of the pin through the nick at right-angles to the long axis of the limb and parallel to the floor, with the limb in the anatomical position. Avoid obliquity in either plane.

> ▶ KEY POINTS Care inserting pins

> ■ Drill the pin through both cortices of the bone with a hand drill until the point just bulges under the skin on the opposite side of the limb.
> ■ Take care that the pin does not suddenly penetrate the skin to impale your hand or the opposite limb. This is particularly likely if the bone is thin and porotic.

4 Incise the skin over the exit point and gently push the pin through until equal lengths are protruding on either side. When using the Denham pin the threaded section should be screwed into the cortex a further 6–8 mm so that the thread engages the bone.

5 Make sure that the skin is not distorted where the pin passes through. Make tiny relieving incisions if necessary.

6 Dress the punctures with small squares of gauze soaked in tincture of benzoin.

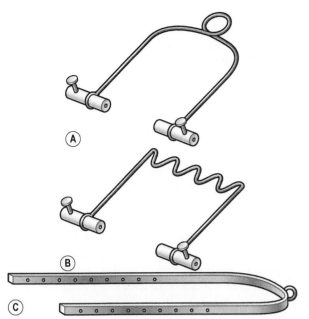

Fig. 30.3   Traction loops: (A) the Bohler stirrup; (B) the Nissen stirrup; (C) the Tulloch-Brown 'U' loop.

7 Attach traction cords or a traction stirrup to the pin. Three types of stirrup are available (Fig. 30.3):
   ■ The Bohler stirrup, for general use
   ■ The Nissen stirrup, for more accurate control of rotation
   ■ The Tulloch-Brown 'U'-loop for Hamilton Russell traction.

8 Put guards on the ends of the pin.

9 Attach a length of cord to the centre of the stirrup, through which the traction will be applied.

Aftercare

1 Keep the pin tracks clean and free of scabbing and incrustation as described above.

2 Continually monitor the position of the fracture and adjust the traction as necessary so as to maintain an accurate reduction.

3 Monitor the condition of the patient as the enforced prolonged period of recumbence predisposes them to chest infection and pressure sores.

SIMPLE SKELETAL TRACTION

1 Simple skeletal traction over a pulley fixed to the end of the bed usually suffices for relatively stable fractures (e.g. of the tibial plateau).

2 Unstable fractures need the support of a splint. Support the calf on two or three pillows with the point of the heel clear of the bed. Have the traction string horizontal and apply sufficient traction weights so as to reduce the fracture and restore alignment and length of the bone. Usually 4–5 kg is sufficient, depending upon the weight of the patient.

HAMILTON RUSSELL TRACTION

This is a convenient method for fractures and other conditions around the hip (e.g. dislocation or acetabular fractures). It controls

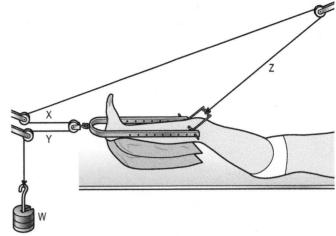

Fig. 30.4   Hamilton Russell skeletal traction.

the natural tendency of the leg to roll into external rotation and avoids the use of a Thomas splint, the ring of which causes discomfort if the hip is tender.

Action

1 Set up the apparatus as in Figure 30.4, passing the cord through the pulleys as indicated. The sections of string 'x' and 'y' must be parallel to the horizontal and the section 'z' must lead in a cephalic direction. Support the calf either on two ordinary pillows or on slings of Domette bandage attached to the 'U'-loop with safety pins.

2 Attach between 2 and 5 kg of weight to the end of the cord and make sure that it is clear of the floor. Remember that the effective traction is doubled as a result of the pulley arrangement.

3 Keep the point of the heel clear of the bed to avoid pressure sores.

4 Place a foot rest between the bars of the loop to maintain the foot at a right-angle to the leg.

5 A separate cord running from the Nissen stirrup through the more proximal pulley can be attached to a handle, so facilitating knee flexion exercises.

SLIDING SKELETAL TRACTION

Sliding skeletal traction with the leg supported on a Thomas or similar splint is a standard method of conservative treatment for femoral shaft or supracondylar fractures.

Action

1 Set up the apparatus as shown in the diagram in Figure 30.5. Apply 4–8 kg of weight for traction ('W').

2 The splint should have a Pearson's or equivalent knee attachment so that the knee may be flexed (20° for shaft fractures and 40° or more for supracondylar fractures). Tie the distal end of this attachment to that of the main splint with traction cord. Only the cord 'X' is concerned with traction. Cords 'Y' and 'Z' and weights 'S1' and 'S2' merely suspend the splint to aid nursing.

3 Support the limb from the sides of the splint with Domette bandage held in place with safety pins. Pad the underside of the limb with sheets of cotton wool.

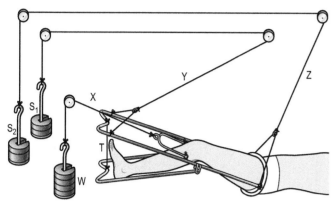

Fig. 30.5   Sliding skeletal traction with a Thomas splint.

CALCANEAL TRACTION

1   Use calcaneal traction with the leg supported on a Bohler-Braun frame in the conservative treatment of unstable fractures of the tibia.

2   It may be combined with a padded plaster cast to provide more lateral stability.

3   Set up the apparatus as shown in the diagram in Figure 30.6.

4   Apply 2–4 kg of weight (W'). Support the calf and thigh from the side-bars of the frame with slings of Domette bandage. Pad under the limb with cotton wool.

Aftercare

As above, but with any tibial fracture constantly check on the neurovascular status of the limb looking for compartment syndrome.

SKULL TRACTION

Appraise

1   Skull traction is often employed to immobilize the cervical spine after injury (fracture, subluxation or dislocation) and sometimes after operations on the neck.

2   The traction is applied through skull tongs inserted under local anaesthetic prior to the administration of any general anaesthetic. The anaesthetist then has the benefit of the added security of the traction.

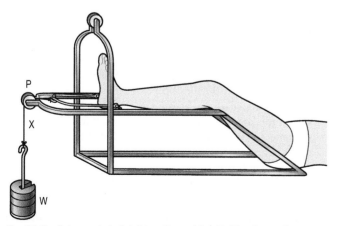

Fig. 30.6   Calcaneal skeletal traction with a Bohler-Braun frame.

3   The common devices available for skull traction are either the Crutchfield tongs or a Cone skull caliper. I have found the Cone caliper easier to apply and less likely to slip than the Crutchfield device.

Access

1   The patient lies supine with the head carefully supported so as to avoid sudden and unexpected movement.

2   Establish the insertion point for the caliper, which is at the point of maximal diameter of the skull in a line running across the vertex of the skull from one mastoid process to the other. In practice, this is usually 2–3 cm above the top of the ear.

3   Shave a small area of the scalp at the proposed insertion points and moisten the surrounding hair to keep it flat.

4   Place a waterproof layer and sterile towel under the head and drape off the bared area. Prepare the skin with a suitable antiseptic agent. Leave the face of the conscious patient uncovered.

5   Infiltrate the scalp down to the pericranium with 5 ml of 1% lidocaine and 1:200 000 adrenaline (epinephrine) on each side, anaesthetizing an area about 1.5 cm in diameter.

6   Open the Cone calipers to their fullest extent and place the points symmetrically on either side of the midline of the scalp. Mark the position of the points with a skin marker.

7   Make a stab incision down to the pericranium on either side. Bring the caliper back into position and introduce the pin through the conical end of the caliper.

8   The caliper is then tightened such that the tips of the cones abut the outer table of the skull. The pins are then tightened down through the outer table to a predetermined depth.

Aftercare

1   Usually no dressing is required, but keep the pin sites clean.

2   Apply traction or proceed to manipulation as desired. Tie the traction cord to the ring on the caliper and not to the screw.

PERIPHERAL NERVE REPAIR

1   Complete disruption of a peripheral nerve may be associated with both open and closed injuries and recovery will not take place unless continuity is re-established surgically.

2   Peripheral nerve repair (Fig. 30.7) is a specialist technique but, faced with it in the field, you should be aware of the principles. If you feel unable to attempt a primary repair then mark the nerve ends with a non-absorbable suture to assist their location at the time of the definitive operation.

Appraise

1   Always assume that a peripheral nerve injury in the presence of an open wound is the result of a complete division of the nerve fibres (neurotmesis). You must therefore identify the nerve when the wound is treated and satisfy yourself as to its integrity. If it is divided, either mark or appose the ends in their correct orientation for secondary repair later.

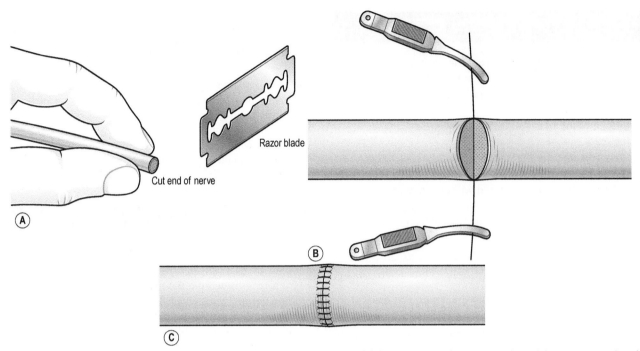

Fig. 30.7 Nerve suture: (A) cutting back to pouting fibres with a razor blade; (B) first and second sutures in place; (C) sutures completed.

2 Some form of magnification is essential in repairing a peripheral nerve. While an operating microscope may not be available, simple magnifying loupes will usually suffice.

3 It is entirely acceptable to treat a peripheral nerve injury conservatively in the absence of an open wound. A neuropraxia (block to conduction of nerve impulses without disruption of the axon or its supporting cells) will usually recover spontaneously in days or weeks, and an axonotmesis (the axon undergoes Wallerian degeneration) in the time it takes for the axons to regenerate. This is calculated by measuring the distance from the site of injury (e.g. a fracture) to the point at which the motor nerve enters the first muscle innervated distal to the lesion. Axons regenerate at a rate of 1 mm/day and so it will take approximately 90 days, for example, for re-innervation of the brachioradialis to occur following an injury to the radial nerve at the distal end of the spiral groove of the humerus. Electrophysiological studies (EMG, nerve conduction) may give some pointers as to the likely nerve lesion and will help in documenting recovery.

4 If recovery fails to occur in the predicted time and if the nerve conduction studies show no improvement, then explore the course of the nerve and treat any lesion appropriately.

▶ KEY POINTS When to repair?

- Primary repair undoubtedly gives the best results and may sometimes be undertaken in specialist centres.
- If the patient is stable and fit for transfer, then do so.
- Secondary repair is safer and sometimes easier when the wound is soundly healed and the danger of infection has passed.

Prepare

1 Do not attempt immediate primary nerve repair unless you have adequate magnification (loupes or operating microscope) and are sufficiently experienced in the techniques involved. If there is any doubt, it is safer to mark or appose the nerve ends for later exploration and repair.

2 Prepare the skin.

3 Apply a tourniquet.

Access

1 Clean and explore the wound.

2 If there is a previous wound that has healed, excise the previous scar if necessary, and extend the wound proximally and distally along the course of the nerve.

3 If there was no wound, make an incision 15 cm long along the course of the nerve centred at the site of injury. Use a 'lazy-S' incision if the incision crosses the flexor crease of a joint.

4 Always begin by exposing the nerve in normal tissue on either side of the site of injury and then work towards the site of the injury, carefully dissecting along the course of the nerve. In the case of an open wound there may be extensive scar tissue and adhesions.

Assess

1 Decide whether repair is possible or not.

2 If repair is possible but beyond your competence, what action should you take?

■ Free the ends of the nerve from the surrounding soft tissues and place a marker suture of 4/0 nylon or other non-absorbable material through the perineurium 2–3 cm proximally and distally from the site of injury to facilitate later alignment of the ends.

■ If possible, appose the ends now, with two or three stitches for ease of later identification.

■ If the ends cannot be apposed without tension, tack them to the underlying soft tissues to prevent retraction until definitive repair can be undertaken.

Action

1 If this is a delayed repair there may be fibrous scar tissue at the cut ends, or joining the ends.

2 If necessary, cut transversely across fibrous scar tissue that may be joining the ends together.

3 Hold one end of the nerve firmly, using a special nerve-holding clamp (a finger and thumb will suffice in extremis) and carefully cut thin slices of tissue from the exposed end with a sharp razor blade at right-angles to the long axis of the nerve until all the scar tissue has been excised and the nerve bundles can be seen pouting from the cut surface (Fig. 30.7A).

4 Repeat the procedure on the other end of the nerve. It may be necessary to resect a centimetre or more from each end of the nerve because of the intraneural fibrosis (neuroma) caused by the initial injury.

5 If this is a primary closure, place the nerve ends in their correct rotational orientation. If this is delayed closure, similarly identify the correct rotational alignment.

6 Mobilize the nerve from the surrounding soft tissues proximally and distally as far as is necessary to bring the ends together without tension, carefully preserving and dissecting out the main branches. Flex a neighbouring joint if necessary. If it proves impossible to appose the nerve ends then an interposition graft may be necessary.

7 Release the tourniquet and achieve perfect haemostasis.

8 Ensure again that the ends of the nerve are correctly orientated.

9 Place an 8/0 nylon stitch through the perineurium on one side of the nerve. Cut the suture 3 cm from the knot and hold the ends in a small bulldog clip (Fig. 30.7B).

10 Place a second suture directly opposite the first and place another bulldog clip on the ends. These act as stay sutures and facilitate rotation of the nerve while placing further sutures.

11 Place further sutures through the perineurium, 1.5 mm or so apart, around the circumference of the nerve.

12 After completing the repair of the superficial surface, turn the nerve over by passing one bulldog clip suture under and the other over the nerve.

13 Complete the repair. Cut the first pair of sutures and turn the nerve back to the correct position (Fig. 30.7C).

14 Close the soft tissues and skin without altering the position of the limb if there is any danger of putting tension on the suture line.

15 Apply a padded plaster without increasing the tension on the repair.

16 Remove plaster and skin sutures after 3 weeks and gently mobilize the limb. If joints were flexed to avoid tension they must only be extended gradually over the next 3 weeks, if necessary by applying serial plasters at weekly intervals, or by incorporating a hinge with a locking device to allow flexion but no more than the set amount of joint extension.

TENDON SUTURE

Appraise

Tendons are relatively avascular structures and heal by the ingrowth of connective tissue from the epitenon. When the tendon is divided within a fibrous sheath on the flexor surface of the hand, for example, the sheath is also damaged and the connective tissue from the healing sheath grows into the healing tendon, causing adhesions. For this reason, injuries to the digital flexor tendons within the sheath should preferably be treated by experienced hand surgeons. Tendons may also require suturing as part of another procedure such as tendon transfer.

■ It is entirely safe to perform a delayed primary repair of a divided flexor tendon up to 14 days post-injury without adversely affecting the final outcome.

ASSESS

1 Examine the wound. As with nerve injuries, if it is in the vicinity of a tendon and there is no distal action, assume that the tendon is divided until it is shown to be intact on clinical examination.

2 If no action is demonstrated or if there is doubt, explore the wound.

Action

1 Prepare the skin.

2 Apply the tourniquet.

3 Explore the wound and extend it if necessary in order to identify any divided tendons.

4 If the wound is suitable for primary closure then proceed to repair the tendons. If not, delay the repair until the wound is healed and is no longer indurated, maintaining full mobility of the joints in the meantime by physiotherapy.

5 When several tendons are divided (e.g. at the wrist), make sure that the cut ends are correctly paired. It is not unheard of to suture the proximal end of one tendon to the distal end of another or even to the cut end of a nerve!

6 Draw the cut ends together after picking up the paratenon round each end of the tendon with fine mosquito forceps, flexing neighbouring joints if necessary.

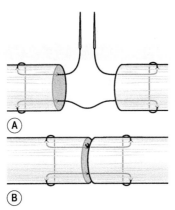

Fig. 30.8   End-to-end suture of a tendon. (A) Modified Kessler suture; (B) Complete knot, cut and bury within tendon.

7 Secure the cut ends of the tendon by passing one needle into an exposed tendon end and bring it out of the side of the tendon about 1.5 cm from the cut end. Now pass this needle transversely through the tendon 3–4 mm nearer to the cut end. Re-insert this needle on the other side of the tendon to create a mirror image and bring it out through the cut end (Fig. 30.8A).

8 Freshen the ends of the tendon by cutting them with a no. 15 blade.

9 Use a 3/0 braided non-absorbable (Ethibond) suture with a 15-mm straight needle at both ends, using a modified Kessler core stitch (Fig. 30.8A). Repeat this process using the second needle on the other tendon end.

10 Make a half-hitch and approximate the tendon ends till they just meet. Complete the knot with at least six throws. Cut the knot flush; this should now have been buried within the tendon (Fig. 30.8B).

11 Complete the repair with a simple running suture of 6/0 monofilament nylon with a small curved needle. It is helpful to begin the running stitch on the posterior face, leaving the cut end of the suture long with which to turn the tendon through 180° for ease of access. The final repair must be smooth, with no bunching at the repair site.

12 Release the tourniquet and secure haemostasis.

13 Close the wound with suction drainage if necessary.

14 Apply a padded plaster so that the suture line is not under tension and remove after 3 weeks in the upper limb and 6 weeks in the lower limb.

BIOPSY

Biopsy of bone or soft tissue may be taken at an open operation or by aspirating material through a needle (closed biopsy). Closed biopsy is now usually performed by interventional radiologists, who are able to take specimens with extreme accuracy aided by the modern imaging techniques at their disposal. In both cases material is taken from the margin of the lesion, for the tissue in the centre is often necrotic and difficult to identify. Take at least two specimens – one for culture and the other for histological examination.

OPEN BIOPSY

Appraise

Bone biopsy is indicated in order to investigate a potential bone tumour (benign or malignant) or where infection is suspected.

▶ KEY POINT Advice on technique and siting

■ In the case of a potential malignant tumour, ask the advice of a surgeon experienced in bone tumour management on the technique and siting of the biopsy and scar so that it will not interfere with any later surgery.

Action

1 Apply a pneumatic tourniquet if possible. In the case of possible infection, do not exsanguinate the limb.

2 Incise the skin over the most superficial aspect of the lesion, taking care to place the incision in such a way that it will be excised if later surgery is required.

3 Incise the deep fascia and split the muscle in the line of its fibres until the margin of the lesion or the bone is reached.

4 Take a wedge-shaped piece of tissue from the margin of the lesion approximately 1 cm long by 0.5 cm thick and 0.5 cm deep. Place it in formal saline unless specific staining techniques are required. Consult the pathologist beforehand if in doubt.

5 Take a further similar specimen for immediate culture.

6 If pus is present, aspirate as much as possible and take a swab for culture.

7 Take a further specimen for microscopic examination and a further specimen for culture from a different part of the lesion if it is large enough.

8 If the lesion is in bone, remove the specimen with a sharp osteotome and include the periosteum.

9 If the lesion is not obvious, drill a Kirschner wire or a thin twist drill into the suspected site and examine the area under the image intensifier, or take plain X-rays in two planes at right-angles. Note the relationship of the lesion to the marker before taking the specimens.

10 Examine radiologically once more to ensure that the specimen has indeed been removed from the lesion.

11 Label each specimen immediately and accurately.

12 Release the tourniquet and secure haemostasis.

13 Close the wound and apply a pressure dressing.

14 Ensure that the specimens are sent to the pathological laboratory.

OSTEOMYELITIS

In a developing country where antibiotics are limited and in the presence of malnourishment, malaria and anaemia, haematological spread of osteomyelitis is common.

Presentation is usually by acute abscess formation or a chronically discharging sinus. A developing abscess in the upper limb may initially present with pain and a periosteal reaction that may be confused with a healing greenstick fracture until the infection has declared itself.

Treatment of an abscess is surgical drainage and the wound is packed and left open. The wound is redressed if necessary under GA until it is clean and begins to granulate. This may not prevent the subsequent development of a sequestrum but will give symptomatic relief.

Sequestra in the upper limb can be removed with impunity and the wounds left open. In the lower limb, the timing of the sequestrectomy is more subtle. This will depend on the maturity and strength of the new bone formation. Too early sequestrectomy may result in the fracture of the residual tibia or femur. In the case of the tibia where there is bone loss, the fibula can be transferred and if necessary protected by an external fixator. Once the infection has settled and the sinus healed, bone grafting may be indicated.

In a child with multiple sequestra and abscesses who is systemically unwell and anaemic, it is prudent to remove the sequestra and drain the pus sequentially. For instance, a distal femoral sequestrum may be removed initially and the wound left open and regularly dressed until the child is systemically better. An associated upper tibial sequestrum can then be removed once the child is no longer toxic.

DRAINAGE OF ACUTE OSTEOMYELITIS

Appraise

1. Assume that any unwell infant or child with an area of local bone tenderness has osteomyelitis until proved otherwise and treat as such. For drainage of joints in the case of septic arthritis, see the appropriate chapter.

2. If an abscess is present on initial clinical examination, or if pain, temperature, local swelling and tenderness fail to improve within 12 hours of starting antibiotic therapy, undertake operative treatment immediately.

3. Do not wait until there is radiological (X-ray) evidence of infection. It is then too late. However, an isotope bone scan may be helpful in determining the site of infection. Magnetic resonance imaging (MRI) can show the extent of the problem.

Prepare

1. Take blood for culture, haemoglobin, ESR (erythrocyte sedimentation rate), CRP (C-reactive protein), WBC (white blood cell count) and differential white cell count.

2. Give cloxacillin 100–200 mg/kg of body weight daily in divided doses intravenously until there is clinical improvement, usually apparent within 24 hours. If the patient is intolerant of penicillins give cefradine 100 mg/kg of body weight daily.

3. Change antibiotic as necessary when sensitivities are known, as a result of blood culture or operation. Otherwise continue with oral flucloxacillin 50–100 mg/kg, when there is clinical improvement.

4. If operation proves to be necessary (see above), perform it under a general anaesthetic. Mark the tenderest point on the limb before premedication.

Action

> **KEY POINT** Tourniquet?

> ■ Apply a tourniquet if possible but do not exsanguinate the limb for fear of propagating the infection.

1. Prepare the skin and apply the drapes.

2. Centre the skin incision over the tenderest point on the bone and extend proximally and distally for 2.5–3 cm.

3. Incise the deep fascia and retract the soft tissues until the periosteum is exposed.

4. Pus may already have escaped into the soft tissues, but, if not, incise the periosteum and take specimens for culture. Excise obvious dead tissue.

5. If frank pus is not visible, swab the bone surface.

6. Drill a single hole with a 2-mm twist drill, 5 mm proximal to the epiphyseal line, which is easily identified under the periosteum. If pus emerges, drill a second and, if necessary, a third hole 5 mm proximal to the preceding hole. Usually, a single drill hole is sufficient to ensure that there is no pus in the medullary cavity.

7. Irrigate the wound with saline and insert a suction drain through normal skin. Plan to remove the drain after 24 hours or when drainage ceases.

8. Close the skin and apply a padded back splint so that the limb is immobilized and the wound can be inspected. Remove the slab when the wound is healed.

Aftercare

Continue antibiotics for 10 days, or longer if necessary, until the clinical signs of infection subside and the inflammatory markers (ESR, CRP) fall.

CHRONIC OSTEOMYELITIS

Appraise

Chronic pyogenic infection of bone may give rise to a recurrently discharging or permanent sinus and be associated with an underlying sequestrum. Identify a sequestrum radiologically by tomography, CT scanning or MRI. In the case of a chronically discharging wound a sinogram may determine the extent of the sinus. It is the sequestrum (a piece of dead bone) that is generally the source of the chronic infection. Therefore, operative treatment is not indicated in the absence of a sequestrum or sinus.

Action

1. Under general anaesthetic apply a tourniquet to the elevated limb, but do not exsanguinate it.

2. Prepare the skin and apply the drapes.

3. It is helpful to identify the extent of the sinus by injecting methylthioninium chloride (methylene blue) solution into its opening until it oozes from the sinus. Remove excess dye with a swab.

4 Centre the skin incision on the mouth of the sinus and excise it. Extend the incision in the direction of any sequestrum, excising any previous scars.

5 Carefully dissect around the track of the sinus down to the bone. The sinus track is usually visible through the surrounding cuff of normal tissue. Excise the sinus track.

6 The entrance of the sinus into the bone will be stained blue. Strip the periosteum proximally and distally to expose any dead underlying bone, which has a white appearance.

7 Remove dead bone with an osteotome and/or bone nibblers and open the medullary cavity.

8 Remove the sequestrum if present, and unroof the part of the cavity stained blue. Curette out all granulation tissue that has been stained by the dye.

9 Irrigate the cavity thoroughly with a mixture of half-strength hydrogen peroxide and alcoholic Betadine and then physiological saline.

10 Place one or more chains of gentamicin-impregnated methyl methacrylate beads into the cavity so that it is completely filled. The chains must not be kinked or intertwined, which would make their subsequent removal difficult. Leave the last bead of each chain protruding above skin level to facilitate later removal.

11 Place a perforated drain under the skin before closure, and connect it to a non-evacuated suction bottle.

12 Close the skin, leaving the terminal bead of each chain protruding from the wound, and dress the wound.

Aftercare

1 Remove the drain after 24–48 hours, or when the discharge ceases.

2 Remove beads by gentle traction on the protruding bead after 10–14 days. An anaesthetic is not usually required.

3 If the chain breaks, leave the beads in situ and remove them subsequently under a general anaesthetic or sedation when the wound is well healed.

COSTO-TRANSVERSECTOMY FOR TUBERCULOUS ABSCESSES IN CHILDREN

In developing countries there may be malnutrition, no immunization against TB, and no anti-tuberculous drugs. In such an environment, the possibility of a tuberculous paraspinal abscess must be borne in mind in a child who develops advancing neurology in the lower limbs or paraplegia (Pott's paraplegia). Schistosomiasis may be a differential diagnosis if this is endemic locally and can be diagnosed by the presence of ova in the urine.

Appraise

1 Suspect TB spine in a patient with progressive debility and gradual onset of paraplegia. An abscess may be palpable externally, depending on its size and the vertebrae involved.

2 The procedure must be performed as soon as is practical following the diagnosis and can be followed by a remarkable improvement in neurology.

Assess

1 Absolute indications for surgery include:
  ■ Severe, rapid onset paraplegia
  ■ Onset of paraplegia during conservative (antibiotic) treatment
  ■ Progressive paraplegia despite appropriate treatment
  ■ Complete loss of motor power for one month despite appropriate treatment
  ■ Paraplegia with associated uncontrollable spasticity.

2 Relative indications for surgery include:
  ■ Recurrent paraplegia
  ■ Paraplegia in old age
  ■ Paraplegia with pain and spasm
  ■ Complications, e.g. recurrent UTI, renal stones.

3 Plain radiology may show erosion of a rib and adjacent thoracic vertebra. There may also be radiological soft tissue evidence of a collection.

4 CT scanning, if available, will confirm the level and extent of the lesion.

Prepare

1 Surgery is ideally performed under general anaesthesia or local anaesthesia with sedation.

2 The operation is performed with the patient prone.

Action

1 Prepare the skin.

2 Make a mid-line dorsal incision over the length of three spinous processes with any kyphos at the apex.

3 Using a periosteal elevator (Cobb, Bristow) reflect the periosteum laterally from the spinous processes to expose the transverse processes.

4 Resect the transverse process at its base using a bone nibbler.

5 Reflect the periosteum from the affected rib, exposing the medial 5 cm, which is then resected using a small bone cutter. Carefully trim and bevel the proximal end of the remaining bone, taking care not to puncture the pleura.

6 Following removal of the rib the abscess should drain and all its contents should be evacuated using a sucker and copious irrigation. If it does not drain spontaneously simply use a finger to perforate the cavity, break down any loculi and evacuate any necrotic material.

7 Occasionally it may be necessary to resect a second rib.

8 Instil antibiotic powder into the cavity.

9 It may be necessary to insert a chest drain if the pleura is damaged.

10 Close the wound in layers without drainage.

Aftercare

Initially nurse the patient on bed rest, taking care to avoid pressure sores, especially if there is sensory impairment. Postoperative mobilization will depend upon the extent of the bony damage. The patient can be mobilized gradually, depending on the rate of motor recovery. If there has been excessive bony involvement a plaster jacket or similar may be used to prevent the onset of late spinal deformity. Anti-tuberculous drugs should be given if available.

ACUTE SEPTIC (PYOGENIC) ARTHRITIS

Appraise

1 In all cases of acute arthralgia, especially in children who are systemically unwell, suspect septic arthritis.

2 If possible, attempt to aspirate the joint (it may be difficult to aspirate a hip) when the signs and symptoms of infection are present in association with a leucocytosis or a raised ESR. A negative aspiration, however, does not exclude infection.

Prepare

1 Take blood for culture, haemoglobin, CRP, WBC count and ESR.

2 X-ray the joint, but remember that these are generally normal in the presence of acute infection.

3 Give cloxacillin and methicillin intravenously.

4 Administer a general anaesthetic.

5 Clean and drape the skin.

Action

1 Insert a wide-bore needle attached to a syringe into the joint through the site of easiest access, maximum tenderness or fluctuation. Do not pass needles through an area of cellulitis because of the risk of infecting a sterile effusion.

2 Aspirate any fluid present for culture, cell counts, Gram stain and an immediate microscopy. If the aspirate is free from pus and no organisms are seen on the smear, treat by antibiotics and immobilization alone, until the results of cultures and all cell counts are available. Do not be confused by a report of 'pus cells' being present – these are merely inflammatory cells and are themselves diagnostic of infection.

3 Open the joint in all doubtful cases involving the hip, if the aspirate is obvious pus, if organisms are visible on the smear or are subsequently grown and if the cell counts exceed 100 000/mm^3.

4 Make an incision 2.5–3.5 cm long at the site of aspiration and approach the joint, if possible through a standard approach (see sections on individual joints).

5 Make a cruciate incision in the capsule and irrigate the joint thoroughly with physiological saline, removing all pus, fibrin or other debris.

6 Insert a suction drain and close the skin only.

Aftercare

1 Immobilize the joint in a stable position in a padded plaster with access to the wound, or skin traction for the hip.

2 Change the antibiotic if necessary when the cultures of the blood or aspirate are available. Change from intravenous to oral administration after 24–48 hours in the light of clinical improvement.

3 Remove the suction drain after 24–48 hours or when drainage ceases.

4 Continue antibiotics and immobilization for 6 weeks.

FURTHER READING

Brown KLB, Cruess RL. Bone and cartilage transplantation in orthopaedic surgery. J Bone Joint Surg Am 1982;64A:270–9.

Dixon RA. Nerve repair. Br J Hosp Med 1978;20:295–305.

Gelberman RH, Berg JSV, Lundborg GN, et al. Flexor tendon healing and restoration of the gliding surface. J Bone Joint Surg Am 1983;65A:70–9.

Johnson KD, Cadambi A, Seibert GB. Incidence of adult respiratory distress syndrome in patients with multiple musculoskeletal injuries: effect of early operative stabilization of fractures. J Trauma 1985;25:375–84.

Klenerman L, Miswas M, Hughland GH, et al. Systemic and local effects of the application of a tourniquet. J Bone Joint Surg Am 1980;62B:385–8.

Lowbury EJL, Lillie HA, Bull JP. Disinfection of the skin of operative sites. Br Med J 1960;2:1039–44.

Müller ME, Allgower M, Schneider R, et al. Manual of Internal Fixation. Techniques Recommended by the AO Group. 2nd ed Berlin: Springer-Verlag; 1979.

Nade S. Clinical implications of cell function in osteogenesis. Ann R Coll Surg Engl 1979;61:189–94.

Nade S. Acute haematogenous osteomyelitis in infancy and childhood. J Bone Joint Surg Am 1983;65B:109–20.

Nade S. Acute septic arthritis in infancy and childhood. J Bone Joint Surg Am 1983;65B:234–42.

Patzakis MK, Gustilo RV, Chapman MW. Management of open fractures and complications. In: Frankel VH, editor. Instructional Course Lectures. American Academy of Orthopaedic Surgeons, vol. 31. St Louis: Mosby; 1982. p. 62–88.

Seddon H. Surgical Disorders of the Peripheral Nerves. 2nd ed. Edinburgh: Churchill Livingstone; 1975.

Shipley JA, van Meerdervoort HF, van den Endej. Gentamicin polymethyl methacrylate beads in the treatment of chronic bone sepsis. S Afr Med J 1981;59:905–7.

Stewart JDM, Hallet JP. Traction and Orthopaedic Appliances. Edinburgh: Churchill Livingstone; 1983.

Orthopaedics and trauma: upper limb

N. Goddard

CONTENTS

THE ANTERIOR (DELTOPECTORAL) APPROACH TO THE SHOULDER

Appraise

1 The glenohumeral joint may be exposed through anterior, posterior or transacromial approaches, but most procedures can be carried out satisfactorily through the anterior approach (Fig. 31.1).

2 This is a straightforward approach through muscle planes and is truly 'extensile' in the manner described by Henry. It is particularly suited for exposure of the upper humerus for internal fixation or draining a potentially infected joint.

Prepare

1 Operate under a general anaesthetic.

2 Place the patient supine on the operating table in a semi-reclining (beach chair) position with a long narrow sandbag between the shoulder blades or alternatively with the head supported in a neurosurgical head ring.

3 Have your unscrubbed assistant elevate the arm.

4 Clean the skin from the scapula posteriorly, round the axilla and over the chest wall to the midline anteriorly, and from the angle of the jaw to the costal margin and down the arm to the elbow.

5 Towel the head separately (see Chapter 20).

6 Carefully tuck a large drape, backed by a waterproof sheet, between the table and the trunk. Cover the trunk with another large sheet, the upper edge of which reaches the lower margin of the head towels. Wrap the arm in a medium-sized towel, from the fingertips to the midpoint of the upper arm, and secure this towel firmly with an open-weave bandage or stockinette.

7 Cover the exposed skin with a transparent adhesive skin drape, taking care to seal the axilla.

Access

1 Incise the skin and subcutaneous fat in an arc from the clavicle above, downwards over the tip of the coracoid process to the anterior axillary fold following the anterior border of the deltoid muscle. Raise the flaps of skin and fat medially and laterally to expose the deltopectoral groove running obliquely across the wound (Fig. 31.1A).

2 Identify the cephalic vein in the deltopectoral groove and incise the investing fascia throughout the length of the vein.

> ▶ KEY POINTS Cephalic vein
>
> ■ While it may be possible to preserve the vein by retracting it medially it is often damaged during the course of an operation.
> ■ It is therefore preferable to ligate the cephalic vein.
> ■ Take care at the lower end where the vein is often duplicated, and then ligate it proximally before it penetrates the clavipectoral fascia immediately below the clavicle.

3 It is not necessary to remove the ligated segment of vein, but cauterize its tributaries as you encounter them.

4 Separate the deltoid from the pectoralis major by blunt dissection and retract the muscles with a large self-retaining retractor, exposing the coracoid process and the underlying short head of biceps and coracobrachialis (Fig. 31.1B).

5 In a simple operation for drainage of the joint it is not necessary to divide the coracoid process, but be willing to do so if you require more extensive exposure.

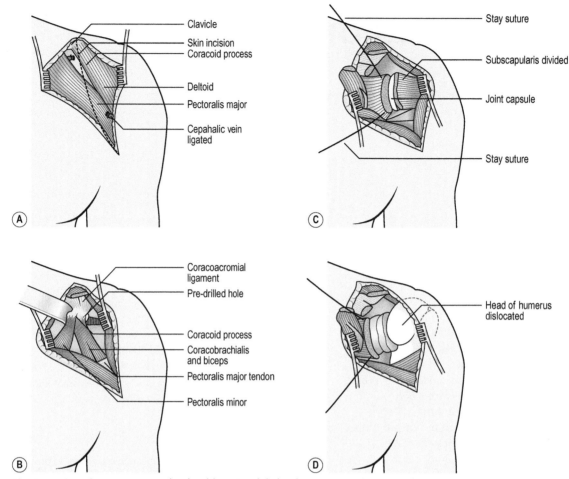

Fig. 31.1 Anterior exposure to the shoulder joint: (A) the skin incision – location of the deltopectoral groove and coracoid process; (B) division of the coracoid process with its attached muscle; (C) division and retraction of the subscapularis and the capsule; (D) dislocation of the head of the humerus.

6 Retract the bulk of the coracobrachialis and short head of biceps medially, so exposing the underlying subscapularis. It is possible to extend the approach distally along the lateral border of the biceps, so exposing the entire humeral shaft (see below).

7 Externally rotate the arm and identify the lower border of the subscapularis by seeing the branches of the anterior circumflex humeral vessels lying on its surface. Divide these between ligatures.

8 Identify the upper margin of the subscapularis and place stay sutures at the upper and lower margins at the musculotendinous junction. Divide the muscle just lateral to the stay sutures (Fig. 31.1C).

9 The underlying capsule is usually adherent to the deep surface and is frequently divided at the same time, opening the joint as the subscapularis is retracted medially.

10 If necessary, now dislocate the head of the humerus by external rotation and extension of the arm.

Closure

1 Internally rotate the arm. Apply gentle traction on the stay sutures to draw together the divided subscapularis muscle. Suture the muscle with 2/0 synthetic absorbable sutures.

2 Insert a suction drain.

3 Draw the margins of the deltoid and pectoralis major muscles together with two or three absorbable sutures.

4 Close the skin and dress the wound.

Aftercare

1 A simple dressing usually suffices, with the arm supported in a collar-and-cuff-type sling.

2 Remove the drain at 24 hours and begin early assisted motion of the shoulder.

APPROACHES TO THE UPPER ARM

Orthopaedic operations on the upper arm are infrequent but access to the humerus is occasionally required for internal fixation of fractures or exposure of the radial nerve.

ANTEROLATERAL APPROACH

Appraise

This approach to the humeral shaft avoids the major neuromuscular structures.

Prepare

1 Have 2 units of cross-matched blood available.

2 Operate under general anaesthesia.

3 Place the patient supine on the operating table with a large arm table in place.

4 An unscrubbed assistant elevates the arm so that it can be cleaned from the neck to the wrist.

5 Place a small triangular towel or split sheet in the axilla and take it over the tip of the shoulder. Fasten with a towel clip.

6 Place a waterproof sheet and covering towel over the arm board and tuck under the trunk.

7 Place a large sheet over the trunk and head.

8 Wrap the forearm and hand in a small towel and bandage firmly to the forearm with an open-weave bandage or stockinette.

9 Cover the exposed upper arm with a large transparent adhesive drape.

Access

1 Palpate the moveable mass of the biceps muscle overlying the fixed mass of the brachialis.

2 Make a longitudinal skin incision along the lateral border of the biceps from the deltoid above to the elbow below. Note that the upper part of the incision takes in the inferior limit of the anterior approach to the shoulder. Once again this is an extensile approach.

3 In the proximal part of the wound retract the deltoid laterally and the biceps and cephalic vein medially, dividing the lateral tributaries to expose the shaft of the humerus.

4 Distal to the insertion of the deltoid expose the brachialis muscle and split it longitudinally down to bone with the scalpel directed obliquely towards the midline of the humerus anteriorly (Fig. 31.2).

5 If necessary, extend the wound proximally by incising the skin in the line of the deltopectoral groove to the clavicle.

6 Detach the deltoid from its origin to the clavicle as far laterally as the acromioclavicular joint with the cutting diathermy. Leave sufficient tissue attached to the clavicle to take the sutures when closing.

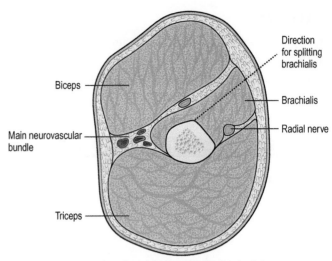

Fig. 31.2 Cross-section through the middle third of the arm showing the lateral part of the brachialis that is not covered by the biceps. This is split in the direction of the dotted line to expose the front of the distal half of the humerus. The cut slopes in to reach the midline of the shaft.

7 Turn back the detached deltoid laterally to expose the tendon of pectoralis major. This may then be cut to allow retraction of the muscle medially, exposing the long and short heads of the biceps and the neurovascular bundle.

8 The anterior surface of the lower third of the humerus can be exposed by extending the skin incision distally along the lateral border of the biceps, curling medially and then distally again, to cross the elbow crease in the midline of the forearm (Fig. 31.3).

9 Split the brachialis as far as the elbow joint and flex the elbow to open the wound.

Closure

1 Re-attach the deltoid and approximate the margins of the brachialis with 2/0 absorbable sutures.

2 Place a suction drain in a subcutaneous layer.

3 Suture the skin.

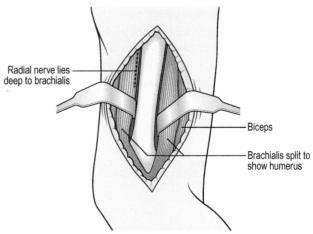

Fig. 31.3 The distal exposure of the humerus.

Aftercare

1 Apply a firm dressing and elevate the arm for 24 hours.

2 Use a sling until the wound has healed.

3 Encourage the patient to exercise the fingers, elbow and shoulder as soon as postoperative pain permits.

APPROACHES TO THE ELBOW

Appraise

1 The elbow joint may be exposed from the anterior, posterior, medial or lateral aspects.

2 Avoid the anterior approach except for very special circumstances.

3 The posterior approach gives access to the whole of the lower end of the humerus, while the medial and lateral approaches give a more limited access to the corresponding side of the joint, which is sufficient for more limited procedures.

> **KEY POINTS** Anatomy: avoid nerve damage
>
> ■ For simple drainage of a joint the posterolateral approach is the most straightforward.
> ■ But take care to avoid damaging the posterior interosseous branch of the radial nerve.

POSTEROLATERAL APPROACH (FIG. 31.4)

Appraise

This approach is particularly suitable for draining the elbow or for exposing the head of the radius. If necessary, it can be extended distally to expose the upper proximal third of the radius and adjoining ulna.

Prepare

1 With the patient under general anaesthetic, apply a pneumatic tourniquet high on the upper arm.

2 Position and prepare the arm as if the humerus were to be exposed, leaving 12 cm of skin exposed above and below the tip of the olecranon.

3 Have an assistant flex the elbow and hold the arm across the chest or on a side table.

Access

> **KEY POINT** Again, protect the nerve
>
> ■ Pronate the forearm so as to move the posterior interosseous nerve away from the operative field and to minimize the risk of accidental injury.

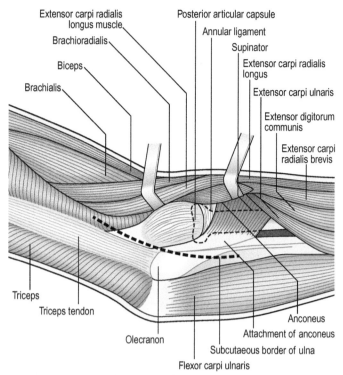

Fig. 31.4 Exposure of the head of the radius.

1 Begin the skin incision 3 cm proximal to the tip of the olecranon and continue distally between the olecranon and the lateral epicondyle down to the subcutaneous border of the ulna.

2 Divide the subcutaneous tissue and cut the deep fascia between the ulna and the anconeus and the extensor carpi ulnaris muscles (the Kocher interval).

3 Strip the anconeus from the ulna subperiosteally. Retract it laterally to expose the capsule covering the radial head and in the distal part of the wound the supinator muscle.

4 Incise the capsule over the radial head, so entering the joint. Extend this down to the annular ligament if you require greater access.

5 If necessary, irrigate the joint with physiological saline.

Closure

1 Release the tourniquet.

2 Secure haemostasis.

3 Re-attach the anconeus.

4 Close the skin.

Aftercare

Support the arm in a collar-and-cuff sling.

SUPRACONDYLAR FRACTURES

Appraise

No matter how experienced you are, be circumspect when treating a displaced supracondylar fracture, especially in a child. It always remains a cause for concern and anxiety because of the potential for damage to the adjacent neurovascular structures and consequent long-term complications.

> ### KEY POINTS Treatment options

- Look for signs of ischaemia and then for nerve damage.
- There is no optimal treatment for this injury in children. Cast immobilization is appropriate for an undisplaced fracture, but continually monitor the position lest it drifts into varus.
- Traction is very safe but requires hospitalization.
- Do not attempt percutaneous pinning unless you are very experienced, and have access to an image intensifier.
- Open reduction is occasionally indicated when the fracture is seemingly irreducible by closed means.

In the presence of potential ischaemia, splint the arm in extension to avoid further compressing the brachial artery.

CONSERVATIVE TREATMENT

1 This fracture can be treated conservatively by manipulation or olecranon traction in children.

2 Take anteroposterior radiographs of both elbows in a comparable position, usually acutely flexed, after closed reduction.

3 Draw a line along the epiphyseal surface of the lower humeral metaphysis and measure the angle between this and a line perpendicular to the long axis of the humerus. Compare this angle (Baumann's angle) on the two sides (Fig. 31.5).

4 Residual varus (Latin: = bent, towards the midline) or valgus (Latin: = originally meant bow-legged; now means bent away from the midline) tilt of more than 10° requires operative correction.

5 Circulatory impairment, either before or after closed reduction, demands immediate exploration of the brachial artery if the circulation cannot be restored by allowing the elbow to extend. Unless you are experienced, seek advice if at all possible (see Chapter 23).

POSTERIOR APPROACH

This gives the widest access to the lower end of the humerus and the elbow joint.

Prepare

1 With the patient under general anaesthetic, apply a pneumatic tourniquet high on the upper arm.

2 Position and prepare the arm as if exposing the humerus, leaving 12 cm of skin exposed above and below the tip of the olecranon.

3 Have an assistant flex the elbow and hold the arm across the chest.

Access

1 Start the skin incision in the midline 10 cm proximal to the tip of the olecranon and extend it distally in a gentle curve to pass just lateral to the tip of the olecranon, ending 5 cm distal to it over the subcutaneous border of the ulna.

2 Dissect the skin and subcutaneous tissues medially and laterally as far as the epicondyles and hold the edges apart with a self-retaining retractor.

3 Identify but do not disturb the ulnar nerve as it lies in its groove on the posterior surface of the medial epicondyle.

4 Identify the attachment of the central portion of the triceps tendon to the olecranon. Turn down a tongue-shaped flap, 7 cm long, based on the olecranon attachment by incising the tendon and the underlying muscle down to the bone (Fig. 31.6).

5 Sweep the residual attachments of the triceps muscle medially and laterally off the posterior surface of the condyles in continuity with the common flexor and extensor attachments, so exposing the distal humerus.

Action

1 Drill a 1-mm Kirschner wire (K-wire) through the fracture surface of the distal fragment at approximately 45° to the long axis of the

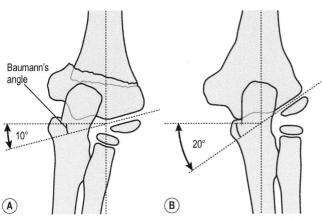

Fig. 31.5 Measurement of Baumann's angle. (A) Injured limb. (B) Controlateral normal limb

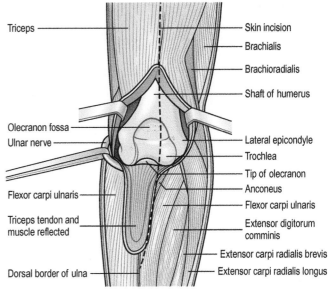

Fig. 31.6 Posterior approach to the elbow joint.

499

humerus, so that it emerges through the medial epicondyle and the overlying skin. Take care to avoid the ulnar nerve.

2 Withdraw the wire until only 1–2 mm protrudes from the fracture.

3 Reduce the fracture under direct vision, freeing any interposed soft tissue.

4 Flex the elbow to 90° and drill the K-wire back across the fracture to engage the lateral cortex of the shaft of the humerus (Fig. 31.7).

5 Through a small stab wound over the lateral condyle, drill a second wire across the fracture site to engage the medial cortex of the shaft.

6 Occasionally, a third wire needs to be introduced from either the medial or lateral side, if the fixation is not stable.

7 Confirm the accuracy of the reduction and the position of the wires by X-rays to check the accuracy of the reduction. Do not accept any position that is less than perfect.

8 If satisfactory, cut the wires leaving the ends just beneath the skin.

Closure

1 Suture the long head of the triceps back into place with interrupted absorbable sutures through the aponeurosis.

> KEY POINT Is the circulation intact?

> ■ Check the circulation and leave instructions that the radial pulse is to be taken every hour for the next 12 hours.

2 Release the tourniquet and stop the bleeding.

3 If necessary, place a suction drain under the skin before closing it.

Aftercare

1 If the fixation is stable immobilize the arm in a collar-and-cuff sling. If you are doubtful, apply a padded plaster back slab.

2 Remove the Kirschner wires at 3–4 weeks.

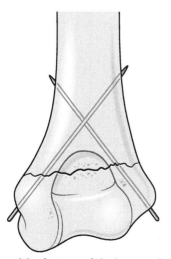

Fig. 31.7 Supracondylar fracture of the humerus held by crossed Kirschner wires.

DECOMPRESSION OF THE ULNAR NERVE (CUBITAL TUNNEL)

Appraise

1 Decompression of the ulnar nerve may be carried out for relieving ulnar neuritis or nerve entrapment. In most cases simple in situ decompression is sufficient but occasionally the nerve needs to be transposed anteriorly to the medial epicondyle if it is unstable, to gain length to repair the nerve following injury, or as part of another procedure (e.g. internal fixation of a distal humeral fracture).

2 If operating for a compression neuropathy, it is advisable to obtain preoperative nerve-conduction studies.

Action

1 Position the patient supine, with a tourniquet applied to the upper arm as high as possible.

> KEY POINT Sufficient access?

> ■ Preoperatively, check that the shoulder will externally rotate sufficiently to allow access to the medial aspect of the elbow, i.e. can the patient place the hand behind their head?

2 Attach an arm table to the side of the operating table. If the shoulder is stiff, place the patient in a lateral position or, alternatively, prone with the arm behind the back in a 'half-Nelson' position.

3 Use a medial approach (Fig. 31.8), regardless of the position of the patient.

4 Flex the elbow to a right angle. Begin the skin incision 3 cm proximal to the medial epicondyle and carry it just anterior to the epicondyle for a further 3 cm.

5 Identify the ulnar nerve in the groove on the posterior aspect of the medial epicondyle. It is usually easier to find the nerve at the proximal end of the incision. Incise the investing fascia in the line of the nerve, preserving its blood supply.

6 Do not be too assiduous in mobilizing the nerve, as excessive dissection can result in late scarring and predispose to recurrent compression.

7 Follow the nerve proximally up to the medial intermuscular septum, where there may be a tight band, which if present should be released.

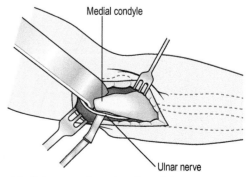

Medial condyle

Ulnar nerve

Fig. 31.8 Medial approach to the elbow joint.

8   It is important to decompress the nerve distally as it passes between the two heads of the flexor carpi ulnaris. Several short small articular branches may be divided, but preserve the branch to the flexor carpi ulnaris. This is usually sufficient in the majority of cases of ulnar neuritis, so that transposition is not necessary.

9   If the nerve is unstable (dislocatable) or if additional length is required, then transpose it anteriorly and proceed as follows (submuscular transposition).

10 Divide the common flexor origin anterior to the ulnar nerve, leaving a cuff of tissue attached to the bone for later re-attachment.

11 Place the nerve deep to the common flexor muscle mass and ensure there are no kinks in its course.

Closure

1   Re-attach the common flexor muscles with three or four absorbable mattress sutures.

2   Release the tourniquet and close the wound.

Aftercare

1   Immobilize the elbow in a collar-and-cuff sling until the patient is comfortable.

2   Remove the stitches and mobilize the elbow at 10–12 days.

APPROACHES TO THE FOREARM

Preferably approach the shafts of the radius and ulna through separate incisions – the ulna from behind and the radius from the front.

POSTERIOR APPROACH TO THE ULNA
(FIG. 31.9)

Prepare

1   The patient, under general anaesthesia, lies supine. Have a large arm table attached to the operating table.

2   Apply a pneumatic tourniquet around the upper arm.

3   Prepare the skin from above the elbow to the fingertips.

4   Cover the arm board with a waterproof sheet and towel.

5   Drape off the arm just proximal to the elbow with a triangular towel.

6   Cover the head and trunk with a large sheet.

7   Cover the fingers and hand with stockinette that can be extended up to the tourniquet if necessary.

8   Pass the arm through a large sheet with a hole in the centre.

Action

1   Much of the ulna, like the tibia, is immediately subcutaneous, so exposure is generally simple, straightforward and safe. Incise the skin along the subcutaneous border of the ulnar over that part of the forearm to be exposed.

2   Divide the common aponeurosis, which attaches to the bone the flexor carpi ulnaris and flexor digitorum profundus medially, and the extensor carpi ulnaris laterally.

3   Separate the muscles from the bone with a periosteal elevator to expose the shaft of the ulna.

THE ANTERIOR (HENRY) APPROACH TO THE SHAFT OF THE RADIUS (FIG. 31.10)

Prepare

1   Prepare the arm as above.

2   Supinate the forearm.

Access

1   Incise the skin, beginning at the radial styloid in the interval between the brachioradialis and the flexor carpi radialis muscles, and extend this proximally in a straight line as far as the lateral side of the biceps tendon, to expose the whole radial shaft. More limited exposure to any part of the radius is gained by using an appropriate part of this incision.

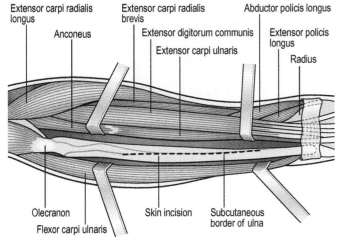

Fig. 31.9   **Exposure of the shaft of the ulna.**

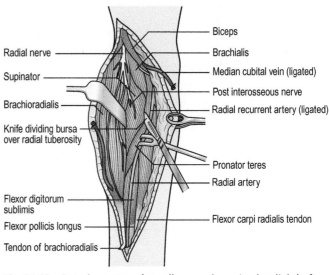

Fig. 31.10   **Anterior approach to elbow and proximal radial shaft.**

2 Starting at the distal end of the incision, identify and protect the sensory branch of the radial nerve as it lies beneath the brachioradialis.

3 Mobilize the flexor carpi radialis and the radial artery and vein. Retract them medially to expose the flexor digitorum superficialis, flexor pollicis longus and pronator quadratus in the floor of the wound.

4 Pronate the forearm and elevate the flexor pollicis longus and pronator quadratus subperiosteally from the outer edge of the radius. Strip them medially to expose the distal two-thirds of the anterior aspect of the radius.

5 To expose the proximal third of the radius, supinate the forearm and extend the incision proximally. Divide and tie the large superficial vein crossing the middle part of the wound.

6 Expose the biceps tendon and divide the deep fascia on its lateral side with blunt-nosed scissors.

7 Retract the belly of the brachioradialis and the long and short radial extensors of the wrist laterally, and the flexors medially, to expose the radial artery. Divide and carefully ligate the fan-shaped leash of vessels passing laterally from the artery (Fig. 31.11).

8 Flex the elbow to 90° to expose the belly of the supinator.

9 Cut down to the tuberosity of the radius immediately lateral to the attachment of the biceps tendon.

> ▶ **KEY POINTS** Protect the nerve

- From this point sweep the supinator laterally off the bone with a periosteal elevator.
- Supination of the forearm protects the posterior interosseous nerve, which lies within its substance.

10 Pronate the forearm to expose the lateral aspect of the radius.

Closure

1 Replace the muscles that have been stripped from the bone and tack them into place with absorbable sutures as appropriate.

2 Release the tourniquet and stop the bleeding.

3 Insert a suction drain if necessary.

4 Close the skin.

APPROACHES TO THE WRIST

ANTERIOR (VOLAR-RADIAL) APPROACH
(FIG. 31.12)

Prepare

1 Position the anaesthetized patient with the affected limb on a large arm table.

2 Use a pneumatic tourniquet on the upper arm.

3 Clean the forearm and fingers and drape the limb as described for the upper arm, but leave the fingers and hand exposed.

Access

1 Incise the skin in line with the tendon of the flexor carpi radialis as far as the midpoint of the transverse palmar crease. If necessary, cross the wrist crease either transversely in the skin crease for 1 cm or with a small zigzag incision.

2 Retract the skin edges with skin hooks, exposing the sheath of the flexor carpi radialis (FCR) and the median nerve.

3 Incise the FCR tendon sheath and retract the tendon along with the radial artery to the radial side and the flexor pollicis longus and median nerve to the ulnar side. Insert a small self-retaining retractor into the interval, so exposing the pronator quadratus.

4 The pronator quadratus lies in the floor of the wound. Identify the distal border (the white line), which is just proximal to the volar lip of the radius and then carefully elevate this from its radial border to expose the lower end of the radius and the radiocarpal joint.

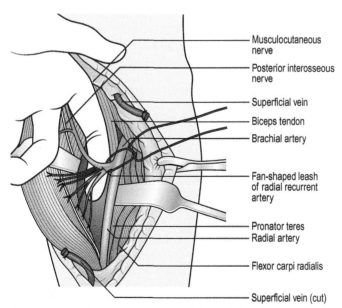

Fig. 31.11 Division of the branches of the radial artery.

Labels:
- Musculocutaneous nerve
- Posterior interosseous nerve
- Superficial vein
- Biceps tendon
- Brachial artery
- Fan-shaped leash of radial recurrent artery
- Pronator teres
- Radial artery
- Flexor carpi radialis
- Superficial vein (cut)

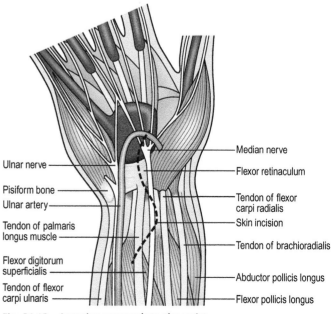

Fig. 31.12 Anterior approach to the wrist.

Labels:
- Ulnar nerve
- Pisiform bone
- Ulnar artery
- Tendon of palmaris longus muscle
- Flexor digitorum superficialis
- Tendon of flexor carpi ulnaris
- Median nerve
- Flexor retinaculum
- Tendon of flexor carpi radialis
- Skin incision
- Tendon of brachioradialis
- Abductor pollicis longus
- Flexor pollicis longus

5 This provides a good exposure of the distal radius for open reduction and internal fixation of a fracture and application of a volar plate.

Closure

1 Remove the tourniquet and stop bleeding.
2 Repair the pronator quadrates if possible.
3 Allow the FCR and FPL to resume their normal position.
4 Close the skin.

POSTERIOR (DORSAL) APPROACH

Prepare

As for anterior approach to the wrist.

Access

1 Pronate the forearm.
2 Make a straight incision 10 cm long on the dorsum of the wrist centred on Lister's tubercle (the bony prominence on the dorsum of the distal radius).
3 Retract the skin edges with skin hooks and expose the extensor retinaculum. Divide this along the line of the sheath of the extensor carpi ulnaris tendon (ECU) and turn it towards the radial side of the wound to sequentially expose the extensor tendons in their respective compartments (Fig. 31.13).
4 Continue elevating the extensor retinaculum as far as Lister's tubercle. This provides access to the distal and radio-ulnar joint, radiocarpal joint and carpal bones.

Closure

1 Pass the extensor retinaculum deep to the extensor tendons and suture it back to the ECU sheath.
2 Release the tourniquet and stop the bleeding.
3 Close the skin.

LATERAL APPROACH (FIG. 31.14)

This is a particularly useful approach to the distal radius, especially for internal fixation of a fracture or for decompression of the first extensor compartment (De Quervain's tenosynovitis).

Prepare

As for anterior approach to the wrist.

Access

1 Make a longitudinal oblique incision 5 cm long centred on the tip of the radial styloid.
2 Extend the incision in a palmar direction towards the tendons of the extensor pollicis brevis and abductor pollicis longus and then proximally, parallel to the radius. Curve the distal limb towards the extensor pollicis longus and then parallel to it.

> ▶ KEY POINTS Anatomy: dorsal radial nerve branches
>
> ■ Identify the dorsal branches of the superficial radial nerve immediately deep to the skin.
> ■ Protect them throughout to avoid causing a painful neuroma ('the meanest nerve in the body').

3 Retract extensor pollicis brevis and abductor pollicis longus, the radial artery and the dorsal branch of the radial nerve towards the palm. The tubercle of the scaphoid and the lateral capsule of the wrist joint are exposed distally and the lower end of the lateral aspect of the radius proximally.

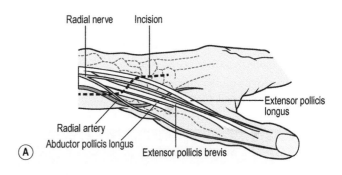

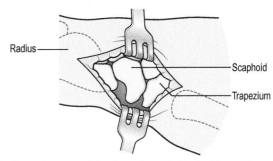

Fig. 31.14 Lateral approach to the wrist: (A) skin incision; (B) approach completed.

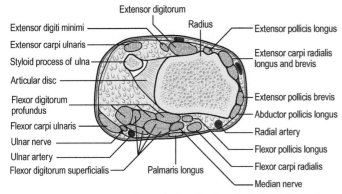

Fig. 31.13 Cross-section through the distal end of the right radius and the styloid process of the right ulna.

Closure

1 Close the capsule with interrupted absorbable sutures.

2 Release the tourniquet and stop the bleeding.

3 Close the skin.

DECOMPRESSION OF THE EXTENSOR POLLICIS BREVIS AND ABDUCTOR POLLICIS LONGUS TENDONS

Appraise

Described by the Swiss surgeon (1868–1940), tenosynovitis of the extensor pollicis brevis and abductor pollicis longus tendons (De Quervain's syndrome) usually resolves following local steroid injections or immobilization of the wrist and thumb. When conservative treatment fails, operation may be required.

Action

1 Use the lateral (radial) incision, taking great care to avoid damage to the superficial branches of the radial nerve.

2 Divide the extensor retinaculum covering the tendons on the lateral aspect of the radius – first extensor compartment.

3 Open the tendon sheaths of the abductor pollicis longus and extensor pollicis brevis in the line of the tendon and lift each tendon in turn from its bed with a small, blunt tendon hook. It is not unusual to find an accessory tendon lying in a third compartment; if you miss this it will cause persistent symptoms.

4 Remove as much of the inflamed synovium as possible from the surface of the tendon using a small pair of curved scissors or fine bone nibbler.

Closure

1 Release the tourniquet and stop bleeding.

2 Close the subcutaneous fat and skin.

3 Immobilize the thumb and wrist in a padded plaster until the sutures are removed at 10 days.

GANGLION OF THE DORSUM OF THE WRIST

Appraise

1 A simple ganglion is the result of cystic degeneration of fibrous tissue. They commonly arise from a synovial joint or less frequently from a tendon sheath (pearl seed ganglion).

2 The commonest site is on the dorsal aspect of the wrist in the midline at the level of the radio-carpal joint where they nearly always originate from the scapholunate joint.

3 Recurrence is common unless you carefully remove the neck of the ganglion.

4 Simple needle puncture (19G) under local anaesthetic provides rapid resolution but the ganglion frequently recurs, although often not to the same extent. This technique often buys time

and if repeated (up to three times) may make surgery unnecessary.

5 There is an increasing vogue to resect the ganglion arthroscopically, which results in less scarring and minimizes the risk of stiffness and recurrence.

Prepare

1 As for anterior approach to the wrist. The operation can be performed under local anaesthetic, but this does not permit the use of a tourniquet.

2 My preference, therefore, is to perform the operation under either a regional block or general anaesthetic, which allows a tourniquet to be used and permits a better exposure of the neck of the ganglion, so theoretically reducing the risk of recurrence.

Action

1 Make a transverse incision in a skin crease over the apex of the swelling.

2 Deepen it carefully until you see the bluish-grey surface of the ganglion.

3 Carefully dissect around the ganglion with small curved scissors.

4 Do not grasp the cyst with toothed forceps, to avoid puncturing it.

5 The swelling is often multilocular and passes between the tendons. Carefully identify its attachment to the capsule of the joint.

6 Trace the ganglion down to its origin and remove the small portion of the capsule (or tendon sheath) to which the ganglion is attached, as well as the ganglion itself.

7 Remove the tourniquet and close the skin.

Aftercare

1 Apply a compression dressing for 24 hours and then replace this with a small adhesive dressing.

2 Remove the stitches at 10 days.

MEDIAN NERVE DECOMPRESSION IN THE CARPAL TUNNEL

Appraise

1 Decompress the median nerve if conservative treatment with night splints, steroid injections and diuretics fails to relieve the symptoms of carpal tunnel syndrome, or if abnormal neurological signs are present, especially wasting of the thenar muscles, loss of sensation and dexterity. Look in particular for wasting and weakness of the thenar muscles and dryness of the skin over the radial two-thirds of the hand.

2 I advise preoperative nerve conduction studies prior to surgical decompression.

3 Combine decompression with flexor tendon synovectomy in rheumatoid arthritis when the proliferating synovium is the cause of nerve compression.

Prepare

As for anterior approach to the wrist. This procedure can normally be carried out using local anaesthetic and adrenaline infiltration (1% lidocaine with adrenaline (epinephrine) 1:200 000). 5 ml is usually sufficient and should be injected at the site of the proposed incision and 1–2 cm proximally to the distal palmar crease.

Action

> **KEY POINT** Preserve the palmar cutaneous branch of the median nerve

> ■ Incise the skin in line with the radial border of the ring finger as far as the midpoint of the transverse palmar crease. This avoids potential damage to the palmar cutaneous branch of the median nerve.

1 Deepen the incision down through the longitudinal fibres of the palmar aponeurosis to expose the transverse fibres of the flexor retinaculum.

2 Insert a small self-retaining retractor (West's). This not only facilitates the exposure but acts as an excellent haemostat. It may need to be adjusted 3-4 times as you deepen the incision.

3 Incise the flexor retinaculum longitudinally with a scalpel to expose the median nerve. Pass a McDonald dissector deep to the retinaculum to protect the nerve while the remaining transverse fibres are divided.

4 Ensure that the proximal part of the retinaculum has been adequately released where it disappears under the skin at the proximal end of the wound, by passing a dissector along the surface of the median nerve. This is a common site of inadequate decompression, which can result in persistent symptoms.

5 Take care not to damage the transverse palmar arch at the distal end of the incision.

6 If there is an associated hypertrophic synovitis affecting the flexor tendons, as in rheumatoid disease, perform a flexor synovectomy by stripping the synovium with a fine pair of bone nibblers.

Closure

1 Release the tourniquet; the nerve will 'blush' at the site of compression.

2 Stop any bleeding using bipolar diathermy.

3 Close the skin with interrupted 4/0 non-absorbable sutures.

Aftercare

1 Apply a firm compression dressing and then replace it with an adhesive dressing after 24 hours.

2 Instruct the patient to exercise the fingers immediately after the operation.

3 Remove the stitches at 10 days.

APPROACHES TO THE HAND AND FINGERS

The unique sensibility and mobility of the hand and fingers call for special care whenever surgical treatment is contemplated.

PALMAR APPROACH (FIG. 31.15)

Appraise

> **KEY POINTS** Palmar skin creases

> ■ Incisions may be made anywhere in the palm of the hand provided that they do not cross the skin creases at right-angles.
> ■ Cross skin creases obliquely (Brunner incisions) or, as far as possible, parallel to, but not within, the creases (Fig. 31.15).
> ■ Take the creases into account with any pre-existing lacerations or injuries.

Prepare

1 Use a general anaesthetic or regional block.

2 Attach the arm table to the operating table.

3 Apply a pneumatic tourniquet to the upper arm.

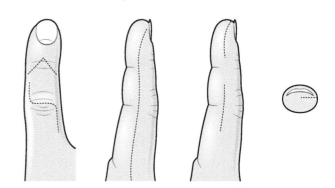

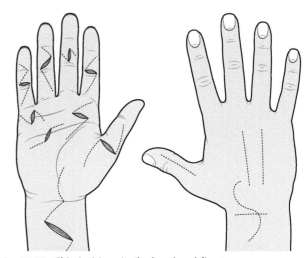

Fig. 31.15 Skin incisions in the hand and fingers.

4 Have an unscrubbed assistant grasp the forearm immediately below the elbow while you clean the skin from the assistant's forearm to the patient's fingertips.

5 Place the towels as if the operation were to be on the wrist.

6 Place the hand on the hand table in a supinated position and secure the fingers and thumb with a 'lead hand'.

Action

1 As a rule, avoid making longitudinal incisions which may result in a late scar contracture. Mark the line of the proposed incision with a skin marker. Then incise the skin and subcutaneous tissue obliquely, crossing the skin creases at their apices (Brunner incision). Extend the incision proximally and distally over the structure to be exposed.

2 Carefully dissect the skin and subcutaneous tissue from the underlying fascia. Retract the edges with skin hooks or 2/0 nylon stay sutures attached to clips.

3 Expose the deeper structures with incisions made according to anatomical considerations and not necessarily following the skin incisions.

? DIFFICULTY

If there is a pre-existing contracted scar, or if additional length is required, consider using a Z-plasty of the skin (Fig. 31.16) or full thickness (Wolff) skin graft.

Closure

1 Release the tourniquet and control bleeding.

2 Close the skin.

3 Apply a non-adherent dressing such as tulle gras or Jelonet, and padded dressing, leaving the fingers mobile.

Aftercare

1 Reduce the dressing as soon as is practical and commence early mobilization.

2 Remove the sutures at 7–10 days.

DORSAL APPROACH TO THE HAND

Appraise

1 The direction and placement of incisions on the dorsum of the hand are not so critical as those on the palm. They may be longitudinal, sinuous or transverse, whichever is most appropriate (see Fig. 31.15).

2 Take care, though, to preserve the veins, which are predominantly dorsal. If you damage them you risk causing excessive swelling of the fingers.

Prepare

As for the palmar approach.

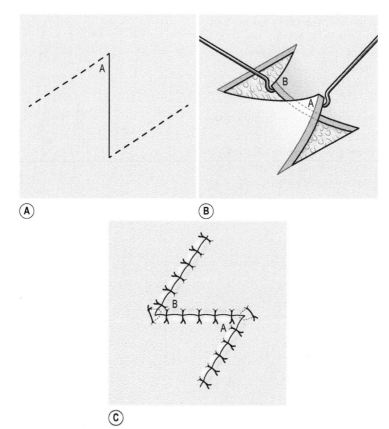

Ⓐ   Ⓑ

Ⓒ

Fig. 31.16 Simple Z-plasty to release a long narrow contracture: (A) the central limb of the Z is made along the line of the contracture, and the other two limbs (broken lines) are made as shown; (B) the flaps are shifted; (C) the flaps are sutured in their new positions.

Access

1. Incise the skin over the structure to be exposed.
2. Retract the skin edges.
3. Avoid damaging the superficial nerves and veins.
4. Employ simple periosteal dissection to expose the underlying bone.

Closure

1. Release the tourniquet.
2. Close the skin.

Aftercare

1. Apply a non-adherent and padded dressing. Elevate the arm in the roller towel if the patient is in hospital, or in a sling for 24 hours.
2. Instruct the patient to move the fingers as soon as possible after the operation, even though this may be painful.

MID-LATERAL INCISIONS ON THE DIGITS

Appraise

You may create a mid-lateral incision (Fig. 31.17) on either the radial or ulnar side of the digit, giving access not only to the corresponding side but also to the palmar and dorsal aspects of the fingers or thumb. In general, incisions on the radial side are more convenient.

Prepare

1. As for approaches on the hand and wrist.
2. Place the hand on the arm table with the forearm in mid-rotation and the thumb uppermost.

Access

1. Flex the interphalangeal joints to 45°.
2. Incise the skin longitudinally on the radial side of the digit from the apex of the proximal interphalangeal joint skin crease to the apex of the distal interphalangeal skin crease.
3. Extend the incisions proximally or distally in the same lateral line as required.

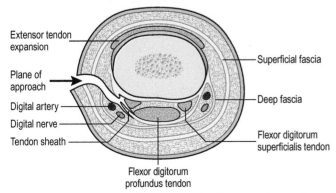

Extensor tendon expansion
Plane of approach
Digital artery
Digital nerve
Tendon sheath
Superficial fascia
Deep fascia
Flexor digitorum superficialis tendon
Flexor digitorum profundus tendon

Fig. 31.17 Lateral approach to expose the flexor tendons and phalanges.

4. Carefully deepen the incision towards the shaft of the phalanx between the dorsal and palmar neurovascular bundles, which are in the respective flaps.
5. Deepen the wound towards the anterior or posterior aspect of the phalanges as required.

Closure

1. Release the tourniquet.
2. Suture the skin only.

Aftercare

1. Apply a pressure dressing.
2. Mobilize the fingers as soon as the underlying condition will allow.

RELEASE OF TRIGGER FINGER OR THUMB (Fig. 31.18)

Appraise

The thickening in the tendon and the flexor sheath usually lies deep to the distal palmar crease or over the metacarpophalangeal (MCP) joint of the thumb and is easily palpable. This represents the opening of the flexor tendon sheath (the A1 pulley).

Prepare

1. As for any hand procedure.
2. A tourniquet is desirable for this operation.
3. It may be possible to perform this procedure using a local anaesthetic infiltration, provided that you are reasonably quick and

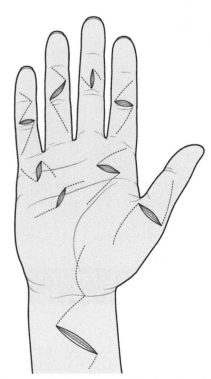

Fig. 31.18 Exposures for the suture of divided flexor tendons. Lacerations (solid lines) may be extended along the dotted lines to provide additional exposure.

that the patient can tolerate the discomfort of the tourniquet for the 5–7 minutes of the operation.

4 If you are performing the operation under pure local anaesthesia, delay inflating the tourniquet until the skin is prepared and drapes are in place.

> ▶ KEY POINT Diabetic?

■ A significant proportion of patients with trigger fingers have diabetes mellitus, which may complicate the perioperative management.

Action

1 Make a transverse or short oblique incision in the skin over the thickened tendon sheath 1.5 cm long. This is usually just distal to the distal palmar crease.

> ▶ KEY POINTS Trigger thumb? Preserve the radial digital nerve

■ Take particular care when releasing a trigger thumb as the radial digital nerve has a tendency to lie immediately subcutaneously over the tendon sheath in the midline or 12 o'clock position.
■ This is not the case with trigger fingers.

2 Deepen the incision down through the palmar fascia using blunt dissection to avoid damaging the digital nerves and vessels.

3 You immediately encounter the flexor tendon sheath. Incise the thickened portion of the A1 pulley longitudinally.

4 Deliver both flexor tendons into the wound with a tendon hook and ensure that they both move freely. If there is any residual tightness it may be necessary to excise a small portion of the sheath.

Closure

1 Release the tourniquet and secure haemostasis.

2 Suture the skin.

Aftercare

1 Apply a non-adherent dressing and elevate the hand for 24 hours.

2 Reduce the dressing after 24 hours and commence active mobilization of the fingers.

3 Remove the sutures after 10 days.

PERCUTANEOUS FASCIOTOMY FOR DUPUYTREN'S CONTRACTURE

Appraise

Whilst the more extensive procedures for Dupuytren's contracture (fasciectomy, dermo-fasciectomy) are beyond the remit of this chapter, there may be a role for the 'general' surgeon to undertake a simple percutaneous fasciotomy under certain circumstances. A significant proportion of patients with Dupuytren's disease present with a

mature pre-tendinous cord in the palm resulting in a flexion contracture of the MCP joint. These patients may be suitable for percutaneous fasciotomy. This technique will usually result in a full correction of any MCP joint contracture; proximal interphalangeal (PIP) joint contracture requires formal surgery.

Prepare

1 As for any hand procedure.

2 Local anaesthetic infiltration is sufficient (1–2 ml 2% plain lidocaine).

3 A tourniquet is not required for this operation.

Action

1 Make a single stab incision in the palm over the mature cord using a 21 or 23 G needle. At this level there is virtually no danger of damaging the digital nerves and vessels which lie deep to the transverse fibres of the palmar aponeurosis.

2 Use the needle effectively as a mini scalpel, sweeping gently back and forth through the thickened cord whilst gently maintaining some slight extension on the finger. You should be able to feel a grating sensation as you gradually cut through the cord until it suddenly gives way, often with a satisfying 'pop', which may surprise the patient.

Closure

1 No suture is necessary.

Aftercare

1 Apply a non-adherent dressing and elevate the hand for 24 hours.

2 Reduce the dressing after 24 hours and commence active mobilization of the fingers.

3 Instruct the patient on simple stretching exercises; occasionally a resting splint may be required for the first 3–4 weeks.

PYOGENIC INFECTIONS OF THE HAND
(Fig. 31.19)

Appraise

1 Pyogenic infections of the hand are common and often present with cellulitis alone. Most resolve with antibiotics, elevation and rest.

2 Incise and drain as soon as an abscess develops or you detect the presence of pus, either visually or because of increasing pain and tenderness.

3 Open subcuticular, intracutaneous and subcutaneous infections where they are most superficial.

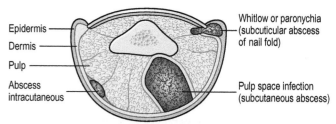

Fig. 31.19 Superficial and deep infections of the digits.

4 Take a swab for bacteriological analysis.

5 Local anaesthetic is not always necessary and many abscesses can be incised using a freezing spray of ethyl chloride, or no anaesthetic at all.

6 Web and palmar space infections are rare. Very little swelling is obvious in the palm, but the back of the hand is oedematous and pain is severe.

7 Tendon sheath infections cause swelling and tenderness along the line of the sheath, and the finger cannot be extended passively because of excruciating pain.

Action

Superficial infections

1 Accurately localize the tenderest point with the tip of an orange stick before inducing anaesthesia.

2 Prepare the hand for a palmar approach but do not exsanguinate the limb.

3 When the infection is superficial, make a cruciate incision over the tenderest point and cut away the corners of the skin to saucerize the lesion. Take a swab for bacteriological analysis.

4 If pus extends under the nail, remove only that portion of the nail that has been raised from the nail bed.

5 Incise in the line of the skin crease over the tenderest part when a web or palmar space is infected. Do not incise the web itself.

6 Carefully explore between the deeper structures (Fig. 31.20) by blunt dissection and follow the track to the abscess cavity.

7 Insert a small latex drain.

8 Cut back the skin edges to ensure adequate drainage but do not insert a drain.

9 Leave the incision open to ensure drainage.

Tendon sheath infections

1 Drain tendon sheath infections through transverse incisions at either end of the sheath (Fig. 31.21).

2 Irrigate the sheath with antibiotic solution through a fine ureteric catheter until the effluent is clear.

3 Leave the catheter in place for subsequent irrigation if necessary. Local anaesthetic can also be instilled for postoperative pain relief.

Palmar space infections

1 When the infection is superficial, make a cruciate incision over the tenderest point and cut away the corners of the skin to saucerize the lesion. Take a swab for bacteriological analysis.

▶ KEY POINTS Dorsal approach?

■ Deep palmar space infections can be drained through a dorsal approach between the first and second metacarpals.
■ Make a small stab incision and simply bluntly dissect with a clip or curved scissors to open the deep palmar space.

---

2 Leave a soft latex drain in situ until the drainage ceases.

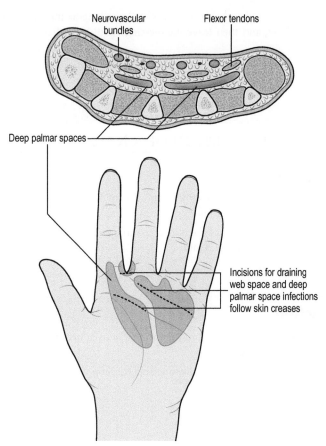

Fig. 31.20 Incisions for the drainage of web and deep palmar space infections.

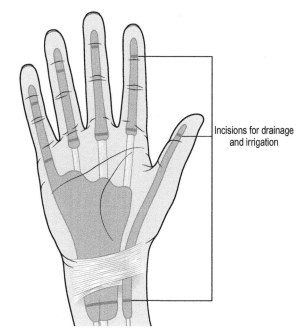

Fig. 31.21 Drainage of tendon sheath infections.

Aftercare

1 Place the corner of a gauze dressing in the wound to keep it open.

2 Apply Tubigrip to the fingers or a fluffed-up pressure dressing to the palm as appropriate and immobilize the hand with a plaster-of-Paris back slab with the fingers in semiflexion.

3 Elevate the hand and re-dress it daily so long as the wound is draining and then leave the dressings until epithelialization is complete.

OPERATIONS ON THE NAILS

PARTIAL AVULSION OF A NAIL

Appraise

1 It may be necessary to remove a portion of the nail in the presence of infection or trauma.

2 Preserve as much of the nail as possible to splint any associated soft tissue or bony injury.

Action

1 Remove only that part of the nail that is separated from the nail bed, using fine scissors.

2 Apply a non-adherent dressing and Tubigrip.

EVACUATION OF A SUBUNGUAL HAEMATOMA

Appraise

1 The diagnosis is usually obvious, generally the result of a crushing injury to the fingertip.

2 It is frequently associated with a fracture of the distal phalanx, which in theory renders this an open fracture, so you should prescribe antibiotics.

3 Check that the nail is not dislocated from the nail bed; if it is, it should be reduced.

Prepare

No specific preparation is necessary.

Action

1 Although there are more sophisticated devices available, it is a simple matter to trephine the nail.

2 Use a red-hot needle or paper clip and the blood spurts out under pressure.

3 Cover the hole with a sterile dressing.

Orthopaedics and trauma: lower limb

N. Goddard, N. Maruthainar

CONTENTS

APPROACHES TO THE HIP AND PROXIMAL FEMUR

1 The hip joint is deeply placed and relatively inaccessible.

2 It may be exposed by several routes that are variations of the anterior, posterior and lateral approaches, which themselves afford good access for most purposes.

3 The anterolateral approach is an extensile approach and provides adequate access for drainage of a potentially septic hip, as well as more complex procedures such as total hip arthroplasty.

4 The lateral approach is usually used for open reduction and internal fixation of femoral fractures.

ANTEROLATERAL APPROACH

Prepare

1 Order 2 units of cross-matched blood.

2 A general anaesthetic is preferable, especially in a child. However, if the general condition of the patient precludes it, use an epidural or spinal anaesthetic.

3 Place the patient supine on the operating table with a sandbag under the buttock of the side to be operated on.

4 Have an unscrubbed assistant elevate the leg.

5 Clean the skin distally from the umbilicus to the knee, including the anterior abdominal wall, perineum and as much of the buttock as possible.

6 Place a waterproof sheet under the affected leg and over the opposite leg, tucking it under the buttock.

7 Place a large drape over the waterproof sheet so that the whole of the unaffected leg and foot and the lower part of the operating table are covered. Pull the top edge firmly into the groin to exclude the genitalia from the field.

8 If possible, use a split sheet to shut off the groin. If this is not possible, fold a medium-sized towel corner-to-corner and place the centre of the long side firmly in the groin. Take one corner under the leg and the other over the iliac crest, and clip the corners together onto the skin at the posterior end of the iliac crest.

9 With the scrubbed assistant, hold a medium towel outstretched by the corners under the leg from the lower third of the thigh to beyond the foot. Direct that the leg be lowered carefully into it and turn the bottom end over the foot before carefully wrapping the lower thigh, leg and foot in the towel. Bandage the towel firmly on to the leg with an open-weave bandage or stockinette.

10 Cover the patient's head and trunk with a large drape.

11 Place the leg through the hole in a large split sheet. Pull the sheet firmly into the groin and around the buttock but leaving the anterolateral aspect of the thigh exposed from the iliac crest distally.

12 Cover the exposed skin with a large adhesive drape wrapped around the thigh.

Access (Fig. 32.1)

1 Make a straight incision extending from the anterior superior iliac spine directed towards the tip of the greater trochanter. This follows the junction between the gluteus medius and the tensor fascia lata.

2 Incise the fascia overlying the interval between the two muscles and develop the plane proximally towards the anterior superior iliac spine. Insert a self-retaining retractor, such as the Norfolk and Norwich type, between the two.

> ▶ KEY POINT Anatomy
>
> ■ Identify the interval between the gluteus medius posteriorly and tensor fascia lata muscle anteriorly. It is often easier to separate the two muscles immediately proximal to the anterosuperior corner of the greater trochanter.

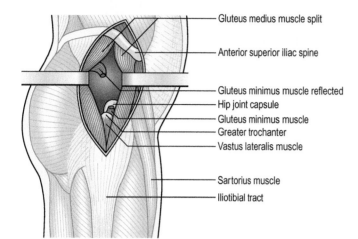

Fig. 32.1 Diagrammatic view of anterolateral approach to the right hip, viewed from the patient's right side. After identifying the opening up of the interval between the tensor fascia lata and gluteus medius muscles, retract them. You may not see the gluteus minimus muscle beneath the gluteus medius, but if you do, you may retract it posteriorly. Below is the joint capsule and greater trochanter.

Labels in Fig. 32.1:
- Gluteus medius muscle split
- Anterior superior iliac spine
- Gluteus minimus muscle reflected
- Hip joint capsule
- Gluteus minimus muscle
- Greater trochanter
- Vastus lateralis muscle
- Sartorius muscle
- Iliotibial tract

3 It should now be possible to see the tendon of the gluteus minimus and the capsule of the hip joint.

4 Retract the gluteus minimus posteriorly and incise the capsule of the hip joint, draining any accumulated intra-articular fluid. Send a sample for bacteriological analysis.

Closure

1 Remove the self-retaining retractor, allowing the gluteus medius and tensor fascia lata muscles to fall back into place, requiring only a few interrupted absorbable sutures to appose the edges.

2 Insert a suction drain.

3 Suture the subcutaneous fat and skin.

LATERAL APPROACH TO THE PROXIMAL FEMUR

1 This exposure may be carried proximally to expose the hip joint if required.

2 Use the distal part of the approach alone for access to the proximal part of the femur and the femoral neck, when treating fractures in this region.

Prepare

1 Cross-match 2 units of blood.

2 Operate with a general anaesthetic if possible, or with epidural or spinal anaesthesia.

3 If you are operating for fixation of a femoral neck fracture, place the patient supine on the orthopaedic operating table with a radiolucent perineal post to allow access for an image intensifier or portable X-ray machine. Operative fixation of femoral neck fractures is, however, beyond the scope of this chapter.

4 Straightforward exposure of the femur is usually carried out with the patient in the lateral position. A traction table and X-ray control are not necessary.

5 Clean the skin from the level of the umbilicus to the knee, including the perineum and buttock and the circumference of the thigh.

6 Hang a large drape over the sound side from the groin to beyond the toes.

7 Hang another large drape over the affected leg from the mid-thigh to beyond the toes.

8 Cover the trunk above the iliac crest with a third large sheet.

9 Cover the remaining part of the thigh with two small towels, leaving only a rectangle of skin 30 cm long by 20 cm wide exposed on the lateral side of the thigh. The anterior superior iliac spine is situated at the top corner of this rectangle.

10 Hold the towels in place with a transparent adhesive drape.

Access (Fig. 32.2)

1 Palpate the posterosuperior corner of the greater trochanter and make a straight longitudinal incision from that point for 15 cm distally, through the skin and subcutaneous fat.

2 Split the fascia lata longitudinally, posterior to the insertion of the tensor fascia lata muscle, in the line of the incision. Insert a self-retaining retractor to expose the vastus lateralis.

3 Identify the aponeurotic attachment of the vastus lateralis to the anterolateral surfaces of the femur, just below the greater trochanter.

4 Identify the posterior attachment of the vastus lateralis. Insert two Trethowan bone spikes and lift the body of the vastus lateralis forwards, releasing it from its attachment to the linea aspera (Latin: *asper* = rough), cauterizing vessels as you go.

5 Reflect the muscle subperiosteally from the anterolateral aspect of the femur and strip the muscle from the anterior and lateral aspects of the femur with a periosteal elevator. Insert the tip of your index finger between the vastus lateralis and the anterior surface of the femur and palpate the lesser trochanter on the posteromedial aspect of the bone.

6 Pass a Lane's lever carefully around the femoral shaft with the tip absolutely in contact with the bone, so that it lies between the lesser trochanter and the femoral neck. This exposes the anterior and lateral surface of the upper femoral shaft and the base of the femoral neck.

7 Strip the posterior portion of the muscle from the bone in similar fashion and insert a second Lane's lever around the underside of the femoral shaft.

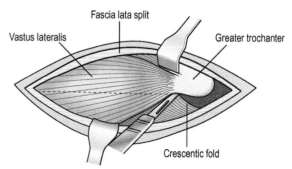

Labels in Fig. 32.2:
- Fascia lata split
- Vastus lateralis
- Greater trochanter
- Crescentic fold

Fig. 32.2 Cutting down on to the femoral shaft.

Closure

1 Insert a suction drain.

2 Allow the vastus lateralis to fall back into its resting position; it is not necessary to insert any sutures at this point.

3 Repair the fascia lata with a continuous absorbable suture.

4 Close the subcutaneous fat and skin.

APPROACHES TO THE UPPER LEG

1 The femoral shaft may be approached from the anterior, medial or lateral aspects.

2 The posterolateral approach is the most convenient and most commonly used.

POSTEROLATERAL APPROACH (Fig. 32.3)

Appraise

1 Use the posterolateral approach to the femoral shaft unless you specifically require access to the medial side of the femur.

2 The approach may be extended proximally and distally if necessary and is most commonly employed to reduce and internally fix fractures of the femoral shaft.

Prepare

1 Have 2 units of cross-matched blood available.

2 Use a general anaesthetic.

3 For operations on the distal two-thirds of the thigh, it may be possible to use a tourniquet but this may compromise the exposure.

4 Place the patient supine on the operating table with a sandbag under the buttock of the affected side.

5 Elevate the leg and clean the skin from the iliac crest and buttock – or the tourniquet, when used, to the upper tibia.

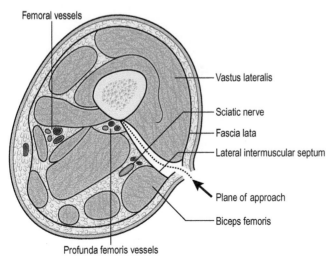

Femoral vessels

Vastus lateralis

Sciatic nerve

Fascia lata

Lateral intermuscular septum

Plane of approach

Biceps femoris

Profunda femoris vessels

Fig. 32.3 **Transverse section of the mid-thigh showing the posterolateral approach to the femoral shaft along the dotted line.**

6 Place a large sheet across the operating table and over the sound leg, and pull the upper edge firmly into the groin to cover the genitalia.

7 Place the long edge of the 'shut-off' towel in the groin, or immediately below the tourniquet, and pull it firmly round the thigh; fasten it with a towel clip on the lateral side.

8 Place a medium-sized drape on the table with its upper edge at the level of the knee joint and carefully lower the leg on to the towel.

9 Fold the distal edge of the towel proximally over the foot and then wrap the towel around the leg.

10 Bandage the towel firmly to the leg with an open-weave bandage or stockinette.

11 Cover the trunk with a large sheet and clip it to the underlying sheet on either side of the thigh.

12 Pass the leg through the hole in a split sheet. Clip the margins of the split to the skin at the upper limit of the operating field.

13 Wrap a large transparent adhesive drape round the thigh to cover the exposed skin.

Access

1 Palpate the tendon of the biceps femoris at the level of the lateral femoral condyle and also the posterior margin of the greater trochanter.

2 Incise the skin along the whole or part of the line joining these two points to gain access to the appropriate part of the thigh.

3 Incise the fascia lata in the line of the incision and locate the lateral intermuscular septum immediately anterior to the biceps femoris.

4 Insert a finger between the septum and the bulk of the vastus lateralis lying anteriorly and continue the dissection down to the bone in this plane with a knife.

5 Ligate the perforating branches of the profunda femoris vessels as you encounter them.

Closure

1 Insert a suction drain.

2 Close the fascia lata with 0 absorbable sutures.

3 Close the skin, dress and bandage the wound.

APPROACHES TO THE KNEE

1 Most operations on the knee joint are carried out from the front, but many do not require a full and formal exposure of the whole joint, and a more limited exposure is adequate.

2 The posterior approach is used to gain access to the popliteal fossa and occasionally to the posterior part of the knee joint.

ANTERIOR APPROACH (Fig. 32.4)

Appraise

1 Use this approach for operations on the extensor mechanism of the knee joint and to gain wide access to the inside of the joint itself.

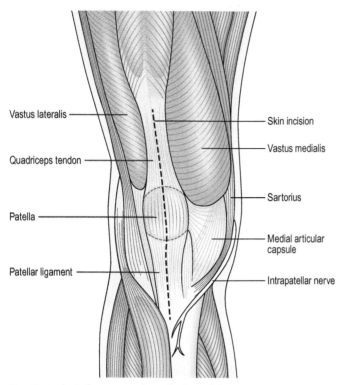

Fig. 32.4   Anterior approach to the knee joint.

2 Use the anterolateral and anteromedial approaches when you re-quire limited access, for example to carry out meniscectomy or removal of loose bodies.

Prepare

1 Use a general anaesthetic.
2 Apply a tourniquet to the mid-thigh.
3 Place the patient supine on the operating table.
4 Drape the leg as if the distal femoral shaft were being exposed, leaving the skin exposed from the tibial tubercle to the tourniquet.
5 Cover the exposed skin with a transparent adhesive drape.

Access

1 Make a straight incision 15 cm long in the midline, extending proximally from the upper margin of the tibial tubercle.
2 Deepen the incision to expose the patellar ligament, the anterior surface of the patella and the quadriceps tendon, and the distal fibres of the rectus femoris (Fig. 32.4).
3 Reflect the skin and subcutaneous fat as a single layer medially, to expose the junction of the quadriceps tendon and the vastus medialis, the medial border of the patella and the patellar ligament.
4 Make an incision along the medial edge of the quadriceps tendon and through the capsule along the medial margin of the patella and medial edge of the patellar ligament into the joint.
5 If required, evert the patella, retract it laterally, and flex the knee at the same time (Fig. 32.5). Extend the incision proximally into the rectus femoris if this proves to be difficult.

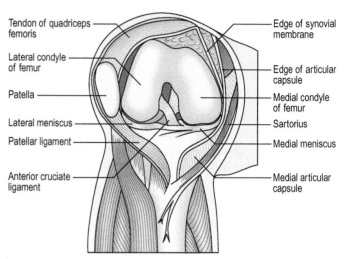

Fig. 32.5   The knee exposed through the anterior approach and flexed.

Closure

1 Extend the knee and return the patella to its normal position.
2 Close the incision in the capsule and the quadriceps tendon with interrupted absorbable synthetic sutures.
3 Close the subcutaneous fat and skin.

POSTERIOR APPROACH (Fig. 32.6)

Appraise

1 Use this approach to gain access to the popliteal fossa.
2 Use it to gain access to the posterior compartment of the knee joint, for example to repair the torn posterior cruciate ligament or to expose the popliteal vessels.
3 Use the medial or lateral part of the full approach for more lim-ited exposure.

Prepare

1 Use a general anaesthetic.
2 Apply a mid-thigh tourniquet.

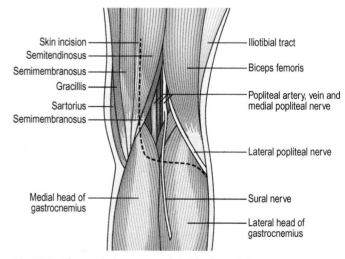

Fig. 32.6   The posterior approach to the knee joint.

3 Place the patient prone on the operating table.

4 Have an assistant flex the knee to 90° and raise the thigh off the table.

5 Place the drapes as described for the anterior approach.

Access

1 Start the skin incision 7 cm proximal to the medial femoral condyle and extend it distally to the transverse skin crease; then curve it laterally and distally again, along the medial side of the head of the fibula.

2 Reflect the skin and subcutaneous tissue to expose the popliteal fascia.

3 Identify the posterior cutaneous nerve of the calf (Latin: sural = calf), lying beneath the fascia between the two heads of the gastrocnemius muscle.

4 Incise the fascia and trace the nerve proximally to its origin from the posterior tibial nerve.

5 Trace the posterior tibial nerve distally and identify its branches to the calf muscles; then trace it proximally to the apex of the popliteal fossa where it joins the common peroneal nerve.

6 Follow the common peroneal (Greek: perone = fibula) nerve distally along the medial border of the biceps tendon.

7 Expose the popliteal artery and vein lying anteriorly and medially to the posterior tibial nerve. Gently retract them to expose the superior lateral and superior medial genicular vessels passing beneath the muscles just proximal to the origin of the two heads of the gastrocnemius.

8 If you require access to the knee, then retract the semitendinosus medially and expose the attachment of the medial head of the gastrocnemius to the joint capsule, incising it longitudinally at this point.

9 Retract the gastrocnemius laterally, using it to protect the nerves and vessels, and enter the posteromedial compartment of the joint.

10 Approach the posterolateral compartment between the tendon of the biceps femoris and the lateral head of the gastrocnemius.

Closure

1 Release the tourniquet.

2 Suture the capsule with interrupted synthetic absorbable sutures.

3 Close the deep fascia and the skin.

SIMPLE KNEE ARTHROTOMY

Appraise

1 If it becomes necessary to open a knee for drainage of a possible infection, carry out open meniscectomy, or remove a loose body.

2 It is not necessary to perform a full approach. All that is required is a limited anterolateral or anteromedial approach.

Prepare

1 Use a general anaesthetic.

2 Apply a tourniquet to the exsanguinated limb.

3 Drape the leg for the anterior approach.

Access

1 It is easier to use an anterolateral incision for ease of access. Incise the skin on the lateral side of the knee from the lateral margin of the patella, downwards and slightly backwards to a point 1 cm below the articular margin of the tibia.

2 Incise the capsule in the line of the incision.

3 Pick up the synovium with forceps and nick it with a knife. In the presence of an effusion it bulges forwards into the wound.

4 Obtain a specimen for bacteriology and irrigate the joint.

Closure

1 Retract the edges of the capsule and pick up each end of the synovium with fine curved artery forceps.

2 Close the synovium with a continuous 2/0 absorbable synthetic suture on a round-bodied needle.

3 Extend the knee and close the capsule with 0 interrupted absorbable synthetic sutures.

4 Close the subcutaneous tissue and skin.

5 Apply a compression bandage from the ankle to the lower thigh. Extend the bandage to the upper thigh after removing the tourniquet.

Aftercare

1 Begin static quadriceps exercises immediately the patient recovers from the anaesthetic and progress to straight leg raising exercises as soon as possible. Allow weight-bearing as tolerated by the patient.

2 Remove the sutures at 7–10 days.

3 Bandage the knee so long as there is any tendency to swell, usually 3–4 weeks, and continue quadriceps exercises until the bulk of the muscle recovers.

ARTHROSCOPY OF THE KNEE

Appraise

1 The arthroscopic technique is now the treatment of choice for the treatment of meniscal tears and for retrieval of loose bodies from the knee.

2 Knee arthroscopy may also be employed in the treatment of chondral lesions and for washout and synovectomy of septic arthritis.

3 Reconstruction of the anterior cruciate ligament and of the posterior cruciate ligament may also be assisted by arthroscopy.

Prepare

1 Check that the necessary equipment and instruments are available and functioning. These include:
   - A 4.5-mm arthroscope with 30 degree angle of view
   - A high luminescence tungsten filament light source (or equivalent) with fibre-optic light delivery cable
   - A camera system

- Sterile isosmotic irrigation fluid
- Arthroscopy instruments including trocar, probe and punches.

2 Operate under general anaesthesia and infiltrate the proposed arthroscopy portals with local anaesthetic and adrenaline (epinephrine) to minimize postoperative pain and bleeding.

3 Examine the knee under anaesthetic. Determine if there is any effusion. Note any fixed flexion deformity and determine the limit of flexion.

4 Apply a thigh tourniquet and exsanguinate the limb.

5 Prepare and drape the skin as if the distal femoral shaft were being exposed, leaving skin exposed from the tibial tuberosity to the tourniquet.

Action

1 Flex the knee to 90 degrees.

2 Make an anterolateral portal for introduction of the arthroscope. Employing an initial landmark, 1.5 cm lateral to the patella tendon and 1.5 cm proximal to the level of the lateral tibial plateau, create a stab incision of approximately 1 cm running horizontally away from the patella tendon.

3 Using a blunt introducer pass the trocar through the portal, aiming towards the intercondylar notch.

4 Remove the introducer and replace with the arthroscope. Visualize the compartments of the knee. Whilst directing the arthroscope to visualize the anteromedial wall, make a further incision to create another portal. Take care not to damage the meniscus.

5 The second portal may be used to pass the probe, punches or other instruments into the cavity of the knee. This portal may also be employed to introduce a further trocar for the drainage of fluid in the case of washout of a septic arthritis.

6 When negotiating instruments about the knee, take care not to damage the chondral surfaces.

7 After addressing any pathology, express excess irrigation fluid from the knee.

Closure

1 Close the portals with 3/0 non-absorbable sutures.

2 Apply a pressure dressing around the knee.

3 Release the tourniquet.

Aftercare

1 Observe for any compartment syndrome, which may arise from extravasation of irrigation fluid into the tissues of the calf.

2 Reduce the dressing after 24–48 hours.

3 Allow mobilization as pain allows (unless the particular intervention undertaken requires further protection of weight-bearing or limitation of knee range of movement).

4 Remove the suture after 10–14 days.

APPROACHES TO THE LOWER LEG

The shafts of the tibia and fibula are subcutaneous and may therefore be exposed by incisions through the overlying skin.

ANTERIOR APPROACH (Fig. 32.7)

Appraise

1 Use the anterior approach for access to the shaft of the tibia and the anterior compartment of the lower leg.

2 Expose the fibula through a separate lateral incision if required.

Prepare

1 Cross-match 2 units of blood.

2 Use a general anaesthetic.

3 Exsanguinate the leg and apply a pneumatic tourniquet to the thigh.

4 Place the patient supine on the operating table.

5 The unscrubbed assistant grasps the calf and elevates the leg.

6 Clean the skin from the ankle proximally.

7 Have a scrubbed assistant apply a stockinette to the foot and continue to support the leg while it is further prepared as far as the tourniquet.

8 Place a large sheet across the operating table and over the sound leg.

9 Place the shut-off towel or split sheet immediately distal to the tourniquet.

10 Continue to drape the leg as described above.

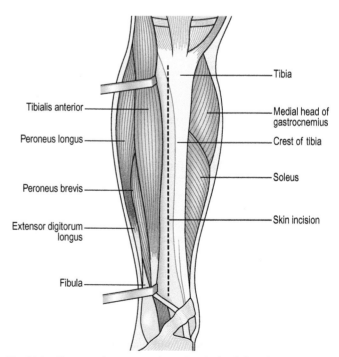

Fig. 32.7 The anterior approach to the shaft of the tibia.

Access

1 Incise the skin longitudinally 1 cm lateral to the crest of the tibia, from the tibial tubercle to the ankle.

2 Reflect skin flaps medially and laterally to expose the subcutaneous surface of the tibia and the tibialis anterior muscle.

Closure

1 Release the tourniquet.

2 Insert a suction drain.

3 Close the skin with 2/0 interrupted sutures.

TIBIAL COMPARTMENT FASCIOTOMY

Appraise

1 Decompression of the fascial compartments of the leg may be indicated in the following circumstances:
- After extensive closed soft-tissue injuries of the lower leg
- After proximal vascular reconstruction following arterial injury
- For chronic exertional compartment syndrome.

▶ KEY POINTS Compartment pressures

- Measure the individual compartment pressures prior to operation.
- Suspect impending ischaemia when the compartment pressure reaches 10–30 mmHg below the diastolic pressure.
- Higher pressures indicate an urgent need for fasciotomy.
- Impending or established compartment syndrome is a surgical emergency.

2 To measure the compartment pressure, you require a slit catheter (14G intravenous cannula), a length of plastic manometer tubing connected to a pressure transducer (a sphygmomanometer suffices if necessary). Prepare and sterilize the skin. Instil 2 ml of 1% lidocaine into the skin and insert the catheter into the anterior compartment. When it is satisfactorily positioned withdraw the trocar. Inject a small quantity of saline into the catheter to fill the dead space. Prefill the manometer tubing with saline and connect this via a three-way tap to the slit catheter and the pressure monitor, ensuring that there are no air bubbles in the system. Now connect the three-way tap to the pressure recorder and measure the compartment pressure.

Prepare

Prepare as for the anterior approach.

Access

1 The anterior and lateral compartments can be decompressed through a full-length longitudinal anterolateral skin incision lateral to the crest of the mid-tibia extending from the level of the tibial tuberosity to just proximal to the ankle.

2 Incise the fascia covering the tibialis anterior muscle and extend the incision in the fascia subcutaneously both proximally and distally, so completely decompressing the anterior muscle group. By slightly undermining the skin it is also possible to decompress the lateral compartment, avoiding damage to the superficial peroneal nerve. In cases of exertional compartment syndrome only, it may be possible to perform a limited decompression through a short skin incision and then extend the fascial incision with a Smillie meniscectomy knife.

3 The superficial and deep posterior compartments can be decompressed in a similar fashion using a single longitudinal posteromedial incision made just medial to the posteromedial border of the tibia.

4 Incise the deep fascia and extend the incision proximally to the level of the tibial tuberosity and distally to a point 5 cm proximal to the medial malleolus, using the same technique.

▶ KEY POINT Emergency decompression

- In an emergency excise the middle half of the fibula; this provides decompression of all compartments.

Closure

1 It is possible to close the skin only following release of chronic exertional compartment syndrome.

2 In acute compartment syndrome leave the wounds open and plan to suture the skin 3–5 days later when the swelling has subsided. If necessary, apply a split skin graft.

3 Be willing to inspect the wound in the interim period.

Aftercare

1 Apply a compression dressing.

2 Elevate the leg.

3 Ability to mobilize the patient depends on the underlying reason for the fasciotomy.

FASCIOTOMY OF THE FOOT

Appraise

1 Decompression of the fascial compartments of the foot may be indicated after trauma to the foot with crush injury, fracture or midfoot dislocation.

2 In the responsive patient, symptoms of compartment syndrome include swelling, pain out of proportion to the antecedent injury and pain on dorsiflexion of the toes.

Prepare

1 Operate under general anaesthesia.

2 Avoid any local anaesthetic regional block.

3 Do not use a tourniquet.

4 Prepare the skin and drape to allow access to the ankle and foot.

Action

1 Incise medially with a longitudinal incision through the skin, starting approximately 2 cm distal to the tip of the medial malleolus and extending to the distal shaft of the 1st metatarsal.

2 Taking care to retract the medial neurovascular structures, employ blunt dissection to decompress the compartments on the plantar aspect of the lesser metatarsals.

3 Consider also two further incisions on the dorsum of the foot. Longitudinal incisions lateral to the 4th metatarsal and medial to the 2nd metatarsal with further blunt dissection should ensure decompression of the interosseous, lateral and central compartments.

Closure

1 Do not close the skin.

2 Loosely apply a pressure dressing.

Aftercare

1 Monitor for clinical response to the decompression.

2 Inspect the wound in the operating theatre, under aseptic conditions after 48 hours. Consider washout and closure of the fasciotomy wounds or split skin grafting, if the tissues are healthy.

APPROACHES TO THE ANKLE

1 Operations on the ankle joint itself can usually be accomplished through an anterior approach.

2 Separate incisions are required to gain access to the malleoli and to the posterior aspect of the joint.

ANTERIOR APPROACH (Fig. 32.8)

Appraise

Use this approach to gain access to the ankle joint itself and for arthrodesis or arthroplasty.

Prepare

1 Use a general anaesthetic.

2 Exsanguinate the leg and apply a pneumatic tourniquet to the thigh.

3 Have an unscrubbed assistant hold the leg just below the knee joint and elevate it.

4 Clean the skin from the assistant's hands to the tip of the toes, paying particular attention to the skin between them.

5 Grasp the foot in a stockinette and then drape the limb as described above.

Access

1 Make an incision in the skin 10 cm long in the midline, centred over the middle of the ankle joint.

2 Incise the superficial fascia, avoiding the superficial peroneal nerve, which crosses the wound diagonally. Retract it laterally.

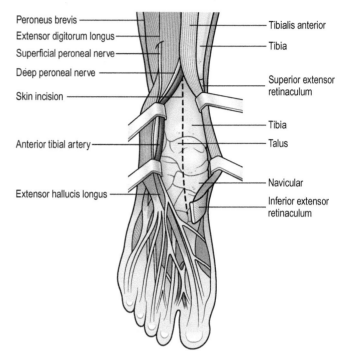

Peroneus brevis — Tibialis anterior
Extensor digitorum longus — Tibia
Superficial peroneal nerve — Superior extensor retinaculum
Deep peroneal nerve —
Skin incision — Tibia
Anterior tibial artery — Talus
Extensor hallucis longus — Navicular
Inferior extensor retinaculum

Fig. 32.8 The anterior approach to the ankle joint.

3 Incise the deep fascia and the extensor retinaculum and identify the anterior tibial artery and the deep peroneal nerve between the tendons of the tibialis anterior and extensor hallucis longus.

4 Retract the neurovascular bundle, extensor hallucis longus and extensor digitorum laterally and the tibialis anterior medially.

5 A pad of fat frequently obscures the anterior capsule of the ankle joint. Excise it.

6 Incise the joint capsule longitudinally and open the ankle joint.

▶ KEY POINT Anatomy

■ Do not confuse the ankle joint with the talonavicular joint, which is unexpectedly close to it.

Closure

1 Release the tourniquet and stop the bleeding.

2 Insert a suction drain.

3 Close the deep fascia.

4 Close the skin.

POSTERIOR APPROACH (Fig. 32.9)

Appraise

Use the posterior approach to gain access to the Achilles tendon and the posterior aspect of the ankle joint and distal end of the tibia.

Prepare

1 Use a general anaesthetic.

2 Exsanguinate the leg and apply a pneumatic tourniquet to the thigh.

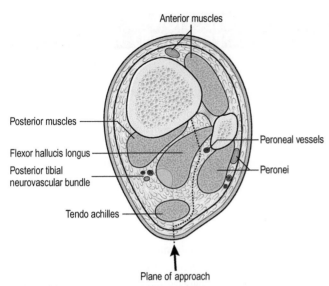

Fig. 32.9 Transverse section of the lower leg just above the ankle joint showing the posterolateral approach to the lower tibia along the dotted line.

3 Place the patient prone on the operating table with the foot hanging over the end.

4 Have an unscrubbed assistant hold the leg just distal to the flexed knee.

5 Clean the leg from the toes to the assistant's hands.

6 Grasp the foot in a stockinette and then drape the limb as described above.

7 Extend the knee and cover the trunk and thighs with a large sheet.

Access

1 Make an incision 15–20 cm long in the midline of the calf, ending at the calcaneum.

2 Expose the lateral side of the Achilles tendon, retracting the sural nerve and short saphenous vein laterally with the skin flap.

3 Deepen the incision through the fascia into a fat-filled space crossed by a branch of the peroneal artery; identify, doubly ligate and divide it.

4 Locate the peroneus brevis laterally and the flexor hallucis longus medially. Separate these muscles proximally, dividing part of the fibular attachment of the flexor hallucis longus if necessary, taking care to preserve the peroneal vessels running down the back of the fibula.

5 Retract the peroneus brevis laterally and the flexor hallucis longus medially to expose the posterior aspect of the ankle joint and the distal tibia.

Closure

1 Release the tourniquet and stop the bleeding.

2 Insert a suction drain.

3 Close the deep fascia.

4 Close the skin.

REPAIR OF RUPTURED ACHILLES TENDON (Fig. 32.10)

Appraise

Ruptures of the Achilles tendon are frequently missed.

▶ KEY POINTS Decisions

■ There is a debate as to whether surgical repair of ruptured Achilles tendon is preferable to plaster immobilization.
■ There is probably very little to choose between the two as far as the end result and re-rupture rate are concerned.
■ Surgical repair may be preferable in young patients with sporting aspirations.
■ If you decide on operation do not delay.
■ If the diagnosis is delayed, wait to allow swelling and bruising to subside.
■ If you have any doubt about the diagnosis, prefer to plaster the leg with the foot in full equinus for 8–10 weeks.

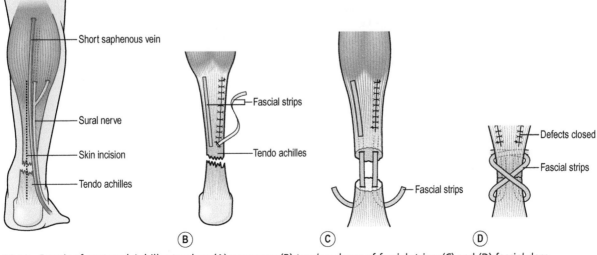

Fig. 32.10 Repair of ruptured Achilles tendon: (A) exposure; (B) turning down of fascial strips; (C) and (D) fascial darn.

Prepare

1 Operate using general anaesthesia.

2 Exsanguinate the leg by elevation only, and apply a pneumatic tourniquet to the thigh.

3 Clean and drape the ankle for the posterior approach.

Action

1 Incise the skin in the midline from the mid-calf to the proximal transverse skin crease. Never use curved or flapped incisions (Fig. 32.10).

2 Carefully elevate the skin for 2 cm on either side of the midline and retract the skin gently with skin hooks.

3 Identify and retract the sural nerve and the short saphenous vein laterally.

4 Open the paratenon and expose the ends of the ruptured tendon, which are usually very ragged, like a shaving brush.

5 Plantar-flex the foot and insert an absorbable size 0 core suture in a modified Kessler pattern, as described in Chapter 30 for tendon suture or use an endogenous fascial strip technique (Fig 32.10). Pull the suture tight to close the gap in the tendon.

6 Insert a 4/0 running suture around the ragged ends of the repaired tendon and then suture the paratenon.

Closure

1 Release the tourniquet and stop the bleeding.

2 Insert a suction drain.

3 Suture the skin with fine interrupted subcuticular sutures and Steri-Strip tapes.

Aftercare

1 Apply a padded compression dressing with the ankle in full plantar flexion.

2 Apply a plaster-of-Paris slab to the front of the ankle from the upper tibia of the toes and bandage it in place. Elevate the leg.

3 Remove the drain and inspect the wound after 24–36 hours.

4 The skin overlying the tendo achilles has a tendency to heal badly and to slough. Avoid pressure over the wound by nursing the patient on the side.

5 Change the plaster at 10–14 days and inspect the wound. By this stage the skin should have healed; apply a below-knee plaster with the foot in full plantar flexion. Allow up, non-weight-bearing.

6 At 2 weeks, replaster the leg with the foot in 50% plantar flexion and again 2 weeks later with the foot in neutral position. Encourage full weight-bearing at this stage. Remove the plaster after a further 2 weeks and encourage ankle mobility.

7 Do not allow full sporting activities for at least 3 months after the repair.

RADICAL RESECTION OF THE NAIL BED (ZADEK'S OPERATION) (Fig. 32.11)

Appraise

1 This operation is suitable for chronic ingrowing toenails.

2 Do not undertake the operation in the presence of sepsis, but merely remove the nail and wait for about 2 months until the sepsis has subsided.

3 Do not perform the operation in the presence of peripheral vascular disease.

Prepare

1 The operation may be performed under local ring-block anaesthesia with a rubber band as a digital tourniquet.

2 Clean and drape the lower leg and foot as described above, placing a shut-off towel around the instep.

Action

1 Remove the nail, if present, by separating it from the underlying nail bed with a McDonald elevator.

2 Make two incisions, 1 cm long, extending proximally from each corner of the nail to the transverse skin crease just distal to the interphalangeal joint.

3 Lift the skin and subcutaneous tissue as a flap and dissect this proximally.

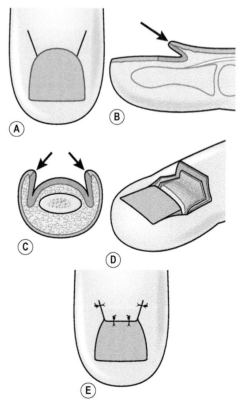

Fig. 32.11 Radical resection of the nail bed: (A) the incisions; (B) proximal flap dissection; (C) lateral flap dissection; (D) excision of the nail bed; (E) suturing the skin flap.

4 Carry the dissection under the edges of the skin incisions on either side of the terminal phalanx to the midlateral line to complete the clearance of the germinal matrix of the nail.

5 Cut across the nail bed transversely at the site of the lunula (Latin: diminutive of *luna* = moon; the opaque whitish half-moon at the root of the nail) and join this transverse incision to the dissections under the nail folds.

6 Remove the block of nail bed from the surface of the proximal phalanx as far back as the insertion of the extensor tendon.

7 Check that you have not left behind any fragments of germinal matrix.

Closure

1 Draw the skin flap distally and carefully insert and tie one or two stitches to attach it to the nail bed. The tissues are fragile and the sutures easily cut out.

2 Close the incisions on either side.

Aftercare

1 Dress the wound with a non-adherent dressing.

2 Apply pressure with Tubigrip bandage.

3 Release the tourniquet.

4 Elevate the foot for 24 hours.

5 Allow weight-bearing with or without crutches as pain permits.

6 Remove the dressings and the stitches after 12–14 days.

FURTHER READING

Antrum RN. Radical excision of the nail fold for ingrowing toenails. J Bone Joint Surg Br 1984;6B:63–5.

Henry AK. Extensile Exposure Applied to Limb Surgery. 2nd ed. Edinburgh: E&S Livingstone; 1957.

Müller ME, Allgower M, Schneider R, et al. Manual of Internal Fixation. Techniques Recommended by the AO Group. 2nd ed. Berlin: Springer-Verlag; 1979.

Nistor L. Surgical and non-surgical treatment of Achilles tendon rupture. J Bone Joint Surg Am 1981;63A:394–9.

Rorabeck CH, Bourne RB, Fowler PJ. The surgical treatment of exertional compartment syndrome in athletes. J Bone Joint Surg Am 1983;65A:1245–51.

Zadik FR. Obliteration of the nail bed of the great toe without shortening the terminal phalanx. J Bone Joint Surg Br 1950;32B:66–7.

33

Plastic surgery

A. Mosahebi, P.E.M. Butler

GENERAL PRINCIPLES

Plastic surgery (Greek: *plassein* = to mould) is concerned with the restoration of form and function of the human body. It is used in the repair and reconstruction of defects following damage or loss of tissue from injury or disease or from the treatment and correction of congenital deformities. It also includes aesthetic or cosmetic surgery, which involves the treatment of developmental or naturally acquired changes in the body.

There have been many advances in plastic surgery in recent years, giving rise to a multitude of new methods of reconstruction. These include improved techniques in microsurgery, tissue expansion, liposuction, craniofacial surgery and a very comprehensive understanding of tissue blood supply. Several hundred cutaneous, myocutaneous and other flaps have now been identified but only those used more commonly will be described in this chapter.

Prepare

▶ KEY POINTS Planning repair

■ Plan for repair and reconstruction of tissue defects well in advance of operation.
■ Carry out the simplest procedure to achieve wound healing.
■ If you need to reconstruct a defect in stages ensure that one stage does not jeopardize a subsequent one.

1 In the region of the proposed operation, identify the lines of tension within the skin described by the Professor of Anatomy in Vienna, Carl Ritter von Langer (1819–1887). Try to make all incisions parallel to these lines. When this is not possible, consider using a Z-plasty or local flap in closing the wound to help prevent the formation of scar contracture postoperatively.

2 When planning a large flap or a sophisticated reconstruction, mark out a plan of the flap on the patient with a skin marker the day before operation. For smaller flaps and simple incisions, mark out the area of incision on the patient after preparing the area, before incising the skin. Use a fine pen and ink for marking out the lines of incisions on the face. Use a broad proprietary marking pen in other areas. Try to follow these lines, as they provide a useful guide once the skin has been incised and tension in the surrounding skin has changed. Be prepared, however, to make adjustments on occasions according to the circumstances.

3 While general anaesthesia is now very safe, do not forget that many operations can be carried out under regional anaesthesia or local anaesthesia (see Chapter 2), especially on the hand, including cases of replantation. Large areas of split skin graft can be taken from the lateral aspect of the thigh by infiltrating the lateral cutaneous nerve of the thigh in the region of the inguinal ligament with local anaesthetic. Many other procedures can be carried out under regional anaesthesia, if necessary with the assistance of a sedative. Many simple skin lesions can be excised under local anaesthesia with 1% lidocaine. To excise small lesions in the head and neck region, where the skin is highly vascular, use 2% lidocaine with 1:80 000 adrenaline (epinephrine). Wait 5 minutes after injecting the mixture, to provide a relatively avascular field as well as anaesthesia. When carrying out extensive excisions of the face or scalp under general anaesthesia, inject a dilute solution of 0.5% lidocaine with 1:200 000 adrenaline (epinephrine).

Technique

Sutures

1 On the face, approximate the deep dermis of the skin edges with interrupted 5/0 polyglactin sutures. Accurately appose the skin edges with 6/0 interrupted nylon sutures. Remove them on the third or fourth postoperative day. If they remain longer, suture marks form, which are unsightly and may prove impossible to remove.

2 Elsewhere on the body, approximate the deep dermis of the wound edges with 3/0 polyglactin sutures and use subcuticular polypropylene sutures whenever possible, tying a knot at either end to prevent slipping. Leave these sutures in for 10 days, or longer if there is a tendency for the scar to stretch because of its site.

Instruments

1 Respect tissues and their viability by handling them with care and using the appropriate instruments. Control and steady the skin with skin hooks or fine-toothed forceps. Do not crush it by grasping it with non-toothed forceps.

2 For accurate suturing, use a fine needle-holder with a clasp that feels comfortable. Practise using needle-holders with their own cutting edges for cutting sutures so you can use them effectively. They are particularly useful when you are inserting many interrupted sutures, the accuracy of which is not crucial to the overall result.

3 Microvascular surgery requires specialized instruments.

Drains

1 When moving large flaps introduce large suction drains at the donor site, which has a large potential cavity.

Diathermy

1 Beware of unipolar diathermy when coagulating vessels near the skin. The burnt tissue may be visible and painful.

2 Always use a bipolar coagulator for fine work and flaps. The current from a unipolar machine could destroy the vessels in the base of a flap as it is being raised.

SKIN COVER

1 Close skin wounds primarily to provide ideal skin cover following incisions of the skin, excisions of skin lesions and simple lacerations.

2 Use split skin grafts to repair wounds with significant skin loss, to avoid skin closure with tension, or following trauma with an appreciable degree of crush injury to the local tissues. Skin graft survival depends on adequate vascularity of the base of the wound.

3 Use skin flaps, which carry their own blood supply and are temporarily self-sufficient, in primary or secondary repair or reconstruction. Use them as primary cover for vital structures such as exposed neurovascular bundles or for structures that have an inadequate blood supply to support a graft, such as bare bone, bare cartilage, bare tendons and exposed joints.

SKIN CLOSURE

Appraise

1 Employ primary skin closure following simple skin incisions, surgical excision of small skin lesions and to repair simple lacerations.

2 Do not carry out primary closure if the tension in closing the wound causes blanching of the skin.

Action

1 Whenever possible, make incisions following the direction of the tension lines, particularly on the face.

2 For excisions, mark the skin in ink, planning to excise the minimal necessary amount of tissue. Draw an ellipse with pointed ends around this mark, parallel to the tension lines (Fig. 33.1A).

3 On the face, inject the surrounding tissue with 2% lidocaine and 1:80 000 adrenaline (epinephrine) and wait 5 minutes for both components to take effect.

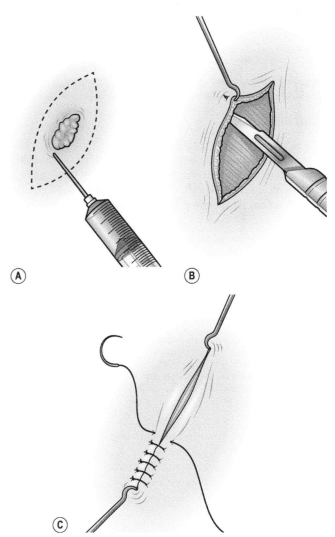

Fig. 33.1 Simple excision of skin lesion: (A) the skin is marked and surrounding skin infiltrated with local anaesthetic; (B) undermining the lateral skin margin; (C) the wound ends are distracted with skin hooks to help approximate the edges of the wound.

4. Make a vertical cut through the skin along the lines of the ellipse. Ensure that you adequately clear the lesion in depth.

5. Undermine the skin edges beneath the layer of subcutaneous fat to facilitate approximating the edges without tension (Fig. 33.1B).

> ▶ KEY POINTS Skin viable?
>
> ■ If the skin edges have been crushed, do not further insult them by inserting sutures, but carefully trim away dead skin and apply a simple dressing. Close the skin after a delay of 24–48 hours.
> ■ Beware of skin that has been degloved or torn from its fascial base. Resect it primarily.
> ■ If damaged skin is possibly viable, replace it, re-examine it at 48 hours, and then resect it if it does not bleed when it is cut.

6. Place a skin hook in each end of the wound and ask your assistant to draw them apart. This manoeuvre approximates the edges (Fig. 33.1C).

7. Close the wound in layers.

8. Apply a small dressing, or use no dressing at all if practical.

SKIN GRAFTS

Appraise

1. A skin graft (Greek: *graphion* = a style; something inserted) is a piece of skin detached from its donor site and transferred to a recipient site. It may contain part of the thickness of the skin (a split skin graft, described by the German surgeon Karl Thiersch in 1874) or the full-thickness graft of skin, described in 1874 by the Austrian ophthalmologist John Wolfe, who settled in Glasgow.

2. A skin graft depends for its survival on receiving adequate nutrition from the recipient bed. Thus, thin split skin grafts survive more readily than thick split skin grafts or full-thickness grafts.

3. If there is a poor vascular bed, or infection, no graft will survive. In these cases prepare the graft bed appropriately with dressings (see below), or consider using a flap.

4. Choose an appropriate donor site for each individual patient.

SMALL SPLIT SKIN GRAFT

Appraise

1. A split skin graft is a sheet of tissue containing epidermis and some dermis taken from a donor site. It is obtained by shaving the skin with an appropriate knife or blade. A layer of deep dermis is preserved at the donor site and, when dressed appropriately, this is re-epithelialized from residual skin adnexae.

2. Use a small split skin graft to repair traumatic loss of small areas of skin from the hand or fingers, and occasionally in other parts of the body. Avoid using them on the tips of the thumb and index fingers since they tend to become hyperaesthetic.

3. Choose the donor site carefully. On the upper limb prefer skin from the medial aspect of the arm where the donor site is inconspicuous; on the forearm an ugly resultant scar may be visible.

Action

1. Mark out on the medial aspect of the arm an area of skin which is more than sufficient to cover the recipient site.

2. Inject 2% lidocaine and 1:80 000 adrenaline (epinephrine) intradermally into and beyond the marked area and wait for 5 minutes.

3. Lubricate the marked area with liquid paraffin.

4. Grip the arm on the lateral aspect with your left hand so that the skin which is marked out becomes tense, with a convex surface.

5. Cut the graft from the marked area using a Da Silva knife (Fig. 33.2).

6. Dress the donor site with a calcium alginate dressing, one layer of paraffin gauze, several layers of dressing gauze and a crepe bandage.

7. Apply the split skin graft directly on to the recipient site, spread it and anchor it using a minimal number of sutures.

8. Apply paraffin gauze, dressing gauze and a crepe bandage.

9. Re-dress the graft at 5 days.

10. Re-dress the graft donor site at 10 days.

LARGE SPLIT SKIN GRAFT

Appraise

1. Use these grafts following extensive skin loss from burns, trauma or radical excisional surgery.

2. Adequately prepare the recipient site to ensure a good 'take' of the graft. Grafts take best on exposed muscle or well-prepared granulation tissue. They do not reliably survive on exposed fat where there is a poor vascular supply.

3. The take of a graft can be improved in certain circumstances by meshing it, quilting it, or by delaying its application and then exposing it. These are described below.

4. Use an electric dermatome, if available, to harvest the graft using the same principles outlined below.

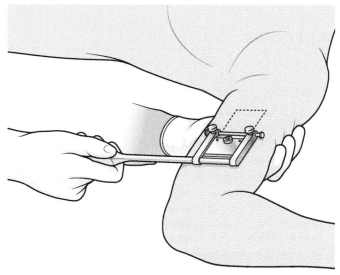

Fig. 33.2 Taking a small split skin graft with a Da Silver knife.

Prepare

1 Following 'cold' surgical excisions apply pressure to obtain haemostasis. Avoid diathermy if possible since skin grafts do not take over diathermy burns.

2 Where subcutaneous fat is exposed, suture the overlying skin down to the muscle or deep fascia to cover it.

3 For infected wounds, take swabs for bacterial culture and prepare the recipient site with dressings of Eusol (Edinburgh University solution of lime) and paraffin. Change them 3–4 times a day. The recipient site is ready to receive a graft when it appears healthy and compact and has red granulation tissue with minimal exudates.

> ### ▶ KEY POINTS Haemolytic streptococci
>
> ■ Do not apply grafts in the presence of Group A beta haemolytic streptococci.
> ■ First eradicate the infection with regular dressing changes and appropriate systemic antibiotics.

4 Choose the donor site most readily available to provide a large area of skin graft; this is usually the thigh. In young people, use the inner aspect of the thigh, where the donor site will be hidden. In elderly people, use the outer aspect of the thigh, where the skin is slightly thicker, so that if healing is delayed the wound is accessible and is easily managed.

Action

1 Prepare both recipient and donor sites by applying skin antiseptic.

2 Have your assistant spread a large swab on the side of the thigh opposite to the proposed donor site. With a hand on the swab it is possible to support the thigh and tense the skin at the donor site by gripping the skin firmly with the swab.

3 Set the blade on the Watson knife to take the appropriate thickness of skin graft. Use a medium setting at first and then adjust it accordingly.

4 Apply liquid paraffin on a swab to the donor site and along the knife blade.

5 Ask your assistant to hold the edge of a graft board at the starting point with the other hand (Fig. 33.3).

6 Cut a skin graft with the Watson knife, holding a board in your non-cutting hand and advancing this a few centimetres in front of the knife. Start with the knife at 45° to the skin and once the blade has entered the dermis rotate it axially so that it runs just parallel with the skin surface. Use a 'sawing' action with the knife, advancing the blade only a few millimetres at a time. When you have harvested an adequate length of skin, turn the blade upwards and cut the graft off with one firm movement. If the graft is not detached with this movement, cut along its base with a pair of scissors.

7 Place the skin graft, outer surface downwards, on a damp saline swab and make sure that you have obtained sufficient skin; in case of doubt, take another strip of split skin.

8 Dress the donor site with calcium alginate dressing, one layer of paraffin gauze, dressing gauze, cotton wool and a crepe bandage.

9 Apply the skin graft to the recipient defect, ensuring that it is placed with its cut surface applied to the wound. The outer

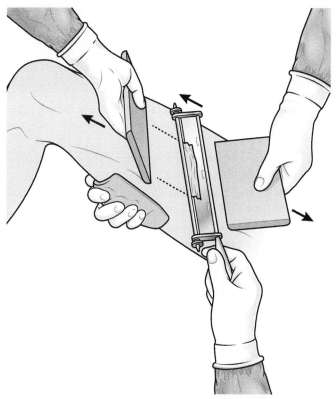

Fig. 33.3 Taking a large split skin graft from the thigh, the surgeon advances board A in front of the knife as it progresses along the thigh. The assistant tenses the skin of the thigh in his right hand, using a large swab to prevent his hand from slipping, and tenses the skin behind the knife using board B.

surface is opaque, the inner surface is shiny. Spread it, using two pairs of closed non-toothed forceps.

10 Cut off the surplus skin at the wound edge, leaving a margin of 3 mm around the periphery.

11 If the skin has been applied on a site to which you can apply a satisfactory compression dressing, do not use sutures.

12 Dress with several layers of paraffin gauze, dressing gauze, wool and crepe bandage, immobilizing the joints above and below the graft with a bulky dressing.

13 In areas where it is difficult to apply a compression dressing, immobilize the graft with interrupted sutures at the edge or insert a circumferential continuous suture around the graft.

14 Dress with paraffin gauze, dressing gauze, wool and strips of adhesive dressing.

15 Keep the graft site elevated postoperatively.

16 For grafts on the lower limb below the knee, do not allow the grafted area to be dependent for 7 days; fluid will collect between the graft and the base unless the graft is meshed. Then arrange progressive mobilization with compression support to the leg and foot, including the graft.

DELAYED EXPOSED GRAFTS

Appraise

1 Use a delayed graft when the graft in its recipient site can be exposed indefinitely by the patient without being disturbed.

2 Apply a delayed graft to surgical wounds when haemostasis is difficult to establish perioperatively. Since the graft is exposed, it can be monitored regularly to ensure that it has taken.

Action

1 Prepare the recipient site during the operation to excise all dead or doubtful tissue and any foreign material, after achieving haemostasis.

2 Dress with several layers of paraffin gauze, dressing gauze, wool and a crepe bandage.

3 Harvest large split skin grafts adequate to cover the defect and dress the donor site (see below).

4 Spread the split skin graft on paraffin gauze with the external opaque surface on the gauze. Fold and wrap this in a saline-soaked swab and place it in a sterile jar to be stored in a refrigerator at 4 °C.

5 On the following day, remove the dressing from the recipient site.

6 Apply the skin graft to the defect and spread it to cover all areas. Trim and store any excess skin at the margin.

7 Remove the paraffin gauze and leave the skin graft exposed.

8 Observe the graft at regular intervals. If serum collects beneath it, roll this out with cotton wool budded sticks soaked in saline, either to the edge or through a small incision made in the graft.

9 Be sure that the exposed area is well protected from any injury, particularly while the patient is asleep.

MESHED GRAFTS

Appraise

1 Meshed grafts are useful for providing skin cover to large areas, particularly when there is limited availability of donor skin, as often occurs in extensive burns.

2 They survive more reliably, as any underlying seroma that collects escapes through the interstices of the graft, leaving the graft elements intact.

3 They are effective in covering irregular surfaces as they can be moulded to these.

4 Unfortunately the resultant appearance is less satisfactory than a sheet graft.

Action

1 Prepare the donor site in the usual way.

2 Harvest long, thin strips of split skin graft, as described above.

3 Dress the donor site.

4 Pass the skin graft through the skin mesher. It may need to be placed on a carrier for this, depending on the type of instrument (Fig. 33.4).

5 Apply the mesh graft directly on to the recipient site using two pairs of non-toothed forceps.

6 Spread the skin out appropriately to cover all suitable recipient areas.

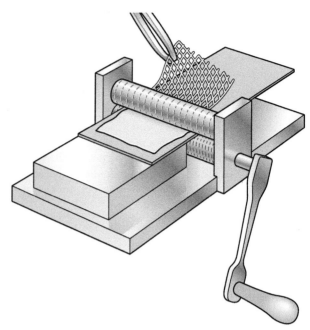

Fig. 33.4 Meshing a split skin graft. The skin graft has been placed on a plastic carrier and is being passed through the skin mesher. The cut skin, elevated at one corner by a pair of forceps, can be stretched to three times its original size or more, depending on the carrier used.

7 Suture the graft with continuous sutures at the periphery only if the area is difficult to dress.

8 Dress the area with a calcium alginate dressing, one layer of paraffin gauze, dressing gauze, cotton wool and crepe bandage.

9 Re-dress at 4 or 5 days.

10 Continue to re-dress at approximately 3-day intervals until the interstices have epithelialized.

QUILTED GRAFTS

Appraise

These are most usefully applied to large areas of the tongue or any other highly vascular area. Any method of graft fixation is liable to cause bleeding beneath the graft. However, at each suture site a small area of graft take is ensured, and epithelialization subsequently spreads out from each of these.

Action

1 Prepare the donor site.

2 Harvest the skin graft.

3 Put two large sutures in the anterior aspect of the tongue and pull it forwards.

4 Apply the skin graft to the tongue and trim the excess at the edges.

5 Place multiple 3/0 absorbable sutures at the edge of the graft and throughout its surface (Fig. 33.5).

6 No dressing is required.

7 Remove the traction sutures.

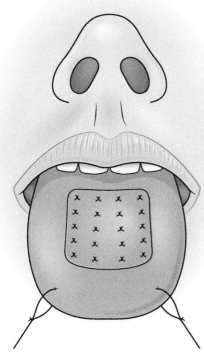

Fig. 33.5 Quilted graft. The graft is fixed to a defect on the dorsum of the tongue with multiple sutures.

FULL-THICKNESS GRAFTS

Appraise

1 These give better cosmetic results than split-thickness grafts as they contract less. The quality of the skin is better but they need a very good vascular bed in order to survive.

2 Their most common application is on the face following excision of small lesions, and the best results are achieved in the eyelid region and around the medial canthus.

3 They can occasionally be used on the hand, but are not generally used elsewhere, as large grafts leave a large primary defect.

4 The best donor sites are those with surplus skin so that the skin can be closed primarily with an insignificant scar. The most common donor areas are post-auricular, pre-auricular, upper eyelid, nasolabial and supraclavicular skin.

Action

1 Mark the area of skin to be removed and measure it.

2 Mark out a similar area in the donor site, allowing an extra 2.5 mm or more at each margin for the contour difference that will be present at the recipient site.

3 Plan an ellipse at the donor site around the proposed graft to allow primary closure.

4 Inject local anaesthetic at the excision and donor sites.

5 Create the defect at the recipient site.

6 With a size 15 blade, cut around the margins of the planned donor skin.

7 Raise the full ellipse of skin and subcutaneous tissue.

8 Undermine the skin edges at the donor defect and close this primarily.

9 Place the skin graft on to a wet saline swab, skin surface down.

10 Using small, curved scissors cut the subcutaneous fat off the skin graft and excise the redundant skin.

11 Place the skin graft into the defect and suture the edges at the periphery. Leave the suture ends long.

12 Use tie-over sutures to fix the dressing of paraffin gauze and proflavine wool.

13 Apply a pressure dressing for 24 hours, if possible.

14 Dress the donor site.

15 Plan to re-dress the recipient site at 1 week.

COMPOSITE GRAFTS

Appraise

1 Composite grafts consist of skin and other tissue, usually subcutaneous fat and some underlying cartilage.

2 They are most commonly used where there is significant loss of a nostril rim.

3 Occasionally, they are used for defects at the periphery of the pinna.

Action

1 Mark out the defect that will be left after excision of diseased or damaged skin, with excision of traumatized or contaminated wound edges, if necessary.

2 Identify a site on either pinna that corresponds in both size and shape to the planned defect.

3 Mark out this area with ink.

4 Prepare both ears.

5 Plan the reconstruction of the donor defect.

6 Inject 0.5% lidocaine and 1:200 000 adrenaline (epinephrine) into both sites and wait for 5 minutes.

RANDOM PATTERN SKIN FLAPS

Introduction

1 Skin flaps are used to repair or reconstruct defects where there is an inadequate blood supply to support a skin graft. They survive on their own blood supply, which they bring with them, and this may be beneficial to the recipient site. It may help by introducing a new blood supply to an avascular area following irradiation, or to a fracture site where there is delayed union.

2 The quality of the skin in a skin flap is almost normal and its texture and cosmetic appearance are much better than a graft. A skin flap may, however, lose its nerve supply and have its vascular supply and lymphatic drainage partly compromised in the transfer.

3 Until relatively recently, all skin flaps were based on a random vascular pattern. It was recognized that flaps with a length greater than their base would survive in certain areas. It is now realized that the reason for this survival is that these flaps had, unknowingly, been based on an axial pattern basis. If a flap is designed

around a recognized artery and vein, with these vessels passing down its central axis, it may be safely transferred with a very large length-to-breadth ratio. Indeed, the breadth need be the artery and vein alone, providing they remain patent.

4   Many of the superficial muscles of the body have one principal vascular hilum, and these muscles can be rotated about the hilum on a single pedicle. It has further been realized that the skin overlying these superficial muscles receives its vascular supply from them. Consequently, the muscle with its overlying skin can be transposed as a single unit, forming a myocutaneous flap. A large number of these flaps have been described, but the more commonly used ones alone will be described below.

5   Special terms are traditionally used in relation to flaps. Delay indicates partial division of a flap at its base and re-suturing. This procedure encourages an improved blood supply to the flap from the opposite attachment. Complete division at the base carried out a few days later is then usually safe. After a flap has been transferred safely, the bridging portion may be divided. The two ends are trimmed and one is sutured into the new recipient area while the other is replaced in the donor site. This is referred to as in-setting.

6   When planning a flap, it is useful to employ a sheet of sterile paper or other similar material to act as a template. This can be cut to shape and used as a trial flap.

Z-PLASTY

Appraise

1   Z-plasties are used for releasing linear contractions. These usually develop along linear scars that traverse Langer's lines.

2   These linear contractions are often most evident when crossing the concavity of the flexor aspect of a joint, but they can occur on extensor surfaces and in other areas unrelated to joints.

> ▶ KEY POINT Breadth taken into length
>
> ■ In effect, skin is drawn in from the sides to increase the length.

Action

1   Draw a line along the full extent of the contracture (Fig. 33.6).

2   From one end, draw a line at 60° to the first line and of the same length.

3   From the opposite end, draw a line at 60° on the opposite side of the line for the same length.

4   Incise along the central line and excise any scar tissue.

5   Incise along the two lateral lines through the full thickness of skin and subcutaneous tissue.

6   Raise the flaps so formed, lifting the skin and subcutaneous tissue as one, holding the tip of each flap with a skin hook.

7   Interchange the two skin flaps.

8   If the flaps do not meet comfortably, undermine the skin and subcutaneous tissue around the periphery of the wound to allow them to lie correctly.

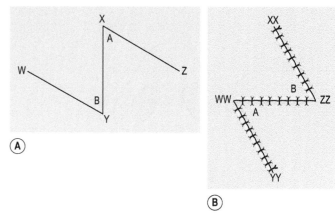

Fig. 33.6   Z-plasty. Contracture along X–Y is released to XX–YY by raising and interchanging flaps A and B. The distance W–Z is shortened to WW–ZZ.

9   Suture the tips of the two flaps into place first.

10   Suture the remaining edges of the flaps.

11   Dress the wound.

Technical points

1   The angle of the Z-plasty can be varied according to circumstances.

2   If the scar contracture is particularly long, use two or more Z-plasties, either in series or at intervals along the length of the contracture.

3   For scar contractures across a web space, use a W-plasty (Fig. 33.7). This consists of two Z-plasties, placed in reverse direction to each other, meeting at the base of the web space.

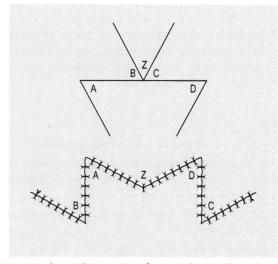

Fig. 33.7   W-plasty. This consists of two Z-plasties along the same contracture placed in reverse direction and meeting at the central point. Flaps A and B are interposed and flaps C and D are interposed. Flap Z stays in the same place but is raised during surgery to permit undermining at its base to allow it to stretch.

TRANSPOSITION FLAP

Appraise

1 Small transposition flaps on the face have long been used. It is well recognized, that in this region, because of the vascularity of the skin, flaps with a large length-to-breadth ratio can be used safely.

2 Transposition flaps allow skin from an area of abundance to be moved to a defect where primary closure is inappropriate.

3 On the face, there is an abundance of skin appropriate for transposition flaps in the nasolabial area, the glabellar area and the upper eyelid.

4 In other parts of the body, many axial pattern flaps are used as transposition flaps.

Action

1 Mark out the defect in ink.

2 Plan the transposition flap in an adjacent area with superfluous skin and mark this out (Fig. 33.8).

3 Check that the margin of the flap most distal from the defect is long enough from the fulcrum at its base to reach the most distal part of the defect. This is the limiting factor of the flap.

4 Excise the lesion to create the defect.

5 Raise the flap, including skin and subcutaneous tissue, and support the tip of the flap on a skin hook.

6 Transpose the flap into the defect and check that it fits.

7 Undermine the edges of the donor site defect and also the edges of the excision area to allow the flap to sit more comfortably in the defect.

8 Close the donor defect in layers.

9 Suture the flap in place.

10 Leave the flap exposed if possible, so you can monitor it.

RHOMBOID FLAP

Appraise

1 A rhomboid flap is, as its name suggests, a flap with the shape of an equilateral parallelogram – a lozenge shape.

2 The rhomboid flap is most useful when the appropriate ellipse for excision of a defect is at right-angles to Langer's lines. It has a similar effect to a transposition flap carried through 90°.

Action

1 Mark out the area of the defect.

2 Around this, draw the smallest possible rhomboid with equal sides.

3 Draw two further lines of equal length as shown in Figure 33.9.

4 Excise the lesion.

5 Transpose the flap, as shown in the diagram.

6 Undermine the edges.

7 Close the donor defect.

8 Suture the flap in place.

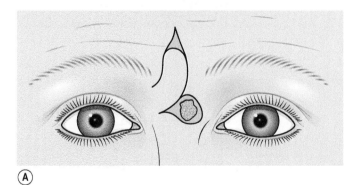

(A)

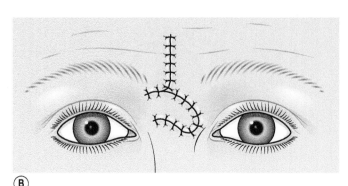

(B)

Fig. 33.8 Transposition flap. (A) A lesion in the region of the medial canthus is excised and a transposition flap from the glabellar region is used to reconstruct the defect. (B) A small triangle of skin at the apex of the flap is discarded and the donor site is closed primarily.

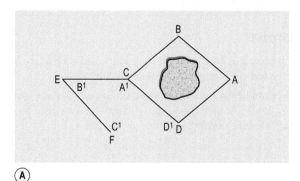

(A)

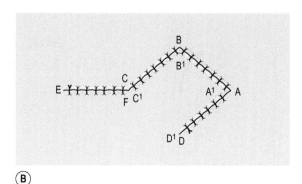

(B)

Fig. 33.9 Rhomboid flap. (A) A rhomboid defect is created: ABCD. CE and EF are drawn with equal length, making a smaller rhomboid: A'B'C'D'. (B) After transposition of the flap to the defect, the donor defect is closed primarily by approximating F to C.

ROTATION FLAP

Appraise

1. These are large flaps used to close relatively small defects.
2. They use excess skin at a distance from the defect and borrow small amounts of skin from a large area.
3. They are principally used to borrow skin from the neck to take up to the face. They can be used on the scalp and for treating sacral pressure sores.

Action

1. Mark out the skin defect.
2. Draw an isosceles triangle around the defect, with the apex of the triangle at or pointing towards the centre of the arc of rotation of the flap (Fig. 33.10).
3. Draw the arc of the rotation flap.
4. Raise the skin and subcutaneous tissue of the flap.
5. Undermine the skin at the edge of the defect and along the skin margin opposite the flap.
6. Rotate the flap into the defect.
7. Suture the flap.
8. If necessary, excise a wedge of tissue along the skin edge opposite the flap to assist rotation. If necessary, 'cut-back' into the flap at the opposite end of the arc of the flap from the defect, to create a better fit.

ADVANCEMENT FLAP

Appraise

1. Advancement flaps are most commonly used on the face to preserve feature lines or structures of the face.
2. They can be used on the forehead or for defects of the eyebrow. Frequently, in these situations, bilateral advancement flaps are used simultaneously to reconstruct one defect.

Action

1. Mark out the defect.
2. Mark out the smallest possible square or rectangle enclosing this defect, with lines parallel and at right-angles to Langer's lines.
3. Extend the marks of the sides running parallel to Langer's lines in each direction from the defect, thus delineating two flaps (Fig. 33.11).
4. Create the defect.
5. Elevate the flaps and advance them towards each other.
6. Suture them together.
7. Suture their sides.

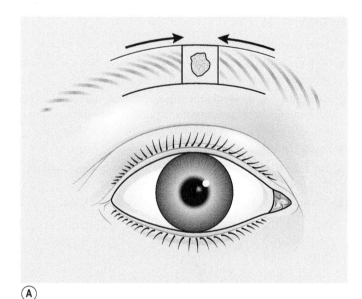

(A)

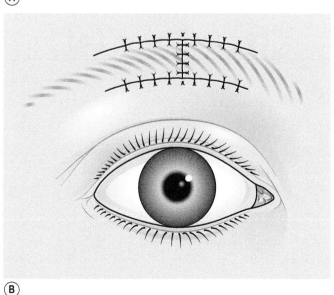

(B)

Fig. 33.11 Advancement flap. (A) A defect in the eyebrow is excised and (B) two advancement flaps, one from each side, are raised and advanced to meet each other over the defect. The natural lines of the eyebrow are preserved.

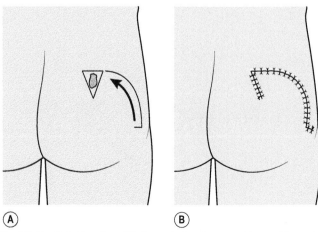

(A)   (B)

Fig. 33.10 Rotation flap. (A) A sacral ulcer is created into a triangular defect and a flap from the buttock is rotated into this. (B) A small cut-back allows greater mobility in rotation.

EXPANSION FLAP

Appraise

1. These flaps are used specifically for repairing and reconstructing defects of the scalp.

2. Flaps on the scalp are notorious for their inability to stretch because of the inelasticity of the galea (Latin: =a helmet).

3. Division of the galea allows some stretching of the skin to take place, especially in younger patients.

Prepare

1. Pay particular attention to the preoperative planning of the flap. Remember that the scalp flap will move in three dimensions.

2. Shave the patient's hair over the whole scalp to a length of 1 cm. Leave long locks of hair only if you can confidently cope with these during the operation.

3. Make a careful plan of the flap to be used, and mark the outline of this.

4. Completely shave the hair for 1 cm on either side of this line and for 1 cm around the outline of the defect.

5. Wash the hair thoroughly to remove all cut and shaved hairs.

Action

1. Place the patient, face downwards, on the operating table. Use a neurosurgical head-rest to support the head, if this is available.

2. Mark out the defect on the scalp.

3. Mark out the flap as previously planned. The flap may be of transposition, rotational or advancement design.

4. Plan a wide base to the flap around the periphery of the scalp to ensure that at least one principal vascular system enters its base.

5. Inject the planned outline of the flap with 0.5% lidocaine and 1:200 000 adrenaline (epinephrine) and wait at least for 5 minutes.

6. Excise the lesion and create the defect.

7. Incise along the margins of the flap to elevate it with the underlying galea so that this is included with the flap.

8. Reflect the flap backwards, exposing the galea.

9. Support the flap on the palm of the hand and make multiple incisions just through the galea with a no. 15 blade, across the full width of the flap (Fig. 33.12).

10. Identify the principal vessels beneath the surface of the galea and avoid dividing them.

11. Make multiple transverse incisions at right-angles to the first set, along the whole length of the flap.

12. Reflect the flap back into the defect.

13. Suture the flap into place with one layer of 3/0 non-absorbable sutures.

14. Always insert suction drains under the flap.

15. Dress with paraffin gauze, dressing gauze, cotton wool and crepe bandages.

16. Re-dress after 48 hours and, if possible, leave exposed.

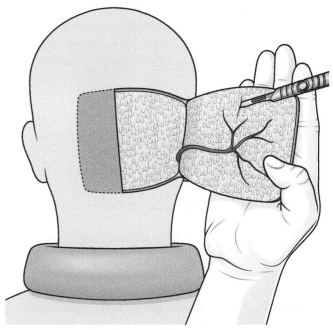

Fig. 33.12 Expansion flap. A knife is used to make multiple incisions in the galea of a scalp flap based on the posterior branch of the superficial temporal vessels which has been reflected back to its base. Following these multiple incisions, the flap can be advanced to cover the defect on the vertex of the scalp.

CROSS-LEG FLAP

Appraise

1. This used to be the most commonly used flap to cover open (compound) fractures of the tibia and fibula with extensive soft tissue loss.

2. There are now many fascio-cutaneous and free flaps described that are more suitable but, on rare occasions, cross-leg flaps may be useful.

3. Cross-arm flaps and cross-thigh flaps can be created using the same principle.

Prepare

1. Mark out the minimal defect on the leg.

▶ KEY POINT Pre-plan the procedure

■ Plan the whole operation meticulously 24 hours beforehand.

2. Plan a flap from the calf of the donor leg, based medially, preserving the long saphenous vein superiorly. Do not exceed a 1:1 length-to-breadth ratio.

3. Enlarge the defect to a size that will receive a safe flap; that is, make the defect fit the flap.

4. Using tapes, ensure that with the legs kept closely together, the flap when hinged on its medial axis will stretch to the distal part of the defect, allowing enough tissue to create a bridge between the two legs.

5 Place the patient's legs on top of a bead bag and apply vacuum so the patient's legs are fixed in what will be their postoperative position.

6 Maintain the patient's legs in this bead bag for as much of the next 24 hours as is practical so that he becomes used to the position preoperatively.

Action

1 With the patient under general anaesthesia, apply a tourniquet to reduce bleeding.

2 Create the planned defect, obtain haemostasis, then remove the tourniquet from the leg.

3 Elevate the planned flap from the opposite leg, raising the deep fascia with the flap.

4 Check that with the legs in the appropriate position, the flap fits the defect.

5 Take a split skin graft from the thigh of the recipient leg and dress the donor area.

6 Apply and suture the split skin graft to the flap donor site and to the back of that part of the flap which will form a skin bridge between the two legs (Fig. 33.13).

7 Suture the four corners of the flap into place and subsequently suture the edges.

8 Dress the skin graft at the flap donor site and use minimal other dressings.

9 Splint the two legs in the bead bag and apply vacuum.

10 Ensure that there is no tension or torsion on the flap and that it is viable.

11 Monitor the flap postoperatively for any changes.

Complete

1 Perform a 'delay' procedure after 2 weeks using local anaesthesia only, partially dividing the base and then re-suturing this wound.

2 Take the patient back to the operating theatre after the third week and divide the flap completely under general anaesthesia, allowing a generous portion to be in-set at the recipient site.

3 Suture the flap into place avoiding tension.

4 Suture the proximal portion to its donor site.

CROSS-FINGER FLAP

Appraise

1 Cross-finger flaps are a convenient means of obtaining good-quality skin cover for defects on the flexor aspects of the fingers, where split skin grafts would contract.

2 Take them from the dorsum of an adjacent finger.

Action

1 Mark out the defect on the flexor aspect of the finger.

2 Apply a tourniquet and create the defect.

3 Mark out a flap on the dorsum of the adjacent finger opposite the defect, or as near as possible, avoiding the skin over the joints.

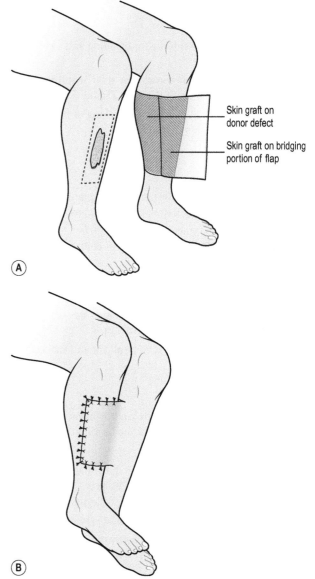

Skin graft on donor defect

Skin graft on bridging portion of flap

Fig. 33.13 Cross-leg flap. (A) A skin defect on the front of the right leg is enlarged to accommodate the flap from the calf of the left leg. After the flap has been raised from the left leg, the donor defect and a portion of the bridging part of the flap are grafted before suturing the flap in place. (B) The cross-leg flap is sutured in place.

4 Elevate the rectangular flap with its base adjacent to the injured finger.

5 Place the flap over the defect (Fig. 33.14).

6 Increase the size of the defect to fit the flap.

7 Remove the tourniquet and achieve haemostasis.

8 Take a small split skin graft with a Da Silva knife.

9 Apply the skin graft to the donor defect.

10 Suture the flap into the defect.

11 Dress the wounds and splint the two fingers together after inserting some dressing gauze between the fingers.

12 Plan to divide the flap at 2 weeks, in-setting the skin bridge at both recipient and donor sites, and re-dress the wounds.

13 Remove all sutures 1 week later.

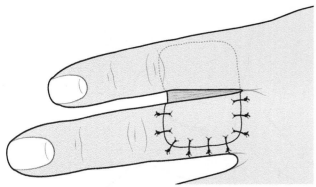

Fig. 33.14 Cross-finger flap. A flap from the dorsum of the ring finger is used to cover a defect on the flexor aspect of the proximal interphalangeal joint of the little finger. The donor site is repaired with a split skin graft sutured in place.

REVERSE DERMIS FLAP

Appraise

1 This flap is similar to the cross-finger flap but is used for defects on the dorsum of the finger.

Action

1 Mark out the defect.
2 Use a tourniquet to control bleeding and create the defect.
3 Mark out an appropriate flap on the dorsum of an adjacent finger, as with a cross-finger flap.
4 Shave the planned flap with a Da Silva knife, removing a thin sheet of epidermis and superficial dermis.
5 Elevate the rectangular flap with subcutaneous tissue, leaving it attached at its base adjacent to the finger with the defect.
6 Increase the size of the defect to fit the flap.
7 Remove the tourniquet and achieve haemostasis.
8 Suture the flap in place.
9 Take a small split skin graft and apply this to the donor site and the flap.
10 Splint the two fingers together with some gauze dressing between the fingers.
11 Plan to divide the flap at 2 weeks, and in-set the bridge portion of the flap at both donor and recipient sites.
12 Remove all sutures 7 days later.

ABDOMINAL TUBE PEDICLE FLAP

Appraise

1 These flaps were formerly used as the standard technique for transferring a large amount of skin and subcutaneous tissue from the abdomen to a distant site such as the foot, the face, or elsewhere where there was extensive loss of tissue. They have been superseded almost totally by the introduction of axial pattern flaps, applied either as pedicle flaps or transferred as free flaps using microvascular surgical techniques. However, they may be useful in a few isolated situations.

2 Raise a planned rectangular area of abdominal skin and subcutaneous tissue by dividing along each side and, while still attached at each end, form the middle part into a tube. After a delay procedure, detach one end and transfer it to a wrist. When it has established a local blood supply, detach the other end and transfer it to the side of the defect. In further stages the whole flap is transferred to the defect and spread over it.
3 The patient requires approximately 5 months of hospitalization, with many operations, and failure is not uncommon at some stage.
4 Tube pedicle flaps can be raised from other sites, including the back and thigh.

ACTION

Raising the tube pedicle

1 Mark out a rectangular area 20 cm x 8 cm obliquely on the lower abdomen.
2 Incise along the long edges down to the deep fascia.
3 Dissect along the deep fascia between the two edges to elevate a bridge of skin and subcutaneous tissue.
4 Approximate the two skin edges of the bridge beneath the subcutaneous tissue to form a tube and suture as far as possible in each direction.
5 At either end suture the skin down to the base to create a closed tube (Fig. 33.15A).
6 Apply a large split skin graft to the residual raw area beneath the skin tube if this defect cannot be closed primarily.

Delay of the flap

1 At 2 weeks, under local anaesthesia, partially divide the base of the flap at one end, dividing through three-quarters of the skin and subcutaneous tissue, ligating and dividing the underlying vessels.
2 Re-suture the wound and apply a small dressing.

Division of the tube

1 Three weeks after raising the tube, divide the base of the tube completely, passing through the delay incision.
2 Close the residual defect on the abdomen using a split skin graft if necessary.
3 Place the patient's contralateral arm on to the abdominal wall and find a suitable recipient site at the level of the wrist to insert the tube pedicle.
4 Mark out an appropriate sized circle on the wrist.
5 Elevate the skin and subcutaneous tissue from half of this circle and reflect it backwards as a flap. This produces a circular defect.
6 Suture the free end of the abdominal tube pedicle to the circular defect (Fig. 33.15B).
7 Splint the arm to the chest wall after applying plenty of padding beneath the axilla.

Delay of abdominal tube pedicle

1 This is carried out under local anaesthesia 2 weeks after insertion to the wrist.

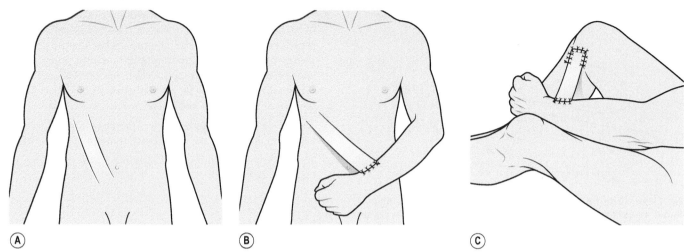

Fig. 33.15   Abdominal tube pedicle flap: (A) the flap is raised on the abdomen; (B) the lower end is transferred to the wrist; (C) after 3 weeks the abdominal end is detached and sutured around the defect on the contralateral leg.

2   Make an incision at the base of the flap still attached to the abdominal wall.

3   The technique is the same as that used in the first delay procedure.

Transfer of flap to defect

1   Free the abdominal tube flap from the abdominal wall by dividing the tube at its residual attachment to the abdomen, passing through the delaying incision.

2   Close the donor defect with a split skin graft if necessary, and dress the wound.

3   Transfer the arm with its attached pedicle to the site of the defect.

4   Mark out a recipient site for the tube pedicle, preferably on the distal side of the defect, so that the seam of the flap overlies the defect.

5   Create a circular defect with a healthy skin margin at the edge of the main defect.

6   Excise any scar tissue from the end of the tube pedicle, and insert the tube pedicle into the skin defect (Fig. 33.15C).

7   Immobilize the limbs appropriately.

Delay of tube pedicle

Carry out a delay of the tube pedicle at the wrist end using the same technique as before.

Transfer of whole flap to defect

1   Divide the flap from the wrist, incising through the site of the delay incision.

2   Return the original skin flap from the wrist to its former site, thus leaving a residual semicircular wound, and suture this.

3   Mark out a circular area on the opposite side of the defect from the initial attachment of the tube pedicle.

4   Create a circular surdect with healthy skin margins at this site.

5   Insert the free end of the tube pedicle into this defect, keeping the seam over the defect.

Insert the flap

1   Allow the flap to 'soften' before in-setting. This may involve waiting for 4 or 5 weeks or more.

2   Excise any doubtful tissue in the base to ensure that it is healthy.

3   Excise the seam of the tube pedicle and spread the skin of the tube pedicle over the defect.

4   Suture the edges into the edge of the defect.

5   Do not carry out any further revisions of the flap until it has been allowed to settle for at least several weeks and preferably for several months.

AXIAL PATTERN SKIN FLAPS

SCALP FLAP

Appraise

1   Scalp flaps are most commonly used for reconstructing defects of the hair-bearing skin on the face. They are usually used for reconstructing the upper lip, lower lip and chin areas in males, but there are many other occasional applications.

2   The flap is based on the posterior branch of the superficial temporal artery.

Prepare

1   Plan the flap on the day before operation.

2   Cut all the hair in the area of the operation to less than 1 cm in length.

3   Shave the hair completely in the area of the planned incisions.

4   Check that the posterior branch of the superficial temporal artery is palpable and that there are no significant scars on the scalp, suggesting previous damage to this vessel.

5   Wash the head thoroughly to remove all cut and shaved hair.

Action

1   Mark out the defect.

2 If appropriate, increase the defect to the shape of a whole cosmetic unit.

3 If appropriate, increase the defect to make it symmetrical on either side of the midline.

4 Make a template of the defect with sterile paper.

5 With one end of a tape attached to the template, and a second fixed on the zygomatic arch below the point where the artery was palpated, swing the template up on to the vertex of the scalp using the point on the zygomatic arch as the pivot.

6 Mark out an appropriate area on the scalp behind the anterior hairline around the template.

7 Infiltrate the scalp along the marked line with 0.5% lidocaine and 1:200 000 adrenaline (epinephrine), and wait for 5 minutes.

8 Elevate the flap together with the underlying galea, starting at its distal extremity.

9 Identify the posterior branch of the superficial temporal vessels in the pedicle of the flap as it is raised, and adjust the shape of the pedicle if necessary to include these vessels (Fig. 33.16).

10 Taper the pedicle to 2 cm at its base, so that it can be rotated.

11 Transpose the flap into the defect, and in-set.

12 Cover the posterior aspect of the flap with paraffin gauze.

13 Close the donor defect primarily if possible. If it is too large, cover it with a split skin graft.

14 Plan to divide the flap at 2 weeks, providing there is a large inset. If you are in doubt, divide the flap at 3 weeks and return the pedicle.

FOREHEAD FLAP

Appraise

1 The forehead flap has been used extensively in the past to provide lining of the oral cavity after major resections for tumour. It is occasionally used for resurfacing defects of the scalp and of the cheek. It is the best flap available for total nasal reconstruction.

2 It has been largely superseded by other myocutaneous and free flaps in its use for oral lining, but it remains an easy, safe and reliable flap to use, especially in the elderly and debilitated patient.

3 Its main disadvantage is the relatively poor cosmetic defect of its donor site.

4 It is not a true axial pattern flap, but it simulates one, surviving on the anterior branch of one superficial temporal artery and its accompanying vein. The distal part of the flap normally acquires its vascular supply from the opposite anterior branch of the superficial temporal artery and the supraorbital and supratrochlear vessels. When these vessels to the flap are divided, the vascular network between the branches of the various vessels is adequate to allow the flap to survive on the supply from the single vascular pedicle.

Action

1 Create the defect and measure its dimensions.

2 Mark out the flap on the forehead, making this symmetrical and preferably including the whole of the forehead skin as a cosmetic unit.

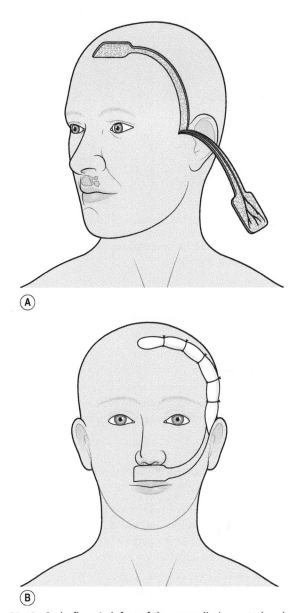

(A)

(B)

Fig. 33.16 Scalp flap. A defect of the upper lip is created and a matching area from the vertex is swung down on a pedicle based on the posterior branch of the superficial temporal artery. (A) The flap is pivoted above the zygomatic arch and turned to fill the defect. (B) A split graft is applied to the donor defect with a tie-over dressing.

3 Increase the defect to accommodate the flap.

4 If the flap is to be used for intraoral lining, excise the coronoid process of the mandible to allow the flap to pass inside the zygomatic arch.

5 Elevate the flap, commencing at the margin distal to the flap pedicle.

6 Identify and ligate the anterior branch of the contralateral superficial temporal artery and the supraorbital and supratrochlear vessels on both sides.

7 Lift the flap in the plane beneath the frontalis muscle.

8 Identify the anterior branch of the superficial temporal artery and its accompanying veins on the undersurface of the flap, and taper the pedicle to a 2-cm margin, including these vessels (Fig. 33.17).

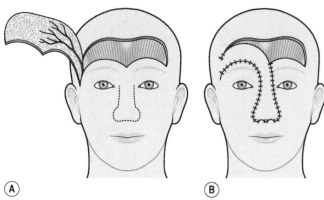

Fig. 33.17 Forehead flap: (A) the forehead skin elevated on the anterior branch of the superficial temporal vessels of one side; (B) forehead flap being used for total nasal reconstruction. The flap is divided and in-set at 3 weeks.

9 If the flap is to be used intraorally, pass this through to the mouth beneath the zygoma.

10 If there is inadequate space to carry this out, excise a segment of the zygomatic arch.

11 To avoid a further operation some 2 weeks later, shave the epidermis and superficial dermis from that part of the pedicle that will remain buried between the skin surface and the intraoral surface.

12 Suture the flap in place.

13 Use 3/0 polyglactin sutures to elevate the skin of the eyebrows on either side symmetrically.

14 Lay several layers of paraffin gauze on the donor site.

15 Harvest a large split skin graft to cover the defect in one sheet. In a young person, use the inner aspect of the arm in preference to the thigh as this gives a better colour match.

16 Store the skin.

17 Apply this skin as a delayed graft 24 hours later.

18 After 2 weeks, divide the pedicle and return it, to provide symmetry to the face.

TONGUE FLAP

Appraise

1 Tongue flaps are used for repairing large palatal fistulae, providing mucosa in lip reconstruction and reconstructing defects of the pharynx and oral cavity.

▶ KEY POINT Take care

■ Suture these flaps very carefully otherwise they readily dehisce. This is because of the difficulty in splinting them.

2 They are not easily tolerated by young children since they are unable to co-operate. Tongue flaps are, therefore, rarely useful below the age of 6 years.

3 Most tongue flaps are not true axial pattern flaps but rely on the rich vascular network within the muscles of the tongue.

4 Flaps for palatal fistulae are taken from the dorsum, those for lining the oral cavity or the pharynx are taken from the lateral aspect, and those providing a vermilion border are taken from the anterior part. In all cases close the defect primarily.

Action

1 Create the defect and measure the dimensions.

2 Insert a large stay suture in the tip of the tongue and pull it forwards.

3 Place two large stay sutures as far to the back of the tongue as possible and use these as the principal stay sutures.

4 Plan and mark out the flap on the tongue. Flaps for palatal fistulae can be based anteriorly or posteriorly, but this depends on the position of the defect.

5 Elevate the flap of mucosa together with a sheet of muscle approximately 4–5 mm thick.

6 Check that the flap fits the defect.

7 Close the donor defect primarily (Fig. 33.18).

8 Suture the most inaccessible part of the flap into the defect first with interrupted sutures.

9 Work proximally, leaving the easiest, most anterior, suture until last.

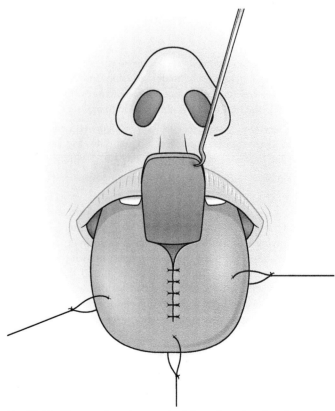

Fig. 33.18 Tongue flap. A posteriorly based tongue flap from the dorsum has been raised for closing a palatal fistula. The donor defect has been closed primarily.

10 Observe the flap carefully; it may require re-suturing at any time.

11 Divide the flap at 2 weeks, and in-set.

DELTOPECTORAL FLAP

Appraise

1 This flap, sometimes known as a Bakamjian flap after its innovator, is used for providing skin flap cover to the chin, the cheek, the region of the pinna and the neck. It can be used to provide lining to the oral cavity and pharynx but may require the development of a temporary oral or pharyngeal fistula, which is unsatisfactory.

2 When raised conventionally there is necrosis of the tip in approximately 15% of cases. Because of this and its unsightly donor defect, it has been superseded by other flaps for mucosal replacement but is occasionally useful for large skin defects.

Action

1 Create the defect.

2 Mark out the flap based on the second, third and fourth perforating branches of the internal thoracic artery (Fig. 33.19).

3 Mark the upper margin of the flap along a line parallel with the clavicle, along its inferior margin. Use a line along the superior margin if a block dissection of the neck has been carried out with a McPhee incision.

4 Mark the inferior border of the flap parallel to and 10 cm below the upper border.

5 Mark the distal end of the flap as a semicircle extending to the midlateral line over the deltoid muscle.

6 Elevate the flap from its lateral margin including the fascia overlying the deltoid and pectoralis muscle.

7 Divide the branch from the acromiothoracic artery, as this perforates the clavipectoral fascia.

8 Divide and ligate the cephalic vein at the margin of the flap.

9 Reflect the flap medially to within 4 cm of the midline.

10 Dissect further medially, very carefully, to avoid dividing the perforating branches on which the flap survives.

11 Pass the flap up to the defect.

12 If the flap passes directly to the defect on the external surface, tube the intervening bridge over the neck.

13 If a block dissection has been carried out and the flap is for intraoral use, shave the epidermis from the central portion of the flap and pass the flap subcutaneously up to the defect. This manoeuvre converts the reconstruction into a one-stage operation.

14 Suture the flap into the defect.

15 Establish haemostasis on the donor site and cover it with paraffin gauze.

16 Take a split skin graft, store it and apply it to the donor site at 24 hours as a delayed graft.

17 At 3 weeks, divide the pedicle if exposed and in-set the flap.

18 Return the remainder of the pedicle to the donor site after excising the split skin graft in the appropriate area.

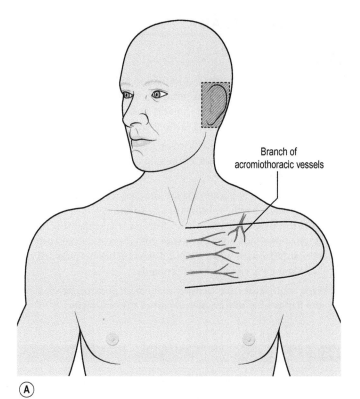

Branch of acromiothoracic vessels

(A)

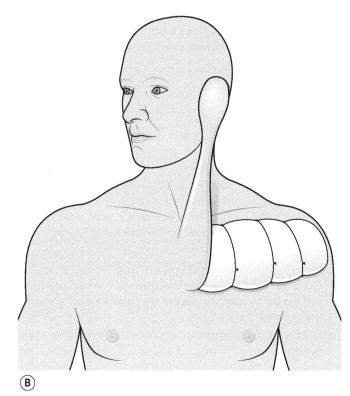

(B)

Fig. 33.19   Deltopectoral flap: (A) the flap is based on the second, third and fourth branches of the internal thoracic artery; (B) the flap being used to reconstruct the skin in the region of the pinna after a pinnectomy. The donor defect in this case is covered with a split skin graft and a tie-over dressing. The pedicle is divided and returned at 3 weeks.

PECTORALIS FLAP

Appraise

1 This is a versatile flap for reconstruction following excision of tumours in the head and neck region. It will reach the pharynx, the lower cheek, the neck and shoulder and will just reach the floor and lateral walls of the oral cavity as well as the area of the pinna.

2 It is a myocutaneous flap based on the pectoral vessels supplying the pectoralis major muscle. These in turn supply skin overlying the muscle.

3 Its most useful application is for intraoral reconstruction, where an island or paddle of skin the size of the defect is transferred from the lower chest wall on the distal part of the flap. The muscle is transposed subcutaneously with this island of skin and protects the carotid vessels when a block dissection has been carried out. The donor site can be closed primarily.

4 Web contractures may develop in the neck postoperatively when the flap is used in the anterior part of the oral cavity.

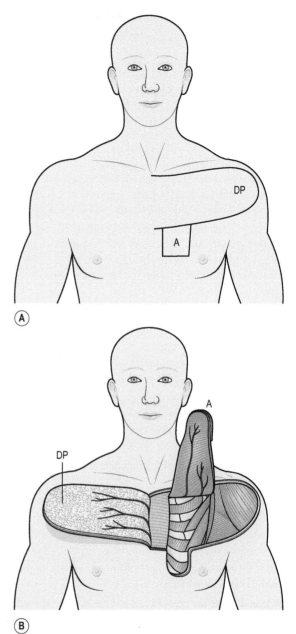

Fig. 33.20 Pectoralis flap: (A) the pectoralis muscle is used to transfer a cutaneous island of skin (A) from the chest wall into the neck; (B) to help exposure, a deltopectoral flap (DP) is reflected medially. The pectoralis muscle with its attached paddle of skin (A) is dissected free to the clavicle where it can be passed directly or subcutaneously to a defect above this level.

> ▶ **KEY POINTS** Caveats
>
> ▪ Hesitate to use this flap in hirsute males, where transposing hairy skin to the oral cavity may prove disadvantageous.
> ▪ In addition, the skin island is cumbersome and less reliable in obese individuals and in women with large breasts.

Action

1 Create the defect.

2 Measure the size of the defect.

3 Measure and mark an appropriate area of skin overlying the distal inferior portion of the pectoralis major muscle just above the costal margin (Fig. 33.20). Do not include skin across the midline or skin more than 2 cm below the lower margin of the pectoralis muscle.

4 Mark out a deltopectoral flap (see above) above the skin paddle.

5 Elevate the deltopectoral flap medially; you can omit this step if you are experienced, by passing the pectoralis flap under the deltopectoral flap.

6 Identify the lateral margin of the pectoralis muscle and elevate its border.

7 Dissect this distally to the sternal attachment, freeing the muscle from its attachments to the chest wall.

8 Dissect the distal element free from the midline.

9 Elevate the muscle with its attached skin island up to the clavicle. In doing this, look for and protect the two vascular pedicles on the undersurface.

10 Divide the attachment of the muscle to the humerus at the margin of the deltoid muscle.

11 Pass the flap subcutaneously beneath the neck skin if a block dissection has been carried out and pass the island of skin into the defect. Some rotation of the muscle pedicle may be necessary. Make sure the flap sits comfortably in place, and suture the skin paddle into the defect.

12 Suture the edges of the muscle to adjacent tissue to support it when the patient sits up.

13 If neck skin has been incised or excised to accommodate the muscle pedicle, take a split skin graft and apply this to the exposed muscle.

14 Close the donor defect primarily. This may require wide undermining to allow approximation of the skin edges.

15 Return and suture the deltopectoral flap.

LATISSIMUS DORSI FLAP

Appraise

1. The most useful application of this flap is as a myocutaneous flap in breast reconstruction and reconstruction of chest wall defects. It can be used in pharyngeal reconstruction and for defects of the back up to and just above the nape of the neck.

2. It can be used as a muscle flap alone to cover a large defect, or the muscle can be used to transfer a small island of skin, as in breast reconstruction, or a large island of skin. If a large island is transferred, primary closure of the donor site is not possible.

3. The flap has wide application in free tissue transfer (see below).

4. The flap is based on the thoracodorsal vessels, and these enter the muscle just below its insertion into the humerus.

Action

1. For an anterior chest wall defect, lay the patient on the table in the lateral position.

2. Create and measure the defect on the anterior chest wall.

3. Mark out the island of skin on the back overlying the latissimus dorsi muscle appropriate to the defect (Fig. 33.21).

4. Check that the island will reach the defect, using a tape based in the region of the vascular hilum at the lower margin of the posterior axillary fold. Remember, the most posterior point of the flap has to reach the most anterior point of the defect.

5. Incise the skin along the marked lines around the island down to the muscle.

6. Dissect the skin and fascia off the upper surface of the whole muscle proximal and distal to the skin paddle.

7. Identify the anterior border of the muscle.

8. Separate the muscle from the underlying serratus muscles and ribs.

9. Divide the muscle from its attachment, distally and posteriorly.

10. Separate the muscle up to its pedicle, identifying and preserving the principal vessels on the underlying surface.

11. Dissect gently at the hilum to avoid damaging the principal vessels.

12. Identify the vessels to the serratus anterior muscle arising from the thoracodorsal vessels, and divide them.

13. Develop a subcutaneous tunnel between the defect of the flap and the anterior chest wall defect.

14. Pass the flap subcutaneously through this tunnel into the anterior wall defect.

15. Close the donor site defect primarily, if possible, even if this means extensive undermining. Insert a large suction drain.

16. Change the patient to the supine position, re-towelling if necessary.

17. Undermine the skin edges of the defect where appropriate.

18. Suture the latissimus dorsi muscle to the chest wall.

19. If this is a breast reconstruction, insert a prosthesis beneath the latissimus dorsi muscle.

20. Suture the skin paddle of the flap to the skin defect.

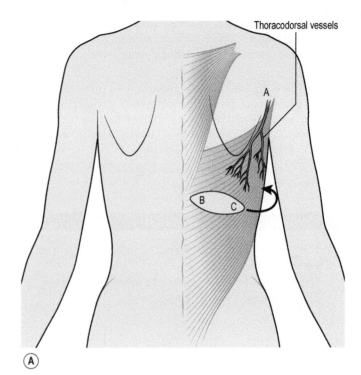

Thoracodorsal vessels

(A)

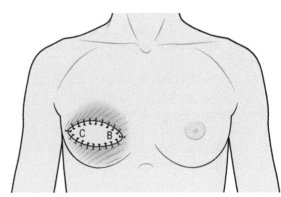

(B)

Fig. 33.21 Latissimus dorsi flap. The skin overlying the right latissimus dorsi flap is elevated from the muscle, leaving a central elliptiform island of skin attached to the muscle. The muscle is freed from its peripheral and underlying attachments and passed subcutaneously to the defect on the anterior chest wall, pivoted on its insertion (A) where the thoracodorsal vessels enter the muscle (A). In breast reconstruction, the muscle is sutured into the region of the reconstructed breast and the island of skin inserted into the mastectomy scar. A prosthesis is inserted beneath the flap (B).

TRAM FLAP

Appraise

1. The transverse rectus abdominis muscle (TRAM) provides an alternative flap for breast reconstruction to the latissimus dorsi muscle. It has the advantage that it can normally transfer sufficient autologous tissue to avoid the necessity of using an implant.

2. The flap can also be used for reconstructing chest wall defects and defects of the perineum. In either of these circumstances the skin paddle may be taken in the vertical plane (a vertical rectus abdominis muscle or VRAM flap), with the skin paddle lying completely over the muscle.

3 The flap may be used as a pedicled flap based either on the superior deep epigastric vessels for breast reconstruction or chest wall defects, or on the inferior deep epigastric vessels for perineal defects.

4 When used as a free flap, most commonly for breast reconstruction, prefer to use the inferior deep epigastric vessels, which are larger and more reliable. These vessels can be dissected through the muscle, avoiding harvesting of the muscle to raise a deep inferior epigastric perforator (DIEP) flap.

5 The abdominal skin wound closure is similar to that of an abdominoplasty (see below).

> **KEY POINTS** Two disadvantages

- The first is the loss of muscle and usual need to replace this with a prosthetic mesh.
- The second is the unreliability of survival of the skin paddle beyond the muscle boundaries.

Action

1 Mark the patient preoperatively in the standing position.

2 For breast reconstruction plan to excise the mastectomy scar if possible.

3 Avoid large skin flaps if the patient has been treated by radiotherapy.

4 Mark the midline and edges of the rectus abdominis muscles.

5 Plan and mark the skin island to be transferred centrally over the contralateral muscle just below the level of the umbilicus. If you are an experienced surgeon, you will centre the flap in the midline.

6 Mark a symmetrical ellipse to be excised that includes the planned skin island of the flap.

7 In the operating theatre, excise the mastectomy scar and raise the adjacent skin flaps to accommodate the flap.

8 Shave the epidermis off the skin adjacent to the planned skin island but within the marked outer ellipse. The residual dermis protects the subdermal pedicle, which in turn contributes to the viability of the subcutaneous flap beyond the boundaries of the skin paddle. Excise the residual skin of the symmetrical ellipse, the skin paddle and the subcutaneous fat (Fig. 33.22).

9 Cut through the deep fascia around the base of the subcutaneous fat to be included on the flap. Include in this the perforating vessels close to the midline both below and just above the umbilicus.

10 Gently pass your finger around the rectus abdominis muscle distal to the flap until the whole muscle is isolated. Cut through it with a cutting diathermy, identifying and ligating the inferior epigastric vessels when you encounter them on the undersurface.

11 Cut vertically through the middle of the anterior sheath of the muscle superiorly.

12 Elevate the muscle with the overlying subcutaneous fat and skin up to the costal margin.

13 Create a subcutaneous tunnel from the abdominal wall cavity through to the mastectomy wound and pass the skin paddle through this.

14 Orientate the skin paddle and fat and tack the base into place, checking there is no tension on the pedicle.

15 Suture the flap into place in layers and insert a Redivac drain.

16 Close the donor defect by suturing the upper part of the anterior rectus sheath first with a continuous 1 polypropylene suture.

17 Repair the residual defect in the anterior sheath with Marlex mesh sutured firmly in place with a continuous 1 polypropylene suture.

18 Close the abdominal wall in layers, transposing the umbilicus to its new site as appropriate. Insert two Redivac drains.

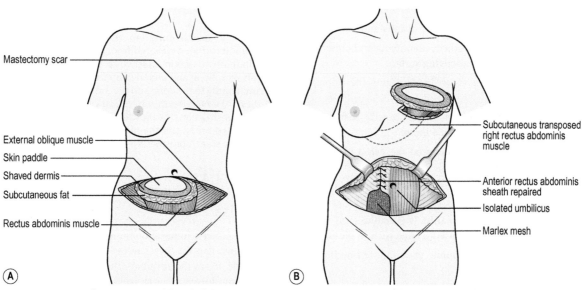

Mastectomy scar

External oblique muscle
Skin paddle
Shaved dermis
Subcutaneous fat
Rectus abdominis muscle

Subcutaneous transposed right rectus abdominis muscle

Anterior rectus abdominis sheath repaired
Isolated umbilicus
Marlex mesh

(A) (B)

Fig. 33.22 TRAM flap. Being used for a left breast reconstruction, the flap is isolated in the abdomen with a skin paddle, a surrounding area of shaved dermis and subcutaneous fat lying over and adjacent to the right rectus abdominis muscle. The remaining skin and subcutaneous fat from the larger ellipse is excised (A). After division of the lower part of the right rectus abdominis muscle, the flap is transferred on the upper part of the muscle and passed subcutaneously into the opened mastectomy wound. The anterior rectus sheath of the upper part of the muscle is closed and the defect of the anterior sheath below this is repaired with Marlex mesh (B).

19 Support the abdomen with a pressure garment and lightly dress the breast wounds.

20 Remove the drains when the drainage has diminished and remove the sutures at 3 weeks.

GROIN FLAP

Appraise

This can be used for defects of the lower abdominal wall, but its greatest application is providing skin cover for severe injuries to the hand or wrist. It is therefore most useful when the skin over the iliac crest is relatively thin.

> KEY POINTS Study the vascular patterns

- The groin flap is an unusual axial pattern flap as the vascular pattern is variable.
- The flap is based on either the superficial circumflex iliac vessels or the superficial epigastric vessels or a combination of the two. Details of these variations need to be known only if the flap is to be used as a free flap.

Action

1 Create the defect on the hand.

2 Identify the femoral artery by palpation.

3 Mark a point over this 2 cm beneath the inguinal ligament.

4 Draw a line from this point to the anterior superior iliac spine, which acts as the axis of the flap.

5 Mark an area over the iliac crest close to the mid-axillary line, which is to be used for the definitive skin cover.

6 Mark the flap to include this with parallel lines on either side of the central axis at an equal distance from it (Fig. 33.23).

7 First incise the skin laterally down to the deep fascia and include the fascia with the flap.

8 Reflect the flap medially.

9 At the edge of the sartorius muscle include the fascia, overlaying it with the flap, and so ensure that the superficial circumflex vessels are retained within the flap.

10 Dissect the flap free to within 3 cm of the femoral vessels.

11 Check that the defect on the hand will accommodate the flap.

12 Close the donor defect primarily up to the pedicle of the flap, if necessary flexing the knee and hip.

13 Tube the portion of the flap that will bridge the gap between groin and hand by suturing the two skin edges together.

14 Suture the distal part of the flap into the defect.

15 Immobilize the limb against the trunk after placing padding between the limb and the trunk.

16 Perform a delay procedure at 2 weeks by incising half of the skin at the base of the pedicle opposite the suture line.

17 Identify the axial vessels; ligate and divide them.

18 Re-suture the wound.

19 Three weeks after the initial procedure, divide the pedicle completely at its base and in-set it into the groin wound.

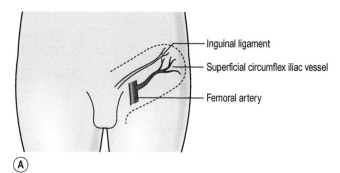

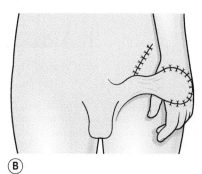

Fig. 33.23 Superficial groin flap. The inguinal ligament is marked in the groin and the position of the projected line of the superficial circumflex iliac vessels is also drawn. This line acts as the axis of the groin flap to be raised (A). After raising the flap the distal portion is sutured into the defect on the hand and the proximal portion is tubed (B). The donor defect is closed primarily.

20 In-set the flap into the hand defect with a few sutures. If tension is apparent in the skin, do not suture it at all, but cover the exposed part of the flap with a paraffin gauze dressing.

21 Insert the flap 2 days later.

22 Thin the flap 3 months later, if necessary, by excising the subcutaneous tissue in stages.

TENSOR FASCIA LATA FLAP

Appraise

1 This flap is useful in treating trochanteric pressure sores and defects of the groin, particularly when the femoral vessels are exposed.

2 It can also be used for ischial pressure sores and defects of the upper thigh and lower abdominal wall.

3 It is a myofasciocutaneous flap and is based on the vessels to the tensor fascia lata muscle.

4 Inclusion of the lateral cutaneous nerve of the thigh within the flap allows it to be used as a sensory flap.

Action

1 Place the patient supine on the table, rotate the pelvis through 30 degrees and support this and the leg on the side of the defect.

2 Create and measure the defect in the groin.

3 Identify the site of entry into the muscle of its vascular pedicle, the transverse branch of the lateral femoral circumflex artery. This point is 8 cm distal and just lateral to the anterior superior iliac spine.

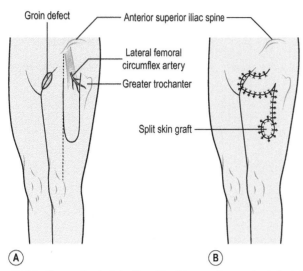

Fig. 33.24 Tensor fascia lata flap. Used to repair a groin defect, the anterior margin of the flap is marked on a line from the anterior superior iliac spine to the lateral border of the patella (A). After transposition of the flap, the donor site is closed primarily although the distal portion may require a split skin graft (B).

4 Keep this point in the base of the flap.

5 Draw a line from the anterior superior iliac spine to the lateral margin of the patella and use this as the anterior margin of the flap.

6 Mark the posterior margin of the flap using a width of 6–10 cm (Fig. 33.24).

7 Mark the distal extremity of the flap so that it is not more than two-thirds of the length of the thigh. Check that the flap will reach the defect.

8 Incise the skin distally down to the deep fascia.

9 Incise the skin on the anterior and posterior margins and elevate the flap together with the fascia lata.

10 As the flap is reflected proximally, the tensor fascia lata muscle comes into view. If necessary, divide any small distal vascular pedicle into the muscle after first identifying the large vascular pedicle proximally.

11 Check that the flap will rotate into the defect.

12 Incise the skin between the flap and the defect, and undermine it on either side, allowing the flap to lie in this defect.

13 Excise any excess thigh skin to allow the flap to sit comfortably.

14 Suture the flap into place.

15 Close the donor defect primarily as far as possible.

16 Take a skin graft from the opposite thigh and apply it to the residual flap donor defect.

17 Dress the graft and its donor site with paraffin gauze, dressing gauze, cotton wool and crepe bandage.

18 Leave the flap exposed and nurse the patient on his contralateral side.

BICEPS FEMORIS FLAP

Appraise

1 This flap is particularly useful for ischial pressure sores.

2 It is a myocutaneous flap but can be used as a simple muscle flap.

3 The biceps femoris muscle receives a segmental blood supply from several vessels which are branches of the profunda femoris artery. In order to preserve all these vessels the flap is transferred as an advancement flap.

4 An advantage of this flap is that it can be advanced more than once.

Action

1 Place the patient prone on the table.

2 Create the defect by excising the whole lining to the ischial pressure sore cavity. With an osteotome reduce the prominence of the ischial tuberosity.

3 Draw a line from the ischial tuberosity to the head of the fibula. Use this as the axis of the flap and mark an elliptiform flap, 8–10 cm broad around this, extending proximally to the defect and distally to within 5 cm of the crease of the knee joint (Fig. 33.25).

4 Incise along the lines down to the margins of the biceps femoris muscle.

5 Divide the origins of the biceps femoris, semitendinosus and semimembranosus muscles at the ischial tuberosity.

6 Divide the biceps femoris tendon at the distal margin of the flap. Divide the semimembranosus and semitendinosus distally if necessary to provide greater mobility of the flap.

7 Advance the flap into the defect and suture the muscle to obliterate the dead space.

8 Suture the skin of the flap into the skin defect after inserting a large suction drain.

9 Suture the distal portion of the flap defect primarily and apply minimal dressings.

10 Nurse the patient on the contralateral side.

11 Leave the sutures in place for at least 3 weeks.

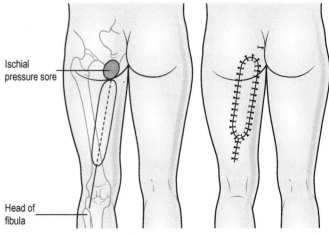

Fig. 33.25 Biceps femoris flap. The flap is drawn with its axis on a line between the ischial tuberosity and the head of the fibula (A). After excising the pressure sore and trimming the bone, the origins and insertion of the long head of the biceps femoris, semitendinosus and semimembranosus are divided. The skin and underlying muscle are advanced into the defect, closing the distant donor site primarily (B).

GASTROCNEMIUS FLAP

Appraise

1. Both heads of the gastrocnemius muscle can be used separately for covering defects on the anterior aspect of the leg.

2. They can be used as simple muscle flaps or as myocutaneous flaps.

3. The flaps are used for covering exposed bone in the upper third of the tibia and for covering the exposed knee joint, sometimes even in the presence of a metal prosthesis.

4. The muscle flap alone is more malleable and versatile than a myocutaneous flap.

5. Although the lateral head is slightly longer, use the nearest muscle head to the defect. Do not use both heads simultaneously.

Action

1. Place the patient in the lateral position, with the affected leg uppermost.

2. Mark out and create the defect.

3. Make a vertical incision through skin and subcutaneous tissue down the midline of the calf, posteriorly.

4. Identify the muscle bellies of gastrocnemius and their relevant attachments to the tendo calcaneus (Fig. 33.26).

5. Separate the fascia overlying the respective belly of the muscle to be used.

6. Incise the tendon just distal to the muscle attachment.

7. Elevate the muscle belly proximally by dissecting laterally and medially, dividing its attachment to the opposite belly.

8. Free the muscle belly to the level of the popliteal fossa, preserving the vascular pedicle passing into it.

9. Create a subcutaneous tunnel from the base of the muscle belly to the defect and enlarge to accommodate the muscle flap.

10. Pass the muscle belly through this tunnel into the defect.

11. Suture the muscle to the edges of the defect.

12. Close the donor defect in layers and insert a suction drain.

13. Take a thick split skin graft from the thigh and apply it to the exposed muscle in the defect.

14. Splint the leg for 10 days.

15. Allow weight-bearing at 10 days and mobilize progressively. Fit an elastic support stocking to cover the graft overlying the muscle. This should be worn for 3 months.

FASCIOCUTANEOUS FLAP

Appraise

1. These flaps have their greatest use in providing skin cover to exposed bone in the middle third of the leg.

2. When based proximally, they may not be true axial pattern flaps but depend on preserving the rich vascular network lying superficial to the deep fascia.

3. You may use flaps with a 3:1 or more length-to-breadth ratio.

4. With intimate knowledge of the anatomy of the vessels which perforate the deep fascia, long flaps based distally can be designed and may be useful in covering the exposed distal third of the tibia.

Action

1. Mark out and create the defect.

2. Mark out the flap based proximally with a 2:1 ratio.

3. Check that the flap will reach the defect when transposed (Fig. 33.27).

4. Incise the flap distally, passing through skin, subcutaneous tissue and deep fascia.

5. Elevate the flap proximally, incising along the lateral margins and preserving the deep fascia with the flap.

6. Transpose the flap into the defect.

7. Suture the flap into the defect in layers.

8. Take a split graft from the opposite thigh.

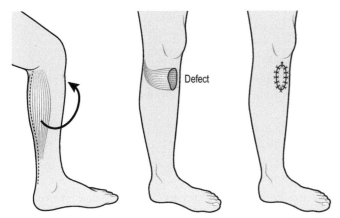

Fig. 33.26 Gastrocnemius flap: (A) a defect in the region of the tibial tuberosity can be covered with the medial head of the gastrocnemius; (B) the flap is raised through a posterior midline incision and passed subcutaneously into the defect; (C) a split skin graft is placed over the muscle within the defect.

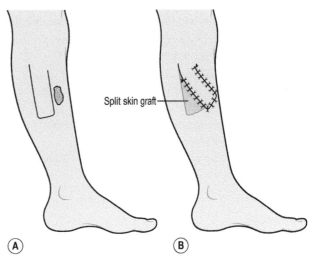

Fig. 33.27 Fasciocutaneous flap: (A) a small defect on the anterior aspect of the leg can be covered with a medially based fasciocutaneous flap; (B) the flap is transposed into the defect and a split skin graft is placed on the donor defect.

9 Apply the split skin graft to the flap donor defect. Dress with paraffin gauze and dressing gauze and retain with tie-over sutures.

10 Leave the flap exposed so that it can be monitored.

TISSUE EXPANSION

Appraise

1 The principle of tissue expansion is exemplified by the stretched abdominal wall resulting from pregnancy.

2 A tissue expander (Fig. 33.28) is inserted beneath the deep fascia or superficial muscle and expanded serially by injections of saline into an attached reservoir to stretch the overlying skin.

3 Following expansion, the expander is removed and the surplus skin used to cover the adjacent defect.

4 Expanders are most effective when placed on a bone base. They are particularly effective when placed on the calvaria (Latin: = skull) to expand scalp, and on the chest wall to expand skin for breast reconstruction. They have limited value in limbs.

> ► KEY POINT Is the skin healthy and normal?

> ■ Do not use tissue expanders under badly scarred or irradiated skin.

5 There are some more sophisticated tissue expanders available specifically designed for breast reconstruction. Some of these have a double lumen, one of which is filled with silicone. Others have a reservoir that can be detached from a valve linking it to the expander, allowing the expander to be left in situ.

Action

1 Identify an area of normal skin to be expanded which is adjacent to the defect.

2 Choose an appropriate tissue expander whose base will lie within the boundaries defined.

3 Make an incision beyond the chosen area in a radial direction.

4 Attach the reservoir to the expander and insert saline. Remove air from the system and check its patency.

5 Make an appropriate pocket for the expander and insert it. This pocket should be submuscular or subfascial, but may be subcutaneous.

6 Make a separate pocket for the reservoir in a suitable accessible adjacent subcutaneous area and insert it.

7 Recheck the patency of the system and close the wound.

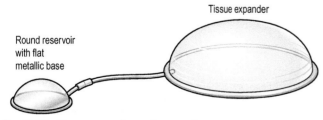

Tissue expander

Round reservoir
with flat
metallic base

Fig. 33.28 Tissue expander and reservoir.

8 Serially inject saline into the reservoir as an outpatient procedure.

9 When sufficient expansion or more has been achieved, re-admit the patient for the second stage.

10 Remove the expander and stretch the expanded skin over the defect.

GRAFTS OF OTHER TISSUES

CARTILAGE GRAFTS

1 Cartilage grafts are used in reconstructing cartilaginous defects of the nose, large defects of the lower eyelids and major defects of the ear.

2 Total reconstruction of an ear is technically extremely challenging. Do not attempt it if you are not experienced in this form of operation.

NOSE

1 Composite defects of skin and cartilage at the nostril margin can be reconstructed using composite grafts from the ear, as described under composite skin grafts (see above).

2 Most other small cartilaginous defects of the nose can be reconstructed using cartilage from other parts of the nose during a corrective rhinoplasty.

3 If there is extensive cartilaginous loss and the nasal tip requires support, take an L-shaped bone graft from the iliac crest and insert it through a midcolumellar incision.

4 More sophisticated techniques include the insertion of homograft cartilage (see below) or calvarial bone graft inserted from above after reflecting a bicoronal scalp flap.

EYELIDS

1 You rarely need to provide cartilage support for the upper eyelid.

2 Large defects of the lower eyelid often require the introduction of cartilage for support and the best donor site for this is the septum of the nose. This provides a composite graft of cartilage and mucous membrane. The latter is used to reconstruct the conjunctival surface.

Action

1 Create the defect and measure it.

2 Mark an appropriate area of the septum using a nasal speculum, commencing at least 3 mm behind the anterior limit of the septum.

3 Infiltrate the marked area with 0.5% lidocaine and 1:200 000 adrenaline (epinephrine).

4 Infiltrate the septum on the opposite side with the same preparation.

5 After allowing at least 7 minutes for the adrenaline (epinephrine) to take effect, incise the mucosa, passing through this and the underlying cartilage but avoid penetrating the nasal mucosa on the contralateral side.

6 Separate the contralateral nasal mucosa from the cartilage using a mucosal elevator.

7 Cut around the full margin of the graft and remove it.

8 Stop the bleeding with pressure for 5 minutes timed by the clock.

■ Avoid diathermy; it can cause necrosis and subsequent perforation in the residual mucosal surface.

9 Insert the graft into the defect and stabilize it with an absorbable suture through the cartilage at each margin.

10 Suture the conjunctival surface with 6/0 absorbable suture.

11 Suture the skin with 6/0 nylon.

EAR

1 Costal cartilage is used for total ear reconstruction.

2 Reconstruction of a major portion of the ear may be difficult. It is sometimes justifiable to discard those cartilaginous segments already present and perform a total ear reconstruction.

3 If there is inadequate skin available, you must employ pre-operative tissue expansion (see above) or use a temporoparietal flap.

Action

1 Measure the normal ear and make a template for the new ear.

2 Make a straight, oblique incision over the medial end of the seventh and eighth costal cartilages.

3 Retract the skin and subcutaneous tissue and expose an area of cartilage equivalent to the size and shape of the ear.

4 Mark out an outline of cartilage from the template using the seventh and eighth costal cartilages and excise this.

5 Close the donor defect in layers.

6 Place the graft on a wooden board on a table and carefully shape the cartilage, creating a well-defined helical rim and an antihelical fold.

7 Make an incision along the hairline of the posterior margin of the auricular skin where it meets hair-bearing scalp skin.

8 Create a subcutaneous pocket beneath the auricular skin to accommodate the cartilage graft.

9 Insert the graft and close the skin.

10 Insert sutures through the skin in the region of the scaphoid fossa and concha, to highlight the contour of the grafts.

11 After 6 months, reflect forwards the cartilage graft together with the underlying subcutaneous tissue and insert a split skin graft on to the posterior surface of the reconstructed ear and the postauricular region to create a postauricular sulcus.

VASCULAR GRAFTS

Appraise

1 Large vascular grafts are described in Chapter 23. Employ small-vessel grafts for replanting and free-flap transfer. They are occasionally used when limb vessels have been injured.

2 Vein grafts are used to replace both damaged arteries and veins.

3 Choose a vein graft that matches the vessel that has been destroyed.

4 Use magnification for the repair and a microscope when repairing grafts under 2 mm in diameter.

Action

1 Identify the length of vessel that has been damaged.

2 Place an appropriate size clamp on normal vessel on either side of the damaged section and resect this damaged section.

3 Inspect the cut ends under magnification and check that the endothelium is normal. If it is not, resect further.

4 Check that there is good flow of blood from the cut proximal arterial stump, or the cut distal venous stump, by holding the adventitia of the vessel with jeweller's forceps, and temporarily releasing the clamp.

5 Select a superficial vein of appropriate size and length for insertion as a graft into the defect. For vessels greater than 2 mm diameter, use the long saphenous vein, which is the best available vein graft for both arteries and veins. For vessels smaller than this, use veins from the dorsum of the foot or from the flexor aspect of the forearm.

6 Make an incision through the skin directly over the full length of the chosen vein.

7 By blunt dissection, isolate the full length of the vein to be used.

8 Ligate all branches of the vein graft or use the bipolar coagulator to seal minute branches. Do not use unipolar diathermy, which will damage the graft.

9 Isolate a segment of vein graft longer than that required. Ligate and divide the vessel proximally and distally.

10 Remove the graft and irrigate it gently with warm heparinized Hartmann's solution or saline to exclude leaks.

11 Place the graft in the site of the defect, ensuring that the blood flow in the graft will be in the usual direction.

12 Choose an appropriate double clamp. Place one portion of this clamp on the proximal end of the divided normal vessel and the other on the vein graft.

13 Under magnification, clean the adventitia from the vessel walls of both stumps using small scissors.

14 Flush the stumps with heparinized Hartmann's solution, being careful not to grasp the endothelium with forceps.

15 Dilate the vessel with vessel dilators and approximate the ends.

16 Suture the anterior wall with interrupted 8/0 or 10/0 nylon sutures. Turn the clamp over and suture the opposite wall.

17 Before inserting the final two sutures, check that the anastomosis is patent.

18 Carry out a similar anastomosis at the distal end, checking that the graft has been stretched to its original length and that there is no torsion.

19 Remove the distal clamps first and then remove the proximal clamps.

20 If there is small leak at either anastomosis, cover it with a warm swab but do not occlude the vessel.

21 If there is a gross leak, reapply a single clamp to obstruct the flow and insert extra sutures. Remove the clamp and observe.

22 If flow is not established, resect the anastomosis and repeat.

OTHER GRAFTS

1 Nerve grafts, tendon grafts and bone grafts are described in Chapter 30.

2 Homograft (Greek: *homos* = same; from the same species) bone, xenograft (Greek: *xenos* = strange, foreign; from a different species) cartilage and xenograft collagen are all used, after appropriate preparation, in reconstruction. Theoretically, they act as a scaffold into which the patient's own tissue grows. The benefit with xenograft cartilage and xenograft collagen may be only temporary as the graft tends to be absorbed.

3 Homograft and xenograft skin may be used as temporary biological dressings in burns, but they are eventually rejected.

MICROVASCULAR SURGERY

1 Microvascular surgery involves the anastomosis and repair of small vessels.

2 It has clinical application in cases of re-plantation and free tissue transfer.

3 The surgery is highly specialized. Operations may take many hours and require special instruments in addition to an appropriate microscope.

4 This type of operation should be carried out only in specialized units.

REPLANTATION

Appraise

Consider re-plantation following accidental amputation or devascularization of any of the following parts:
- Limbs proximal to the ankle or wrist joints: this is called macroreplantation
- Parts of limbs distal to the ankle or wrist joint: this is called microreplantation
- The ear
- The scalp
- The penis
- Composite pieces of facial tissue.

Action

1 Control bleeding from the amputation stump by simple pressure and elevation.

2 Avoid clamping vessels to stop haemorrhage unless essential, as this may cause unnecessary damage.

> ▶ KEY POINTS Care of the amputated part to be replanted

- The part to be re-implanted should have been placed in a polythene bag, which is laid on ice.
- Cool but do not freeze the amputated part since freezing prevents successful re-plantation.
- If a part is devascularized and not fully amputated, cool this part by placing polythene bags containing ice around it.

3 Contact the nearest microvascular surgery unit and take advice.

4 Prepare the patient and amputated part for urgent transfer.

MACROREPLANTATION

Appraise

1 The force required to sever a major portion of a limb is considerable and patients who have suffered such an injury may have other injuries to their body which may take priority in treatment.

2 Criteria for attempting re-plantation are:
- The patient should be relatively fit
- The amputated portion should not be too severely damaged
- The 'warm ischaemic time' of the amputated part should not exceed 6 hours. Muscle is unlikely to recover after this period and if it is revascularized it could infuse a fatal dose of nephrotoxic substances, including myoglobin, into the circulation
- There should be a reasonable prospect of some functional recovery.

Action

1 Debride and clean both the proximal stump and the wound of the amputated part.

2 Shorten the skeletal structures and fix these. This should allow primary anastomosis of vessels and nerves.

3 Revascularize the amputated part by anastomosing the appropriate artery, or arteries, using vein grafts if necessary.

4 If the warm ischaemic time has been relatively long, revascularize the part prior to skeletal fixation. Allow perfusion of the amputated part for several minutes, discarding the venous blood. Transfuse the patient appropriately. Revise the anastomoses after skeletal fixation if necessary.

5 Anastomose twice the number of veins as the number of arteries repaired, again using vein grafts if necessary.

6 Repair the tendons and muscles.

7 Repair the nerves.

8 Carry out extensive fasciotomies, incising through skin, subcutaneous tissue and deep fascia on the proximal stump and on the amputated part.

9 Harvest a split skin graft and apply this to the fasciotomy sites and any other residual raw areas where there has been skin loss.

10 Monitor the limb carefully postoperatively, and be prepared to return the patient to theatre at any time if there is doubt about viability of the replanted or revascularized part.

FREE TISSUE TRANSFER

Appraise

1 Free tissue transfer is used in many forms of reconstruction. It consists of transferring tissue from one part of the body to another.

2 Isolate the tissue on a recognized vascular pedicle and, after transfer to its distant site, anastomose the vessels of the vascular pedicle to appropriate nearby vessels, either directly or with vein grafts.

3 The arterial supply to the tissue is usually established with an end-to-side anastomosis to an adjacent artery, so that the distal flow of this artery is not terminated.

4 The venous drainage of the tissue is usually established via end-to-end anastomoses to superficial veins or to venae comitantes of a nearby artery. Occasionally, if the venous drainage is inadequate, you can apply leeches to the compromised tissue temporarily until adequate venous drainage is established.

5 Most free flaps currently used in reconstruction consist of cutaneous or myocutaneous flaps. Apart from the flaps described above there are many other cutaneous and myocutaneous flaps which are occasionally used.

6 Other free tissue transfers include the following:
- Vascularized bone grafts from rib, iliac crest, fibula, radius and metatarsal
- Osseocutaneous flaps from the iliac crest, fibula, radius or metatarsal with overlying skin
- Sensory cutaneous flaps
- Muscle flaps with motor innervation
- Fascial flaps
- Small bowel, for oesophageal reconstruction
- Omentum, for soft tissue defects
- Testis, re-siting a high undescended testicle in the scrotum
- Digits or parts of digits from toe to hand.

7 One of the most common free flaps used in reconstruction is the radial forearm flap. It is based on the radial artery and either the venae comitantes or superficial veins, usually the cephalic, can be used for venous drainage.

8 The flap can be raised as a fasciocutaneous flap providing a small, thin, pliable flap useful in intraoral reconstruction, as an osseo-cutaneous flap for bone reconstruction, or simply as a fascial flap with a skin graft for covering small soft tissue defects on the limbs.

9 It is only occasionally used as a pedicled flap, although in these circumstances it may be based distally for use in the hand. Its elevation for use as a free flap is described below (Fig. 33.29).

Action

1 Perform an Allen's test prior to surgery to confirm that the ulnar artery alone will provide sufficient blood flow to the hand. The

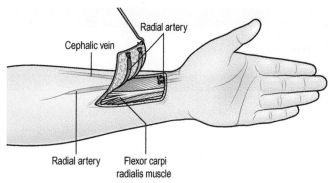

Fig. 33.29 Radial forearm flap. In elevating the flap from the medial aspect, the radial artery (RA) is identified distally, lateral to the flexor carpi radialis muscle (FCR) and divided. As the flap is raised the cephalic vein (CV) is also divided distally.

radial and ulnar arteries are occluded to the raised, fisted hand, which then appears pale on opening it if either artery is released. The whole hand should flush within 10 seconds.

2 Use a template of the defect to determine the size and shape of the flap to be harvested. Mark this out on the ventral aspect of the forearm with the distal limit extending to within 2 cm of the wrist joint. Check that the flap overlies the radial artery, which can be palpated. Confirm that the distal end of the cephalic artery also lies within the area of the flap.

3 Exsanguinate the limb with elevation alone and apply the tourniquet.

4 Raise the flap from the medial side first and include the underlying fascia.

5 Dissect laterally, raising the fascia but being careful not to remove the paratenon of the flexor tendons.

6 Beyond the flexor carpi radialis retain the loose areolar tissue passing down to the radial artery and its accompanying venae comitantes and include these with the flap.

7 Isolate and divide these vessels distally beyond the distal limit of the flap.

8 Continue the dissection laterally by dividing the flap at its distal and then its lateral border preserving, if possible, the branches of the radial nerve by dissecting these out from the under surface of the flap.

9 Identify the radial artery and cephalic vein in the proximal attachment of the flap. Divide the skin proximally with one longitudinal incision, keeping these in sight.

10 Dissect the cephalic vein up to the cubital fossa.

11 Dissect the radial artery up to its origin from the brachial artery if this length of artery is required.

12 When appropriate, divide and clamp the artery and vein and transfer the flap.

13 Ligate the stumps of the two vessels.

14 Repair the donor defect with a split skin graft and immobilize.

15 If you are experienced you may wish to use a transposition, rotation or other local flap to close the donor defect primarily.

16 Dress the donor site and subsequently remove sutures as appropriate.

BURNS

Appraise

> ▶ KEY POINTS Special circumstances
>
> ■ Treat patients with burns involving 15% of the body surface area (10% in children), or severe burns of the face or hands in a specialized burns unit.
> ■ Treat patients with any significant inhalation burn in a specialized unit.

1 The treatment of patients with extensive burns is complex and ideally these patients should also be treated initially in an intensive care unit.

2 Either colloid or crystalloid can be used in fluid replacement but the principle of using the former is described below.

Assess

1 Take a careful history, paying attention to the time and nature of the accident. Was smoke present and did the accident occur in an enclosed space? Note what kinds of clothes were worn by the patient and what first aid was given.

2 Find out the patient's normal medication.

3 Examine, looking for signs of an inhalation burn. Record the extent and distribution of superficial and full-thickness burns. Pinprick sensation is usually preserved in superficial burns but do not rely on it.

4 The best guide to the depth of burn is found by taking an accurate history of the mechanism of the burn:
   ■ Thermal burns with gases usually cause superficial burns.
   ■ Thermal burns with liquids usually cause deep dermal burns. Boiling water and fat cause full-thickness burns. Boiling water that has cooled for 5 minutes causes superficial burns.
   ■ Contact with hot solids and flames usually causes full-thickness burns.
   ■ Electrical burns usually cause full-thickness skin loss.
   ■ Radiation burns are usually superficial.
   ■ Chemical burns are usually superficial.

5 Estimate the area of the burn using a Lund and Browder chart or 'the rule of nines'.

6 Examine the patient to exclude other injuries.

7 Weigh the patient.

Action

1 Give oxygen if you suspect an inhalation burn. Consider ventilation, particularly if the blood PO_2 is low (normal range 10.5–13.5 kPa).

2 Set up a reliable intravenous line after taking blood for a full blood count and biochemical profile.

3 Catheterize and record the urine output hourly.

4 Give PPF (plasma protein fraction) using a Muir and Barclay formula as a guide to the volume to give to replace plasma lost through the burn. This involves giving a volume in millilitres of half the weight in kilograms multiplied by the percentage burn

in each of six periods. These periods start at the time of the burn and include three of 4 hours, two of 6 hours and one of 12 hours. Use the packed cell volume (PCV), urinary output and clinical state of the patient to adjust the volume of PPF given.

5 Prescribe appropriate medication, including:
   ■ Adequate analgesia
   ■ Adequate anti-emetics
   ■ H_2-receptor antagonists
   ■ Adjust the doses of insulin, steroids or anticonvulsants if given previously.

6 Do not give antibiotics for the burn per se but reserve these for use later.

7 Treat the burn wounds according to their depth.

SUPERFICIAL BURNS

Action

1 Clean the burn wound and remove the roof of all blisters.

2 Expose superficial burns of the face but apply sterile liquid paraffin to reduce crusting.

3 For burns of the perineum, clean these and expose but apply silver sulfadiazine (Flamazine) cream. Nurse the patient without dressings on a sterile sheet on a low-air-loss or water bed but keep him warm.

4 Cover superficial burns of other areas with two layers of paraffin gauze and a bulky absorptive dressing. Leave this dressing for 1 week unless it becomes soaked, whereupon you should change it. Change the dressing at 1 week and subsequently twice per week until the wound is healed.

DEEP DERMAL BURNS

1 Tangentially shave with a graft knife between the second and fifth day.

2 Continue to shave until you observe punctate bleeding from the surface.

3 Achieve haemostasis with pressure and apply a split skin graft.

4 Re-dress at 4 days.

5 When fully healed, measure and apply a pressure garment. This is an elasticated garment specifically measured for the individual to cover the area of the burn wound. Advise the patient to wear this for 6 months or longer if necessary, to minimize hypertrophy and contracture of the resulting scars.

6 If you do not have facilities or expertise for this management, treat the burn conservatively and re-dress twice each week.

7 Treat areas that are not healed at 3 weeks as full-thickness burns.

EXTENSIVE FULL-THICKNESS BURNS

ESCHAROTOMY

1 Note the areas of full-thickness burns that are circumferential around digit, limb or trunk. If the viability of the distal part is jeopardized, or if respiration is hindered, as with partial

circumferential burns of the chest wall, carry out an escharotomy (Greek: *eschara* = a hearth; the mark of a burn).

2 Give an appropriate intravenous dose of diazepam.

3 Take a scalpel and incise along the full length of the full-thickness burn, allowing subcutaneous fat to bulge out of the escharotomy wound.

4 Repeat the longitudinal escharotomy at different sites of the circumference until you have restored satisfactory perfusion of the distal part.

5 Dress the wounds with paraffin gauze or silver sulfadiazine (Flamazine).

ACTION

1 Identify a suitable area, not exceeding 20% of the body area, to treat primarily.

2 Identify a suitable donor site for the skin graft.

3 Excise the chosen area of full-thickness burn with a scalpel and be sure that the resultant bed consists of viable tissue. It is often safer to excise all subcutaneous fat to leave a graft bed of deep fascia. Achieve haemostasis.

4 Harvest a split skin graft and mesh this (see above).

5 Apply the mesh graft to the burn wound site and dress with several layers of paraffin gauze and an absorbent dressing.

6 Re-dress after 4 days.

> ▶ KEY POINT Importance of timing
>
> ■ Do not excise burn tissue between the fifth and the twelfth day post-burn, as the patient may be in an unsuitable catabolic state.

7 Do not excise further burn until the donor site has healed and is ready for reharvesting, or another donor site is available.

SMALL AREAS

1 Operate between the second and fifth day.

2 Excise all burn tissue and apply a split skin graft.

3 If the viability of subcutaneous fat is in doubt, excise this down to the deep fascia.

4 If the viability of the tissue is still in doubt, dress the wound and bring the patient back to the theatre 48 hours later. Re-assess viability at this second operation. Excise further if necessary and graft.

5 Re-dress after 4 days.

OTHER WOUNDS

1 Do not close infected wounds primarily. They arise in a multitude of different situations.

2 Two common causes presenting to plastic surgeons include pressure sores and necrotizing fasciitis. Their management is described below.

WOUNDS FROM PRESSURE INJURIES

Appraise

1 Pressure injuries are common and difficult to detect in the early stages of development. The tissues between the skeleton and an external surface are compressed, causing a variable degree of ischaemia, which may be sufficient to cause necrosis. Necrosis may involve the superficial skin, the full thickness of skin or all the tissues overlying the skeleton.

2 Pressure injuries can occur in many sites but are most frequently found in well-recognized 'pressure areas' over the backs of the heels and around the pelvis, over the ischial tuberosity, the sacrum and the greater trochanter.

3 They result from the patient lying on or against a hard surface for a prolonged period. They may occur when the patient is comatose or under general anaesthesia or when the area is insensate, as in diabetic neuropathy or paraplegia. They are more likely to occur in these circumstances if the patient is thin, poorly nourished, cachectic and relatively immobile. Some surgical patients are therefore at particular risk.

4 There may be no significant evidence of the injury for some time after the event. Usually the first sign is erythema in the damaged area. Blistering usually indicates a superficial injury only. If the damage is deep the skin colour changes to blue and then to black as a thick eschar develops over a period of many days. This remains dry for several weeks before the necrotic tissue starts to separate.

5 Spontaneous separation of the underlying necrotic tissue may take many weeks or even months. When the necrotic tissue has separated, the wound will heal by secondary intention. A residual sinus will persist if necrotic tissue remains buried or if the underlying bone becomes infected.

6 As many patients with these injuries are debilitated, the above process may take many months and treatment is aimed at accelerating the healing process without insulting the patient further with unnecessary surgery.

Action

1 Avoid these injuries by identifying those patients particularly at risk.

2 Attend to their general health, specifically their nutrition and other medical disorders.

3 Take appropriate precautions when they are on the operating table and when in bed on the ward. Use one of the many specialized mattresses or beds to distribute the weight of the patient where possible. If these are not available the nursing staff may need to assist a change of position of the patient at least every 2 hours.

4 Cover superficial wounds with non-adherent dressings such as paraffin gauze and change on alternate days until healed.

5 Cover hard eschar with simple protective dressings only, or leave exposed if appropriate.

6 When the eschar starts to separate use a debriding agent such as Eusol and paraffin dressings changed daily.

7 Assist separation of the eschar by using a forceps and scissors during a dressing change. Repeat this with every change of dressing and avoid formal debridement in theatre and an unnecessary general anaesthetic.

8 Take wound swabs at regular intervals to monitor the organisms present but use antibiotics sparingly, for example if there is evidence of surrounding cellulitis.

9 Advise the patient to have a regular bath or shower, if appropriate, to help clean the wound and improve the patient's morale.

10 When a cavity is established use a vacuum dressing. After irrigating and cleaning the wound with saline, insert the foam dressing, introduce the drain and cover with an occlusive dressing. Apply negative pressure to the drain via the pump and leave for 2–3 days before repeating.

11 If a vacuum pump is not available, change the dressings to calcium alginate when the necrotic tissue has separated and a surface layer of red granulation tissue is evident. Change this daily.

12 If a large cavity persists consider introducing a large cutaneous or myocutaneous flap (see above, Rotation flap, Biceps femoris flap, Tensor fascia lata flap).

13 Also consider continuing with dressings until healed, avoiding surgery and allowing uninterrupted mobilization.

NECROTIZING FASCIITIS

Appraise

> **KEY POINT** Recognize and act

- If the patient is to survive you must make an early diagnosis and act immediately.

1 This is a rare condition but you must recognize it immediately as serious and life-threatening.

2 There is a focal point where the infection commences, and this often arises from a surgical intervention.

3 The condition results usually from the symbiotic effect of the co-incidental occurrence of an aerobic staphylococcus and an anaerobic streptococcus.

4 The bacteria appear to spread initially and preferentially along fascial planes. The overlying subcutaneous fat and skin are subsequently rendered ischaemic and necrotic.

Action

1 Look out for:
- Unexpected local cellulitis
- Rapidly expanding cellulitis
- Deteriorating general condition.

2 Take wound swabs and blood specimens for culture of organism and sensitivities.

3 Commence on appropriate antibiotics.

4 Mark the edge of the area of erythema on the skin.

5 If the area of erythema is seen to progress beyond the marked line within a few hours, take the patient to theatre immediately.

6 Use a cutting diathermy to remove all skin showing erythema as well as underlying subcutaneous fat and deep fascia.

7 Remove any tissue suspicious of being involved in the infective process.

8 Dress the wound with gauze soaked in saline and further absorbent dressings, leaving the skin adjacent to the wound available for inspection.

9 Take the patient back to theatre after 24 hours, or earlier if there are signs of progression of the disease.

10 Carry out further debridement of infected tissue.

11 Repeat this after a further 24 hours, remaining vigilant until all signs of infection have been eradicated.

12 When the patient is stable, consider covering the residual defect with split skin grafts or skin flaps or a combination of these.

FACIAL CLEFTS

> **KEY POINTS**

- These descriptions are reminders for surgeons working in isolation but who have been trained in the procedures. They are also included for trainees helping at operations who can offer intelligent and effective assistance at these highly skilled procedures.
- Do not attempt them if you are inexpert because you may create disastrous results.

CLEFT LIP

Appraise

1 The treatment of clefts of the lip and palate may be very complex. Refer patients for treatment at specialist centres with a paediatrician, a paediatric anaesthetist, an orthodontist, an ENT surgeon, an oral surgeon, a dentist, an audiologist and a speech therapist as well as the plastic surgeon.

2 The extent of the cleft of the lip is variable and ranges from a slight notch in the vermilion border to a complete cleft of the whole lip.

3 The cleft may be bilateral and there may be an associated cleft of the palate.

4 Midline clefts of the lip, with absence of philtrum (Greek: *philtron* = love potion; median groove of upper lip) and columella (Latin: = a little column) and associated hypoteleorism, are rare. Refer patients to a specialized unit, as also those with rare oblique clefts of the face involving the lip.

5 Repair clefts of the lip at 3 months of age or soon after birth.

6 If the cleft is bilateral, repair the two sides separately with a 1-month interval between operations. Repair the more severe cleft first.

7 A prominent philtrum, particularly obvious in bilateral cleft lips, can be corrected preoperatively with orthodontic appliances. If these are not available, apply simple Elastoplast strapping from cheek to cheek across the prominent philtrum, to help reduce it before operation.

8 There are many techniques for repairing a cleft of the lip, but the Millard repair as described below is popular. The steps are outlined.

Prepare

1 Identify the midpoint of the philtrum on its vermilion border, and mark (Fig. 33.30, point 1).

2 Identify the vermilion border at the base of the normal philtral column and mark (point 2).

3 Mark the corresponding point on the vermilion border at the base of the projected contralateral philtral column (point 3).

4 Mark the midpoint of the junction of the columella with the philtrum (point 4).

5 On the lateral segment of the lip, mark the vermilion border at a point where the white roll disappears (point 5).

6 On the lateral segment, mark the most medial point of normal skin, horizontally level with the base of the nostril (point 6).

7 Draw a straight line between points 5 and 6 and a curved line between points 3 and 4 of equal length.

8 Infiltrate the area with local anaesthesia using 0.5% lidocaine and 1: 200 000 adrenaline (epinephrine).

Action

1 With a size no. 11 blade, cut through the full thickness of the lip along the curved line of the medial segment.

2 Excise the mucosal surface lateral to this, preserving a small triangular flap of normal skin (the 'C' flap).

3 Excise the mucosa medial to the straight line on the lateral segment.

4 Incise the lateral segment from point 6 laterally around the base of the ala.

5 Reflect back the skin and identify the muscles inserted into the alar base.

6 Divide these muscles and dissect them free from their attachment to the alar base.

7 Identify and dissect free the muscle in the medial segment.

8 Suture together the orbicularis oris muscle from each segment with 4/0 absorbable suture.

9 Approximate the skin using 6/0 polyglactin as a subcutaneous suture.

10 Approximate point 6 to point 4.

11 Approximate point 5 to point 3.

12 Use the 'C' flap to create a nostril sill.

13 Suture the skin with 6/0 nylon.

14 Suture the skin and mucosa within the nostril with 6/0 polyglactin.

15 Adjust the mucosa of the lip and suture. If necessary incorporate a small Z-plasty.

16 Remove sutures at 3–4 days.

CLEFT PALATE

Appraise

1 A cleft palate often occurs in conjunction with a cleft lip, but may occur separately.

2 The extent of the cleft palate varies from a complete cleft to a submucous cleft, where the palate is apparently intact but there has been failure of fusion of the levator palati muscles across the midline.

3 Repair the muscle in submucous clefts of the palate to ensure satisfactory function of the palate during speech.

4 Repair clefts of the palate at about 6 months of age to restore the speech mechanism to normal as early as is practical.

5 The bone defect may be constructed with a bone graft after the secondary dentition has erupted.

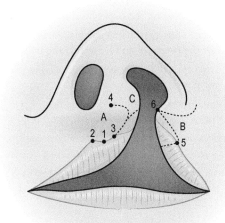

(A)

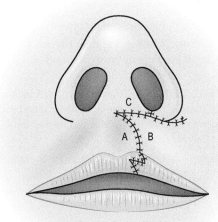

(B)

Fig. 33.30 Cleft lip—the Millard repair: point 1 is the centre of the Cupid's bow; point 2 is the peak of the Cupid's bow on the normal side; point 3 is the projected point of the peak of the Cupid's bow on the cleft side; point 4 is the junction of the midpoint of the philtrum and columella; point 5 is the start of the mucosal thickening of the cleft side; point 6 is the medial extremity of the alar base on the cleft side. The dashed lines indicate the incisions (A). Flaps A and B have been sutured into place and flap C is used to create the nostril sill. A Z-plasty has been introduced into the vermilion mucosa (B).

Prepare

1. Insert a suitable mouth gag such as the Dingman.
2. Pack the pharynx with ribbon gauze.
3. Mark out bilateral flaps on the palate passing from the uvula along the side of the cleft to its apex and anteriorly along the midline to within 3 mm of the alveolus (Fig. 33.31).
4. Continue marking laterally, keeping just within the margin of the alveolus and passing backwards behind the hamulus to the anterior pillar of the fauces.
5. Infiltrate the flaps with 0.5% lidocaine and 1:200 000 adrenaline (epinephrine).

Action

1. Incise along the marked edges of one flap, commencing at the tip of the split uvula.
2. Elevate the flap from its anterior margin as a mucoperiosteal flap.

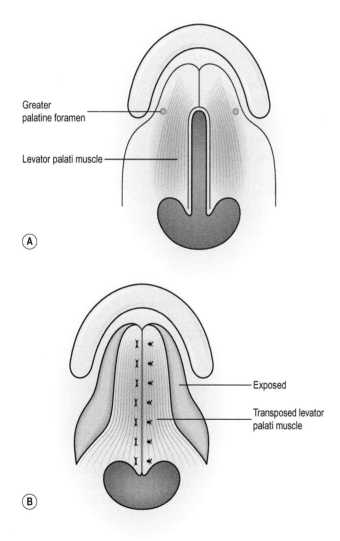

Fig. 33.31 Cleft palate repair. (A) The flaps of the two-flap repair. Note the attachment of the levator palati into the hard palate. This muscle should be dissected off the hard palate and sutured together in the midline. The subsequent repair of the mucosa of the soft palate leaves a residual exposed area laterally, which epithelializes spontaneously during the first postoperative week (B).

3. Scrape the periosteum off the palate using a Mitchell trimmer.
4. On approaching the greater palatine artery, identify this as it emerges through its foramen and dissect the flap away from the bone around its perimeter.
5. Using the Mitchell trimmer, separate the nasal mucosa from the palatal bones.
6. Identify the levator palati muscle inserted into the posterior margin of the hard palate and place a spatula between this attachment and the nasal mucosa.
7. Cut down through this attachment on to the spatula, freeing the levator palati muscle completely from the hard palate.
8. Dissect the levator palati free from both underlying nasal mucosa and its covering palatal mucosa.
9. Repeat the dissection on the opposite side.
10. Repair the nasal mucosa with 4/0 polyglactin, commencing anteriorly and work posteriorly to reconstruct the uvula.
11. Suture the two ends of the levator palati together in the midline with 4/0 polyglactin sutures.
12. Repair the oral mucosa in the midline using 4/0 polyglactin sutures. Use deep mattress sutures in the central portion.
13. The anteriors tips of the two flaps when sutured together may protrude into the mouth. They need not be sutured down as they adhere to the palate very early in the postoperative phase if left free.

ANTERIOR CLEFT PALATE

Appraise

1. A cleft of the anterior palate co-exists with a cleft of the lip.
2. It can be partially closed at the time of the lip repair but is usually closed at the time of the palate repair when this is also present.
3. Repair in specialized centres is usually achieved in layers by mobilizing the nasal mucosa on the cleft side first and suturing this to the vomerine mucosa. The lateral and medial mucoperiosteal flaps are closed over this.
4. For the inexperienced or isolated surgeon a more reliable closure is achieved by overlapping and suturing the mucoperiosteal flap of the cleft side to the vomerine flap.

Action

1. Insert a Dingman gag.
2. Mark out a flap on the vomer with its base at the vomerine margin (Fig. 33.32).
3. Mark out a lateral flap as for repair of a cleft palate. Infiltrate both flaps with 0.5% lidocaine and 1:200 000 adrenaline (epinephrine).
4. Elevate both flaps.
5. Oppose and suture the raw surface of the two flaps together.

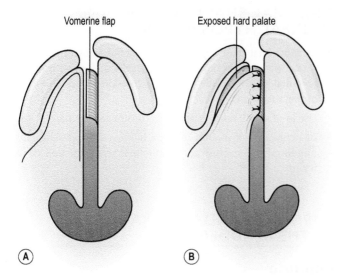

Fig. 33.32 Anterior palate repair. A superiorly based vomerine flap is raised off the septum (A). A palatal flap is raised laterally and mobilized. The two flaps are sutured raw surface to raw surface using mattress sutures (B).

PHARYNGOPLASTY

Appraise

1 A pharyngoplasty is necessary to reduce the velopharyngeal space when this is responsible for nasal escape during speech. This is usually due to the soft palate being too short to reach the posterior pharyngeal wall.

2 Carry out preoperative assessment with a nasendoscope wherever possible.

3 There are many different kinds of pharyngoplasty. Most provide a reduction in the anatomical size of the velopharyngeal space.

4 A few, including the Ortichochea repair described below, attempt not only to reduce the anatomical size of this space but also to provide a dynamic sphincter, which helps closure during speech.

Action

1 Insert a Dingman gag.

2 Mark a rectangular pharyngeal flap, based inferiorly and reaching as high as can be visualized on the posterior pharyngeal wall.

3 Infiltrate the flap with 0.5% lidocaine and 1:200 000 adrenaline (epinephrine).

4 Identify the palate-pharyngeus muscle within the posterior pillar of the fauces, and insert a McIndoe scissors behind this after penetrating the mucosa.

5 Separate the blades of the scissors and dissect free the muscle along its length. Dissect it free to its lower limit and divide it at this point.

6 Dissect the opposite muscle free in the same manner, preserving some overlying mucosa.

7 Raise the posterior pharyngeal flap down to its base and achieve haemostasis of its bed.

8 Suture the muscle belly of each of the two flaps to the raw surface of the pharyngeal flap with 4/0 polyglactin sutures.

9 Improve the attachment by suturing the mucosa of the muscle flap to the mucosa of the pharyngeal flap along the various attachments with 6/0 polyglactin.

CRANIOFACIAL SURGERY

Appraise

1 Craniofacial surgery involves correction of abnormalities of the facial and cranial bones and overlying soft tissues.

2 Many cranial abnormalities occur as part of well-recognized syndromes. Others result from premature fusion of one or more of the cranial sutures.

3 This surgery was pioneered by Tessier, who has classified the different types of facial cleft.

4 Craniofacial surgery is now recognized as a specialty in its own right. It often involves combined expertise from several specialists, including a neurosurgeon, ophthalmic surgeon, maxillofacial surgeon, ENT surgeon and paediatric surgeon, as well as the plastic surgeon.

5 These cases are rare but often much can be done to help these patients in specialized centres where this surgery is carried out.

GENITALIA

HYPOSPADIAS

Appraise

1 The male urethral meatus may appear on the surface at any point in the midline between its normal position at the tip of the glans penis and the perineum.

2 In many cases of hypospadias (Greek: *hypos* = under + *span* = to draw), a tight fibrous band, the chordee, is evident distal to the ectopic meatus, which causes curvature of the penis when in the erect position.

3 Reconstructive surgery to place the meatus in its normal position at the tip of the glans is intended to produce an apparently normal penis without urethral fistula.

4 Many operations have been designed to treat the condition but none consistently fulfils the above criteria.

5 Experienced surgeons advocate a one-stage procedure, but if you are an inexperienced surgeon, proceed with a staged reconstruction.

6 Ideally, carry out operation in infancy. Some surgeons prefer to wait until the child is continent of urine to release the chordee and then reconstruct the urethra just before the child starts school.

Release of chordee

1 Under general anaesthesia, carry out a Horton test. Place some rubber tubing around the base of the penis and pull it tight. Inject the corpora with physiological saline to produce an erect penis and note the extent of chordee. Release the rubber tubing.

2 Mark the extent of the chordee in ink. Mark out a Z-plasty for reconstruction following excision of the chordee.

3 Incise down the central line overlying the chordee.

4 Excise all underlying fibrous tissue.

5 Use a bipolar coagulator to achieve haemostasis.

6 Raise the flaps of the Z-plasty, transpose them and suture them with 6/0 polyglactin. Do not dress the wound.

Distal shaft correction

1 Under general anaesthesia, carry out a Horton test as above.

2 If any chordee is still evident, excise this and defer reconstruction for a further 6 months.

3 If no chordee is apparent, mark out a rectangular flap proximal to the meatus with its base at the meatus. The flap should be 1 cm broad and long enough to reach the glans when turned distally (Fig. 33.33).

4 Mark out a strip of skin distal to the meatus from the meatus to the glans.

5 Catheterize the urethra with a small Foley catheter.

6 Elevate the flap and reflect it distally.

7 Cut along the margins of the strip of skin and elevate the edges.

8 Suture the flap to the cut edges of the strip of skin using 6/0 absorbable suture.

9 Elevate lateral flaps of skin by incising around the attachment of preputial skin to the glans. Mobilize the flaps round to the dorsal surface.

10 Suture the flaps across the reconstructed urethra, so that the suture line between the two flaps traverses the reconstructed urethra. Use 6/0 polyglactin.

11 Suture a foam dressing around the reconstructed penis. This prevents interference from the patient. Suture or strap the catheter to the upper thigh.

12 Remove the dressing and catheter at 10 days.

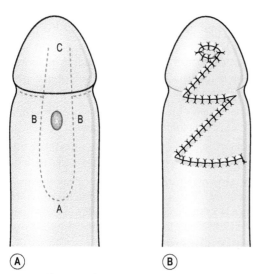

(A)   (B)

Fig. 33.33 Distal hypospadias repair. A plan of the incisions should be marked preoperatively. The proximal flap must have adequate length for A to reach C when hinged at point B adjacent to the external meatus (A). After suturing the lateral margins of this flap, lateral flaps are mobilized using the redundant preputial skin and closed in a Z-plasty fashion (B).

PROXIMAL SHAFT, SCROTAL AND PERINEAL HYPOSPADIAS

1 As with distal shaft hypospadias, there are many operations to correct these deformities. Reconstruct the urethra with flaps of preputial skin from the redundant foreskin or use a free graft of preputial skin.

2 Use local skin flaps to cover the reconstructed urethra.

3 In perineal hypospadias, use the hairless strip of skin in the middle of the scrotum for the urethral reconstruction in this region.

EPISPADIAS AND ECTOPIA OF THE BLADDER

Appraise

1 Epispadias and ectopia of the bladder represent different expressions of the same basic embryological defect.

2 These rare conditions require highly specialized treatment, where one-stage correction is advocated.

Action

1 If specialized treatment is not available do not carry out a pelvic osteotomy.

2 Close the bladder wall with abdominal flaps.

3 Tighten the bladder neck at a second stage.

4 In a third stage, close the residual epispadias by passing a funnel of mucosa through the base of the penis to the ventral surface and reconstruct the resultant hypospadias.

SCARS

HYPERTROPHIC SCARS

Appraise

1 These present as red, raised, broad, hard, itchy scars that are unsightly and uncomfortable. They develop a few months after the wound has healed.

2 Beware of excising or revising them unless there was failure of primary healing or unless a marked contraction has developed. Simple excision of the scar alone will probably cause a larger one to develop.

Action

1 Inject the scar tissue only with triamcinolone.

2 Repeat the injections at monthly intervals for 3–6 months, or longer if necessary, until the scar is soft.

3 Avoid excessive injections and avoid injecting the triamcinolone into the surrounding skin. This may cause skin atrophy.

4 If the scars are extensive, fit and apply a pressure garment as early as possible. Advise the patient to wear this garment for 6–12 months.

Pressure garments

1 A pressure garment is a synthetic elastic garment that is specifically measured to fit part of an individual.

2 In applying pressure to a scar, it modifies the maturation and limits hypertrophic scar formation, provided it is applied early.

3 Pressure garments are most useful in reducing hypertrophic scar formation and preventing the development of contractures, particularly from burn wounds.

4 They are also used in controlling progressive lymphoedema.

KELOIDS

Appraise

1 Keloids (Greek: *kelis* = scar + *eidos* = like) have a different histological appearance from hypertrophic scars.

2 They are most commonly found in patients of African origin but can be found in all races.

3 Excision of keloids, like excision of hypertrophic scars, only temporarily cures the problem. A larger lesion will develop in its place and this treatment is to be condemned.

4 Treatment with triamcinolone, as used for hypertrophic scars (see above), reduces the size of most keloids but does not eliminate them. This may, however, be the best treatment.

5 Excision of the whole keloid followed by radiotherapy to the resultant scar can be very effective. This requires expertise in radiotherapy but may not be suitable for young patients.

Action

1 Identify the boundaries of the keloid.

2 Excise its central bulk, keeping the margin of excision at the lateral borders and in depth within the keloid tissue. Close the wound primarily, preserving a rim of keloid tissue at all margins. Keep all sutures within this rim.

3 Give monthly injections of triamcinolone into the residual scar as for a hypertrophic scar (see above).

4 Apply pressure to the area for at least 3 months afterwards with a pressure garment specifically fitted for the patient if appropriate.

5 If the keloid is extensive, take a split skin graft from the surface of the keloid and apply to the raw surface after removing the major bulk of the keloid. Again, keep all sutures within the keloid tissue and apply pressure postoperatively.

AESTHETIC SURGERY

1 You should undertake these operations only if you are an expert. Aesthetic (Greek: *aisthanesthai* = to feel, perceive) operations demand specialist management, since they are intended to be pleasing to the patient.

2 These operations can nearly always be deferred until specialist treatment is available, but a brief outline of the more common operations is given below.

3 Careful preoperative assessment and full explanation of the expectation of the results of surgery and all potential complications are vital parts of management of patients in this field of surgery.

FACELIFT

Appraise

1 The principal aim of a facelift is to resuspend the soft tissues of the face, which have fallen as a result of gravity and other factors. This may involve tightening or reducing muscles and removal or replacement of subcutaneous fat and skin.

2 There are many different types of facelift, some involving the use of an endoscope.

3 There are also many associated procedures that can be carried out at the same time, such as an endoscopic brow lift to elevate and stretch the forehead skin and a platysmaplasty to increase the cervicomental angle.

4 In the cheek, the skin may be elevated by dissecting in the subcutaneous plane or in the plane of the superficial musculoaponeurotic system (SMAS) or in both.

Action

1 Make a vertical incision in the temple hairline down to the pinna. Extend this around the lower two-thirds of the pinna and backwards horizontally into the lateral occipital hairline (Fig. 33.34).

2 Raise the skin anterior to this incision and undermine it halfway to the nasolabial fold and an equivalent distance towards the chin and the neck. Avoid dividing branches of the facial nerves.

3 Plicate the superficial fascia (the SMAS layer) to reduce subsequent tension on the skin.

4 Retract the skin flap towards the incision line and excise the excess tissue.

5 Suture the flap into place along the original incision margin.

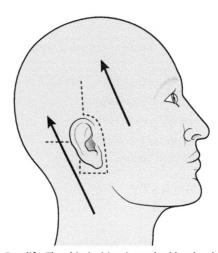

Fig. 33.34 Facelift. The skin incision is marked by the dotted line. After undermining and SMAS plication, the skin is pulled in the direction of the arrows and, after excision of excess skin, the wound is closed.

6 Insert a small corrugated drain beneath the postauricular skin.

7 Repeat the process on the opposite side to produce symmetry.

RHINOPLASTY

Appraise

1 Compare and contrast the patient's assessment of his or her nose with your own assessment of the nose.

2 Establish exactly what the patient wants.

Action

1 Shave or cut the vibrissae in the nostrils.

2 Make an intercartilaginous incision on each side through mucosa between the alar and lateral cartilages.

3 Extend this incision over the vault of the nostril down to the front of the septum.

4 Through this incision separate the skin on the top of the nose from the underlying septum.

5 Incise the mucosa along the roof of each nostril and divide the upper lateral cartilages from the septum.

6 Reduce the upper lateral cartilages as necessary.

7 Reduce the septal hump with a knife.

8 Remove the hump of the nasal bones with an osteotome and hammer.

9 Make a small incision in each pyriform fossa.

10 Insert a periosteal elevator through this incision on the lateral margin of the nose and elevate the periosteum from the lateral margin of each nasal bone.

11 Insert a nasal saw along each incision in turn and cut halfway through the nasal bone.

12 Insert an osteotome along each incision in turn and complete the nasal osteotomy.

13 Manipulate the nasal bones into the new position.

14 Rasp the nasal septum as necessary.

15 Through the intercartilaginous incision, evert the alar cartilages and reduce as necessary.

16 Expose the anterior margin of the nasal septum and adjust as necessary.

17 Suture the nasal mucosa with 3/0 absorbable thread.

18 Pack each nostril with paraffin gauze.

19 Dress with tape and a nasal splint.

20 Remove the nasal packs at 24 hours.

21 Remove the splint at 10 days.

BLEPHAROPLASTY

Appraise

1 This operation is carried out to reduce the skin and fat tissue in the upper and lower eyelids (Greek: *blepharon* = eyelid).

2 Identify before operation the site and volume of the underlying pads of fat.

Action

1 Under local or general anaesthesia, mark the excision margins of the skin of the upper eyelid as a crescent with an accessory tail laterally.

2 Mark the excision margin on the lower eyelid with a minimal reduction in height.

3 Infiltrate with local anaesthetic, if indicated.

4 Excise the skin from the upper eyelid and excise the underlying fat pads from beneath the orbicularis muscle if any are present. Achieve haemostasis and suture with subcuticular 5/0 polypropylene.

5 Raise the lower eyelid skin and, with a skin hook, pull the skin upwards and laterally.

6 Excise a triangle of skin at the lateral margin and a minimal amount of skin along the eyelid margin.

7 Reflect the skin flap and excise the fat pads from beneath the orbicularis muscle.

8 Suture the skin with 6/0 nylon.

9 Remove the sutures at 3–4 days.

CORRECTION OF PROMINENT EARS

Appraise

1 This operation is carried out to reduce prominence of the ears ('bat ears'), which may be due to a deep concha, but is more commonly due to an absence of the antihelical fold.

2 The principle of the operation is to remould the shape of the cartilage.

3 Operations that depend on skin and cartilage excision are unsatisfactory.

4 Defer surgery in children until the age of 6 years, as the cartilage is thin and children do not normally appreciate or suffer from any psychological problem before this age.

Action

1 Use general or local anaesthesia.

2 Infiltrate the pinna with local anaesthesia.

3 Mark the site of the proposed antihelical rim and tattoo the underlying cartilage by passing a needle covered with ink through the full thickness of the pinna at several points along this line.

4 Excise a narrow vertical ellipse of skin from the posterior surface of the pinna.

5 Incise the cartilage posteriorly along the tattoo marks.

6 Dissect the cartilage away from the anterior skin of the pinna.

7 Score the anterior aspect of the cartilage with circumferential and radial incisions, to allow the cartilage to fold backwards.

8 When you have obtained adequate reduction, re-drape the skin over the cartilage and suture the skin wound with subcuticular polypropylene.

9 Repeat the process for the opposite ear to provide symmetry.

10 Dress both ears with proflavine wool to ensure apposition of skin to cartilage.

11 Cover both ears with cotton wool and a supportive bandage.

12 Remove the dressing at 10 days and remove the sutures.

13 Maintain a protective dressing over the ears at night for 4 weeks.

BREAST AUGMENTATION

Appraise

1 Breasts can be augmented in size by inserting prostheses in the submammary plane or in the subpectoral plane.

2 The most common complication is the development of a fibrous capsule around the prosthesis. When this contracts appreciably, the prosthesis feels hard and uncomfortable and the breast becomes distorted.

3 The size of prosthesis to be used is dependent on the size of the patient and the breast size. A history of previous surgery, previous pregnancy and lactation and weight changes all influence the choice of the size of prosthesis to be used.

Action

1 Incise the skin along the submammary fold.

2 Dissect a pocket in the submammary plane sufficient to accommodate the prosthesis.

3 Insert the prosthesis.

4 Close the wound in layers.

5 Keep the breasts well supported in the postoperative phase and for the subsequent 3 months.

6 If a capsular contracture develops, carry out a closed capsulotomy by compression of the capsule in the first instance.

7 If this fails, carry out an open capsulotomy.

BREAST REDUCTION

Appraise

1 Breast reduction is carried out most commonly for physical symptoms.

2 Large breasts may be of sufficient weight to affect the posture of the patient and to cause backache.

3 Pressure marks over the shoulders may be evident where the straps of the brassiere rest.

4 The aim of surgery is to produce an aesthetic breast shape with a viable, sensitive nipple and areola. Preserve the areola on a vascular pedicle.

5 Breast feeding may be possible after breast reduction but warn the patient not to expect this.

6 There are many operations designed to reduce the mass of the breasts. The inferior pedicle technique devised by Robbins is described below.

Action

1 Mark the breasts preoperatively with the patient sitting.

2 Choose a suitable site for the new position of the nipple near the midclavicular line.

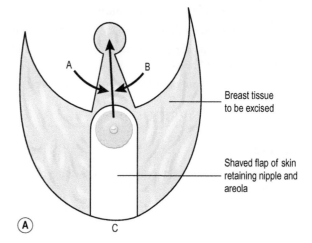

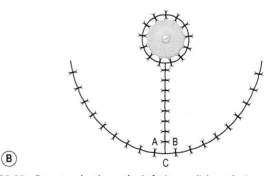

Fig. 33.35 Breast reduction—the inferior pedicle technique. The nipple and areola are preserved on a flap of skin in which the epidermis has been removed. This flap of skin helps to protect the underlying breast tissue which contains the vessels and nerves supplying the nipple. Breast tissue and overlying skin on either side and above this flap are excised (A). The nipple is transferred upwards and flaps A and B, after reflection outwards, are brought together in the midline below the nipple (B).

3 Use a keyhole-type breast reduction pattern based on this site and mark the lateral and medial skin flaps (Fig. 33.35).

4 Mark the medial and lateral ends of the submammary crease and the submammary crease itself.

5 Perioperatively, make an intradermal incision through the skin along the patterns marked out preoperatively so that the skin marks are not lost.

6 Shave off the epidermis from the skin between the normal areola and the inframammary fold, and from a rim of skin around the areola.

7 Excise the lateral and medial segments of skin between the lower margin of the skin flaps and the inframammary fold, together with the underlying breast tissue.

8 Excise breast tissue beneath the new site of the nipple and areola.

9 Dissect the inferior pedicle to its base.

10 Elevate the medial and lateral skin flaps with their underlying breast tissue.

11 Support the inferior pedicle by anchoring it to the pectoralis muscle superiorly.

12 Suture the nipple and areola into its new site.

13 Approximate the skin flaps in the midline below the new nipple site.

14 Insert a suction drain.

15 Close the wounds in layers, using subcuticular sutures to the skin.

16 Repeat the operation on the opposite side to provide symmetry.

17 Support the breast postoperatively with light dressings and remove the sutures at 3 weeks.

18 Keep the breasts well supported for 3 months postoperatively.

DERMAL MASTOPEXY

Appraise

1 The breasts of all women have a tendency to become ptotic with increasing age.

2 Ptosis tends to be greater when there has been considerable weight reduction or excessive involution following lactation. It is also marked when the breasts have not been supported with a brassiere over a long period.

3 Dermopexy or correction of the ptosis is appropriate when the nipple can be re-sited at a higher level and the skin envelope of the breast tissue can be reduced without any change in the volume of breast tissue.

Action

1 Mark the patient as for a breast reduction.

2 Carry out the stages as enumerated in a breast reduction, but do not excise breast tissue.

3 In advancing the inferior pedicle to its new site, incise breast tissue at the new site and undermine the skin edges around the new nipple site appropriately.

4 Manage the patient postoperatively as for a breast reduction.

ABDOMINAL REDUCTION

Appraise

1 An abdominal reduction or lipectomy is most appropriate when a patient has lax abdominal skin following multiple pregnancies or substantial weight loss.

2 It is not normally an operation to produce weight reduction.

Action

1 Mark out a symmetrical line traversing the lower abdomen. Start beneath the anterior superior iliac spine on one side and pass through the upper part of the site of the pubic hair to the other.

2 Incise along this mark and cut down to the fascia overlying the muscles.

3 Dissect upwards in this plane.

4 Incise the skin around the umbilicus and separate this from the skin flap.

5 Undermine the skin up to the costal margin on either side.

6 Stretch the skin downwards.

7 Excise the redundant skin and subcutaneous fat.

8 Identify the new site on the skin flap for the umbilicus and excise an oval piece of skin to accommodate it.

9 Break the operating table at the level of the pelvis to flex the hips.

10 Close the lower abdominal wound in layers and suture the umbilicus.

11 Insert a suction drain on each side.

12 Close the skin of the umbilical scar, if still present, in the vertical plane.

13 Postoperatively, keep the hips flexed to reduce tension on the lower abdominal wound for a few days.

14 Remove the sutures at 3 weeks.

LIPOSUCTION

Appraise

1 This technique of removing subcutaneous fat has a useful but limited place in aesthetic surgery.

2 It is occasionally used in refining a reconstructive procedure.

3 The technique is sometimes used alone but only a limited amount of fat can be removed without the need for excising further redundant skin.

4 The technique is often used as an adjunct to other surgery when skin is being removed, particularly in abdominoplasty and thigh and buttock reduction.

5 It can be used to remove lipomata from prominent sites on the trunk or limbs, avoiding an ugly scar and leaving a small discreet scar at some chosen distant inconspicuous site. In these circumstances excision is likely to be incomplete and the procedure may need repeating later for recurrence.

Action

1 Identify a suitable site for insertion of the liposuction cannula which is both discreet and within range of the area to be treated.

2 Make a small stab incision in the skin.

3 Through this insert the appropriate cannula and infiltrate the area with fluid made from adding 1 ml of 1:1000 adrenaline (epinephrine) and 20 ml of 0.25% bupivacaine to 500 ml of Hartmann's solution. Then wait at least 5 minutes.

4 Insert the chosen liposuction cannula and pass it into the deepest plane of subcutaneous fat.

5 Apply suction as the cannula is passed up and down the channel formed.

6 Repeat in multiple other deep subcutaneous channels.

7 Avoid passing the cannula superficially as this may cause pitting of the skin surface.

8 Suture the incision on removal of the cannula.

9 Apply a pressure garment immediately to the area treated and retain for 3 months.

LASER SURGERY

Lasers are being used to treat an increasing number of skin lesions. These fall into four principal groups:

1 *Vascular lesions.* Many cutaneous vascular lesions can be eradicated without leaving any significant scarring. These include all types of telangiectasia, capillary haemangiomata, including port

wine stains, pyogenic granulomata and other small vascular lesions. Many of the small lesions can be treated successfully with a single treatment with one of the pulsed dye lasers. While the larger lesions can be eradicated, treatment may leave a residual area of variable pigmentation.

2 *Pigmented lesions.* Several lasers with short wavelengths, such as the Q-switched lasers, remove pigmented lesions limited to the epidermis and basal layer, such as lentigo simplex, solar lentigines and ephilides. They also remove pigment from the superficial dermis. Pigment in the deeper dermis requires a laser with a longer wavelength, but treatment of these lesions is less satisfactory and surgical excision may be the better option of treatment.

3 *Tattoos.* Removal of professional as well as accidental tattoos with lasers is now much more effective than surgical excision because of the absence of scars. The Q-switched ruby, Nd-YAG and Alexandrite lasers are all effective in removing blue-black pigment, but complete excision can be difficult to achieve even with multiple treatments and pigmentation changes may occur.

4 *Skin resurfacing.* The carbon dioxide laser in effect causes a predetermined superficial burn to the skin and has a similar effect to dermabrasion, which causes a physical burn, and a chemopeel, which causes a chemical burn. Treatment of wrinkles and irregular scarring of the skin surface with the carbon dioxide laser is more accurate and predictable than these treatments and is therefore replacing them. The occasional complication of a change in pigmentation remains unresolved.

ENDOSCOPIC PLASTIC SURGERY

Appraise

Endoscopic surgery was very limited until the development of fibreoptics and fibreoptic instruments. This allowed investigation and treatment of lesions of hollow viscera. By insufflation of air the peritoneal cavity becomes accessible to endoscopic surgery, and injection of saline into joints such as the knee has rendered these accessible to this type of surgery.

With refinements in the instrumentation it is now possible to explore soft tissues, allowing plastic surgeons to use the techniques that others have hitherto pioneered, with the benefit of reducing the extent of scars on the skin surface. The latissimus dorsi muscle flap (see above) can now be raised and transposed into the breast area using only a small incision in the axilla and a periareolar incision. Nerve, vein or fascial grafts can be harvested. The carpal tunnel can be released and subcutaneous lesions can be removed. Tissue expanders and prostheses can be inserted. In the aesthetic field endoscopic brow lifts have replaced the conventional brow lift involving an extensive coronal scar and endoscopic surgery is used for some types of facelift.

PROSTHETIC IMPLANT MATERIALS

Appraise

1 All implants must be inserted under strict aseptic techniques.
2 Implants require good-quality soft tissue cover to prevent ulceration of the overlying skin.

3 If subsequently exposed, most implants will become infected and require removal. It may be possible to replace the implant when the infection has been eradicated.

4 All implants develop a surrounding fibrous capsule. This may be useful but is a disadvantage with a breast prosthesis as the fibrous capsule may contract and distort the prosthesis.

5 Several inert metals are used in reconstruction:
- Titanium plates are used in cranioplasty
- Gold weights are inserted into the upper eyelid in facial palsy to improve function by assisting closure
- Stainless steel, vitallium and tantalum are occasionally used.

6 Hard plastics used in reconstruction include: methyl methacrylate, used in cranioplasty; polyethylene, used as a mesh in abdominal wall repair; and polypropylene. Proplast, a combination of two polymers (polytetrafluoroethylene and pyrolytic graphite), is used to augment the cheek and the chin.

7 Silicone is a general term for a class of polymers with long chains of dimethylsiloxane units [$-CH_3-Si-O-CH_3$]. These are manufactured in many forms, including liquids, gels, resins, foams, sponges and rubbers.

8 Silicone implants are used in facial bone augmentation, small-joint replacement in the hand and as a stent to reconstruct tendon sheaths prior to tendon grafting.

9 Silicone implants are commonly used in breast augmentation or reconstruction. Some breast implants consist of a silicone gel contained within a silicone elastomer shell. Others are made using a cohesive gel that maintains their shape. A textured surface modifies the fibrous reaction of the body and capsule contracture is reduced. There is no scientific evidence to show that any silicone breast implant has a significant carcinogenic risk and, although these implants may leak, there is no evidence that the silicone that does leak causes any serious complication.

STEM CELL THERAPY

The name is derived from the German word *stammzelle*, which could either mean the original cell of the origin of species or the cell of the origin of an organ (http://www.nature.com/stemcells/2009/0906/090625/full/stemcells.2009.90.html). For therapeutic purposes they are divided into embryonic and adult stem cells. Stem cell transplantation is still not in routine clinical practice and its use in clinical surgery is experimental.

Stem cell therapy has shown potential in wound healing by modulating scar formation, which is a fundamental aspect of surgical practice. Almost every surgical field would lend itself to this use: orthopaedic surgery (cartilage repair), neurosurgery (spinal cord and nerve regeneration) and ophthalmology (retinal and cornea regeneration), to name a few. It is a fast-changing field and one that may have a major impact on all aspects of practice in the future.

BIOLOGICAL THERAPY

Biological therapy refers to the use of larvae (maggots) and leeches in surgery.

Larval therapy[1]

1 The main indications include a necrotic wound that is difficult to surgically debride and/or a patient who is not suitable for surgery. It may also be used in a sensitive area where precise debridement is required. The advantage of larval debridement is that it only removes dead tissue without affecting healthy living areas. The wound must be open and moist: cavities and dry wounds are not suitable.

2 Prepare the patient psychologically: patients and staff are often poorly tolerant of larval therapy. Maggots have a short lifespan and have to be ordered freshly. Once the maggots are introduced into the wound, use a breathable dressing to cover the area to avoid them escaping as well as hiding them from sight.

3 Use larval therapy prior to negative pressure therapy to prepare the bed and remove necrotic tissue.

Leech therapy[2]

1 The European medicinal leech (Hirudo medicinalis), is commonly commercially produced and used. Indications for their use are:

- Following a microsurgical procedure that is showing evidence of venous insufficiency and congestion, especially post re-implantation or revascularization. Use leeches to relieve this congestion, thus giving time for venous outflow to improve secondarily.

- Replants such as fingers or ears where venous return from the organs is compromised and venous return is small enough for leeches to cope with.

2 Use prophylactic antibiotics for *Aeromonas hydrophila* (contained in the leech).

3 Using gloves, apply the leeches over the raw area of the organ and cover it with moist gauze. When leeches are engorged and fall off, discard in a biological waste bin.

NEGATIVE PRESSURE WOUND THERAPY (VAC-PUMP™)

1 Application of sub-atmospheric pressure to the wound was originally applied for burn wounds, but any exudating wound which is difficult to close primarily or to cover with a skin graft is often suitable. Avoid application directly over bowel and vessels, and in the presence of malignancy. The decision to commence negative pressure wound therapy (NPWT) should be made in consultation with the tissue viability team and/or plastic surgeon.

2 Ensure the wound is free from necrotic material, as NPWT has no debriding effect on the wound (cf. larval therapy). Apply the dressing (either foam or gauze dressing, depending on the manufacturer); this needs to be covered by the airtight film (usually supplied), which is then connected by a length of tubing to the manufacturer's pump device. The value and the pattern of negative pressure can be adjusted to the comfort of the patient and also to the type of the wound, the most common setting being 125 mmHg continuous suction.

3 Aim to continue the treatment for 1–3 weeks (although longer periods are possible), and change the dressing every 3–4 days depending on the type of the wound and the volume of exudate. Mobile, pocket-sized and even disposable machines are available to enable outpatient use of NPWT.

THE FUTURE

- When greater control of the immune response has been achieved, it will be possible to use many different parts of cadavers for reconstruction using microvascular surgery.

- Tissue culture is in an embryonic phase of development and has great potential in reconstruction. Cultured keratinocytes have been grafted on to open wounds.

- In-utero surgery has been carried out and may have a role in treating congenital deformities.

- Better understanding and control of wound healing will improve the quality of plastic surgery and will help all branches of surgery, but the most important advances will most likely be in the field of tissue engineering and in harnessing the potential of stem cells.

FURTHER READING

Aston SJ, Beasley RW, Thorne CHM. Grabb and Smith's Plastic Surgery. 5th ed. Philadelphia: Lippincott-Raven; 1997.
A concise guide to clinical practice in plastic surgery in one volume. It is packed with information.
McCarthy JG. Plastic Surgery. Philadelphia: Saunders; 1990.
Whilst this, in its eight volumes, remains the commonly accepted authoritative reference book in plastic surgery, it now requires updating.
McGregor AD, McGregor IA. Fundamental Techniques of Plastic Surgery and their Surgical Applications. 10th ed. Edinburgh: Churchill Livingstone; 2000.
An excellent manual of basic techniques in plastic surgery, ideal for young trainees in the specialty and general surgeons.
Richards AM. Key Notes on Plastic Surgery. Oxford: Blackwell; 2002.
Settle JAD. Principles and Practice of Burns Management. Edinburgh: Churchill Livingstone; 1996.
A comprehensive guide to the management of patients with burns, indicating many of the difficulties and controversies in treating these cases.
Strauch B, Vasconez LO, Hall-Findlay EJ. Grabb's Encyclopaedia of Flaps. 2nd ed. Philadelphia: Lippincott-Raven; 1998.
Published in three large volumes, this is a comprehensive guide to flaps, with over 500 chapters, each describing one or more flaps in detail.

---

[1]Reames MK, Christensen C, Luce EA. The use of maggots in wound debridement. Ann Plast Surg 1988;21(4):388–91.
[2]Porshinsky BS, Saha S, Grossman MD, Beery Ii PR, Stawicki SP. Clinical uses of the medicinal leech: a practical review. J Postgrad Med 2011;57(1):65–71.

34

Paediatric surgery

N.J. Hall, E. Kiely

CONTENTS

GENERAL CONSIDERATIONS IN PAEDIATRIC SURGERY

INTRODUCTION

1 In many countries the general surgery of children from birth to early teenage years is the preserve of specialist paediatric surgeons. As these surgeons work in centres with paediatric anaesthetic care and paediatric nursing, together with a wide spectrum of paediatric medical expertise, a high level of specialist care is possible.

2 This model of care is not, however, universally available and in exceptional circumstances, in all countries, an adult general surgeon will be called upon to act. Because of unfamiliarity, general surgical junior and senior staff may be intimidated when faced with a young child with a significant surgical problem. There is justifiable concern about the evaluation of a sick child, assessment of respiratory and cardiovascular status and, of course, consideration of an unfamiliar range of potential diagnoses.

3 Attending paediatricians may be accustomed to dealing with sick children but are not usually familiar with the details of surgical disease, nor the likely effects of intervention on the child's physiology. Although young children and adults differ in their response to surgery, the impact of surgical disease or a surgical procedure are broadly similar and predictable in all age groups.

4 Your assessment of the child prior to and following operation is critical to success.

ASSESSMENT OF THE 'SURGICAL' CHILD

1 Assessing a 3-day-old infant is clearly different from assessing a 12-year-old child. Nonetheless, certain features of acute surgical diseases are common throughout the paediatric age group.

2 Assess the child's general demeanour, respiratory rate, level of activity and response to intervention. They all give an initial impression of severity of illness.

3 First assess the cardiovascular status. Ensure the peripheries are warm with palpable peripheral pulses. If you cannot palpate the radial, ankle or foot pulses, impairment of the circulation is likely and needs volume replacement. Give this either as colloid – human albumin or gelatin solution, or as crystalloid – normal (0.9%) saline or Ringer's lactate. Give 20 ml/kilogram rapidly (<1 hour), repeated two or three times depending on the response. Confirm restoration of circulatory volume by detecting an improved pulse volume or a falling pulse rate. Institute more invasive intravascular monitoring if there is a failure to respond to two such boluses.

4 Examine the abdomen in the standard manner – each quadrant in turn. Palpate gently only in children. Do not perform deep palpation – it is unhelpful. Never seek to test for rebound tenderness; this is quite unreliable. Be patient but persistent when dealing with anxious young children.

5 Digital rectal examination is, for the most part, quite useless. Reserve it usually for those in whom you suspect an anorectal abnormality. In this case have it performed only once by the most senior person available. You rarely gain useful or important information by this manoeuvre.

6 Opinions vary on the usefulness of listening to bowel sounds. We remain convinced that auscultation consistently yields useful information on what is happening within.

7 It is impossible to stop nurses and paediatricians from measuring abdominal girth. We have never seen a patient of any age in whom this information was useful.

ASSESSMENT OF THE 'SURGICAL' NEWBORN

Surgical problems presenting in the newborn comprise a group of conditions unique to this period of life which are almost never seen in older children. The following list includes the commoner symptoms and signs with which these conditions present:

1 Respiratory distress or cyanosis at birth in a full term infant may be a consequence of congenital diaphragmatic hernia or oesophageal atresia. Order a chest X-ray as an aid to diagnosis. Diagnose choanal atresia (Greek: choane = funnel; funnel-shaped narrowing of the posterior nares) by your inability to pass a nasogastric tube beyond the nasopharynx.

2 Consider bile-stained (green) vomiting to be the result of mechanical intestinal obstruction until proven otherwise. Always order an abdominal X-ray and carry out a surgical evaluation.

3 Consider abdominal distension as pathological, particularly if it is associated with bile vomiting or a failure to pass meconium (the dark green faeces passed by neonates).

4 All but 3% of full-term infants pass meconium in the first 24 hours. Carefully inspect the perineum if meconium does

not appear within this period. If you see a normally sited anus, gently insert a little finger to confirm patency – one of the few indications for this intervention.

5 Failure to pass urine in the first 24 hours is always abnormal. In a male infant, the presence of an associated distended bladder indicates the presence of urethral obstruction, most commonly caused by posterior urethral valves.

6 The majority of abdominal masses in the newborn are renal in origin. Almost all are benign.

7 The passage of blood per rectum is always significant. When the bleeding occurs on the first day of life test the blood to see whether it is fetal or maternal in origin. Subsequent bleeding is almost always from the baby and indicates the presence of intestinal disease.

PRE-NATAL DIAGNOSIS

1 Routine ultrasound examination of the fetus is part of antenatal care. This results in detection of a wide variety of structural abnormalities, often in the first trimester.

2 Detection of an abnormality early in the pregnancy may affect the subsequent management of the pregnancy or the timing and mode of delivery: detection of a lethal abnormality such as anencephaly (Greek: an = no + encephalos = brain) or bilateral renal agenesis raises the question of termination.

3 If you detect an abnormality which can be successfully treated postnatally (e.g. unilateral hydronephrosis) it changes neither the timing nor mode of delivery. Elective caesarean is the likely mode of delivery in the presence of a sacro-coccygeal teratoma or a large exomphalos (Greek: ek = out + omphalos = navel). Occasionally, subsequent scanning reveals not only the persistent abnormality but also deterioration in the condition of the fetus. This is particularly true with chest masses, such as cystic adenomatoid malformations of the lung, where progressive enlargement may result in venous obstruction, and hydrops fetalis (severe oedema of the fetus). Under these circumstances, premature delivery may be the only option available to try to save the baby.

NEONATAL TRANSPORT

1 With appropriate support, newborn infants can be safely transferred over very long distances.

2 You require transport incubators with facilities to monitor heart rate, body temperature and provide mechanical ventilation.

3 You also need facilities to allow endotracheal intubation, insertion of a chest drain and vascular access.

4 For general surgical transfer, insert an 8 or 10Fr nasogastric tube and leave on free drainage.

5 Ensure that a signed consent form for operation accompanies the baby, together with details of the pregnancy, delivery and postnatal course.

6 Finally, send 10 ml of the mother's blood with the baby to facilitate cross-matching.

7 If the baby is significantly compromised, as a general rule undertake resuscitation prior to transfer. Only exceptionally should the baby be transferred with ongoing intensive resuscitation.

▶ KEY POINT

■ Most importantly, ensure that an experienced neonatal nurse travels with the baby and, if possible, also a neonatal or intensive care paediatrician.

INTRAVENOUS FLUIDS — THE STANDARD MAINTENANCE

1 The standard maintenance intravenous fluid available in the UK is 0.45% saline in 5% dextrose. This is adequate for most children, although premature infants may need the dextrose level to be raised to 10%.

2 In the newborn, you may use the umbilical vein but prefer peripherally sited cannulae.

3 Replace fluid losses – nasogastric aspirate or vomiting – using 0.9% saline with 20 mmol of potassium chloride per litre.

The standard daily requirements are shown in Table 34.1.

Postoperative fluid requirement

1 In the initial 48 hours after operation, give one half of maintenance requirements.

2 On the third and fourth days, give two-thirds of maintenance requirements and full maintenance fluids from the fifth day onwards.

3 After major surgery there are substantial hidden losses within the tissues and the peritoneal cavity. Assess and replace these losses. Standard replacement fluids for this purpose include normal saline, Ringer's lactate solution, human albumin or gelatin solutions.

4 Assess the need for such additional fluid on the basis of heart rate, pulse volume, peripheral temperature and urine output. In general, give one or two boluses of 20 ml/kilogram in the first 12–18 hours after major surgery. Calculate such losses and replacement separately from the maintenance fluid which is given in the manner noted above. Calculate nasogastric losses separately and replace them ml for ml.

TABLE 34.1 Daily intravenous fluid requirement		
	Weight	Daily requirement
Neonates	Up to 1500 g	180 ml/kg
	1500–2500 g	150 ml/kg
	Over 2500 g	120 ml/kg
Infants and children	Up to 10 kg	100 ml/kg
	10–20 kg	1000 ml + 50 ml/kg for each kg above 10 kg
	Over 20 kg	1500 ml + 25 ml/kg for each kg above 20 kg

Examples:

An 8-kg infant requires 8 × 100 = 800 ml/day.

A 14-kg child requires 1000 ml plus 4 × 50 ml = 1200 ml/day.

A 25-kg child requires 1500 ml plus 5 × 25 ml = 1625 ml/day.

GENERAL PAEDIATRIC SURGICAL TECHNIQUES

THE ABDOMINAL OPERATION IN INFANTS AND CHILDREN

Many conditions require an abdominal operation. Traditionally, laparotomy is used but laparoscopy is becoming a popular alternative in centres with suitable facilities, equipment and expertise. We describe a general purpose approach to both laparotomy and laparoscopy in children and infants.

Prepare

1 Cross-match 1 unit of fresh packed cells.

2 Administer vitamin K, phytomenadione 1 mg intramuscularly, if this was omitted in the immediate postnatal period.

3 Check the blood glucose using Dextrostix. Correct hypoglycaemia by giving 10% glucose intravenously.

4 Correct any fluid and acid–base imbalance (most acid–base imbalances will self-correct with adequate resuscitation).

5 In all emergencies, keep the stomach empty through a large (8FG) nasogastric tube.

6 Ensure good intravenous access through a cannula conveniently sited for the anaesthetist.

7 Use ECG, pulse, blood pressure and oxygen saturation monitors. Monitors for measuring partial pressures of oxygen and carbon dioxide in inspired and expired gases are also available.

8 For very sick infants, continuously record blood pressure through a transduced intra-arterial cannula, which also facilitates intermittent blood gas analysis and assessments of serum electrolyte and haemoglobin concentrations.

9 Use a central venous cannula when blood loss is expected to be massive or when peripheral venous access is limited, but measurements of central venous pressure are of limited value in this age group.

10 Keep the infant normothermic. Radiant heat losses, especially from the head, must be limited by wrapping the head and swaddling the infant in warm gamgee. A thermostatically controlled warm air blanket should be placed below the patient. The ambient temperature of the theatre should be kept at 26°C with doors closed to prevent draughts.

▶ KEY POINTS Incision

■ Because of the relatively wide, truncated abdomen of the young child, greater access is afforded by transverse rather than longitudinal incisions.

■ A recommended 'general purpose' incision is a transverse, muscle-cutting, supra-umbilical incision extending across right and left rectus abdominis muscles.

Access

1 Place the prepared infant supine on the operating table.

2 Make an adequate, transverse skin incision, 1–2 cm above the umbilicus, with a scalpel.

3 Divide the subcutaneous fat and fascia with cutting diathermy to limit blood loss.

4 Similarly, divide the anterior sheath of the left and right rectus abdominus muscles and then divide the muscle bellies.

5 Coagulate the superior epigastric vessels on the deeper surface of each rectus abdominus muscle.

6 Divide the posterior sheath and fascia down to the peritoneum.

7 Open the peritoneum on either side of the midline.

8 Identify, clamp and divide the relatively large umbilical vein. Ligate both ends of the vein with 4/0 polyglycolic acid ties.

9 After assessment, the incision may be readily extended, using cutting diathermy, into the oblique muscles of the abdominal wall at either or both ends.

Closure

1 It is unnecessary to close the peritoneum separately.

2 Close the muscles and fascia *en masse* with either continuous or interrupted sutures of 3/0 or 4/0 polyglactin, polyglycolic acid or polydioxanone.

3 Close the skin with a continuous subcuticular 4/0 or 5/0 suture.

4 Do not use tension sutures or through-and-through skin sutures because the cosmetic results are unacceptable.

LAPAROSCOPY IN INFANTS AND CHILDREN

With instruments of suitable size for use in infants (including neonates) and children being widely available, many abdominal and thoracic procedures are being performed using minimally invasive surgery. A recommended general purpose approach to laparoscopy is described. The operation itself is usually performed using identical operative steps to the open procedure, with the exception of inguinal hernia repair.

Preoperative preparations (in addition to those for laparotomy)

1 Inform your anaesthetist of your intention to perform the case laparoscopically.

2 Check that the camera and light source are working correctly.

3 Check that you have an adequate supply of insufflation gas and that your insufflator is working correctly. Select your maximum intra-abdominal pressure (start with 6–8 mmHg in an infant and 8–10 mmHg in an older child). Select a low initial flow rate 0.2 L/min in an infant, 0.5 L/min in an older child.

4 Ensure that equipment and access ports of the correct size are available to you. Use 3 mm equipment for infants and 5 mm for older children. Laparoscopy in infants (e.g. inguinal hernia repair, pyloromyotomy) may be performed without access ports, passing the instruments directly through the thin abdominal wall. Occasionally a larger access port (10 or 12 mm) will be required to remove an operative specimen (e.g. appendicectomy, cholecystectomy).

5 Ensure that a full set of open operating equipment is ready in the event that conversion is required.

Access

1 Make a short transverse incision using a scalpel in the upper margin of the umbilicus long enough for the intended access port.

2 Divide the subcutaneous fat with scissors down to the linea alba.

3 Clear a short (approximately 1 cm long) section of the linea alba so that you can see it clearly. Pick up the linea alba with two artery forceps, one just above the umbilicus, the other 1 cm cranial to this.

4 Incise the linea alba transversely between the artery forceps with a knife, taking care not to incise the underlying peritoneum or umbilical vein.

5 Pick up the peritoneum with two pairs of toothed forceps, ensuring that you have not picked up bowel or omentum, and incise it with a scalpel.

6 At this stage insert a 3/0 (infant) or 2/0 (older child) polyglycolic acid suture in a purse-string around the edges of the muscular layer. A suture mounted on a 'J' shaped needle is preferable for this. Inserting the suture at this stage improves the seal and security of the access port.

7 Insert the access port mounted with a blunt trocar.

8 Tighten the purse-string suture around the access port, place one throw of a knot on the suture and use the long end of the suture to secure the access port in the wound.

9 Attach the gas tubing to the access port and begin insufflation. Ensure that a pneumo-peritoneum is developing by abdominal examination. There should be free flow of gas into the peritoneal cavity up to the pre-set insufflation pressure. If a pneumo-peritoneum is not developing or if the flow of gas is not free then cease insufflation, check that the access port is correctly located in the peritoneal cavity and restart.

10 Perform a laparoscopic examination of the abdominal cavity to confirm the preoperative diagnosis and identify optimal sites for working port insertion. As a general rule, these should be on either side of the camera with an adequate angle between them to allow easy vision and comfortable dissection.

11 Insert the working ports under direct vision. Make a short transverse skin incision with a scalpel. Insert a port mounted with a cutting trocar and advance it into the peritoneal cavity using a back and forth screwing type movement. Watch carefully via the laparoscope to avoid damage to abdominal viscera. Once the port is within the abdominal cavity, remove the trochar and insert a working instrument.

Closure

1 Remove all working instruments and working ports. Approximate the muscle edges using a 4/0 or 5/0 polyglycolic acid suture. Observe the inside of the incision through the laparoscope to ensure adequate closure and avoid damage to viscera with the needle.

2 Once working ports are closed, cease insufflation, remove the laparoscope and primary port and allow gas to escape.

3 Undo the single throw on the purse-string suture and tighten the suture, approximating the edges of the wound. Tie the suture, ensuring that the defect is completely closed with no viscera (especially omentum) extruding.

4 Close the subcutaneous tissue with a 4/0 polyglycolic acid suture.

5 Close the skin with skin glue.

INTESTINAL ANASTOMOSIS (Fig. 34.1)

An anastomosis may be required in the treatment of a number of conditions, including correction of congenital anomalies, such as duodenal or ileal atresia, following intestinal resection or when closing an enterostomy.

Prepare

1 An anastomosis may be created between two intestinal ends following resection so long as there is a healthy blood supply. Discrepancy in the size of the two ends is not a contraindication to anastomosis. However, in case of doubt it is often safer to fashion a stoma.

2 Identify the ends to be anastomosed, ensuring their orientation is correct.

3 Trim each end so that the margin is straight and clean. Clear the mesentery from the serosal surface of the bowel for a few millimetres from the cut edge to create a clean margin for anastomosis, ensuring that you do not impair the blood supply.

4 Take an appropriately sized monofilament suture – 4/0 in a child, 4/0 to 6/0 in an infant.

Action

1 Starting on the mesenteric border, place a single extramucosal, seromuscular suture approximating the two edges. Place this suture adjacent to the mesentery, taking care not to damage

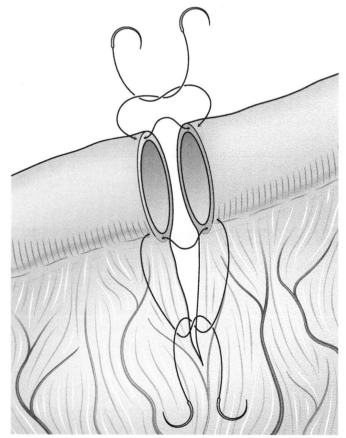

Fig. 34.1 Intestinal anastomosis.

the vessels. Leave the end of this suture long and grasp it with artery forceps to aid manipulation.

2 Place an additional single interrupted suture on either side of, but close to the first suture.

3 Place a single suture approximating the edges on the ante-mesenteric border. Leave the end long and grasp it with artery forceps.

4 Using the artery forceps to lay the anastomosis out in front of you, complete the anterior wall of the anastomosis using a single layer of interrupted extramucosal sutures. Ensure that they are adequately spaced to make a water-tight anastomosis, but not so tight as to cause ischaemia. If there is a discrepancy in size between the two ends you will need to leave a wider space between each suture on the wider end of bowel than the other.

5 Use the artery forceps to turn the bowel over, laying out the posterior wall in front of you. Complete the anastomosis as for the first side.

STOMA FORMATION

1 An ileostomy or colostomy may be required in a number of scenarios whenever it is desirable or essential to divert the faecal stream. The loop colostomy is one of the most commonly used stomas in paediatric surgery and is suitable in the infant with obstruction such as Hirschsprung's disease or anorectal malformations, as well as some conditions in older children. End stomas may be created in small or large intestine.

2 When creating an ileostomy it is prudent to evert a section of the bowel to create a luminal orifice away from the skin so as to protect the skin from effluent. We describe the techniques of loop colostomy and end ileostomy. Prescribe preoperative antibiotics giving anaerobic cover.

LOOP COLOSTOMY (Fig. 34.2)

Action

1 Make a V-shaped incision, either in the left iliac fossa for a sigmoid colostomy, or in the right hypochondrium for a transverse colostomy. The latter colostomy has the advantage of leaving sufficient distal colon for secondary surgery to be performed in conditions requiring mobilization of the distal colon.

2 Carry the V incision through skin and subcutaneous tissue.

3 Raise the flap of the V, exposing the underlying muscle.

4 In an older child you may need to extend the incision in the skin and subcutaneous layer to allow adequate room for passage of the colon. Turn a V-shaped incision into a W (see Fig. 34.2).

5 Split the muscle transversely, perpendicular to the V incision.

6 Open the peritoneum in the same direction as the muscle.

7 Locate the part of the intestine that will form the colostomy. Remember that the sigmoid loop may be greatly dilated and may appear in the right upper quadrant where it is easily confused

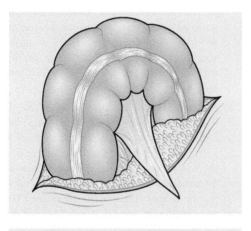

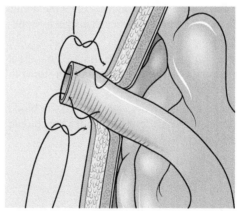

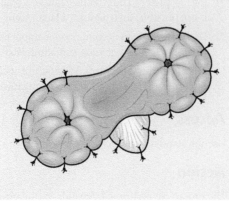

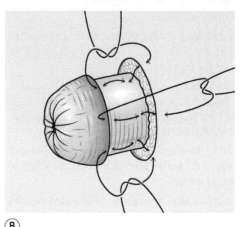

(A)   (B)

Fig. 34.2 (A) Loop colostomy; (B) terminal ileostomy.

with the transverse colon. The lack of an attached omentum serves to differentiate it from the transverse colon.

8 Ensure that the bowel is not twisted as it is drawn to the surface. Twisting may produce intestinal obstruction.

9 Make a small opening in the colonic mesentery.

10 Pass the apex of the V skin flap through the mesenteric defect and suture it to its original position with two or three loosely tied 4/0 polydioxanone sutures.

11 Incise the colon longitudinally with cutting diathermy.

12 Suture the full thickness of the opened colon to the surrounding skin with interrupted 4/0 polyglycolic acid sutures.

Aftercare

1 Consider the continuing need for antibiotics and the duration of postoperative starvation. In general terms, the child can take oral fluids and then a light diet once the stoma begins to function. At this point place a stoma bag.

2 This technique may also be used to form a loop ileostomy. In this case you should attempt to evert the proximal limb using the technique described below for terminal ileostomy.

TERMINAL ILEOSTOMY

Prepare

1 Identify a suitable location on the abdominal wall for the stoma. This should be on flat skin, with a wide enough margin for application of a stoma bag.

2 Consider where you will place the mucous fistula to the distal bowel. Ideally this should be beside the functioning stoma in order to facilitate eventual stoma closure.

3 Ensure that the bowel end is healthy with an adequate blood supply and that the mesentery is long enough for the cut end to reach the anterior abdominal wall.

Action

1 Excision of a disc of skin is not usually necessary: a simple transverse incision is usually satisfactory.

2 Carry the incision through the subcutaneous tissue and split the muscle. Ensure that the peritoneum is divided adequately to avoid obstruction of the intestine.

3 Place grasping forceps through the incision and grasp the end of the bowel to be made into a stoma. Pull the bowel through, ensuring that it does not become twisted and that the entire thickness of the bowel wall passes through the opening.

4 Draw the bowel out of the wound and suture the peritoneum or deep muscular fascia to the serosa, leaving an adequate length to form a mature everted stoma.

5 Place a suture through the skin, through the adjacent serosa, then take a full-thickness bite of the cut end of the bowel and tie the knot snug with the skin, everting the bowel. Repeat this circumferentially using 4 or 6 sutures to form a spout.

6 This technique may also be used to form a terminal colostomy. In this case you do not need to evert the bowel forming a spout, but can simply suture the bowel flush with the skin edge.

Aftercare

As for loop colostomy above.

Complications

1 Stenosis, which may cause partial or even complete obstruction and require dilatation or revision of the stoma.

2 Prolapse usually involves the distal limb of a loop stoma. An attempt at reduction should be made, but this is sometimes difficult and revision may be necessary. A small degree of uncomplicated prolapse is well tolerated and is best left alone.

CONDITIONS PRESENTING MAINLY IN THE NEWBORN OR NEONATAL PERIOD

NEONATAL INTESTINAL OBSTRUCTION

The commonest causes of intestinal obstruction in newborns include Hirschsprung's disease (1:5000 live births), intestinal atresia (1:8000 live births) and meconium ileus (1:15 000 live births).

Appraise

1 Proximal small-bowel obstruction is usually associated with bile-stained vomiting, a failure to pass meconium and an absence of abdominal distension. Mid-small-bowel obstruction or distal intestinal obstruction is usually associated with abdominal distension from early in life and subsequently with bile-stained vomiting. Frequently, there is a failure to pass meconium.

2 Abdominal X-ray confirms whether the obstruction is high or low, depending on the number of gas-filled loops seen on the X-ray film. If the anus is present, perform a digital examination to confirm that the anus is patent and also to see if the baby subsequently passes flatus and stool. Obviously, in the presence of intestinal atresia or meconium ileus, no flatus will be passed but the reverse is true in the presence of Hirschsprung's disease, when explosive decompression may occur.

3 Ideally, prefer to transfer the child to a regional centre, but if this is not possible, then perform a laparotomy without undue delay.

4 Do not hesitate to decompress the upper gastrointestinal tract by passing a nasogastric tube and administer intravenous fluids.

5 Administer broad-spectrum antibiotics, including cover for gram-negative organisms and anaerobic organisms.

Access

Use the standard transverse laparotomy incision.

Action

The procedure performed depends on the operative findings:

1 If duodenal atresia is encountered, tack together the two duodenal segments with three or four seromuscular sutures. Then open

the two segments with parallel incisions and complete an anastomosis.

2 For jejunal atresia, the best option is an end-to-end anastomosis but this is not a straightforward anastomosis for a non-specialist surgeon as it necessitates tapering of the very dilated proximal bowel. Under these circumstances a side-to-side anastomosis may be safer.

3 For distal small-bowel atresia, either a double-barrelled stoma or end-to-end anastomosis is possible.

4 Construct all anastomoses using fine monofilament sutures – nothing larger than a 5/0 suture – using the standard anastomosis technique previously described.

5 In meconium ileus, the distal small bowel is plugged with inspissated pale meconium pellets. Proximal to this, the small bowel is dilated and filled with tenacious meconium. Preferably perform an enterotomy in the dilated bowel and patiently evacuate all intestinal content with the help of saline irrigation. Close the enterotomy.

6 With complicated meconium ileus – in the presence of a twisted gangrenous segment or an associated atresia – resect the compromised bowel, evacuate intestinal contents and, ideally, anastomose the remaining intestine. If this is not possible, then create a double-barrelled stoma.

7 In Hirschsprung's disease, the intestine is in continuity but there is usually a change of calibre in the sigmoid colon. Under these circumstances, the best option is to perform either a right transverse colostomy or an ileostomy in the terminal ileum. This allows the baby to be fed and the length of affected bowel can be assessed at leisure.

OESOPHAGEAL ATRESIA

▶ **KEY POINTS** Refer to specialist?

- Surgery for the repair of oesophageal atresia is seldom an emergency so there is adequate time for referral to a specialist centre.
- In the absence of other severe congenital anomalies (especially cardiac malformations) nearly all infants weighing over 1500 g survive.

Appraise (Fig. 34.3)

1 The diagnosis may have been suspected antenatally in a fetus with polyhydramnios (Greek: high level of amniotic fluid), and a small stomach bubble. However, the majority of cases of oesophageal atresia are not diagnosed before birth.

2 Establish the diagnosis with a plain X-ray to reveal arrest of a radio-opaque nasogastric tube in the upper oesophagus. Include the abdomen on the radiograph. Air in the stomach indicates a distal tracheo-oesophageal fistula, for which primary repair is usually possible.

3 Absence of an abdominal gas shadow usually indicates isolated oesophageal atresia in which the distance between the proximal and distal segments is too long to permit primary oesophageal anastomosis, so a feeding gastrostomy and an end cervical oesophagostomy may be required.

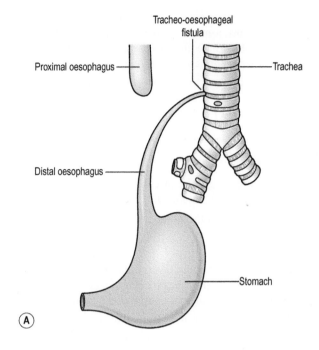

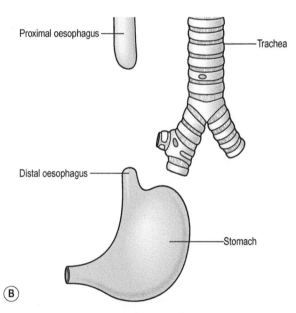

Fig. 34.3 The two main varieties of oesophageal atresia: (A) the most frequent (90%) condition with distal tracheo-oesophageal fistula; (B) the infrequent (5%) state of isolated oesophageal atresia.

Prepare

1 Insert a tube into the upper oesophageal pouch to allow for suctioning of secretions and swallowed saliva. A Replogle™ tube is ideal as it has a second channel which can be flushed to ensure that the tube does not become blocked.

2 If the infant is stable, contact your regional specialist centre and arrange for urgent transfer.

3 If the infant requires intubation and ventilation for respiratory distress then there is a risk that ventilation will be further impaired by the passage of gas through the fistula under pressure into the stomach and distal intestine. Gas preferentially follows

this path rather than enter the lungs, until the stomach becomes so distended that ventilation becomes impossible. Stomach rupture is very likely under these circumstances. Emergency ligation of the tracheo-oesophageal fistula may be life saving.

4 Cross match a unit of blood and arrange for emergency surgery.

LIGATION OF TRACHEO-OESOPHAGEAL FISTULA

Anaesthesia

1 Institute intubated general anaesthesia with the infant in the left lateral position and arm raised.

2 Mark the tip of the scapula once the infant is secured in position.

Access

1 The incision is a right posterolateral thoracotomy. Make a transverse incision just below the tip of the scapula with one third of the incision in front of your mark and two-thirds behind.

2 Incise the subcutaneous tissue with diathermy.

3 Divide the muscles with diathermy to minimise blood loss. Be careful to avoid damage to the long thoracic nerve running in the mid-axillary line.

4 Elevate the scapula and palpate the ribs to identify the fourth or fifth intercostal space.

5 Divide the external and internal intercostal muscles just above the rib to avoid damage to the neurovascular bundle.

6 Having exposed the pleura, incise the pleura with a scalpel avoiding damage to the underlying lung, and insert a suitably sized self-retaining rib retractor, e.g. Finochietto. Open the retractor and place a non-abrasive flat retractor into the thorax to retract the lung anteriorly allowing access to the posterior mediastinum.

7 Identify the azygos vein which crosses the fistula, incise the overlying pleura on either side of the vein and gently isolate the vein. Ligate it twice with 4/0 absorbable ties and divide.

8 Next identify the distal oesophagus. Look for the vagus nerve which lies on the surface of the distal oesophagus.

9 Trace the distal oesophagus to its proximal connection with the trachea.

10 Isolate the fistula and temporarily occlude it whilst asking the anaesthetist to continue ventilation. Ensure that the right lung continues to expand with the fistula occluded. This avoids inadvertent division of the right main bronchus.

11 Divide the fistula. Suture the defect in the trachea with interrupted 5/0 or 6/0 polypropylene sutures. Ensure that the repair is airtight by submerging the repair with saline: bubbles arising from the repair indicate a leak requiring closure. Aspirate the saline before closure.

12 Do not attempt definitive repair of the oesophageal atresia. This is not an emergency and is best performed by trained specialists. Close the chest and transfer to a specialist centre.

Closure

1 Allow the lung to re-expand fully. A chest drain is not required.

2 Close the intercostal muscles if possible with interrupted 3/0 or 4/0 polyglactin sutures. If there is not enough muscle to hold the suture place the suture around the rib, taking care not to bring the ribs too close together.

3 Close the muscles anatomically with interrupted 4/0 polyglactin sutures.

4 Close the skin with a subcuticular suture.

EXOMPHALOS AND GASTROSCHISIS

Appraise

1 Exomphalos is herniation of abdominal viscera into the persistent fetal umbilical hernia. The viscera are covered by a thin transparent membrane consisting of an outer layer of amniotic membrane lined by peritoneum, with Wharton's jelly between the two.

2 Gastroschisis is evisceration of the intestine through a defect in the anterior abdominal wall immediately to the right of an apparently normal umbilical cord. The intestine rapidly becomes oedematous and exudes a proteinaceous fluid that cocoons and mats together the intestinal loops.

3 Exomphalos is often associated with other major abnormalities such as serious cardiac and renal defects. Lethal chromosomal abnormalities such as Patau and Edward's syndrome are not uncommon.

4 Gastroschisis (Greek: gaster = belly + schisis = cleft; abdomen remains open) is not associated with extra-abdominal anomalies but atresias may occur in the intestine. Do not attempt definitive treatment of associated intestinal atresias prior to abdominal wall closure. Allow the abdomen to heal, maintain the infant on parenteral nutrition and perform a laparotomy after 4–6 weeks to treat these.

> ▶ KEY POINTS Abdominal wall closure?
>
> ■ Neonates with gastroschisis and ruptured exomphalos have a better prognosis if the abdominal wall can be closed, or placed into a silo, within a few hours of birth.
> ■ This implies either in-utero transfer or urgent transfer to the regional unit.

Transfer

1 As soon as possible after birth pass a nasogastric tube and aspirate the stomach. Leave the tube on free drainage.

2 Insert an intravenous cannula, replace the volume of fluid aspirated from the stomach with replacement fluid (0.9% saline with 10 mmol KCl; per 500 ml bag) and give the infant a further 20 ml/kg of plasma. Ongoing fluid losses in abdominal wall defects are large and usually underestimated.

3 Check the blood sugar and correct with 10% dextrose if necessary.

4 Before transfer, wrap the herniated bowel with Clingfilm to limit fluid losses and protect the intestine. This is best done by wrapping Clingfilm around the entire abdomen. In addition, support the intestine using rolled up nappies or sheets of gamgee to prevent it moving from side to side and kinking on its mesentery, causing ischaemia. Nursing the baby on its side may help this.

5 Transfer the baby as per neonatal transport guidelines, ensuring that further fluid is given as required and that the nasogastric tube is regularly aspirated.

Principles

Exomphalos minor

1 If very minor (herniation into the umbilical cord), reduce the intestine into the abdominal cavity and ligate the base of the cord with a thick ligature, thereby avoiding operation. The alternative is to twist the cord to reduce the contents and strap the cord on to the abdomen for a few days. Only do this if you are entirely sure that all of the viscera are reduced into the abdomen.

2 If operative repair is necessary, close the defect with a purse-string suture of 3/0 or 4/0 polyglycolic acid. The sac may be used as part of the repair or excised. If part of the sac is adherent to the liver, do not try to separate it. Leave it in situ and return the liver to the abdomen.

3 Perform an upper gastrointestinal contrast study before or after surgery as 30% of infants with exomphalos will need a laparotomy and Ladd's procedure (see below).

Unruptured exomphalos major

1 Non-operative treatment is achieved by applying a dressing to the sac, which promotes healing. An antiseptic such as silver sulfadiazine may also be used. As the sac dries out an eschar forms which separates after many weeks, leaving an epithelialized defect that grows at a slower rate than the rest of the infant. A large ventral hernia may result and this can be repaired during the second year of life.

2 Operative treatment is by application of a Prolene mesh silo to cover the unruptured exomphalos, with gradual reduction of the contents over the subsequent days or weeks. Suture the Prolene mesh to the abdominal muscles at the edges of the defect. When full reduction has been achieved, remove the Prolene mesh and close the defect.

Ruptured exomphalos major

1 Primary repair is usually impossible.

2 Repair the sac and treat as an unruptured exomphalos.

Gastroschisis

There are two options:

Either routine placement of a preformed silo

Or attempted reduction of the bowel under general anaesthesia with placement of a surgical silo if this proves impossible.

Action: preformed silo placement

The aim is to cover the eviscerated bowel with a pre-made silo of flexible silicone rubber (Medicina™ silo). First ensure that the bowel is free from the edge of the defect around its circumference. Then estimate the diameter of the defect in the abdominal wall and select an appropriately sized silo. Identify the apex of the loop of eviscerated bowel and insert this into the silo first, followed by the remaining loops of bowel. Finally, insert the flexible rubber ring into the abdominal cavity.

Action: abdominal wall closure

Gently attempt to return the eviscerated organs to the peritoneal cavity. You may need to enlarge the defect in the midline cranially and/ or caudally to do this. Separate the skin from the muscle layers at the

end of the defect and close the defect in the abdominal wall longitudinally with 3/0 or 4/0 polyglycolic acid or polydioxanone. An attempt should be made to recreate the umbilicus in the repair.

Postoperative mechanical ventilation and parenteral nutrition are invariably required. If it is not possible to return the eviscerated bowel to the abdomen then separate the muscle from the overlying skin and apply a silo. To do this, take a sterile bag (e.g. a bag of intravenous fluid cut in half), place the bag over the bowel and tuck the edges inside the peritoneal cavity. Then take a piece of prolene mesh and tack this to the fascia around the bag using 4/0 polyproylene, completely encircling it. Finally, close the edges of the mesh together at the top.

Aftercare

1 The intestine does not function immediately, so maintain the infant on parenteral nutrition.

2 If a silo has been placed, gradually reduce the size of the silo, compressing the bowel into the abdominal cavity over a period of 7–10 days. Once the bowel is returned to the abdomen the defect can be closed using adhesive dressings in the case of a preformed silo. If a silo has been attached surgically then general anaesthesia and formal closure are necessary.

3 Once the bowel has been returned to the abdomen, start trophic feeds and increase enteral feeds as tolerated. Infants with gastroschisis will have impaired gastrointestinal motility and take a long time to achieve full enteral feeds.

Prognosis

1 In the absence of other serious anomalies, the prognosis for exomphalos minor is excellent.

2 The survival rate for gastroschisis is now over 90%. A small percentage of infants are born with loss of their herniated midgut ('closed gastroschisis') and these children have a much poorer outcome.

3 Because of operative difficulties and the presence of serious associated anomalies, the prognosis of exomphalos major is poorer.

CONGENITAL DIAPHRAGMATIC HERNIA

Appraise

1 Most cases of congenital diaphragmatic hernia are diagnosed antenatally in centres with such facilities.

2 Presentation is otherwise with respiratory distress in the newborn period. About 10% of patients present after the newborn period with either recurrent respiratory symptoms or, occasionally, acute gastrointestinal symptoms.

3 A chest radiograph reveals intestinal gas shadows in the involved hemithorax with displacement of the mediastinal structures to the contralateral side.

Action

1 Do not ventilate the infant with a face-mask as this will blow air down the oesophagus and into the intestine, resulting in rapid deterioration.

2 Pass a large (8 or 10F) nasogastric tube to keep the stomach empty and to limit the amount of air passing into the intestine.

3 Pass an endotracheal tube and use positive-pressure mechanical ventilation.

4 Ventilatory pressures should ideally not exceed 12 cmH$_2$O to avoid alveolar rupture and pneumothorax. Treat tension pneumothorax by inserting a chest drain attached to an underwater seal.

5 Insert an intravenous cannula for expansion of circulating volume.

6 Insert an arterial cannula for assessment of blood gases.

> ▶ KEY POINTS Resuscitation
>
> ■ Once resuscitation is under way, arrange urgent rapid transfer to a regional surgical unit.
> ■ Resuscitation must be undertaken rapidly and effectively, but operative intervention should not be performed until cardiorespiratory stability has been achieved. This may take several days.
> ■ Respiratory support has developed significantly and now includes oscillatory ventilation, permissive hypercapnia and nitric oxide. Inspiratory pressures should be kept as low as possible to avoid barotrauma.
> ■ The timing of operation is best assessed by an experienced regional team.

Principles

1 Laparotomy is performed using the 'general purpose' incision but confining it to the side of the hernial defect.

2 Gently withdraw the intestines, stomach and finally the spleen from the chest.

3 Identify the diaphragmatic defect and excise the sac if present.

4 If small, primarily repair the diaphragmatic defect with non-absorbable sutures.

5 If the defect is so large that the diaphragm hardly exists, repair the defect using a prosthetic patch of woven Dacron^{TM} (polyester) sutured with non-absorbable sutures to the chest wall.

6 Close the abdomen.

Aftercare

1 Postoperative assisted ventilation is mandatory. Respiratory status usually deteriorates temporarily following closure.

2 Nurses experienced in neonatal intensive care are essential.

Complications

1 Pleural effusion is extremely common but rarely requires treatment.

2 Chylous effusion may occur if posterior medial dissection has been necessary, due to damage to lymphatic trunks. Treat with medium chain triglyceride feeds ± octreotide ± TPN.

3 Recurrence of the hernia occurs in 10% of cases, more if a patch is required.

Prognosis

1 About 50% of all fetuses with antenatally detected diaphragmatic hernias have associated lethal malformations which will preclude independent existence. Overall survival for infants diagnosed at birth is about 80%. Those with a right-sided hernia have a worse prognosis.

2 Death occurs almost entirely from pulmonary hypoplasia and pulmonary hypertension.

3 A small number of infants with adequate lung size but refractory pulmonary hypertension may be saved by extracorporeal membrane oxygenation (ECMO).

4 Long-term respiratory outcome is determined by the extent of pulmonary hypoplasia.

5 Feeding problems and gastro-oesophageal reflux are common, often requiring medical treatment and sometimes fundoplication.

ANORECTAL MALFORMATIONS

These occur in about 1:5000 newborns. There are over forty different types of anorectal malformation but they are commonly grouped into two categories – high and low malformations.

The high malformations comprise those where the bowel terminates above the pelvic floor and opens either into the urinary tract in boys or the urogenital tract in girls.

In those with low malformations, the bowel traverses the pelvic floor but becomes stenosed or ectopic lower down. In general terms, children with low abnormalities have a better outlook in terms of bowel control.

Appraise

1 Undertake a detailed inspection of the perineum. It may be difficult to distinguish between high and low anomalies in the first 24 hours of life. In girls, assess the number of openings. If there is a single orifice, the baby probably has a cloacal malformation whereby the urinary, genital and gastrointestinal tracts open into a common cavity. This is the most complicated form of high anomaly in girls.

If only urethra and vagina are visible in a female infant, seek a tiny opening in the posterior fourchette. This is the commonest malformation in girls. The safest management for such infants is to perform a colostomy. Use the loop colostomy technique previously described.

2 In boys, a stenosed, ectopic anus may only become evident after 24 hours. If no meconium is seen at this time or if meconium is seen in the urine, the lesion is high and a stoma is needed.

3 All these babies need ultrasound examination of the urinary tract because of the common association of urinary anomalies and imperforate anus.

4 Once a defunctioning stoma has been fashioned, refer the infant to a specialist centre for definitive surgery.

MALROTATION WITH OR WITHOUT MIDGUT VOLVULUS

Development

The midgut develops within the physiological umbilical hernia in early intrauterine life. Between the tenth and twelfth weeks of development, the midgut loop returns to the peritoneal cavity, rotating in an orderly manner beginning with the jejunum and ending with the ileocaecal region. The duodenum rotates into its C-loop and the ileocaecal loop undergoes counter-clockwise rotation of 270 degrees, resulting in fixation of the proximal duodenum and ascending colon in the right retroperitoneum and the duodenojejunal flexure on the left. As a result, the root of the mesentery of the small intestine is obliquely attached across the posterior abdominal wall over a relatively long distance.

Malrotation results when this process of rotation and fixation is incomplete and the duodenum and caecum lie close together with the superior mesenteric vessels between. The base of the small bowel mesentery is thus very narrow and is prone to volvulus.

Volvulus may occur at any age but occurs most commonly during the first few months of life.

Appraise

1 Consider the diagnosis of malrotation in any infant manifesting bilious vomiting. This may be intermittent, indicating twisting and untwisting of the bowel.

2 Plain abdominal radiographs may reveal a dilated stomach and duodenum with the rest of the abdomen relatively gasless when volvulus has occurred.

3 A child in whom malrotation with or without volvulus is suspected must undergo confirmation of the diagnosis by means of urgent upper gastrointestinal contrast radiography.

4 Treatment is urgent when volvulus has occurred, as untreated volvulus results in shock and gastrointestinal haemorrhage. The blood supply to the entire midgut may be compromised and delay in treatment serves only to increase the amount and extent of intestinal necrosis. Nevertheless, a short (1–2 hours) intensive period of active resuscitation to correct fluid and electrolyte loss and acid–base imbalance may be worthwhile.

Prepare

1 Correct dehydration with intravenous fluid (0.9% saline, 20 ml/kg) as rapidly as possible.

2 Administer broad-spectrum antibiotics.

3 Effect urgent transfer to a specialized paediatric surgical unit, ensuring that full resuscitative measures continue en route.

4 Where regional specialized facilities are unavailable, operation will have to be performed locally.

Anaesthesia

Use general endotracheal anaesthesia with the infant in the supine position.

Access

Open the abdomen using the 'general purpose' incision.

Assess

1 Inspect the bowel for obvious areas of gangrene. These should be handled very gently as the intestinal wall is extremely friable and prone to perforation.

2 Assess the direction of rotation and untwist the volvulus. This is usually in an anti-clockwise direction.

3 If extensive intestinal gangrene is present as a consequence of the volvulus, the bowel should be de-rotated, the abdomen closed and urgent transfer to a regional centre arranged. We generally recommend the use of tissue plasminogen activator (tPA) when compromised bowel has been untwisted and no return of colour seen. A second laparotomy is performed 36 to 48 hours later and any necrotic bowel removed. Remarkable return of perfusion may occur with the use of tPA.

4 Whilst awaiting return of circulation to compromised bowel, inspect the root of the mesentery for evidence of malrotation.

5 In a typical case, the root of the mesentery between the duodenojejunal flexure and the ileocaecal junction is very narrow and fibrotic. The caecum lies below the liver and may even be attached to the gallbladder by peritoneal bands.

Action

1 Ladd's procedure is recommended.

2 Divide the avascular peritoneal bands arising from the caecum and attaching to the liver, gallbladder and the lateral abdominal wall.

3 Once all the bands are divided, the caecum may be placed in the left upper quadrant of the abdomen.

4 Mobilize the duodenum by Kocher's manoeuvre and divide all peritoneal folds so that all kinks in the duodenum are straightened.

5 Incise what is now the anterior layer of peritoneum at the root of the mesentery and divide all fibrous bands so that the caecum may be moved as far to the left as possible, away from the duodenojejunal flexure, broadening the base of the mesentery.

6 Inspect the duodenum carefully, searching for areas of duodenal stenosis. This is uncommon except in patients presenting in early infancy. Correct duodenal stenosis by performing a duodenoduodenostomy.

7 Return attention to the small bowel. Measure the length of the ischaemic bowel and assess the blood supply.

8 Resect all truly gangrenous areas unless this would leave the child with less than 30 cm of small bowel. Consider whether it would be better to perform a primary anastomosis or to bring out both ends as temporary stomas. If the ends of resected intestine are viable it is preferable to perform a primary anastomosis.

9 When most of the intestine is ischaemic, return it to the abdomen, having untwisted the volvulus and divided constricting bands and adhesions. Close the abdomen en masse. Continue intensive medical treatment, and re-explore after 24–48 hours. At the 'second-look' laparotomy in young infants, one is often surprised at how the blood supply has improved. At the second operation, resect all bowel that is obviously gangrenous, but retain all bowel of doubtful viability. Bring the two ends out as temporary stomata. An anastomosis in compromised bowel is not advised as it is prone to disruption.

10 If all the bowel is viable, consider performing an appendicectomy, because the appendix would otherwise lie below the left costal margin and could cause diagnostic confusion at a later date.

Appendicectomy is best performed by the inversion method so as not to spill intestinal bacteria in an otherwise 'clean' operation.

Closure

1 Close the abdomen en masse.
2 Suture the skin with a continuous subcuticular suture.

Aftercare

1 Postoperative mechanical ventilation and cardiovascular support with inotropes may be necessary in the infant with massive intestinal necrosis.
2 Even in uncomplicated malrotation with or without volvulus, ileus commonly occurs for up to 2 weeks and parenteral nutrition is often necessary.
3 After massive intestinal resections, prolonged parenteral nutrition will be required. Oral nutrition is re-introduced with considerable caution as there is frequently intolerance to lactose, lipids and proteins.

CONDITIONS TYPICALLY PRESENTING OUTSIDE THE NEWBORN PERIOD

INGUINAL HERNIA

Appraise

1 In the paediatric age range, inguinal hernia is generally due to failure of closure of the processus vaginalis. The hernia may be complete (to the scrotum) or incomplete (confined to the inguinal region). Operation is indicated in all cases.
2 Inguinal hernias become irreducible in up to 30% of infants, the peak incidence being between the ages of 6 and 12 weeks. Strangulation is rare in the neonatal period, but, when it does occur, there is appreciable postoperative morbidity and a high mortality rate.
3 If the hernia becomes irreducible, pressure upon the spermatic cord causes testicular ischaemia, and infarction may occur after as little as 4 hours. Up to 25% of neonates with an irreducible hernia develop severe testicular ischaemia.
4 Most 'irreducible' inguinal herniae can be reduced following sedation and 'taxis' – gentle to-and-fro pressure applied to the neck of the hernial sac at the level of the external inguinal ring. Following reduction, it is recommended that elective repair of the hernia is carried out about 48 hours later once the oedema has subsided.
5 Premature babies are particularly prone to develop complications. Herniotomy should be carried out at a stage when the infant has gained sufficient weight to warrant discharge from hospital or as soon as complications occur. These small infants often have co-existing medical problems including chronic lung disease. The help of an experienced paediatric anaesthetist is invaluable and sometimes the operation can be performed only by using spinal or epidural anaesthesia. These patients are prone to all of the complications associated with 'persistent fetal circulation', and postoperative deaths do occur, even with elective operation in a regional centre.

6 In infants under the age of 6 months, the tissues are thin and friable so operative difficulties are common. Treatment is best left to paediatric surgeons.
7 If the ipsilateral testis is not in the scrotum do not attempt to bring it into the scrotum in a child below 6 months of age. Leave the testis in position and re-assess when the child is approaching 1 year. Above 6 months of age a simultaneous orchidopexy may be performed.
8 Except in children with neuromuscular disorders, herniotomy rather than herniorrhaphy is the treatment of choice.

Action: herniotomy through the inguinal canal

1 Make an incision 2 cm long in a skin crease midway between the deep ring and pubic tubercle.
2 Divide the subcutaneous fat and Camper's fascia using scissors.
3 Incise Scarpa's fascia with scissors and retract it.
4 Clear a small patch of external oblique aponeurosis over an area of 2 cm^2, at least 1 cm above the inguinal ligament.
5 Incise the external oblique aponeurosis along its fibres with scissors or a scalpel and retract the edges. Do not open the external inguinal ring.
6 Dissect into the inguinal canal, keeping close to the posterior surface of the external oblique aponeurosis.
7 Soon the ilio-inguinal nerve will come into view, and this provides a useful landmark.
8 Using a mosquito artery forceps, split the fibres of the cremaster muscle overlying the spermatic cord just inferior to the ilio-inguinal nerve. If you have difficulty identifying the spermatic cord, pull gently on the ipsilateral testis within the scrotum. The cord will move, helping you to identify its location within the layers of muscle.
9 Gently grasp the internal spermatic fascia with a mosquito forceps and use this to deliver the spermatic cord from its bed whilst pushing away the adherent fibres of the cremaster muscle with a delicate non-toothed dissecting forceps.
10 Create a 'window' behind the cord using blunt dissection ensuring that you have all of the cord anteriorly. Pass the index finger of the non-dominant hand behind the cord and use it and the thumb to rotate the cord so that its posterior aspect comes into view.
11 Using a non-toothed dissecting forceps, split the internal spermatic fascia overlying the vas and vessels in a longitudinal direction.
12 Gently sweep the vas and vessels away from the sac. Do not hold the vas or vessels with the forceps because a crush injury may occur.
13 Ensure that the sac is empty. If you have any doubt it is safest to place artery forceps on one edge to secure it and then open it. Having confirmed it is empty, place an artery forceps across the sac (proximal to the opening if you have made one) and divide the sac distal to the forceps. Allow the distal part of the sac to fall back into the wound.
14 Dissect the vas and vessels from the proximal part of the sac, until the inferior epigastric vessels are seen.
15 Rotate the artery forceps to twist the neck of the sac, so ensuring that there is no bowel or omentum within it.

16 A transfixion ligature of 4/0 absorbable suture is used to close the neck of the sac.

17 Allow the vas and vessels to drop back into the inguinal canal.

18 Close the inguinal canal with two or three sutures.

19 Approximate Scarpa's fascia with one or two sutures.

20 Close the skin with a subcuticular stitch.

21 Gently pull the testis to the bottom of the scrotum to ensure that it does not become caught in the superficial inguinal pouch, necessitating later orchidopexy.

? DIFFICULTY

1. Do not panic: think rationally.
2. The ilio-inguinal nerve is a good landmark.
3. If lost, keep close to the deep surface of the external oblique, and track down to the inguinal ligament; the cord lies between the ligament and the ilio-inguinal nerve. Traction on the testis will move the cord, enabling you to identify it.
4. Remember that the inguinal canal has definite boundaries and the cord must lie between the external ring, which is palpable, and the deep ring that is delineated medially by the inferior epigastric vessels, which should be visible.
5. If still in doubt, check that you are in the inguinal canal, and check that the incision is placed between the landmarks of the deep and superficial inguinal rings.
6. As a last resort, extend the incision, identify the external inguinal ring and proceed from there, possibly by incising the ring and laying open the entire inguinal canal.

Action: laparoscopic inguinal hernia repair

1 Use the laparoscopic approach described previously with a 5-mm supra-umbilical access port.

2 Make a full thickness 'stab' incision on the left side of the abdomen (assuming you are right handed), lateral to and just above the umbilicus under direct vision. Insert an atraumatic grasper.

3 Gently move the bowel up from the pelvis with the grasper bringing the deep inguinal rings into vision (tilting the patient's head down may help).

4 Confirm the preoperative diagnosis of a suspected open deep inguinal ring and examine the other side. If open, you will close both sides. Identify the limits of the internal ring, the vas deferens heading medially towards the bladder and the testicular vessels heading up the retroperitoneum.

5 Make a second stab incision on the right side of the abdomen under direct vision. Cut a length of 4/0 non-absorbable suture 12cm long, grasp the suture (not the needle) with a 3-mm needle-holder and pass this directly through the abdominal wall into the peritoneal cavity.

6 Mount your needle.

7 Pick up a fold of peritoneum at the edge of the deep inguinal ring at the 3 o'clock position. Pass the needle and suture through this fold leaving an adequate 'tail'.

8 Create a 'purse-string' suture in the peritoneum around the deep inguinal ring by picking up the peritoneum and passing the needle through it. Work in a clockwise direction ensuring that you do not pick up the testicular vessels or the vas deferens nor include them in the purse string. At some point in the purse string include a deeper bite into the muscle well away from the vas, vessels and inferior epigastric vessels. This helps to prevent the suture in the internal ring from herniating down the inguinal canal after you have closed it.

9 Lift the knot away from the tissues and take up all the slack before tightening the suture. Cut the suture and remove the short cut end from the abdomen. If there is any doubt, place a second purse string or a Z-stitch over the top of the first. A 12-cm suture should allow you to tie two purse strings.

10 If the contralateral PPV is patent close it in an identical fashion. This will help to prevent metachronous hernia.

11 Close the incisions as previously described.

Aftercare

1 Except in infants less than 50 weeks' post-gestational age, the procedure is carried out on a day-case basis and there are no special postoperative precautions.

2 A slight fever on the first postoperative night may be a normal response to surgery.

Complications

1 Recurrence of the hernia occurs in 1–2% of cases, but more frequently in ex-preterm infants.

2 Unrecognized damage to the testicular vessels may result in testicular atrophy following up to 1% of repairs.

3 Following repair of a hernia that has been incarcerated, testicular atrophy may occur due to ischaemia.

PYLORIC STENOSIS

Appraise

1 This occurs predominantly in male infants (male-to-female ratio = 6–8:1) around the second to sixth week of life.

2 The cardinal features are projectile non-bilious vomiting, failure to thrive and constipation.

3 The diagnosis is established by palpating the pyloric 'tumour' in the right hypochondrium.

4 Confirm by ultrasound examination when you remain in doubt about the diagnosis after examining the baby.

Prepare

1 Measure serum urea, electrolytes and acid–base status.

2 Correct hypochloraemia and hypokalaemia with intravenous infusion of half-normal saline with 10% dextrose, adding potassium (10–15 mmol KCl per 500 ml of 0.45% saline/10% dextrose).

3 It is unnecessary to correct the alkalosis, which resolves spontaneously with the saline infusion. Surgery should not be performed until the serum bicarbonate is 26 mmol/L or less.

4 Prohibit all feeds and leave a nasogastric tube on free drainage, replacing losses millilitre for millilitre with normal saline and potassium (10 mmol KCl per 500 ml of 0.9% saline).

5 Check that serum potassium levels are above 3.5 mmol/L before arranging operation.

> ### ▶ KEY POINTS Resuscitate
>
> ■ The operation for pyloric stenosis is NEVER an emergency.
> ■ Delay it for 24–48 hours or even longer until you have corrected dehydration and electrolyte disturbances.

Anaesthesia

1 Arrange general anaesthesia with endotracheal intubation by an experienced paediatric anaesthetist.

Access

1 The infant lies supine on the operating table protected from cold.

2 There are two possible incisions:
Either a transverse incision, 3–4 cm long, in the right hypochondrium midway between the costal margin and the palpable inferior margin of the liver; the medial end of the incision ends 1–2 cm from the midline
Or a supra-umbilical incision of adequate length to allow delivery of the 'tumour'.

Note: The operation can also be performed laparoscopically with equally good results.

3 Having incised the skin with the scalpel, divide the subcutaneous tissue and muscles using cutting diathermy to limit blood loss.

4 Open the peritoneum.

5 Retract the inferior margin of the liver superiorly by means of a broad malleable retractor protected by a moist gauze swab (not required with a supra-umbilical incision).

6 Identify the greater curvature of the stomach directly or after applying gentle traction on the omentum.

7 Do not attempt to withdraw the pyloric tumour by applying direct traction on the mass; this results in serosal tears and haemorrhage.

8 Deliver the greater curvature of the body of the stomach into the wound.

9 Apply gentle traction on the greater curvature until the firm, white, glistening pyloric tumour is brought into view. Ease it out of the peritoneal cavity and into the wound.

10 Identify the pyloric vein of Mayo. This marks the distal end of the pyloric canal.

Action: pyloromyotomy (Fig. 34.4)

1 Make an incision 1–2 mm deep with a scalpel on the anterior surface of the pyloric tumour in the relatively avascular plane midway between the superior and inferior borders. Extend the incision from the pyloric vein of Mayo, through the pyloric canal and onto the hypertrophied body of the stomach.

2 Using firm but gentle pressure on the incised pylorus with a McDonald dissector, the blunt handle of a scalpel or a blunt

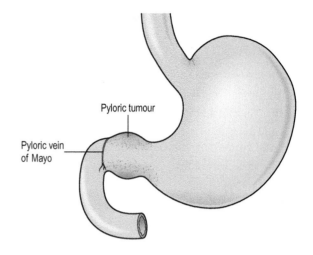

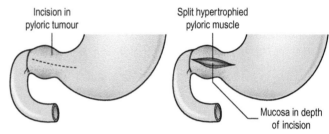

Fig. 34.4 Ramstedt's pyloromyotomy.

artery forceps, split the hypertrophied muscle down to the submucosa.

3 Split the pyloric mass from end to end using a pyloric spreader (Denis Browne) or blunt artery forceps. Ensure that all the fibres of the pyloric tumour are split.

4 Bubbles of air or bile at the duodenal end of the incision signify a perforation of the mucosa, most common in the duodenal fornix.

5 Close a perforation with a few interrupted 5/0 absorbable sutures and cover with omentum.

6 Haemorrhage from the incised pylorus is mainly due to venous congestion. Bleeding usually ceases once the pylorus is returned to the abdominal cavity. If bleeding persists, use diathermy coagulation.

Closure

1 Close the wound en masse using interrupted 4/0 polyglycolic acid sutures.

2 Approximate the skin with a continuous subcuticular 5/0 absorbable suture.

Aftercare

1 Feeds can be commenced 6 hours after the operation. Start with 15–20 ml of milk and, if tolerated, increase to a full volume of feed. Warn the parents that postoperative vomiting is common.

2 Continue intravenous fluids until feeding is established.

3 The infant should be ready for discharge from hospital on the first or second postoperative day.

4 If a perforation of the mucosa occurred, withhold feeds for 24 hours while continuing nasogastric decompression and intravenous fluids. Then introduce feeds as above.

Complications

In addition to perforation, pyloromyotomy is incomplete in approximately 1% of cases. This may be more common with the laparoscopic approach. Presentation is with recurrence of symptoms between 1 and 10 days following the procedure. The diagnosis is difficult as symptoms are similar to the preoperative state and to gastro-oesophageal reflux. Contrast studies are not helpful as even after a successful pyloromyotomy the appearance is like an unoperated pyloric stenosis. As a result it usually takes some weeks to be certain of the diagnosis. Repeat pyloromyotomy is necessary if confirmed.

INTESTINAL OBSTRUCTION

Causes of intestinal obstruction which occur primarily in older infants and children (but may also occur in the newborn) include intestinal volvulus as a consequence of malrotation, intussusception, adhesional obstruction and incarcerated inguinal hernia. Abdominal pain is a prominent feature. Vomiting also occurs and becomes bile-stained. Dark blood per rectum is a feature of intestinal compromise from volvulus. Red blood per rectum may occur in a child with intussusception. Diagnosis is primarily based on features from the history, physical examination and abdominal radiograph.

INTUSSUSCEPTION (Fig. 34.5)

Appraise

1 Between the ages of 6 months and 2 years, most intussusceptions are 'idiopathic', possibly caused by viral infections. The vast majority originate in the ileocaecal region. The condition is less common after the age of 2 years and rare in the neonatal period.

2 The sick infant should be resuscitated and then transferred to a specialized unit, resuscitation continuing during the journey. The usual volumes of resuscitation fluids are given – 20 ml/kg – and repeated as necessary. These infants often deteriorate rapidly after operation and may not survive unless there are adequate facilities for intensive care.

3 In the 'idiopathic age group', and in the absence of radiological evidence of intestinal obstruction or perforation, initial treatment is attempted using either pneumatic or hydrostatic reduction, the latter by means of a barium enema. Such facilities are usually only available in specialist centres. If this is unsuccessful, operation is required.

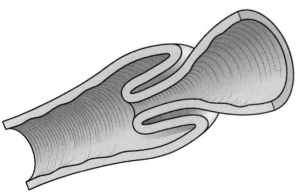

Fig. 34.5   Intussusception.

4 Outside the usual age range there is more likely to be a leading point such as a Meckel's diverticulum, polyp, duplication cyst or tumour causing the intussusception, and operation should be advised at an early stage.

5 If the infant is in good condition and regional facilities for non-operative reduction are not available, prepare for operation.

> **KEY POINT** Resuscitation

- Infants and children with intussusception are often significantly hypovolaemic and require aggressive fluid resuscitation.
- Administer at least 20 ml/kg of normal saline at presentation and insert a large bore nasogastric tube.
- Replace all gastrointestinal losses ml per ml and repeat the fluid bolus if necessary.

Prepare

1 Set up a well-placed, adequately running, intravenous infusion.

2 Most infants will have reduced intravascular volume and will need preoperative rehydration. Many will require replacement of 10% or more of blood volume with plasma, plasma expanders or whole blood.

3 Once anaesthetized, the peripheral vascular resistance falls and the child may deteriorate suddenly.

4 Administer preoperative antibiotics.

5 Pass a large nasogastric tube.

Access

1 An expert may be able to reduce an intussusception through a short Lanz incision, as for appendicectomy.

2 In the absence of such skills, it is wise to use the 'general purpose' supra-umbilical transverse incision.

Assess

1 There should be an obvious sausage-shaped mass, usually in the midline, but possibly along the course of the right or left colon.

2 The anatomy of the right colon will be distorted, being drawn towards the transverse colon.

3 The appendix may not be visible.

Action

1 Withdraw the colon distal to the mass and gently attempt to push out the intussusceptum by squeezing the intussuscipiens in an antiperistaltic direction towards the caecum.

> **KEY POINT** Gentleness

- Never try to pull out the intussusceptum by traction upon it, for if the bowel is ischaemic it will perforate or tear away in your hand.

2 Patience and gentleness will succeed in the majority of cases.

3 Reduction becomes increasingly difficult as it proceeds towards the starting point (apex), the last few centimetres being the most difficult. Proceed very slowly if the serosa of the intussuscipiens begins to split.

4 Continue assessment during reduction. If the reduced intussusceptum is obviously gangrenous or perforates, abandon the reduction and proceed to a limited right hemicolectomy.

5 If the reduction is successful, examine the distal ileum to ensure there is no ileo-ileal element to the intussusception. The anti-mesenteric border of the ileum 5–10 cm from the ileocaecal valve is the usual starting point of the intussusception and it is to be expected that there will be a thickened patch in the bowel wall 2–3 cm long at that site. This is not an indication for intestinal resection. This patch of oedematous bowel is an enlarged Peyer's patch and is not to be confused with a polyp or tumour.

6 If the bowel is viable, some surgeons perform an appendicectomy (especially if the Lanz incision is used), by either the inversion or the routine method. If there is doubt about the viability of the caecum, leave the appendix in situ. The intestine has remarkable powers of healing in this age group.

7 If the bowel is non-viable, resect the affected length. A standard right hemicolectomy is rarely necessary. Excise only the gangrenous areas and perform an end-to-end ileocolic anastomosis as previously described.

8 Check for a Meckel's diverticulum. If present, excise it using a simple intestinal resection and anastomosis.

9 Ensure that there is no polyp, duplication cyst or tumour acting as a 'lead-point'.

Closure

As for standard laparotomy.

Aftercare

1 Observe closely for hypovolaemic or bacteraemic shock following gangrenous intussusception.

2 Hyperpyrexia is not uncommon in the first 24–48 hours. Measures to reduce body temperature may be required.

3 Approximately 10% of non-operatively reduced intussusceptions will recur. The parents usually recognize the cry immediately.

ADHESION OBSTRUCTION

Appraise

1 Adhesion obstruction as a consequence of previous surgery occurs in about 5% of children who have undergone laparotomy.

2 The majority of such episodes occur within 12 months of the previous operation but the risk is lifelong.

3 Typically, symptoms begin with abdominal pain which becomes more severe and is associated with vomiting. In the presence of strangulation, the pain becomes relentless.

4 Young children frequently have obstruction by peritoneal bands and intestinal strangulation is an early feature.

5 In children with intestinal obstruction, there may be visible bowel loops and peristalsis on inspecting the abdomen. Obstructive bowel sounds are heard on auscultation. Tenderness occurs when the bowel is severely compromised.

6 Abdominal X-ray usually shows multiple dilated loops of bowel with no gas in the rectum. The presence of visible jejunal loops is almost diagnostic in this setting.

7 The treatment of adhesion obstruction in infants and children is surgical. There is very limited, if any, role for non-operative treatment.

Prepare

1 Pass a large bore nasogastric tube for gastric decompression.

2 Children with obstruction may require aggressive fluid resuscitation. Administer intravenous fluids and monitor.

3 Administer broad-spectrum antibiotics prior to surgery.

Access

Use the standard upper transverse incision. If there has been a previous incision resulting in adhesion obstruction then that incision can be used, but it will need to be enlarged.

Action

1 Taking great care not to cause a perforation, divide the obstructing adhesions.

2 If an ischaemic loop of bowel is encountered, perform a resection and anastomosis as necessary.

Aftercare

1 Intravenous fluids are given until the ileus resolves.

2 It is common for these children to need extra boluses of fluid to replace ongoing occult losses in the abdomen.

APPENDICITIS

Appraise

1 Appendicitis is the commonest surgical cause of abdominal pain in children. The estimated lifetime risk of appendicitis is approximately 8%. The commonest age of presentation is between 8 and 14 years.

2 The diagnosis may be difficult to make. Classical features are worsening abdominal pain migrating from umbilicus to right iliac fossa, nausea, vomiting and malaise. Examination findings include fever, tachycardia, localized peritonism in the right iliac fossa and generalized peritonism in advanced cases.

3 The diagnosis is clinical. Measurements of neutrophil count, white cell count and C-reactive protein are neither sensitive nor specific. Imaging modalities including ultrasound and CT scanning are being used increasingly to assist in diagnosis.

4 If the diagnosis is uncertain and the child is stable then serial observation is employed to detect changes in clinical status over time. If the child improves then the diagnosis is excluded. If clinical features progress then the diagnosis is confirmed.

Prepare

1 Assess degree of dehydration and resuscitate if necessary with 20 ml/kg of normal saline as a bolus.

2 If the child is vomiting insert a nasogastric tube and discontinue all oral intake. Replace any nasogastric losses ml per ml with normal saline with 10 mmol potassium chloride per 500 ml.

3 If advanced appendicitis is suspected based on abdominal examination and general clinical features, administer broad-spectrum antibiotics.

4 Consider the need for appendicectomy. Localized perforated appendicitis may be preferentially and successfully treated with broad-spectrum intravenous antibiotics, intestinal rest and analgesia.

Anaesthesia

1 Induce general anaesthesia with the child supine.

2 After the induction of general anaesthesia examine the abdomen to determine the presence of a firm, fixed mass arising from the right side of the pelvis. If present, abandon the procedure, wake the child up and treat with broad-spectrum intravenous antibiotics until fever and abdominal pain subside.

Access

1 There are two options:
Either open appendicectomy: make a transverse incision 4–5 cm long in the right iliac fossa centred on McBurney's point which lies one third of the distance along a line drawn from the anterior superior iliac spine to the umbilicus
Or laparoscopic appendicectomy: use a 5-mm supra-umbilical port in a younger child or a 10–12-mm port in an older child. Further port positioning depends on the size of the child and location of the appendix. Open appendicectomy is described further.

2 Divide the subcutaneous tissues and Scarpa's fascia using cutting diathermy.

3 Identify and clear the external oblique aponeurosis for the length of the wound.

4 Incise the aponeurosis parallel to the fibres and split the fibres.

5 Split the internal oblique and transverse muscles in the direction of their fibres using blunt dissection and spread them using retractors.

6 Divide the transversalis fascia and grasp the underlying peritoneum. Open it with a scalpel. Suction any free fluid and send any pus for culture. Enlarge the peritoneal opening with scissors.

7 Insert your finger into the peritoneal cavity and identify the appendix and caecum by palpation and vision.

8 Deliver the caecum into the wound using a rocking motion. You may need to divide lateral adhesions under direct vision. If this proves difficult extend the wound.

9 Having delivered the caecum, deliver the entire appendix.

Action: open appendicectomy

1 Divide the meso-appendix using clips and ties down to the base of the appendix.

2 Crush the appendix 5 mm above its base using a straight crushing clamp and then re-apply the clamp a few millimetres distally. Tie the crushed area with a 3/0 polyglactin tie then cut along the proximal edge of the clamp with a scalpel, thereby excising the appendix.

3 Invert the stump of the appendix and secure it with a purse string or Z-suture of 3/0 polyglactin through the serosal layer of the caecum only.

4 Return the caecum to the abdomen and suction the paracolic gutters and pelvis.

5 Close the wound in layers using absorbable sutures. Close the peritoneum using a continuous suture. Approximate the transverse and internal oblique muscles with a couple of interrupted sutures. Close the external oblique and then Scarpa's fascia, both with a continuous suture.

6 Close the skin with a subcuticular suture.

Aftercare

1 In the case of simple inflamed appendix provide intravenous antibiotic cover for 24 hours and introduce oral fluids once the child has recovered from anaesthesia.

2 In more advanced cases, treat with broad-spectrum intravenous antibiotics for 3–5 days, changing to oral only once the child is making clinical progress and is taking oral diet. Use intra-operative microbiology swab results to guide antibiotic use. Use a nasogastric tube to decompress the intestine until the ileus has resolved, at which point diet can be introduced.

Complications

1 Intra-abdominal collection/abscess may present with prolonged postoperative fever with or without prolonged ileus and abdominal pain. The diagnosis is confirmed with ultrasound. Treatment is initially with prolonged intravenous broad-spectrum antibiotics but percutaneous image-guided abscess drainage may be required.

2 Adhesion small-bowel obstruction is a risk following any intra-abdominal procedure, including appendicectomy.

35

Neurosurgery

L.W. Thorne, C.E.G. Uff

INTRODUCTION

Neurological surgery encompasses surgical disease of the central nervous system (the brain and spinal cord) and the peripheral nervous system. It is a specialty in its own right and is fast subdividing into sub-specialties such as neuro-oncology, vascular, paediatrics and spine. Neurosurgeons operate on every part of the body as the nervous system extends into every part of the body. There is extensive crossover with other specialties: ENT for skull base approaches; cardiothoracics for anterior approaches to the thoracic spine, thoracic sympathectomy and deep hypothermic cardiac arrest (DHCA) for complex neurovascular cases; general vascular for carotid disease; orthopaedics for spine and peripheral nerve; plastics for peripheral nerve repair. The only barrier intentionally breached by a neurosurgeon and by no other specialist is the dura mater.

Referrals stem from neurology, the emergency department, general practice, any surgical specialty, paediatrics and even obstetrics, both for the management of neurosurgical disease occurring during pregnancy and the prenatal diagnosis of congenital conditions such as spinal dysraphism that require neurosurgical management as soon as the child is born. There have even been recent forays into intra-uterine surgery for open spina bifida but these operations are currently beset by unacceptably high maternal mortality rates and are not recommended. Neurosurgical patients range from 25-week premature babies with intraventricular haemorrhage or spina bifida to 100-year-olds with chronic subdural haematoma. Many patients are unconscious preoperatively and many require intensive care postoperatively, hence strong links with the intensive care unit are essential.

Pituitary surgery and spinal surgery are intentionally not discussed since they fall outside the scope of this chapter and should only be undertaken by experts in the field.

THE ETHOS OF NEUROSURGERY

1 Damage to the brain will result in disability at remote sites which is not always proportional to the extent of brain damage: a massive lesion in a non-eloquent area such as the right frontal lobe can cause virtually no disability whereas a lesion no larger than a few millimetres in the internal capsule or brainstem can cause hemiplegia. Modern neurosurgical approaches make ingenious use of corridors through the skull base or non-eloquent areas of the brain: it is always preferable to remove more skull and retract the brain less.

2 Although the brain is 2% of the body weight, it receives 15% of cardiac output. It depends on this massive blood supply to support its extremely high metabolism and tolerates any disruption poorly. It can also bleed catastrophically and the usual haemostatic measures of applying firm pressure and ligating vessels cannot be used due to the risk of causing neurological injury.

3 Emergency neurosurgery generally involves removing pressure from some point of the neuroaxis to prevent extension of injury. This can ameliorate secondary injury, and if the primary injury can be survived this allows some chance of recovery:
   - Primary injury relates to structural neurological damage caused by transfer of kinetic energy, pressure, shearing, etc. This injury is static, but may be overwhelming; for example, a high-velocity bullet wound.
   - Secondary injury arises from local and systemic events that follow. There will be a local inflammatory cascade and subsequent oedema. In the enclosed space of the skull and spine this will create raised pressure resulting in impaired perfusion. Systemic hypotension and hypoxia will be equally deleterious.

In some patients the primary injury may be trivial: an extradural haematoma usually arises from a low-velocity injury. There is often no injury to the brain from the blow, but the expanding blood clot will produce a rapidly fatal secondary injury unless decompressed.

As a general principle, the speed of the surgical remedy needs to be proportional to the speed of onset. Trauma and haemorrhage require rapid intervention, whereas a slow growing tumour has a less dramatic effect on the brain despite occupying a similar volume.

TRAUMA

Trauma is the most likely emergency to be encountered but the same principles can be applied to most other neurosurgical problems:
1 The head is vulnerable to injury due to its position and its weight. Under normal conditions it is supported by powerful muscles in the neck, but in high-speed deceleration its weight results in massive forces acting on it about the moment of the top of the chest. Most assaults include blows to the head.

2 Patients with a severe head injury frequently have neck injuries and this must be assumed and the cervical spine protected unless the patient is fully conscious and the neck can be cleared of injury by clinical examination according to ATLS protocol.

3 Patients with severe head injury frequently require immediate surgery to save their life; however, adequate resuscitation is of greater importance: operating on a hypoxic hypotensive patient with an unprotected fractured cervical spine is far more likely to result in the patient's death than delaying whilst they are resuscitated: an intubated, oxygenated patient with a sustainable blood pressure and a protected cervical spine is in a far better condition to tolerate a trauma craniotomy. Specific management must be preceded by adequate resuscitation.

INTRACRANIAL PRESSURE

Intracranial pressure (ICP) is defined as the pressure of CSF in the frontal horn of the lateral ventricle. The relationship between ICP and the volume of an expanding mass lesion within the brain is given by the Monro-Kellie doctrine (Fig. 35.1). This divides the intracranial contents into compartments: brain, CSF, venous blood, and arterial blood. There may be an extra compartment in the form of a mass lesion such as haematoma. The doctrine states that since the intracranial volume is fixed, an increase in one compartment must be compensated by a decrease in another or ICP will rise. In effect this means that normal ICP can be maintained with an expanding haematoma by displacing CSF and venous blood (the total volume is approximately 100 ml). Thereafter, ICP will rise steeply, clinically manifest by a sudden and often catastrophic deterioration in the patient's conscious level. This explains the lucid interval seen in extradural haematoma (see below). Subsequent decrease in the volume of the arterial blood compartment will produce ischaemia, with further injury and swelling. As a haematoma expands, the brain is displaced towards the foramen magnum, and pressure builds up in the conical posterior fossa causing the brainstem to herneate through the foramen magnum, compressing the respiratory and cardiac centres in the medulla – this is 'coning'. Ischaemia and herniation are the mechanisms of death from raised ICP.

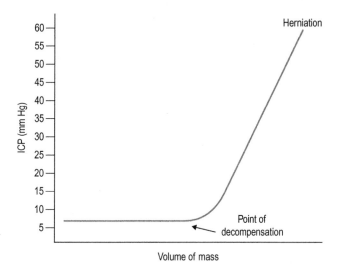

Fig. 35.1 Monro-Kellie doctrine.

CEREBRAL BLOOD FLOW

Cerebral blood flow (CBF) is the volume of blood that supplies the brain. At 15% of cardiac output (5 L/min), the brain receives 750 ml/min. The weight of the brain is approximately 1500 g so cerebral blood flow is 50 ml/100 g/min (grey matter receiving approximately thrice the blood flow of white matter). In a normal brain, a process called cerebral autoregulation maintains this blood flow over a mean arterial pressure (MAP) ranging from 50 to 150 mmHg. In the damaged brain, this relationship is lost and a more linear relationship develops (as MAP increases so does CBF). With this linear relationship, a MAP of 90 mmHg corresponds to a (normal) CBF of 50 ml/100 g/min. CBF is also affected by blood CO_2 levels: as CO_2 rises, CBF increases and so will ICP. Hence hyperventilation (which reduces $PaCO_2$) can be used in an emergency to reduce ICP by reducing CBF. Care must be taken to avoid prolonged hypocapnia since a $pCO_2 < 4.0$ KPa can cause ischaemia from excessive vasoconstriction.

CEREBRAL PERFUSION PRESSURE

Cerebral perfusion pressure (CPP) is the net blood pressure within the cranial cavity. Because the skull is a closed compartment, the ICP works against MAP to slightly reduce the blood pressure to the brain. CPP = MAP – ICP. Under normal conditions, MAP (~ 80 mmHg) – ICP (~ 5 mmHg) = CPP (~ 75 mmHg). If intracranial pressure increases, CPP decreases. A minimum CPP of 55 mmHg is required. Sustained CPP below this level is liable to result in global cerebral ischaemia. In basic terms, if the pressure in the head is too high, the heart cannot squeeze blood into it and the brain will die.

The management of raised ICP is based on the practical use of the Monro-Kellie doctrine. Venous blood is encouraged to flow from the intracranial compartment by positioning and reducing impedance, such as avoiding positive end expiratory pressures (PEEP). The volume of the arterial blood compartment can be regulated physiologically. CSF can be drained to reduce the volume of this compartment. Mass lesions can be excised to remove that compartment from the equation. If these measures have been exhausted and ICP is still a problem due to a swollen brain, the doctrine can be defeated with a radical change in the physiological parameters: the box can be opened. An extensive craniectomy (removal of skull bone) changes the rigid box of the intracranial space to a space with an elastic boundary: the scalp. This can allow expansion of the swollen brain without compromise of perfusion.

INITIAL MANAGEMENT OF THE OBTUNDED HEAD INJURED PATIENT

The intracranial pressure must be reduced immediately:

1 Secure the airway with endotracheal intubation and hyperventilate to a $PaCO_2$ of 4–4.5 KPa, or double the minute ventilation if ABGs are not immediately available. This causes a reduction in $PaCO_2$ resulting in reduced cerebral blood flow. Although this is ultimately bad for the brain, it results in an immediate drop in intracerebral pressure and can save the patient's life.

2 Sit the patient up to between 30 and 45 degrees. This can still be accomplished with a fractured cervical spine. Make sure that nothing is compressing the neck veins: if blood cannot leave

the head venous congestion will needlessly raise ICP. Cervical collars should be removed as soon as the patient has been transferred to a trolley. Bolsters either side of the head, with tape across forehead and chin, anchored either side of the trolley, will hold the neck still and prevent unnecessary compromise of the neck veins. Collars should only ever be used for transferring patients.

3 Administer Mannitol: accurate dose calculations are time consuming and based on a (usually wildly inaccurate) estimate of the patient's weight. Give 200 ml of 20% over 20 minutes (or 400 ml of 10%, etc.). This dose is easy to remember when the patient's pupil has just fixed. Insert a urinary catheter since a massive diuresis will occur within 15 minutes.

4 As soon as the patient is stable obtain cross sectional imaging, if available. There is no place for skull X-rays when CT scanning is available.

The above measures can buy you up to 4 hours. Transfer to a neurosurgical unit for definitive treatment is the most desirable option. If the anticipated transfer time (including packaging the patient for a critical care transfer) exceeds 4 hours then you may have to operate yourself. A definitive operation (craniotomy) can be delayed until the patient reaches a neurosurgeon, but a burr hole or craniectomy to partially decompress a haematoma can save the patient's life if death from raised ICP is imminent.

ANAESTHETIC CONSIDERATIONS

The same principles should be applied to neurosurgical anaesthesia as are applied to any anaesthetic, with particular emphasis on an understanding of neurophysiology, and neuropharmacology, including the effect of anaesthetic drugs, posture, etc., on cerebral perfusion. This includes relevant medical and surgical history and examination, test results, explanation of the procedure and informed consent. Most patients should be starved, but clear fluids are allowed up to 2 hours before surgery/anaesthesia. Depending on the urgency and condition of the patient intravenous (I.V.) access and physiological monitoring (non-invasive/invasive) is established prior to induction of anaesthesia.

A typical anaesthetic for elective craniotomy may be given with the following:

1 I.V. induction of anaesthesia with Propofol with or without a strong opiate (fentanyl/alfentanil/remifentanil).

2 A muscle relaxant is given and the trachea is intubated with a reinforced/armoured endotracheal tube.

3 The response to laryngoscopy may be obtunded using adjuvant drugs.

4 Anaesthesia is maintained with either ≈ 1 MAC of volatile agent ± analgesia or total intravenous anaesthesia (TIVA). A non-depolarizing muscle relaxant is used.

5 Normotension and normocarbia are usually maintained, but certain surgical procedures may require relative hypotension.

6 At the end of the operation, if the patient is to be woken up, the muscle relaxant is reversed and the volatile agent/TIVA is turned off. Once the patient is able to breathe they are allowed to wake up. Analgesia is given as required. Some patients are electively intubated and ventilated after surgery to protect the brain using anaesthesia or maintain strict blood pressure control.

Specific considerations for anaesthetic drugs

- Induction agents: propofol can cause hypotension (given slowly to minimize effect). Thiopentone may be useful to reduce $CMRO_2$ (cerebral metabolic rate of oxygen) and seizure activity.

- Narcotics/opiates: (fentanyl, morphine and alfentanyl) may reduce CBF and ICP, but can raise ICP in patients with brain trauma.

- TIVA: remifentanil is usually given as an infusion.

- Inhalational agents: isoflurane, desflurane or sevoflurane are preferred. Halothane, enflurane and nitrous oxide all affect cerebral autoregulation and can raise ICP.

- Paralysis: non-depolarizing drugs are preferred (e.g. atracurium, vecuronium, rocuronium).

Specific considerations for craniotomy

The head is away from the anaesthetic machine and is covered with drapes. Access to the head and airway is therefore restricted during surgery, so the airway and all components of the circuit must be secured.

The patient is always positioned in such a way as to minimize pressure damage.

The eyes must be protected. They are very close to and sometimes within the operative field and can be damaged. The cornea should be covered with sterile ointment, the eyelids taped shut and a protective paraffin gauze and protective pad placed on top and secured with a clear waterproof dressing. These steps minimize the risk to the eyes from trauma and (alcoholic) skin preparations which may damage the cornea.

SCALP LACERATIONS

Appraise

1 An unsutured small scalp laceration can bleed profusely, so arrest bleeding from the scalp as soon as is practicable after injury, using a temporary single layer of through-and-through sutures.

2 If the patient has been struck on the head with a heavy object, X-ray the skull to ensure that the laceration does not cover a depressed skull fracture.

Action

1 Shave adequately and closely round the laceration before exploring it.

2 The scalp is vascular, heals well and seldom gets infected, so do not excise the contused edges of the laceration too enthusiastically which will produce a scalp defect requiring apposition of the edges under tension.

3 If the galea has been breached, always close the scalp laceration in two layers, one for the galea and a second through-and-through skin layer, as previously described.

4 If possible, transfer a patient with severe scalp loss to a special unit where plastic and neurosurgical facilities are available.

DEPRESSED SKULL FRACTURE

Appraise

1. The purpose of elevating a depressed skull fracture is to reduce the risk of infection, so elevate only compound depressed skull fractures.

2. Leave alone depressed fractures with intact overlying scalp. Occasionally, the dislocation of the skull contour may be so great that elevation is required for cosmetic reasons, but these more severe injuries are invariably compound, so that the customary indication for operation is also present.

Access

1. Excise the overlying scalp laceration if it is badly contused. Extend the incision to give access to the whole depressed area. Scrape the scalp off the underlying bone and hold the incision wide open with self-retaining retractors.

2. Clear the pericranium away with a periosteal elevator to reveal the whole depressed area.

3. The inner table will have been driven in over a much wider area than the visible area of depressed outer table. Make a single burr hole just outside the edge of the visibly depressed region in order to expose dura not involved in the depression.

Action

1. Insert a periosteal elevator into the burr hole, slide it gently between the bone and the dura and ease out the depressed fragments so that the dura beneath them is fully exposed. Remove dirt, debris and any small flakes of bone from the wound and send them for bacteriological culture.

2. If the dura is intact, do not open it. If it is lacerated, carefully extend the laceration to inspect the brain beneath. If the brain surface is torn, probe gently in the tear for any in-driven debris and bone and remove them.

3. Remove pulped and clearly necrotic brain tissue by a combination of gentle suction and irrigation with 0.9% saline at body temperature.

4. Coagulate bleeding points in the brain with low-intensity diathermy coagulation, and diffuse oozing by applying patches of surgical cellulose compressed into place beneath lintine strips.

5. If the depressed bone fragments have been driven through the dura, their removal may tear large cerebral vessels as the fragments are extracted. A large cerebral vessel, not visible on the brain surface, may be picked up and held in the tip of a fine sucker under fairly strong suction while it is coagulated with diathermy or occluded with a metal clip.

▶ **KEY POINTS** Beware venous sinuses

- Be very cautious about elevating a depressed fracture overlying the superior sagittal, transverse or sigmoid sinuses.
- If the dura over the sinus is torn there will be torrential bleeding as you remove the bone.

6. If a sinus is torn, do not try to close it with sutures. Reduce the pressure in the sinus by tilting the patient feet-down, then cover the sinus with several layers of surgical cellulose and hold them firmly in place under lintine strips for 5–10 minutes. When you release the pressure and remove the lintine, the bleeding should not recur. Do not now disturb the surgical cellulose.

? DIFFICULTY

- If the bleeding is absolutely uncontrollable, you may suture a surgical gauze in place beneath the scalp, which is closed over it as a temporary measure to reduce bleeding while you arrange transfer of the patient to a special centre.

Closure

1. Before closing, irrigate the whole wound with hydrogen peroxide solution and 20 ml of 0.9% saline containing 20 000 units of penicillin and 50 mg of streptomycin.

2. Close the dura with interrupted 3/0 silk sutures. Cover any gaps in the dura with two layers of surgical cellulose.

3. Unless the wound has been neglected and is obviously infected, replace the removed bone fragments on the dura to fill in the skull defect. Scrub them thoroughly in aqueous Savlon before replacing them.

4. Close the scalp in two layers without drainage.

EXTRADURAL HAEMATOMA

Extradural haematoma is a blood clot between the inside of the skull and the dura. It is usually caused by a skull fracture lacerating a meningeal artery (typically the middle meningeal artery (MMA) in the temporal region) but it can result from a simple skull fracture. The injury often causes little or no underlying brain injury and so there is the potential for full recovery.

The urgency to evacuate these clots cannot be overstated. There is frequently a lucid interval where the patient has no symptoms other than the history of head injury. As the haematoma expands, rapid clinical deterioration occurs and the patient will lose consciousness. The brain is displaced medially by the clot and as the temporal lobe is compressed against the brainstem it causes pressure on the oculomotor nerve and the pupil on the affected side becomes fixed and dilated.

EMERGENCY BURR HOLE/CRANIECTOMY FOR EXTRADURAL HAEMATOMA

Appraise

1. This operation can be performed by any competent surgeon whether or not you have any prior experience in neurosurgery. If you have never done this before, stay in telephone contact with a neurosurgeon who can talk you through the operation. In our unit, all junior medical staff (including physicians) are strongly encouraged to learn this simple and life-saving skill.

2 It can be performed concurrently with surgery for other imminently life-threatening injuries such as laparotomy or thoracotomy.

3 If available, always obtain CT scans and have these available in theatre. Remember that the sides are reversed when looking at a CT scan so check the side with another doctor.

4 If CT scans and immediate transfer to a neurosurgeon and a CT scanner are unavailable and the patient has a severe head injury with an underlying skull fracture and a fixed pupil, the diagnosis is not in significant doubt.

5 Operate on the side of the fixed pupil.

6 If both pupils are fixed, operate on the side of the pupil that fixed first. The patient is on the verge of death and you can do no harm.

Prepare

1 Unless the cervical spine has been cleared, position the patient on the operating table with the head and neck in alignment with the rest of the spine. Secure the patient to the table with the strongest tape available. Use extra arm supports on the side that is going to be tilted down. Side-tilt the whole table to 30 degrees. Use a head ring, or even better, a horseshoe table attachment to keep the head clear of the table to permit access. If the spine has been cleared place the patient supine, with the head on a ring or a horseshoe and turned to the side. This can be aided by placing a bolster under the ipsilateral shoulder.

2 Ask the anaesthetist to give an intravenous dose of broad-spectrum antibiotics.

3 Shave the side of the head you are going to operate on generously.

Access

1 Mark a linear incision starting 1 cm anterior to the pinna and 2 cm above the zygoma running superiorly towards the vertex for 10 cm. Prep and drape the scalp in the way that you would prep any wound for surgery (Fig. 35.2a).

2 Using a scalpel, cut sharply down to bone for the entire length of the incision. The wound edges will probably bleed briskly but this can be controlled by an assistant pressing on the wound edges.

3 Insert a periosteal elevator or similar sharp scraping instrument and quickly scrape all layers of the scalp and muscle back from the bone.

4 Insert a self-retaining retractor with the blades under the periosteum and muscle. This will stop bleeding from the wound edges.

5 Using a drill with the largest round burr available (if no burr is available any attachment that can cut bone will suffice), fashion a hole in the centre of the wound. Use both hands and work quickly but carefully. Try to avoid plunging into the skull; however, this is not a problem with an extradural haematoma since there is a blood clot between the skull and the brain. In the temporal region, the skull is rarely more than 5 mm thick but may be half this (Fig. 35.2b).

Action

1 Once you are through you will see the surface of a dark solid blood clot. Use bone rongeurs to enlarge the craniectomy. Bite away the thin temporal bone to the margins of your incision.

2 Insert an atraumatic sucker (glass or plastic) into the hole and work on the surface of the clot, carefully removing as much of it as access permits. It is usually fairly tough but continue sucking at the clot, angling the operating lights (or using a head light) obliquely into the hole to afford greater access until you cannot reach any more under direct vision, or until you see a tough white membrane (the dura). Do not press onto the dura and do not insert the sucker blindly under the edges of the burr hole. Gentle irrigation with saline into the hole will often yield more of the clot.

3 If fresh blood is welling up from the inferior limit of the craniectomy, bite off more of the thin squamous temporal bone inferiorly. This exposes the intracranial course of the middle meningeal artery and you may find the bleeding point and be able to stop it (Fig. 35.2c).

Closure

1 Leave the self-retaining retractor in and secure a simple dressing such as a large swab over the open wound.

2 If transfer is not possible, convert to craniotomy (see below).

Postoperative

1 The patient is now safe for transfer to your local neurosurgical unit.

2 If you have cross-matched any blood, send it with the patient.

3 Please don't forget a copy of the scans.

CRANIOTOMY FOR EXTRADURAL HAEMATOMA

Appraise

Because blood clots into a solid state within a few minutes, an acute haematoma on the outside of the brain requires craniotomy for definitive treatment. Although a burr hole can decompress the haematoma in an emergency when timely transfer to an experienced neurosurgeon is not possible, this is not a substitute for craniotomy.

Prepare

1 Ask for emergency burr hole or craniectomy.

2 Crossmatch 6 units of blood.

Access

1 Mark the incision starting at the zygoma 1 cm anterior to the pinna, running up and curving posteriorly over the pinna. Go as far posteriorly as you can before curving upwards and then anteriorly as far as the hairline (or 8 cm from the bridge of the nose), 1 cm lateral to the midline without crossing it (Fig. 35.3a).

2 Prep and drape. Infiltrate the wound with local anaesthetic with 1 in 200 000 adrenaline (epinephrine).

3 Start at the anterior extent of the incision near the midline cutting sharply down to bone, opening the incision in 5-cm increments. If you have scalp clips (such as Raney or Leroy) available then use them. Otherwise catch the galea (the deepest white layer of the scalp) with artery clips at intervals of 1 cm. Use straight clips on the flap side, curved clips on the scalp side. Gather them together in groups of four with elastic bands. They can be retracted once the wound is open.

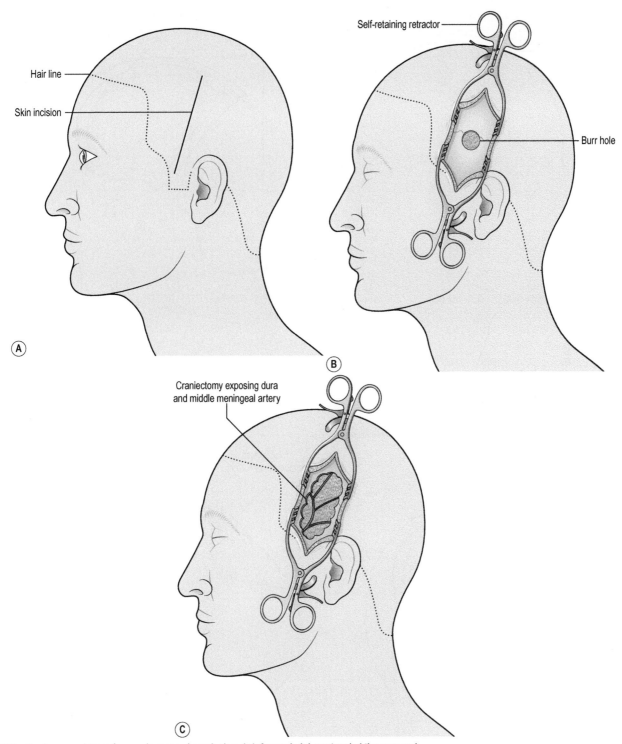

Fig. 35.2 Surface markings for exploratory burr holes: (A) frontal; (B) parietal; (C) temporal.

4 Once you are anterior to the pinna, you will encounter the superficial temporal artery. Do not worry about cutting it but stop the brisk haemorrhage quickly. Bipolar rarely works so grasp the artery with forceps and use monopolar on the coagulation setting.

5 Begin retracting the flap forwards with an assistant keeping it under constant tension. Start working from the posterior limit and use a sharp periosteal elevator to retract all layers of the scalp as one. Once you encounter the temporalis muscle, switch to monopolar diathermy on the cutting setting, with a medium to high current. Hold the tip on the bone and strip the muscle fibres from their attachment. You will have to incise the temporalis along the line of the scalp incision: this is best done with cutting diathermy, dividing a few fibres then deepening a self-retaining retractor until you reach bone. This way blood loss from this extremely vascular muscle will be minimized (Fig. 35.3b).

6 Push it as far forward as you can and wrap the flap in a wet swab, retracting it with towel clips or heavy sutures placed through the temporalis connected to elastic bands.

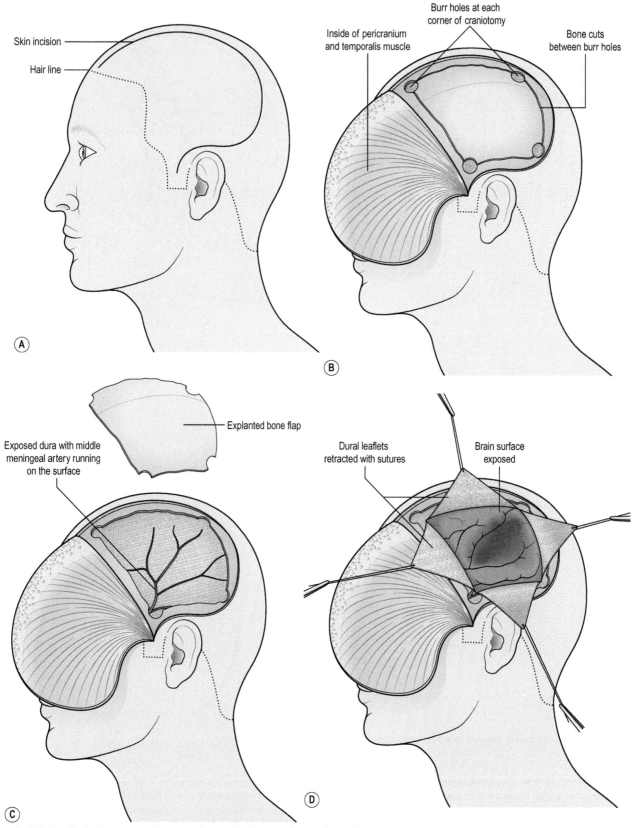

Fig. 35.3 (A) the skin incision starts 1 cm anterior to the pinna and 1 cm above the zygoma, running up and back behind the ear before curving anteriorly to finish just in front of the hairline 2 cm medial to the midline; (B) all layers of the scalp are retracted forward including temporalis. Burr holes are fashioned at each corner of the exposure and cuts are made between them; (C) the bone flap is explanted exposing either an extradural haematoma, or the dura (as shown); (D) the dura has been opened in a cruciate fashion and the leaflets are retracted with a suture attached to a clip. This exposes an acute subdural haematoma or the surface of the brain (as shown).

7 Drill several burr holes using either the automatic perforator or a high-speed drill with a round burr or acorn attachment. The automatic perforators have a gear that cuts out automatically once the skull has been breeched, leaving a thin rim of bone that can be removed using forceps: always run it at full speed and do not stop, since they are notoriously difficult to restart if they cut out half way through. The high-speed burr requires a little more skill but is easily mastered: again, run it at full speed and using firm but controlled pressure, drill through the skull holding it perpendicular to the bone. It will run smoothly through the outer table and diploe and start kicking back or juddering as it breeches the inner table.

8 Use the craniotome attachment to join up the burr holes. The craniotome is a side-cutting drill that incorporates a base plate that is used to strip the dura from the inside of the skull as the bone is cut in a line. Make the largest craniotomy that your bone exposure will permit (Fig. 35.3c).

▶ KEY POINTS

■ An experienced surgeon may use a single burr hole to reduce operation time and improve the cosmetic result, but the default should be to make a minimum of three. The first two should be placed one above the other in the slight depression behind the frontal process of the zygomatic bone. This will give you access to the anterior and middle cranial fossae, spanning the sphenoid ridge which is a frequent sticking point for the drill. Place the third burr hole at the posterior edge of the bone exposure.

■ If you have any difficulty identifying landmarks for the burr holes, simply make one at each corner of the bone exposure (Figure 35.3b,c).

■ If there is a skull fracture, do not drill a burr hole directly into the fracture line.

Action

1 As soon as a burr hole that has solid clot at the bottom has been made, use the suction to quickly aspirate as much of the clot as can be reached under direct vision. Do not spend long doing this (a few seconds should suffice) since you are about to perform a craniotomy.

2 As soon as the bone is removed, an extradural haematoma will immediately be visible.

3 Evacuate the haematoma using gentle suction and copious saline wash. Once the entire clot has been removed and the dura can be seen, identify the bleeding point. It will be either from the middle meningeal artery (MMA) or from a fracture. The MMA can be easily identified on the surface of the dura running superiorly and posteriorly. It can usually be controlled with bipolar but if there is any doubt about haemostasis, lift the dura with toothed forceps and encircle the artery with a suture.

4 If blood is welling up from the inferior edge of the craniotomy, it is likely to be coming from the MMA at, or just distal to, the foramen spinosum (where the MMA enters the skull). As you follow the artery under the temporal lobe, use bone rongeurs to remove the thin squamous temporal bone down to the floor of the middle fossa, then retract the dura up gently. This will give you good access to the intracranial course of the MMA. If there is still solid clot here, remove it with suction since it will be impossible to find the bleeding point until the clot has been removed. If bleed is coming from the foramen spinosum itself, plug the foramen with a suitable tamponade: anything from a small piece of temporalis muscle to bone wax covered in surgical cellulose will do. The MMA is a terminal branch of the external carotid so bleeding will be brisk. Hold the tamponade firmly in place for at least 5 minutes and leave it in situ.

5 If blood is coming from a fracture line, pack the fracture line with bone wax. Work the bone wax between your fingers to soften it as much as possible before using it. It is almost impossible to apply it using anything except your finger.

Check

1 A gentle ooze from under the bone edge can stopped by packing the extradural space with surgical cellulose and placing hitch stitches: place the stitch (we use 3/0 Vicryl) through only the outer layer of the dura (this prevents the risk of lacerating the brain) as flush with the bone edge as possible, and suture it to periosteum. You may need to place these at 1 cm intervals around the edge of the entire craniotomy to achieve haemostasis.

2 If there is any suspicion that there is an associated subdural haematoma, open the dura in the centre of the craniotomy: lift the dura with a small sharp hook and incise it with a new blade. Once you are through, extend the incision to about 1 cm in length. If there is no haematoma, then close the dura with a running suture.

Closure

1 Replace the bone flap using either a purpose-built plating system or a heavy suture through drill holes in the bone flap and the skull. Take care that the bone flap is not dropped on the floor at this stage.

2 Re-oppose the edges of the temporalis and insert a wound drain bringing it out behind the hairline (take care that it does not pierce the pinna). If the dura has not been opened, this can be on gentle suction, otherwise leave it on gravity.

3 Close the scalp using an interrupted inverted, absorbable suture through the galea. Remove the scalp or artery clips in sections rather than all at once. The scalp may bleed profusely at this stage and the best way of stopping it is to close the galea tightly. Make sure that you place one or two sutures in the centre of the wound first so you do not end up with a mismatch.

4 Close the skin with staples or a running stitch.

Postoperative

1 If the brain was slack at closure, the patient should have an ICP of 0–5 mmHg and should wake up. This allows for early neurological assessment.

2 If the patient cannot be woken up immediately, or fails to wake, insert an ICP monitor if available. Alternatively, arrange for an early postoperative scan.

3 If the ICP is greater than 10 mmHg, rescan them *immediately*: they may have a re-collection or a contralateral haematoma, both requiring immediate evacuation (the pressure from a haematoma on one side can tamponade an injury on the contralateral side which starts bleeding as soon as the tamponade is released).

Complications

1 Infection.
2 Re-collection of haematoma.

> ### KEY POINTS Hudson brace and Gigli saw

- If no high-speed drill is available, use a Hudson brace to drill the burr holes: this is a hand drill with two attachments: the perforator is flat with a shallow-tapered point which cuts sideways.
- Check frequently to see if you have perforated the inner table. This is accompanied by a sensation of progression once the point of the drill is no longer engaged.
- Once you are through and can see a tiny area of dura (or clot if it is an extradural haematoma), change the bit to the burr. This is used to widen the burr hole at the deep end.
- Make enough burr holes so that the Gigli saw's guide can safely be passed between the burr holes.
- Have an assistant hold the head firmly and with the handles held widely apart, pass both hands from left to right rather than up and down.

CRANIOTOMY FOR ACUTE SUBDURAL HAEMATOMA

Appraise

1 Acute subdural haematoma (ASDH) is associated with bleeding from an injury to the surface of the brain and is almost always associated with a severe head injury with underlying damage to the brain. Due to an injury mechanism called *contra coup* where an impact on one side of the head causes the brain to impact diametrically opposite, the haematoma may well be on the opposite side of the head to the injury.

2 ASDH may also be associated with traumatic intracranial haemorrhage or haemorrhagic contusions.

3 The patient will usually be unconscious from the start. There is rarely a lucid interval (as there is in extradural haematoma). Motor vehicle accidents, assaults and falling down stairs are common injury mechanisms. Alcohol is seldom far from the cause.

Prepare

As for Extradural haematoma.

Access

As for Extradural haematoma.

Action

1 As soon as the bone flap has been removed, the dura will be exposed. If there is a large subdural haematoma it will be discoloured and tense. Use a sharp hook to tent it in the centre and carefully incise it with a new blade.

2 You can open the dura in a cruciate (Fig. 35.3d) or peripheral manner, leaving an adequate anterior pedicle.

3 Gently irrigate the clot from the cortical surface using saline warmed to body temperature.

4 Remove as much clot as is required to achieve decompression.

5 Do not chase clot under the edges of the bone flap as this runs the risk of bleeding that you cannot control.

6 Once the cortex has been exposed, look for obvious bleeding points. Although you need to coagulate vessels that are bleeding profusely, you may be able to control less profuse bleeding with surgical cellulose and gentle pressure which will preserve the vessel. This is particularly important in eloquent areas such as the left superior temporal gyrus (receptive speech) or the precentral gyrus (motor cortex).

7 Occasionally, haemorrhagic contusions will present to brain surface and spontaneously express haemorrhagic brain when the dura is opened and the clot removed. If this happens, remove the expressed material but do not explore the cavity since it will be extremely friable and you are likely to cause further bleeding.

> ### KEY POINTS

- Occasionally, devastating injuries can result in massive and uncontrollable brain swelling as soon as the dura is opened. The brain will herniate out of the craniotomy with astonishing speed and unless immediate action is taken, you will not be able to close the wound. If this starts to happen, you cannot close the wound fast enough.
- Replace the scalp flap over the wound and have an assistant hold it in place. This may require firm pressure and if necessary, push the brain back in.
- Use a heavy monofilament suture to close the wound using an all layer interlocked running suture as fast as possible.
- In this situation the patient has a clearly unsurvivable brain injury and your priority is to get them off the operating table alive and with a closed wound.
- Amputation of the herniated brain is likely to result in cardiac arrest.
- A decompressive craniectomy for cerebral oedema should never be attempted by anyone other than an expert for this very reason.

Closure

1 If the brain is slack, close the dura using a running suture. If you have opened it in a cruciate fashion, first place a suture in the centre to aid opposition of the flaps.

2 If the dura will not close easily, do not put interrupted sutures across the deficit since these can damage the brain if swelling occurs later. Leave the dural flaps lying on the brain surface and cover the entire craniotomy with a dural substitute: pericranium

(from the outside of the bone flap), fascia lata, or a commercially available dural graft. We often use a sheet of surgical cellulose. This is of paramount importance if the bone flap is left out or subsequently removed.

3 If there are obvious contusions (the brain is discoloured – anything from the red tinge of traumatic subarachnoid haemorrhage to black–blue haemorrhagic contusion), if the brain is clearly swollen, or if brain swelling is anticipated, do not replace the bone flap but store it in a subcutaneous pouch in the abdominal wall rather than perform a craniectomy later.

4 Replace the bone flap and close the wound as you would for an extradural haematoma (see above).

5 ASDH is high-velocity injury and more likely to require prolonged periods in intensive care. Always insert an ICP monitor.

Postoperative

1 Brain swelling is common. Keep the patient under anaesthesia on intensive care for 24–48 hours before gradually weaning off sedation.

2 Blood pressure should be supported by intravenous filling and inotropic support to ensure adequate CPP, 60–70 mmHg.

Complications

1 As for Extradural haematoma.

2 If the ICP rises due to brain swelling and you have replaced the bone flap, you may need to remove it (it can be stored in a subcutaneous pouch in the abdominal wall). Although ideally performed in the operating theatre, if the patient is too unstable to be moved or if the patient has just fixed their pupils, this can easily be performed on the ITU with minimal surgical equipment.

BURR HOLE FOR TAPPING CEREBRAL ABSCESS

Appraise

The diagnosis is supported by symptoms of raised intracranial pressure developing in a patient with neglected otitis media or frontal sinusitis.

Access

1 Make a burr hole (Figure 35.4) according to the clinical situation, either through a vertical incision in the temporal region just above the top of the pinna in line with the external auditory meatus or through a horizontal incision in the forehead just above the line of the affected frontal sinus.

2 Frontal sinuses vary considerably in size and configuration, so have a preoperative anteroposterior skull X-ray available so you can place your burr hole avoiding entering the sinus.

Action

1 Diathermy the tense brain surface, avoiding any vessels, and incise the coagulated cortex.

2 Hold the widest available brain cannula between thumb and index finger and gently run it towards the expected position of the

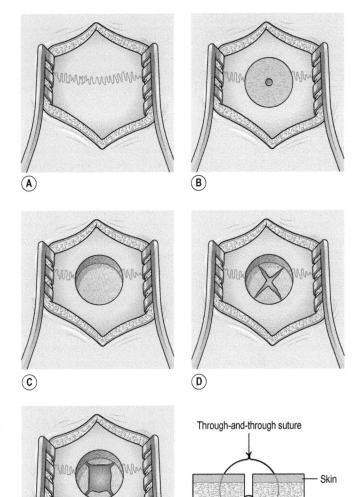

Fig. 35.4 Stages of making a burr hole: (A) scalp cut down to bone; (B) after use of perforator to expose a small area of dura; (C) after use of conical burr to expose dura more widely; (D) dura opened in cruciate fashion; (E) dura burnt back with the diathermy; (F) closure of the scalp.

abscess. This is either just behind the frontal sinus or just above the tegmen tympani.

3 The wall of the abscess is rubbery and offers a definite resistance to the cannula tip. Push the cannula through into the centre of the abscess.

4 Remove the stylette and gently suck out the pus, using moderate suction until no pus comes out freely. Inject 5 ml of 0.9% saline containing dissolved 200 000 units of penicillin and 50 mg of streptomycin, into the empty cavity. Also inject 1 ml of sterile barium sulphate to outline the cavity.

Closure

Withdraw the cannula and close the scalp in two layers of interrupted silk as already described, without drainage.

HYDROCEPHALUS

Hydrocephalus is an easily treatable condition that can rapidly kill if not recognized. The brain produces 450–500 ml of cerebrospinal fluid (CSF) per 24 hours. The total volume of CSF is 150 ml so the entire volume is replaced every 8 hours. Approximately 50 ml is in the ventricles and 100 ml in the lumbar cistern. CSF is produced by the choroid plexus and the ependymal lining of the ventricles and drains through the aqueduct of Sylvius into the IV ventricle then out of the foramina of Luschka and Magendie. From here it drains over the surface of the spinal cord (which has a large reservoir around the cauda equina called the lumbar cistern) and over the surface of the brain. It is reabsorbed into the superior sagittal sinus via the arachnoid granulations. CSF is actively secreted and the rate of production is not affected by increased pressure in the head. An expanding CSF compartment will cause damage by raised ICP as per the Monro-Kellie doctrine. Treatment is simple: excess CSF is drained to restore the compartment to its normal size. Definitive treatment is by shunting CSF, usually from the ventricles to the peritoneal cavity, where it can be resorbed, but simple techniques are used in emergency situations with good effect.

Hydrocephalus can be classified into obstructive and communicating. In communicating hydrocephalus, the obstruction is at the level of the arachnoid granulations and the pressure is raised but similar in all the CSF spaces. This has a more insidious onset since the increase in volume in 24 hours is a factor of 4 (150 ml + 450 ml) and the lumbar cistern can accommodate a large volume of CSF. This can always be treated by lumbar puncture. Do not be put off by the high pressure measured when you tap the subarachnoid space. The pressure on the end of your needle is the same as that in the ventricle. You want to return this to normal so don't be afraid to drain large amounts of CSF until your manometer is showing a normal figure. The excess CSF drained will be replenished all too soon.

In obstructive hydrocephalus, obstruction of the aqueduct of Sylvius or the III ventricle results in increased pressure in the brain which forces the cerebrum into the posterior fossa where it compresses the brainstem. The increase in volume in 24 hours is a factor of 10 (50 ml + 450 ml). Onset can be very rapid and will result in the patient's death if not treated immediately. Treatment by lumbar puncture is hazardous and best avoided. There will be a pressure gradient across the foramen magnum. Removing lumbar CSF will increase this gradient and facilitate coning.

If the hydrocephalus is non-communicating, or you cannot establish whether it is communicating or not, CSF should be removed from the ventricle directly.

EXTERNAL VENTRICULAR DRAIN (VENTRICULOSTOMY)

Appraise

1 A patient exhibits progressively worsening morning headache and vomiting, blurred vision, papilloedema and impaired upgaze. The absence of papilloedema does not exclude raised ICP. Papilloedema may take hours or even days to develop.

2 If a CT scan is available it will show enlarged lateral and III ventricles. You may well see the cause of the problem, such as intraventricular tumour or haemorrhage.

3 If a parent tells you their child has a dysfunctioning CSF shunt, they are right until disproved by an experienced neurosurgeon, usually after surgical exploration of the shunt.

Prepare

1 Place the patient supine on the operating table. It is advisable to shave the head to facilitate identification of anatomical landmarks.

2 Make sure the head is perfectly straight as this helps with orientation.

3 Mark the midline, the mid-pupillary line and the coronal suture (this is easily palpable 10 cm back from the nasion).

4 Mark a 3-cm incision running parallel to the midline in the midpupillary line, centred on the coronal suture.

Access

1 Open the scalp: cut sharply down to bone, scrape all layers back and insert a self-retaining retractor.

2 Fashion a burr hole using any means described above.

3 Coagulate the dura in the centre of the burr hole and make a cruciate incision in the centre. Do not worry about damaging the underlying brain – indeed, if the pia is breached with the dura this merely speeds up the operation.

4 Coagulate the dural edges so that the hole easily admits the catheter and also supports it.

5 Coagulate the underlying cortical surface (this is the pia) and make a cruciate incision to a depth of 2 mm, avoiding any visible vessels. If there is any bleeding, use bipolar forceps to coagulate the edge of the incision (the pia).

Action

1 Hold the catheter like a dart in the right hand with the stylette in situ, orientated so that you can see the depth markers (most catheters have a black marker every 5 cm).

2 Aim for the intersection of the midline and the external auditory meatus. This is often easier said than done and in practice many surgeons simply aim perpendicular to the cortical surface: if the ventricles are large enough to obtund the patient you will not miss using this method.

3 Advance it slowly and gently. As it enters the ventricle you will feel a slight pop and be rewarded by CSF gushing out of the catheter. Advance it to the 5-cm mark and withdraw the stylette. Allow CSF to flow until normal pressure is restored. Keeping the end of the drain 10 cm above the burr hole will prevent over-drainage.

4 Holding the catheter in non-toothed forceps, connect the catheter to the tunneller and tunnel it laterally through the temporalis muscle as far as you can. Infection travels up the outside of the catheter at approximately 1 cm per day so you must tunnel at least 7 cm for the drain to last a week.

5 Secure it at the exit wound. Most catheters are supplied with a silicone collar that fits snugly around the catheter and can be sutured to the skin. We then secure a loop of the catheter to the scalp. Pay particular attention to securing it well. Regardless of how it is accidentally pulled out, you will be putting it back in, which subjects the patient to further risks and demoralizes you, especially if you struggled to insert the first one.

6 If you have not hit CSF by 5 cm then your trajectory is wrong. Withdraw the catheter, wash it with saline and try again. You are usually aiming too lateral and too posterior so aim more medial and

anterior. Never advance it further then 5 cm: you will probably hit a CSF space eventually but will cause untold neurological damage in the process. There are many vital neurological structures less than a centimetre away from the intended insertion point.

7   If you have not hit CSF after three attempts, call for senior help. If you are the senior help, check placement of the burr hole, check the orientation of the patient's head, check the scans. If you have still not hit the ventricle, consider operating on the contralateral side or closing the wound and obtaining a CT scan (with the patient asleep): the ventricles may have reduced in size or may have moved due to rapidly enlarging haematoma. If available, a stereotactic scan should also be performed (see below).

Check

1   Check that the drain is draining CSF after everything you do to tunnel and secure it: never close the wound on a drain that you are not absolutely sure is draining freely.

Closure

1   Taking care not to suture in the EVD catheter, place interrupted inverted absorbable sutures (we use 2/0 Vicryl) through the galea. Close the skin with clips unless an MRI is planned, in which case use a continuous suture.

2   Set it to drain connected to a manometer set at 10 cm CSF, with zero at the level of the external auditory meatus. This equates to a normal ICP. CSF will only drain when the ICP exceeds this and over-drainage will be prevented. If such a system is not available, aim to drain 15–20 ml/hour to match normal production of CSF.

Complications

1   Failure to hit the ventricle (vide supra).

2   Intracranial haemorrhage (1% risk).

3   Blockage: get a CT scan to confirm that the catheter is within the ventricle then flush the catheter with not more than 5 ml 0.9% saline. This may be repeated as required, especially if there is an intraventricular blood clot.

4   Displacement of the catheter: if the catheter has been partially pulled out, do not push it back in. Take the patient to theatre and insert a fresh catheter in a sterile environment.

5   Over-drainage: can result in the brain collapsing (especially in the elderly) and development of an acute subdural haematoma.

6   Infection: the investigation of pyrexia in any patient with an EVD must include CSF sampling from the drain. If organisms are seen on gram stain or if the cell count is suspicious (white cells >20 with a high proportion of polymorphs, allowing for 1 white cell for every 1000 red cells), start antibiosis with good CSF penetrance. Consider changing the EVD catheter and intrathecal antibiotics (Gentamicin or Vancomycin are most commonly used: seek expert advice for preparation and dosing).

7   Accidental use of EVD catheter for I.V. medications or radiological contrast (anecdotes abound with horrific consequences): label it and make sure the nursing staff know what it is.

▶ **KEY POINTS**

■   Patients with obstructive hydrocephalus may clinically deteriorate very rapidly. Deep coma with fixed dilated pupils must be treated immediately and unless the patient responds rapidly to Mannitol (see above), there is no time to transfer the patient to a neurosurgical unit in another hospital. Occasionally, hydrocephalus can cause cardiorespiratory arrest and in this situation the ventricles must be drained immediately as part of the resuscitation.

■   Many patients with hydrocephalus have pre-existing burr holes, and in an emergency the ventricles can be accessed percutaneously: wherever the burr hole is, insert the needle perpendicular to the contour of the head to a depth of 4–5 cm, allow 50 ml CSF to drain passively, withdraw the needle and arrange for a formal operation immediately.

■   If the patient does not have a burr hole, the ventricles can be accessed via the orbital roof (the thinnest part of the skull): prep the right cornea with aqueous antiseptic (alcohol will cause severe corneal damage), depress the globe and puncture the orbital roof via the conjunctiva with a spinal needle 1–2 cm back from the orbital rim. Aim for the coronal suture in the midline. CSF in the frontal horn should be encountered by 4 cm. Drain 50 ml CSF passively, withdraw the needle and arrange for a formal operation immediately. Of historical note, this approach was popularized in the 1940s for the transorbital frontal leukotomy.

POSTOPERATIVE OBSERVATIONS

All patients who have had craniotomy must have regular (15-minute) neurological observations for the first 6 hours. This is because after 6 hours the chance of a postoperative haematoma reduces significantly.

Neurological observations must include the following:

■   Conscious level (GCS including full breakdown)

■   Limb movement using the MRC grade (0–5)

■   Pupil size, shape and reactivity

■   Physiological parameters (HR, BP, (if an arterial line is available, use it) respiration rate, SpO_2, temperature)

■   Output from EVD

■   Output from surgical drains.

OUTCOMES FROM NEUROSURGERY

The outcome from neurosurgery can often surprise. Patients with severe injuries can make remarkable recoveries, where others with relatively trivial injuries can fail to do well. The former is a function of plasticity. The brain can repair over anything up to 24 months. Even though anatomical changes stop at this point, patients can continue to improve as a result of unconscious functional changes that maximize their abilities. For severely injured patients, outcome should not be judged until these processes have run their course. Good rehabilitation is essential. It can be a pleasant surprise to see a patient again after a long interval. Those who were at first minimally responsive can sometimes have returned to work. A good example of plasticity is the child who has had a hemispherectomy for epilepsy. Two years down the line you may notice a slight limp only when the child is running, seemingly in defiance of all neuro-anatomical knowledge. This plasticity can be included in surgical strategy. If tumour resection is limited by functional cortex, delayed functional imaging may show the area of function to have moved to the contralateral side after some months, and allow for further resection.

Many patients who have suffered moderate head injuries or survived relatively minor haemorrhages suffer a catalogue of complaints. Headaches are common; they complain of fatigue, irritability and may struggle in their work or relationships. Suicide is more common in survivors of subarachnoid haemorrhage. These problems are in part due to difficulties with higher executive function, but are sometimes in part due to the terrifying nature of the experience, a problem akin to post-traumatic stress disorder. Differences in perception of these issues can illuminate the difference in outcome as perceived by patient and doctor. While patients may be independent and have full limb function, thinking is what we use our brains for more than anything else. These problems should never be trivialized. Although early intervention with information and counselling may help, some patients may never reclaim the lives they had.

FURTHER READING

Samandouras G, editor. The Neurosurgeon's Handbook. Oxford: OUP; 2010. A satisfactory primer for a neurosurgical post.

36

Upper urinary tract

G. Smith, S. Pridgeon

CONTENTS

INTRODUCTION

1 Urology has developed as a separate surgical specialty over the last few decades and sub-specialization within the discipline is now common. Urological surgery requires open, laparoscopic and endoscopic skills and urologists have readily incorporated new technology into their daily practice, including the use of lasers, minimally invasive techniques and, more recently, robotic surgery.

2 It is common for core surgical trainees to rotate through a number of surgical specialties during their training, including urology, and it is therefore important to be familiar with the common urological operations. In addition to major life-saving surgery, urology offers a variety of day-case procedures, which provide ideal training opportunities for the surgeon-in-training.

3 Not all general hospitals have a urology department and general surgeons may be required to assess patients with acute urological problems or even operate to save life or prevent severe morbidity. It is important for surgeons to be aware of emergency urological procedures and how to recognize when urgent intervention is required in the absence of specialist colleagues.

4 Be aware of the potential benefits of specialist procedures.

ACUTE PYONEPHROSIS (OBSTRUCTED INFECTED KIDNEY)

Appraise

1 The treatment of an acutely obstructed infected kidney is a urological emergency as patients will become very unwell with septicaemia and can die if left untreated. Obstruction may be due to a stone, congenital pelvi-ureteric junction (PUJ) obstruction or tumour within or outside of the ureter. Diabetic and immunologically compromised patients are particularly at risk. The diagnosis is made by ultrasound or CT scanning, which will show hydronephrosis and may demonstrate the underlying cause of the obstruction. The urine contains organisms that can also be cultured from the blood.

2 Decompression of the obstructed kidney using ultrasound guided percutaneous nephrostomy is the optimum treatment. Infected urine or frank pus may be drained and should be cultured.

3 Carefully secure the nephrostomy tube to the patient's skin. When the patient has recovered from the acute illness, address the underlying cause of obstruction. Temporary drainage with a ureteric stent inserted antegrade via the nephrostomy tract will allow definitive treatment to be planned in an elective setting with the appropriate expertise.

4 Open operation is indicated only if you are sufficiently expert and it is impossible to introduce a satisfactory percutaneous drain, or if the pus in the kidney is too thick to be aspirated through the small-calibre tube used for percutaneous nephrostomy. This is not a simple procedure, so do not undertake it lightly.

5 If you undertake open operation when the cause of obstruction is a stone in the upper ureter or renal pelvis, remove it.

OPEN NEPHROSTOMY FOR ACUTELY OBSTRUCTED KIDNEY

Prepare

1 Aggressively resuscitate the patient with intravenous fluids and broad-spectrum antibiotics. If necessary, manage a severely ill patient in an intensive care unit for monitoring, and respiratory and circulatory support.

2 Review the imaging and mark the side to be operated upon.

3 Position the patient in a lateral position with the side to be operated on uppermost.

4 Have the break in the table under the 12th rib to open the flank fully. Flex the uppermost hip and knee and place a pillow between the legs. Maintain the position using a back support behind the thorax and fix the arm to an armrest with a wide adhesive bandage.

5 Check that the lowermost arm is not compressed by the patient's body.

Access

Make an incision below the 12th rib of sufficient length to expose the convex border of the kidney. Perirenal tissues appear oedematous and the kidney is swollen.

► KEY POINTS Handle gently

- Tissues are friable and bleed easily on dissection.
- Take extra care to handle the tissues gently.

Action

1 Occasionally, the pus-filled calyces 'point' on the surface of the kidney like ripe abscesses. Make an incision through the parenchyma at this point to release the pus.

2 More commonly, the calyces are impalpable because the overlying renal tissue is oedematous. Enter the collecting system through the renal pelvis. Follow the capsule over the convex posterior border of the kidney, keeping towards the lower pole. Find the renal sinus and gently clear away the fat by blunt dissection to reveal the posterior surface of the renal pelvis. It is not necessary to mobilize the kidney fully.

3 Make a small transverse pyelotomy (Greek: *pyelos* = trough, pelvis + *tome* = a cutting).

4 Introduce a malleable silver probe with an eyehole at the end through the pyelotomy and manoeuvre it to puncture the cortex from within a lower pole calyx.

5 Tie the tip of a size 18 F tube drain or a Foley catheter to the probe with a suture and pull it back into the renal pelvis (Fig. 36.1). Use a Willschner nephrostomy tube with a built-in malleable stylet if it is available.[1]

6 Close the pyelotomy using 3/0 or 4/0 absorbable sutures. Tie these sutures gently and with just enough tension to approximate the edges, as there is risk of these sutures cutting through. Anchor the catheter to the capsule using absorbable sutures.

► KEY POINTS Anatomy

- Take care to puncture the renal parenchyma near the convex border of the kidney and not on the anterior or posterior surface.
- This minimizes the risk of injury to large intra-renal vessels.

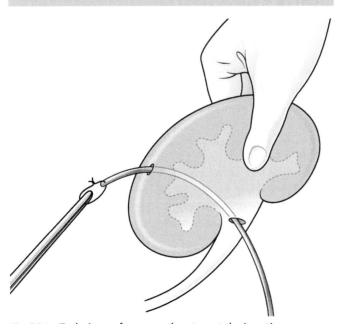

Fig. 36.1 Technique of open nephrostomy tube insertion.

7 Bring out the nephrostomy tube through the abdominal wall with as straight a course as possible, to facilitate changing the tube if necessary.

Aftercare

1 Perform gentle saline wash-outs if the percutaneous nephrostomy does not drain adequately, or insert a larger calibre tube after dilating the track.

2 If side-holes of the nephrostomy tube slip outside the parenchyma, urinary extravasation occurs. Re-adjust it under radiographic control.

3 A nephrostomy can be left in place for weeks or months, but it has a tendency to fall out however carefully it is anchored.

4 As soon as possible, refer the patient to a urologist for definitive management.

REFERENCE

1. Noble M. Miscellaneous renal operations. In: Novick AC, Streem SB, Pontes JE, editors. Stewart's Operative Urology. 2nd ed. Baltimore: Williams & Wilkins; 1989. p. 240–9.

OBSTRUCTED KIDNEY CAUSED BY A STONE

Appraise

1 Common sites for stone impaction are at the pelvi-ureteric junction, the pelvic brim or at the vesico-ureteric junction.

► KEY POINT Danger of septicaemia

- An obstructed infected kidney is a potent cause of septicaemia and represents a urological emergency.

2 The diagnosis is usually made with a non-contrast CT scan (CT-KUB) or an intravenous urogram.

3 Renal function will become acutely impaired in patients with a solitary kidney obstructed by a stone, bilateral ureteric stones, or with unilateral ureteric obstruction in patients with pre-existing renal disease. These patients need urgent intervention.

4 In the absence of sepsis or impaired renal function, the majority of patients with a ureteric calculus can be managed with an initial period of watchful waiting to allow for spontaneous stone passage.

5 Obstruction of a kidney for a short period does not usually cause serious harm. However, if there is infection or if there is poor function in the contralateral kidney, there is an urgent need to drain the kidney.

6 Unilateral obstruction lasting for over 6 hours leads to a gradual decrease in renal blood flow and after 24 hours it is reduced to 55%. Following relief of 7 days of unilateral ureteric obstruction, full recovery of renal function occurs within 2 weeks. However, obstruction of 14 days, duration results in a permanent decline in renal function to 70% of control levels. An obstructed kidney is at risk of infection and pyonephrosis (Greek: *pyon* = pus + *nephron* = kidney + *-osis* = production). In cases of incomplete

ureteric obstruction, watchful waiting for spontaneous stone passage is usually limited to about 4–6 weeks.

7 Relieve obstruction in patients where pain is not controlled by oral analgesia.

8 In the absence of a trained urologist, an acutely obstructed kidney is best relieved using a percutaneous nephrostomy. If you do not have an expert radiologist available, perform an open nephrostomy in an emergency.

9 When the patient is not critically ill but needs decompression of an obstructed kidney, a urologist will opt to insert a retrograde ureteric stent. This is usually performed under general anaesthesia.

CYSTOSCOPIC INSERTION OF A URETERIC STENT

Prepare

1 Review the imaging and mark the side to be stented.

2 Arrange for a radiographer to be present in the operating theatre to operate an image intensifier for on-table fluoroscopy.

Action

1 Pass a cystoscope and carefully inspect the bladder.

2 Locate the ureteric orifice on the obstructed side.

3 Pass the floppy tip of a guide-wire through the working channel of the cystoscope and direct it into the distal end of the ureter.

4 Advance the guide-wire slowly into the ureter using the image intensifier to screen the wire as it is advanced.

5 Resistance will be met when the wire reaches the obstructing stone. Gently probe the stone with the guide-wire until it slides past the stone. Advance the wire into the renal pelvis, where you will see it curl.

6 Confirm that you are in the kidney by passing a 6 Fr ureteric catheter over your guide-wire. Again, use X-ray guidance to observe the catheter advancing over your wire.

7 When the catheter is near the tip of your wire, remove the guide-wire. Attach an empty 10- or 20-ml syringe to the end of the ureteric catheter and aspirate urine. Send a sample for culture.

8 Inject radiological contrast into the ureteric catheter to outline the renal collecting system.

9 Replace the guide-wire through the ureteric catheter then remove the catheter leaving just the guide-wire in the collecting system.

10 Choose a double J stent based on the height of the patient (26 cm for tall patients, 22 cm for short patients and 24 cm for the average patient).

11 Feed the stent over the guide-wire and advance it towards the kidney. Keep the cystoscope close to the ureteric orifice as you do this and direct the radiographer to screen the stent as it passes up the ureter. Insert a stent pusher over the wire to advance the stent through the cystoscope.

12 When there is an adequate length of stent in the renal pelvis, remove the wire completely, which will allow the proximal end of the stent to curl in the renal pelvis and the distal end to curl in the bladder.

▶ **KEY POINTS**

If your guide-wire is unable to advance beyond the obstructing stone:

■ Pass the ureteric catheter over the wire to the level of the stone and continue to probe the stone gently with the wire. The ureteric catheter will provide some stiffness to the wire and prevent it from curling beneath the stone;

■ Failing this, exchange the wire for a hydrophilic 'slippery' wire. Remember to prime the slippery wire by flushing it with saline;

■ If you are unable to pass a guide-wire beyond the stone, insert a nephrostomy rather than cause ureteric damage with repeated attempts at retrograde passage.

DEFINITIVE STONE MANAGEMENT

1 Leave a stent *in situ* for 4–6 weeks before attempting stone removal. This will allow any infection to be treated completely and ureteric inflammation to settle. A stent will also result in ureteric paralysis and dilatation facilitating subsequent ureteroscopy.

2 Prior to stone surgery, obtain a plain KUB X-ray to locate the position of the stone alongside the stent.

3 Ureteroscopy should be performed by a urologist. A semi-rigid ureteroscope is used for ureteric stones with laser stone fragmentation. Occasionally, a ureteric stone is pushed back into the kidney during stent insertion and will require flexible ureteroscopy for fragmentation and removal.

RENAL TRAUMA

Appraise

1 Renal injuries are most commonly due to blunt trauma from falls, road traffic accidents or sporting injuries. Penetrating injuries may result from stabbings or gunshot wounds. Renal injuries are rarely isolated, as the mechanism of injury commonly results in damage to other organs, e.g. bowel and spleen.

2 Aggressive resuscitation of the patient is required and a full clinical assessment of all the injuries should be performed.

3 Blunt abdominal or loin trauma with associated visible haematuria is suggestive of a renal injury and a contrast enhanced CT scan is required (CT urogram). If that is not available, order intravenous urography (IVU), combined with angiography if you suspect involvement of the renal pedicle. Blunt trauma with associated non-visible haematuria has a low incidence of significant renal injury and imaging is only required if the patient is haemodynamically compromised, other injuries are suspected or if the mechanism of injury involves significant forces.

4 The majority of blunt renal injuries can be managed conservatively. The availability of renal angiography and selective embolization of bleeding renal vessels has positively altered the management of renal injuries so that even a severely shattered kidney can be managed initially using non-operative measures.

5 If there is parenchymal disruption associated with extravasation of contrast from the collecting system, conservative management is still possible but be ready to operate quickly if the patient's condition deteriorates. Poor visualization, even on CT scan, suggests injury to the renal pedicle. If the patient is stable, perform angiography.

6 Massive and potentially life-threatening haemorrhage from a renal injury is an indication for immediate surgical exploration. Patients who are unstable despite a trial of conservative management will require exploration. Other indications for surgery include extensive urinary extravasation, an expanding retroperitoneal haematoma or a pulsatile haematoma.

▶ KEY POINTS Surgical exploration

- If the patient has not had a preoperative IVU and you discover renal trauma at exploration, perform IVU on the operating table to determine the status of the uninvolved kidney.
- If you suspect associated bowel and pancreatic injury perform a laparotomy through a midline incision. If the kidney is irretrievably damaged, remove it after ligating the renal artery and vein.
- Explore and complete the bowel, pancreatic, splenic and other intra-abdominal surgery (see Chapter 4) before opening the retroperitoneal space, provided there is no major bleeding.
- If you have excluded any other abdominal visceral injury preoperatively, you may explore the kidney through a loin incision. However, a trans-peritoneal approach through a midline incision gives excellent access to the renal pedicle and the great vessels in the abdomen.

NEPHRECTOMY FOR TRAUMA

Access

1 Place the patient in the supine position.

2 Employ a midline trans-abdominal incision, which provides complete access to abdominal organs, vasculature and kidneys.

3 Perform a careful and systematic survey of the intra-abdominal organs.

4 Mobilize the bowel and peritoneum off the aorta and vena cava.

5 Palpate the retroperitoneal structures. If you encounter a large pulsatile expanding haematoma, gain control of the renal pedicle before opening the peri-renal fascia of Gerota. Eviscerate the small intestine and incise the peritoneum over the aorta, exposing the vena cava and aorta. Isolate the renal artery(ies) and vein(s). Place vessel loops around the vessels of the injured kidney to gain control. If the vascular anatomy is obscured by a large retroperitoneal haematoma, then identify the inferior mesenteric vein and incise the retroperitoneum medial to this land mark and the aorta is located in the lower part of the incision.

? DIFFICULTY

1. Bleeding can be terrifying. Do not blindly clamp vessels. You may cause collateral damage that is difficult to repair. Instead, insert a pack and apply direct pressure for 10 minutes or more before taking another look at the vessels.
2. When the anatomy is distorted and obscured by haematoma, you might commit the disastrous mistake of ligating the vessels of the undamaged, contralateral kidney in error. Take care!

6 When you have the bleeding under control, open the fascia of Gerota (Dumitru Gerota, 1867–1939, Professor of Surgery in Bucharest) and expose the kidney. If you have the necessary skill, and the parenchymal damage is not great, repair the kidney. Close the defects in the collecting system with continuous sutures of 4/0 Monocril or any other available absorbable suture. Carefully excise devitalized tissue, preserving as much capsule as possible. If the collecting system is injured, always leave a drain in the perinephric space.

7 If the contralateral kidney has been confirmed as intact, perform a nephrectomy rather than exposing the patient to unnecessary risk by attempting a difficult repair.

8 Double ligate the artery(ies) and the vein(s) with 2/0 Vicryl suture in continuity and then divide the vessels. If the right renal vein is very short, perform suture ligation using 2/0 Vicryl on a round-body needle for extra safety.

9 Carefully ligate and divide any adrenal vein and artery(ies) arising from the main renal vessels.

10 In the case of the left kidney, also ligate and divide the gonadal vein draining into the renal vein.

▶ KEY POINTS Anatomical variations

- A lumbar vein frequently drains into the left renal vein on the posterior aspect. Carefully ligate and divide it.
- Remember that accessory arteries are present in about 25% of people and that there are frequent variations of venous anatomy.

11 The fascia of Gerota has already been dissected off the kidney for exploration and assessment of renal injury. Complete any required remaining dissection to free the kidney from the surrounding tissues.

12 Remove the kidney by dividing the ureter between clamps. Ligate the distal ureteric stump with a 2/0 Vicryl suture.

13 After removing the kidney, carefully check the haemostasis, particularly of the hilar vessels and the adrenal area. Control any bleeding by suture ligation.

14 Place a wide bore Silastic tube drain with its tip in the most dependent point of the cavity.

15 Close the abdominal wound in a single layer using 1/0 looped monofilament PDS.

REPAIR OF A DAMAGED URETER

Assess

1. If you operate in the vicinity of the ureter, always check for damage. If you recognize inadvertent surgical ureteric injury at the operation, repair it immediately.

2. Iatrogenic ureteric injury may become apparent in the postoperative period. Clinically, this may present with loin pain or sepsis, urine might be identified in an abdominal drainage bag or occasionally leaking from an abdominal wound.

3. The mechanism of ureteric injury in cases of delayed presentation is usually a result of ischaemic injury to a segment of ureter from placement of haemostatic clips or sutures in the proximity of the ureter or inadvertent diathermy injury. Diagnosis is confirmed with either an intravenous urogram or CT urogram with delayed phase images. Where a ureteric injury is diagnosed postoperatively, consult with a urologist. Radiological placement of a nephrostomy to divert urine from the injury is usually a good holding measure whilst reconstruction is planned.

END-TO-END ANASTOMOSIS OF A DIVIDED URETER

Action

1. Consider end-to-end anastomosis for injuries of the mid and upper ureter providing the defect can be breached without tension. For injuries of the distal ureter, reimplantation with or without a psoas hitch or Boari flap (see below) is the procedure of choice.

2. Mobilize both ends of the divided ureter to make sure that they are accessible for anastomosis.

3. Place a double pigtail stent with one end in the renal pelvis and the other in the urinary bladder. If you do not have available a double pigtail stent, splint the anastomosis with a small-calibre (6F or 8F) paediatric feeding tube.

4. Open out the ends like a broad, flat-bladed spatula (Greek: *spathe*=broad blade) and hold the ends between stay sutures (Fig. 36.2). Anastomose them using fine interrupted sutures of 4/0 or 5/0 Monocril or any other available absorbable suture.

? DIFFICULTY

1. If you cannot repair the ureter, and if the patient's prognosis is poor, perform nephrectomy, provided that the contralateral kidney is normal. It is sometimes safer in such patients to sacrifice the kidney than to be committed to multiple repair operations.

2. If the patient's prognosis is good, pass a simple tube through the proximal ureter into the renal pelvis, bringing it out through the skin. Ligate the distal end with a marker suture for identification. Alternatively, ligate the distal ureter and place a percutaneous nephrostomy. When the patient has recovered, arrange a referral to a specialist centre for reconstruction.

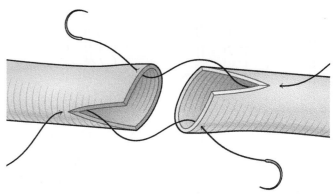

Fig. 36.2 Spatulated uretero-ureterostomy.

5. Leave a size 18F tube drain in the vicinity of the ureteric anastomosis.

6. Remove the stent or tube splint after about 10 days.

BOARI FLAP (BLADDER FLAP URETEROPLASTY)

Appraise

1. The Boari flap operation (originally described in 1894 by Casati and Boari) of replacing the distal ureter with a bladder flap is used where the distal ureter is irreparably damaged or where it has been removed due to stricture or a distal ureteric tumour in a patient who is not suitable for nephro-ureterectomy.

Action

1. Position the patient in the supine position. Prepare the abdomen and genitalia and insert a urinary catheter.

2. Place a curved incision over the iliac fossa starting near the midline over the pubic tubercle and extend it over the surface marking of the linea semilunaris (Fig. 36.3).

3. Use a muscle cutting incision using monopolar diathermy to open the rectus muscle and rectus sheath.

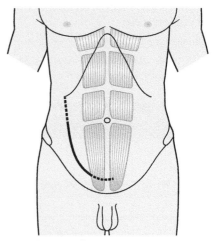

Fig. 36.3 Incision for Boari flap operation.

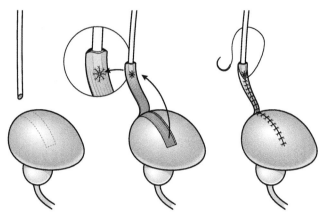

Fig. 36.4 Boari flap operation.

4 Sweep the peritoneum medially and superiorly to expose the retroperitoneal structures.

5 Locate the ureter. Remember that it crosses the pelvic brim at the bifurcation of the common iliac vessels.

6 Excise the diseased segment of ureter. If the diagnosis is a ureteric tumour, excise a small cuff of bladder with the distal ureter. Close the bladder defect in two layers with a 2/0 Vicryl suture.

7 If the procedure is being performed for a distal ureteric injury, locate the end of the ureter and debride any necrotic tissue.

8 Spatulate the distal end of the ureter by making a 2-cm longitudinal incision and place a stay suture at the apex of the spatulation.

9 Distend the bladder by instilling 200–300 ml of sterile saline via the urethral catheter.

10 Use a marker pen to draw three sides of a rectangle 10 cm long and 4 cm wide (Fig. 36.4) and incise along your mark to raise a bladder flap.

11 Create a submucosal tunnel using blunt dissection with scissors and create an opening about half way down the flap.

12 Pull the distal ureter through your submucosal tunnel using the stay suture and anastamose the ureter to the bladder mucosa using a fine Vicryl suture (Fig. 36.4).

13 Insert the floppy tip of a guide-wire through the distal ureter and slide a ureteric catheter over the wire.

14 Run a continuous Vicryl suture to tubularize your flap and close the bladder defect (Fig. 36.4).

15 Leave a drainage tube in the pelvis before closure.

16 A urinary catheter should be left for 2 weeks and a cystogram performed before removal of the catheter.

DRAINAGE OF A PERINEPHRIC ABSCESS

Appraise

▶ KEY POINTS Have you identified the cause?

■ Is the patient diabetic? Immunocompromised? Debilitated?
■ Is the patient suffering from renal cortical abscess or pyonephrosis?

1 The safest procedure is preliminary drainage followed by nephrectomy.

2 Percutaneous drainage by a trained interventional radiologist is the best option. If this is not available then undertake open drainage.

Action

1 Position the patient as for nephrectomy.

2 Make a small incision below the 12th rib or where the abscess is pointing on the surface.

3 Deepen the incision to the perinephric space. Pus usually starts to pour out as you reach the space.

4 Sweep your forefinger around in the perinephric space to break down all the septa.

5 Leave a wide-bore soft plastic tube drain in the cavity and secure it to the skin.

6 Close the wound lightly with interrupted monofilament nylon sutures.

OPERATIONS FOR PELVI-URETERIC JUNCTION OBSTRUCTION

Appraise

1 Obstruction at the level of the pelvi-ureteric junction (PUJ) causes hydronephrosis without evidence of ureteric dilatation.

2 The underlying cause can be classified according to intrinsic or extrinsic obstruction.

3 In paediatric patients, the most common cause is a functional obstruction due to a non-dynamic segment of ureter or atresia of the tissue at the PUJ.

4 Extrinsic compression can be due to a peri-ureteric fibrous band or a crossing vessel.

5 Patients may present with loin pain, urinary tract infections, abdominal mass or incidentally on abdominal imaging.

6 A MAG3 renogram will confirm an obstructed dilated system.

PYELOPLASTY

1 This procedure can be performed with an open loin incision or laparoscopically. The procedure can also be performed using robotic surgery.

2 Mobilize the proximal ureter and the renal pelvis and identify the PUJ. Take care when dissecting the ureter; leave adequate peri-ureteric tissue to preserve its blood supply.

3 Place stay sutures anteriorly though the renal pelvis and the proximal ureter to aid with orientation of the anastomosis and minimize handling of the tissues.

4 Transect the ureter at the level of the PUJ (Fig. 36.5A).

5 If the obstruction is secondary to a crossing vessel, pass the ureter around the vessel. If the obstruction is due to a stricture/scarred PUJ then excise the diseased segment.

6 Spatulate the cut end of the ureter using a 2-cm longitudinal incision on the opposite side to the stay suture. If a ureteric stent has not been placed preoperatively, insert one by placing an antegrade guide-wire to the bladder and passing a double J stent over the wire.

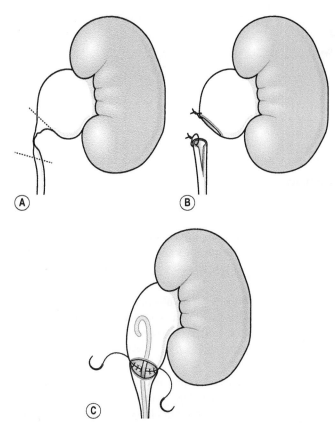

Fig. 36.5 Pyeloplasty for pelvi-ureteric junction obstruction: (A) transection of ureter; (B) spatulation of ends; (C) pelvi-ureteric anastomosis.

7 Spatulate the cut end of the renal pelvis with a 2-cm incision (Fig. 36.5B).

8 Perform the anastomosis using a fine absorbable suture. Place the first suture at the apex of the ureteric spatulation by passing the needle from outside to in and opposed to the renal pelvis by placing the suture from inside to out and tie.

9 Run a continuous suture along the posterior side of the spatulated ureter to anastamose it to the posterior spatulated edge of the renal pelvis so that the two stay sutures are aligned (Fig. 36.5C). Once one side is completed, place the proximal loop of the stent into the renal pelvis. Use a second suture starting again from the apex of the spatulated ureter to close the anterior side over the stent. The two sutures are tied together to complete the anastomosis.

10 Leave a tube drain in the area of the anastomosis.

11 Leave the stent in situ for 6 weeks and perform a MAG3 renogram 12 weeks after surgery to assess drainage.

FURTHER READING

Camunez F, Echenagusia A, Prieto ML, et al. Percutaneous nephrostomy in pyonephrosis. Urol Radiol 1989;11:77.

Ghali AM, El-Malik EM, Ibrahim AI, et al. Ureteric injuries: diagnosis, management, and outcome. J Trauma 1999;46:150–8.

Krane RJ, Siroky MB, Fitzpatrick JM, editors. Operative Urology: Surgical Skills. London: Churchill Livingstone; 2000.

Santucci RA, Wessells H, Bartsch G, et al. Evaluation and management of renal injuries: consensus statement of the Renal Trauma Subcommittee. BJU Int 2004;93:937–54.

Lower urinary tract

G. Smith, S. Pridgeon

CONTENTS

SUPRAPUBIC CATHETER INSERTION

Appraise

1 Suprapubic catheterization is indicated in both emergency and elective settings. A suprapubic catheter (SPC) may be required to drain a bladder in acute urinary retention when urethral catheterization is not possible, e.g. in the presence of a urethral stricture, or to divert urine following injury to the lower urinary tract such as from a pelvic fracture.

2 An SPC may also be used to divert urine following complex reconstructive urological surgery.

3 SPCs are the preferred option for long-term catheterization. By bringing out the catheter through a clean part of the anatomy it is easier to maintain hygiene around the catheter site. Changing an SPC is a clean and technically easy procedure. The risk of infection is reduced, although not completely eliminated. An SPC leaves the genitals free for sexual activity.

Anatomical considerations

1 The bladder lies in the anterior part of the pelvic cavity behind the fat-filled retropubic space. As the bladder fills, it rises above the pubic crests and comes into contact with the lower part of the anterior abdominal wall.

2 The distended bladder intervenes between the parietal peritoneum and the abdominal wall and access can be gained without breaching the peritoneum.

3 The layers of the anterior abdominal wall are firstly the skin and subcutaneous fat. Scarpa's fascia is the next layer. It is well defined and can be thick in obese patients. Deep to Scarpa's fascia, in the midline, below the level of the umbilicus, the rectus sheath forms a single fibrous layer which passes anterior to the rectus abdominis muscles. The posterior surface of the rectus muscles is in direct contact with the transversalis fascia, beneath which is the extraperitoneal fat.

Action

1 There are three types of suprapubic catheter – one where the catheter is introduced over its own needle (the Bonanno™ catheter); the second relies on a Seldinger technique of placing a guide-wire, dilating the track and then introducing the catheter; the third type is introduced via a trocar and cannula placed blindly.

2 The Bonanno™ catheter (BD Biosciences) is a fine-bore catheter tube that can be used as a temporary method of draining the bladder. Due to the narrow calibre of the catheter it is prone to blocking and is not suitable for medium or long-term use.

3 Foley balloon catheters are preferred for suprapubic drainage and are generally available in kits for insertion. Prepare the patient's abdomen in the supine position. Place the drapes to ensure that the midline of the abdomen is identifiable.

4 Locate the site for insertion, two finger-widths above the pubic symphysis in the midline. Use ultrasound to localize the bladder, if available. Infuse local anaesthetic into the skin and the subcutaneous tissues. Continue to advance the needle through all the layers of the anterior abdominal wall until urine is aspirated.

5 Introduction of a suprapubic catheter can only be safely performed following aspiration of urine.

6 Place a 1-cm incision at the site of injection using a blade and deepen it through the subcutaneous fat.

7 Insertion of an SPC using the Seldinger method is considered to be the safest method due to the higher degree of control and accuracy of placement.

8 Attach a long 18-gauge needle to a syringe for deep local anaesthetic infiltration and aspiration of urine from the bladder (Fig 37.1A). Once aspiration is confirmed, detach the syringe leaving the needle in place with its tip still in the bladder. Insert the floppy tip of a guide-wire through the long needle into the bladder (Fig 37.1B). Remove the needle over the guide-wire. Feed the stiff end of the guide-wire through the aperture in the tip of the trocar (Fig 37.1C) and advance the trocar along the guide-wire into the bladder (Fig 37.1D). Remove the trocar leaving the sheath in situ. Introduce a Foley catheter through the sheath and inflate the balloon (Fig 37.1E).

9 If using a blind trocar, push the trocar in its sheath through the skin incision angled at 90° to the skin. Apply constant pressure with rotational movements as you advance the trocar. A sudden loss of resistance will indicate penetration of the rectus sheath. This does not indicate access to the bladder. The trocar will need to be advanced further to enter the bladder.

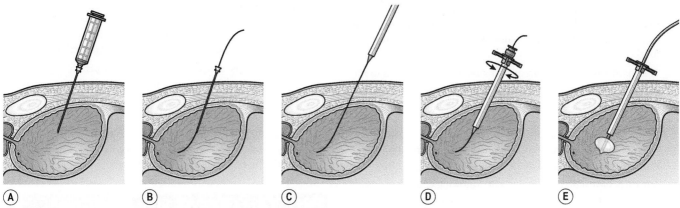

Fig. 37.1 Insertion of suprapubic catheter using the Seldinger technique. (A) Cannulation of bladder (B) Insertion of guidewire (C) Threading trocar over guidewire (D) Introduction of trocar into bladder (E) Insertion of Foley catheter.

10 Confirm access to the bladder by withdrawing the trocar from its sheath to observe a flow of urine. If no urine is seen, replace the trocar in the sheath and advance further until urine is obtained. Insert the catheter quickly through the sheath into the bladder and inflate the balloon. Remove the sheath and secure the catheter with a non-absorbable suture.

11 Where suprapubic catheterization is required electively for long-term catheterization, perform this under direct vision by filling the bladder with a flexible or rigid cystoscope. The cystoscope is used to watch the safe placement of the instruments from within the bladder.

> ### ▶ KEY POINTS

- Blind placement of an SPC can only be performed safely when the bladder is full.
- If the bladder is not palpable, placement may be possible using ultrasound guidance.
- If the patient has had previous abdominal surgery, this increases the risk of bowel injury. Open insertion may be required.

CYSTOSCOPY

Appraise

1 There are very few indications for you, as a general surgeon, to cystoscope a patient.

2 However, you may be forced to pass an instrument, usually a rigid one, in order to relieve clot retention. The procedure is very similar to passing a metal urethral dilator (see below).

3 If you are a junior doctor working on a urological firm you will be expected to undertake this procedure safely as a core skill.

Action

1 Use general anaesthesia when possible.

2 Place the patient in the lithotomy position.

3 Clean and appropriately drape the patient.

4 Check the cystoscope for lighting and irrigation.

5 Insert the lubricated cystoscope under direct vision, using a 0° or 12° rod lens telescope, with the irrigation running. In a male patient, stretch the penis and hold it straight at an angle of about 45° to the horizontal. Slowly advance the scope, visualizing the whole urethra. As you approach the external sphincter lower your hands so the scope is approaching the horizontal. Carefully advance the scope through the sphincter. You will see the verumontanum (a small raised structure in the 6 o'clock position). At this point, do not advance any further; drop your hands further so the scope is now pointing upwards and you can see the two lobes of the prostate. When the scope is pointing upwards at about 45°, advance the scope into the bladder.

6 There is no justification for passing the cystoscope blindly. This is particularly important immediately following prostatectomy, when 'blind' passage of the cystoscope can be extremely difficult and its tip may undermine the trigone.

7 Inspect the bladder using a methodical approach to ensure that it is inspected in its entirety. You may need to exchange the telescope for a 30° or 70° lens for complete inspection.

8 When the bladder is full of clot, it is often necessary to pass the larger 27 F resectoscope sheath in order to evacuate the clots effectively. Use a visual obturator to insert the resectoscope under vision using the principles described above for passing the cystoscope. If the visual obturator is not available and you have to insert the resectoscope sheath 'blind', obtain a preliminary view of the urethral anatomy with the cystoscope to help you know where you are going. Clots can be evacuated from the bladder using an Ellik's evacuator.

OPERATIONS FOR URETHRAL STRICTURES

Appraise

1 Urethral strictures commonly cause symptoms of bladder outflow obstruction and are the most common cause of urinary obstruction in young and middle aged men.

2 Any injury to the epithelium lining the urethra or to the underlying corpus spongiosum which results in healing by scar formation may cause a urethral stricture.

3 The aetiology may be infective (Chlamydia, gonococcal), traumatic (usually blunt or iatrogenic), inflammatory (e.g. lichen sclerosus et atrophicus), ischaemic (secondary to distraction injury) or idiopathic.

4 Traumatic strictures may occur after straddle injuries, kicks to the perineum or pelvic fractures. Iatrogenic trauma is a common aetiology and any form of urethral instrumentation resulting in urethral epithelial damage may subsequently result in stricture formation. This can range from minor instrumentation such as urethral catheterization to bladder neck strictures resulting from transurethral resection of the prostate.

5 Strictures have a high recurrence rate following endoscopic treatment. Recurrence is more common with longer and denser strictures.

URETHRAL DILATATION

The principle of urethral dilatation is to pass blunt instruments of increasing calibre through the stricture to achieve dynamic stretching without inducing epithelial damage, which would result in a further scarring process.

Action

1 Choose a dilating instrument to suit the site of the stricture. Use generous amounts of lubricating gel.

2 For distal or meatal strictures, use short female dilating instruments, for example Canny Ryall dilators.

3 For more proximal strictures, use curved Clutton dilators. With the patient in lithotomy, hold the penis vertically. Introduce the dilator, point the penis towards the patient's head and slowly advance the dilator. Push the curve of the dilator against the bulbar urethra and lower your hands. As you do this, the dilator will slide into the bladder. To confirm that you are in the bladder, rotate the dilator; if it rotates easily then you are in the right place.

OPTICAL URETHROTOMY

1 Use an optical urethrotome.

2 Pass the instrument to the level of the stricture. Pass a guide-wire via the side channel through the stricture into the bladder to define the direction of the stricture.

3 Extend the cutting blade from the urethrotome sheath through the stricture. Aim to incise the stricture in the 12 o'clock position. Advance the blade through the stricture, lower your hands to apply upward pressure and pull the blade back through the stricture.

4 Repeat this action if necessary in the same position until the stricture opens up. The incision must be full thickness through the depth of the scar.

5 Advance the urethrotome sheath through the stricture into the bladder and remove the inner working element to leave the outer sheath in place. Advance a urinary catheter through the outer sheath and inflate the catheter balloon before removing the sheath.

6 Leave a urethral catheter *in situ* after the urethrotomy for 24–72 hours.

URETHROPLASTY

1 For recurrent strictures, excision of the diseased urethra will provide a better long-term outcome than optical urethrotomy.

2 Urethroplasty is a specialist urological operation performed through a perineal incision. An anastamotic urethroplasty involves excision of the strictured segment, mobilization of the urethra and primary anastamosis of the two cut ends of the urethra.

3 Free graft urethroplasty involves excision of the stricture, laying a tissue graft and tubularization over a catheter. Buccal mucosa is currently the favoured tissue for grafting.

PROSTATECTOMY FOR BENIGN PROSTATIC ENLARGEMENT

Appraise

1 Prostatectomies are usually performed to treat bladder outflow obstruction secondary to benign prostatic enlargement (BPE). The majority of prostatectomies are carried out endoscopically (transurethral resection of prostate – TURP). Where the prostate volume is estimated to be above 100 cc, an open retropubic or transvesical prostatectomy is preferred. Recently, laser vapourization of the prostate or laser enucleation have become popular. Holmium laser enucleation can be used to treat very large (>100 cc) glands, avoiding the need for open surgery.

2 Indications for prostatectomy are: failed medical management of BPE, chronic urinary retention, high pressure retention with renal impairment, recurrent haematuria secondary to BPE, recurrent urinary tract infections or bladder stone formation due to outflow obstruction. TURP is sometimes performed to manage lower urinary tract symptoms (LUTS) in patients with prostate cancer.

3 Consider long-term catheterization as an alternative to surgery where patients have a poor performance status or where severe dementia or Parkinson's disease would render the patient susceptible to postoperative incontinence.

4 Beware of patients with severe storage LUTS which may be due to detrusor over-activity. These symptoms may not improve with bladder outlet surgery. Preoperative urodynamic assessment may be valuable in patients with mixed storage and voiding symptoms to confirm whether there is evidence of obstruction or concomitant detrusor over-activity.

5 Do not approach clinically malignant prostates through the open route.

6 Very small prostates, often amounting only to a tight unrelaxing bladder neck, are far better approached transurethrally. The operation of choice may be a bladder neck incision.

7 When obtaining consent from a patient for prostatectomy, warn him of the risk of retrograde ejaculation (70–80% for TURP), erectile dysfunction (10–15% for TURP) and permanent incontinence (1% for TURP). Tell the patient he may experience residual urinary symptoms or temporary urinary incontinence (3% for TURP). There is around a 4% incidence of postoperative urethral stricture or bladder neck contracture, which may require further surgery. Bleeding and infection should also be mentioned as perioperative complications as well as TUR syndrome if monopolar glycine resection is being used.

RETROPUBIC PROSTATECTOMY

Prepare

1 Perform a preliminary cystoscopy to establish that the gland is suitable for enucleation and that there is no urethral or bladder pathology.

2 Place the patient in the supine position.

3 Position yourself on the left side of the patient; clean the lower abdomen, genitalia and upper thighs. Apply drapes so that you have access to the genitalia.

Access

1 Make either a 10 cm Pfannenstiel incision or an infraumbilical lower midline incision.

2 Expose the rectus sheath.

3 Incise the rectus sheath in the direction of your skin incision, exposing the muscle belly.

4 Grasp the midline of cut edges of the rectus sheath with long artery forceps, and with finger dissection free the rectus sheath from both muscles. Use scissors for the linea alba; carry this incision downwards to the symphysis and upwards for about 6 cm, exposing the rectus muscles (Fig. 37.2).

5 Gently dissect with scissors between the rectus muscles, developing the longitudinal gap between them.

6 Retract the rectus muscles laterally and develop the prevesical space with the peritoneum swept superiorly.

7 Sweep your right index finger beneath the symphysis to clean the retropubic space. Position a long-bladed Millin self-retaining retractor that depresses the bladder while holding the wound open.

Action

1 With diathermy forceps, coagulate all the veins coursing across the prostatic capsule. After this, clean the capsule of fatty tissue.

2 Have your assistant depress the lower part of the bladder downwards and backwards with a sponge in a sponge-holder, exposing the upper border of the prostate gland (Fig. 37.3A).

3 Place a stay suture in the upper border of the capsule and a second stay suture just distal to the first.

4 Make a 2-cm transverse incision through the capsule of the prostate between the two stay sutures using cutting diathermy (Fig. 37.3B). The capsule may be up to 0.5 cm thick, and there are vessels within it that need to be coagulated. The two lobes of the prostate bulge into view. Insert long dissecting scissors between the two lobes into the prostatic urethra and open them longitudinally. Remove the retractor and other instruments.

5 Insert your right index finger into the prostatic urethra. You feel it gripped between the two lobes. Push your finger downwards until it reaches the back of the prostatic urethra and curl it laterally towards yourself. You will be able to break into a plane between the urethra and the left lobe of the 'adenomatous' gland. Extend

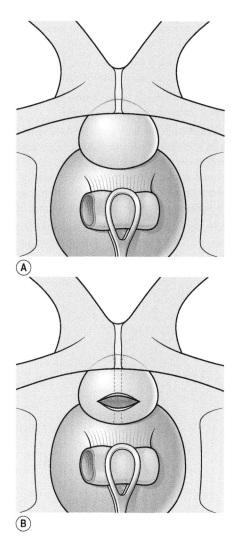

(A)

(B)

Fig. 37.3 (A) Exposure of prostatic capsule, (B) Incision into prostatic capsule.

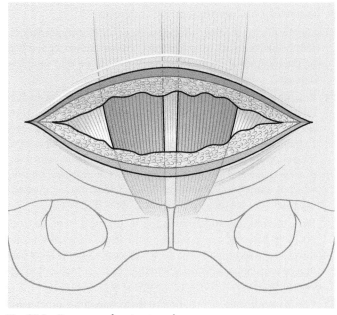

Fig. 37.2 Exposure of rectus muscle.

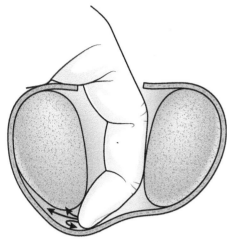

Fig. 37.4 Enucleation of prostatic adenomas.

this plane to the apex of the prostate and backwards to the bladder neck (Fig. 37.4).

6   Next, come back to the apex (distal end) of the prostate. With your index finger under the lobe and your thumb on the outside of the capsule, you can nip through the apex and so free it. Continue to work your index finger round the front and lateral border, so freeing the lobe completely except for that part attached to the bladder neck.

7   Repeat the process on the opposite lobe. Use the index finger of each hand to facilitate enucleation of the gland.

8   Dislocate the two lobes out of the capsule and nip them off at the bladder neck, using thumb and forefinger.

9   Insert a bladder neck spreader (e.g. the Badenoch spreader) into the bladder. Get an assistant to hold it in position (Fig. 37.5). This reveals the bladder neck, and middle lobe if present, both of which must be totally excised. Pack a swab into the prostatic cavity to prevent the field from being obscured by blood, and likewise into the bladder to stop the bladder urothelium folding upwards.

10 The bladder neck can now be grasped with long-toothed forceps and excised with a diathermy point. Do not be tempted to excise just a small 'V'.

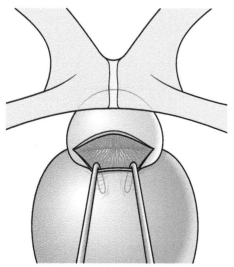

Fig. 37.5 Bladder neck retractor in position.

11 Insert a wide-bore (24 F) three-way irrigating catheter.

12 Close the prostatic capsule using a continuous 2/0 absorbable suture. Start the sutures from both ends of the incision in the prostatic capsule using two different lengths of the suture and meet in the middle tying the two together. Complete the closure by tying the 2 stay sutures together.

13 Wash out the bladder to ensure your suture line is watertight.

14 Use a wide-bore drain placed in the retropubic space.

15 Close the rectus sheath with a 2/0 or 0/0 PDS suture and select a skin closure that you are familiar with.

16 Finally wash the bladder out again and ensure that your irrigation is running freely.

TRANSURETHRAL RESECTION OF PROSTATE

Prepare

1   Place the patient with his legs in the lithotomy position.

2   You may wish to perform a digital rectal examination of the prostate to assess the size before embarking on endoscopic resection, although this information should have been obtained preoperatively.

3   If you are using monopolar resecting equipment place a diathermy pad on the patient's skin and ensure that the irrigation fluid is glycine 1.5%. For bipolar equipment use saline for resection.

Action

1   First perform a cystoscopy to assess the urethra, sphincter, prostatic urethra, prostatic lobes and verumontanum. A systematic inspection of the bladder is essential, paying particular attention to the position of the ureteric orifices in relation to the bladder neck.

2   Introduce the resectoscope sheath into the bladder with a visual obturator. Once in the bladder, replace the obturator with the working element of the resectoscope with resecting loop attached.

3   Ensure the diathermy cables are connected and the inflow and outflow for bladder irrigation are both open.

4   Start by placing the tip of the resectoscope at the verumontanum. This is the landmark for the external urethral sphincter and will be the most distal extent of your resection to prevent sphincter damage.

5   Resection usually begins in the 6 o'clock position of the median lobe. Extend the resecting loop and apply the cutting diathermy pedal as you retract the loop (Fig 37.6A). Repeat this to create a channel between the two lateral lobes from the bladder neck to the verumontanum. Resect the adenomatous tissue, which appears granular and 'bread-like'. Stop when you reach the capsule, which is a smooth fibrous layer. At the bladder neck stop resecting when you see the circular muscle fibres (Fig 37.6B).

6   Next resect the lateral lobes starting at either the 10 or 2 o'clock position. Resect in one position to the level of the capsule and move your resection towards the 6 o'clock position. Achieve haemostasis using coagulation diathermy. Apply a methodical approach to achieve a smooth resection (Fig 37.6C).

7   Check your position in relation to the verumontanum regularly to avoid excessive resection near the sphincter.

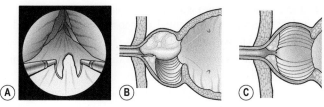

Fig. 37.6 Transurethral resection of prostate. (A) The resectoscope in action (B) Resection of median lobe (C) Completed resection

8 Place the tip of the scope at the verumontanum and look up towards the bladder. If the resection is complete you will be able to see into the bladder from here with an unobstructed view.

9 Evacuate the prostate chips using an Ellik device. Inspect the bladder carefully to ensure that all chips are removed.

10 Re-inspect the prostatic bed for further bleeding before inserting a three-way catheter using a catheter introducer in the same way as introducing a curved metal urethral dilator (above).

11 Ensure the irrigation is running freely.

FORMATION OF ILEAL CONDUIT

Appraise

1 An ileal conduit is a form of urinary diversion where the ureters are anastomosed to a segment of small bowel, which is fashioned as a stoma to the skin of the anterior abdominal wall (Fig. 37.7).

2 Other forms of urinary diversion exist which can be continent or incontinent; the ileal conduit is the most common diversion procedure.

3 Urinary diversion is required when the bladder is removed either for malignant disease (radical cystectomy) or for benign disease (simple cystectomy). It can also be carried out leaving the native bladder *in situ*, for example for severe lower urinary tract symptoms or to palliate symptoms in patients with locally advanced bladder malignancy.

Action

1 Mark a stoma site preoperatively by assessing the patient in the supine, seated and standing positions to avoid the appliance being located in a skin fold.

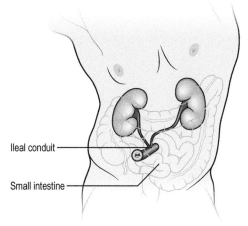

Ileal conduit

Small intestine

Fig. 37.7 Ileal conduit formation.

2 A lower midline abdominal incision is usually used for cystectomy. This allows adequate access to the bladder and pelvic organs as well as the bowel.

3 The posterior peritoneum is incised on both sides and the large bowel reflected to expose the iliac vessels.

4 Identify the ureters by locating the bifurcation of the common iliac arteries where the ureters cross over the vessels. Dissect the ureters distally to the vesico-ureteric junctions and divide them close to the bladder. Clip or tie the cut ends to allow dilatation of the ureters. When dissecting the ureters, leave adequate peri-ureteric tissue to preserve its blood supply.

5 Prepare a segment of distal small bowel by firstly locating the ileo-caecal junction and, using a tape measure, select a 15-cm length of ileum 20 cm from the ileo-caecal valve. When selecting the bowel, trans-illuminate the small bowel mesentery to identify a length of ileum that can be isolated on a pedicle without compromising the blood supply.

6 Apply non-crushing bowel clamps at the boundaries of the isolated loop and divide the bowel. Place a stay suture at the distal end of the bowel segment to allow ante-peristaltic orientation of the conduit. Flush the conduit bowel segment with sterile water. Re-establish bowel continuity by joining the free ends of the small bowel with either a hand-sewn or stapled anastomosis.

7 Prepare the distal ends of the ureters for the ureteric-bowel anastomosis. Pass the left ureter through an opening created in the sigmoid mesentery to swing it to the right side of the abdomen. For a Wallace anastomosis, the distal ends of the ureters are spatulated with a 2-cm longitudinal incision. The ureters can be joined using a 66 or 69 technique with a fine absorbable suture. The joined ureters can then be anastomosed to the proximal end of the ileal segment. Alternatively, the ureters can be anastomosed separately in an end-to-side Bricker anastomosis. Ureteric catheters should be fed to the kidney on each side and passed through the loop of bowel and out of the stoma.

8 Create a stoma by excising a plug of skin at the predetermined site and dissect down to the rectus fascia. Make a cruciate incision in the fascia and bluntly dissect through the peritoneum. Pass the distal end of the small-bowel conduit through the aperture, taking care not to displace the ureteric catheters. Pull the bowel 2–3 cm above the level of the skin in order to facilitate the fashioning of a spout. The stoma is anchored to the rectus fascia with four sutures applied between each of the four leaves of the cruciate incision and the bowel serosa. Absorbable sutures are used to create the stoma by everting the bowel to form a spout.

9 Leave the ureteric catheters in place for 10 days.

TRAUMATIC RUPTURE OF THE BLADDER

Appraise

1 Extraperitoneal rupture can follow blunt trauma to the lower abdomen when the bladder is full. It can be diagnosed by a cystogram, using aqueous contrast medium, which may also demonstrate associated urethral injury.

2 Extraperitoneal bladder rupture can be treated conservatively by inserting a urethral catheter, giving broad-spectrum antibiotics and monitoring the patient.

3 Operative repair of the bladder is indicated if there is a failure to drain urine through the catheter, increasing lower abdominal distension or evidence of intra-peritoneal rupture.

4 Rupture of the bladder into the peritoneal cavity is an unusual injury in isolation, though it may occur as a complication of transurethral surgery to a bladder lesion. If it results from external trauma, there are commonly associated injuries that need attention.

Action

1 Expose the bladder intra- and extraperitoneally. This enables you to perform an exploratory laparotomy at the same time.

2 Clean the peritoneal cavity using saline lavage.

3 Open the bladder anteriorly to detect other bladder injuries that may have escaped notice.

4 Close the bladder incision and injuries in two layers using an absorbable suture. Drain the bladder urethrally if there is no urethral injury, and suprapubically if there is any doubt.

5 Before closure of the abdomen instil 100–200 ml of sterile saline into the bladder via the catheter to test your bladder closure and check for other sites of bladder injury.

RUPTURE OF THE POSTERIOR URETHRA

Appraise

1 Injuries to the urethra that result from pelvic trauma require expert attention if the patient is to avoid lifelong disability.

2 If the patient cannot pass urine following lower abdominal or pelvic trauma, the differential diagnosis lies between bladder rupture and posterior urethral injury.

3 Urethral injury is more likely if there is significant bony deformity of the pelvis.

4 Stabilize the urinary tract by inserting a suprapubic catheter while life-threatening injuries receive attention.

5 The operative management of posterior urethral rupture is often complex and beyond the scope of this book, so seek expert urological advice.

FURTHER READING

Blandy J. Cystoscopy. In: Blandy J, editor. Operative Urology. 2nd ed. Oxford: Blackwell Scientific; 1986. p. 6–9.

Blandy J. Dilatation of a stricture. In: Blandy J, editor. Operative Urology. 2nd ed. Oxford: Blackwell Scientific; 1986. p. 216–9.

Blandy J. Suprapubic cystostomy. In: Blandy J, editor. Operative Urology. 2nd ed. Oxford: Blackwell Scientific; 1986. p. 117–20.

Blandy J, Fowler C. Bladder: trauma. In: Blandy J, Fowler C, editors. Urology. 2nd ed. Oxford: Blackwell Scientific; 1996. p. 265–71.

Blandy J, Fowler C. Urethra and penis: trauma. In: Blandy J, Fowler C, editors. Urology. 2nd ed. Oxford: Blackwell Scientific; 1996. p. 460–71.

Chapple C, Barbagli G, Jordan G, et al. Consensus statement on urethral trauma [review]. BJU Int 2004;93:1195–2002.

May F, Hartung R. Surgical atlas: transurethral resection of prostate. BJU Surgery Illustrated 2006;98:921–34.

Millin R. Retropubic prostatectomy: new extravesical technique. Report on 20 cases. Lancet 1945;ii:693.

Nesbit RM. Transurethral Prostatectomy. Springfield: Charles C Thomas; 1943.

Renvall S, Nurmi M, Aho A. Rupture of the urinary bladder: a potentially serious condition. Scand J Urol Nephrol 1989;23:185.

Webster GD, Mathes GL, Selli C. Prostatomembranous urethral injuries: a review of literature and a rational approach to their management. J Urol 1983;130:898.

38

Male genitalia

G. Smith, S. Pridgeon

CIRCUMCISION

Appraise

1 At birth and in very young boys, the normal foreskin is non-retractile because of glanulo-preputial adhesions but the preputial orifice is unscarred and pliant. This normal appearance is clearly distinguishable from a pathological phimosis (tight non-retractile foreskin).

2 As boys mature, the glanulo-preputial adhesions separate and the foreskin becomes retractile.

3 Pathological phimosis in boys is usually caused by lichen sclerosus. The preputial orifice is pale, scarred, and non-pliant. This condition affects less than 1% of boys, peaks in incidence at age 11 and is rarely encountered before the age of 5. The condition is the main medical indication for paediatric circumcision. Recurrent balano-posthitis is a further relative indication.

4 In adults, the medical indications for circumcision are phimosis, paraphimosis (inability to reduce a retracted foreskin over the glans penis to its naturally occurring position), recurrent balano-posthitis and suspected or established penile cancer. Some men with recurrent cracking or tearing of the foreskin or frenulum and certain skin conditions refractory to medical treatment (e.g. genital warts) also benefit from circumcision.

5 In many cultures, circumcision is performed for ritual or religious reasons.

6 Patients and parents seeking circumcision should be counselled fully about the short and long-term risks and benefits of the procedure.

7 Consent should include the risk of bleeding and superficial infection as well as alteration in sexual sensation.

8 In addition to surgical circumcision, there are several non-surgical methods using a variety of clamps or constriction devices which aim to cause ischaemic necrosis of the foreskin.

Prepare

1 Adult circumcisions can be performed under general anaesthesia or with a local anaesthetic penile ring block using a combination of short-acting (lidocaine) and long-acting (bupivicaine) local anaesthetics. Calculate the dose according to the patient's body weight and never use adrenaline. Inject a good bolus just under the pubic symphysis in the midline where the dorsal nerves pass. Inject further anaesthetic around the base of the penis in a ring.

2 Perform paediatric circumcision under general anaesthesia.

Action

Various surgical techniques can be employed. Two methods are described below, the first being more suited for paediatric patients and the alternative method useful for adults:

1 Firstly, retract the foreskin to clean the glans. If the phimosis is severe, this can be done by placing an artery clip through the preputial opening and opening the clip to widen the orifice. If this is not possible, the tight band can be incised with tissue scissors.

2 Once the foreskin is retracted, use a probe to release the adhesions from the glans and define the coronal margin. Use antiseptic wash to thoroughly clean the glans and remove any inspissated smegma.

3 Replace the foreskin and apply two straight artery forceps side by side in the midline on the dorsal surface of the foreskin (Fig. 38.1A). Divide between these two forceps with scissors, taking care not to cut the glans with the inner blade of the scissors (Fig. 38.1B). Continue the incision until about 0.5 cm short of the corona (depending on the age of the child or the size of the penis), which leaves a cuff of tissue below the corona (Fig. 38.1C).

4 From the apex of this incision cut laterally around the base of the glans creating an even cuff of tissue all the way round to the frenulum on one side and then the other (Fig. 38.1D). Ensure that both the inner and outer layers of the foreskin are cut together to give a good cosmetic outcome.

5 Use bipolar diathermy to achieve haemostasis. The small artery of the frenulum may need to be tied.

6 Reconstruct the frenulum with a fine absorbable suture (Fig. 38.1E) and leave one end long to act as a stay. Place the second suture on the dorsal side in the midline and again create a stay stitch. The penis can be manipulated between the two stay sutures and the two layers of the foreskin can be opposed with fine absorbable interrupted sutures (38.1F).

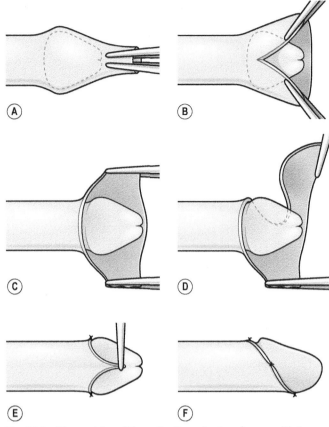

Fig. 38.1   Circumcision: (A) application of artery forceps; (B) the dorsal slit; (C) dorsal slit completed; (D) resection of prepuce; (E) reconstruction of frenulum; (F) the completed circumcision.

ADULT CIRCUMCISION

Action

1. With a pen, mark the line of incision just above the level of the corona on the foreskin. On the ventral aspect of the penis follow the natural tapering of the corona.

2. Use a blade to incise the skin over your marked line. Take care not to sever the large veins that lie just beneath the skin. Divide the veins between clips and tie them.

3. Retract the foreskin to expose the glans. If the phimosis is very tight, use scissors to make an incision through the dorsum of the foreskin to allow retraction. Then make a second circumferential incision with the knife on the inside surface of the retracted foreskin about 0.5 cm from the corona.

4. Excise the skin between the two circumferential incisions.

5. Apply careful haemostasis with bipolar diathermy and ties where appropriate.

6. Approximate the two cleanly cut skin edges with interrupted fine absorbable sutures as described above.

FRENULOPLASTY

Appraise

1. A tight frenulum may present clinically as a non-retractile foreskin or pain on retraction, painful erections or pain on intercourse.

2. A tight frenulum may be congenital or it may result from scarring.

3. Obtain consent including possible alteration in sexual sensation, persistent symptoms and the possible need for subsequent circumcision.

Action

1. Perform this procedure under general anaesthesia or under local anaesthesia with a penile block.

2. Retract the foreskin fully and this will usually define the tight band of the frenulum.

3. Incise the frenulum transversely over the tight band, releasing the subcutaneous tissues as well as the skin. Do not incise too deeply as this may result in a urethral injury.

4. Use bipolar diathermy to achieve haemostasis.

5. Close the incision longitudinally with a fine absorbable suture. This lengthens the frenulum by 0.5–1 cm.

HYDROCELE REPAIR

Appraise

1. A hydrocele is an abnormal collection of fluid contained within the tunica vaginalis and usually surrounds the testis.

2. The testis cannot be palpated separately from the hydrocele collection.

3. Undertake surgical repair if the hydrocele produces troublesome symptoms. Asymptomatic or minimally troublesome hydroceles are best left alone.

4. Three commonly practised surgical repairs are the Lord's plication, the Jaboulay procedure and hydrocele excision. There is minimal dissection of the hydrocele sac with Lord's plication, resulting in a relatively bloodless procedure. This technique works well with thin-walled hydroceles that are not too large. Jaboulay eversion and excision of the hydrocele sac require more dissection of the sac, with increased opportunities for bleeding but are more suited to thick-walled hydroceles.

Prepare

1. Image the scrotum with ultrasound to confirm the diagnosis and rule out an underlying malignancy.

2. Warn the patient of the risks of bleeding and haematoma formation, superficial skin infection and the possibility of recurrence.

Action

1. Check the imaging and mark the side to be operated on.

2. Incise either along the midline raphe or use a transverse scrotal incision, avoiding small vessels in the skin.

3. Use a hand-held diathermy point to deepen the incision through the dartos layer.

4. For Lord's procedure, incise the tunica to drain the hydrocele fluid and then extend the incision in the tunica using scissors.

Make the incision large enough to deliver the testis. Note that in Lord's procedure the hydrocele sac is not dissected from the dartos layer.

5 To perform the plication, use interrupted absorbable sutures to gather together the tunica in several small bites, starting from the cut edge and working towards the testis. Avoid placing the suture through the epididymis. After all the sutures have been placed, the tunica vaginalis appears bunched around the testis, thus obliterating the hydrocele sac (Fig. 38.2).

6 For a Jaboulay procedure, the hydrocele sac is dissected from the overlying dartos and the hydrocele and testis delivered through the incision.

7 Incise the tunica vaginalis, evert it behind the testis and re-approximate the edges around the cord and epididymis posterior to the testis, using a continuous absorbable suture.

8 Alternatively, excise the tunica vaginalis close to the testicle and achieve haemostasis by running a fine continuous absorbable suture around the cut edge.

9 Before returning the testis to the scrotum, apply meticulous haemostasis using diathermy or ties where appropriate.

10 Close the dartos using a continuous absorbable suture, taking large bites of this muscle layer to aid haemostasis.

11 Close the scrotal skin with absorbable interrupted mattress sutures.

12 A scrotal support minimizes swelling and reduces the risk of scrotal haematoma formation.

EXCISION OF EPIDIDYMAL CYSTS

Appraise

1 Excise epididymal (Greek: *epi* = upon + *didymos* = twin; upon the testes) cysts only when they become uncomfortably large.

2 Removal of epididymal cysts is relatively contraindicated in young males as it may cause epididymal damage leading to reduced fertility.

3 The condition is multiple, so warn patients that recurrent cysts are likely.

Action

1 Check any imaging and mark the side to be operated on.

2 Incise the scrotal skin as described for excision of a hydrocele sac. Deepen the incision through the scrotal layers using a handheld diathermy point or knife.

3 Deliver the testis along with its appendages, including the cysts. Remember that cysts are often multiple and commonly occur in the upper pole of the epididymis.

4 Combine blunt and scissor dissection. Hold the testis with one hand, or have an assistant hold it, while you clean off all the adventitial tissue surrounding the cyst.

5 With scissors, completely excise the cyst or else de-roof it by cutting off the whole protruding surface.

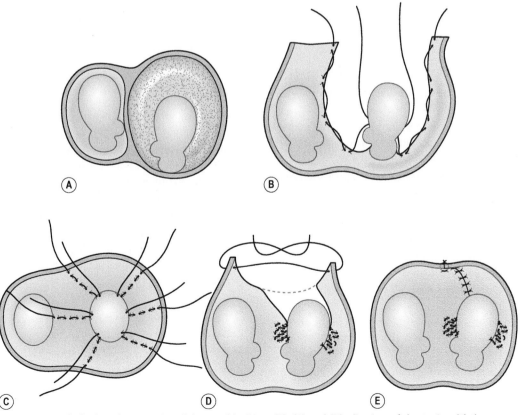

Fig. 38.2 Lord's hydrocele operation: (A) scrotal incision; (B), (C) and (D) plication of the tunica; (E) the completed repair.

6 If there are very many cysts, excise that part of the epididymis bearing them.

7 Oversew the raw area left following this, using fine absorbable sutures.

8 Return the testis to the scrotum and close as described for hydroceles.

INGUINAL ORCHIDECTOMY

Appraise

1 Removal of a testis through a groin incision is indicated where a malignancy of the testis has been diagnosed or is suspected. This approach is taken to prevent potential seeding of tumour cells into the scrotal skin.

2 Testicular tumours usually present with a painless testicular lump which is firm and irregular on palpation, often found incidentally by the patient or his partner. When a testicular tumour is suspected, order urgent scrotal ultrasound imaging. Serum tumour markers help in the diagnosis, to predict tumour bulk and act as a marker of residual tumour after surgery. However, normal markers do not exclude malignancy.

3 Once diagnosed, testicular tumours require prompt surgery. Perform orchidectomy on the next available operating list.

4 Before surgery, offer patients the opportunity for cryogenic sperm banking, since subsequent oncological treatment may render the patient infertile.

5 If the patient requests a testicular prosthesis, this can be inserted at the time of orchidectomy or delayed until a later opportunity.

6 Warn patients of the risk of scrotal haematoma.

Action

1 Check the imaging and mark the side to be operated on.

2 Position the patient in the supine position and prepare the lower abdomen and external genitalia.

3 Make an incision 1–2 cm superior to the surface markings of the inguinal ligament from above the pubic tubercle extending laterally to a point just beyond the deep inguinal ring.

4 Deepen the incision through the subcutaneous tissues to expose the fibres of the external oblique aponeurosis. Clean the external oblique aponeurosis using blunt dissection, allowing clear demarcation of the inguinal ligament and external inguinal ring.

5 Use a knife to make a small incision in the external oblique aponeurosis in the direction of the fibres and, using scissors, open the inguinal canal from the deep inguinal ring to the superficial ring, exposing the spermatic cord. Locate and preserve the ilio-inguinal nerve.

6 Bluntly dissect the spermatic cord from the floor of the inguinal canal. Doubly clamp the cord close to the deep ring. The testis can then be manipulated safely.

7 Apply traction on the cord with simultaneous pressure on the scrotum to deliver the testis through the incision with its surrounding tunical coverings. The most inferior part of the testis is attached to the scrotum by the gubernaculum (Latin: rudder, from the belief it steers the line of descent of the testis). Divide and tie it.

8 Divide the cord between the double clamps thus excising the testis and cord.

9 Transfix the stump of the cord. Leave an artery clip on the surgical tie so that the stump does not retract into the abdominal cavity before complete haemostasis is achieved.

10 Control any points of bleeding in the wound and scrotal cavity to minimize the risk of scrotal haematoma.

11 Close the external oblique with a continuous 2/0 Vicryl suture and reconstruct the superficial ring. Be careful not to catch the ilio-inguinal nerve in your suture line. Scarpa's facia can be opposed with interrupted sutures and skin closure can be with clips or a subcuticular suture.

12 A scrotal support will help to tamponade any intrascrotal bleeding.

SIMPLE ORCHIDECTOMY

Appraise

1 The indications for simple orchidectomy are:
- Severe or recurrent attacks of acute epididymitis
- Chronic epididymitis, including tuberculous epididymitis
- Severe testicular trauma when the testis is not salvageable
- Testicular infarction from a neglected torsion
- Hormonal treatment for advanced prostate cancer (although a subcapsular orchidectomy is often preferred in this situation).

Prepare

1 Remember to discuss the possibility of inserting a testicular prosthesis if appropriate, but avoid inserting a foreign body in an infected/inflamed area. Delay inserting a prosthesis until the inflammatory process has resolved.

Action

1 Check any imaging and mark the side to be operated on.

2 If the condition is inflammatory and involves the skin, then make the incision in the scrotum so as to excise the overlying attached infected skin if necessary. The incision, therefore, varies in shape and size according to the condition.

3 Leave the involved skin attached to the underlying structures. Enter the scrotal sac away from the inflamed area.

4 Deliver the testicle with the overlying attached area of skin. Do not hesitate to remove all the involved surrounding skin. The scrotal skin has amazing powers of regeneration.

5 Apply gentle traction to the testicle and clean the cord structures to free about 5 cm of cord.

6 Cross-clamp the cord at this level with two strong artery forceps, dividing it between them.

7 Tie the clamped upper end with strong absorbable suture, but do not release the forceps before applying a second tie. If the cord is very thick, tease it into two structures and cross-clamp each, to avoid creating a bulky pedicle with a tie that is not secure.

8 Use finger dissection and traction on the lower divided cord to remove the testicle.

9 In the presence of severe infection, leave the scrotal wound unsutured to drain freely. Otherwise, place a corrugated Yates' drain through the most dependent part of the scrotum and insert a few interrupted absorbable sutures to approximate the skin edges.

10 Apply loose dressings only.

TESTICULAR TORSION

Appraise

1 Torsion (Latin: torquere = to twist) of the testis usually presents with acute hemi-scrotal pain in adolescents and young adults. It is rare after the age of 35 years.

2 Pain is usually severe and of sudden onset. There may be associated lower abdominal pain and vomiting.

3 The testis can become swollen and may sit high in the scrotum.

4 The testis is acutely tender on palpation.

5 The diagnosis is obvious if the patient presents with classical symptoms and signs but atypical presentation is well recognized. Always consider it when assessing any patient with acute scrotal pain.

6 Differential diagnoses include epididymo-orchitis, incarcerated inguino-scrotal hernia and, in children, torsion of the hydatid of Morgagni and idiopathic scrotal oedema.

> ▶ KEY POINTS
>
> ■ A painful, swollen testis in a child or young man is torsion until proven otherwise.
> ■ Do not delay surgery. Be prepared to perform a negative exploration rather than to miss a testicular torsion.

Prepare

1 Obtain consent from the patient (and parents) for scrotal exploration, bilateral testicular fixation and possible orchidectomy for infarcted testis.

2 Inform the patient that, in the event of orchidectomy, a prosthesis can be inserted. In a child, delay this until he has reached full maturity. For an adult, a prosthesis is usually inserted at an interval after acute surgery to avoid the infective risk of inserting a foreign body into an acutely inflamed surgical site.

3 Mark the affected side preoperatively.

Action

1 Use a midline scrotal incision to allow access to both testes through the same incision. Deepen it through the dartos layer. Grasp the tunica vaginalis between two clips and open it with a knife or scissors.

2 Use scissors to further open the tunica vaginalis longitudinally. Avoid damaging the epididymis.

3 Deliver the testis and inspect it carefully. A torted testis appears dusky in colour, whilst a necrotic testis is black. Untwist the torsion and wrap the testis in a pack soaked in warm saline.

4 While you are waiting for the torted testis to recover, deliver the contralateral testis through the midline septum. Inspect it carefully and fix it using a non-absorbable prolene suture. Check the orientation of the testis before placing three sutures (medial, lateral and lower pole) between the tunica albuginea and the scrotal side wall. Avoid placing sutures in the epididymis.

5 Remove the packs from the torted testis and examine it carefully to assess viability. Remove a necrotic testis by placing heavy clips around the cord, excising the dead testis and transfixing the cord. If the testis recovers, fix it using the three-point technique as described above.

6 If the diagnosis is not torsion, look for another cause. The presence of hydrocele fluid when the tunica vaginalis is opened may suggest an intrascrotal pathology. The epididymis appears inflamed and engorged in acute epididymitis. A torted hydatid of Morgagni is recognizable as a small inflamed or necrotic piece of tissue at the upper pole of the testis. Excise it.

7 Perform careful haemostasis using diathermy before closure. Close the dartos layer with a continuous absorbable suture taking bites of the left side, the septum and the right hemiscrotum. Close the skin with interrupted undyed mattress sutures.

8 A scrotal support will help to reduce haematoma formation.

TESTICULAR TRAUMA

Appraise

1 Significant testicular trauma is uncommon and is usually a result of sporting injuries or assaults.

2 The immediate pain may be excruciating; however, the effect of adrenaline during contact sports or a brawl may lead to delayed presentation.

3 Carry out an ultrasound scan to assess for rupture of the tunica albuginea of the testis.

4 If rupture is confirmed, undertake scrotal exploration.

5 When there is no rupture and the degree of pain and swelling are stable, treat conservatively with scrotal support, rest and analgesia.

6 If ultrasound is not available, decide whether or not to explore the scrotum on clinical grounds. Recognize increasing pain and swelling as this may indicate increasing haemorrhage within the tunica vaginalis, which may compress and damage the testis.

Action

1 If the testis is completely disrupted, perform simple orchidectomy.

2 However, the testis can often be salvaged by simply evacuating the haematoma, excising any devitalized tissue and loosely tacking the split and torn tunica albuginea together. Allow plenty of space for the blood to escape. Insert a small drain if necessary.

3 Administer prophylactic antibiotics and fit a scrotal support.

VASECTOMY FOR STERILIZATION

Appraise

1. Bilateral vasectomy is a reliable and convenient method of contraception and can be performed under local anaesthesia.

2. Vasectomy is the most common cause of medical negligence claims against urologists. The most common reason for complaint is failed sterilization, but failure to warn of possible complications or to inform the patient of a positive postoperative semen analysis can also lead to claims.

3. Counsel the patient carefully before performing the procedure and document this discussion in the case notes. Enquire into the size of the patient's family and whether the family is complete. Advise the patient that the procedure must be considered irreversible.

4. A failure rate of 1:2000 is recognized due to re-canalization of the vas.

5. Sterilization is not immediate so tell the patient to use other forms of contraception until he has been informed that two sets of semen analysis at around 12 and 14 weeks postoperatively are free of sperm (azospermia). These tests also identify the small proportion of patients with early failure due to incomplete vasal occlusion.

6. Warn the patient of a 1 in 20 risk of chronic scrotal pain. This is often caused by small sperm leaks leading to local inflammation and irritation. Sperm granulomas may cause palpable lumps as well as chronic scrotal pain.

7. Risks also include bleeding with haematoma formation and superficial skin infection.

8. Examine the scrotum and cord preoperatively to assess the accessibility of the vas. A short cord length may make a local anaesthetic procedure difficult especially in a nervous patient in a cold operating theatre.

Action

1. Palpate the cord structures through the scrotum and using your thumb, index and middle fingers identify the vas and bring it towards the scrotal skin (Fig. 38.3).

2. With the vas securely positioned, inject local anaesthetic into the scrotal skin and subcutaneous tissues over the vas.

3. Make a 0.5 cm incision in the scrotal skin directly over the vas and use a sharp tipped clip to spread the subcutaneous tissues. Use vasectomy ring forceps to grasp the vas and pull it through the skin opening. As an alternative, consider using the no-scalpel technique for this step. An extracutaneous fixation ring clamp is used to secure the vas and a sharp curved haemostat is used to puncture the scrotal skin. The no-scalpel technique is associated with a lower risk of haematoma.

4. Carefully dissect the tissue layers covering the vas using the sharp curved haemostat. When the bare white muscular coat of the vas is exposed, reposition the ring forceps so that it holds only the vas without any of the covering tissue layers.

5. Place two clips on the vas and excise a small segment for histological examination. Vasal occlusion is the next step. A number of techniques are described, for example cautery to the cut ends

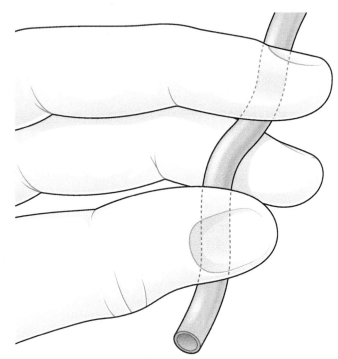

Fig. 38.3 Vasectomy: identifying the vas.

of the vas, tying the cut ends of the vas either simply or by doubling the vas back on itself and placing a tie around the 'U'. Many urologists replace the two cut ends in the scrotum in separate tissue planes by suturing the loose adventitial tissue over one of the ends (fascial interposition). The choice of technique depends on the facilities available, but intra-luminal cautery of the cut end in combination with fascial interposition is associated with the lowest failure rates.

6. Apply meticulous haemostasis to reduce the incidence of haematoma formation.

7. Close the skin with one or two fine absorbable mattress sutures.

FRACTURED PENIS

Appraise

1. A fractured penis occurs as a result of blunt trauma to the erect penis with subsequent rupture of the tunica albuginea around the corpus cavernosum.

2. In Western society this is commonly due to blunt sexual trauma where the erect penis slips out of the vagina during intercourse and the penis is thrust against the partner's perineum. If there is adequate force the erect penis will buckle and the tunica albuginea ruptures.

3. Patients often report hearing a cracking or popping noise and a sudden loss of erection. There is usually significant swelling and bruising, manifested as the 'aubergine deformity'. Blood at the urethral meatus suggests an associated urethral injury.

4. Patients may be embarrassed to seek help, so delaying presentation.

5 Prompt repair reduces adverse long-term outcomes such as impotence or penile curvature.

6 If the diagnosis is not clear, an MRI scan may help to locate the tunical defect. Ultrasound of the penis can also be used to define the site of rupture.

Prepare

1 Examine the penis carefully. If the haematoma is localized and a discrete defect can be palpated this may facilitate your subsequent exploration.

2 Catheterize the patient if there is no suspicion of urethral injury.

Action

1 If preoperative imaging has been utilized to locate the tear in the tunica albuginea, make a 2-cm longitudinal incision over this location.

2 To explore the penis in the absence of preoperative imaging, make a distal circumferential degloving incision. This provides optimal exposure.

3 Dissect through the subcutaneous tissues, tying off any large vessels as you go. The tissues are oedematous. Keep dissecting until you reach the pale tunica albuginea. Stay in this plane and deglove the penis completely at this level.

4 You can see a haematoma at the site of the rupture. Evacuate the haematoma completely to reveal the defect in the tunica.

5 Close the laceration using a continuous or interrupted absorbable suture.

6 Perform careful haemostasis, replace the penile skin over the shaft and close the skin with fine interrupted absorbable sutures.

> ### ▶ KEY POINTS
>
> ■ If you cannot locate the tunical defect place a large-bore butterfly needle into the corpora and inject about 20 ml of sterile saline to create an artificial erection. Saline leaks from a tunical tear if present.

PRIAPISM

Appraise

1 Priapism (Greek: Priapos was an ancient god personifying male virility and sexuality), is a persistent, often painful, erection in the absence of sexual stimulation. Since it is frequently due to underlying medical conditions, consider it both as a medical and surgical emergency.

2 Whatever the cause, commence treatment as soon as possible. Involve the appropriate medical specialty; for example, if the priapism is due to a sickle cell crisis then consult the haematologists.

3 If there is delay, the resulting stasis of blood in the corpora and subsequent fibrosis lead to impotence. Even with early treatment, impotence is common.

4 Carry out the simplest procedure to obtain detumescence (Latin: de-=reversal+tumere=to swell) and then refer the patient to a specialist centre.

Aspiration

1 Initial attempts at detumescence are carried out under local anaesthesia. Perform a penile ring block as described above for circumcision.

2 Use a 20-ml syringe with a wide-bore butterfly needle. Insert the needle into the base of one of the corpora in the 3 o'clock or 9 o'clock position.

3 Aspirate blood from the penis. You may need to adjust the position of the needle for optimum results. You may need to aspirate several hundred millilitres of blood to achieve detumesence. Aspiration alone has a success rate of 30%.[1]

Irrigation

1 Insert a wide-bore aspiration needle into the distal end of one corpus cavernosum and another into the proximal end of the opposite one.

2 Irrigate with 100–200 ml of physiological saline or heparin saline into the proximal needle.

3 Eventually, the fluid emerging from the opposite needle is reasonably clear. Each injection of fluid causes a considerable hardening of the priapism.

4 Massage the corpora to facilitate escape of the fluid, making them flaccid. If necessary, insert four needles into the corpora.

Intracavernosal vasoconstrictors

1 For persistent priapism make up a 100 µg/ml solution of phenylephrine in normal saline (1 ml containing 10 mg, diluting it to 100 ml with normal saline). Inject 3–5 ml into the corpora, repeated at 10-minute intervals until the erection subsides.

2 Be aware of possible adverse sympathomimetic effects – hypertension, headache, reflex bradycardia, tachycardia, palpitations and arrhythmia. Monitor the patient's blood pressure, pulse and, in patients with high cardiovascular risk, the electrocardiogram.

3 Apply a firm bandage and return the patient to the ward. This technique is highly effective if carried out within the first 12 hours of onset.[2]

4 It may be necessary to repeat this process three or four times over the ensuing 48 hours before the corpora remain flaccid.

5 If the priapism persists despite these measures, refer to a specialist.

REFERENCES

1. Montague DK, Jarow J, Broderick GA, et al. American Urological Association guideline on the management of priapism. J Urol 2003;170:1318–25.
2. Kulmala RV, Tamella TL. Effects of priapism lasting 24 hours or longer caused by intracavernosal injection of vasoactive drugs. Int J Impot Res 1995;7:131–6.

FURTHER READING

Blandy J. Radical cure of hydrocoele. In: Blandy J, editor. Operative Urology. 2nd ed. Oxford: Blackwell Scientific; 1986. p. 246–7.

Blandy J, Fowler C. Circumcision. In: Blandy J, Fowler C, editors. Urology. 2nd ed. Oxford: Blackwell Scientific; 1996. p. 445–7.

Blandy J, Fowler C. Orchidopexy. In: Blandy J, Fowler C, editors. Urology. 2nd ed. Oxford: Blackwell Scientific; 1996. p. 553–6.

Blandy J, Fowler C. Torsion of the testis. In: Blandy J, Fowler C, editors. Urology. 2nd ed. Oxford: Blackwell Scientific; 1996. p. 569–71.

Dittrich A, Albrecht K, Bar-Moshe O, et al. Treatment of pharmacological priapism with phenylephrine. J Urol 1991;146:323.

Rickwood AMK. Medical indications for circumcision. BJU Int 1999;83 (Suppl. 1):45–51.

Whitfield HN, Hendry WF, Kirby RS, Duckett JW. Textbook of Genitourinary Surgery. 2nd ed. Oxford: Blackwell Scientific; 1998.

Gynaecological surgery

A. Magos, B. Thomas

GENERAL CONSIDERATIONS

INTRODUCTION

1 Unexpected gynaecological pathology may be found at an emergency abdominal operation or as an incidental lesion during surgery for an unrelated presentation. It is therefore advisable for the general surgeon to become familiar with this pathology and the operations that may need to be performed in an emergency. However, most *elective* gynaecological operations are of a specialized nature and should not be tried on an occasional basis.

2 Handle the pelvic organs especially gently when operating on premenopausal women. Careless surgery in the female pelvis will result in adhesions, which may considerably decrease a woman's fertility.

3 Gynaecologists use the Pfannenstiel incision for many operations, but in emergencies dealt with by the general surgeon a midline or paramedian incision will often have been chosen because of the uncertain nature of the diagnosis. If access proves difficult, incise the medial one-third of the rectus abdominis muscles bilaterally, or ligate the inferior epigastric vessels and incise the full width of the rectus muscles (Maylard incision), or divide the rectus aponeurosis ½ cm above the symphysis pubis (Cherney incision).

4 Laparoscopy has been used as a diagnostic tool in acute pelvic pain for many years, as in general surgery. Minimal access surgery now includes a growing range of operative procedures, with the advantages of less postoperative pain, faster recovery and discharge, but it has not replaced laparotomy for many indications. It requires expertise and expensive equipment.

5 Ultrasound is well established as a diagnostic aid in gynaecological conditions, and in many cases exploratory surgery may be avoided where this is available.

6 Perform a pregnancy test on any female aged 12–50 with abdominal pain (with or without vaginal bleeding), as ectopic pregnancy is an important cause of maternal mortality.

Perioperative care

> ### KEY POINTS Special considerations in gynaecology

- Ensure that your patient is thoroughly informed about the proposed procedure, and clearly document that consent has been given. Give a full explanation of expected (and rare) consequences, particularly if future fertility is likely to be affected. If the woman wishes, keep her partner informed as well. Use drawings, as they aid understanding (and file them in the hospital notes for medico-legal purposes).
- Keep shaving of pubic and vulval hair to a minimum; it is particularly uncomfortable when it is re-growing.
- Menstruation is not a contraindication to gynaecological surgery, nor indeed to thorough examination. ALWAYS have a female chaperone accompany you during intimate examinations.
- Remember that pelvic surgery and pregnancy predispose to thromboembolism, so use prophylactic low-molecular-weight heparin readily. Patients are advised to stop taking the combined oral contraceptive pill 6 weeks before elective major gynaecological surgery.

Prepare

1 *Positioning of patient.* Vaginal operations are carried out in the lithotomy position. Laparoscopy is best carried out with the patient in Lloyd-Davies stirrups, with steep head-down tilt. Laparotomy is carried out with the patient supine and with 5–10° of head-down tilt.

2 *Catheterization.* Empty the bladder by catheterization before all open abdominal procedures and, if the patient has not passed urine immediately prior to surgery, before laparoscopy as well. Separate the labia and swab the urethral meatus with antiseptic

solution. Without allowing the labia to close again, pass a silver or plastic catheter well into the bladder. Now let the labia approximate and press firmly and continuously suprapubically. When the urine flow ceases, gradually withdraw the catheter, taking care not to allow air to be sucked into the bladder.

BARTHOLIN'S ABSCESS (OR CYST)

Appraise

1. An abscess of the glands described in 1677 by the Copenhagen Professor Caspar Bartholin (1655–1738). It is an acutely painful condition, so deal with it as an emergency.

2. A sterile cyst may be dealt with electively by excision. Aim to remove (enucleate) the entire cyst, but if rupture occurs continue to remove the whole cyst cavity before obliterating the remaining space and closing the skin with interrupted 2/0 synthetic absorbable sutures.

3. The operation of marsupialization (Greek: *marsypion* = a pouch) is the procedure of choice for an abscess, since resection of the abscess cavity (as above) may cause considerable bleeding and recurrence is very likely following simple incision and drainage.

4. Ensure that the patient understands that the perineum is likely to be unsightly and very sore for a couple of weeks postoperatively.

Action

1. Make a vertical incision 1 cm long between the ipsilateral labium minor and hymenal remnants. Take a microbiological swab from the discharging pus.

2. Remove an elliptical area of skin and cyst wall from each side of the incision.

3. Break up loculations digitally.

4. Insert half a dozen or so fine synthetic absorbable sutures circumferentially to bring the cyst wall and skin into apposition, so leaving a wide ostium to the gland. Leave a gauze ribbon drain in the cavity for several hours.

Postoperative

1. Discharge the patient home the same day, with simple oral analgesia and encourage her to bathe or shower regularly.

2. Prescribe antibiotics and arrange for contacts to be traced if gonorrhoea or *Chlamydia* is confirmed.

REMOVAL OF PRODUCTS OF CONCEPTION FROM THE CERVICAL CANAL

Appraise

1. This simple procedure may help avoid surgery, and is highly effective at stopping the heavy vaginal bleeding of a miscarriage.

2. Removing products which distend the cervix will correct bradycardia and resultant hypotension.

Action

1. After taking a gynaecological history, where a woman is pregnant and has vaginal bleeding or abdominal pain, examine her sensitively with a bright focused light source and Cusco's bivalve speculum, with gauze and metal sponge-forceps to hand.

2. Open the speculum after full insertion (applying pressure to keep it in place), allowing the cervix to be displaced into the area between the speculum blades.

3. Do not abandon the examination here if there is a lot of blood clot in the vagina. Use gauze held with sponge-forceps to sweep blood and clots from the vagina, and repeat with dry gauze until the vagina is dry, and you obtain a clear view of the vagina and cervix.

4. Look for purple or whitish material in an open cervix. These are products of conception, signifying an inevitable miscarriage. Stop heavy bleeding promptly by grasping this material firmly with the sponge forceps and applying continuous traction, removing the products.

5. Empty the vagina of blood again.

6. Observe the extent of bleeding onto a fresh sanitary pad for the next hour. The heavy bleeding almost always resolves with this intervention, but if not, perform dilatation and curettage (D&C) or evacuation of retained products of conception (ERPC).

DILATATION AND CURETTAGE (D&C), AND EVACUATION OF RETAINED PRODUCTS OF CONCEPTION (ERPC)

Appraise

1. You may need to perform a diagnostic dilatation and curettage (D&C) on a patient with intermenstrual or postmenopausal vaginal bleeding. Therapeutic D&C – or alternatively evacuation of retained products of conception (ERPC) – is performed for heavy prolonged bleeding associated with retained products of conception (RPOC) in the uterine cavity.

2. In women with persistent (greater than 1 week) light vaginal bleeding after the heavy bleeding of a miscarriage, ultrasound is generally of limited use in distinguishing endometritis with altered blood in the uterine cavity from RPOC. Give antibiotics, e.g. co-amoxiclav for 1 week, and only if bleeding persists perform D&C or ERPC.

3. If there are obvious substantial RPOC on ultrasound associated with fever, septic miscarriage/abortion is likely, and in this circumstance the myometrium will be at its softest and most liable to be perforated by ERPC. Give antibiotics intravenously for 1–2 days prior to ERPC unless *in extremis*.

Prepare

1. Gynaecologists usually perform hysteroscopy prior to a *diagnostic* D&C, as it allows visualization of the endometrium, polyps and submucous fibroids *in situ*. For gynaecologists skilled in its use, the operating hysteroscope allows resection of submucous fibroids, polyps or endometrium in the treatment of menorrhagia.

2. Any woman in the reproductive age group (12–50 years) who has heavy bleeding could have a threatened or an incomplete

miscarriage. Order a pregnancy test on urine or blood and a transvaginal ultrasound scan of the uterus before she is taken to theatre. Also order a full blood count, and group and save. Blood transfusion is rarely necessary.

3 If the D&C is for missed or threatened miscarriage, give misoprostol 400 µg vaginally 1 hour preoperatively to prime (soften) the cervix. This may also cause uterine contraction and vaginal bleeding which will resolve once the D&C is completed.

4 Ask the anaesthetist to give 5–10 units of synthetic oxytocin (Syntocinon) intravenously immediately before commencing the operation, to reduce bleeding.

5 Thoroughly wash the vagina and perineum with iodine or chlorhexidine to prevent the introduction of infection. This may be achieved by using soaked gauze held by sponge-forceps. Drape the patient.

Access

1 Take great care to perform a thorough bimanual examination to determine the axis and size of the uterus (and to detect any adnexal swellings).

2 Insert a Sims' speculum into the vagina posteriorly and grasp the anterior lip of the cervix with two vulsellum forceps.

3 Hold the cervix under tension. This straightens the axis of the uterus slightly and helps prevent uterine perforation.

Action

1 *Gently* pass a curved uterine sound in the direction of the uterine axis to confirm this axis and to determine the length of the uterine cavity. This step is best avoided in a pregnant uterus as the soft pregnant uterus is easily perforated by a sound.

2 Dilate the cervix progressively, increasing by 1 mm at a time, by passing metal dilators devised by Alfred Hegar (1830–1914, Professor of Gynaecology in Freiburg). You may need to press firmly to pass through the internal cervical os, but then be careful to reduce the pressure as soon as you overcome the resistance so as not to continue on and perforate the uterine fundus. This is achieved by holding the dilator not more than 2 cm from the cervix when applying pressure to overcome the resistance of the internal os, or by holding each dilator such that less of the dilator protrudes from your hand than the length of the sound measurement. If insertion of a dilator is difficult, go back to the previous dilator or consider using half-size dilators. Dilate up to 8 mm for a diagnostic D&C; 10 mm for a therapeutic D&C.

3 Pass a pair of polyp forceps, open them, twist through 180°, close them and withdraw any tissue present. Repeat two or three times in different planes or more frequently if there are retained products of conception.

4 Pass a curette, small and sharp in a non-pregnant woman, large and blunt in a patient who has been pregnant, until you reach the fundus of the uterus. With firm pressure on the uterine wall, withdraw the curette and collect the specimen on a swab. Repeat the manoeuvre by going systematically around the uterus, ensuring the cavity is completely empty. The surface of the cavity should feel like a fine sandpaper at the end. Send the curettings for histology.

5 ERPC using a suction curette is the method of choice to remove retained products of conception. It replaces steps 3 and 4 above, results in fewer introductions of instruments into the uterus and, therefore, may reduce the risk of perforation. Measure the suction curette against the sound measurement as in step 2, and insert gingerly between finger and thumb until any resistance is felt (this will tally with the sound measurement). The curette is now at the uterine fundus. Activate the suction and then rotate the suction curette rapidly whilst slowly withdrawing, thus tracing a spiral within the uterine cavity. Performing this a few times is almost always sufficient to empty the cavity safely without the need for further instrumentation.

6 If bleeding is heavy during therapeutic D&C or ERPC, then either the uterus is not yet empty, it is failing to contract, or a uterine perforation has occurred. Try ergometrine 500 µg intramuscularly, (or syntometrine if closer to hand), and if you are confident that perforation has not occurred, continue to check the cavity is empty with either a blunt curette or suction curettage. Very light bleeding signifies that the cavity is empty.

7 Give analgesia and metronidazole 1 g rectally at the end of the procedure, and azithromycin 1 g orally on the ward.

> ### ► KEY POINTS Preventing and managing uterine perforation
>
> ■ If you are unsure whether the uterus is anteverted or retroverted, pass the sound with great care, holding it between a finger and thumb. Alter the ante- or retroverted angle of the end of the sound. When you have the correct angle, it will be admitted with minimal pressure.
>
> ■ If you think you have perforated the uterus with a blunt instrument (such as a Hegar dilator, sound or diagnostic hysteroscope) abandon the procedure and observe the patient on the ward for 24–48 hours. Signs of peritonism or significant haemorrhage merit laparotomy.
>
> ■ If a sharp instrument (such as forceps or a curette) has perforated the uterus, it may also have damaged or perforated bowel, so perform laparoscopy to check that there is no other injury. (When an operative hysteroscope such as a resectoscope has been used and perforation is suspected, laparotomy is essential to exclude thermal injury to bowel; laparoscopy should only be considered by highly experienced surgeons).
>
> ■ If the uterus is bleeding, you may be able to control it with diathermy but suturing is often required, particularly in the pregnant uterus.

Postoperative

1 Discharge the patient with simple analgesia the same day in the absence of complications.

2 If there is evidence of infection such as offensive tissue, pyrexia or raised inflammatory markers, treat with broad-spectrum antibiotics in hospital.

3 If there is endometrial hyperplasia or likely carcinoma, refer the patient as soon as possible to a gynaecologist for staging and probable hysterectomy and bilateral salpingo-oophorectomy.

4 Remember to give anti-D within 48 hours to women whose blood group is Rhesus-negative after a miscarriage.

VAGINAL LACERATION

Appraise

Profuse vaginal bleeding in any sexually active (or psychiatric) patient may be due to vaginal laceration.

Action

1 After following steps 1 to 3 in the "Removal of products of conception from the cervical canal – Action" section above, use a continuous 2/0 polyglactin 910 suture to close the laceration and achieve haemostasis.

2 Unlike the removal of products of conception from the cervix, this usually requires a general anaesthetic.

LAPAROSCOPY

Appraise

1 This is a very useful and important diagnostic procedure where there is pelvic pain, both acute and chronic. It is particularly valuable in cases of suspected ectopic pregnancy.

2 You may find diagnostic laparoscopy useful in many situations, including the acute abdomen, the diagnosis of ascites, for direct liver biopsy and for peritoneal biopsy.

3 Do not attempt operative laparoscopy unless you are appropriately trained and suitable equipment is available, such as a light source, camera, optic, laparoscopic instruments, diathermy and irrigation.

4 It is contraindicated in the presence of generalized peritonitis, intestinal obstruction or ileus. Be particularly cautious when you suspect extensive adhesions. Pre-existing severe cardiorespiratory disease may also be a contraindication as the sustained increased intra-abdominal pressure of a pneumoperitoneum may further compromise the patient.

Prepare

1 Order a full blood count, group and save, pregnancy test and transvaginal ultrasound scan.

2 Ensure the patient understands that despite the small size of abdominal incisions, laparoscopy should still be regarded as major surgery, and has a small risk of serious complications (bowel, large vessel and ureteric injury requiring conversion to laparotomy and occasionally stoma formation).

Access

1 Place the patient flat in a semi-lithotomy position, with the legs in Lloyd-Davies stirrups.

2 Empty the bladder if the patient has not urinated in the previous hour, and perform a bimanual examination. Apply forceps and a Spackman cannula (or similar) to the cervix in order to allow manipulation of the uterus intraoperatively.

3 Make an incision in or just below the umbilicus; for a 5-mm diagnostic laparoscope a 5-mm incision is sufficient, but if operative laparoscopy is a possibility we prefer a 10-mm laparoscope and incision.

? DIFFICULTY

■ If there are extensive lower abdominal scars from previous surgery it is safer to insert the Veress needle and trocar in the left upper abdomen 3 cm below the ribs in the midclavicular line (Palmer's point).

■ The open Hasson technique of peritoneal cut-down has not been shown to be safer than the 'closed' technique using the Veress needle as described above, but use it prior to insertion of the primary port if you feel more comfortable with this approach.

Action

1 Palpate the lower limit of the aorta prior to its bifurcation.

2 Grasp the Veress needle in the right hand with the fingers lying along the shaft of the needle to act as a stop to insertion of excessive needle length. Introduce almost vertically (but slightly towards the pelvis, away from the aortic bifurcation) through the umbilical skin incision. Take care not to allow the needle to deviate laterally so as not to injure the iliac vessels. It is helpful to hold up the lower abdominal wall between the left fingers and thumb to provide counter-traction to the introduction of the Veress needle; the left hand should also be used to elevate the anterior abdominal wall in thin patients. Two clicks are felt as the blunt spring-loaded obturator springs forwards to guard the cutting edge on breaching the rectus sheath and then the peritoneum. As soon as the tip is through the peritoneum, insert the needle only a little further, towards the pelvis.

3 Aspirate the needle with a syringe to check that neither a blood vessel nor a viscus has been entered. Then attach a syringe with 10 ml of physiological saline and remove the plunger to check that the saline passes into the peritoneal cavity by gravity alone.

4 Connect the needle to the carbon dioxide insufflator and start the gas flow. Ensure the initial pressure created is no greater than 10 mmHg (Pressure test). If not, immediately stop the gas flow.

5 Continue to insufflate such that the intra-abdominal pressure rises steadily to 20–25 mmHg, and then remove the Veress needle.

6 With your left hand pressing firmly down on the upper abdomen pass the large trocar and cannula into the peritoneal cavity, in the same direction as used for the Veress needle with a twisting motion. Ensure that the trocar is not inserted too deeply into the peritoneal cavity thereby endangering bowel or the retroperitoneal vessels.

7 Remove the trocar and insert the optic through the cannula; attach the fibreoptic light cable and, whenever possible, the video camera.

8 Insert a second port (5 mm) in order to pass a probe or atraumatic grasper to assist in demonstrating pelvic anatomy clearly. This may be suprapubic or well lateral of the inferior epigastric vessels. Injury to the epigastric vessels is the commonest complication of laparoscopy. Transilluminate the abdomen from within to identify the superficial vessels, and identify the inferior vessels lateral to the medial umbilical ligaments on a laparoscopic view of the anterior abdominal wall. If identification of these vessels is difficult, place the port either in the 'safe triangle' (area of the anterior abdominal wall between the symphysis pubis and umbilicus bounded laterally by the umbilical ligaments) or 2–3 cm medial to the anterior superior iliac spine of the pelvic bone.

9 The uterus can be moved by an assistant grasping the Spackman cannula to facilitate visualization of all parts of the pelvis. Ensure that both tubes including their distal ends, ovaries, ovarian fossae, the pouch of Douglas, and anterior and posterior surfaces of the uterus have been visualized.

10 If you detect no disease, look at the appendix, caecum and upper abdomen.

11 Make a decision as to whether operative laparoscopy, laparotomy or no further surgical procedure is necessary.

12 Insert further accessory ports if operative laparoscopy is required.

13 Decrease the pressure relief on the insufflator to 15 mmHg once all ports have been inserted.

14 Perform any necessary procedure. See below for how laparoscopy may be used to treat various conditions. Remove any necessary biopsies with biopsy forceps, using diathermy coagulation to obtain haemostasis.

15 When the procedure is completed, let out as much of the carbon dioxide as possible, remove the trocar and insert one skin suture in each incision.

OVARIAN OPERATIONS

Appraise

1 Ovarian cysts may cause acute abdominal pain because of rupture, haemorrhage or torsion, but a cyst of less than 5 cm diameter rarely causes pain unless secondary to endometriosis (ask about dyspareunia and dysmenorrhoea). Polycystic ovaries are not painful unless there is torsion.

2 Ovarian torsion is characterized by nausea in addition to pain, and infarction by raised inflammatory markers. Endometriotic cysts rarely undergo torsion as they are often stabilized by adhesions.

3 On other occasions you may discover a cyst incidentally on imaging, or whilst operating. If symptomatic at all, ovarian cancer usually presents with only mild non-specific abdominal symptoms.

4 Consider the differential diagnosis of pelvic tuberculosis in a patient from the developing world.

▶ KEY POINTS Decision making

■ Obtain a transvaginal ultrasound (which gives better images than an abdominal scan) if you suspect an ovarian cyst clinically. If confirmed, obtain a CA-125 serum, CEA (a differential diagnosis of a pelvic cyst is colorectal cancer), CA 19-9 (a differential diagnosis of ascites is pancreatic cancer), CRP, FBC, G&S, even if some of these results may only be available postoperatively. Also measure serum AFP (suggestive of a germ-cell tumour) and HCG (suggestive of choriocarcinoma when very high) in a young woman.

■ Decide whether ovarian cancer is the likely diagnosis: postmenopausal patient, complex appearance of the ovarian cyst on ultrasound, presence of ascites and/or bowel adhesions, neovascularization demonstrated on colour Doppler scan, high CA-125. Poor blood-flow may represent torsion and critical ischaemia.

■ If diagnostic laparoscopy has revealed an ovarian cyst, consider removing it laparoscopically if you have sufficient experience, or through a Pfannenstiel incision (or by midline laparotomy if you have a high suspicion of cancer).

■ It is wise to call a gynaecologist to help in the assessment.

Prepare

▶ KEY POINT Importance of informed consent

■ In no other gynaecological operation is informed consent more important, particularly when one or both ovaries may need to be removed once the abdomen is open and the clinical findings apparent. Counsel the patient about this possibility.

Access

1 Unless you have had considerable laparoscopic experience, you will need to perform laparotomy to remove most ovarian tumours.

2 Use a transverse suprapubic incision only if preoperative ultrasound or laparoscopy has provided strong evidence that the tumour is benign. In all other cases, employ a vertical incision.

Assess

1 You must recognize physiological cysts which should be left alone: a mature Graafian follicle (simple, straw-coloured fluid-filled cyst up to 2 cm in diameter) or a corpus luteum (Latin: yellow body) cyst. A luteal cyst may develop in early pregnancy; it secretes progesterone to support the early pregnancy and unnecessary removal may result in miscarriage. Simply use diathermy or oversew it if bleeding.

2 Do not operate for an ovarian cyst under 5 cm in diameter without evidence either that it is neoplastic or that it has undergone haemorrhage or rupture, giving rise to acute abdominal pain.

3 If you find an endometrioma, check the pelvis for other evidence of endometriosis (especially the uterosacral ligaments and ovarian fossae).

4 It is of great importance for you to be able to distinguish a benign cyst from ovarian cancer visually. In a woman of reproductive age it is better to err on the side of conservatism, even if a further laparotomy will be required, rather than risk sacrificing healthy ovaries. In general, a smooth ovarian surface indicates a benign cyst. These may be very large. Features of malignancy are an irregular ovarian surface, papillary growth, neovascularization, ascites, adhesions between ovary and bowel and peritoneal, omental or palpable liver surface metastases. Bilaterality is no guide to the likelihood of malignancy.

5 Ovarian cystectomy is the preferred treatment for benign ovarian cysts, but carry out salpingo-oophorectomy if:
- The patient is postmenopausal (bilateral)
- There is evidence of malignancy (bilateral if cancer is obvious)
- The cyst has undergone torsion and is gangrenous
- The tumour is very large and little normal ovarian tissue can be conserved.

6 If you suspect malignancy, explore the whole abdomen, including the diaphragmatic surface of the liver and the undersurface of the diaphragm. Palpate the para-aortic and pelvic lymph nodes and biopsy them if enlarged. Send ascitic fluid or peritoneal washings for cytology. Further treatment depends upon accurate staging. If there are no metastases and the contralateral ovary is grossly normal, split it open and send a slice for histology or frozen section if it is available, before closing the ovary with fine absorbable synthetic or fine non-absorbable sutures.

7 If the ovarian tumour is obviously malignant, remove the uterus, both ovaries and tubes (see Hysterectomy, below), the infracolic omentum, palpable lymph nodes and as much metastatic tumour bulk as possible. Record the extent of residual disease, an important predictor of survival. Adjuvant chemotherapy is generally required. The only exceptions to such radical surgery are in a young woman with disease confined to one ovary and no sign of abdominal metastases, or in a patient who has very extensive disease when primary chemotherapy or even palliative treatment should be considered.

Action

Ovarian cystectomy

1 Separate the tumour from adhesions and draw it out of the wound.

2 Surround the operation site with large gauze packs, and have suction ready in case the cyst is accidentally ruptured.

3 Make a very superficial incision on the medial aspect of the ovary over the cyst.

4 Find the plane of cleavage and shell out the tumour, using blunt dissection with scissors and gauze swab. If the cyst ruptures, remove all the cyst fluid, ensure that you remove all the cyst lining, and thoroughly irrigate the area, and again wash out the peritoneal cavity prior to closure of the abdomen. Dermoid cyst fluid and endometrioma 'chocolate fluid' are highly irritant, and leakage of malignant cyst fluid may result in peritoneal metastases.

5 Repair the residual ovarian tissue, using a fine prolene suture; good haemostasis is important to prevent future adhesion formation.

Salpingo-oophorectomy

1 If you decide to remove the whole ovary, skeletonise the ovarian pedicle (infundibulopelvic ligament) taking care to identify the ureter. Place a clamp across this pedicle, and a second across the ovarian ligament and fallopian tube, adjacent to the uterus. Resect the ovary together with the tube and broad ligament between the clamps.

2 Doubly ligate each pedicle with 1-polyglactin 910. Use a transfixion suture or gently release and re-apply the clamp while tying the ligature. At the end of the operation check the pedicles before closing the abdomen.

Closure

1 The parietal peritoneum does not have to be closed.

2 Close the rectus sheath with 1-polyglactin if a transverse incision and 1-nylon or polydioxanone if a vertical incision has been employed, incorporating the peritoneum as part of the 'mass closure' technique.

3 Close the skin with sutures or clips.

Postoperative

1 If both ovaries have been removed, consider starting the patient on hormone replacement therapy.

? DIFFICULTY

1. If you come across a malignant ovarian tumour that is fixed in the pelvis, perhaps with matted adherent omental metastases, it is better to remove a small biopsy and carefully record the site and size of the metastases and close up, rather than perform a very inadequate debulking operation. If at all possible, refer the patient to a gynaecological oncology team for full radiological investigation in order for decisions to be made regarding preoperative chemotherapy.

SURGERY FOR ECTOPIC PREGNANCY

Appraise

1 A classic ruptured ectopic pregnancy is easily diagnosed by the findings of severe abdominal pain and shoulder pain, guarding and rebound tenderness, and hypovolaemic shock. (There is usually little or no vaginal bleeding; if bleeding is heavy the diagnosis of miscarriage is more likely.) A failing ectopic pregnancy or slowly bleeding ectopic pregnancy is less easy to diagnose.

2 The appearance on transvaginal ultrasound scan is of an empty uterus and free pelvic fluid if there is intra-abdominal bleeding. It is much less common to see an adnexal mass. If the serum βHCG is greater than 1500 IU/L, a *correctly sited* pregnancy should

be visible on vaginal ultrasound scan, and so this combination often helps to make the diagnosis.

3 In uncertain cases (e.g. patient haemodynamically stable, βHCG<1500 IU/L and normal ultrasound scan with empty uterus, no free fluid or adnexal mass in the pelvis), repeat the βHCG in 48 hours. Suboptimal increase or decrease of βHCG may signify ectopic pregnancy and should be investigated by serial βHCG testing or laparoscopy. If a non-surgical approach is taken, discharge when the pain settles, with instructions to return urgently if the pain returns or she feels unwell. Very early ectopic pregnancies may be managed medically with a single intramuscular dose of methotrexate.

4 Laparoscopy is required to confirm the diagnosis of unruptured ectopic pregnancy when HCG is greater than 1500 with an empty uterus, or if there is any doubt about the diagnosis.

5 Once the diagnosis of ruptured ectopic has been made, take the patient to the operating theatre as soon as possible. Do not wait for blood to be cross-matched and do not delay for resuscitation. Your patient will improve only when the bleeding fallopian tube is clamped.

6 If the patient is shocked, perform a laparotomy – via a Pfannenstiel incision if you can perform this as rapidly as a midline incision – and never laparoscopy.

Prepare

1 Order a full blood count, group and save serum if not cross-matching, and secure intravenous access as soon as you suspect ectopic pregnancy.

2 Gain consent for laparoscopy and laparotomy, and for salpingectomy and salpingotomy.

3 If the patient is shocked, take her to the operating theatre for immediate laparotomy. In less acute forms arrange for laparoscopy.

4 Remember to give anti-D immune globulin within 48 hours to women whose blood group is Rhesus-negative.

LAPAROSCOPIC SALPINGECTOMY OR SALPINGOTOMY

Access

1 Use a 10-mm laparoscope if available as this gives better visualization in the presence of a haemoperitoneum.

2 Ensure that a suction/irrigation device is available if you contemplate laparoscopic surgery.

3 Have monopolar electro-diathermy equipment available for incising the tube and if possible use bipolar diathermy for obtaining haemostasis.

4 Having introduced the laparoscope, insert a lateral port so that a probe or forceps can be used to demonstrate and manipulate the fallopian tube.

5 If there is copious blood in the peritoneal cavity, aspirate it using the suction/irrigation apparatus to improve the view of the tube.

Assess

1 Make a careful inspection of the uterus and of both tubes and ovaries, in order to decide the most appropriate operation.

2 Decide whether to proceed to laparotomy or complete the operation laparoscopically. Laparotomy is appropriate if there is major bleeding preventing good visualization, the patient becomes shocked or you are not experienced in laparoscopic surgery.

3 The second decision is whether to perform salpingotomy to conserve the tube, or salpingectomy. Salpingectomy is generally the preferred option (as the incidence of persistent trophoblast and future ectopic pregnancy is less, without significantly affecting the future pregnancy rate when the contralateral tube is normal). Even if the contralateral tube is abnormal, salpingectomy should also be performed when:
- The bleeding is substantial
- The tube is badly damaged by the tubal rupture
- The patient does not wish to become pregnant in the future.

Action for operative laparoscopy

1 Insert lateral ports.

2 Grasp the affected tube as close as possible to the tubal swelling with grasping forceps near the uterine end.

3 Apply bipolar diathermy to the mesosalpinx parallel and just inferior to the Fallopian tube, and coagulate the tissue with its blood vessels. Divide the mesosalpinx with laparoscopic scissors. Coagulate the proximal tube well, prior to dividing it 1-2 cm from the uterus.

4 Alternatively, partial salpingectomy can be done using an 'Endoloop' ligature to occlude the vessels and then remove the tube with scissors.

5 Remove the fallopian tube through a lateral port, enlarged to 10 mm, using a bag if necessary.

6 Irrigate and aspirate the peritoneal cavity to remove as much blood, clot and trophoblast as possible.

7 If you decide that salpingotomy and conservation of the tube is more appropriate make a 10-mm linear incision over the ectopic pregnancy on the antimesenteric border of the fallopian tube using diathermy needle, scissors or hook (Fig. 39.1).

8 Use the suction/irrigation cannula to separate the trophoblast tissue from the tube and then remove the tissue with grasping forceps. If the ectopic pregnancy is aborting through the fimbrial end of the tube, it may be possible to aspirate and remove it through the fimbrial ostium.

9 Extract the tissue from the abdomen through a 10-mm port, unless it is very small, using an extraction bag if necessary.

10 It is not necessary to close the salpingotomy incision but, if there is any residual bleeding after applying pressure, use the diathermy forceps to complete haemostasis.

> ### ▶ KEY POINTS Decisions
>
> - Shocked patient=immediate laparotomy
> - If it is difficult to gain access to the tube because of adhesions or visualization is poor, proceed to laparotomy.

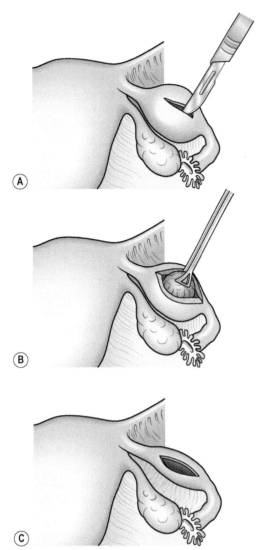

Fig. 39.1 Conservative management of an ectopic pregnancy; a similar technique applies to both a laparoscopic and an open approach: (A) incision over antimesenteric border of tube with needle diathermy; (B) removal of the trophoblast tissue with grasping forceps and suction/irrigation cannula; (C) salpingotomy left to heal without suturing after ensuring haemostasis.

- Inspect the contralateral tube and record its condition.
- It is usually better to perform a salpingectomy rather than a salpingotomy unless the contralateral tube is also damaged, e.g. by chronic pelvic inflammatory disease, or the ectopic pregnancy is very early and can be aspirated.

Closure

Close the laparoscopic incisions, using a deep sheath suture if 10- or 12- mm operating ports have been used.

Postoperative

See below.

SALPINGECTOMY OR SALPINGOTOMY BY LAPAROTOMY

Access

1 Make a generous incision: either midline or Pfannenstiel, provided you are familiar with this incision.

Action

1 As soon as the peritoneal cavity is open, aspirate blood with the sucker.

2 Pass a hand into the pelvis and bring the uterus with its appendages up into the wound. Identify the ruptured tube. Place one or more clamps across the mesosalpinx and another clamp across the cornual end of the tube, then excise the damaged tube. In most cases it is neither necessary nor desirable to remove the ovary. Doubly ligate the pedicles beneath the clamps, using 1-polyglactin 910.

3 You can decide to conserve the tube if the other tube is also damaged or has previously been removed and the tubal pregnancy is small. The pregnancy can be removed by aspiration or salpingotomy.

4 If the ectopic pregnancy is small and distal you may aspirate it through the fimbrial end.

5 If not, create a salpingotomy with a 1-cm linear incision using a scalpel or needle diathermy over the swollen portion of the tube (see Fig. 39.1) and remove the pregnancy with a combination of forceps traction and hydrodissection. You do not need to close the tube, but ensure that haemostasis is complete using diathermy coagulation.

6 Inspect the contralateral tube and ovary. The other tube may have a hydro-salpinx or haemato-salpinx but do not be tempted to tamper with it. Bilateral tubal pregnancy is exceedingly rare. Carefully record the state of the pelvis.

7 Before closing the abdomen, aspirate and swab out as much blood as possible, and estimate the volume of blood loss. Washing the peritoneal cavity with normal saline may help to reduce adhesion formation.

▶ KEY POINTS Inspect and react to findings

- If the tubal pregnancy is greater than 4 cm in diameter, elect to perform a salpingectomy rather than a salpingotomy.
- Inspect the contralateral tube and record its condition.

Postoperative

1 Obtain as accurate an estimate as possible of the amount of blood aspirated from the peritoneal cavity, and replace it with blood transfusion if the loss exceeds 1 Litre.

2 Use central venous pressure monitoring to gauge blood and fluid replacement if there has been severe shock.

3 Administer prophylactic antibiotics such as co-amoxiclav for three doses if tubal rupture and substantial haemoperitoneum have occurred.

4 If salpingectomy has been performed when the other tube was absent or badly damaged, counsel the woman that assisted conception (e.g. IVF) will be required to try and achieve a pregnancy.

5 If salpingotomy and aspiration of the ectopic have been carried out, perform follow-up serum HCG levels weekly until it is certain that levels are declining, because of the small risk of persistent trophoblast.

6 Counsel the patient about the increased risk of future ectopic pregnancy. Advise early medical assessment in any subsequent pregnancy.

TUBAL LIGATION

Appraise

1 You may be asked to carry out a sterilization procedure either in the course of a caesarean section (see below) or as an additional procedure during the course of an abdominal operation.

2 Sterilization may be carried out by one of the modifications of Pomeroy's method as described below, or laparoscopically by the simple application of Hulka or Filshie clips across the whole diameter of each tube.

3 Gain informed consent, by ensuring the patient understands that the procedure should be considered irreversible, but that it has a failure rate (<1%) in the same way as other methods of female contraception. Should there be a pregnancy, the risk of it being ectopic is great after female sterilization. Explain other methods, which are reversible and may treat dysmenorrhoea and menorrhagia (e.g. Mirena IUS). Male sterilization is more reliable. Avoid sterilizing a woman under the age of 30 years unless there is a good medical reason.

Action

1 Pick up a loop of fallopian tube with a Spencer Wells forceps 2–3 cm from the uterus (Fig. 39.2A).

2 Tie an absorbable synthetic ligature tightly around the base of the loop and excise the end of the loop. You may seal each end of the tube with the diathermy needle as an additional precaution (Fig. 39.2B).

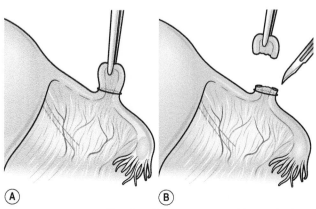

(A)   (B)

Fig. 39.2 Pomeroy sterilization: (A) ligature round loop of tube; (B) excision of loop of tube.

HYSTERECTOMY

Appraise

1 You may need to perform a hysterectomy – for example, as part of a larger surgical procedure such as the removal of a rectal cancer, because of fibroids or other benign uterine disease causing severe menorrhagia, or for ovarian carcinoma that had not been diagnosed preoperatively. Do not be tempted to carry out a hysterectomy during the course of another operation because of the incidental finding of large uterine fibroids, unless you have discussed this with the patient preoperatively. Even when they have large fibroids, most women are fertile.

2 Unless there is gynaecological malignancy, conserve at least one ovary whenever possible in premenopausal women.

3 Vaginal hysterectomy and radical hysterectomy, described in 1900 by the Viennese gynaecologist Ernst Wertheim (1864–1920), are not likely to fall within your competence.

Prepare

1 Give heparin 2 hours preoperatively unless there is a significant risk of intraoperative bleeding.

2 Give a dose of antibiotics on induction and continue for 5 days.

Access

1 Empty the bladder by catheterization and cleanse the vagina with an antiseptic. Added Bonney's blue or methylthioninium chloride (methylene blue) dye has the advantage of staining the vaginal skin, making it more easily recognized at operation.

2 A Pfannenstiel incision is suitable for many hysterectomies, but avoid it if you suspect malignancy, if the uterus is larger than the size of a 16-week pregnancy or if the diagnosis is in doubt. In these cases use a vertical incision.

3 Carefully pack off the intestines, both large and small, to render the operation easier and safer. It is well worth spending a few minutes displacing all the intestines from the pelvis and packing them above the pelvic brim.

4 Insert a self-retaining retractor of the Balfour type, preferably one with a third blade.

Action

1 If the adnexae are to be preserved, place a strong straight clamp such as Kocher's type as close to the uterus as possible across the fallopian tube, round ligament, ovarian ligament and upper part of the broad ligament. If these structures are held on the stretch, an avascular window is visible at a depth of about 3 cm into the broad ligament. Aim to put the tip of the clamp into this avascular window. In the case of oophorectomy, the infundibulopelvic pelvic ligament and round ligament pedicles are taken separately.

2 Place a second straight clamp just lateral to the first clamp, again with the tip in the avascular window.

3 Divide the tissue between the clamps down to their tips, and ligate the lateral pedicle with No 1 absorbable synthetic suture material, doubly tied (Fig. 39.3).

4 Repeat this procedure on the opposite side.

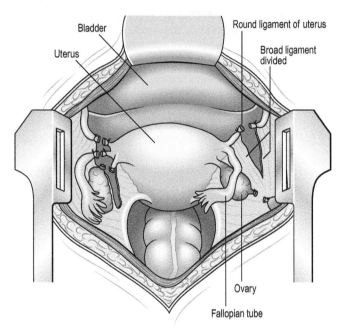

Fig. 39.3   Hysterectomy: incision of broad ligament, with conservation of adnexae (left), with adnexae removed (right).

5 Open the layers of the broad ligament below the sutured pedicle by inserting closed scissors and gently opening them. Incise the anterior leaf of the broad ligament and gradually continue opening the broad ligament, until you reach the loose fold of uterovesical peritoneum.

6 Now pass the closed scissors in a medial direction, open them and cut the loose uterovesical peritoneum. Carry out the same manoeuvre on the other side until the bladder peritoneum is completely incised in front of the cervix.

7 Pick up the bladder flap with dissecting forceps and apply tension. This manoeuvre displays the loose connective tissue between bladder and cervix, which can be carefully cut with scissors while keeping their points angled towards the cervix.

8 Now push the bladder off the cervix with a swab wrapped around your thumb. Apply pressure on to the cervix rather than the bladder. Once the longitudinal fibres of the vagina are visible, no further displacement of the bladder is necessary. Adequate displacement of the bladder may also be checked by gripping the cervix between thumb and forefinger until you can feel that you are below the level of the cervix.

9 Identify the ureters, either visually or, more often, by palpating the medial leaf of the broad ligament. The ureters feel like whip-cords and typically 'snap' as you move your thumb and index finger over them. If required, push the ureters caudally so that the uterine vessels can be clamped (see step 10).

10 Now clamp the uterine vessels. Apply a strong straight or curved hysterectomy clamp (e.g. Maingot's) at right-angles to the uterus at the level of the utero-cervical junction. Make sure that the tips of the clamp are as close as possible to the uterus. Divide the uterine vessels by cutting with a knife close to the clamp and around its tip and doubly ligate with a 1-synthetic absorbable suture.

11 If the cervix is relatively long, clamp the paracervical tissue by applying a straight clamp medial to the uterine pedicle towards the vagina. Divide the pedicle and tie with a single suture.

12 Now open the vagina by inserting a scalpel transversely in the midline through the vaginal fascia and then into the vagina itself. Extend the vaginal incision towards the vaginal angles by pulling the opened scissors in the vagina out through the incision. Apply Maingot clamps (or similar) to the vaginal vault by placing one blade inside and the other outside the vaginal angles to include the uterosacral ligaments behind the vagina. Cut off the uterus and cervix from the vagina to complete the hysterectomy.

Closure

1 The two vaginal angle pedicles are sutured ensuring that the full thickness of the vaginal wall is included. Having tied the suture, leave long and hold with Spencer Wells forceps (Fig. 39.4).

2 Close the vaginal vault with a series of interrupted absorbable sutures. Alternatively, leave it open and arrest oozing by inserting a running suture around the vault (Fig. 39.5).

3 Check that there is no bleeding from the vaginal vault or uterine vessels. Many surgeons now do not close the pelvic peritoneum provided haemostasis is good. If there is oozing it is worth tacking it across with continuous 2/0 synthetic absorbable stitches, starting at one ovarian pedicle and concluding at the other.

4 The parietal peritoneum need not be closed, but carefully close the rectus sheath with 1-polyglactin 910, before closing the skin with clips or sutures.

5 Consider carrying out a cystoscopy if there is any concern about the integrity of the bladder or ureters. Indigo carmine can be

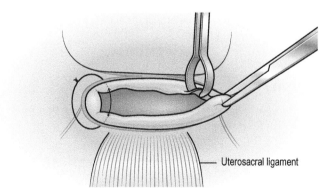

Fig. 39.4   Closure of vault: tying of vaginal angle.

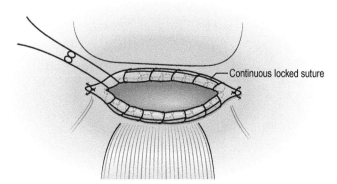

Fig. 39.5   Vaginal vault circumsuture, leaving vagina open for drainage.

given intravenously to make identification of normal ureteric function easier. Consult a urologist if injury is suspected.

Postoperative

If both ovaries have been removed discuss the use of hormone replacement therapy with the patient.

Complications

1. Reactionary or secondary haemorrhage from the vaginal angle may occur and presents as profuse vaginal bleeding. It can be dealt with through the vagina, applying a figure-of-eight suture to the bleeding points.

2. Ureteric or bladder injury are unwelcome complications which will present either as urinary leakage and fistula formation, or loin pain if the ureter is completely tied off. Get expert urological assistance if there is any suggestion of such complications.

? DIFFICULTY

1. Occasionally, if there are very dense pelvic adhesions and the uterus remains fixed deep in the pelvis, it may be difficult to remove the cervix. It may then be safer to perform subtotal hysterectomy.

2. Proceed exactly as described, but there is no need to apply a clamp to the paracervical tissue (step 11). At this stage, cut across the stump and close the cervical canal. Cover the stump with the pelvic peritoneum.

MYOMECTOMY

Appraise

1. Do not contemplate the surgical treatment of fibroids unless they are likely to be the cause of the patient's severe symptoms. Fibroids are common, usually asymptomatic, and almost always benign. Fertility is improved only by the removal of *submucous* fibroids which substantially protrude into the uterine cavity.

2. As a general surgeon you are unlikely to be called upon to carry out myomectomy. If fibroids are multiple, the operation can be more time-consuming and hazardous than hysterectomy.

3. On the other hand, it is preferable to conserve the uterus in a young woman who has not completed her family, and a solitary pedunculated subserous fibroid which can undergo torsion is easily removed.

Prepare

1. Bear in mind that this is the gynaecological operation with the greatest expected blood loss, so optimize the haemoglobin concentration preoperatively. Cross-match 4 units of blood.

2. Ensure the patient is aware that there is a risk of requiring hysterectomy if bleeding is uncontrolled, and clearly document this on the consent form. Most gynaecologists would not perform myomectomy on a patient who refuses blood products in an emergency.

3. Give intravenous antibiotics on induction, and continue until eating, when a 5-day course may be completed orally.

Access

1. Perform a bimanual examination under anaesthetic to decide on the abdominal incision.

2. In general, if the uterus is mobile and it extends no further than the umbilicus, use a Pfannenstiel incision. Otherwise, use a lower midline incision, which may be extended around or even above the umbilicus if necessary.

3. Once the abdomen is open, deliver the uterus into the wound.

Assess

1. Plan the uterine incision(s): The aim is to remove as many fibroids through as few uterine incisions as possible. Try to avoid incisions in the posterior wall of the uterus, since these often give rise to bowel adhesions.

2. You can remove a posterior fibroid through an anterior incision by crossing the uterine cavity, or via an inverted 'U' hood incision in the posterior uterine wall.

3. Generally, it is best not to breach the endometrium if possible, as the risk of uterine rupture during a future labour is thought to be increased.

Action

1. Unless removing a few subserous or pedunculated fibroids, bluntly fenestrate an avascular area of parametrium bilaterally. Through these apply a Bonney's myomectomy clamp or a rubber pericervical tourniquet to compress the uterine arteries, and bilateral rubber touniquets around the infundibulopelvic ligaments (the ovarian vessels lie within) to reduce haemorrhage during the procedure. These will need to be re-tightened during the procedure should they loosen. An alternative to rubber tourniquets to the ovarian vessels are ovarian artery clamps which can be placed medial to the ovaries, thereby avoiding ovarian ischaemia during surgery (Fig. 39.6).

2. If there are anterior fibroids, try to remove all of them through a single anterior midline incision. To facilitate manipulating the fibroids, extend the cut into each fibroid by about 1 cm.

3. Grasp the fibroid with tissue-holding forceps (e.g. Lane's). The required plane of cleavage lies directly on the fibroid. Shell it out either digitally or using blunt dissection with Mayo scissors. Remove as many fibroids as possible through this incision. If there are posterior fibroids, continue the myomectomy as described previously.

4. Insert deep 1-polyglactin 910 or other synthetic absorbable sutures to obliterate the cavity left after removal of the fibroids. Several layers of sutures are needed to achieve an adequate repair and achieve haemostasis. If the endometrial cavity has been breached, repair this with a fine 2/0 absorbable suture.

5. Close the serous surface of the uterus with 0-polyglactin 910 or polypropylene sutures.

6. Remove the tourniquets and observe for haemostasis.

7. If there is oozing from the incisions, insert further haemostatic deep figure-of-eight 1-polyglactin 910 sutures.

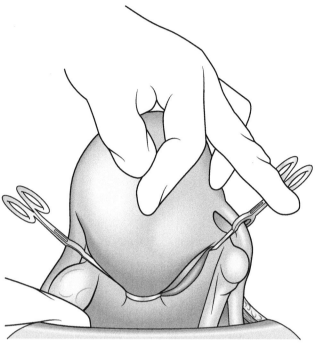

Fig. 39.6 Ovarian artery clamp and pericervical tourniquets in place during open myomectomy.

8 If the uterus is retroverted, you could plicate the round ligaments with non-absorbable suture in order to antevert the uterus. This manoeuvre prevents adhesion formation.

9 Insert a size 16 Robinson drain to the pelvis and close the abdomen.

10 Prescribe prophylactic heparin if there is no sign of ongoing haemorrhage 12 hours postoperatively.

INCIDENTAL GYNAECOLOGICAL CONDITIONS

PELVIC INFLAMMATORY DISEASE

1 Uncomplicated pelvic inflammatory disease (PID) does not require surgery. It is a cause of an acute abdomen and fever. Distinguishing features are of recent sexual activity (which need not be "high-risk"), symmetrical lower abdominal pain, recent vaginal discharge and exquisite deep tenderness on bimanual examination. Take high-vaginal, intracervical and intracervical nucleic acid amplification swabs. Start antibiotics at once, according to local antibiotic guidelines. These usually include a 2-week course of doxycycline to cover *Chlamydia trachomatis*, (the most common cause in the developed world), a single dose of ceftriaxone to treat gonorrhoea, and a 2-week course of either co-amoxiclav or metronidazole to cover anaerobes.

2 Not uncommonly a patient explored for suspected appendicitis is found to have acute salpingitis. The condition is almost always bilateral, although one tube may be more affected than the other. The tubes are oedematous and reddened, and pus is often seen dripping from the fimbrial end. Swab for bacteriological culture, close the abdomen and treat as above.

3 Tubal infection may progress to pyosalpinx, a tubo-ovarian abscess or pelvic abscess. If there has been little improvement in

the patient's condition after 2 days on antibiotics, laparotomy is justified. Adhere to the usual surgical principle of draining pus (sending some for culture), digitally breaking up loculi, irrigating the pelvis and abdomen (some use antiseptic wash-out) and inserting a drain through a separate abdominal incision. Give antibiotics as above.

4 Unlike many general surgical abscesses there is no perforated viscus and resection of the indurated pelvic organ is unnecessary despite the patient's toxic state.

FIMBRIAL CYST AND PARAOVARIAN CYST

1 Small cysts may be seen in relation to the distal end of the fallopian tube or broad ligament. They arise in remnants of the mesonephric (Wolffian) duct and occasionally undergo torsion to produce acute abdominal pain.

2 Remove them only if they have undergone torsion. Tie the pedicle before excision.

ENDOMETRIOSIS

1 Most cases of endometriosis are effectively treated medically with hormones, so avoid first-line surgery if the diagnosis is suspected, and do not be radical if you find pelvic endometriosis unexpectedly.

2 This condition may involve the pelvic peritoneum when it typically appears as small purple or dark-brown nodules, but appearances can be varied. Most women with the incidental finding of peritoneal endometriosis have no symptoms, and therefore require no treatment. If symptoms of abdominal pain, dysmenorrhoea and classically deep dyspareunia are present, ablate these areas of peritoneum with diathermy, taking extreme care not to injure vessels or the ureters deep to this tissue.

3 When involving the ovaries, endometriosis may be seen superficially and treated as above, or may form endometriomata (otherwise known as 'chocolate cysts'). Rupture of a chocolate cyst produces acute abdominal pain. Excise the cyst cavity, ensure haemostasis and repair the ovary with a fine polyglactin 910 suture if the cyst was large. Irrigate the pelvis at the end of surgery.

4 Occasionally, endometriosis involves the intestine. It is a cause of rectal bleeding and the appearance may mimic a carcinoma. In the large intestine it may produce sub-acute obstruction and can be extremely difficult to differentiate from carcinoma.

CAESAREAN SECTION

Appraise

1 You may be asked to perform a caesarean section (said to have been the method of delivery of Caius Julius Caesar) if you work in a hospital where there is no specialist obstetrician.

2 It is likely that the patient has been in labour for some hours, although occasionally it is necessary to perform the operation on a patient who is bleeding heavily from a placenta praevia or severe placental abruption.

3 The lower segment operation is almost universally employed nowadays, being associated with less bleeding and fewer

postoperative complications than the 'classical' (midline longitudinal uterine) section.

Prepare

1 Establish the haemoglobin concentration and group and save the patient. It may be wise to cross-match 4 units of blood preoperatively if blood is not immediately available, if the starting haemoglobin is low, or if blood loss is expected to be higher than usual for any reason.

2 Give ranitidine to decrease the gastric acidity and hence the risk of pneumonitis should the patient aspirate gastric contents.

3 Perform the operation under spinal or epidural rather than general anaesthesia when possible; a regional anaesthetic carries a lower mortality in most circumstances. If a general anaesthetic is employed, a cuffed endotracheal tube is mandatory, to prevent aspiration of gastric contents, which are more liable to reflux in pregnancy.

4 Anti-thromboembolic compression stockings should be worn.

5 Insert an indwelling catheter.

6 Apply about 15° of left lateral tilt to the patient by tilting the operating table, or by placing a wedge under the patient's buttocks to avoid compression of the inferior vena cava prior to emptying the uterus.

7 Give a single dose of a broad-spectrum antibiotic such as co-amoxiclav.

Access

1 A Pfannenstiel incision is suitable, but if you are inexperienced you may find a vertical sub-umbilical midline incision easier. If you are right-handed, it is better to stand on the patient's right so that you can use your right hand to deliver the fetal head.

2 After opening the peritoneal cavity, place a large Doyen retractor into the lower edge of the wound.

Action

1 Identify the loose fold of uterovesical peritoneum. Pick it up with dissecting forceps and incise it with scissors centrally. Extend the incision laterally almost to the broad ligament on each side.

2 Push the bladder downwards with a swab and replace the Doyen retractor over the bladder to retract it well away from the lower uterine segment.

3 Incise the lower segment transversely, beginning in the midline, 2 cm inferior to the original reflection of the uterovecical peritoneum. The lower segment may be very thin, especially if the patient has been in labour for a long time, so take care not to cut too deeply and injure the neonate. Use several shallow incisions, wiping the bleeding edge of the partially cut myometrium with a finger. Once the fetal membranes are seen, insert the index finger of each hand through the myometrial incision and extend it laterally by stretching until the incision is approximately 11 cm in length (Fig. 39.7).

4 Rupture the exposed membranes with scissors while your assistant aspirates liquor and blood with a sucker.

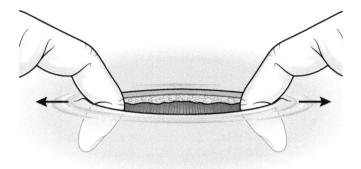

Fig. 39.7 Caesarean section: digital enlargement of incision.

5 Insert all fingers of your right hand into the uterus inferior to the fetal head, remove the Doyen retractor, and displace the fetal head superiorly out of the pelvis.

6 Flex the fetal head on its neck, and deliver the head into the wound, whilst your assistant applies sustained firm fundal pressure (practically speaking, this involves leaning with some of the assistant's weight on the patient's abdomen). Once the head is delivered, displace the fetal head inferiorly, firmly but gently, to deliver the superior shoulder, and then displace the fetal head superiorly to deliver the posterior shoulder. Withdraw the baby from the uterus. Immediately after delivery of the baby, have the anaesthetist give an intravenous injection of synthetic oxytocin (Syntocinon) 10 units.

7 Lay the baby on the mother's thighs and apply two clamps to the umbilical cord. Divide the cord between the clamps and hand the baby to the midwife.

8 Deliver the placenta by firmly massaging the uterine fundus and applying gentle cord traction, taking care to remove all fetal membranes.

9 Use large swabs to remove blood from the wound and again insert the Doyen retractor between the uterovesical peritoneum and uterus.

10 Grasp the lateral ends of the uterine incision with Green-Armytage clamps and also place two of these clamps on the upper and lower edges of the uterine incision where bleeding is greatest. This will control most of the bleeding.

? DIFFICULTY

1. If the fetal head is deeply wedged in the pelvis, have the head pushed up vaginally by an assistant.

2. Sometimes the uterine incision may extend, either laterally to involve the uterine vessels or downwards, where the ureter or bladder may be jeopardized if sutures are inserted hastily to try and secure haemostasis. It is often helpful to deliver the uterus through the incision to obtain better access. Ensure the bladder is well reflected away from the edge of the uterine incision/tear prior to suturing.

3. If the uterine incision continues to bleed after the 2-layer uterine closure, before placing haemostatic sutures

ensure the uterus is well contracted by: (1) rubbing the uterine fundus, (2) giving a syntocinon infusion at 10 units per hour intravenously, (3) ergometrine 500 μg intramuscularly, (4) carboprost 250 μg intramuscularly, and/or (5) misoprostol 800 μg rectally.

4. In exceptional circumstances it may be necessary to carry out a 'classical' upper segment caesarean section. This may be necessary if there is an anterior placenta praevia (Latin: *previus* = leading the way), a fibroid over the lower segment, or if the operation is being performed at an early stage of pregnancy. In this case use a vertical skin incision and make a large midline incision in the upper segment of the uterus. The uterine wall is much thicker in the upper segment and three layers of sutures are needed to close it.

Closure

1 Using an atraumatic 0 or 1-synthetic absorbable suture, include one lateral angle of the uterine incision in a stitch, ensuring that you have also taken the angle on the deep surface of the uterus. Close the incision with a continuous running suture. Insert a second continuous running suture to invaginate the first, so closing the uterus in two layers.

2 Apply a swab firmly over the uterine incision for 2 minutes. When it is removed there may be one or two small bleeding vessels, which need to be dealt with by individual figure-of-eight stitches.

3 Swab out any blood or liquor from the paracolic gutters on each side.

4 Ensure haemostasis of the inferior epigastric vessels running on and perforating the deep aspect of the rectus sheath.

5 Close the rectus sheath and skin incision.

Postoperative

1 Encourage breastfeeding as soon as possible after delivery. It aids contraction of the uterus, thereby decreasing bleeding, keeps the baby warm and helps 'bonding'.

2 Maintain intravenous fluids for 12 hours, but start oral fluids and indeed normal diet as soon as tolerated – often within hours.

3 In most cases give prophylactic subcutaneous heparin from 6 hours postoperatively.

4 Aim to mobilize the patient within 24 hours.

5 Leave a urinary catheter in place until the patient is mobile.

6 The patient should be ready for discharge 2–4 days postoperatively.

Complications

1 Pyrexia may be due to urinary infection, breast abscess, wound infection or endometritis. Examine the patient thoroughly, and take appropriate microbiological samples before starting antibiotics.

2 Excessive bleeding after caesarean section should be initially assumed to be due to uterine atony. Use uterotonic therapy as in the 'Difficulty' box above.

3 Broad ligament haematoma is a rare but important problem. Suspect it if there is excessive pain, fall in haemoglobin and pyrexia, possibly with a mass in the iliac fossa. If bleeding is ongoing, it will require laparotomy and possibly hysterectomy and salpingoooophorectomy on the affected side.

EMERGENCY SURGERY IN PREGNANCY

The presence of a pregnancy may cause considerable confusion in the diagnosis of an acute abdomen and may make access more difficult at laparotomy. It should not, however, deter you from performing emergency abdominal operations when necessary. Semi-urgent surgery is best delayed until the second trimester, as this is when the uterus is least likely to expel the pregnancy on provocation.

APPENDICITIS

The appendix is displaced upwards and outwards throughout pregnancy, and so is the site of maximal tenderness. As the uterus may be interposed between appendix and abdominal wall, focal irritation of parietal peritoneum may not occur to the same extent. Omentum may be prevented from surrounding the appendix and so generalized peritonitis occurs more readily.

Most surgeons have a higher threshold for surgery in pregnancy, and the mortality from appendicitis in pregnancy is higher as a result. Counsel your patient that there is risk to the pregnancy, but that inaction may threaten both her and the pregnancy. Make a gridiron incision over the area of maximal tenderness, above and lateral to the normal site, or consider a midline incision if there is doubt about diagnosis.

CHOLECYSTITIS

Acute cholecystitis are not uncommon in pregnancy, but the symptoms may be atypical, simulating hyperemesis or indigestion of pregnancy. If you make the diagnosis of cholelithiasis, it is preferable to wait until after delivery before carrying out cholecystectomy. If you need to perform the operation during pregnancy, try to do so in the second trimester. If the patient is unwell with acute cholecystitis, immediate surgery is justified as with acute appendicitis.

RED DEGENERATION OF A FIBROID

Fibroids are very common and often grow in pregnancy. A fibroid growing rapidly may undergo red degeneration, an extremely painful condition that has frequently prompted exploratory laparotomy. However, you should manage this condition conservatively.

> ▶ KEY POINTS Danger of myomectomy in pregnancy
>
> ■ Do not attempt to remove fibroids in pregnancy.
> ■ Myomectomy in pregnancy risks catastrophic haemorrhage, and loss of the fetus.
> ■ The only exception to this rule is if a pedunculated fibroid has undergone torsion and is gangrenous.

PLACENTAL ABRUPTION

1. Detachment of the placenta prior to delivery may result in fetal death and cause profound life-threatening maternal shock.

2. The presentation is of severe abdominal pain and bleeding (which may *or may not* be apparent vaginally). The uterus is very tender and classically woody-hard.

3. A lesser extent of abruption may cause diagnostic difficulty.

4. Unless labour occurs spontaneously, if near 37 weeks' gestation induce with prostaglandins and amniotomy – artificial rupture of the fetal membranes.

5. Where shock is present at any gestation or impending fetal demise likely (abnormal fetal heart rate pattern) perform caesarean section immediately. Emptying the uterus will allow it to contract and cease maternal bleeding. This may also save the fetus.

RENAL AND URETERIC CALCULI

Manage urinary tract calculi as in a non-pregnant patient, with analgesics and a high fluid intake, resorting to surgical management if this fails.

URINARY TRACT INFECTION AND PYELONEPHRITIS

Pregnancy predisposes to these conditions due to stasis produced by uterine pressure on the bladder and progesterone-induced ureteric relaxation. Pyelonephritis also causes premature labour. Whenever you investigate an obscure abdominal pain in pregnancy, send urine for culture as symptoms may not be typical. Amoxicillin, cephalexin and erythromycin are safe in pregnancy.

RECTUS SHEATH HAEMATOMA

Very occasionally, a haematoma occurs in the rectus sheath as a result of spontaneous haemorrhage from the inferior epigastric vessels in pregnancy. A tender mass appears in the abdominal wall. Treat conservatively.

FURTHER READING

Hudson CN, Setchell ME. Shaw's Textbook of Operative Gynaecology. 6th ed. New Delhi: Elsevier; 2004.

Monaghan JM, Lopes T, Naik R. Bonney's Gynaecological Surgery. 10th ed. Oxford: Blackwell Science; 2004.

Monson J, Duthie G, O'Malley. Surgical Emergencies. Oxford: Blackwell Science; 1999.

Rock JA, Jones HW, editors. Te Linde's Operative Gynecology. 10th ed. Philadelphia: Lippincott Williams & Wilkins; 2008.

Setchell ME. Gynaecological surgery. In: Kirk RM, editor. General Surgical Operations. 5th ed. London: Elsevier Science; 2006.

Sutton CJ, Diamond MP. Endoscopic Surgery for Gynaecologists. Philadelphia: Saunders; 1998.

Ear, nose and throat

M.P. Stearns

INTRODUCTION

Otolaryngological emergencies need to be managed on occasion by generalists. You may need to decide if that treatment can await later specialist care (e.g. a foreign body in the ear canal), or may even be unnecessary. Avoid acting inexpertly in such circumstances. Remember the maxim 'Primum non nocere (Latin: = First do no harm).

If a patient presents a challenge outside your personal experience but the operative techniques are familiar to you, then you may feel equipped to proceed if qualified aid is unavailable. If these conditions are not met, it may be wiser to accept the role of general practitioner and temporize. If you are a generally trained surgeon, lacking ENT training and with no ENT colleague at hand, you may find some of the procedures described are within your competence, such as incision of retropharyngeal abscess, removal of foreign bodies from the throat and relief of upper airway obstruction.

As a junior doctor faced with an ear, nose or throat condition in the Accident and Emergency Department, you may be able to remove a foreign body from the nose or ear and control nasal bleeding and institute initial management of a fractured nose.

FOREIGN BODY IN THE EAR

Appraise

1 The patient, usually a child, may complain of pain in the ear if the foreign object is irritating or has caused infection in the external ear canal.

2 A live insect may cause noise in the ear.

3 Most foreign bodies in the external auditory canal are found by chance.

Action

1 Remove insects to relieve pain. Fill the ear with olive oil to asphyxiate it, or kill it with alcohol. Gently remove it by syringing the ear with water at body temperature.

2 Inanimate foreign bodies may yield to gentle syringing, but those that occlude, or nearly occlude, the meatus cannot be removed by syringing so they need to be extracted with an instrument. Commonly inserted small pieces of sponge rubber can be removed using crocodile forceps if they lie close to the external auditory meatus. Unless you are expert, do not attempt to remove solid foreign bodies, since you risk damaging the middle ear, including the ossicular chain. A general anaesthetic may be required.

3 If the child is cooperative, examine the ear in a good light, initially without, then with, an auroscope. When the child is relaxed and quiet, touch the foreign body with a fine probe to confirm its shape and texture. You may not need to insert an aural speculum to do this. Look for a graspable edge; if you can seize it with very fine Hartmann's crocodile forceps you may be able to remove it.

? DIFFICULTY

1. If the object is smooth and rounded, such as a bead, do not apply forceps; they cannot grasp the object, and risk pushing it deeper into the meatus, through the drum, ossicular chain and possibly into the facial nerve and labyrinth.
2. The safest way to remove an occluding foreign body is under general anaesthesia, using an operating microscope. If this is not available, use illuminating loupes and the largest aural speculum the meatus will accept. Insinuate a stapedectomy hook beyond the object anteroinferiorly unless there is an obvious space above it, turn the hook to engage it, and ease it out by rolling or sliding. Alternatively, try the effect of using a small sucker.
3. *Golden rules:*
   - Do nothing that could push the foreign body further into the ear canal.
   - Pass hooks or probes anteroinferiorly, where the obliquity of the tympanic membrane allows you to insert the instrument more deeply without risk of injury.

REMOVAL OF NASAL FOREIGN BODY

Appraise

1 Suspect a self-inserted foreign body in any young child with unilateral nasal discharge. The discharge is usually foul smelling, causing obstruction and often contains blood.

2 The foreign body is commonly a screwed-up fragment of paper, vegetable matter, a plastic or metal bead, or rubber sponge.

Prepare

1 As with aural foreign bodies, first gain the child's cooperation. You may succeed if the foreign body is graspable and if you have appropriate instruments, clear visibility, a headlight, and are skilful in using a nasal speculum. If any of these are lacking, it needs to be removed under general anaesthesia by a specialist with oral, not nasal, intubation.

2 Ask the anaesthetist to avoid inflating the lungs with a face-mask, since this could force a nasal foreign body backwards.

3 Alternative positions:
- Place the patient in the tonsillectomy position, which is supine with the neck extended. Use a Boyle-Davis gag to prevent the foreign body slipping backwards into the nasopharynx, where it will stay because this is the most dependent part.
- Alternatively, insert a firm oropharyngeal pack around the tube to entrap the foreign body if it slips backwards. Have the head of the table raised so that you can look along the floor of the nose.

4 If the object is graspable use fine forceps; otherwise, use a small hook that can be passed above the foreign body, easing it downwards and forwards for delivery.

> KEY POINT Do not operate 'blind'

- Retain full visibility throughout.

MANIPULATION OF FRACTURED NOSE

Appraise

1 Realignment of displaced nasal bones is not only a cosmetic operation. Nasal fractures are frequently associated with nasal obstruction and many nasal fractures have an associated fracture of the nasal septum.

2 Nasal fractures may be associated with other facial injuries such as a fractured maxilla or 'blow-out' fracture of the orbit. Do not fail to examine the patient for other facial injuries.

3 Try to manipulate nasal fractures within 2 weeks of the injury. The most suitable times to do so are either very early, before there has been much nasal swelling, or at about 7 days when much of the swelling around the fracture site has subsided. If you try to manipulate the nasal bones while there is much swelling, it is difficult to see whether or not the nose is straight.

Action

1 It may be possible to straighten the nose by digital pressure, easing the nasal skeleton back into the midline. You can often manipulate it without anaesthesia within the first hour or two after injury. Alternatively re-align the nasal bones under local anaesthesia. You may feel a click as the fragments move into place.

2 If you cannot reduce the fracture in these ways you need the aid of general anaesthesia.

> KEY POINTS General anaesthetic precautions

- You may either have the patient intubated or have the facility of using a laryngeal mask.
- The nasal bones, if quite mobile, may be manipulated with an intravenous induction agent alone.

3 First, attempt manual reduction, pressing with your thumbs against the more prominent of the nasal bones. If this succeeds, over-reduce the fracture, and then mould the mobilized fragments into the desired symmetry.

4 If this fails, insert one blade of a Walsham's forceps into the nostril and grasp one nasal bone. The rubber cuff on the other blade of Walsham's forceps should lie on the skin, protecting it from damage by the forceps. Rotate and displace the nasal bone laterally to disimpact the fractured nasal bone. Then grasp the other nasal bone with the other Walsham's forceps and rotate it laterally also. The nasal fragments are now mobile and can be centralized with digital moulding. Take great care to protect the skin from injury during manipulation with these instruments.

5 If the septum is displaced, or the bridge-line is depressed, pass the blades of Asch forceps into the nostrils, grasp the septum, and bring it into the midline, while lifting up the dorsum.

> KEY POINT Gentleness

- Use only minimal force or the nasal mucosa will be torn, causing bleeding which may even require nasal packing.

Postoperative

1 If the reduced fracture is stable do not cover it with a splint.

2 Grossly comminuted, unstable fractures require a plaster-of-Paris splint secured with adhesive strapping. Mould the splint and the underlying nose beneath, while the plaster sets. Leave the splint in place for 7 days.

FOREIGN BODIES IN THE THROAT

Appraise

1 Fish bones lodge at any level, often in the tonsil or vallecula (diminutive of Latin: *vallis* = valley). More substantial bones (e.g. from chicken, rabbit or chops) usually stick in the postcricoid region or upper oesophagus.

2 Rarely, occluding foreign bodies such as sweets or a meat bolus can cause airway obstruction, leading to sudden death.

3 Dentures, which are often broken, impact in the mid-oesophagus.

4 A benign or malignant stricture may become occluded by a small bolus such as a pea or piece of potato.

Action

1 Inspect the throat carefully, using a headlight and tongue depressor. Look for the tip of a buried fish bone in the tonsil or base of tongue. Remove it with a fine pair of angled forceps, if necessary anaesthetizing the throat with a lidocaine topical spray.

2 If you cannot see the foreign body directly, use a laryngeal mirror, in the same manner as in indirect laryngoscopy, to examine the back of tongue and laryngopharynx. You can often retrieve a bone in these sites under indirect vision, using angled forceps. Have the patient grasp his own tongue with a gauze swab and draw it forward as far as possible. Hold the mirror in your non-dominant hand and the forceps in your dominant hand.

> ▶ KEY POINT Do not operate 'blind'
>
> ■ You must grasp the foreign body in the forceps under vision or you risk causing serious damage.

3 If on examination with a mirror you see the foreign body deep in the pyriform fossa or postcricoid space, or if a radiograph demonstrates that it is in the hypopharynx or upper oesophagus, then you need to remove it by direct endoscopy under general anaesthesia. Use a laryngoscope or short oesophagoscope and suitable forceps to bring the foreign body into the lumen of the endoscope. Take care not to push a sharp object through the visceral wall. Try to rotate it so that its most traumatic aspect is disimpacted and either trails harmlessly or can be drawn within the endoscope as it is withdrawn.

> ? DIFFICULTY
>
> 1. Do not attempt to remove a denture bearing exposed sharp hooks from the oesophagus. Safe removal may be facilitated by passing a cutting forceps through the endoscope and cutting the denture into pieces.
> 2. In some cases the foreign body can be removed safely only by thoracotomy and oesophagotomy (see Chapter 8).

INCISION OF QUINSY (PERITONSILLAR ABSCESS)

Appraise

1 Suspect the diagnosis of quinsy (Greek: *kynos* = dog + *anchien* = to throttle) or peritonsillar abscess from a history of an extremely sore throat in a toxic patient. The patient has trismus (Greek: *trizein* = to grate, gnash) and dysphagia for solids and liquids, often with drooling because swallowing saliva is too painful.

2 Although inspection may be difficult because of the trismus, a swelling of the soft palate may be seen in association with a contralateral tonsillitis.

3 Although incision of peritonsillar abscess is frequently described in textbooks, it is rarely performed because it usually responds to broad-spectrum systemic antibiotics. Treat early disease with high-dose antibiotics given intravenously, and reviewed after 24–36 hours. Incise it only if the swelling is not subsiding or if there is a fluctuant peritonsillar abscess.

Action

1 Inject local anaesthetic into the palatal mucosa at the intersection of a horizontal line through the base of the uvula with a vertical line along the anterior pillar of the fauces. Preferably use a dental syringe and needle with 2% lidocaine and 1:80 000 adrenaline (epinephrine). Allow at least 5 minutes for it to take effect.

2 Use a Bard-Parker handle with a no. 15 blade which can be wrapped in adhesive tape with only the last 1 cm exposed, preventing too deep penetration of the pharynx. Insert the knife blade backwards through the mucosa to a depth of 1 cm (Fig. 40.1). When pus gushes out, widen the track with sinus forceps.

3 Take a swab for culture. Quite often, however, no pus is obtained, because the quinsy is not sufficiently mature.

> ▶ KEY POINT Caution
>
> ■ Do not insert the blade more deeply than 1 cm, or you risk damaging the internal carotid artery.

4 As an alternative to incising the abscess use a large-bore hypodermic needle. You can dispense with local anaesthesia.

INCISION OF RETROPHARYNGEAL ABSCESS

Appraise

1 As a cause of acute illness with respiratory obstruction in infants and toddlers, this abscess tends to be to one side of the midline.

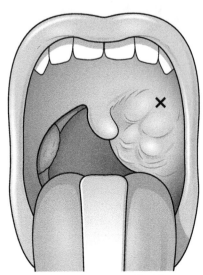

Fig. 40.1 Quinsy. 'X' shows the point of incision.

2 In older patients the abscess may be truly prevertebral, strictly midline and, usually, tuberculous in nature, secondary to tuberculous osteomyelitis of a cervical vertebra, in which case treatment is not primarily surgical.

3 If significant respiratory obstruction develops in spite of intravenous versatile antibiotic treatment in a young child or infant, you should incise a pyogenic abscess.

4 Lateral retropharyngeal abscesses in particular are often associated with a foreign body. Consequently, carry out a careful search for one when incising the abscess.

Action

Lateralized pyogenic abscess

1 Have the child anaesthetized by an experienced anaesthetist because, if the abscess is ruptured during intubation, the patient may inhale the pus. Have the patient held in a head-down position when being intubated and until the airway is protected by a cuffed endotracheal tube.

2 When the tube is in place the abscess contents can be aspirated with a per-oral needle. Alternatively, it can be incised through a pharyngoscope or using a Boyle-Davis gag.

3 Having incised the abscess send specimens of the abscess wall for histology and culture.

RELIEF OF UPPER AIRWAY OBSTRUCTION

Appraise

1 Immediately relieve respiratory obstruction from major facial or laryngeal trauma, laryngopharyngeal tumours and impacted foreign bodies.

2 Ensure that there is a clear airway if the patient is comatose. If necessary, assist respiration with mouth-to-mouth breathing, Ambi bag, a laryngeal mask or endotracheal intubation. If necessary, ventilate the patient.

3 An obstructed airway can frequently be expanded using positive pressure by mouth-to-mouth respiration or through a face-mask or oral tube, thus providing an adequate passage for air or oxygen.

> ▶ KEY POINTS Managing airway obstruction
>
> ■ Identify the cause of obstruction.
> ■ Eliminate the cause if possible.
> ■ Or pass an endotracheal tube through or past it.
> ■ Or perform laryngotomy or tracheotomy to get below the obstruction.
> ■ A totally obstructed patient can be partially relieved by inserting one or more large-bore hypodermic needles through the cricothyroid membrane.

LARYNGOTOMY

1 Lie the patient supine with extended neck.

2 Make a horizontal stab incision between the cricoid and thyroid cartilages. Press the blade backwards until you feel the point enter

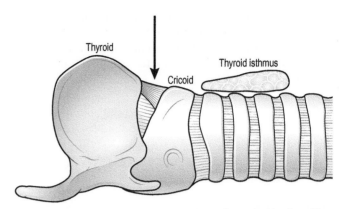

Fig. 40.2 Emergency laryngotomy: incision through cricothyroid membrane.

the airway and air begins to hiss in and out through the wound with respiration (Fig. 40.2).

3 With no loss of time, remove the knife and insert a small tube, curved downwards, inside the tracheal lumen. A correctly designed laryngotomy tube is flattened somewhat, so as to lie neatly between the cartilages, but if none is available use any type of tube – metal, rubber or plastic – even unsterile, if it maintains the airway.

4 An improvised tube is difficult to keep in a correct position so control it manually until you can establish a stable airway.

5 Unless the cause of acute asphyxia is quickly curable by removing an impacted foreign body or reducing angioneurotic oedema, perform an elective tracheostomy within 48 hours and close the laryngotomy incision.

EMERGENCY TRACHEOSTOMY

Appraise

1 Always prefer laryngotomy to tracheostomy because the former can be performed more quickly with less haemorrhage.

2 Rarely, if, for example, a subglottic lesion makes it impossible to perform laryngotomy and defies attempted incubation even through a rigid bronchoscope, you must perform emergency tracheostomy.

Prepare

1 Lie the patient supine with extended neck by placing a sandbag or a 1-L bag of fluid for intravenous infusion beneath the shoulders. Ensure the head is in a central position.

2 Deliver oxygen by face-mask to give a few more minutes of operating time.

3 If there is time, inject local anaesthetic such as 1% lidocaine with 1:100 000 adrenaline (epinephrine).

Action

1 Cut vertically from the lower border of the thyroid cartilage in the midline, to the suprasternal notch. Deepen the incision and extend it between the strap muscles. Feel the first tracheal ring with the left index finger.

2 Then divide the thyroid isthmus to expose the anterior tracheal wall. Control bleeding, which can be profuse, by pressure from an assistant. Decide quickly whether there is time to clamp major bleeding points before incising the trachea vertically through the second, third and fourth rings.

3 Insert a tracheal dilator to secure an airway. Introduce a tracheostomy tube. A cuffed tube prevents further aspiration of blood and allows ventilation, but is slightly more difficult to insert.

4 Now control the worst of the bleeding. Use a tracheal suction catheter through the tube to clear blood that has already been aspirated into the trachea.

Postoperative

1 Subsequent decisions and procedures depend upon the cause of the obstruction and the patient's general condition.

2 Monitor respiration and pulse during, and for several hours after, such a crisis.

3 Institute assisted ventilation and/or cardiac resuscitation immediately postoperatively if necessary.

ELECTIVE TRACHEOSTOMY

1 This procedure is considerably easier to perform in controlled conditions on an appropriately prepared and anaesthetized patient. Use either local or general anaesthesia.

2 Ensure that you have available a correct-sized tracheostomy tube. If it has a cuff, test it for leaks. If you intend to ventilate the patient, use a plastic cuffed tube, not a metal one. Check the patency and security of connections from tube to anaesthetic equipment.

Action

1 Inject the surgical area with a solution of 1:200 000 adrenaline (epinephrine) to help achieve haemostasis. Make a horizontal skin crease incision halfway between the cricoid cartilage and the suprasternal notch.

2 Separate the pretracheal muscles vertically and divide the thyroid isthmus between artery clips. Seal with diathermy the pretracheal vessels just below the cricoid. Ligate the inferior thyroid veins, since diathermy is unreliable. Ligate or oversew the edges of the thyroid isthmus and expose the anterior tracheal wall.

3 Having established haemostasis, make a 1–2-cm vertical incision, centred on the third or fourth tracheal ring (Fig. 40.3). Do not excise segments or cut flaps because there is a risk of subsequent stenosis or obstruction from a displaced tracheal cartilage flap. In addition, a tracheal flap may obstruct the passage of a tracheostomy tube.

▶ KEY POINTS Avoid extubation

■ If a patient is accidentally extubated and the tube cannot be rapidly replaced, fatal respiratory obstruction can occur.

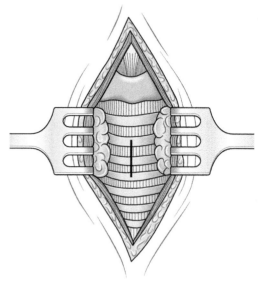

Fig. 40.3 Elective tracheostomy.

■ Insert a strong stitch through the cut tracheal edge on each side and leave the ends long, protruding through the skin wound. These can be used to draw the trachea forwards and open the incision in it to facilitate the reintroduction of a tube. This is particularly useful in paediatric tracheostomies.

4 Hold the tracheal incision open with a tracheal dilator. Ask the anaesthetist to remove the endotracheal tube to the subglottic level. Now insert, for example, a cuffed plastic tracheostomy tube. Inflate the cuff just sufficiently to prevent leakage around it when the anaesthetist inflates the patient's lungs. Overinflation of the cuff can lead to subsequent tracheal stenosis. The anaesthetist can now connect the tubing to the tracheostomy tube and withdraw the endotracheal tube. Have the endotracheal tube left in situ until now, so that if there is any difficulty in inserting the tracheostomy tube, or if the cuff bursts, the anaesthetist can continue to ventilate the patient through the endotracheal tube.

5 Close the skin loosely around the tube. Loose suturing allows drainage of any blood and also helps prevent air emphysema around the incision.

Complications

1 Haemorrhage can occur from the thyroid isthmus and the inferior thyroid veins. Ensure that the surgical field is dry before closing up.

2 In young infants the brachiocephalic vein may rise above the suprasternal notch, so take care to avoid injuring it.

Oral and maxillofacial surgery

P. McDermott

CONTENTS

GENERAL PRINCIPLES OF ORAL SURGERY

This chapter is limited to oral surgical procedures that you may need to perform when an appropriately trained colleague is not available. Whenever possible obtain the advice of a maxillofacial surgeon.

▶ KEY POINTS Can you see and manoeuvre within the mouth?

■ The oral cavity is small, dark, sensitive and has a slippery surface.
■ Patients may be nervous. They may tend to move their tongue or close their mouth at an inopportune moment.
■ Anxious patient? Consider giving intravenous sedation in adults.

Preparation

1 Ensure you have good illumination.
2 Arrange for adequate suction apparatus.
3 Make sure your assistant is efficient and can anticipate possible difficulties.

Anaesthesia

▶ KEY POINTS Anaesthesia

■ For general anaesthesia, an endotracheal tube or laryngeal mask and a throat pack are required to prevent inhalation of blood and debris.
■ Remember to remove the pack at the end of the operation.

1 Most minor procedures such as tooth extraction, biopsy, removal of salivary calculi and suturing of lacerations can be carried out using local analgesia. Local anaesthetics are available in 2-ml glass cartridges, the most common of which contain 2% lidocaine with adrenaline (epinephrine). Use 3% prilocaine with felypressin for patients sensitive to adrenaline (epinephrine). These cartridges fit into a syringe with a disposable needle.

2 In the upper jaw, deposit 1.5 ml of solution over the apex or apices of the offending tooth on the buccal side and about 0.5 ml on the palatal side. In the lower jaw, a similar technique may suffice for the anterior teeth. For the posterior teeth, an inferior alveolar and lingual nerve block is required at the lingula of the mandible, along with a long buccal nerve block at the anterior edge of the ramus of the mandible. Regional nerve block can also be used in the maxilla but, before attempting this, refer to appropriate literature.

▶ KEY POINTS Failure of local anaesthesia?

■ Test the tissues at the operation site and ask the patient if the area feels numb.
■ Adequate analgesia may not be achieved in the presence of inflammation.
■ If so, try depositing a few drops of anaesthetic solution into the periodontal membrane of the tooth.

3 General anaesthesia is often preferable in the treatment of children, patients who have fluctuant abscesses and if there is a history of allergy to local anaesthetic.

4 Hold the jaws apart with a prop or gag and stabilize the head in a rubber ring or horseshoe. Do not dislocate the jaw or tear the lips, which tend to be dry following preoperative fluid restriction.

5 Lightly coat the lips with petroleum jelly to keep them moist.

Haemostasis

1 Remove excess clot. Suture tightly across the socket and repair any lacerations. Apply pressure with a damp gauze pad for 10 minutes, timed by the clock.

2 If bleeding continues, infiltrate local anaesthetic with adrenaline around the area and lightly press a resorbable haemostatic material, such as oxidized cellulose, into the socket.

3 Sit the patient up at least 45° and if necessary give a sedative.

4 Control secondary haemorrhage with pressure, treat infection with systemic antibiotics. A 5-day course of metronidazole and amoxicillin will cover most oral infections. Prescribe 6% hydrogen peroxide mouthwashes.

5 Treat medical causes for prolonged bleeding appropriately, such as haemophilia, thrombocytopenia or hepatic cirrhosis.

In patients with haemophilia it is essential to liaise with their haematologist to ensure appropriate factor replacement over the course of the treatment. When dealing with patients on warfarin or antiplatelet medications (e.g. clopidogrel, aspirin) give 5% tranexamic acid as a mouthwash. Flush the socket with the liquid then insert some oxidized cellulose and suture the socket. Prescribe the mouthwash four times a day for 5 days.

6 If the prothrombin time is within the normal therapeutic range, you need not stop the warfarin in order to remove only a few teeth.

> ### KEY POINTS Post-extraction haemorrhage?
>
> - Post-extraction bleeding is often due to torn mucosa or unsupported mucosa.
> - Did you identify and correct pre-existing medical causes of bleeding?

Suturing

1 Use a half-circle 22–24-mm needle with a reverse cutting edge.

2 Use 3/0 sutures. Silk is easy to use but must be removed. Nylon is uncomfortable and also needs to be removed. Polyglactin 910 remains intact in the mouth for 3–4 weeks and produces minimal reaction but the knots and ends are irritating.

3 Use a needle-holder with a ratchet to avoid dropping the needle into the pharynx.

4 Insert the needle into the mucosa 3–5 mm from the edge, taking greater care on the more friable lingual edge.

5 The mucosal edges can rarely be approximated over a socket without excessive removal of bone. If you wish to apply even tension, insert mattress sutures.

6 Tie knots with the needle-holder rather than fingers: this is easier if you keep the end of the suture material short.

7 Remove non-resorbable sutures after 5–7 days.

Aftercare

1 Warn the patient that, until healing is complete, there may be constant discomfort because of the need to eat, swallow and speak.

2 If necessary, prescribe moderate analgesics such as ibuprofen or paracetamol. Aspirin mixture, used as a gargle, relieves a sore throat caused by an endotracheal tube and packing and ensures more comfortable swallowing. Ice packs applied to the skin for the first 4–6 hours reduce the swelling and subsequent discomfort.

3 Advise the patient that there may be difficulty in opening the mouth wide and chewing may be painful so that a soft diet may be beneficial.

4 Patients who have had their fractured jaws fixed together require special care in the early postoperative hours to avoid inhaling vomit. Swallowed blood may cause vomiting. To avoid this ensure that the stomach is empty preoperatively and administer an antiemetic. Keep a suction machine and wire-cutters by the bedside and show the nurses which wires to cut in an emergency.

5 When carrying out an operation on bone, many surgeons prescribe prophylactic antibiotics.

TOOTH EXTRACTION

Appraise

1 Is the extraction urgent or will antibiotics give relief until a specialist is available?

2 Tooth removal is indicated when there is a large cavity in a painful tooth, a painful loose tooth resulting from periodontal infection, an alveolar abscess or a loose tooth following trauma that could be inhaled.

Prepare

1 Extraction forceps: there are three basic pairs (Fig. 41.1), although many more specialized forceps are available.

2 Elevators (levers) enable you to remove broken roots or to loosen teeth before using forceps.

3 Prepare yourself by obtaining a radiograph before tooth removal to display unfavourable curved root patterns, buried roots, impacted teeth and latent pathology.

4 As a rule, have the patient seated, although the supine position is sometimes appropriate. Use local or general anaesthesia.

Action

1 Stand in front of the patient for most extractions. If you are right-handed, it is most convenient to stand behind the patient's right shoulder to remove lower right teeth.

2 Position the forceps blades on the buccal and lingual aspects of the tooth and push them under the gum as far as they will go along the root.

3 Grip the tooth and move it to expand the socket.

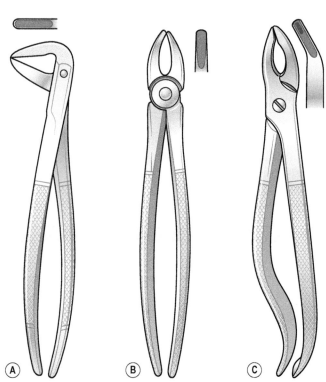

Fig. 41.1 Extraction forceps: (A) for mandibular teeth; (B) for maxillary anterior teeth; (C) for maxillary posterior teeth.

4 Deliver the tooth in the direction of the weakest wall – generally the buccal.

> **KEY POINTS** Gently as possible

- Avoid excessive force or you may fracture the roots or the jaw.
- Tooth extraction varies enormously in difficulty and root removal can be unexpectedly complicated.

5 Squeeze the socket with your fingers to reduce the dead space and position a damp gauze pad for the patient to bite on until the clot has formed.

6 Instruct the patient to avoid touching the clot for 24 hours and then bathe the wound frequently with warm saline mouth washes until it heals.

7 Leave small broken roots but attempt to remove large superficial roots using fine forceps or elevators.

8 If possible, refer patients with unerupted or impacted teeth to a specialist. Extraction may necessitate removing sufficient bone to allow elevation of the tooth. Use a small chisel or drill to remove the bone.

Aftercare

1 Inspect the socket if infection and pain develop a few days following extraction.

2 If the blood clot has disappeared, the empty socket fills with debris and pus.

3 Syringe out the socket and insert an antiseptic, which usually cures the osteitis. Although the socket closes slowly, a protective epithelial layer soon covers it.

JAW INFECTIONS

DENTAL ABSCESS

1 Once pus has escaped from bone, its direction of spread is influenced by gravity and muscle attachments.

2 Antibiotics given before there is significant fluctuation may suppress it.

3 Order radiographs.

Action

1 If there is no swelling, remove the tooth. Antibiotics are rarely required.

2 Treat a non-fluctuant swelling with antibiotics. The bacteria may be anaerobic.

3 Remove the source of infection if you can provide adequate anaesthesia.

4 When the tooth is partly erupted, clean the underside of the gum flap with an antiseptic solution or 6% hydrogen peroxide.

5 A sharp upper wisdom tooth may traumatize the cheek or the gum over a lower tooth. Removal of the upper is usually simple and gives relief of pain until the more complex lower can be extracted.

6 When fluctuation is present in the mouth, remove the offending tooth if accessible and incise the swelling in the buccal sulcus or palate to release pus that has not emptied into the socket.

7 Pus around the muscles of mastication produces trismus and prevents easy access to posterior teeth. This usually presents as a submandibular abscess. Under general anaesthesia, incise the skin of the neck at the most dependent point of the swelling and parallel to the lower border of the mandible. Extend the wound by blunt dissection then open up the loculi. Pass a pair of sinus forceps to the full depth of the cavity. Open the jaws of the forceps and remove them to enlarge the opening. Repeat this manoeuvre in a plane at right-angles to the original. In large cavities, the septae can be broken down with a finger.

8 Insert a drain for 24–48 hours. If the abscess is extensive, pass the drain from the skin through the abscess cavity and lingual mucosa into the mouth lateral to the submandibular duct. Draw it out of the mouth and fix it to the other end of the drain.

9 Remove the diseased tooth if possible during the anaesthetic period.

CELLULITIS

1 Cellulitis involving the sublingual and submandibular spaces and the cervical fascial plane is named Ludwig's angina after the German surgeon who described it. It is usually caused by streptococcal infection, making breathing and swallowing difficult.

2 Inspect an X-ray of the neck and mediastinum, looking for gas bubbles.

Action

1 Administer parenteral penicillin and metronidazole and a steroid such as dexamethasone every 8 hours for 24 hours, which will produce rapid improvement in early cases.

2 If the infection is established, you may need to make multiple superficial incisions of the skin of the neck to relieve pressure on the glottis. Deeper incisions and blunt dissection may cause additional, dangerous oedema.

3 Perform tracheostomy (see Chapter 40) if dyspnoea threatens. If the source of infection is accessible, remove it.

OSTEOMYELITIS/OSTEONECROSIS OF THE JAW

1 This rarely occurs in well-nourished populations, except those patients who have undergone previous radiotherapy to the jaws or have been on parenteral or long-term bisphosphonates.

2 The mandible is more frequently involved than the maxilla.

3 Most patients respond to long-term treatment with antibiotic therapy or in the case of osteoradionecrosis, hyperbaric oxygen can be used if available. If infection persists operation may be required.

Action

1 In the acute phase, expose the lateral cortex of the mandible through a submandibular incision. Remove the cortex with a dental drill. If a large drill is not available, make multiple

perforations and prise off segments with a chisel. Remove loose sequestra. Insert drains and close the wound.

2 In the chronic stage, expose the outer cortex of the mandible and dissect out the inferior alveolar neurovascular bundle. Remove the area of involved bone in a block and plan to graft the defect at a later date. Gentamicin beads or foam may be helpful.

3 Osteonecrosis following radiotherapy is difficult to treat and may require a microvascularized graft from a distant donor site. Referral to a specialist unit is necessary.

FACIAL SINUS

1 A sinus on the face, such as the chin, cheek or nasolabial fold, may be caused by a chronic low-grade dental infection. Multiple or recurring sinuses suggest the possibility of actinomycosis.

2 Clinical and radiographic examination usually shows a tooth is involved.

Action

1 If the sinus is recent, remove the tooth or refer to a dental surgeon for root canal treatment.

2 Excise the sinus with an ellipse of skin if it is retracted. Encourage a small sinus to heal by cauterizing the track with a crystal of silver nitrate.

3 If you suspect actinomyces infection, give an antibiotic such as penicillin for 6 weeks.

TEMPORO-MANDIBULAR JOINT DISLOCATION

1 The temporo-mandibular joint (TMJ) has an upper and lower joint space divided by a disc of fibrocartilage. The cartilage moves with the condyle to ensure smooth passage as it passes down the articular eminence to increase mouth opening.

2 There are many problems associated with this joint, ranging from acute myofascial pain syndrome to generalized systemic disorders, e.g. gout or rheumatoid arthritis, which are best treated by appropriate specialists.

3 Dislocation is an alarming and stressful condition for the patient. Oral sedation followed by manipulation is frequently cited as the method to reduce the condition but often results in failure and great stress to the patient.

Action

1 A simple and reliable method is to inject 1–2 ml of 2% lidocaine solution into the TMJ space which lies just anterior to the tragus. A hollow in the tissues can be palpated when the joint is dislocated.

2 In addition, infiltrate a further 2 ml of 2% lidocaine into the sulcus high above the 2nd and 3rd upper molars on the affected side. This procedure blocks the proprioceptive feedback and reduces spasm in the lateral and upper part of medial pterygoid muscles which hold the disc and joint in the dislocated position.

3 Wait for 10 minutes and then place each thumb onto the posterior buccal aspect of the last mandibular molar area.

4 Press downwards and backwards to unlock the condylar head over the articular eminence. If the local anaesthetic is correctly placed, the procedure is not usually painful and will reduce most dislocations.

5 In the last resort, reduce the jaw under general anaesthesia.

6 If the TMJ repeatedly dislocates, as may occur in stroke patients, then selective botulinum toxin injections or surgical reduction of the articular eminence can be tried. Refer the patient to a specialist.

FACIAL FRACTURES

Appraise

1 Facial injuries involve the nose, maxilla, zygoma and mandible. Fractures of the nose are dealt with in Chapter 40.

2 *Respiration.* Posterior and inferior displacement of the maxilla and blockage of the nose with blood clot cause respiratory distress. Bilateral fractures of the body of the mandible may result in lack of support for the tongue, which then falls back against the pharynx if the patient lies on his back.

3 Bleeding from facial injuries may appear copious, but is rarely life-threatening. If there are signs of shock, check other injured sites such as ruptured internal organs and fractured limbs. Fixation of fractures reduces haemorrhage.

▶ KEY POINTS Exclude other injuries

- Fractures of the skull and other bones are often associated with facial injuries.
- Cervical fractures are also often present.

Emergency action

1 Respiratory obstruction from posterior displacement of the maxilla will be relieved by pulling the maxilla forwards with a finger hooked around the back of the palate.

2 Relieve obstruction following bilateral mandibular fractures by placing the patient in the recovery position. This allows the tongue to fall forward under gravity and prevents blood and debris from being inhaled. If necessary, insert a tongue stitch to pull the bulk of the tongue forwards.

3 Remove foreign bodies, such as broken teeth or dentures, from the mouth and pharynx. Plastic dentures are radiolucent and may not be apparent on a chest X-ray.

4 Unconscious patients with severe facial injuries may require an elective tracheostomy if oral or nasal intubation proves difficult.

5 Control persistent bleeding from the nose with posterior nasal packs.

Assess

1 Mandibular fractures are often bilateral. A mandibular body fracture is often accompanied by a contralateral condylar fracture. Unilateral condyle neck fractures may not require treatment if the occlusion can be maintained. Bilateral condyle neck fractures combined with a fractured maxilla may require complex treatment.

2 Most fractures through the tooth-bearing areas are compound.

3 Carefully look for deformity or loss of facial symmetry.

4 Assess the number and position of teeth, and note any wear facets, in order to determine if the relationships have been altered.

5 Note the proximity of a fracture line to apex of tooth, as a devitalized tooth may become infected and delay healing.

6 Identify and record the presence and site of skin lacerations.

7 Test for sensory loss to assess the possibility of nerve damage, including loss of smell, indicating possible olfactory nerve damage.

8 Look for possible complications of fractures, such as diplopia and trismus.

9 Carefully check for cerebrospinal fluid leakage from the nose or ear.

Appraise

1 If the teeth meet correctly, the mandibular fractures are probably reduced.

2 Maxillary fractures need to be splinted to the skull or zygomatic arches if they are intact.

3 Intermaxillary fixation of maxillary fractures needs to maintained for 3 weeks and 4–6 weeks for the mandible.

4 Remove teeth if they are in the line of the fracture and loose.

5 Give appropriate antibiotics.

6 Treat the patient under general anaesthesia unless the displacement is minimal.

7 If a general anaesthetic is administered, remember to remove the throat pack before finally tightening the intermaxillary fixation.

8 Consider the need for anti-emetics and nasogastric tube gastric aspiration.

MANDIBLE

Appraise

Plating is rigid and reduces the need for intermaxillary fixation and time off work. The technique is not difficult but intraoral access can make it complex. The plates are placed across the fracture line and where possible along the known stress lines in the jaw. Titanium is the ideal material and does not need to be removed unless it becomes infected or exposed (rarely). The plate, drill, screws and screwdriver should be made of the same metal to avoid electrolytic action.

> ▶ KEY POINTS Plating fractured facial bones

- Plating is the method of choice, but you should not attempt it unless you are properly trained in the various techniques and a specialist is not available.
- The anatomy of the area may be distorted by haematoma and the displacement of bone fragments. Identify the large neck blood vessels, which may have been displaced.

- The inferior alveolar neurovascular bundle is easily damaged when manipulating the jaw or when drilling into the bone, resulting in a numb lower lip.
- Avoid the roots of teeth and main nerves. Drilling or inserting a screw into a tooth root risks loss of vitality, subsequent loss of the tooth and infection in the fracture line.

Action

1 Plating:
  - If appropriate, expose the fracture through the mouth or a skin laceration.
  - Remove an unerupted posterior tooth if it is in the fracture line.
  - Reduce the fracture.
  - Apply temporary intermaxillary fixation to hold fragments accurately.
  - Mould the plate to lie flush against the bone, with at least two holes on each fragment. In atrophic mandibles apply the plate external to the periosteum to minimize damage to an already compromised blood supply.
  - Drill holes, starting with an end one.
  - Insert screws (Fig. 41.2).
  - Close the wound.
  - Remove the intermaxillary fixation at the end of the operation for safety, replacing it with elastic bands or wire for a few days when the patient is fully conscious.

2 *Eyelet wiring.* This may be possible when there are sufficient occluding teeth. Stretch soft, stainless steel wire of 0.5 mm diameter by 10%. Fold 15 cm of wire in half and bend round the shaft of a dental burr to form a loop in the middle. Pass the two ends between adjacent teeth so that the eyelet is on the buccal side. Separate the ends and pass them back around each tooth. Thread one end through the eyelet and twist off with the other. The wire should be between the gum margin and the most bulbous part of the tooth (Fig. 41.3). When sufficient wires have been placed in both jaws and on all fragments, place the teeth in occlusion. Pass a tie wire through an eyelet in the lower jaw and one in the upper jaw and twist them together. Ensure the ends of the twisted wires are tucked between a pair of teeth to protect the lips and cheeks (Fig. 41.4). By convention, all wires are

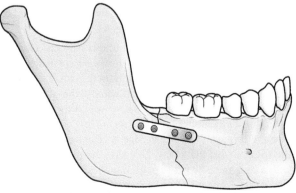

Fig. 41.2 Bone plate in position across mandibular fracture.

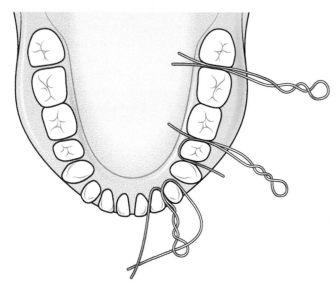

Fig. 41.3　Steps in the placement of eyelet wires.

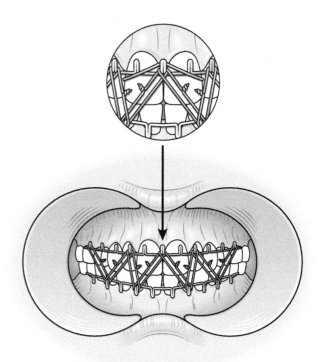

Fig. 41.5　Arch bars and intermaxillary fixation. The inset shows the intermaxillary wires and some of the wires fixing the arch bar to the teeth.

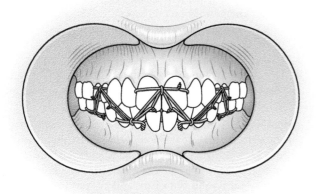

Fig. 41.4　Eyelet wires and intermaxillary wires in place.

twisted in a clockwise direction. Take care when using wires to avoid a needle-stick injury.

3　*Arch bars*. These are an alternative to eyelets, especially when there are missing teeth. Commercially prepared bars are available with loops or cleats attached. Cut a sufficient length of bar and apply it to all the teeth in one jaw. The loops point towards the roots of the teeth. Fix the bar to the jaws with wire twisted round each tooth and the bar. Carry out a similar procedure in the other jaw. Place the teeth in occlusion and twist the wire around the opposing loops of the arch bars (Fig. 41.5).

4　*Gunning splints*. Use these for edentulous patients. Obtain the help of a maxillofacial technician. The splints are made from impressions of the patient's mouth or from the patient's dentures if available. The splints or dentures are wired to the jaws after reducing the fractures. The wires are passed round the splint and the mandible. In the upper jaw the wires are looped round the denture and through the alveolar ridge. A large hole in the palate of the splint makes this easier. The wires are placed using an awl with a hole near the trocar point in which the wire can be held (Fig. 41.6). Take care not to let the wire enter the fracture or damage the submandibular ducts.

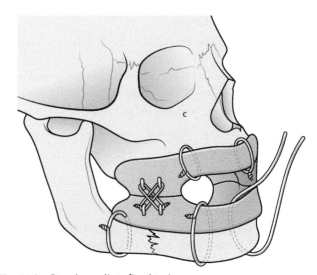

Fig. 41.6　Gunning splints fixed to jaws.

5　*Barrel bandage*. This is normally used only as a temporary measure before the patient can receive the correct treatment. The bandage should be non-stretch material. Apply it to hold the lower jaw against the upper and not to pull the chin backwards (Fig. 41.7). Ensure there is adequate space for easy observation of the pupils and lips.

MAXILLA

1　A fractured maxilla is displaced posteriorly and inferiorly.

2　Disimpaction involves moving the maxilla in the opposite directions after freeing it with disimpaction forceps.

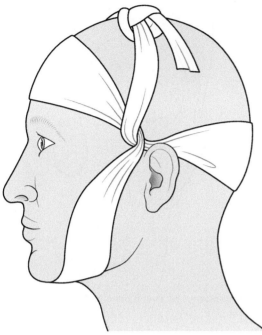

Fig. 41.7 Barrel bandage.

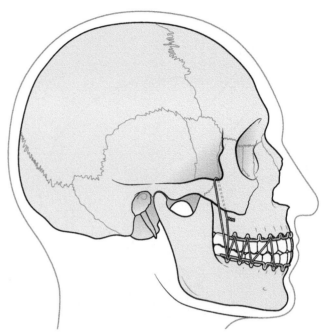

Fig. 41.8 Circumzygomatic wires fixed to arch bars on teeth.

3 After disimpaction, fix the teeth in occlusion with a few wires round upper and lower teeth.

4 By applying pressure under the mandible, reduce the fracture between the maxilla and skull.

5 Cranial fixation is then normally applied.

? DIFFICULTY

1. Reduction of the fracture may be difficult because of impaction of the bones and oedema. Access is easier after 3–4 days when the oedema has subsided.
2. Inadequate reduction results in a concave profile that is difficult to correct.

Fixation

1 *Plating.* Do not embark on this unless you have had special training in the use of plates and are familiar with the anatomy of the maxilla and nose. Plates can be used to fix a fractured maxilla, reducing the need for intermaxillary fixation. They are placed across the fracture lines using a suitably shaped plate. The bone over the zygomatic buttress is thick and will hold a relatively long screw as will the piriform rim of the nose but the anterior wall of the maxilla is thin and the thread of the screw may strip the bone. Avoid placing a screw into the maxillary antrum or a tooth root. Metal plates can interfere with CT (computed tomography) scans. Titanium causes less interference and can be used round the orbit, on the frontal bone and nose.

2 *Halo frame.* This is easy to use, versatile and firm but you should not attempt to use it unless you have had special training. The same warnings apply to the use of pins and screws.

3 *Internal fixation* may be within your capabilities. Using an awl or lumbar puncture needle, pass a loop of wire round the zygomatic arch and into the mouth in the molar region. Pass one end through

an eyelet or round a cleat on splints or arch bars in the upper or lower jaws and twist it with the other end (Fig. 41.8).

Aftercare

1 Administer prophylactic antibiotics where there are compound fractures around the mouth. If you suspect cerebrospinal fluid leakage, amoxicillin or equivalent is mandatory.

2 If you have used a general anaesthetic remove the anaesthetist's throat pack.

3 Patients with intermaxillary fixation need close supervision postoperatively in case they inhale vomit. Keep a suction machine and wire-cutters by the bedside and instruct the nurses how to use them.

4 Give anti-emetics at the end of the general anaesthetic.

5 Elastic bands are safer than wires for intermaxillary fixation but need replacement.

6 Give a fluid or semifluid diet. Six small meals are easier to take than three large ones.

7 Keep the mouth clean with mouthwashes in a syringe and a small toothbrush.

ZYGOMATIC COMPLEX (MALAR)

These are best treated within a week of injury, but allow excessive periorbital oedema to subside first.

Access

1 Use Gillies temporal approach. Make a 2.5-cm incision in the hairline between the main branches of superficial temporal vessels. Cut at 45° to zygomatic arch inclining the incision posteriorly.

2 When you reach glistening temporalis fascia, incise it carefully to avoid damaging the temporalis muscle.

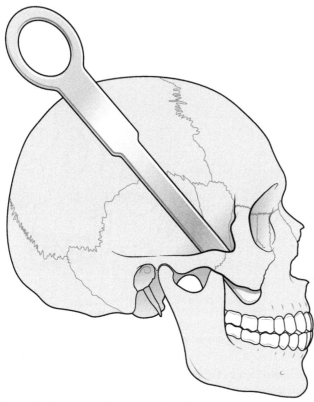

Fig. 41.9   Elevator under zygomatic arch.

3 Slide a Howarth's periosteal elevator or similar shaped instrument under the fascia until it is beneath the zygomatic arch. You should not feel any resistance until you reach the arch.

Action

1 Exchange the Howarth for a Bristow elevator or one of the modifications (e.g. Rowe zygomatic elevator) and lift the displaced bone with an anterior and lateral motion. A slight lateral rotation may also help. Do not lever against the middle cranial fossa. The bone usually jams into place with a click (Fig. 41.9).

2 Suture the skin.

3 Mark the affected cheek and instruct nurses not to lay the patient on that side. Pressure on the bone at this stage may easily displace it.

? DIFFICULTY

1. The reduced fracture may be unstable. Do not attempt to insert plates or wires unless you are specially trained. If you attempt wiring, look for and protect the infraorbital nerve as it comes out of the foramen. The fracture often runs through it. Protect the eye when drilling the holes (Fig. 41.10).
2. Support can be provided by placing a pack into the antrum, but do not attempt to insert a pack into the antrum through a Caldwell-Luc approach unless you have had special training.

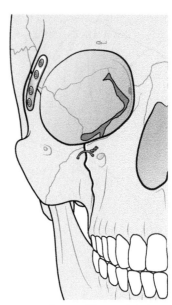

Fig. 41.10   Interosseous wires and bone plate in unstable zygomatic bone fractures.

3. If there are trapped orbital contents and the patient displays marked diplopia with unequal pupil levels, you should make every effort to obtain specialist help and advice.

FURTHER READING

Banks P, Brown A. Fractures of the Facial Skeleton. Oxford: Wright; 2000.

Burkitt HG, Quick CRG. Essential Surgery. 3rd ed. Edinburgh: Churchill Livingstone; 2002.

Ferraro JW. Fundamentals of Maxillofacial Surgery. New York: Springer; 1997.

Hawkesford J, Banks JG. Maxillofacial and Dental Emergencies. Oxford: Oxford University Press; 1994.

Hutchison I, Lawlor M. Major maxillofacial injuries. Br Med J 1990;301:595–9.

Kaban LB, Pogrel MA, Perrott DH. Complications in Oral and Maxillofacial Surgery. Philadelphia: Saunders; 1996.

Langdon JD, Patel M. Maxillofacial Surgery. London: Chapman & Hall Medical; 1998.

McGowan DA. An Atlas of Minor Oral Surgery: Principles and Practice. London: Martin Dunitz; 1999.

Miloro M. Peterson's Principles of Oral and Maxillofacial Surgery. 2nd ed. New York: Marcel Decker; 2004.

Moore UJ. Principles of Oral and Maxillofacial Surgery. 5th ed. Oxford: Blackwell Science; 2000.

Moore JR, Gilbe GV. Principles of Oral Surgery. 4th ed. Manchester: Manchester University Press; 1991.

Pedlar J, Frame JW. Oral and Maxillofacial Surgery. Edinburgh: Churchill Livingstone; 2001.

Robinson PD, Pitt Ford TR, McDonald F. Local Anaesthesia in Dentistry. Oxford: Wright; 2000.

Ward-Booth P, Hausaman J, Schendel SA. Maxillofacial Surgery. Edinburgh: Churchill Livingstone; 1999.

Wray D, Stenhouse D, Lee D, et al. Textbook of General and Oral Surgery. Edinburgh: Churchill Livingstone; 2003.

Ophthalmology

C.C. Davey

CONTENTS

INTRODUCTION

The procedures described here are semi-expert but do not require extraordinary technical skills. Examination of patients that might need these procedures is likely to take place without the full facilities available to the ophthalmologist. A non-specialist using a torch and a loupe and some means of assessing visual acuity will be able to decide on the necessity for treatment in emergency circumstances.

> ► KEY POINT Anatomy

> ■ Do not embark on ophthalmic procedures without first revising the anatomy.

Prepare

1 Many of the procedures described in this chapter can be carried out with small instruments available in a general surgical theatre.

2 Ideally, however, a selection of special instruments will render these eye operations easier to perform:
   - *Lid specula:* right and left, guarded, to keep the eyelashes away
   - *Forceps:* plain (Moorfields); and fine-toothed (e.g. Lister, Jayles or St Martin's)
   - *Scissors:* straight iris scissors; blunt-nosed straight and curved; spring conjunctival scissors; corneal scissors; and fine intraocular scissors
   - *Knives:* disposable knife for entry into the anterior chamber (Alcon or Weiss) or diamond knife if available; Bard-Parker scalpel handles with no. 11 and 15 blades
   - *Needle-holder:* coarse (Castroviejo); fine (Barraquer)
   - *Sutures:* black silk 4/0, 6/0; synthetic absorbable such as Vicryl 5/0, 6/0, 8/0; nylon 9/0, 10/0; all these are available on atraumatic needles
   - *Squint muscle hooks*
   - *Viscoelastic* (*sodium hyaluronate*) is useful to protect the corneal endothelium and create space in the anterior chamber, for all intraocular operations
   - *Eye drops and ointments:* antibiotics chloramphenicol 0.5% (for postoperative) and ofloxacin 0.3%, drops (for suspected corneal ulcer) and fusidic acid gel (fucithalmic), useful in children. Local anaesthetic drops are tetracaine 1% (previously known as amethocaine) and benoxinate (oxybuprocaine hydrochloride 0.4%), or proxymetacaine 0.5% (does not sting but does require refrigeration).

PROTECTING THE EYE

Assess

1 Take particular care when there is exposure of the cornea and there is risk of corneal ulceration. This is present when there is a seventh nerve palsy, trauma including burns causing eyelid damage, proptosis or herpes zoster ophthalmicus in which the cornea may also be anaesthetic, or in the unconscious patient.

2 When the problem is likely to be temporary, it may simply be necessary to apply copious artificial tear drops and ointment until recovery occurs.

3 When the problem is likely to be longstanding, arrange to cover the cornea with the eyelid, either by keeping the lid over the eye with paraffin gauze or an eye-covering gel, or by dropping the lid with botulinum toxin (see below).

4 Alternatively, suture the eyelids together with a tarsorrhaphy.

TARSORRHAPHY

Appraise

1 Stitching the lids together may be done either centrally, which of course obscures vision, or laterally, where the protection given is due to the shortening and consequent narrowing of the palpebral fissure.

2 Central tarsorrhaphy is advised where there is inability to close the lids (lagophthalmos) and there is drying of the cornea, or when ulceration is actually present. It is indicated also when severe or protracted ulceration occurs for other reasons, for example in an anaesthetic cornea.

3 In ectropion of the lower lid, in particular that occurring in facial palsy, a lateral tarsorrhaphy suffices.

4 A bandage soft contact lens may be useful in a non-healing corneal ulcer; if it is not available, copious lubricants and daily observation are required.

5 Temporary protection of the cornea can be achieved by inducing
a ptosis. Inject 100 pg of botulinum A toxin into the levator pal-
pebrae superioris through the upper lid, entering above the tarsal
plate. Keep close to the orbital roof to avoid injecting the toxin
into the superior rectus muscle, which would cause diplopia.

6 Superglue closure is dangerous because of the risk of the hard-
ened glue rubbing on the cornea.

Action

1 In all cases, use local anaesthesia with tetracaine (amethocaine)
1% drops to the conjunctiva and 1% lidocaine with adrenaline
(epinephrine) infiltration into the lid substance, both subcutaneously and subconjunctivally.

2 In tarsorrhaphy proper, raw surfaces of the lid margins are prepared. The easiest way to do this is simply to divide the lid into
anterior and posterior layers through the 'grey line' (Fig. 42.1A).
This is the midline of the edge of the lid between the roots of the

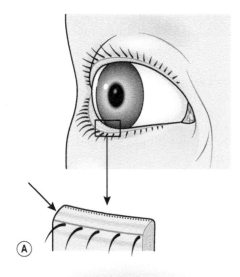

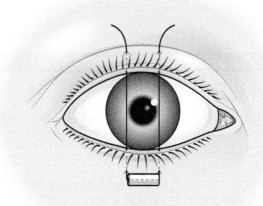

(B)
Fig. 42.1 (A) Tarsorrhaphy: (A) division through the 'grey line';
(B) inserting the sutures.

eyelashes in front and the mouths of the meibomian glands behind. The trouble is that in many patients it does not exist as a
defined line, and when preparing the lid it is important to keep
away from the roots of the lashes as this could distort them and
lead to their growing inwards.

3 Start with the lower lid. Hold it up vertically with toothed forceps
while an assistant holds it up with similar forceps some way along.
Sink the blade (no. 15BP) of a scalpel in about 3–4 mm through
the grey line in the plane of the lid, and take the cut the required
length along the lid. If the initial stretch of lid grasped by yourself
and your assistant is not long enough, both of you move along and
continue the incision. Deal similarly with the upper lid opposite
the raw area in the lower. In a lateral tarsorrhaphy make sure
the two raw areas are continuous round the outer canthus.

4 Now insert the sutures (Fig. 42.1B). Use double-armed 4/0 black
silk and pass the needle through the bore of a 3-mm length of
rubber tube so as to prevent it cutting out. Grasp the edge of
the lower lid with one blade of the toothed forceps in the raw area
in the lid margin, the other in the substance of the lid 3–4 mm
from the margin. Enter the needle through the skin 4 mm from
the lid margin and come out in the raw area. Now grasp the upper
lid similarly and pass this needle through the raw area and out on
the skin 4 mm from the lid margin. Repeat this procedure with
the other needle, entering the skin of the lower lid about
4 mm laterally or medially from the entry of the first.

5 Now pass one needle through a second similar piece of rubber tube
and either tie it or, according to the length of lid closure required,
put in as many more of these mattress sutures as are indicated.

6 Before tying, wipe away any clot from the raw edge of the lids. Do
not buckle the lids when tying; moderately firm apposition is all
that is needed as postoperative swelling will add further tension.

7 Put on antibiotic ointment and bandage the eye over paraffin
gauze or non-adherent dressing and a pad only if bleeding has
been excessive. Uncover the next day. Inspect again in a week
and remove the sutures after 2 weeks.

EYELID INJURIES

1 Lacerations heal well, but there are important points to
remember.

2 If the lid margin is involved, try to appose the edges as accurately
as possible. Use 6/0 Vicryl for the skin but try to insert a suture of
6/0 silk through the lid margin itself. Enter the needle on one side
through the grey line 2–3 mm from the cut edge, emerging in the
latter a similar distance down the cut and then in reverse through
the other edge. After tying the suture, leave the ends 3 cm long
and strap them down, then check that they do not abrade the
cornea. Use the skin sutures to tie over the long ends of the lid
margin sutures to keep them out of the eye.

3 If the lids are widely split, suture the tarsal plate before tackling
the skin. Do this with interrupted 6/0 absorbable stitches. Insert
the sutures at 2-mm intervals, placing the knots anteriorly in the
substance of the lid, not facing backwards where they will be
uncomfortable and again may abrade the cornea.

4 In cases where the inner third of the lower lid is lacerated, or there
is a deep horizontal cut of the upper lid, call in the experts immediately. Restoration of continuity of a possibly divided lower

lacrimal canaliculus or levator repair is too specialized a procedure to be covered here. Simply suture the tarsal plate, orbicularis and skin, then refer for later surgery.

5 Massive loss of the substance of the lids may give rise to an immediate problem of ocular (particularly corneal) protection. A protective contact lens may be indicated. Immediate plastic procedures may be advisable, if possible, finishing with some form of tarsorrhaphy or even a purse-string conjunctival flap to protect the cornea. This creates a moist chamber. This entails making a circular incision around the ocular conjunctiva well away from the limbus, mobilizing the ocular conjunctiva off the sclera, then inserting a purse-string suture around the margin, drawing it together to form a closed chamber protecting the cornea.

INJURIES OF THE GLOBE

LACERATIONS

Appraise

1 *Conjunctiva.* Leave small cuts (less than 5 mm) alone. Suture larger ones under local anaesthesia with interrupted 8/0 synthetic absorbable sutures at 4-mm intervals, removing any prolapsed Tenon's capsule, if excessive, or burying it.

2 *Cornea and sclera.* Insert a speculum, and find and remove foreign bodies. Glass from windscreens is especially difficult. Put a drop of fluorescein in the eye; it may help to show small particles as well as corneal epithelial loss.

> ▶ KEY POINT Foreign bodies
>
> ■ For removal of metal foreign bodies, see page 650, but always X-ray a lacerated eyeball as a matter of routine.

3 If obvious foreign bodies are present in the anterior chamber, only, attempt to remove them with the finest small-bladed forceps under high magnification after re-forming the anterior chamber with Viscoelastic. Do this only during a procedure for a lacerated cornea. There is no substitute for Viscoelastic, so do not attempt to re-form the anterior chamber if none is available.

4 Try to preserve iris and ciliary body if practical to do so, lens and vitreous, if coming out of the would will need to be removed. If the iris cannot be replaced then, pick it up with iris forceps etc. Pick them up with iris forceps and withdraw a little in an attempt to free them from an incarcerated position in the wound. Make a cut with De Wecker scissors to remove the tissue, flush with the plane of the globe at the site of the penetration. Gently replace any intraocular tissue remaining in the wound, using an iris repositor. In an emergency, leave alone incarcerated material that is not prolapsed externally, particularly if the anterior chamber is not lost.

Closure

1 Wound closure varies in difficulty. Insert sutures into clean lacerations of less than 5 mm only if aqueous humour is leaking.

2 As a general surgeon, you may not wish to undertake direct corneal or scleral suture. If you do undertake it, however, remember

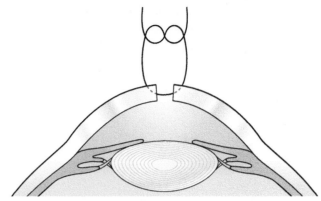

Fig. 42.2   Corneal and scleral sutures.

that, although the stitches should be almost full thickness, they must not penetrate into the eyeball (Fig. 42.2). Use magnification, if it is available, to ensure this.

> ▶ KEY POINT Placing sutures
>
> ■ You must place the stitches in, but not through, the tissue.

3 Enter and emerge about 1–1.5 mm from the wound edge. Grasp each edge lightly with the finest-toothed forceps you have, such as Jayles, St Martin's, or finer. Use 9/0 or 10/0 nylon and keep the sutures in a line perpendicular to the wound. In suturing scleral wounds it may be necessary to dissect the conjunctiva back from the edge.

4 It may, however, be unwise to attempt direct suture, either because you lack experience or because the wound is too irregular. In such cases, and particularly if the anterior chamber is shallow or absent, prefer to cover the wound with a conjunctival flap. In a corneal wound, for example, carry out a partial peritomy. Thus if, for example, the wound is in the 4 o'clock meridian, cut the conjunctiva at the limbus (Latin: = border; between the sclera and the cornea) from 1 o'clock to 7 o'clock in the lower left half of the globe (Fig. 42.3). If it is possible to choose the origin and direction of the flap, remember that the upper and temporal conjunctiva is the loosest and easiest to mobilize. Undermine the conjunctiva so freed back, for at least 15 mm. Insert one needle of a double-armed 8/0 absorbable suture in the paralimbal connective tissue at 8 o'clock and, using a second suture, do the same at 12 o'clock.

5 To insert these sutures, try to get a reasonable bite without going right through the sclera into the eye. Aim for a 2-mm track, parallel to and 1 mm from the limbus. To steady the eye use fine-toothed forceps such as Jayles, to grasp the episcleral tissue close to the point of suture insertion.

6 Now put the two arms of one suture through the edge of the freed conjunctiva at an appropriate place and repeat this with the other suture. Figure 42.3 indicates suitable insertion points. Tie each suture while an assistant, using two pairs of plain forceps, draws the edge of the flap well over the site of the penetration. If the penetration is central, it should still be possible to cover it in this way.

7 Finally, give a subconjunctival injection of cefuroxime 125 mg in 1 ml of water. Give the injection by passing the needle tangentially through the conjunctiva in a horizontal direction 1 cm back from the limbus, into the quadrant opposite to that of the penetrating injury.

the cornea 2 mm inside the limbus (corneoscleral junction) with the plane parallel to the presumed plane of the iris, which you cannot see.

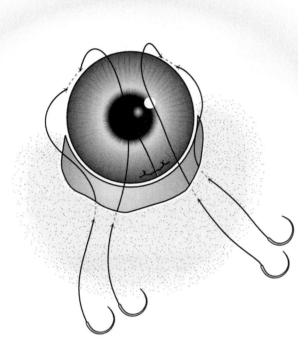

Fig. 42.3 Conjunctival flap.

BLUNT INJURIES

EVACUATION OF HYPHAEMA

Appraise

1 Hyphaema (bleeding into the anterior chamber) is invariably treated conservatively initially, with bed rest and topical steroids to reduce the risk of further bleeding, such as dexamethasone (Maxidex) 0.1% four times a day. Patients with sickle cell disease or trait may have severe hyphaemata, which is very slow to resolve.

2 Removal of the blood from the anterior chamber is very rarely indicated. Undertake it only when:
- The anterior chamber is full of blood and
- There is a considerable rise in the intraocular pressure, which is unresponsive to acetazolamide (Diamox) and oral glycerol or mannitol infusions over a 3-day period or
- The patient is in severe pain.

Action

1 Anaesthetize the eye with topical 4% benoxinate (oxybubicaine), tetracaine (amethocaine) drops given at 5-minute intervals. A general anaesthetic is unnecessary.

2 Insert an eye speculum. Have available a disposable or diamond knife, otherwise use a Bard-Parker scalpel with a no. 11 blade.

3 Grasp the medial rectus muscle with a 2-in-3 forceps and gently lift the eye ceiling-wards, to fix its position. Hold the knife like a pencil and steady your hand by placing your fourth and fifth fingers on the patient's temple. Pass the tip of the blade through

> ### ▶ KEY POINTS Correct plane
>
> - Keep in the plane of the limbal 'ring' (the corneoscleral junction; Fig. 42.4).
> - Enter at 3 o'clock or 9 o'clock on the corneal dial.

4 You cannot see the tip of the knife once it is within the anterior chamber because it disappears in blood. Do not push on any further than 2 mm once this happens. Withdraw the knife gently but rapidly in its own plane. If you withdraw it correctly, nothing escapes from the anterior chamber even if the ocular tension is very high.

5 Now press gently on the posterior (peripheral) lip of the incision and some blood-stained aqueous should escape. Do not press for longer than a second at a time initially, since a rapid drop in intraocular pressure may re-start the bleeding. Repeat intermittent pressure until you note some clearing of the anterior chamber. Do not persist until all blood has been evacuated.

6 Inject subconjunctival cefuroxime, remove the speculum and cover the eye with a plastic shield.

7 Very little blood may appear if the anterior chamber contains a solid clot. A larger incision is then needed.

8 Paracentesis is also a standard emergency procedure for arrest of the retinal circulation (central retinal artery occlusion). Carry it out within 2–3 hours of the onset. This condition justifies a much more rapid evacuation of the clear normal aqueous humour.

RUPTURED GLOBE

Appraise

1 A totally disrupted eyeball may require enucleation, either immediately or within a few days of the injury, and the same applies to

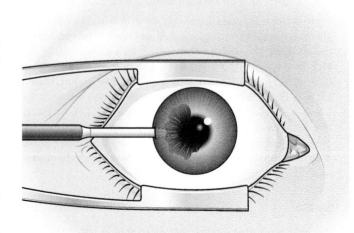

Fig. 42.4 Evacuation of hyphaema. Fixation of globe not shown.

badly lacerated and collapsed eyes. It is usually better, from a psychological point of view, to suture the eye as best you can then discuss removal of the eye, if it is not viable, with the patient over the next few days.

2 Take the decision for enucleation, bearing in mind the possibility of the dreaded complication of sympathetic ophthalmia. Months, or even years later, the unaffected eye and the affected eye develop panuveitis with sight-threatening sequelae including glaucoma and cataract.

3 Smaller posterior ruptures with some preservation of function may be diagnosed by the finding of a deep anterior chamber and chemosis (Greek: cheme – a yawning; the swelling around the cornea from oedema of the conjunctiva) resulting from loss of the vitreous humour. An ophthalmic surgeon might explore the eye. You should manage the rupture conservatively.

FOREIGN BODIES

Appraise

Intraocular foreign bodies

▶ KEY POINTS Management

- These require specialist intervention if it is available.
- It is important that you recognize the possibility of the condition.

1 A foreign body is easily missed when the entry wound is small and the initial disturbance minimal. Metallic foreign bodies must be removed within a week because of the risk of the metallic ions causing toxicity to the retina. Copper is particularly dangerous.

2 If there is a history of something going into the eye, especially while hammering and chiselling, and you cannot detect a foreign body on superficial inspection, promptly order an X-ray of the orbit.

3 Most small intraocular foreign bodies are sterile. Be willing to wait if this allows more favourable conditions for treatment.

4 A large foreign body may cause a penetrating injury that requires to be dealt with in itself.

Subtarsal foreign bodies

1 Remove these by everting the upper eyelid after instilling proxymetacaine, tetracaine (amethocaine) or oxybuprocaine. Have a cotton-wool swab to hand before starting. Ask the patient to look down and keep doing so. Grasp the upper lid lashes with the thumb and forefinger of one hand and pull the lid down and forwards. With an orange stick, press the upper edge of the tarsal plate downwards (some 4 mm from the lid margin) and then lift the lashes so as to rotate the lid over the orange stick, which pushes the tarsal plate down and under the lid margin at the same time.

2 Once the eyelid is everted, keep hold of the lashes and press them against the eyebrow, instructing the patient meanwhile to keep looking down. Remove the orange stick and use your freed hand to remove the foreign body with the cotton-wool swab. Return the lid to its normal position by withdrawing both hands and asking the patient to look up.

Corneal foreign bodies

1 If you suspect the foreign body to be deep within the cornea, manipulation may push it into the anterior chamber. Unless you are expert, with available equipment, avoid tackling it.

2 Superficial corneal foreign bodies can be removed after anaesthetizing the cornea. Make sure you have a good light focused on the cornea and magnification.

3 Corneal foreign bodies are best removed with a green (19 G) disposable needle. Insert the needle tangentially to the cornea to get behind the foreign body. Do not insert the needle directly at the foreign body, but enter the cornea a little to the side. Lever the foreign body out. If any rust is left behind, attempt to pick it out, but do not persist too long. Rust that is slight and milk-chocolate in colour will disappear itself. Remove as much dark rust as is easily possible. You may be able to remove more after a few days of softening up.

4 Insert chloramphenicol antibiotic ointment into the conjunctival sac then pad the eye. Put in atropine drops only if the foreign body was very hard to remove. Monitor the patient daily, if possible, until the conjunctiva has healed and no longer stains with fluorescein. If daily monitoring is not possible, advise the patient to use chloramphenicol ointment three times a day until symptoms resolve.

BURNS

1 *Chemical burns.* Immediately concentrate on removing any matter mechanically and, in particular, copiously irrigate the eye using any harmless fluid you have at hand. Keep irrigating for at least 20 minutes. Do not hunt for specific antidotes. If the cornea is affected, apply antibiotic/steroid ointments such as Maxitrol (containing dexamethasone 0.1%, neomycin sulphate 0.35%, hypromellose 0.5%, polymyxin B sulphate 6000 IU) drops, or Sofradex (containing dexamethasone 0.05%, framycetin sulphate 0.5% and gramicidin 0.005%) drops, and atropine 1%. Keep the conjunctival fornices patent to prevent symblepharon (adhesion of the eyelids to the eyeball), by twice-daily passing a glass rod between the lids and the eyeball after anaesthetizing the eyeball with oxybuprocaine 0.4% (Benoxinate) or tetracaine (amethocaine) hydrochloride 0.5% drops. Always admit patients with lime burns for observation as the effects may be delayed and you may need to institute half-hourly drops including vitamin C in high dosage. Also encourage the patient to eat citrus fruits, since vitamin C is an antioxidant and a cofactor in collagen synthesis.

2 *Thermal burns.* Treat those affecting the lids as skin burns elsewhere, but problems of ocular protection may arise. If there is loss of skin following a thermal burn, the ocular surface may also be severely damaged by the injury. If there is exposure of the cornea, apply lubricants such as hypromellose 1.0% and try to produce a moist chamber. In the longer term it will be necessary to reconstruct the lids using tissue from elsewhere, such as skin from behind the ear and hard palate grafts to recreate the tarsal plate.

INFECTIONS AROUND THE EYE

PYOGENIC INFECTIONS

Appraise

1 Eyelids:
   - Infections may occur in the lids. A stye is an infection of a sebaceous gland of the lid, and resolves without treatment in 36 hours.
   - Meibomian cysts (described by Heinrich Meibom in 1666) or chalazia (Greek: = a small tubercle) are common swellings of the meibomian glands, and are usually sterile. They all go away eventually but if they are persistent they may be incised and curetted.
   - Inflammation in the lacrimal ducts that drain tears from the eye to the nose is called dacryocystitis (Greek: dacryon = a tear). Treat with systemic antibiotics such as amoxicillin. Avoid incision wherever possible but, in the presence of a tense abscess causing pain, release it. Local anaesthetic is not always needed and you do not need to insert a drain.

2 Infection of the eyelid, preseptal cellulitis, requires prompt treatment with systemic oral antibiotics such as amoxicillin. Review the patient daily, and admit for intravenous antibiotics if it deteriorates. Incise an abscess. Distinguish preseptal cellulitis from orbital cellulitis, which is a life-threatening illness. In preseptal cellulitis, even if the lid is swollen the eye is not proptosed and is fully mobile, with a normal or near normal visual acuity.

3 Infection of the orbit, orbital cellulitis, usually spreads from a sinus infection. It is usually associated with fever, reduced visual acuity on the affected side, proptosis and gross eyelid swelling and reduced eye movements. The patient needs to be admitted, the organism isolated and treatment started with intravenous antibiotics.

4 Infections of the eyeball itself may be localized, as for example a pyogenic corneal ulcer, or widely disseminated, as when a metastatic infection lodges in the choroid, spreading thence to the vitreous and all parts of the eye:
   - A corneal ulcer may perforate and require a conjunctival flap to cover it and help it to heal. It may also be accompanied by pus in the anterior chamber (hypopyon); if this is unresponsive to intensive local and systemic antibiotics, you may need to perform paracentesis to obtain a specimen for microscopy and culture. Application of superglue to the thin cornea may provide emergency treatment of corneal perforation. Anaesthetize the eye first with amethocaine. Apply 2–3 drops of superglue to the perforation after drying the cornea with a sterile swab. Cover the eye with a bandage contact lens.
   - Treat severe destructive infection or endophthalmitis with local and systemic chemotherapy and steroids. Failure to control it may require removal of the eye.

Action

1 Whenever possible, incise lid abscesses from the inner aspect. Anaesthetize the lid (see Tarsorrhaphy, above). Evert the lid (Fig. 42.5) and incise it at right-angles to its margin, through the tarsal plate.

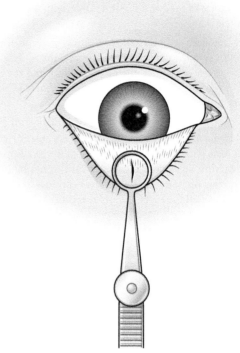

Fig. 42.5 Everting the lower lid, with a chalazion clamp.

2 If incision is needed for abscesses of the eyelid or lacrimal ducts, it should be done directly over the site of where the abscess is pointing.

REMOVING AN EYE

Appraise

1 The main indications for removal of an eye are irreparable injury with loss of sight, total or near total, severe pain in an already blind eye, or neoplasms such as a choroidal malignant melanoma that is too large for local irradiation or laser treatment.

2 There are two surgical approaches: enucleation and evisceration. In the former, the eyeball is removed from within Tenon's capsule – the sheet of connective tissue beneath the conjunctiva that covers both the eye and the insertion into it of the ocular muscles. In evisceration, the eyeball is not removed as a whole but the structural wall – the sclera – is left in situ, the contents being removed; access is obtained by removing the cornea.

3 Evisceration is often reserved for blind eyes with obvious gross intraocular infection but with no evidence of malignancy. Mobility of the prosthetic eye is better following evisceration than following enucleation.

ENUCLEATION

Prepare

1 Decide how sophisticated an operation you are going to do.

2 A general anaesthetic is usual but, in severely ill patients, local anaesthesia, including a retrobulbar injection (see Relief of pain) may be adequate.

Action

1. Sit at the head of the table and put in an eye speculum to separate the lids. Most specula are sprung. There should be adequate access.

2. Carry out a peritomy (incision of the conjunctiva around the rim of the cornea) by first opening the conjunctiva close to the edge of the cornea. Pick up a fold at 6 o'clock on the corneal dial (Fig. 42.6A) with plain forceps (Moorfields) and cut it with sharp-pointed scissors.

3. Undermine both away from the cornea and towards the left (if you are right-handed), keeping close to the cornea. Cut the conjunctiva close to this edge, undermine some more and proceed snipping right round the cornea. The conjunctiva should now be free from the globe (Fig. 42.6B) and sufficiently undermined backwards for you to explore and open Tenon's capsule.

4. This is best done in the lower nasal quadrant, below the medial rectus muscle. If Tenon's capsule is thick you may not be able to see the muscles at all at this stage. If you have opened the correct part of Tenon's capsule you will expose the sclera. This is a lustrous grey-white colour, and you should satisfy yourself that you are really down to it by cutting away any other loose fascial planes (e.g. episcleral tissue) that can be picked up.

> ▶ KEY POINT Bleeding?
>
> ■ Achieve perfect haemostasis using bipolar diathermy forceps. Clear visualization is essential.

5. Next expose and cut off the extraocular muscles, starting with the medial rectus. Take a muscle hook and pass it upwards through the opening in Tenon's capsule, with its blunt point against the sclera deep to this muscle. Test that you have caught the muscle by pulling the hook anteriorly, when it will be stopped short at the insertion and will then move the whole eye. With the point above the level of the muscle, rotate the hook so as to tent Tenon's capsule (Fig. 42.6C).

6. Cut down on this and then brush back Tenon's fascia with a small swab so as to expose a length of the muscle tendon. Cut this off with blunt-nosed scissors, 3–5 mm behind the insertion, in order to leave a stump of muscle.

7. Through the gap in Tenon's capsule above the medial rectus, pass a hook laterally to engage the superior rectus and cut this off, using the same steps described for the medial rectus; then carry on round to the lateral and the inferior recti. Cut off the tendons of the superior, lateral and inferior recti flush with the globe instead of leaving a stump attached to the globe as was done with the medial rectus.

8. If you have any idea where the inferior and superior oblique muscles are, and they can be found, divide them. Usually, however, no formal search need be made for them as they can be dealt with as the globe is removed.

9. Once the rectus muscles have been dissected from the globe, test whether the globe rotates freely by grasping the stump of the medial rectus. If it does not do so, explore backwards beneath Tenon's fascia with blunt-nosed scissors and divide any structures that resist the rotation.

10. Next, dislocate the globe forwards. Loosen the eye speculum and, holding it so as to keep it about 25 mm apart, press it back towards the apex of the orbit (i.e. towards the floor). The eyeball should now come forwards with something of a jerk; its equator will be in front of the plane of the speculum. Now slightly close the speculum and tighten its screw so that the globe is kept in its forward dislocated position. This stretches its remaining attachments, making it easier to divide them.

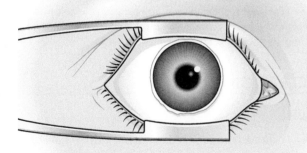

(A)

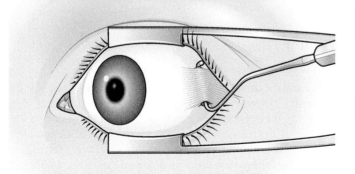

(B)

(C)

Fig. 42.6 Enucleation: (A) opening the conjunctiva; (B) conjunctiva freed; (C) tenting Tenon's capsule.

11 Divide the optic nerve. Any short, but tough, blunt-nosed scissors, preferably slightly curved, will do. First rotate the globe outwards by grasping the stump of the medial rectus with 2-in-3 fixation forceps. Probe the region of the optic nerve, which you cannot yet see, by passing the points of closed scissors from the nasal side to where it should be. Move the scissor tips up and down to feel the cordlike structure. Do this two or three times to make sure of its location. Now withdraw the scissors about 5 mm, open the blades widely enough to flank the nerve, then advance the blades to engage it, making sure you are far enough in to section the nerve with one cut.

> ### KEY POINT Optic nerve section
>
> ■ Avoid too flush a section of the nerve or, even worse, an amputation of the posterior pole of the eye.

12 While the scissors are in position embracing the nerve, dip them about 15 degrees so that the tips of the blades go slightly deeper into the orbit. In this position close the blades, boldly cutting through the nerve.

13 The globe now comes forwards very easily. Trim away from it any remaining attachments such as the oblique muscles and posterior ciliary vessels, allowing you to remove it completely.

14 Bleeding is usually brisk at this stage so proceed immediately to pack the socket with gauze wrung out in hot saline. Keep two or three fingers' pressure on this for 1 minute. Inspect it then and reapply a fresh pack and pressure until bleeding stops. Direct haemostasis is virtually never needed. While applying pressure, inspect the enucleated eye for completeness of removal, especially in the region of the optic nerve. In the most unsophisticated enucleation, simply put on some antibiotic powder, line the conjunctival sac with tulle gras, cover the lids similarly and apply a pressure dressing – two eyepads and a crepe bandage. Fold the deeper pad double.

Suturing the conjunctiva and Tenon's fascia

Do this if it worries you not to do so. Always do it, however, if you implant anything in the orbit (see below). Use a continuous 7/0 or 8/0 synthetic absorbable suture, either in a continuous keyhole or over-and-over pattern; tie at each end.

Orbital implants

Modify your technique as follows:

1 Insert sutures into each of the rectus muscles before cutting them off the globe. If you intend to use an implant to which the muscles will actually be attached, use 6/0 synthetic absorbable sutures. If the implant is simply a ball (glass or plastic) then use 4/0 black silk.

2 The sutures should be 'whipped' or tied so as to give a better grip of the tendons (Fig. 42.7).

3 In all cases where an implant is to be used, dissect back under Tenon's capsule to make a definite layer that can be sutured over the front of the implant. The capsule, described by the Parisian surgeon in 1806, is the connective tissue sheath of the eyeball.

4 If a ball is to be used, after removing the eye and securing reasonable haemostasis, put the implant in and lift up the muscles by their silk sutures. Then sew a purse-string suture of 6/0 absorbable

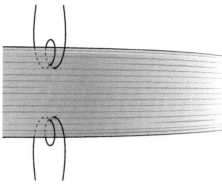

Fig. 42.7 Suturing the rectus muscles when using an implant.

to close Tenon's capsule over the ball and include the muscle tendons in the purse string. Remove the black silk sutures. Finally, close the conjunctiva as a separate layer with 6/0 or 8/0 synthetic absorbable sutures.

5 If the muscles are to be attached to the implant, do this and then pull Tenon's capsule forwards to cover it. Dissect it well enough to avoid much tension. Sew up Tenon's capsule using a continuous 6/0 absorbable suture for both, starting with Tenon's right to left and then coming through to the conjunctiva proceeding left to right.

> ### KEY POINT Capsular closure
>
> ■ Failure to close Tenon's capsule in a separate layer results in late extrusion and infection of the orbital implant.

6 The best cosmesis is obtained by suturing the muscles to a hydoxyapatite orbital implant covered in polyglactin 910 mesh or a Vicryl ball implant covered in Mersilene mesh.

EVISCERATION

Appraise

1 If the vital internal structures of the eye are destroyed by infection, with loss of vision, evisceration (removal of the soft contents from within the sclera), is indicated rather than enucleation, since mobility is better following evisceration.

2 If you have any suspicion of an intraocular tumour, however, choose enucleation to avoid any potential spread of the tumour.

Action

1 Insert a speculum to separate the eyelids.

2 Cut off the cornea. This may be difficult if the eye is very soft, following, for example, perforation of an infected corneal ulcer. Steady the eye by grasping the insertion of a rectus muscle with toothed forceps. Now cut through the periphery of the cornea circumferentially over a 5-mm length by progressively deepening a scalpel incision. Use the belly of a Bard-Parker no. 15 blade or ophthalmic blade.

3 Once you have entered the anterior chamber, cut right round the edge of the cornea with corneal scissors, if they are available; alternatively, use any narrow-bladed, blunt-nosed scissors.

4 Having topped the eye, scoop out all its contents – lens, iris and retina as well as the humours. It is important to do this thoroughly. A special scoop is available, but a large and not-too-sharp curette is adequate. End by wrapping gauze round it to wipe away all the remnants of the uvea. Inspect the cavity to make sure that all that is left is sclera. Recent practice is to sever the optic nerve, split the posterior sclera and insert the implant behind the scleral remnant to reduce the risk of extrusion – a technique for the specialist.

5 Finally, pack the socket with paraffin gauze, apply a pad and bandage. Dress in 48 hours. No suture is required.

ACUTE ANGLE-CLOSURE GLAUCOMA

Appraise

1 Acute glaucoma produces sudden pain, loss of vision, headache, nausea and vomiting. It may be preceded by episodes of seeing haloes in the evenings. The eye appears red, with a swollen conjunctiva and the pupil may be mid-dilated and unresponsive to light. The corneal reflex is often cloudy or glassy in appearance.

2 Surgical intervention is infrequently necessarily indicated because of the availability of effective medications. Treat acute angle-closure glaucoma with miotics such as pilocarpine 2 or 4% 1 drop every hour, the beta-blocker timolol maleate 0.5% (Timoptol-LA) twice daily, dexamethasone 0.1% (Maxidex) four times a day. Oral acetazolamide (Diamox) 500 mg may be given orally twice daily; it may be administered intravenously if the patient has severe nausea and vomiting. When ophthalmological facilities are available, a YAG laser is used to produce a peripheral iridotomy.

3 In primary acute closed-angle glaucoma the pressure can usually be lowered adequately, if temporarily, by acetazolamide (Diamox), 500 mg intravenously, miotic drops and osmotic agents. For this reason, classic iridectomy for glaucoma is hardly ever employed as an emergency procedure. In ophthalmic units laser iridectomy is performed several hours or days after the acute attack has been controlled and the eye is 'quiet', the pressure having been controlled with miotics such as pilocarpine 4%.

4 Chronic open-angle glaucoma is usually asymptomatic in the early stages: the pressure is only moderately raised and loss of vision takes place years after the onset of the condition. It is usually treated medically by pressure-lowering eye drops where such drops are available; if unobtainable, it is treated surgically by a specialist.

Relief of pain

1 Intractable glaucoma with severe pain is one example of the blind, painful eye, and for this sort of glaucoma some relief may be given by a retrobulbar alcohol injection if removal of the eye is impracticable.

Retrobulbar alcohol injection

1 Put 1.5 ml of 1% lidocaine with 1:200 000 adrenaline (epinephrine) in a 2-ml syringe and fit a retrobulbar needle or a 40-mm 23G or 25G needle.

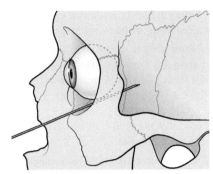

Fig. 42.8   Retrobulbar alcohol injection.

2 Clean the skin of the lower lid after determining the site of entry of the needle, which should be the lower outer angle of the bony orbit.

3 With the patient lying down, ask him or her to keep the eyes open and to look straight ahead.

4 Insert the needle through the skin in the intended direction, which is backwards, and slightly medially and upwards (Fig. 42.8), towards the opposite superoparietal area. There is a tendency to avoid getting too close to the globe for fear of penetrating it; but, if you keep too far away, you will miss the muscle cone, which you want to penetrate through Tenon's capsule between the lateral and inferior recti.

5 Inject very slightly as you go in. You will probably feel resistance when Tenon's is about to be penetrated and you may see the eye roll slightly down and out at this point. Be resolute and push on; the eye will resume its former position. Inject the bulk of the local anaesthetic. When it has had time to work there will be some relief of pain.

6 Now leave the needle in place and detach the syringe. Draw up 1 ml of 75% alcohol and after an interval of 1 minute inject this through the retrobulbar needle still in situ. Withdraw needle and syringe.

7 Warn the patient that relief may not be very long-lasting (it does, however, often last months), and also warn of the possibility of ptosis of the upper lid, which again may not be permanent.

NEOPLASMS

Appraise

The most common important ocular neoplasms affect the lids and the uveal tract.

Small benign lesions of the lid

These can be removed by cautery or a variety of methods of excision under local anaesthetic.

Larger benign and malignant lesions of the lid

1 Carefully decide upon the surgical approach after noting the size of the lesion and its position in relation to the lid margins. You need to remove at least 3 mm beyond the visible margin of the lesion of a malignant lesion, to allow for possible microscopic

extension. Where available, malignant eyelid lesions should be ideally removed using Mohs techniques.

2 For larger lesions away from the lid margin, you may excise the lesion and arrange a local skin flap. Alternatively, insert a free graft of skin from the contralateral upper lid. As you distend the skin with the preoperative anaesthetic injection of 2% lidocaine with added adrenaline (epinephrine) to reduce bleeding, you can ensure that the graft is of adequate size, and also that you can close the donor site.

3 For lesions of the lid margin, employ a pentagonal excision, provided that the gap can be simply closed by direct suture. If this will cause too much tension, facilitate closure by making an outer canthal incision, dividing the lateral canthal tendon mobilizing the lid and gaining horizontal laxity. This allows the lateral portion of the lid to be easily approximated. This is also helpful when shortening the lower lid for senile ectropion. Local anaesthesia is all that is required.

4 Make the excised pentagon at least 2 cm in height with the tarsal edges vertical, the apex being angled. Closure is in two layers, as described in the section on lid injuries.

5 Major reconstructive surgery of the eyelids is beyond the scope of this section. Intraocular malignancies are again a matter for the specialist, but the general principle applies that, for lesions of any size (which to the non-specialist means any degree of obviousness), enucleation is indicated.

FURTHER READING

Collin JRO. A Manual of Systematic Eyelid Surgery. Edinburgh: Churchill Livingstone; 2006.

Leatherbarrow B. Oculoplastic Surgery. London: Martin Dunitz; 2011.

Tyers AG, Collin JRO. Colour Atlas of Ophthalmic Plastic Surgery. Edinburgh: Elsevier Health Sciences; 2008.

Spaeth GL. Ophthalmic Surgery: Principles and Practice. Edinburgh: Saunders; 2003. www.eyetext.net.

Index

NB: Page numbers in *italics* refer to boxes, figures and tables.

D

Printed and bound by CPI Group (UK) Ltd, Croydon, CR0 4YY

08/05/2025

01864795-0001